Feature Papers "Age-Friendly Cities & Communities: State of the Art and Future Perspectives"

Feature Papers "Age-Friendly Cities & Communities: State of the Art and Future Perspectives"

Editors

Joost van Hoof
Hannah R. Marston

MDPI • Basel • Beijing • Wuhan • Barcelona • Belgrade • Manchester • Tokyo • Cluj • Tianjin

MDPI

Editors
Joost van Hoof
Faculty of Social Work & Education
The Hague University of Applied Sciences
The Hague
The Netherlands

Hannah R. Marston
Health and Wellbeing Strategic Research Area
The Open University
Milton Keynes
United Kingdom

Editorial Office
MDPI
St. Alban-Anlage 66
4052 Basel, Switzerland

This is a reprint of articles from the Special Issue published online in the open access journal *International Journal of Environmental Research and Public Health* (ISSN 1660-4601) (available at: www.mdpi.com/journal/ijerph/special_issues/Age_Friendly_Cities).

For citation purposes, cite each article independently as indicated on the article page online and as indicated below:

LastName, A.A.; LastName, B.B.; LastName, C.C. Article Title. *Journal Name* **Year**, *Volume Number*, Page Range.

ISBN 978-3-0365-1227-3 (Hbk)
ISBN 978-3-0365-1226-6 (PDF)

Cover image courtesy of Marion Duimel, GetOud, The Hague.

Contents

About the Editors

Joost van Hoof

Joost van Hoof works as a full professor of Urban Ageing with the Faculty of Social Work & Education of The Hague University of Applied Sciences in The Netherlands. Since December 2017, he has also been affiliated with the Department of Spatial Economy, Faculty of Environmental Engineering and Geodesy, Wrocław University of Environmental and Life Sciences in Poland.

His research interests lie in the domain of age-friendly cities, housing for older people and gerontechnology. He has a background (MSc) in Building Physics and Services (Eindhoven University of Technology), and obtained his doctoral degree (PhD) from the same university in 2010. In addition, he obtained the Eur Ing qualification from the European Federation of National Engineering Associations in 2007. In 2019, he gained his higher doctoral degree (DSc) in the field of engineering and technical sciences from Warsaw University of Life Sciences.

Hannah R. Marston

Dr Hannah R. Marston is a Research Fellow in the Health and Wellbeing Strategic Research Area at The Open University, UK, and her research takes an inter- and multi-disciplinary approach, intersecting across the fields of gerontechnology, social sciences, and technology. She gained her PhD from Teesside University, UK in 2010, focusing on videogame and older adults. Her research projects previously include the Technology In Later Life (TILL) (2015-17); and currently the COVID-19: Technology, Social Connections, Loneliness, and Leisure Activities international study; COVID-19: Dating Apps, Social Connections, Loneliness, and Mental Health in a Pandemic study; the Adapt Tech, Accessible Technology study. She has published over 40 journal papers, 9 book chapters, and has presented her work to policy makers and to national and international audiences. Hannah was a panel member on the 'Game and Interaction design for Older Adults: That Means You (Someday)'-PAXOnline.

Preface to "Feature Papers "Age-Friendly Cities & Communities: State of the Art and Future Perspectives""

The "Age-Friendly Cities & Communities: States of the Art and Future Perspectives"publication presents contemporary, innovative, and insightful narratives, debates, and frameworks based on an international collection of papers from scholars spanning the fields of gerontology, social sciences, architecture, computer science, and gerontechnology. This extensive collection of papers aims to move the narrative and debates forward in this interdisciplinary field of age-friendly cities and communities.

Joost van Hoof, Hannah R. Marston
Editors

International Journal of
Environmental Research and Public Health

MDPI

Editorial

Age-Friendly Cities and Communities: State of the Art and Future Perspectives

Joost van Hoof [1,2,*] and Hannah R. Marston [3]

1 Faculty of Social Work & Education, The Hague University of Applied Sciences, 2521 EN Den Haag, The Netherlands
2 Faculty of Environmental Engineering and Geodesy, Institute of Spatial Management, Wrocław University of Environmental and Life Sciences, 50-357 Wrocław, Poland
3 Health & Wellbeing Strategic Research Area, School of Health, Wellbeing & Social Care, The Open University, Buckinghamshire MK7 6HH, UK; hannah.marston@open.ac.uk
* Correspondence: j.vanhoof@hhs.nl; Tel.: +31-6-23381404

Citation: van Hoof, J.; Marston, H.R. Age-Friendly Cities and Communities: State of the Art and Future Perspectives. *Int. J. Environ. Res. Public Health* **2021**, *18*, 1644. https://doi.org/10.3390/ijerph18041644

Received: 1 February 2021
Accepted: 5 February 2021
Published: 9 February 2021

The number of older adults is increasing rapidly, and this demographic shift places an increased level of strain and tension on the various international healthcare and welfare systems. The vast majority of older adults wish to age in place. Many make use of long-term care services, including homecare, rehabilitation services, and social support, as well as home modifications and technology, although, contrary to popular belief, this is not the majority of older people. One way to support older people to live the lives they wish to live is through the Age-Friendly Cities and Communities initiative, a world-wide programme launched by the World Health Organization (WHO) in 2007 [1] in order to make cities more tuned to the needs and requirements of older citizens [2–4]. The World Health Organization defines Age-Friendly Cities and Communities as follows: *"In an age-friendly community, policies, services and structures related to the physical and social environment are designed to support and enable older people to "age actively"—that is, to live in security, enjoy good health and continue to participate fully in society"* [5].

The WHO published an age-friendly cities guideline that was accompanied by a checklist of essential features of age-friendly cities. This checklist was based on the results of the WHO Global Age-Friendly Cities project consultation in 33 cities in 22 countries [6]. For the checklist to be effective, older people must be involved as full partners. In assessing a city's strengths and deficiencies, older people describe how the checklist of features matches their own experience of the city's positive characteristics and barriers. They should play a role in suggesting changes and in implementing and monitoring improvements [1].

In the second decade of the WHO programme, it is fair to say that it contributed to the emancipation of older people, namely that their voices were heard in urban governance and planning, as well as in the programming of services for older persons all over the world. Yet, there are many unanswered questions and challenges lying ahead. For instance, how is the complex interplay of needs and demands of older persons [7–9] included into the design of age-friendly solutions in every possible domain? In order to create age-appropriate living environments, it is of the utmost importance to involve older people in the design of their living environment, particularly because the importance given to neighbourhoods in old age can vary greatly [10]. Another question is what the age-friendly agenda and its recommendations mean for older people living in such age-friendly cities and communities. In short, what do citizens notice in their everyday lives of the efforts to be or become an age-friendly city? Additionally, how can you really tell that a city is age-friendly, for instance, by measuring the age-friendliness of cities using core indicators [11–17], and that being part of this global network of cities is not just a tokenistic attempt of urban governments to show a friendly image to the outside world? Do age-friendly cities and communities really offer better living conditions and environments to their older citizens and the overall population than non-age-friendly cities? In short, what does it truly mean to be age-friendly in practice? Relevant for various stakeholders is the question whether the programme is still up to date after being in use for nearly a decade and a half.

The WHO published a report in 2018 [18] with the subtitle "*Looking back over the last decade, looking forward to the next*", in which technology is explicitly mentioned as a support for age-friendly environments. In 2019, Marston and van Hoof [19] presented a critique of the WHO's Age-Friendly Cities and Communities model, as *technology is not explicitly considered in this model. Their paper discusses the gaps in the WHO's framework in the field of technology and provides insights and recommendations for expansion of the model for application in the context of countries with a high human development index (HDI) that wish to be fully age-friendly. The question was raised if* the age-friendly programme prepares cities to be truly age-friendly in a world that is increasingly moving towards being a digital or even smart society? How considerate is the age-friendly movement of the inclusion of digital technologies, embracing their potential to the fullest? *Over the decades, technology has become essential for contemporary and future societies, and even more imperative as the decades move on.* Podgórniak-Krzykacz et al. [20] also called for smart cities to seek to ensure meeting the needs of older citizens and promoting solutions tailored to their digital literacy, digital skills, and perception capabilities.

The world of the 2020s needs answers to the abovementioned questions and challenges. These questions, therefore, provide some of the rationales for the Feature Paper Special Issue entitled "*Age-Friendly Cities and Communities: State of the Art and Future Perspectives*" which is published in the section of Health Care Sciences and Services of the International Journal of Environmental Research and Public Health (IJERPH).

The primary focus of this Feature Paper Special Issue is to critically assess the state-of-the-art Age-Friendly Cities and Communities programme. It adds to a previous special issue by van Hoof et al. [21] entitled "Creating age-friendly communities: Housing and technology" of MDPI's Healthcare in the following manner, by providing a wider scope of papers that provides a more diverse set of recommendations for practice and future work. The purpose of this Feature Paper Special Issue was to publish high-quality research papers, commentaries, and review articles addressing recent advances in age-friendly cities. There are eight domains of an age-friendly city, specifically social participation, communication and information, civic participation and employment, housing, transportation, community support and health services, outdoor spaces and buildings, and respect and social inclusion. In addition, this Feature Paper Special Issue also considered the importance of (geron)technology and digital solutions in relation to age-friendly environments.

For this Feature Paper Special Issue entitled "*Age-Friendly Cities and Communities: State of the Art and Future Perspectives*", a total of 29 papers [22–50] were recently published on different topics related to this subject matter. Of the published papers, seven papers [22–28] related to age-friendly neighbourhoods, cities, communities and societies, three papers [29–31] explored innovative approaches to housing, two papers [32,33] concentrated on age-friendly transportation, four papers [34–37] focused on innovative practices in the domain of cure and/or care for older citizens, four papers [38–41] related to respect and social inclusion, and nine papers [42–50] dealt with the consideration of technology in an age-friendly city or community.

Age-friendly neighbourhoods, cities, communities and societies

The seven papers in this section provide a wide range of insights, which add to the current scientific base in the domain of urban ageing [4,51–59]. The role of neighbourhoods is studied through various methodological approaches. In addition, new approaches to evaluating age-friendliness of a city or community are presented, as well as directions for future research policy and practice.

The paper by Versey et al. [22] from the United States of America explored neighbourhoods within age-friendly cities and communities and their role in shaping the everyday lives of older adults. The study explored the impact of gentrification on older adults and explored indirect displacement due to the change in character and social identity of a neighbourhood, which is one of the consequences of gentrification. The perceptions of older people concerning indirect displacement were studied in New York City and were characterised by perceived cultural shifts and housing concerns among adults. The implications of indirect displacement are potential threats to ageing-in-place in age-friendly cities.

Von Faber et al. [23] presented a study on participatory video design as an empowering approach to collect experiences and perceptions of older people focusing on the age friendliness of their city or neighbourhood. They described how this co-creation method can add to specific knowledge about the needs and wishes of older people about the improvement and/or preservation of their environment. Older participants produced short films on the topics that were perceived as important from their own perspective regarding their neighbourhood. Topics of the films included communication and information, outdoor spaces, social relations, and community support.

Sterns et al. [24] presented a survey from the city of Akron in the state of Ohio. In order to provide direction for future ageing initiatives, an assessment of Akron current state was conducted in early 2020. A total of 656 individuals participated and rated Akron from good to excellent. Most Akronites like and use their neighbourhood parks, find their streets well-lit, and feel safe walking in their neighbourhood. Conversely, more than 80% of respondents indicated how they disagree with the notion of them being disconnected from the community. Overall, Akron benefitted from its historical efforts to become age-friendly.

The study by Davern et al. [25] set out with a major critique of the age-friendly community movement, which argued for a more clearly defined scope of actions, the need to measure or quantify results and increase the connections to policy and funding levers. The scholars provided a quantifiable spatial indicators framework to assess local lived environments according to each of the eight domains of the WHO. The selection of the spatial indicators can be applied within local neighbourhoods, census tracts, suburbs, municipalities, or cities with minimal resource requirements other than applied spatial analysis.

Dikken et al. [26] also stressed the need for validated instruments to assess the age-friendliness of cities and communities. They developed and validated a questionnaire measuring age-friendliness, providing full transparency and reproducibility, coined the Age Friendly Cities and Communities Questionnaire (AFCCQ). Their process of development and validation resulted in a valid, psychometrically sound, comprehensive, 23-item questionnaire (Figure 1). Only those people aged 65-years or over (with an exception of 10 people aged between 60 and 65 from an existing database, who identified as older citizens) who lived in their own home were included. The AFCCQ can be used to measure older people's experiences regarding the eight domains of the WHO Age-Friendly Cities model and an additional financial domain. The AFCCQ allows practitioners and researchers to capture the age-friendliness of a city or community in a numerical fashion, which helps monitor the age-friendliness and the potential impact of policies or social programmes.

A commentary by Marston et al. [27] described and presented the existing Blue Zones® checklists and set out initial thoughts and explorations relating to the checklists. Additionally, Marston and colleagues discussed the two age-friendly frameworks by the WHO [1] as well as by Marston and van Hoof [19], and discussed the current gaps associated to the current Blue Zones® checklists. This commentary presented a series of recommendations for a roadmap to be considered by scholars, in conjunction with various industrial and third sector actors, to consider alternative and innovative approaches moving into the 21st century.

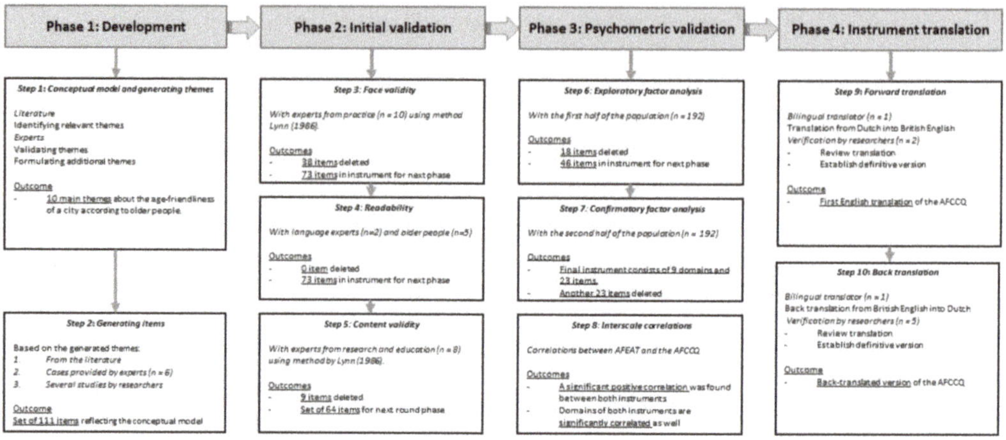

Figure 1. Flowchart representing the phases and steps for developing the Age-Friendly Cities and Communities Questionnaire (AFCCQ). Step 7 had 9 domains and 23 items as the final outcome. Please note that in §2.2.2. of the paper [26] step 2.1 should be step 3, and in §2.2.4 of the paper, step 2.3 should be step 5.

Rémillard-Boilard et al. [28] focused on driving the 'age-friendly' agenda, notably through the WHO's Global Network of Age-Friendly Cities and Communities. Little is known about the progress made by cities developing this work around the world. Therefore, their work addresses this research gap by comparing the experience of eleven cities located in eleven countries. Using a multiple case study approach, the authors explored the key goals, achievements, and challenges faced by local age-friendly programmes. They identified four priorities the age-friendly movement should consider to expand its development: (1) changing the perception of older age; (2) involving key actors in age-friendly efforts; (3) responding to the (diverse) needs of older people; and (4) improving the planning and delivery of age-friendly programmes. These conclusions carry implications for both research and policy in the field of age-friendly cities and communities.

Innovative approaches to age-friendly housing

The three papers in this section provide an additional knowledge base to the wider body of knowledge that exists in the field of age-friendly housing and ageing-in-place [60–66].

The paper by Rusinovic et al. [29] built on a previous contribution [67], which concerned the qualitative investigation of co-housing communities for older people in The Netherlands. Such communities offer an in-between solution for older people who do not want to live in an institutional setting but prefer the company of their age peers. Rusinovic et al.'s study focused on housing initiatives that offer innovative and alternative forms of independent living which deviate from mainstream housing arrangements. The study investigated how the founders dealt with challenges of establishing and governing such 'rebellious' innovative living arrangements for older people in the highly regulated context of housing and care in The Netherlands. Qualitative, in-depth interviews with social entrepreneurs, directors, and supervisory board members were conducted. These founders encountered various obstacles which are often related to governmental and sectoral rules and regulations. Their stories about successes and failures demonstrate dthe opportunities and constraints of innovative entrepreneurship at the intersection of housing and care.

The study by Bennetts et al. [30] dealt with thermal comfort in the homes of older people and is part of a larger project *Improving the thermal environment of housing for older Australians* [68,69]. This paper described the fundamental approach for developing the guidelines, using data from the study participants and the concept of personas to develop a total of six discrete 'thermal personalities'. The thermal personalities represented different approaches to achieving thermal comfort, considering a wide range of factors including personal characteristics, ideas, beliefs and knowledge, house type, and location. Basing the guidelines on thermal personalities highlights the heterogeneity of older people and the context-dependent nature of thermal comfort in the home, making the guidelines more user-friendly and useful.

Sengers and Peine [31] presented an overview of pilot projects in the field of housing, which are referred to as 'sociotechnical experiments'. These experiments embody different kinds of promising futures and provide direction to current developments in the emerging domain of age-friendly homes. The authors provided an overview of 53 ongoing sociotechnical experiments from The Netherlands, France, Ireland, and Poland. Most of the innovations tested in these experiments were not primarily material or technical, but primarily social or conceptual in character, and there were seven distinct innovation pathways in the experiments.

Age-friendly transportation

The following two papers deal with age-friendly transportation, which is becoming increasingly important in the light of smart mobility. At the same time, classic indicators for the quality of transportation, such as affordability, availability, and accessibility, remain important.

The study from Canada by Klicnik and Dogra [32] looked at the active transportation facet as an affordable and accessible form of transportation that facilitates the mobility of older adults in their communities. Age-friendly cities often do not adequately address active transportation. The study set out to identify and understand the constraints to active transportation that older adults experience to inform the development of viable solutions. The study conducted focus groups with community-dwelling older adults. Themes pertaining to environmental, individual, and task constraints, as well as their interactions, were identified. The study showed that constraints to active transportation interact to exacerbate one another, and that there is an opportunity to minimise such constraints by implementing age-friendly policies and practices.

Loos et al. [33] explored older people's (smart) mobility, with a particular interest in public transport, considering digital elements through a narrative literature review. Their study aimed to conceptualise transport as a core element of a smart, age-friendly ecosystem, and to propose a justice-informed perspective for the study of age-friendly smart mobility. Their findings contribute towards a framework for the evaluation of age-friendly smart transport that comprises mobility practices, digital data, digital networks, material/physical geographies and digital devices and access. The authors coined the term 'mobility digital ecosystem' to describe this framework, which comprises mobility practices, digital data, digital networks, material geographies, digital devices, and access to services.

Innovative practices in age-friendly cure and care

The following four papers dealt with innovative practices in age-friendly cure and care, whether it concerns hospital care services, older people's health information needs, the innovation of long-term care services, or models of care. All papers dealt with evidence-based or evidence-informed approaches to practical innovations [7,8].

The study by Ferrari et al. [34] from Italy focused on age-friendly hospital care. Consultation–Liaison Psychiatry Services (CLPS) are significantly involved in providing age-friendly hospital care. Such services perform psychiatric assessment for older people who are hospitalised with suspected medical–psychiatric comorbidities and support ward teams in a biopsychosocial-oriented care management. Changes in features of the population referred to a CLPS over a 20-year course were analysed and discussed, especially comparing older and younger referred subjects. The number of referrals for older patients significantly increased over the past 20 years. The analysis outlined recurring patterns that should guide future clinical, training, and research activities.

A study from the Russian Federation by Ziganshina et al. [35] presented the case of Kazan, the capital of Tatarstan, as a potential age-friendly city. This survey study assessed health information needs of the ageing population and the challenges these older people face in improving their health and longevity. Older people (60+ years) were less positive about their quality of life, who more often took medication on a daily basis, who also encountered age-related health problems and rated their overall quality of life as unsatisfactory. Awareness in evidence-based approaches was higher within health professions, and health information needs did not differ between age or gender groups or people with satisfactory and unsatisfactory quality of life. The minority (10%) were aware of ageism without age or gender differences. The low awareness calls for the need of interventions for both care recipients and professionals in order to move the age-friendly agenda forward.

Luijkx et al. [36] dealt with long-term care organisations for older adults that are expected to provide person-centered care in the complex arena of The Netherlands. In order to address the challenges of the innovative Dutch context, these organisations increasingly use scientific knowledge to evaluate and innovate long-term care. Their paper described how co-creation is a key factor in the success of improving long-term care for older adults, and how scientific knowledge is created by working together with partner organisations and how societal impact is achieved.

De Boer et al. [37] presented the case of alternative care environments for regular nursing homes. Insight is lacking on how to translate evidence-based knowledge from theory into a congruent care model in regular practice. This study reported on the co-creation and redesign of an alternative nursing home model in The Netherlands. A participatory research approach was used to co-create 'the Homestead care model' with researchers, practitioners, and older people, following an iterative process. Achieving positive outcomes for people with dementia, (in)formal carers, and the community is dependent on how well the physical, social, and organisational environments are congruently designed.

Respect and social inclusion in an age-friendly city

The following four papers dealt with the social environment(s) of age-friendly cities and communities, and the inclusion, representation, and participation of older people, as well as the role gender plays in the perception of age-friendliness.

Ronzi et al. [38] focused on the social environment of the age-friendly city's model. Using a photovoice methodology within a community-based participatory research approach, their study drew on photographs, interviews, and focus groups among older residents (60+ years) living in Liverpool to explore how the city promotes respect and social inclusion. Their study provided novel insights into how (i) respect and social inclusion are shaped by aspects of both physical and social environment, and (ii) the accessibility, affordability, and sociability of physical spaces and wider social processes (for instance, neighbourhood fragmentation) contributed to or hindered participants' health, well-being, intergenerational relationships, and feelings of inclusion and connection. Their findings suggested that respect and social inclusion are core to an age-friendly city, and relevant across all eight domains.

Codd [39] presented an interdisciplinary article, bringing together perspectives from gerontology, criminology, penology, and social policy to explore the research, policy, and practice on age-friendly cities and communities for people who are ageing within prison settings across many countries. There is a general omission of consideration of the place of the prison and prisoners within the broader context of age-friendly cities and communities. Codd identifies the potential for integration and for cross-disciplinary research in this context, concluding with recommendations for developing inclusive research, policies, and evaluation frameworks which recognise and include prisons and older prisoners, both during and after incarceration.

Blakey and Clews [40] presented a study from Tāmaki Makaurau Auckland in Aotearoa New Zealand, which houses the largest Polynesian population of any global city.

This case study inquiry applied the bricolage methodology to provide diverse contextual perspectives of this unique Polynesian setting, prior to exploring interview narratives of three Auckland Council's Seniors Advisory Panel members. Service-learning recommendations included co-developing a sustainable co-governance framework for an independent Steering Group to enable empowered active ageing for all residents, and a succession plan enabling the timely transfer of knowledge and skills to empower incoming Auckland Council's Seniors Advisory Panel members.

The study by del Barrio et al. [41] analysed the interaction between age-friendliness (physical and social) and subjective well-being through a survey among people aged 55-years and over in the Basque Country in Spain. The predictive power of age-friendliness over subjective well-being was analysed using linear regression models separated by sex. Among the predictors of well-being in men, the coexistence stood out as a safety and support network. In women, the neighbourhood proved to be a very important resource. The findings may contribute to interventions promoting more effective strategies that enhance older people well-being from a gender perspective.

Technology and the age-friendly city

The following nine papers dealt with technological solutions and ageing built on the foundations laid out by Marston and van Hoof [19], who laid down the importance of technology and digitalisation as a third pillar for age-friendly cities and communities. Aspects of use-friendly and sustainable design, technology acceptance, and aspects of implementation and needs of carers were all acknowledged in the following contributions [8,9,70–77].

The study by Baraković et al. [42] was a deliverable of COST Action CA16226 'Indoor living space improvement: Smart Habitat for the Elderly' and presents the collaborative efforts of researchers from Europe and North America. This review focused on the quality of life through the concept of personalised ageing. Information and communication technologies (ICT) are subject to constant and rapid development and can contribute to the goal of an improved quality of life for older adults. The systematic review of the state-of-the-art literature and patents in this field was based on a framework for the quality of life of older adults. Selected ICT solutions covered by articles and patents were intended for older adults and were validated by them. The study presented several recommendations that can help move the agenda concerning the quality of life of older people and personalised ageing with the use of ICT solutions forward. This paper was related to a comprehensive and structured analysis of the existing literature in the field of the Web of Things, and the user's quality of experience towards used technology [78].

The study by Anghel et al. [43] from Romania set out with the limitations posed by a decreasing workforce in the supply of care and social services. The development of smart, physical, social, and age-friendly environments was part of the solution. The authors conducted a survey of smart environments and robot assistive technologies that offer support for the independent living and providing age-friendly care services. Two cases were presented of services that are innovatively using assistive technologies for the assessment and delivery of timely interventions for polypharmacy management and for social and cognitive activity support in older adults. The study also provided a top-level architectural view of these services focusing, on details about technology usage, end-user interaction flows, and data models.

The study by Liddle et al. [44] from the United Kingdom focused on social connectedness in later life. The authors explored the design opportunities and role of technology for connectedness within a geographically local community context through interviews with older people and a linked ideation workshop. Shared concerns and negative perceptions around local relationships, connections, and characteristics of the geographical area were identified. Local connectedness through technology was largely absent from day-to-day life and even perceived as contributing to disconnection. A thoughtful consideration of the role of technology in optimising social connections within age-friendly communities is needed.

Silvius et al. [45] presented results on the use and acceptance of commercially available technology by home dwelling older citizens. A comparison was made between self-efficacy and perceived physical and mental quality-of-life-related parameters on an intervention location of 279 households and a control location of 301 households located in The Hague in The Netherlands. Technology adoption was significantly associated with perceived physical quality of life, depending on the number of technology interventions used. A higher number of adopted technologies was associated with a stronger effect. The study showed that successful and effective adoption of technology by older people is feasible with commercially available products amongst home dwelling older citizens.

In their study on smart and age-friendly cities in Romania, Ivan et al. [46] compiled an overview of public policy and practice. Smart cities are one of the technological-driven initiatives that may help create an age-friendly city. Few research studies analysed emerging countries in terms of their national strategies associated to smart or age-friendly cities. Through document analysis, current initiatives at the local, regional, and national level addressing the issue of smart and age-friendly cities in Romania were investigated. To date, Romanian smart home initiatives have limited connection to the age-friendly cities agenda.

Freeman et al. [47] studied the intergenerational effects on the impacts of technology use in later life through an online survey. As the use of technology becomes an integral part of daily life for all persons, including older adults, it is important to investigate how the perceptions and use of technology intersect with intergenerational relationships. Descriptive and thematic analyses suggest that older adults are not technologically adverse and leverage intergenerational relationships with family and friends to adjust to new technologies and to remain connected to adult children and grandchildren, especially when there is a large geographical separation between them. The intergenerational support to adopt to new technologies has important implications to support older persons to remain independent and to age-in-place, in both age-friendly cities and in rural geographies.

Pedell et al. [48] presented two case studies, one focusing on older adults using activity wearables for health self-management in the neighbourhood, and one focusing on older adults engaged in social prescribing activities in the community. A co-design and citizen-based approach was applied. Results suggested how the convergence of the often-siloed age-friendly city components based on older adults' goals and input can lead to better social participation and longer-term health outcomes. The authors proposed that the digital, physical, and social aspects need to be considered in all domains of age-friendly cities to achieve benefits for older adults.

Marston et al. [49] presented a theoretical case study to explore how digital technology has played an integral role during COVID-19, assisting various sectors of the community and demonstrating that smart cities can provide opportunities to respond to many future societal challenges. Although we need to create future smart age-friendly ecosystems to meet these needs, technology still does not feature in the WHO eight domains of an age-friendly city. This paper expands upon Marston and van Hoof's [19] 'Smart Age-friendly Ecosystem' (SAfE) framework, and explores how digital technology, design hacking, and research approaches can be used to understand a smart age-friendly ecosystem in a post-pandemic society. By exploring a series of case studies and using real-life scenarios from the standpoint of COVID-19, the authors proposed the 'Concept of Age-friendly Smart Ecologies (CASE)' framework.

Reuter et al. [50] set out by stating that the WHO's age-friendly city initiative emerged as a response to the intersecting global trends of population ageing and urbanisation. A third global trend—digitalisation—is largely overlooked. The authors explored older adults' digital citizenship in an age-friendly city in the north of England through interviewing, observations, and field notes from design workshops as part of an ongoing participatory action research project. The analyses focused on two age-friendly domains, namely communication and information and civic participation. The authors saw the need to reframe the role of digital technologies within the age-friendly city, broadening the scope from accessibility towards enhancing digital citizenship opportunities.

In this special issue, a rich palette of views and studies was presented. After taking notice of this vast and diverse body of knowledge, the question emerges of how to move forward from here. How can this knowledge contribute to the further development of age-friendly cities and communities which benefits people of all ages?

We would like to call upon the wider scientific community, local, regional, and national governments, social enterprises, local and national businesses (such as construction companies, tradesmen etc.), and industry leaders (such as design agencies, manufacturing, fin-tech etc.), architects and urban planners, construction companies, and the creative industries, which can afford citizens of all ages various opportunities for active engagement in various elements of their respective age-friendly cities and ecosystems.

As Wetle ([79], p. 1930), posited, "designing and implementing age-friendly communities, health systems, or ecosystems requires long-term commitment and considerable resources, which necessitates a strong and effective champion who can bring together potential partners, share a compelling vision, and provide energy and leadership to the continuing effort". Therefore, it is laudable that an inclusive and age-friendly society is becoming more mainstream in Western societies through actions of the media. By working together between the disciplines and creating truly multisectoral actions, a genuine age-friendly society may be achieved for current and future generations. Such actions may even go beyond the current borders of the age-friendly movement, covering age-friendly public health and health systems, age-friendly states, and age-friendly universities [80].

The sharing of metrics and outcomes is one of the essential keys for successful action. This Feature Paper Special Issue entitled "*Age-Friendly Cities and Communities: State of the Art and Future Perspectives*" is one of the ways to expand and disseminate the knowledge on age-friendly cities and communities and to facilitate the actual age-friendliness of cities and communities agenda and narrative further. The body of knowledge presented here in this special issue acknowledges the importance of the interplay surrounding ageing, urbanisation, and digitalisation (technology). Additionally, this special issue affords scholars, stakeholders, regional and national policymakers and governments, and various actors within industry to understand, learn, and act upon to ensure the interconnected and adjoining facets associated to the quality of life for both younger and older people are met. Furthermore, this information and knowledge can and should benefit members of the wider communities (for instance, younger generations, people with chronic health/life-limiting conditions etc.) in our respective societies through real actions, instead of holding a mere promise for age-friendliness through the endless development of more tokenistic and policy-oriented age-friendly agendas, models, and frameworks that are based on outdated references from the previous century.

Author Contributions: J.v.H. wrote the first draft of the editorial and approved the final version. H.R.M. expanded the editorial by adding descriptions of the papers that are included in the special issue, in addition to structuring, strengthening, and amending the revisions of the editorial. All authors have read and agreed to the published version of the manuscript.

Funding: This editorial work received no external funding.

Institutional Review Board Statement: Not applicable.

Informed Consent Statement: Not applicable.

Acknowledgments: The authors wish to acknowledge the support of the International Journal of Environmental Research and Public Health staff and the work of the anonymous reviewers, editors and editorial board members.

Conflicts of Interest: The authors declare no conflict of interest.

References

1. World Health Organization. *Global Age-Friendly Cities: A Guide*; World Health Organization: Geneva, Switzerland, 2007; ISBN 9789241547307.
2. Plouffe, L.; Kalache, A. Towards Global Age-Friendly Cities: Determining Urban Features that Promote Active Aging. *J. Urban Health* **2010**, *87*, 733–739. [CrossRef] [PubMed]
3. Buffel, T.; Phillipson, C.; Rémillard-Boilard, S. Age-Friendly Cities and Communities: New Directions for Research and Policy. In *Encyclopedia of Gerontology and Population Aging*; Gu, D., Dupre, M.E., Eds.; Springer Nature: Cham, Switzerland, 2019. [CrossRef]
4. Van Hoof, J.; Kazak, J.K.; Perek-Białas, J.M.; Peek, S.T.M. The Challenges of Urban Ageing: Making Cities Age-Friendly in Europe. *Int. J. Environ. Res. Public Health* **2018**, *15*, 2473. [CrossRef]
5. World Health Organization. *The Checklist of Essential Features of Age-Friendly Cities*; World Health Organization: Geneva, Switzerland, 2007.
6. World Health Organization. Global Age-Friendly Cities Project. Available online: https://www.who.int/ageing/projects/age_friendly_cities/en/ (accessed on 30 January 2020).
7. Van Hoof, J.; Verkerk, M. Developing an integrated design model incorporating technology philosophy for the design of healthcare environments: A case analysis of facilities for psychogeriatric and psychiatric care in The Netherlands. *Technol. Soc.* **2013**, *35*, 1–13. [CrossRef]
8. Van Hoof, J.; Rutten, P.G.S.; Struck, C.; Huisman, E.R.C.M.; Kort, H.S.M. The integrated and evidence-based design of healthcare environments. *Arch. Eng. Des. Manag.* **2015**, *11*, 243–263. [CrossRef]
9. Kort, H.S.M.; Steunenberg, B.; van Hoof, J. Methods for Involving People Living with Dementia and Their Informal Carers as Co-Developers of Technological Solutions. *Dement. Geriatr. Cogn. Disord.* **2019**, *47*, 149–156. [CrossRef] [PubMed]
10. World Health Organization. *Measuring the Age-Friendliness of Cities: A Guide to Using Core Indicators*; World Health Organization: Geneva, Switzerland, 2015; ISBN 9789241509695.
11. Barrie, H.; Soebarto, V.; Lange, J.; Mc Corry-Breen, F.; Walker, L. Using Citizen Science to Explore Neighbourhood Influences on Ageing Well: Pilot Project. *Healthcare* **2019**, *7*, 126. [CrossRef]
12. Van Hoof, J.; Dikken, J.; Buttiġieġ, S.C.; van den Hoven, R.F.M.; Kroon, E.; Marston, H.R. Age-friendly cities in the Netherlands: An explorative study of facilitators and hindrances in the built environment and ageism in design. *Indoor Built Environ.* **2020**, *29*, 417–437. [CrossRef]
13. Flores, R.; Caballer-Miedes, A.; Alarcón, A. Evaluation of an Age-Friendly City and Its Effect on Life Satisfaction: A Two-Stage Study. *Int. J. Environ. Res. Public Health* **2019**, *16*, 5073. [CrossRef]
14. Garner, I.W.; Holland, C.A. Age-friendliness of living environments from the older person's viewpoint: Development of the Age-Friendly Environment Assessment Tool. *Age Ageing* **2019**, *49*, 193–198. [CrossRef]
15. Buckner, S.; Mattocks, C.; Rimmer, M.; LaFortune, L. An evaluation tool for Age-Friendly and Dementia Friendly Communities. *Work. Older People* **2018**, *22*, 48–58. [CrossRef] [PubMed]
16. Buckner, S.; Pope, D.; Mattocks, C.; LaFortune, L.; Dherani, M.; Bruce, N. Developing Age-Friendly Cities: An Evidence-Based Evaluation Tool. *J. Popul. Ageing* **2019**, *12*, 203–223. [CrossRef]
17. World Health Organization. *The Global Network for Age-Friendly Cities and Communities: Looking back over the Last Decade, Looking Forward to the Next*; World Health Organization: Geneva, Switzerland, 2018.
18. Marston, H.R.; van Hoof, J. "Who Doesn't Think about Technology When Designing Urban Environments for Older People?" A Case Study Approach to a Proposed Extension of the WHO's Age-Friendly Cities Model. *Int. J. Environ. Res. Public Health* **2019**, *16*, 3525. [CrossRef]
19. Podgórniak-Krzykacz, A.; Przywojska, J.; Wiktorowicz, J. Smart and Age-Friendly Communities in Poland. An Analysis of Institutional and Individual Conditions for a New Concept of Smart Development of Ageing Communities. *Energies* **2020**, *13*, 2268. [CrossRef]
20. Fabian, C.; Janett, S.; Bischoff, T.; Pardini, R.; Leitner, J.; Knöpfel, C. The Development of 'Age Appropriate' Living Environments: Analysis of Two Case Studies from a Social Work Perspective. *Urban Plan.* **2019**, *4*, 123–133. [CrossRef]
21. Van Hoof, J.; Marston, H.R.; Brittain, K.; Barrie, H. Creating Age-Friendly Communities: Housing and Technology. *Healthcare* **2019**, *7*, 130. [CrossRef] [PubMed]
22. Versey, H.S.; Murad, S.; Willems, P.; Sanni, M. Beyond Housing: Perceptions of Indirect Displacement, Displacement Risk, and Aging Precarity as Challenges to Aging in Place in Gentrifying Cities. *Int. J. Environ. Res. Public Health* **2019**, *16*, 4633. [CrossRef] [PubMed]
23. Von Faber, M.; Tavy, Z.; van der Pas, S. Engaging Older People in Age-Friendly Cities through Participatory Video Design. *Int. J. Environ. Res. Public Health* **2020**, *17*, 8977. [CrossRef] [PubMed]
24. Sterns, A.A.; Sterns, H.L.; Walter, A. Prioritizing Age-Friendly Domains for Transforming a Mid-Sized American City. *Int. J. Environ. Res. Public Health* **2020**, *17*, 9103. [CrossRef] [PubMed]
25. Davern, M.; Winterton, R.; Brasher, K.; Woolcock, G. How Can the Lived Environment Support Healthy Ageing? A Spatial Indicators Framework for the Assessment of Age-Friendly Communities. *Int. J. Environ. Res. Public Health* **2020**, *17*, 7685. [CrossRef] [PubMed]

26. Dikken, J.; van den Hoven, R.F.M.; van Staalduinen, W.; Hulsebosch-Janssen, L.M.T.; van Hoof, J. How Older People Experience the Age-Friendliness of Their City: Development of the Age-Friendly Cities and Communities Questionnaire. *Int. J. Environ. Res. Public Health* **2020**, *17*, 6867. [CrossRef] [PubMed]
27. Marston, H.R.; Niles-Yokum, K.; Silva, P.A. A Commentary on Blue Zones®: A Critical Review of Age-Friendly Environments in the 21st Century and Beyond. *Int. J. Environ. Res. Public Health* **2021**, *18*, 837. [CrossRef]
28. Rémillard-Boilard, S.; Buffel, T.; Phillipson, C. Developing Age-Friendly Cities and Communities: Eleven Case Studies from around the World. *Int. J. Environ. Res. Public Health* **2021**, *18*, 133. [CrossRef]
29. Rusinovic, K.M.; van Bochove, M.E.; Koops-Boelaars, S.; Tavy, Z.K.C.T.; van Hoof, J. Towards Responsible Rebellion: How Founders Deal with Challenges in Establishing and Governing Innovative Living Arrangements for Older People. *Int. J. Environ. Res. Public Health* **2020**, *17*, 6235. [CrossRef]
30. Bennetts, H.; Martins, L.A.; van Hoof, J.; Soebarto, V. Thermal Personalities of Older People in South Australia: A Personas-Based Approach to Develop Thermal Comfort Guidelines. *Int. J. Environ. Res. Public Health* **2020**, *17*, 8402. [CrossRef] [PubMed]
31. Sengers, F.; Peine, A. Innovation Pathways for Age-Friendly Homes in Europe. *Int. J. Environ. Res. Public Health* **2021**, *18*, 1139. [CrossRef]
32. Klicnik, I.; Dogra, S. Perspectives on Active Transportation in a Mid-Sized Age-Friendly City: "You Stay Home". *Int. J. Environ. Res. Public Health* **2019**, *16*, 4916. [CrossRef]
33. Loos, E.; Sourbati, M.; Behrendt, F. The Role of Mobility Digital Ecosystems for Age-Friendly Urban Public Transport: A Narrative Literature Review. *Int. J. Environ. Res. Public Health* **2020**, *17*, 7465. [CrossRef]
34. Ferrari, S.; Mattei, G.; Marchi, M.; Galeazzi, G.M.; Pingani, L. Is Consultation-Liaison Psychiatry 'Getting Old'? How Psychiatry Referrals in the General Hospital Have Changed over 20 Years. *Int. J. Environ. Res. Public Health* **2020**, *17*, 7389. [CrossRef] [PubMed]
35. Ziganshina, L.E.; Yudina, E.V.; Talipova, L.I.; Sharafutdinova, G.N.; Khairullin, R.N. Smart and Age-Friendly Cities in Russia: An Exploratory Study of Attitudes, Perceptions, Quality of Life and Health Information Needs. *Int. J. Environ. Res. Public Health* **2020**, *17*, 9212. [CrossRef] [PubMed]
36. Luijkx, K.; van Boekel, L.; Janssen, M.; Verbiest, M.; Stoop, A. The Academic Collaborative Center Older Adults: A Description of Co-Creation between Science, Care Practice and Education with the Aim to Contribute to Person-Centered Care for Older Adults. *Int. J. Environ. Res. Public Health* **2020**, *17*, 9014. [CrossRef] [PubMed]
37. De Boer, B.; Bozdemir, B.; Jansen, J.; Hermans, M.; Hamers, J.P.H.; Verbeek, H. The Homestead: Developing a Conceptual Framework through Co-Creation for Innovating Long-Term Dementia Care Environments. *Int. J. Environ. Res. Public Health* **2021**, *18*, 57. [CrossRef]
38. Ronzi, S.; Orton, L.; Buckner, S.; Bruce, N.; Pope, D. How is Respect and Social Inclusion Conceptualised by Older Adults in an Aspiring Age-Friendly City? A Photovoice Study in the North-West of England. *Int. J. Environ. Res. Public Health* **2020**, *17*, 9246. [CrossRef]
39. Codd, H. Prisons, Older People, and Age-Friendly Cities and Communities: Towards an Inclusive Approach. *Int. J. Environ. Res. Public Health* **2020**, *17*, 9200. [CrossRef]
40. Blakey, J.; Clews, J. Knowing, Being and Co-Constructing an Age-Friendly Tāmaki Makaurau Auckland. *Int. J. Environ. Res. Public Health* **2020**, *17*, 9136. [CrossRef] [PubMed]
41. Del Barrio, E.; Pinzón, S.; Marsillas, S.; Garrido, F. Physical Environment vs. Social Environment: What Factors of Age-Friendliness Predict Subjective Well-Being in Men and Women? *Int. J. Environ. Res. Public Health* **2021**, *18*, 798. [CrossRef] [PubMed]
42. Baraković, S.; Baraković Husić, J.; van Hoof, J.; Krejcar, O.; Maresova, P.; Akhtar, Z.; Melero, F.J. Quality of Life Framework for Personalised Ageing: A Systematic Review of ICT Solutions. *Int. J. Environ. Res. Public Health* **2020**, *17*, 2940. [CrossRef]
43. Anghel, I.; Cioara, T.; Moldovan, D.; Antal, M.; Pop, C.D.A.; Salomie, I.; Pop, C.B.; Chifu, V.R. Smart Environments and Social Robots for Age-Friendly Integrated Care Services. *Int. J. Environ. Res. Public Health* **2020**, *17*, 3801. [CrossRef] [PubMed]
44. Liddle, J.; Pitcher, N.; Montague, K.; Hanratty, B.; Standing, H.C.; Scharf, T. Connecting at Local Level: Exploring Opportunities for Future Design of Technology to Support Social Connections in Age-Friendly Communities. *Int. J. Environ. Res. Public Health* **2020**, *17*, 5544. [CrossRef]
45. Silvius, H.A.; Tak, E.C.P.M.; Mook-Kanamori, D.O.; Vos, H.M.; Numans, M.E.; Chavannes, N.H. Effects of Technology Use on Ageing in Place: The iZi Pilots. *Int. J. Environ. Res. Public Health* **2020**, *17*, 5052. [CrossRef]
46. Ivan, L.; Beu, D.; van Hoof, J. Smart and Age-Friendly Cities in Romania: An Overview of Public Policy and Practice. *Int. J. Environ. Res. Public Health* **2020**, *17*, 5202. [CrossRef]
47. Freeman, S.; Marston, H.R.; Olynick, J.; Musselwhite, C.; Kulczycki, C.; Genoe, R.; Xiong, B. Intergenerational Effects on the Impacts of Technology Use in Later Life: Insights from an International, Multi-Site Study. *Int. J. Environ. Res. Public Health* **2020**, *17*, 5711. [CrossRef]
48. Pedell, S.; Borda, A.; Keirnan, A.; Aimers, N. Combining the Digital, Social and Physical Layer to Create Age-Friendly Cities and Communities. *Int. J. Environ. Res. Public Health* **2021**, *18*, 325. [CrossRef] [PubMed]
49. Marston, H.R.; Shore, L.; White, P. How does a (Smart) Age-Friendly Ecosystem Look in a Post-Pandemic Society? *Int. J. Environ. Res. Public Health* **2020**, *17*, 8276. [CrossRef] [PubMed]
50. Reuter, A.; Liddle, J.; Scharf, T. Digitalising the Age-Friendly City: Insights from Participatory Action Research. *Int. J. Environ. Res. Public Health* **2020**, *17*, 8281. [CrossRef]

51. Van Hoof, J.; Kazak, J.K. Urban ageing. *Indoor Built Environ.* **2018**, *27*, 583–586. [CrossRef]
52. Buffel, T.; Phillipson, C. Urban ageing: New agendas for geographical gerontology. In *Geographical Gerontology: Perspectives, Concepts, Approaches*; Skinner, M.W., Andrews, G.J., Cutchin, M.P., Eds.; Routledge: London, UK, 2018; pp. 123–135, ISBN 9781138241152.
53. Buffel, T.; Phillipson, C. A Manifesto for the Age-Friendly Movement: Developing a New Urban Agenda. *J. Aging Soc. Policy* **2018**, *30*, 173–192. [CrossRef]
54. Buffel, T.; Phillipson, C. Can global cities be 'age-friendly cities'? Urban development and ageing populations. *Cities* **2016**, *55*, 94–100. [CrossRef]
55. Caro, F.G.; Fitzgerald, K.G. (Eds.) *International Perspectives on Age-Friendly Cities*; Routledge: New York, NY, USA, 2016; ISBN 9780415720717.
56. Szewrański, S.; Świąder, M.; Kazak, J.K.; Tokarczyk-Dorociak, K.; Van Hoof, J.J. Socio-Environmental Vulnerability Mapping for Environmental and Flood Resilience Assessment: The Case of Ageing and Poverty in the City of Wrocław, Poland. *Integr. Environ. Assess. Manag.* **2018**, *14*, 592–597. [CrossRef]
57. Chao, T.-Y.S. *Planning for Greying Cities. Age-Friendly City Planning and Design Research and Practice*; Routledge—Taylor & Francis Group: Abingdon, UK, 2018; ISBN 978-0-367-33190-0.
58. OECD. *Ageing in Cities*; OECD Publishing: Paris, France, 2015; ISBN 9789264231146.
59. Buffel, T.; Handler, S.; Phillipson, C. (Eds.) *Age-Friendly Cities and Communities: A Global Perspective*; Policy Press: Bristol, UK, 2018; ISBN 978-1-4473-3134-6.
60. Van Hoof, J.; Kort, H.S.M.; van Waarde, H. Housing and care for older adults with dementia: A European perspective. *J. Hous. Built. Env.* **2009**, *24*, 369–390. [CrossRef]
61. Van Hoof, J.J.; Kort, H.S.M.; van Waarde, H.; Blom, M.M. Environmental Interventions and the Design of Homes for Older Adults with Dementia: An Overview. *Am. J. Alzheimers Dis. Other Dement.* **2010**, *25*, 202–232. [CrossRef]
62. Van Hoof, J.; Blom, M.M.; Post, H.N.A.; Bastein, W.L. Designing a "Think-Along Dwelling" for People with Dementia: A Co-Creation Project Between Health Care and the Building Services Sector. *J. Hous. Elder.* **2013**, *27*, 299–332. [CrossRef]
63. Kazak, J.K.; van Hoof, J.; Świąder, M.; Szewrański, S. Real Estate for the Ageing Society—The Perspective of a New Market. *Real Estate Manag. Valuat.* **2017**, *25*, 13–24. [CrossRef]
64. Van Hoof, J.; Boerenfijn, P. Re-Inventing Existing Real Estate of Social Housing for Older People: Building a New De Benring in Voorst, The Netherlands. *Buildings* **2018**, *8*, 89. [CrossRef]
65. Kazak, J.K.; van Hoof, J. Decision support systems for a sustainable management of the indoor and built environment. *Indoor Built Environ.* **2018**, *27*, 1303–1306. [CrossRef]
66. Eijkelenboom, A.; Verbeek, H.; Felix, E.; van Hoof, J. The Architectural factors influencing the sense of home in nursing homes: An operationalization for practice. *Front. Arch. Res.* **2017**, *6*, 111–122. [CrossRef]
67. Rusinovic, K.; van Bochove, M.; van de Sande, J. Senior Co-Housing in the Netherlands: Benefits and Drawbacks for Its Residents. *Int. J. Environ. Res. Public Health* **2019**, *16*, 3776. [CrossRef]
68. Soebarto, V.; Bennetts, H.; Hansen, A.; Zuo, J.; Williamson, T.; Pisaniello, D.; van Hoof, J.; Visvanathan, R. Living environment, heating-cooling behaviours and well-being: Survey of older South Australians. *Build. Environ.* **2019**, *157*, 215–226. [CrossRef]
69. Van Hoof, J.; Bennetts, H.; Hansen, A.; Kazak, J.K.; Soebarto, V. The Living Environment and Thermal Behaviours of Older South Australians: A Multi-Focus Group Study. *Int. J. Environ. Res. Public Health* **2019**, *16*, 935. [CrossRef] [PubMed]
70. Meiland, F.J.M.; de Boer, M.E.; van Hoof, J.; van der Leeuw, J.; de Witte, L.; Blom, M.; Karkowski, I.; Mulvenna, M.D.; Dröes, R.-M. Functional Requirements for Assistive Technology for People with Cognitive Impairments and Dementia. *Commun. Comput. Inf. Sci.* **2012**, *277*, 146–151. [CrossRef]
71. Marston, H.R.; Greenlay, C.A.; van Hoof, J. Overview of Nintendo Wii^{TM} use and potential applications for the Microsoft Kinect^{TM} in residential facilities. *Technol. Disabil.* **2013**, *25*, 77–85. [CrossRef]
72. Van Rijn, H.; van Hoof, J.; Stappers, P.J. Designing Leisure Products for People with Dementia: Developing "the Chitchatters" Game. *Am. J. Alzheimers Dis. Other Dement.* **2010**, *25*, 74–89. [CrossRef] [PubMed]
73. Van Hoof, J.; Kort, H.S.M.; Rutten, P.G.S.; Duijnstee, M.S.H. Ageing-in-place with the use of ambient intelligence technology: Perspectives of older users. *Int. J. Med. Inform.* **2011**, *80*, 310–331. [CrossRef] [PubMed]
74. Nieboer, M.E.; van Hoof, J.; van Hout, A.M.; Aarts, S.; Wouters, E.J.M. Professional values, technology and future health care: The view of health care professionals in The Netherlands. *Technol. Soc.* **2014**, *39*, 10–17. [CrossRef]
75. Peek, S.T.M.; Luijkx, K.G.; Rijnaard, M.D.; Nieboer, M.E.; van der Voort, C.S.; Aarts, S.; van Hoof, J.; Vrijhoef, H.J.; Wouters, E.J.M. Older Adults' Reasons for Using Technology while Aging in Place. *Gerontology* **2016**, *62*, 226–237. [CrossRef] [PubMed]
76. Marston, H.R.; Samuels, J. A Review of Age Friendly Virtual Assistive Technologies and their Effect on Daily Living for Carers and Dependent Adults. *Healthcare* **2019**, *7*, 49. [CrossRef]
77. Marston, H.R.; Genoe, M.R.; Freeman, S.; Kulczycki, C.; Musselwhite, C. Older Adults' Perceptions of ICT: Main Findings from the Technology in Later Life (TILL) Study. *Healthcare* **2019**, *7*, 86. [CrossRef] [PubMed]
78. Baraković, S.; Baraković Husić, J.; Maraj, D.; Maraj, A.; Krejcar, O.; Maresova, P.; Melero, F.J. Quality of Life, Quality of Experience, and Security Perception in Web of Things: An Overview of Research Opportunities. *Electronics* **2020**, *9*, 700. [CrossRef]

79. Wetle, T.T. Age-Friendly Ecosystems: An Aspirational Goal. *J. Am. Geriatr. Soc.* **2020**, *68*, 1929–1930. [CrossRef]
80. Fulmer, T.; Patel, P.; Levy, N.; Mate, K.; Berman, A.; Peloton, L.; Beard, J.; Kalache, A.; Auerbach, J. Moving Toward a Global Age-Friendly Ecosystem. *J. Am. Geriatr. Soc.* **2020**, *68*, 1936–1940. [CrossRef]

International Journal of
Environmental Research and Public Health

MDPI

Article

Beyond Housing: Perceptions of Indirect Displacement, Displacement Risk, and Aging Precarity as Challenges to Aging in Place in Gentrifying Cities

H. Shellae Versey [1,*], Serene Murad [2], Paul Willems [1] and Mubarak Sanni [1]

1 Department of Psychology, Wesleyan University, Middletown, CT 06459, USA; pwillems@wesleyan.edu (P.W.); msanni@wesleyan.edu (M.S.)
2 Physicians for Human Rights, New York, NY 10018, USA; smurad@wesleyan.edu
* Correspondence: sversey@wesleyan.edu

Received: 14 October 2019; Accepted: 8 November 2019; Published: 21 November 2019

check for updates

Abstract: Neighborhoods within age-friendly cities and communities are an important factor in shaping the everyday lives of older adults. Yet, less is known about how neighborhoods experiencing change influence the ability to age in place. One type of rapid neighborhood change occurring across major cities nationally and globally is gentrification, a process whereby the culture of an existing neighborhood changes through the influx of more affluent residents and businesses. Few studies have considered the impact of gentrification on older adults, who are among the most vulnerable to economic and social pressures that often accompany gentrification. The current study explores one consequence of gentrification, indirect displacement. While gentrification-induced displacement can refer to the physical (e.g., direct) displacement of residents moving out of a neighborhood due to rising housing costs, it also references the replacement of the unique character and social identity of a neighborhood (e.g., indirect displacement). We examine perceptions of the latter, characterized by perceived cultural shifts and housing concerns among adults aging in place in a gentrifying neighborhood in New York City. The implications of indirect displacement for displacement risk and aging precarity are discussed as potential threats to aging in place in age-friendly cities.

Keywords: age-friendly cities; physical environment/space; urban ageing; gentrification; displacement; aging in place

---

1. Introduction

The number of older adults living in cities and urban areas is expected to increase in the coming years [1–3]. As a result, guidelines developed by the World Health Organization aim to help cities and communities become more age-friendly [3–6]. One central concern in accommodating the growing population of older adults is the availability of and accessibility to affordable housing for adults who desire to remain rooted in their homes and communities [7]. Aging in place—or the ability to live in one's own home and community safely, comfortably, and independently, regardless of age, race, income, or ability—is defined as the ideal by the majority of older adults and seniors [8–10]. However, there are challenges to achieving this goal for all those who desire to age in place that warrant further attention.

Aging in place can be difficult for lower-income adults with limited options for housing, particularly if neighborhood change results in more expensive rental and housing prices. Over the years, efforts to preserve affordable housing has resulted in the construction of Section 202 buildings. The Section 202 program helps expand the supply of affordable housing with supportive services for older adults, and allows them to live independently. Section 8 housing also provides housing assistance to moderate- and low-income households through the United States Department of Housing and Urban Development program [11]. However, in cities experiencing rapid turnover in many of its previous low-income neighborhoods due to gentrification, affordable housing has become increasingly scarce. In addition, the lack of affordable housing in gentrifying areas contributes to homelessness among older adults, which has received less attention in discussions about gentrification effects [12–15]. The current study explores these issues in New York City, a recognized age-friendly city that is undergoing gentrification, to better understand how housing scarcity within gentrifying neighborhoods presents obstacles to fully realizing an age-friendly agenda. Specifically, we aim to fill a gap in the literature about how gentrification can lead to various forms of displacement, highlighting implications for adults aging in place.

1.1. Literature Review

1.1.1. Gentrification

The transformation of lower-income neighborhoods into higher-income neighborhoods is increasingly common, due to what has been called a "back-to-city" movement [16,17]. One result (or perhaps cause) of this movement is gentrification, typically characterized by affluent (often younger and White) residents moving into lower-income (often ethnically-minority) neighborhoods. What qualifies as gentrification has been heavily debated in the academic literature [18]. Gentrification is defined here as a large-scale housing market process in which more affluent residents move into an area of less affluence that results in changes of neighborhood character, sociodemographic composition, and higher prices for goods, services, and housing [17]. This process may lead to the direct and indirect displacement of lower-income residents [17,19–21]. While a growing body of research has given attention to the displaced (e.g., those forced to leave gentrifying neighborhoods), less is known about the people who remain behind [22,23]. Besides qualifying 'what' gentrification is, questions that probe 'who' is affected by it are often secondary. A third question that remains unclear is, what are the effects of gentrification for people who continue to live in these changing neighborhoods, particularly for older adults aging in place?

1.1.2. Displacement: Direct and Indirect

Displacement can take several forms, direct and indirect. In one of the initial reports on neighborhood displacement, Grier and Grier [24] (p. 8) provide three criteria for defining displacement:

Displacement occurs when any household is forced to move from its residence by conditions which affect the dwelling or immediate surroundings, and which:

1. Are beyond the household's reasonable ability to control or prevent;
2. Occur despite the household's having met all conditions of occupancy; and
3. Make continued occupancy by that household impossible, hazardous, or unaffordable.

Therefore, when a household can no longer afford to remain in the same residential unit, residential displacement is a direct consequence (e.g., direct displacement). Direct displacement includes involuntary moves such as evictions, increased rent, and deliberate neglect of dwelling upkeep (by a landlord), all of which threaten a residents' ability to stay put [25]. Subsequent reports note that displacement is the negative outcome of gentrification specifically, not other types of neighborhood upgrading [26]. As a result, affordable housing available to lower-income residents in gentrifying neighborhoods can become scarce, displacing longtime residents as the cost of living in the neighborhood increases.

In New York City, displacement pressures are severe. For example, Figure 1 indicates types of residential displacement across New York City, showing that a number of census tracts in Northern Manhattan, particularly in West and Central Harlem, are undergoing advanced gentrification, defined here as lower-income households experiencing a higher risk of displacement by higher-income households.

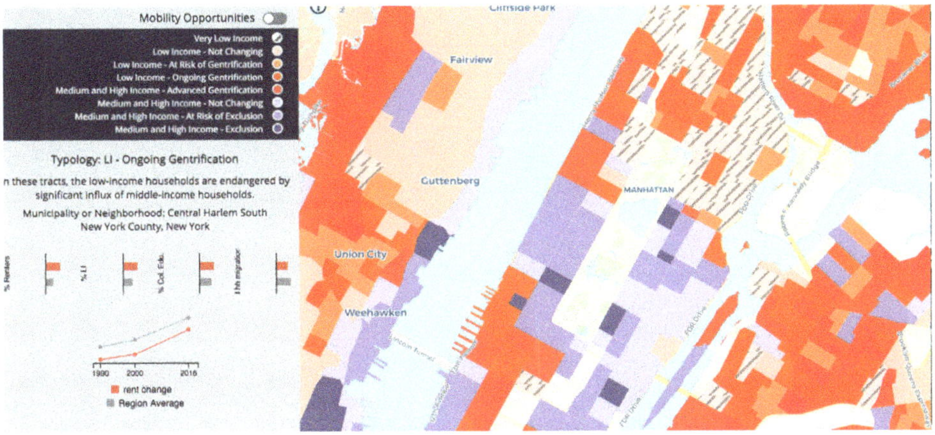

Figure 1. Source: Urban Displacement Project. Accessed October 19 at http://www.udpny.org/map.

In some cases, mobility rates of lower-income people are similar for both gentrifying and non-gentrifying neighborhoods. Several researchers have interpreted this finding as evidence that displacement is not occurring [27–29]. However, an alternate explanation suggests that these patterns represent one type of mobility (e.g., out of neighborhood), and indicates that rates of mobility among lower-income residents are uniformly high across all types of neighborhoods. Rather than no displacement, these trends indicate that lower-income people move more frequently. Furthermore, there are other indirect ways in which individuals continuing to live in gentrifying neighborhoods can be displaced that are important to highlight [16,30].

Scholars suggest that a second consequence of gentrification is indirect displacement [31–34]. While less documented, indirect displacement may have a significant impact on older residents [35,36]. Indirect displacement describes a type of social displacement that occurs when incoming residents and/or businesses:

1. Drive housing demand that inflates costs that make buying or renting property unattainable for existing residents (also called *exclusionary* displacement) [37]; or
2. Change the feel, tastes, norms, and desires of an existing neighborhood, replacing the preferences or desires of existing residents (also called *cultural* displacement) [36,38].

Therefore, although remaining in place, residents staying put may still encounter displacement indirectly, evidenced by the increased cost of goods, services, housing, and a changing neighborhood culture [36,39]. Unlike direct displacement in which residents themselves relocate (voluntarily or involuntarily), indirect displacement is facilitated by moving the people, places, and structures *around* existing residents who are able to remain in the neighborhood, effectively recreating a new space designed to attract newer residents [20].

1.1.3. Indirect Displacement and Aging in Place

Place is an important factor for how older adults see themselves within a community [9,40–45]. Research suggests that connectedness to public and semi-public spaces, community institutions, and landmarks strengthen social bonds, life satisfaction, and neighborhood identity, which are also significant for aging in place [16,39,46–48]. Since gentrification can change the 'feel' of a neighborhood by refashioning spaces in ways that cater to a selective few, neighborhoods can feel unwelcoming, even for longtime residents [5]. The establishment of new shops that feature expensive food or clothing, for example, convey implicit messages about who can and should enter these spaces [49]. In fact, a recent study finds that existing residents in gentrifying communities report feeling suddenly unwelcome in public spaces, playgrounds, and green spaces that should be accessible to everyone [50].

Broadly, if a place changes, feelings of displacement and/or exclusion can also be experienced, even if a person does not move. In this way, feeling unwelcomed in places that used to feel familiar may trigger insecurities and uncertainties about belonging, social exclusion, and the inability to feel 'in-place'. For older adults especially, feeling 'out of place' can have implications for everyday life, perceived isolation, and overall well-being [5,50,51]. While almost no study has investigated links between gentrification, indirect displacement and belonging among older adults specifically, complementary research suggests that losses associated with direct displacement can be traumatic [52]. Atkinson [53] (p. 382) finds that descriptions of gentrification among the forcibly displaced include feelings of resentment, anger, "as well as a deeper sense of nostalgia for changing social relations and lost connections". Studies have also shown that a sense of loss and grief can accompany residents who are forced to relocate to other places unexpectedly [32,47]. Whether the same loss is experienced when longtime residents manage to stay put in gentrifying neighborhoods remains a question.

1.1.4. Opportunities to Expand Aging in Place Research

Age-friendly neighborhoods that offer a sense of safety, belonging, and inclusion can provide additional support for older adults, particularly for those who may have fewer friends and family members living close by. If place can be understood as a source of familiarity where one attributes meaning, identity, and importance, then the loss of places that residents consider 'home' should be explored further. Yet, little research in the United States has explored the importance of place, or how older adults can remain in place as they age.

In global and graying cities such as New York City, a limited affordable housing stock presents challenges for residents living in cities that have high levels of economic inequality [54]. For example, rent burden, or paying 30% or more of household income in rent, creates financial strain that contributes to precarity. Aging precarity represents instability in later life and usually stems from additional care and support needs, combined with limited disposable resources to accommodate such needs [55].

In New York City, rent burden is highest among the most vulnerable–adults over the age of 65, as well as extremely low-income, and very low-income residents (see Table 1, Figure 2). Single, low-income adults over the age of 60 are the most vulnerable, subject to the highest rates of severe rent burden in the city. Yet research connecting aging in place to drivers of affordable housing for seniors, such as gentrification, is surprisingly scarce [5,23].

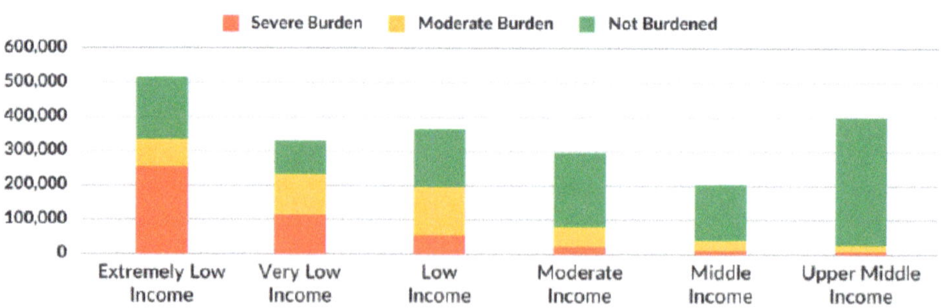

Figure 2. New York City renter households by level of rent burden by income group (2017). Note: Rent burden was calculated using Gross Rent Measure = Gross Rent Paid/Household Income.

Table 1. Renter households by rent-burden type and household characteristics, New York City (2017)

		Low Income Severely Burdened	Share of Low Income Severely Burdened	Share of All Households in Group
Total Households		420,798	100%	20%
Singles		202,644	48%	27%
	29 or younger	14,538	3%	19%
	30 to 59	79,194	19%	22%
	60 and older	100,912	26%	35%
Multiple Adults without Children		114,212	27%	15%
	29 or younger	17,685	4%	11%
	30 to 59	45,010	11%	11%
	60 and older	51,517	12%	24%
Single Parents		32,289	8%	26%
	29 or younger	4834	1%	30%
	30 to 59	25,926	6%	26%
	60 and older	1529	0%	20%
Multiple Adults with Children		71,654	17%	16%
	29 or younger	10,851	3%	20%
	30 to 59	54,673	13%	15%
	60 and older	6129	1%	19%

Source: Citizens Budget Commission staff analysis using U. S. Census Bureau data and New York City Housing and Vacancy Survey, 2017.

Therefore, one aim of this work is to understand how older adults describe the experience of living in a neighborhood that is changing. As many older adults express a continuing desire to age in place, it is important to understand how the ability to do so may be aided or compromised by neighborhood change. The traditional focus of aging in place research has been on physical features of the home that support growing old. This study aims to expand that focus to neighborhoods and communities using guidelines outlined by the Age-Friendly Agenda [56,57]. Since aging happens in a larger social and environmental context, realizing that agenda entails highlighting differential processes that may facilitate thriving, or simply surviving, during later years. The current study focuses on these issues within a gentrifying neighborhood in New York City to address the following research questions: What is the importance of neighborhood for adults aging in place? How do older adults perceive gentrification-induced change in their neighborhood, and do they perceive these changes as beneficial to older adults in the community?

2. Methods

2.1. Research Site: Central Harlem, New York City

Within the five boroughs of New York City, parts of Manhattan have undergone extensive gentrification, particularly in Northern Manhattan, where rentals and home sales have set record highs [58,59]. For example, between 1996 and 2006, home prices increased by 270% in the Central Harlem neighborhood, decreasing the number of affordable housing units during the same period (see Table 2, Figures 2–4). Central Harlem is a mixed-income community in the borough of Manhattan that is currently undergoing gentrification [59,60]. Central Harlem was selected for this study because it is a gentrifying neighborhood and home to a large, yet declining number of long-term and older African American residents. It is also a historical neighborhood and a culturally distinctive place among Black people and people of African descent–both foreign born and African Americans–across the diaspora generally [61,62].

Table 2. Neighborhoods with the largest increases in home sale prices (1996–2006).

Neighborhood	Borough	% Increase
East Harlem	Manhattan (Upper)	499.6%
Morningside/Hamilton Heights	Manhattan (Upper)	398.7%
Washington Heights/Inwood	Manhattan (Upper)	333.4%
Central Harlem	Manhattan (Upper)	270.2%
Fort Greene/Brooklyn Heights	Brooklyn	261.5%

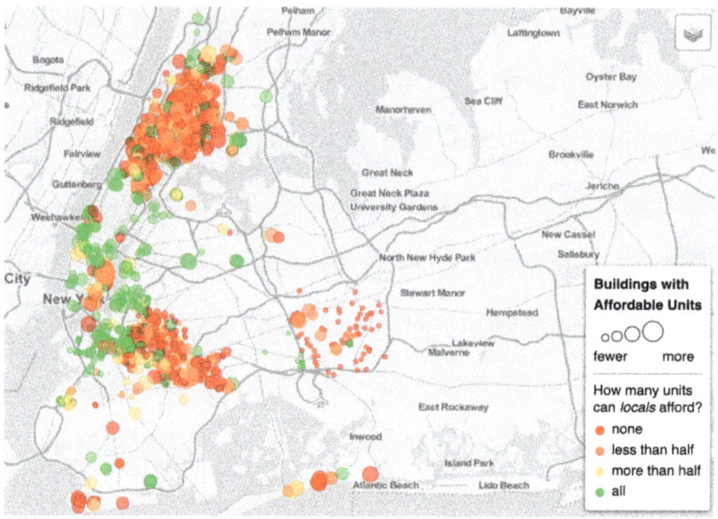

Figure 3. Buildings with affordable units for a typical median household, New York City (2018).

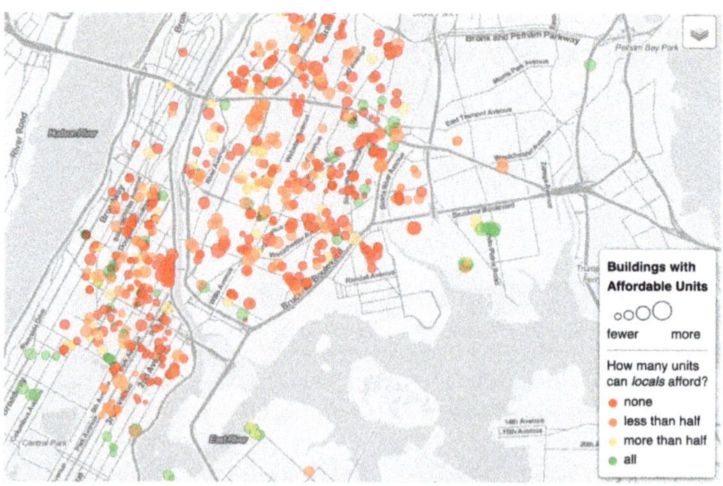

Figure 4. Buildings with affordable units for a typical median household, for the South Bronx and Northern Manhattan, including Central Harlem (2018). Source: Sam Raby's data analysis for Curbed, Vox Media. Data sources: American Community Survey, New York Open Data, Housing and Urban Development Office of Policy Development and Research. Accessed September 30, 2019 at https://voxmedia.github.io/curbed-maps/HNY/

Quantifying the impact of gentrification in numerical terms has numerous challenges, and secondary data analyses may underestimate various types of displacement that occur within and across gentrifying neighborhoods [35,63]. There are few studies that describe the experiences of aging residents in gentrifying areas, and fewer that engage topics of displacement, particularly among communities of color. Therefore, a qualitative approach is used to explore how older African American adults perceive markers of neighborhood change while staying put. All participants are aging in place, and have lived in the same community for the past decade with some level of independence.

2.2. Participants and Demographic Characteristics

Participants were recruited from senior housing residential buildings and senior centers in the Central Harlem neighborhood. Nine focus groups with 98 African American men and women were conducted. Participants were required to have lived in Central Harlem for the past 10 years, be age 55 or older, and English-speaking. The minimum age limit of 55 was set to capture a wider variation of older adults, particularly those considered to be young-old [64–66].

The mean age of participants was 76 years old (SD = 1.64), with ages ranging from 55 to 92 years of age. Men and women were nearly equally represented, with women comprising 52% of participants. According to a short demographic survey administered prior to interviews, most respondents were single, widowed or divorced (82%). The average educational level was "some high school" (45.4%) or "graduated from high school" (16.8%). Eighty-seven percent were either retired (51%), unemployed (27.6%), or unable to work due to disability (8.4%). All respondents identified as Black/African American.

2.3. Participant Recruitment and Focus Group Facilitation

Participants were recruited through word of mouth from residential site managers, social workers, and paper flyers. Leading up to the first session, there was a four-week planning phase with all site coordinators regarding the scope and aims of the project. All (de-identified) data would be available to participants or coordinators following the conclusion of the project, if requested. This planning phase also included training of undergraduate students who would participate in the project.

At the first session, residents were invited to participate after a verbal explanation of the purpose of the study. Residents were informed that participation was voluntary, and all responses would be anonymously reported. Focus groups were held in the community space of each senior housing building, with the exception of one group that was held at a senior center. The research team was led by a trained and experienced African American female focus group facilitator. Three trained undergraduate students—one African American male, one African American female, and one European American female—served as research assistants for the study. Participants were encouraged to respond openly and honestly, regardless if thoughts and attitudes differed from other responses. Undergraduate students served as assistants and note-takers throughout the sessions.

Open-ended questions were posed in such a way to allow participants to be descriptive of the neighborhood, and all participants were encouraged to speak. With the consent of all participants, the discussion was taped and later transcribed verbatim by a third-party transcription service. Each focus group took approximately 60–90 min to complete and participants were paid $20 for their participation.

The focus group guide explored perceived neighborhood change as a function of gentrification. Sample questions included: What is most important about this neighborhood? Has the neighborhood changed in the past 10 to 15 years? If so, do you think of these changes as mostly positive or negative for the people who have been living here? The Human Subjects Research Institutional Review Board reviewed and approved the study, protocols, and materials (2016-0421-sversey-HCS).

2.4. Data Analysis

Thematic analysis was used to identify and organize major themes from discussions [67]. Data analysts listened to audio recordings and read the transcripts several times, developing initial codes and synthesizing them into broader categories [68,69]. Data collected during each focus group were primarily analyzed for mentions of neighborhood importance and neighborhood change, whether it is occurring and to what extent, as well as potential benefits and challenges to aging in place.

Inconsistencies in initial textual coding were discussed and resolved, and a second round of coding was conducted for accuracy and agreement ($\kappa = 0.82$) (95% CI, 0.500 to 0.886). Coding schemes were then categorized and discussed as a group, yielding three major themes—(1) neighborhood importance and identity; (2) perceived cultural displacement; and (3) housing concerns and financial precarity. Cultural displacement was defined according to conventional usage in the literature [48,70].

3. Results

3.1. Descriptive Analysis

The majority of respondents were renters (86.5%), with the highest percentage living in senior housing residences (HUD 202). The Housing and Urban Development (HUD) 202 program the only federal rental assistance program targeted specifically to older adults. In order to qualify for Section 202 housing, applicants must meet age and low-income requirements. Other participants lived in New York City Housing Authority buildings/public housing (15.6%) or rent-stabilized apartments (12.5%).

Results are organized by major themes that emerged in response to study questions—neighborhood importance, neighborhood identity, perceived cultural displacement, housing, and financial precarity. Breaks between quotes indicate responses by different participants. In at least half of the conversations, the notion that the neighborhood had changed over time was spontaneously generated by participants themselves, allowing the facilitator to probe about specific changes, and ways in which these changes were perceived. In other cases (when change was not mentioned), the facilitator asked whether participants thought the neighborhood had changed any since they had been living there.

When participants mentioned neighborhood change or gentrification specifically, the facilitator asked for qualification regarding the meaning of 'change'. Generally, changes referred to the number of new residents moving in, mostly White and higher income people, more African Americans moving out, increased housing/rental prices, the establishment of new businesses, and the provision of better community services, such as park improvement, more policing, and sanitation.

3.2. Neighborhood Importance and Identity

When asked about what is 'relevant' or 'important' about the neighborhood, respondents overwhelmingly noted that it was "the people" that made Harlem special. When asked to elaborate, several participants recounted childhood stories growing up there, or referenced a time when they first moved to the neighborhood. Participants who had migrated to the neighborhood from other cities or boroughs discussed an attraction to the place, its vibrancy, its cultural familiarity, and the warmness of the people. A familiar refrain throughout the interviews was that the central identity of Harlem was a "mecca for Black people", yet it was open and welcoming to all people.

3.2.1. Neighborhood Identity

The notion that Harlem represented the people led to discussions that the neighborhood was changing into a 'new' version of itself, due primarily to gentrification. While some changes were welcomed (e.g., cleaner streets, better maintenance services) others voiced concern that "pushing out the people who made the neighborhood special" meant changing, or perhaps displacing, the culture of the place. For example, one respondent noted that even during the drug era of the 70s and 80s that plagued many urban neighborhoods, those involved in illicit activity were still part of the Harlem community and Harlem's history for better or worse:

But it's the people in Harlem that's important. Now we're not talking about the people that you see down on 123rd Street and Lexington Avenue (a place known for drug activity) . . . even though they're still a part of us. They're still a part of us and they just got lost. But they're not the majority.

Others perceived that the people of Harlem built the neighborhood as it is known today (e.g., as a distinctive place to experience Black culture), and recent changes eroded a sense of what Harlem meant to the Black community.

One thing it does...it drives out the identity of what Harlem was.

I was born in Harlem, I said, "Okay, I'm going to die in Harlem." You know, because regardless of all the crap that goes on in Harlem, these are my people. I love Harlem. And you know, as bad as it is, I still love Harlem.

Especially when you try to change the name [of Harlem], you erase all of what forefathers have done for us. That's exactly what they're trying to do. Not even the next generation, or the next, next generation is going to know what Harlem was.

Speaking of the Harlem Renaissance, we came up on 7th Avenue, on 138th Street. Remember the old Renaissance Ballroom? What is it now? It's being built for luxury condos. And you know we can't afford it, because everybody that I know on 132nd, 133rd, 134th Street—I was looking for them and they're gone.

The final participant observes that not only is the Renaissance Ballroom (a historical structure) no longer standing, but the people who live in the surrounding blocks are also gone—an acknowledgement that if people make places, both have suffered as a result of gentrification. Responses suggest that a loss of place (e.g., displacement) is occurring even though the people themselves are remaining put.

3.2.2. Neighborhood as 'Home'

The second most frequently mentioned sentiment about the importance of Harlem (besides the people) was that it symbolized a sense of 'home'. When probed about the meaning of 'home', respondents noted that they considered the neighborhood to be home. In addition to not wanting to leave the neighborhood, they felt secure in not having to leave, due to the financial housing subsidies provided to older residents that allowed them to remain put. Interestingly, while almost all respondents felt fortunate to have secured a unit within a senior housing building in which they were relatively protected from increasing rents, many participants expressed disappointment in living far from family members who were physically displaced due to not being able to afford to live in the same neighborhood. Perhaps as a result, several respondents expressed that the legacy of the neighborhood as being unique, distinct, and predominantly Black was in danger of being lost and should be preserved.

3.3. *Perceived Cultural Displacement and Black Space Erasure*

Related fears about the erasure of people and historic places led to the expression of more general concerns about the future of Black people and Black spaces that cultivate inclusion, belonging, and ownership among Black people.

Harlem was described as one of the few places where Blacks could enjoy a sense of Black history and be welcomed by other Black people. One participant explains the transition from the way things were to a newer version of the neighborhood in terms of an "assault" on Black people, threatening a larger sense of community through displacement of the culture:

It's like an assault on black people. You know, you don't want to say this, but it's like a huge assault, forever, on black people. And if it's not one thing, it's another. It's always to take us down or take us out altogether.

Another respondent highlights tensions between the economic boom in Harlem and cultural loss, suggesting that the "boom in diversity" may exclude Black residents already living in the neighborhood.

> *Just recently, it's just been a boom in diversity here, of all nationalities. And the people that I growed up with in Harlem for the last 50 years, including now, they have really decreased in numbers. Its upsetting the culture balance. And our culture, as far as I'm concerned, our culture balance has been like drastically changed.*

> *They taking our space. And we can't live—we can't go back to how it used to be.*

The idea that the neighborhood had changed in the past decade was unanimous among participants. Collectively, some participants viewed the neighborhood transition as change for a better community, enabling greater access to certain services. On the other hand, the majority of respondents viewed the changes as eroding a deeper sense of community and neighborhood identity, which were perceived to be at least equally important to, if not more important than, the improvement of amenities, some of which were viewed to accommodate incoming residents more than existing residents.

3.3.1. Church Tourism

Participants also mentioned the unique aspects of the neighborhood were being marketed to others who lived elsewhere, in an attempt to draw them to Harlem. Several participants reported that churches were part of the problem, complicit in gentrification, catering to real estate developers and tourists. Generally, there was a sense of frustration that churches were not doing more to assist older people in the community who were vulnerable to displacement.

Churches were also criticized for profiting from gentrification by selling church-owned property to developers and discontinuing social activities that kept the community connected. Larger churches were described as being in a position to use political and social influence to redirect, and even stop displacement efforts. However, participants perceived that the majority of pastors and church officials were preoccupied with financial gain.

> *Churches have become tourist attractions. People come and fall in love with Harlem and the next thing you know, they move here! That's how come most of the churches in Harlem got two services, because they couldn't accommodate them in one service.*

> *Now, if you go to any church in Harlem you'll notice two-thirds of the churches now are filled with tourists. Yeah, they drop off two busloads of tourists here every Sunday.*

> *Most of us, our churches are three-quarters tourists now. And that's who's coming here now–immigrants from Europe.*

Disagreement among participants regarding whether churches were helping or harming the community was expressed in the majority of interview groups. Some participants maintained that the church was still regarded as a place where community outreach and important charitable functions still took place. For example, most respondents who indicated that they were politically involved primarily participated in church-related efforts.

3.3.2. Outsider/Insider Tensions

Finally, respondents reported feeling 'out of place' when local businesses were replaced by more expensive retail options. Participants described the replacement of mom-and-pop businesses with new businesses that made Harlem more expensive and also made it feel less like a community.

> *You don't have any people, black people, owning stores anymore. It's all Caucasian, different nationalities. We don't have anything. We don't have anything to say that the black people have a store. And all the stores that are opening is not for us.*

Most new businesses were perceived as providing services for newer residents. In addition, participants reported that competition with new businesses put a strain on mom-and-pop stores (primarily Black) that had been long-term establishments in the neighborhood.

When you talk about economy, our people failed, not because they wanted to. They couldn't get loans in the banks. Mom and Pop stores for blacks can't get loans like Mom and Pop stores who are white.

Besides the racial turnover in ownership of local businesses, several participants mentioned being treated "differently" when interacting with new shopkeepers.

We went in there (Korean-owned beauty-supply store) and they were following us around. You know, we didn't have that experience before. And my daughter said, "Mom, what's this here?" She was really upset that it had changed like that. It had changed for me too because, you know, this is my home. This is my home, you know, this is where I grew up.

This participant summarizes recurring tensions between residents and new, incoming businesses. If home is a place in which one feels safe and welcomed, negative neighbor relations may contribute to residents feeling alienated. When asked about other types of businesses in the neighborhood, such as restaurants and new eateries, participants expressed disinterest in entering such establishments, citing that they were "too expensive" and "not intended for them". As one respondent noted:

Well, we accept everybody in Harlem but we're not accepted everywhere we go.

On the other hand, some participants welcomed new businesses into the neighborhood as a sign that Harlem was improving. New supermarkets that provided more fresh fruits, vegetables and food options, for example, were considered amenities worth paying for. In some cases, these businesses and improved services were seen as markers of progress that strengthened the community.

I have nothing against white folks moving in to my neighborhood, okay? Because my garbage is getting picked up better.

While a few participants thought gentrification was positive since it brought selective improvements such as cleaner streets and better public services, others voiced frustration that services such as trash pick-up and community policing seemed to be a priority only when new residents moved in. Since these and other amenities were done in selective areas (i.e., mostly where newcomers lived) they were perceived as serving the needs of the community only when newcomers arrived. Interestingly, some participants expressed the idea that "White people complain more" to get things accomplished as one reason why some amenities had improved.

Overall, participants reported that the neighborhood was important—as a physical 'home', but also as a place that Black people generally could call home due to its history and sense of being welcoming. In all nine focus groups, there were references that a cultural piece of Harlem had been lost, or was in danger of disappearing. Follow-up probes about precisely what has been lost yielded a variety of answers including a sense of history, the Black community, its people, and most of what has made it unique in the past. At the same time, participants across all sites were divided about whether these changes were entirely positive or negative.

3.4. Housing Concerns and Financial Precarity

3.4.1. Housing Concerns

Respondents agreed that Harlem had become a more expensive place to live, and this was a frequent response to the question regarding whether the neighborhood had changed in the past decade. Although several participants agreed that they were not personally impacted by rising housing costs (those living in HUD Section 202 Housing), one participant argued that it was the lack of affordable housing in the neighborhood generally that pushed other longtime residents out, changing who was able to move in and thus, why the neighborhood felt less welcoming. One woman who had been unable to afford her previous rent before finding her current apartment commented:

> *My apartment was also the same thing. I started out paying $500 and before I knew it they want $2500. So, it's crazy. Every time you turn around they open up a new outside restaurant but people got no place to live.*

According to the same participant, rising rental costs are misaligned with the incomes of current residents, particularly seniors on limited budgets.

3.4.2. Housing Precarity

Increasing rents were mentioned as particularly troublesome for residents in the past, creating a cycle of living in multiple places for a period of time, and then moving when the rent was increased. While these moves would not qualify as displacement out of the neighborhood, the need to move multiple times within the same neighborhood represents a type of displacement pressure and housing precarity that is typically not captured in traditional displacement studies.

In addition, respondents mentioned that long waiting lists to get an apartment in senior buildings forced older renters out of the neighborhood who could not afford to wait. Participants reported waiting two to five years on average to be notified about an available unit. Both accounts reference a type of indirect displacement that 'prices out' would-be renters, who, as a function of rising rents and limited affordable housing stock, are no longer able to live within the neighborhood.

Several participants suggested that the increasing rents were intentional, in order to move existing (Black) residents out, incentivize new (White) residents to move in, and encourage new development in the neighborhood.

> *Poor people can't afford it. Therefore, in changing the neighborhood you'll need more white people to sustain it.*

> *When I say housing, [I mean] the accessibility to affordable housing. Okay? So now, if you can afford it, you're taking more of your income to pay rent, as opposed to saving and doing other things with it that you could have been doing.*

While the phrase 'rent burden' was not used in conversations, participants reported that much of their income was devoted to paying rent, leaving fewer resources for recreational or discretionary purposes. Similar examples of rent burden and housing strain were consistent across all study sites.

3.4.3. Homelessness

Conversations about being rent-burdened overlapped with concerns about financial security. Chief among housing-related concerns was the prospect of no longer being able to afford to live in the neighborhood, should a health emergency or some unexpected need arise. Ten participants across three separate groups independently introduced the notion that in such circumstances, they had known family members or acquaintances who had resorted to living in shelters. One participant disclosed that he had previously lived in a homeless shelter. Across several sites, respondents described a variety of financial situations that preceded un-homing friends or relatives, compromising their ability to stay housed.

Mod: *Where do you think people are going?*
Participant P: *Shelters.*
Participant K: *Sleeping on the street.*
Participant L: *Homeless.*
Participant C: *Yeah, sleeping on the street.*

Mod: *Oh?*
Participant K: *Yeah, because even the shelters are getting crowded now.*
Participant P: *Right, they were crowded before, but they're worse now.*

At a different study site, one participant who disclosed having previously worked in the social service system in the city mentioned the hidden elder and working population that lives in homeless shelters, which she believed to be increasing.

The shelter population is ridiculous right now. It's like it's so many people in the shelters. And we're talking working people, working people! Not they're doing drugs on the street. They cannot pay their rent with the money they're asking for rent.

Taken together, while participants felt affordable housing was an issue for the community, discussions focused on the more indirect effects of increasing rents that pushed residents to other precarious housing arrangements, still within the same neighborhood. The idea that Harlem was a more expensive place to live now, however, was only partially directed towards housing. Residents discussed how increased housing costs created additional spillover effects.

3.4.4. Gentrification and Financial Insecurity

The increased cost of living was considered the greatest threat to the ability to remain in the neighborhood. In other words, while participants were not *directly* displaced through eviction or relocation out of the neighborhood, the cost of living was cited as a major challenge to being able to age in place and enjoy a reasonable quality of life. For example, participants mentioned that although they were able to pay rent, they often had difficulty affording other necessities such as food and transportation, coinciding with other citywide changes in public benefits (e.g., reduction in food assistance programs and increases in MTA public transit fares) [71,72].

Several participants reported that rent consumed most of their monthly income. Residents who lived in public housing were concerned by increasing rents that would accompany privatization efforts headed by the New York City Housing Authority (NYCHA) and private interests (e.g., Rental Assistance Demonstration—RAD conversion). When asked whether or not privatizing public housing would be beneficial for older, and lower-income families, responses were mixed.

They want to clean it up. You know, that would be one way of making it safe and better for residents.

Yes, and they want the buildings. And they want the real estate—so now they're pushing them [public housing residents] all to the Bronx or Long Island.

The last point related to "pushing low-income residents out" led to subsequent discussions about the impact of gentrification on outer boroughs, traveling longer distances to visit family, and less frequent visits from family.

3.4.5. Summary of Findings

Overall, participants felt that their neighborhood was important to them and felt like home. Despite some benefits that accompanied neighborhood change, the majority of participants stated that the essence of the neighborhood was being displaced by newcomers. Church tourism and insider/outsider tensions were cited as visible markers of a changing neighborhood feel, while housing scarcity and financial pressures contributed to concerns about aging in place, and aging near family.

4. Discussion

4.1. Indirect Pathways: Gentrification-Induced Displacement

This study examined a sample of older Black adults' experiences aging in place in a gentrifying neighborhood. Our findings highlight the social, financial and mental health consequences of neighborhood change for older adults—neighborhood identity, cultural displacement, housing, and financial precarity. These markers describe how older adults felt displaced despite remaining in the neighborhood, suggesting that there are indirect ways in which gentrification can engender displacement. These results are also notable considering that previous research has found little evidence of displacement in Central Harlem using quantitative indices. Nearly all respondents considered the neighborhood to be 'home' and wanted to remain in the neighborhood in hopes of aging in place. Indirect displacement has received less attention in previous research on gentrification; yet it may have several important consequences, particularly related to aging in place.

In some ways, this research reflects what is known about the effects of gentrification, however, findings related to cultural displacement and older adults specifically illuminate new ideas about how residents understand displacement and relatedly, what makes place (e.g., placemaking). Lefebvre's [73] idea that space is a social production permeates underlying narratives about gentrification and the terminology used to describe it. The language of renewal, revitalization, and reinvestment, for example, suggests a new valuation placed upon a previously devalued space. In fact, this study reveals that the Harlem neighborhood always held value, even in times of economic ruin, based on its cultural significance to the people living there. This set of realities has been called 'Black placemaking', to reflect the ways that Black people have created sites of cultural relevance, endurance, belonging, and resistance in spite of segregation, redlining, disinvestment, and neglect [74].

While this literature has not been linked to gentrification previously, the notion of placemaking extends knowledge about how neighborhoods function as places for how people see themselves in a larger context (e.g., place identity) [75,76]. While certainly not specific to Harlem, Black enclaves and residential communities are one way older residents might connect with a larger community, feel welcomed and appreciated [77]. In this way, Harlem is not simply a neighborhood, it is an example of Black placemaking, evidenced by participants' reflections of how residents were able to transform what others deemed as disorder into authentic experiences, community, and spaces of inclusion and celebration [74,78]. Therefore, in the absence of being welcomed elsewhere, Black neighborhoods provide Black people an opportunity to carve out places where they satisfy the need to belong.

Developing spaces that are inclusive of older residents is a central priority of age-friendly initiatives. However, our study finds that gentrification may increase the invisibility of aging adults by contributing to indirect and direct processes that erase people and places of significance. According to Kelley and colleagues [79] (p. 56) as cited by Buffel and Phillipson [5]:

> *Erasure is a concept used as a social critique of the ways certain groups of people are simply unseen in policy, research, or institutional practices. It is a form of social exclusion so embedded in the cultural assumptions of a society that the absence of these groups is not even recognized.*

Future research may consider how to reconcile new development with preservation efforts in collaboration with the community to increase visibility for all residents. Public, residential, and commercial spaces should be examined further, since together, they shape the way neighborhoods are experienced. Policy that specifically targets older adults and aging in place is one way to include interests that have previously not been recognized. Expanded rent protections for low-income and extremely low-income residents, for example, can make communities accessible to groups with fewer resources.

4.2. Precarious Aging in Place

A primary finding suggests that the ability to afford (and have access to) housing, goods, and services is important in order to remain rooted [23,80]. When new, more affluent residents move in, existing residents may benefit in some ways. Residents may also find it difficult to buy or rent property in the same neighborhood at the same rate, leading to housing precarity, a state of uncertainty and instability [81,82]. Aging precariously in place means that older adults are often managing multiple challenges tied to housing, such as housing-cost burden, financial insecurity, changes to mobility, and/or experiencing social isolation [83].

Lower-income and African American older adults are more likely to be housing cost-burdened than other groups, and are more likely restrict (or skip entirely) meals, food purchases, prescriptions, and transportation services in order to pay for rent [80]. Among older residents already facing severe financial challenges, making decisions between paying for food or housing may mean forgoing important primary or preventive medical care [50]. Housing instability was mentioned as a housing concern in which rising rents led to frequent moves and in some cases, homelessness. While homelessness among the working poor has received little attention in the larger conversation on gentrification, it was mentioned as a real fear (and reality) for several residents. Housing costs also contributed to what participants described as rent burden, leaving fewer resources for food or other expenses. Housing costs also complicated ways to receive and provide assistance to family members, many of whom were displaced to outer boroughs.

4.3. Limitations

There are some limitations to this research worth noting. This study focuses on one neighborhood as a case study to illustrate the effects of gentrification. Therefore, the findings are not necessarily generalizable to other neighborhoods within New York City, or other age-friendly cities generally. Given this, however, we caution against oversimplifying the findings as being unique since similar trends have been found in other metropolitan areas in the United States, including Seattle, San Francisco, and Washington, DC.

Second, although the focus of this study is older adults, it is likely that the issues raised in the current study are not specific to aging in place, but extend to other groups as well, including younger Black Americans and/or other racial-ethnic groups. Since all participants were required to speak English, there may be additional neighborhood dynamics among lower-income, non-English speaking adults that the current study was unable to observe. We do hope this research ignites dialogue and further discussion about the far-reaching implications of gentrification, cultural displacement, and precarity for all socially vulnerable groups.

4.4. Implications for Future Research

4.4.1. Age-Friendly Communities in Gentrifying Cities?

A robust body of research shows that neighborhoods are increasingly important to support health and aging [84–86]. Meaningful social connections become important with age, since older adults are more likely to frame their daily activities and interpersonal interactions within their immediate neighborhoods [87,88]. When a neighborhood changes, new neighbors can create a less-inclusive social environment that can contribute to long-term residents feeling 'pushed out' of one's own neighborhood. Therefore, understanding how gentrification reshapes networks, a sense of belonging, and 'age-friendliness' is important.

Our research finds several consistencies worth noting. One consistency is that participants do not want to lose the essence of their neighborhood, nor feel like strangers in it. Another consensus is that neighborhoods undergoing gentrification are more expensive to live in, and as a result, make some aspects of aging in place more difficult. A lack of affordable housing, the closure of longtime businesses, and feeling socially and financially insecure increased feelings of uncertainty among participants, potentially hurting, rather than helping older adults wanting to age in place.

Future research on age-friendly cities should address the availability of affordable housing, as well as how housing scarcity contributes to secondary effects (e.g., homelessness) mentioned in the current study. Few studies have addressed homelessness as a byproduct of gentrification, and additional research will yield knowledge about how to ensure housing is accessible for all residents, particularly seniors. Similar to other national models that have developed pilot interventions for evaluating and measuring the collective impact of age-friendly community initiatives [89,90], future research should consider assessing indicators of elder displacement and homelessness as metrics of how well age-friendly cities and communities are meeting the needs of its constituents.

4.4.2. Mixed-Methods, Counter Mapping, and Policy Changes

Improved metrics that use standard measures to document gentrification, displacement, and displacement risk would be useful in assessing the broad impact of gentrification on older and long-term residents. For example, the Anti-Eviction Mapping Project combines several mixed-method strategies including data visualization, data analysis, and oral histories to 'counter map' patterns of eviction and displacement across San Francisco and Alameda counties [91]. A similar strategy used by the Urban Displacement Project shows that over 33% of low-income households across a 31-county region in the New York metropolitan area live in low-income neighborhoods at risk of or already experiencing displacement and/or gentrification pressures, representing over 1.1 million low-income households [92]. Mapping techniques are tools that call political attention to high-risk areas and help ensure accountability and equity [93]. While some cities track indices of displacement risk, such as evictions, these audits are not consistently used. As one necessary feature of the Age-Friendly Cities and Communities project is to maintain sufficient and affordable housing, all age-friendly cities should be subject to a citywide displacement risk assessment. Collecting and aggregating city and countywide data will facilitate a review of residential shifts, highlight areas in most need of housing and aging services, and increase the visibility of low-income seniors at risk for housing displacement.

Broadly, additional research is needed to investigate the various forms of displacement that exist in cities and communities globally, particularly in understudied areas, such as global south cities, rural areas, and non-Western, non-European contexts [94]. Anti-displacement efforts typically aim to develop without displacement, consulting community members and establishing advocacy councils that work within the community to fine-tune development strategies. Advocates and city officials might review existing policies that encourage community-led investment initiatives to ensure that they are meeting the needs of older adults and enable existing residents to stay and benefit from renewal efforts. For example, interventions aimed at bridging residential divides can leverage churches, cultural institutions, grassroots planning, and city officials to develop strategies in which resident stakeholders communicate their needs to the broader community, re-envisioning what "revitalization" means [95].

Finally, older adults may be well-served by intergenerational community-building programs that could provide support and increase social engagement. Living in gentrifying neighborhoods increases stress burden for people of color, largely as a function of housing insecurity [96]. Therefore, opportunities to stay rooted and connected with other community members through homeownership, rental protections, and businesses opportunities may mitigate the effects of stress and ultimately stem the tide of displacement.

5. Conclusions

Over a decade ago, Sabiyha Prince [61] wrote about changes in the "New Harlem". Her interviews indicated that residents made a deliberate choice to live there because they "liked living around Black people". One of her respondents commented, "I like living in a place where people say good morning to you and really care. I like the mix of elderly people. I wanted to be a part of our condition whether that be good or bad". Another person noted, "Here you still get folks in the community walking up to you and saying, 'Hi baby ... how you doing?' I want to hear that kind of language in my neighborhood, you know, people talking to me like I am welcome" [61] (p. 21).

While much has changed since then, some things have not. Our findings support what previous research on Harlem has found—Harlem is a culturally significant place where Black people, old and young, want to live precisely *because* it is a Black neighborhood [60,62]. Almost all participants considered Harlem to be home, and wished to remain there. However, recent changes in the neighborhood were reported as threats to staying put.

Growing older has its own challenges and invisibilities. Since gentrification has the potential to displace people and the cultural identity of a neighborhood, eroding a sense of belongingness, indirect displacement is worth highlighting in future studies on gentrification, aging, and neighborhoods. The notion that one can feel out-of-place while remaining in place requires additional theorization about how gentrification reconstructs place, place meanings, and the perception of age-friendliness. Furthermore, aging studies might consider the role of place attachment, neighborhood importance, and housing stability in shaping how older adults engage with others in changing neighborhoods.

Author Contributions: The authors designated for authorship met all criteria according to the CMJE guidelines for authorship. H.S.V. conceived of the study, research question, and study design. She also acquired the data and drafted the final version of the manuscript. S.M., P.W. and M.S. assisted in drafting versions of the manuscript, coding and analyzing the data.

Funding: This research received no external funding.

Conflicts of Interest: The authors declare no conflict of interest.

References

1. Plouffe, L.; Kalache, A. Towards global age-friendly cities: Determining urban features that promote active aging. *J. Urban Health* **2010**, *87*, 733–739. [CrossRef] [PubMed]
2. OECD. *Ageing in Cities*; OECD: Paris, France, 2015; ISBN 9789264231146.
3. Van Hoof, J.; Kazak, J.K.; Perek-Białas, J.M.; Peek, S.T.M. The challenges of urban ageing: Making cities age-friendly in Europe. *Int. J. Environ. Res. Public Health* **2018**, *15*, 2473. [CrossRef]
4. Buffel, T.; Phillipson, C. Can global cities be 'age-friendly cities' Urban development and ageing populations. *Cities* **2016**, *55*, 94–100. [CrossRef]
5. Buffel, T.; Phillipson, C. Ageing in a gentrifying neighbourhod: Experiences of community change in llater life. *Sociology* **2019**, 1–18. [CrossRef]
6. Marston, H.R.; van Hoof, J. Who Doesn't Think about Technology When Designing Urban Environments for Older People? A Case Study Approach to a Proposed Extension of the WHO'S Age-Friendly Cities Model. *Int. J. Environ. Res. Public Health* **2019**, *16*, 3525. [CrossRef]
7. Park, S.; Han, Y.; Kim, B.; Dunkle, R.E. Aging in place of vulnerable adults: Person-environment fit perspective. *J. Appl. Gerontol.* **2017**, *36*, 1327–1350. [CrossRef] [PubMed]
8. Cutchin, M.P. The process of mediated aging-in-place: A theoretically and empirically based model. *Soc. Sci. Med.* **2003**, *57*, 1077–1090. [CrossRef]
9. Wiles, J.L.; Leibing, A.; Guberman, N.; Reeve, J.; Allen, R.E. Meaning of "Aging in place" to older people. *Gerontologist* **2012**, *52*, 357–366. [CrossRef]
10. Van Hoof, J.; Boerenfijn, P. Re-inventing existing real estate of social housing for older people: Building a new De Benring in Voorst, The Netherlands. *Buildings* **2018**, *8*, 89. [CrossRef]
11. Pynoos, J. The future of housing for the elderly: Four strategies that can make a difference. *Public Policy Aging Rep.* **2018**, *28*, 35–38. [CrossRef]
12. Cohen, C.I. Aging and homelessness. *Gerontologist* **1999**, *39*, 5–14. [CrossRef] [PubMed]
13. Dooling, S. Ecological gentrification: A research agenda exploring justice in the city. *Int. J. Urban Reg. Res.* **2009**, *33*, 621–639. [CrossRef]
14. Grenier, A.; Barken, R.; Sussman, T.; Rothwell, D.; Bourgeois-Guérin, V. Homelessness among older people: Assessing strategies and frameworks across Canada. *Can. Rev. Soc. Policy Rev. Can. De Polit. Soc.* **2016**, *74*, 1–39.

15. Kasinitz, P. Gentrification and homelessness: The single room occupant and the inner city revival. *Urban Soc. Chang. Rev.* **1984**, *17*, 9–14.
16. Hyra, D.S. The back-to-the-city movement: Neighborhood redevelopment and processes of political and cultural displacement. *Urban Stud.* **2015**, *52*, 1753–1773. [CrossRef]
17. Lees, L.; Slater, T.; Wyly, E.K. *Gentrification*; Routledge/Taylor & Francis Group: New York, NY, USA, 2013. [CrossRef]
18. Slater, T. The eviction of critical perspectives from gentrification research. *Int. J. Urban Reg. Res.* **2006**, *30*, 737–757. [CrossRef]
19. Glass, R. Introduction: Aspects of change. In *London: Aspects of Change*; MacKibbon and Kee: London, UK, 1964; pp. xiii–xlii.
20. Newman, K.; Wyly, E.K. The right to stay put, revisited: Gentrification and resistance to displacement in New York City. *Urban Stud.* **2006**, *43*, 23–57. [CrossRef]
21. Wyly, E.K.; Hammel, D.J. Gentrification, segregation and discrimination in the American urban system. *Environ. Plan. A* **2004**, *36*, 1215–1241. [CrossRef]
22. Brown-Saracino, J. Explicating divided approaches to gentrification and growing income inequality. *Ann. Rev. Sociol.* **2017**, *43*, 515–539. [CrossRef]
23. Smith, R.J.; Lehning, A.J.; Kim, K. Aging in place in gentrifying neighborhoods: Implications for physical and mental health. *Gerontologist* **2018**, *58*, 26–35. [CrossRef]
24. Grier, G.; Grier, E. *Urban Displacement: A Reconnaissance*; The Grier Partnership: Bethesda, MD, USA, 1978.
25. Davidson, M.; Lees, L. New-build 'gentrification' and London's riverside renaissance. *Environ. Plan. A Econ. Space* **2005**, *37*, 1165–1190. [CrossRef]
26. Zuk, M.; Bierbaum, A.H.; Chapple, K.; Gorska, K.; Loukaitou-Sideris, A.; Ong, P.; Thomas, T. *Gentrification, Displacement and the Role of Public Investment: A Literature Review*; Federal Reserve Bank: San Francisco, CA, USA, 2015.
27. Ding, L.; Hwang, J.; Divringi, W. *Gentrification and Residential Mobility in Philadelphia*; Federal Reserve Bank of Philadelphia Discussion Papers; 2015; Available online: https://www.philadelphiafed.org/discussion-paper_gentrification-and-residential-mobility.pdf (accessed on 15 March 2019). [CrossRef]
28. Freeman, L. Displacement or succession? Residential mobility in gentrifying neighborhoods. *Urban Aff. Rev.* **2005**, *40*, 463–491. [CrossRef]
29. McKinnish, T.; Walsh, R.; White, T.K. Who gentrifies low-income neighborhoods? *J. Urban Econ.* **2010**, *67*, 180–193. [CrossRef]
30. Billingham, C.M. The broadening conception of gentrification: Recent developments and avenues for future inquiry in the sociological study of urban change. *Mich. Sociol. Rev.* **2015**, *29*, 75–102.
31. Clay, P. *Neighborhood Renewal: Middle Class Resettlement and Incumbent Upgrading in American Neighborhoods*; Free Press: New York, NY, USA, 1979.
32. Davidson, M. Displacement, space and dwelling: Placing gentrification debate. *Ethics Place Environ.* **2009**, *12*, 219–234. [CrossRef]
33. Green, R.; Mulusa, J.; Byers, A.; Parmer, C. The indirect displacement hypothesis: A case study in Washington, D.C. *Rev. Black Political Econ.* **2017**, *44*, 1–22. [CrossRef]
34. Twigge-Molecy, A. Exploring resident experiences of indirect displacement in a neighborhood undergoing gentrification: The case of Saint-Henri in Montréal. *Can. J. Urban Res.* **2014**, *23*, 1–22.
35. Atkinson, R.; Wulff, M. *Gentrification and Displacement: A Review of Approaches and Findings in the Literature*; AHURI Positioning Paper No. 115; Australian Housing and Urban Research Institute Limited: Melbourne, Australia, 2009; Available online: https://www.ahuri.edu.au/research/position-papers/115 (accessed on 20 November 2019).
36. Shaw, K.S.; Hagemans, I.W. Gentrification without displacement' and the consequent loss of place: The effects of class transition on low-income residents of secure housing in gentrifying areas. *Int. J. Urban Reg. Res.* **2015**, *39*, 323–341. [CrossRef]
37. Marcuse, P. Abandonment, gentrification and displacement: The linkages in New York City. In *Gentrification of the City*; Smith, N., Williams, P., Eds.; Unwin Hyman: London, UK, 1986; pp. 153–177.
38. Chernoff, M. Social displacement in a renovating neighborhood's commercialdistrict: Atlanta. In *Back to the City: Issues Inneighborhood Renovation*; Laska, S., Spain, D., Eds.; Pergamon Press: Oxford, UK, 1980; pp. 204–219.

39. Versey, H.S. A tale of two Harlems: Gentrification, social capital, and implications for aging in place. *Soc. Sci. Med.* **2018**, *214*, 1–11. [CrossRef]
40. Lewicka, M. Place attachment: How far have we come in the last 40 years? *J. Environ. Psychol.* **2011**, *31*, 207–230. [CrossRef]
41. McHugh, K.E.; Mings, R.C. The circle of migration: Attachment to place in aging. *Ann. Assoc. Am. Geogr.* **1996**, *86*, 530–550. [CrossRef]
42. Rowles, G.D. Place attachment among small town elderly. *J. Rural. Community Psychol.* **1990**, *11*, 103–120.
43. Rubinstein, R.I.; Parmelee, P.A. Attachment to place and the representation of the life course by the elderly. In *Place Attachment. Human Behavior and Environment (Advances in Theory and Research)*; Altman, I., Low, S.M., Eds.; Springer: Boston, MA, USA, 1992; Volume 12. [CrossRef]
44. Scannell, L.; Gifford, R. Place attachment enhances psychological need satisfaction. *Environ. Behav.* **2017**, *49*, 359–389. [CrossRef]
45. Wiles, J.L.; Allen, R.E.S.; Palmer, A.J.; Hayman, K.J.; Keeling, S.; Kerse, N.M. Older people and their social spaces: A study of well-being and attachment to place in Aotearoa New Zealand. *Soc. Sci. Med.* **2009**, *68*, 664–671. [CrossRef]
46. Croff, R.L.; Witter IV, P.; Walker, M.L.; Francois, E.; Quinn, C.; Riley, T.C.; Sharma, N.F.; Kaye, J.A. Things are changing so fast: Integrative technology for preserving cognitive health and community history. *Gerontologist* **2018**, *59*, 147–157. [CrossRef]
47. Fullilove, M.T.; Wallace, R. Serial forced displacement in American cities, 1916-2010. *J. Urban Health* **2011**, *88*, 381–389. [CrossRef]
48. Zukin, S. *The Naked City: The Death and Life of Authentic Urban Places*; Oxford University Press: New York, NY, USA, 2010.
49. Zukin, S.; Trujillo, V.; Frase, P.; Jackson, D.; Recuber, T.; Walker, A. New retail capital and neighborhood change: Boutiques and gentrification in New York City. *City Community* **2009**, *8*, 47–64. [CrossRef]
50. Anguelovski, I.; Triguero-Mas, M.; Connolly, J.T.; Kotsila, P.; Shokry, G.; Pérez Del Pulgar, C.; Garcia-Lamarca, M.; Argüelles, L.; Mangione, J.; Dietz, K.; et al. Gentrification and health in two global cities: A call to identify impacts for socially vulnerable residents. *Cities Health* **2019**, 1–10. [CrossRef]
51. Lim, S.; Chan, P.Y.; Walters, S.; Culp, G.; Huynh, M.; Gould, L.H. Impact of residential displacement on healthcare access and mental health among original residents of gentrifying neighborhoods in New York City. *PLoS ONE* **2017**, *12*, e0190139. [CrossRef]
52. Fullilove, M.T. *Root Shock: How Tearing up City Neighborhoods Hurts America, and What We Can Do about It*; One World/Ballantine Books: New York, NY, USA, 2004.
53. Atkinson, R. Losing one's place: Narratives of neighborhood change, market injustice and symbolic displacement. *Hous. Theory Soc.* **2015**, *32*, 373–388. [CrossRef]
54. Kawachi, I.; Kennedy, B.P.; Lochner, K.; Prothrow-Stith, D. Social capital, income inequality, and mortality. *Am. J. Public Health* **1997**, *87*, 1491–1498. [CrossRef] [PubMed]
55. Grenier, A.; Phillipson, C. Precarious aging: Insecurity and risk in late life. *Hastings Cent. Rep.* **2018**, *48*, S15–S18. [CrossRef] [PubMed]
56. World Health Organization. *Active Ageing: A Policy Framework*; WHO: Geneva, Switzerland, 2002.
57. World Health Organization. *Global Age-Friendly Cities: A Guide*; World Health Organization: Geneva, Switzerland, 2007.
58. New York University Furman Center for Real Estate and Urban Policy (NYU Furman Center). *State of New York City's Housing & Neighborhoods—2008 Report*; New York University Furman Center for Real Estate and Urban Policy: New York, NY, USA, 2008.
59. New York University Furman Center for Real Estate and Urban Policy (NYU Furman Center). *State of New York City's Housing & Neighborhoods—2016 Report*; New York University Furman Center for Real Estate and Urban Policy: New York, NY, USA, 2016.
60. Freeman, L. *There Goes the Hood: Views of Gentrification from the Ground Up*; Temple University Press: Philadelphia, PA, USA, 2006. [CrossRef]
61. Prince, S. Changing places: Race, class, and belonging in the "new" Harlem. *Urban Anthropol. Stud. Cult. Syst. World Econ. Dev.* **2002**, *31*, 5–35.
62. Jackson, J.L. *Harlemworld: Doing Race and Class in Contemporary Black America*; University of Chicago Press: Chicago, IL, USA, 2001.

63. Atkinson, R. The hidden costs of gentrification: Displacement in central London. *J. Hous. Built Environ.* **2000**, *15*, 307–326. [CrossRef]
64. Bozovic Stamenovic, R. "Old, Older, Oldish–NEW elderly and impact on healing design in Singapore". In *Get Better!* Del Nord, R., Ed.; TESIS Inter-University Research Center, Systems and Technologies for Healthcare Facilities, University of Florence: Florence, Italy, 2014.
65. Neugarten, B.L. Age groups in American Society and the rise of the young-old. *Ann. Am. Acad. Political Soc. Sci.* **1974**, *415*, 187–198. [CrossRef]
66. Neugarten, B.L. The future and the young-old. *Gerontologist* **1975**, *15*, 4–9. [CrossRef]
67. Braun, V.; Clarke, V. Using thematic analysis in psychology. *Qual. Res. Psychol.* **2006**, *3*, 77–101. [CrossRef]
68. Braun, V.; Clarke, V. *Successful Qualitative Research: A Practical Guide for Beginners*; Sage: Newbury Park, CA, USA, 2013.
69. Fereday, J.; Muir-Cochrane, E. Demonstrating rigor using thematic analysis: A hybrid approach of inductive and deductive coding and theme development. *Int. J. Qual. Methods* **2006**, *5*, 80–92. [CrossRef]
70. Hyra, D.S. *Race, Class, and Politics in the Cappuccino City*; University of Chicago Press: Chicago, IL, USA, 2017. [CrossRef]
71. Metropolitan Transportation Authority. MTA Unveils Proposed 2019 Budget and Four-Year Financial Plan. MTA Press Release. 2018. Available online: http://www.mta.info/ (accessed on 15 February 2019).
72. Rogers, K, Edmondson, C. Trump Administration Moves to Restrict Food Stamp Access, the Farm Bill Protected. 2018. Available online: https://nyti.ms/2GzUdjr (accessed on 28 February 2019).
73. Lefebvre, H. *The Production of Space*; Blackwell: Malden, MA, USA, 1991.
74. Hunter, M.A.; Pattillo, M.; Robinson, Z.F.; Taylor, K.-Y. Black placemaking: Celebration, play and poetry. *Theory Cult. Soc.* **2016**, *33*, 31–56. [CrossRef]
75. Prochansky, H.M.; Fabian, A.K.; Kaminoff, R. Place identity: Physical world socialization of the self. *J. Environ. Psychol.* **1983**, *3*, 57–83. [CrossRef]
76. Twigger-Ross, C.L.; Uzzell, D.L. Place and identity processes. *J. Environ. Psychol.* **1996**, *16*, 205–220. [CrossRef]
77. Drake, C.S.; Cayton, H. *Black Metropolis: A Study of Negro Life in a Northern City*; University of Chicago Press: Chicago, IL, USA, 1945.
78. Hunter, M.A.; Robinson, Z.F. *Chocolate Cities: The Black Map of American Life*; University of California Press: Oakland, CA, USA, 2018.
79. Kelley, J.; Dannefer, D.; Masarweh, L. Addressing erasure, microfication and social change. In *Age-Friendly Cities and Communities: A Global Perspective*; Buffel, T., Handler, S., Phillipson, C., Eds.; Policy Press: Bristol, UK, 2018.
80. Stone, R.I. The housing challenges of low-income older adults and the role of federal policy. *J. Aging Soc. Policy* **2018**, *30*, 227–243. [CrossRef] [PubMed]
81. Stein, S. Precarity and Gentrification: A Feedback Loop. *Metropolitics*. 2015. Available online: www.metropolitiques.eu/Precarity-and-Gentrification-A.html (accessed on 28 July 2019).
82. Waite, L. A place and space for a critical geography of precarity? *Geogr. Compass* **2009**, *3*, 412. [CrossRef]
83. Bates, L.; Wiles, J.; Kearns, R.; Coleman, T. Precariously placed: Home, housing and wellbeing for older renters. *Health Place* **2019**, *58*. [CrossRef]
84. Greenfield, E.A. Support from neighbors and aging in place: Can NORC Programsmake a difference? *Gerontologist* **2015**, *56*, 651–659. [CrossRef]
85. Stephens, C.; Szabó, A.; Allen, J.; Alpass, F. Livable environments and the quality of life of older people: An ecological perspective. *Gerontologist* **2019**, *59*, 675–685. [CrossRef]
86. Yen, I.H.; Michael, Y.L.; Perdue, L. Neighborhood environment in studies of health of older adults: A systematic review. *Am. J. Prev. Med.* **2009**, *37*, 455–463. [CrossRef]
87. Cain, C.L.; Wallace, S.P.; Ponce, N.A. Helpfulness, trust, and safety of neighborhoods: Social capital, household income, and self-reported health of older adults. *Gerontologist* **2018**, *58*, 4–14. [CrossRef]
88. Emlet, C.A.; Moceri, J.T. The importance of social connectedness in building age-friendly communities. *J. Aging Res.* **2012**. [CrossRef]
89. Kano, M.; Rosenberg, P.E.; Dalton, S.D. A global pilot study of age-friendly city indicators. *Soc. Indic. Res.* **2018**, *138*, 1205–1227. [CrossRef]

90. Orpana, H.; Chawla, M.; Gallagher, E.; Escaravage, E. Developing indicators for evaluation of age-friendly communities in Canada: Process and results. *Health Promot. Chronic Dis. Prev. Can.* **2016**, *36*, 214–223. [CrossRef] [PubMed]
91. Maharawal, M.M.; McElroy, E. The anti-eviction mapping project: Counter mapping and oral history toward Bay Area housing justice. *Ann. Am. Assoc. Geogr.* **2016**, *108*, 380–389. [CrossRef]
92. Urban Displacement Project. Mapping Displacement in the New York City Metropolitan Area. 2016. Available online: http://www.udpny.org/map (accessed on 19 October 2019).
93. Kwan, M. Feminist visualization: Re-envisioning GIS as a method in feminist geographic research. *Ann. Assoc. Am. Geogr.* **2002**, *92*, 645–661. [CrossRef]
94. Gonzalez, S. Looking comparatively at displacement and resistance to gentrification in Latin American cities. *Urban Geogr.* **2016**, *37*, 1245–1252. [CrossRef]
95. National Community Reinvestment Coalition. Shifting Neighborhoods: Gentrification and cultural displacement in American Cities. 2019. Available online: https://ncrc.org/gentrification/#_edn1 (accessed on 17 September 2019).
96. Gibbons, J. Are gentrifying neighborhoods more stressful? A multilevel analysis of self-rated stress. *SSM Popul. Health* **2019**, *7*. [CrossRef]

International Journal of
Environmental Research and Public Health

MDPI

Article

Engaging Older People in Age-Friendly Cities through Participatory Video Design

Margaret von Faber [1], Zsuzsu Tavy [2,3] and Suzan van der Pas [1,4,*]

1. Faculty of Social Work & Applied Psychology, University of Applied Sciences Leiden, Zernikedreef 11, 2333 CK Leiden, The Netherlands; Faber.von.m@hsleiden.nl
2. Chair of Urban Ageing, Faculty of Social Work & Education, The Hague University of Applied Sciences, Johanna Westerdijkplein 75, 2521 EN Den Haag, The Netherlands; Z.K.C.T.Tavy@hhs.nl
3. Faculty of Health, Nutrition & Sport, The Hague University of Applied Sciences, Johanna Westerdijkplein 75, 2521 EN Den Haag, The Netherlands
4. Department of Public Health and Primary Care, Leiden University Medical Centre, Hippocratespad 21, 2333 ZD Leiden, The Netherlands

* Correspondence: pas.vd.s@hsleiden.nl

Received: 28 October 2020; Accepted: 24 November 2020; Published: 2 December 2020

check for updates

Abstract: Participatory video design is a novel approach to collect experiences and perceptions of older people about the age-friendliness of their city or neighborhood. In this article, we describe how this co-creative method can add to specific knowledge about the preferences and needs of older people about the improvement or preservation of their environment. We describe two examples of this approach in the cities of The Hague and Leiden, the Netherlands. Persons of 60 years and older were invited to participate in a "workshop" on filmmaking focusing on age-friendly cities. A professional filmmaker and a researcher of the University of Applied Sciences worked in co-creation with older people, to produce short films on the topics that were perceived as important from the perspective of the participants. The older people worked in couples to produce their short films about the city or their neighborhood. Topics of the films included communication and information, outdoor spaces, social relations, and community support. The use of participatory video design can foster empowerment and social interaction among older participants, and insight into the preferences and needs of older people regarding age-friendly cities.

Keywords: participatory video design; participation; age-friendly cities

1. Introduction

There are two global trends with a major impact on societies in the 21st century: Population ageing and urbanization. World-wide, the proportion of older residents in cities is predicted to increase. Building on the "active ageing" framework, the World Health Organization (WHO) launched the Age-Friendly cities and Communities (AFC) initiative. Eight aspects of city life influencing age-friendliness are specified in a guide: Outdoor spaces and buildings; transportation; housing; social participation; respect and social inclusion; civic participation and employment; communication and information; community support and health services. For a city's self-assessment, a companion "Checklist of Essential Features of Age-Friendly Cities" can be used to chart progress [1]. An age-friendly city should ideally be a place where older people are actively involved, valued, and supported with infrastructure and services that effectively accommodate their needs [2].

In the Netherlands, the percentage of people of 65 years and over is predicted to increase from the current 19.5% of the Dutch population to 23% in 2030, rising to 25.5% in 2040 [3]. The national policy is to enable older people to live as long as possible in their own home and environment [4]. In the Pact on care for older persons [*Pact voor de Ouderenzorg*] launched in 2018 [5], living environment and housing are important topics. Actions are directed at creating age-friendly living environments. On a local level, municipalities have to record the supply and demand on housing and cooperate with housing corporations, private partners, and citizens. Municipalities also have to gather knowledge on the preferences and needs of older citizens, in order to provide for sufficient housing, alternatives if older people want to move, and the livability of neighborhoods for an increasing older population [4]. In the next decades, the largest increase in older people will be in the major cities and the Western part of the Netherlands [6].

The EU and the local and national governments are emphasizing the need for local communities to encourage older people to play an active role in communities and position them at policy levels as contributors in policies dealing with the local and individual needs that citizens encounter. More tailored solutions centered on older adults' needs and circumstances need to be developed in collaboration with older adults. In 2014, The Hague was the first city in the Netherlands to join the World Health Organization's network of age-friendly cities. Together with local stakeholders and various organizations, the city encourages active ageing in the urban environment by stimulating opportunities for activities and social participation in order to enhance quality of life as people age.

In this study, we focus on participation in research, enabling older people to seek their own solutions according to their priorities. The most important difference between participatory research and conventional methodologies is who defines the research problem, and who generates, analyses, owns, and acts on the information that is sought [7]. Participatory research (PR) provides a means to enable older adults to gain ownership over their social and physical environment [8]. PR is used as a term encompassing research approaches such as community-based participatory research, action research (AR), and participatory action research (PAR), which are aimed at engaging community members as co-researchers to guide personal and social change [9].

In participatory research, the target group is actively involved in the research [10]. Different degrees of participation are possible, such as: Identification of themes and relevant research questions, advice on methods and approach of participants, involvement in data gathering, analysis of the data, and dissemination of results. Participatory research as a method is used in several disciplines and academic studies, for example, anthropology, sociology, and psychiatry, but also in the field of health research, education research, and development studies [11]. Moreover, participatory research covers a range of different methodologies in which the role of participants and researcher can be very different. Tangvald-Pedersen and Bongaardt [12] distinguish three different ideologies that have different consequences for user involvement and participation and preferred methodologies. They describe a liberal, market-based ideology; an emancipation-based ideology; and an education-based ideology. In the liberal ideology, the consumer/client is involved as an advisor and consultant. The research design is consultative, the researcher is "in the lead", and the methodology is important. In the emancipation-based ideology, the research is user-led. The methodology is less prescribed, depending on the goal of the research. The goal of the education-based ideology is to explore and understand the perception of the people under study, for example, a patient or client. The involvement of the participants depends on the context and goal of the research. The research design is collaborative and flexible, adjusting methods to the abilities of the participants. This means that participatory research can be considered a continuum of participation, from projects being led by a professional researcher at one end, to a user-led project at the other end [13]. To evaluate the intended results of the specific research approach, it is essential to describe the knowledge that is collected, to be transparent about the ownership and the distribution of the knowledge.

Participatory research with older people has been conducted for several years. Tanner [14] found that it is even possible to involve older people with dementia in a meaningful way in research processes. Older people with dementia participated in planning the research methods, conducting interviews, and making sense of the findings, with the assistance of the researcher. Both co-researchers and participants can benefit significantly from their participation, but they also make a valuable contribution to the research because they present an "insiders" or "emic" perspective, as opposed to an "outsiders" or "etic" perspective of the matter. Baur and Abma [15] found that active participation of a group of older women in a residential home enhanced empowerment and even co-management of their own needs and preferences. According to the authors, participation can foster empowerment and vice versa, whereby power is not given or taken but is a mutual process that emerges through interaction with others on the level of individuals, organizations, and communities [16]. Buffel [17] described that working with co-researchers on the topic of age-friendly communities also poses challenges, for example, managing expectations about the benefits of the research, or ethical issues of confidentiality between co-researcher and interviewee.

Visual methods, like Photovoice and video research, are specific ways of data-gathering in participatory research. Using the method of Photovoice, older people have participated in research on the age-friendliness in their community [18,19] or the sense of home of nursing home residents [20]. This visual method can be combined with interviews to elicit the views of older people who have more difficulty expressing themselves verbally. Moreover, the use of visual imagery to feature a problem can be particularly empowering and effective in communication with policymakers and stakeholders [18].

In participatory video, participants are trained to use video as part of the research. This practice can be linked to the field of visual anthropology, in which collaborative ethnographic filmmaking has a long history in the work of visual anthropologists David MacDougall and Jean Rouch [21]. This visual method also evolved in social action research, and is used, for example, in development projects and programs [22]. Different forms of, and approaches to, participatory video are possible, varying from organizing a video workshop in a local community and collecting data regarding a certain topic, to finding ways for participants to tell, produce, share, and own their own stories using film. Most approaches have in common that they strive to use film to create a means for often more marginalized or underrepresented groups of people to represent their own experiences [22].

Film is perceived as a powerful tool for representing experiences and communication of knowledge in an experiential way [23,24]. Film also has the ability to capture situations in a social and material context [23,24]. In addition to the power of film as a medium, the process of filmmaking itself is often seen as an important part of the method, and it is held to be able to transform and empower the participants [22]. For participants, this process entails among others, the development of skills, interaction and bonding with others, and reflection on certain topics or on their own identity or position in the community or society at large [22].

The main aim of this paper is to describe how participatory video design can add knowledge about the preferences and needs of older people about the improvement and preservation of their local environment. We describe examples of this approach focusing on age-friendliness in two cities in the Netherlands, The Hague and Leiden. We describe how participants are recruited, the topics that participants perceive as important, and their experiences with this method. In the discussion, we reflect on the implications of this method from a participatory perspective.

2. Methodology

Both in The Hague and Leiden, the participatory video design was developed and shaped by a project team, including researchers and filmmakers. In the city of Leiden, representatives of older people were also part of the project team. They decided in which neighborhood the participants would be recruited and assisted in the project. Residents of 60 years or older were eligible for participation, in accordance with the definition of "older persons" of the WHO [1]. As we aimed at a variety of older persons, there were no exclusion criteria on living situation or ethnic background.

2.1. The Hague: Setting, Participants, and Method

As part of the activities of The Hague Age-Friendly City, a workshop on documentary making by older people was organized in 2017 [25]. In total, 21 older people (14 women and 7 men), ranging in age from 63 to 90, took part in these workshops. Participants had a Dutch background. Two persons with a Chinese Surinamese background participated.

Over the period of one week, they went through all the phases of making a documentary, forming duos and together making a documentary on "my age-friendly city". While the topic of "age-friendly city" was chosen by the city council, the participants were free to choose a theme relating to this topic that they further wanted to explore during the workshop. Participants were recruited through an advertisement in *De Posthoorn*, a free local newspaper and via word-of-mouth.

The workshop was conducted over five consecutive days with an introduction starting on Monday and a public premiere at the end of the week on Friday. On the first day, after the introduction, pairs were formed and homework was given for the next day: Decide on a topic and develop a script. On the second day, a test run was done in the studio, with an iPad in hand, to which a hand microphone was connected. On the third day, filming took place at various locations in The Hague, such as a community center, a Chinese co-housing community, and a local gym. The fourth day was devoted to editing the material into short documentaries. Participants were trained in working with Adobe Premiere Pro, and worked on computers in the local movie theater to edit their film.

The workshop was guided by researchers from the University of Applied Sciences Leiden (SP) and The Hague University of Applied Sciences and film professionals with extensive teaching experience, and the latest equipment was used. During the week, they supported the older people in the process of making their films. In the development of the scripts, they gave participants feedback and helped in practicing using the iPads. During the shooting of the film, a film professional was linked to two duos and was there to help and give feedback on the filming and interviewing and to provide technical support if needed. The use of the iPad as a camera posed only a few problems for the older participants. However, editing was more difficult and required more time and work to achieve a coherent end product. During this process, film professionals were there to help. After participants edited their film, the final editing was done by a film professional to create the right sound and volume. On the last day, a premiere took place of the documentaries, where friends and family were invited.

Apart from the individual documentaries that were made, a summary documentary was also made of the entire process of the workshop. All the videos were presented to the municipality, aimed at contributing to aligning policy with the actual needs of older persons when it comes to giving meaning to a (age-friendly) living environment.

2.2. Leiden: Setting, Participants, and Method

The University of Applied Sciences Leiden conducts research on the topic of "Living longer in the own environment". For this topic, researchers (MvF, SP) worked together with the Regional Advisory Board of Older Persons [Ouderenberaad Zuid Holland-Noord] in the city of Leiden. The Regional Advisory Board of Older Persons is a client panel of 15 older persons (aged 60–90 years) who reflect on research proposals/results, housing, and healthcare policy in the Leiden area [26]. In 2017, a participative research on "Vitality and living independently" in the region was conducted. The members of the Regional Advisory Board of Older People were trained as co-researchers and conducted interviews and focus group discussions. However, the report that was presented to the different municipalities with suggestions for improvement did not have the desired impact. In co-creation, the participatory video design was then chosen as a means to focus the attention of policymakers and stakeholders on the perspectives of older people in a specific neighborhood. Members of the board chose the neighborhood for the video project, because it was known that local residents found it important to live and grow older in this place.

Participants were invited to participate by face-to-face contact over a period of three weeks. At a central point in the neighborhood, the local supermarket, members of the Regional Advisory Board of Older Persons, and a researcher (MvF) asked older people to participate in a workshop on filmmaking on the topic of an age-friendly neighborhood. Flyers with an explanation of the goal and content of the workshop were handed out and questions were answered on the spot. In 2019, a group of nine older persons (seven local residents and two members of the Regional Advisory Board of Older People) participated in the project. In total, three women and six men with a Dutch background took part in the workshops. Two other members of the Regional Advisory Board of Older People were present at the meetings.

The workshop was conducted in five half-days. During the first meeting of the workshop, participants received information about the context of the video project, and they explored the topic "Living longer in the own neighborhood". Subtopics were discussed and participants formed duos on the subjects. In the second meeting, attention was directed at interviewing and filming. Participants rehearsed in interviewing and filming each other, with an iPad in hand, to which a hand microphone was connected. After this, participants were instructed in the use of the app Pinnacle Studio Pro and editing. They practiced in editing their first short films. In the third meeting, participants set off with the iPad and microphone, and filmed in their neighborhood. The professional filmmaker was present for support. The films were edited by the participants, with the help of the filmmaker and his assistant, in the 4th meeting. Finally, in the last meeting, the films were shown to the other participants and the workshop was evaluated. Due to Covid-19 and the following lockdown, it was not possible to organize a public gathering for the presentation of the films in Leiden. However, because some participants expressed the desire to receive their own film, we distributed these to those participants.

3. Results

The workshop in The Hague on "My age-friendly city" resulted in 11 mini-documentaries. The workshop in Leiden on "Living longer in the own neighborhood" resulted in 5 mini-documentaries. In the results, we can distinguish the topics that were filmed, and the process of filmmaking.

3.1. Topics of the Films

The topics that were filmed were: Outdoor spaces; housing; social participation; communication and information; and community support. Both in The Hague and Leiden, a film with characteristics of the neighborhood was made.

3.1.1. Outdoor Spaces

In The Hague, one duo showed the accessibility of the city for older people who travel by foot (see Figure 1). They took the viewer on a trip from point A to point B while evaluating the route from their own perspective. In the video, it is shown that in this short route, big and busy roads and viaducts have to be crossed, sometimes without traffic lights or pedestrian crossings. As one participant tells the viewers: *"You have to be on guard all the time"*.

Another video explored the accessibility of the renovated promenade in Scheveningen beach for people in wheelchairs. The video showed the difficulties a participant in a wheelchair encounters while getting to the promenade from her house. She had to ride over cobblestones, which made her back hurt, and sometimes she would get stuck. The pedestrian bridge was no option for her, as it has two steps at the end. The promenade itself has uneven stone paving, which makes driving in a wheelchair difficult. Another duo made a video on older people visiting a shopping mall in their mobility scooter. They wanted to research the driving skills of older people and found contrasting perspectives. Interviewees driving a mobility scooter mentioned it was easy for them to drive and shop in the shopping mall. By contrast, a shop employee talked about older people lacking driving skills, driving too fast, and crashing into the revolving door. In another video, safety in traffic situations was explored by filming different pedestrian crossings or streets the participants themselves found unsafe. Busy intersections and small streets in which trams and bicycles intersect were shown. The video showed little space between the sidewalk and the tram rails, leaving almost no space for bicycles. One interviewee on a bicycle pointed out that people often get stuck in these tram rails.

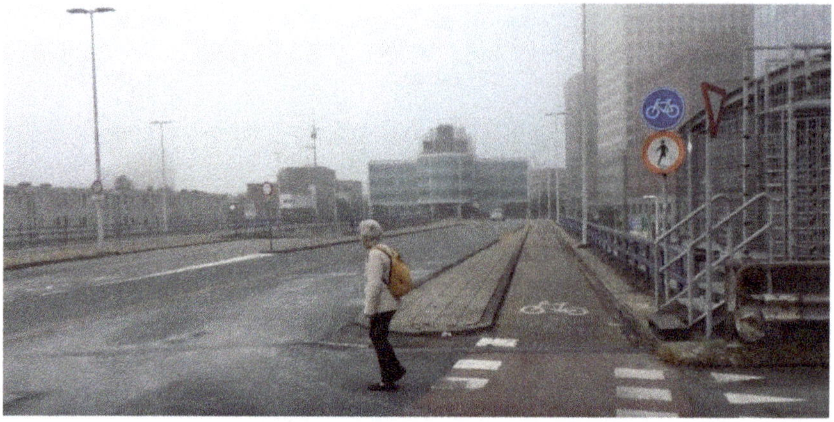

Figure 1. Video fragment: Outdoor spaces in The Hague.

Another duo presented a park in the city center with the title "A green oasis of peace". One interviewee talks about finding peace while walking the small labyrinth in the park. According to the duo and the older people they interviewed in the park, the park provides a pleasant and green space.

In Leiden, the participants that filmed the housing and outdoor spaces reflected on the desire to move to an apartment on the ground level in the same neighborhood. They interviewed a man in a mobility scooter on his view on accessibility. They also filmed bicycles on the pavement and other hindrances, like tree roots, and walking with a walker. With their film, the older participants showed possibilities for improvement in an age-friendly environment.

In another video, participants interviewed a visually impaired woman that also suffered from other physical disabilities. This interviewee experienced difficulties in maintaining her garden. As a solution to this problem, the participants interviewed a young woman who recently started her own small enterprise in helping others with gardening. With the film, they wanted to show this recent opportunity for support in their neighborhood.

3.1.2. Social Participation

In The Hague, one duo portrayed in their video a theater- and dance group for 55+ amateur actors. They showed parts of the rehearsal and performance and interviewed a member of the group. This person explained why she enjoys being part of this group. Another duo investigated what is needed to attract more older people to a community center in the neighborhood, by interviewing people on the street. It becomes clear that people wish to see another ambiance in the center, they want to have good coffee, and they want to participate in other types of activities, like political activities, music, or lectures. In another video, two Chinese participants presented cultural aspects of activities in old age. Filmed in their own house, the viewer sees how they make a religious offering, and also take time to work on calligraphy, which they explain is also a finger exercise. One participant mentioned she was pleased that in The Hague, the Chinese Holidays are celebrated and that she is able to buy Chinese products.

3.1.3. Social Contacts and Community Support

In Leiden, a duo went to the local shops, as shown in Figure 2. They also went to a supermarket and a local restaurant, and discussed social support for older people when they needed assistance in the case of health problems. To their surprise, all interviewees emphasized that they knew their regular customers, that they enquired after their wellbeing when they did not see them for a while, and that they were able to provide services at home (for example, the hairdresser) or deliver food or meals (for example, the catering company and greengrocer) at home.

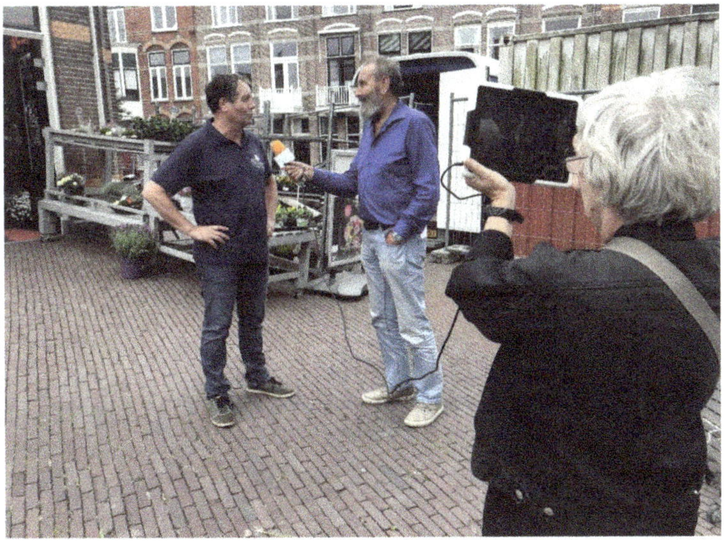

Figure 2. Interviewing a shop-owner in Leiden.

3.1.4. Communication and Information

In Leiden, one duo chose the theme of information. One participant was actually searching for information on meals and a course in working with a computer. The interviews on the street led to the community center, which could indeed provide an answer to these questions.

3.1.5. Housing, Residential Care, and Social Contacts

In The Hague, a participant filmed a man of 90 years old, one of the participants, on his orientation journey to live in a housing facility for older people. Still living by himself, he is followed to the gym, and he explains what he looks for in a new home: A nice green environment together with the dynamics of the city center, a sports club, a spacious apartment, a recreation room, and nice (older) ladies for social contact.

3.1.6. Characteristics of the Neighborhood

In The Hague, one video showed a relatively new district (Leidschenveen). Participants interviewed passers-by on the street. Although there are activities organized for older people, loneliness and isolation were perceived as important topics in this district. An older lady being interviewed explained how she has to walk 20 min to reach the nearest public transport. It is also shown that to get to the tram at the square of the station, many stairs must be climbed. The participants wanted to show that accessibility of public transport could be improved for older people and persons physically handicapped.

In Leiden, one film described the characteristics of the neighborhood, like the demographics and different types of housing. The positive image of the neighborhood prevailed in the film.

Both in The Hague and Leiden, participants filmed topics perceived as important for an age-friendly city. These topics were often interrelated. The topics of public and outdoor spaces were often linked to mobility and safety. Social participation is also connected to activities that may not be exclusively age-specific, like enjoying a good coffee or listening to music. A connection between social support, keeping an eye on older persons, and the presence of shops and small enterprises in the neighborhood are also valued positively by participants. The film in Leiden shows that a community center can fulfil an important role in providing specific information and practical support for those who are less digitally skilled.

3.2. The Process of Participation

In the participation of older persons in the workshops, we can distinguish different aspects: First, participation in the identification of themes and showing what is relevant and important from the perspective of participants; secondly, how the video method itself impacted the empowerment of the participants; thirdly, in making suggestions for improvement; and finally, the follow-up of the films on "owning" the story.

3.2.1. During the Project—Telling the Story

Participants in The Hague had to choose one of the age-friendly city features to explore in their film, whereas in Leiden, the participants were free to choose their own sub-themes. The topics that were picked in Leiden by participants themselves, however, did match the age-friendly city features. They showed what they thought was important. One participant in Leiden stated:

> *"I think this topic [community support] is important. I have experienced that myself. I am alone and I go twice a week to the restaurant. They missed me when I was ill. They enquired after my condition. When I returned, I got coffee for free! It is a kind of social concern"* (woman, Leiden)

In the process of the editing of films, participants could further shape the story they wanted to tell. Participants in The Hague expressed that the support from professional filmmakers during the process was of great value, for it helped them express their views in the best way possible, as some of the participants did find the technical aspects challenging.

Participants in Leiden were more interested in learning how to film and less in the editing process. They wished to have a say in the final product, but the editing itself was perceived as a bit difficult, despite the received support from the filmmaker and his assistant, as shown in Figure 3. In The Hague, the editing was perceived as challenging too, though one of the participants stated afterward that they did not think they would want to hand over the technical aspects of the editing process though, *"for following every step yourself, makes the whole process more rewarding"*.

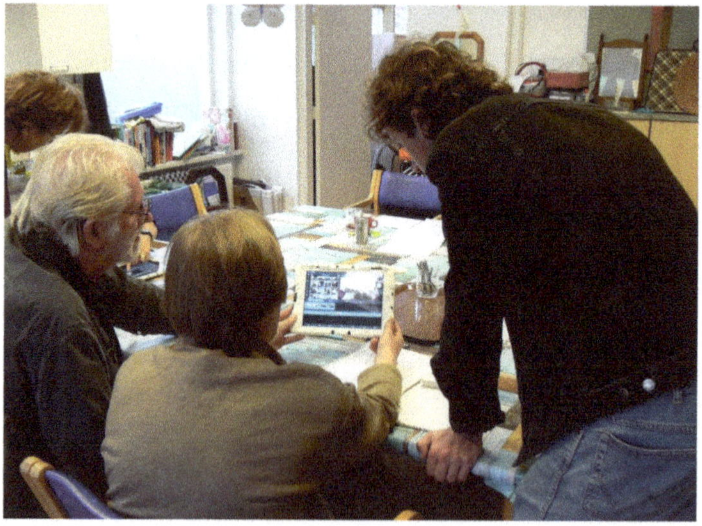

Figure 3. Editing the video fragments in Leiden.

The participants in the workshop also involved other older people in the neighborhood in telling the story as well. Participants interviewed people on the streets, or people they already knew on their topic. In one of the videos in The Hague, we followed an acquaintance of one of the participants as she showed her experiences while driving a mobility scooter in the mall. Local organizations in the community were also involved in the process of exploring a topic. In The Hague, for example, we see a theater group for older people, a Chinese co-housing community, a gym, and a community center.

3.2.2. Filmmaking as a Process

Both the participants in The Hague and Leiden expressed enjoying learning something new together, although there were some participants who had previous experience with making a film. Some participants were happy to see that they could learn to use, film, and edit with iPads, something not all of them were expecting when they started the project as one participant who called herself "digitally illiterate" expressed. One participant in The Hague even emphasized the importance of showing the world that *"older people can learn new things too, even new media."*

During the process, some participants in The Hague formed new friendships. Learning something fun and new together, and experiencing this process during the week together might have attributed to this. Figure 4 shows two participants having fun in rehearsing recording and interviewing. In one of the films, the viewers can see a duo laugh and making jokes together, during a search for housing for older people. This fun is captured and visible for the viewers. Even after the project was finished, this participant and his new friend continued the journey and visited housing for older people together.

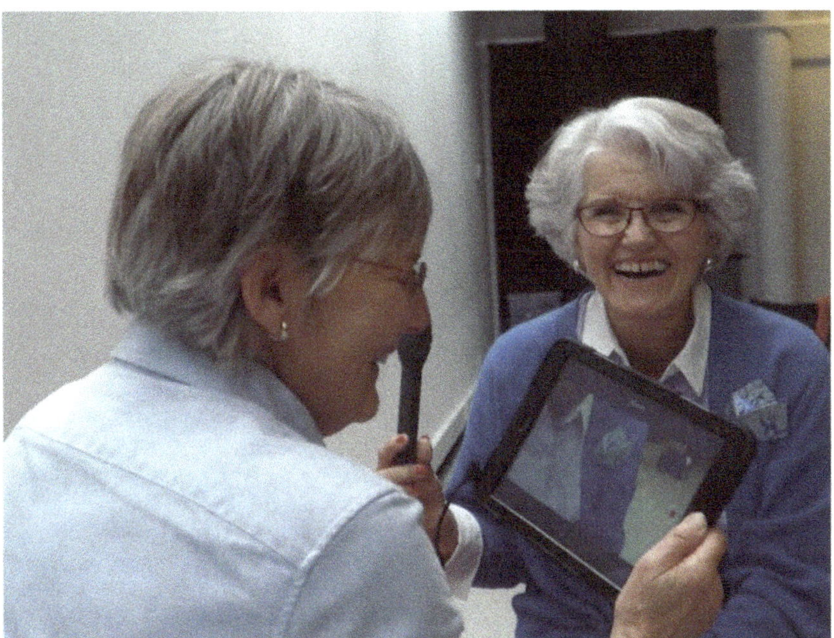

Figure 4. Participants in The Hague having fun together.

Also in Leiden, participants enjoyed working in duos, because they could help and complement each other. They even started filming and interviewing together even outside the scheduled film day, which was possible as they could lend the iPads. One participant was eager to continue in filmmaking, and he kept contact with some of his fellow participants and informed the professional filmmaker afterward. In both cities, several participants kept contact with each other after the workshop finished.

Participants in The Hague expressed being proud of the films they had made, and some of them also expressed feeling good about exploring social themes together. One participant even linked her participation in this project to a newfound drive for societal involvement:

> *"I started to feel young again, to feel involved again, and I started to feel I wanted to be part of society again. I experienced different sides of myself again. Looking back, it was the start of a phase in which I started to follow a new direction."* (woman, The Hague).

3.2.3. Suggestions for Improvement

In Leiden, the films in themselves created awareness among the participants of what could be improved:

> *"I thought the film about the information was the best. "Where do I have to go if I have these questions?". I think the community center is the place, and maybe we could go one step further and make it a center of knowledge [...] there has to be information desk from the municipality. It doesn't have to be put on a higher level, but on an extended level."* (woman, Leiden)

> *"In another neighborhood, they have this fitness for older persons. That could also be initiated here."* (man, Leiden)

The suggestions for improvement were not only directed at stakeholders in the city, but also to older people themselves:

> *"Shop owners stated that they only provided support for regular customers. [... as an older person] you must continue to do your shopping in your own neighborhood and visit the hairdresser, and that kind of things. When you need help, you can call upon them and they will come to you. So this is an advice for older people."* (woman, Leiden).

In the evaluation of the process, participants agreed that it was important to make your voice heard as an older person.

3.2.4. After the Filming: Owning the Story

In The Hague, on the last day of the project, a festive premiere took place in the city's movie theater. Here, the films were proudly shown to friends, family, and involved parties. After the premiere, a group discussion was held about the themes in the films. The themes were further explored and the discussion provided new insights. This process and these insights, however, were not well-documented or included as results. After the project, the films from the project in The Hague were shown on a website and the films were handed over to the municipality by the project team.

After the films were finished, participants in Leiden had little interest in a follow-up by participating in a focus group about the final results and suggestions for improvement. The main aim of the participants was to increase their knowledge on filmmaking. Only two of the older participants were willing to participate in the focus group, which constituted of a member of the Regional Advisory Board of Older People, the chairman of the Neighborhood association, and a representative of the municipality that is responsible for the livability in the neighborhood [the "*wijkregisseur*"]. Suggestions for improvement were discussed on the topics: Information and communication, housing, community health and dementia, mobility, and safety. An example of the latter is to make pavements free of bicycles and other obstructions, and make it wide enough for wheelchairs and walkers.

Participants also made suggestions for relevant stakeholders that could be involved in these improvements. The Neighborhood association could discuss the topic of bicycles on the pavement in the neighborhood-newsletter, and Council officials of the neighborhood and the department of Communication could emphasize the topic of mobility and safety for the city of Leiden. The municipality could also improve the pavements. The Community center could take up a central role as provider of information, together with the Neighborhood-newsletter. Health providers could provide an update of the available printed information on services for older people and informal caregivers. Municipality and social housing associations are important for the improvements in the topics concerning housing and modification. Healthcare providers, welfare organizations, and case managers could provide information on neighborhood level, for example, on dementia and support for informal caregivers. Healthcare providers could offer fitness, Tai-Chi, or other courses in the neighborhood. The primary school in the neighborhood could be involved by offering space for these courses.

Covid-19 and the following lockdown prevented the presentation of the films. Moreover, changes in stakeholders, due to public procurement for welfare organizations, provided an impediment for the discussion on the suggestions for improvement. However, the Neighborhood association and the "*wijkregisseur*" have already taken up the responsibility of improving the mobility and safety on pavements, and the improvement for information and communication.

4. Discussion

By applying the method of participatory video design, the aim of this study was to investigate the preferences and needs of older people about the age-friendliness of their environment. This method enabled older people to show aspects of age-friendliness from their own perspective. The participants chose the following topics: Outdoor spaces, housing, social participation, communication and information, and community support. These topics are in accordance with elements of the model of an age-friendly city of the WHO [1]. The films showed the relation between participants and their environment. Not only did the films show what could be improved, but also what was highly appreciated and what should be preserved as an aspect of age-friendliness, like the support of local shop owners. In relation to improvement of age-friendliness, the activities in the community center were mentioned, as well as communication and information. Most public information is made available in a digital form, and the digital competence of older people is stimulated. However, one of the videos showed that oral and printed information remain essential for older persons that are not (or no longer) digitally skilled. With regard to housing, mobility, and safety, participants showed environmental barriers and risks, such as busy roads without traffic lights or pedestrian crossings, or sidewalk hazards with little space that poses a problem for a person with a walker. As we follow one of the participants in The Hague on her trip from point A to B, we can see she encounters different obstacles. The viewer gets a sense of the whole route, the imposing environment, and the reaction of the participants while being confronted with this environment (Figure 1). This is perceived as one of the strengths of film.

Apart from the insight into the various aspects of age-friendliness, the method of participatory video added to the collection of data that were unexpected and creative. According to MacDougall [23], exploring the neighborhood through the lens of a camera can provide participants with a new view, as one engages with the world in other ways. In this research, participants were conscious or became more aware of the age-friendliness of their environment. For example, in the focus group in Leiden, participants stated that they were unaware of the support for older people living with dementia in their neighborhood.

The process of filmmaking was an important aspect for participants. Moreover, statements on "*feeling part of society*" and "*enabling the voice of older people to be heard*" resembled elements of empowerment. Our research design can be described as consultative, stemming from a liberal ideology. Our stakeholders depart from the standpoint that knowing the preferences of the older citizens leads to better improvements in age-friendliness of the city. However, the results of this research show that they also could tie in with an emancipatory ideology [12].

A potential limitation of visual methods like video research is that it could exclude persons with impairments related to vision, hearing, or mobility. This could introduce a selection bias and under-representation of vulnerable groups [19]. These groups are likely to include a disproportionate share of people from lower socio-economic backgrounds, and people with mental health issues, low self-esteem, and health problems [27]. However, because in visual methods, like video design and photovoice, language is not the only element, it has been documented that it can also be used with populations in different health and living conditions, for example, people with dementia [20], different social economic status, or immigrants [27]. This participatory video design attracted older people that were interested in learning something new, and although participants were sometimes insecure about their ability to make a documentary, they also perceived it as a challenge. Both in The Hague and Leiden, some participants had filmed in their youth, and were eager to learn how to film with an iPad and edit the product. For those who found the editing the most difficult part, professional support was at hand. As mentioned in other participatory research, the training contributed to older participants' "skills and self-esteem and a sense of mastery" [18,22,28]. We found that participants were very proud of their achievements. Working in duos also resulted in mutual learning. This aspect can contribute to a "stronger voice" of older people in processes of co-creation for improvement [15].

The films showed the heterogeneity in older people, challenging the dominant stereotypes of older people as frail and dependent. For future research, it would be interesting to investigate the effects of these images from the perspective of the viewers. For example, exploring the effects on policy makers could reveal to what extent these images would influence policy advice.

Video research is able to change the traditional role of researcher and the "researched" [29]. The participants may act as "reflective insider" and as "active researcher", interviewing other people. New roles arise, for example, the *"director"* and the *"editor"* [30]. Both in The Hague and Leiden, participants took up a role as researcher, eliciting the aspects that they wanted others to see. In the process of editing, some participants in Leiden were leaving out "unwanted" comments, because of strategic reasons. These participants thought the local community center was of major importance and some of the participants were actively involved in activities of this community center. However, in one interview, the interviewee stated that the community center was for "the most vulnerable persons" in the neighborhood and he distanced himself from this negative image. This, as a negative perceived remark, was deliberately left out in the montage by the participants. These findings are relevant because what is deliberately left out of the film might have been used for improvement, and at the same time, it underscores the fear of the participants of depicting negative images of aspects that they find important to keep within the neighborhood.

A challenge for video research is how to "use" the data for improvement of the neighborhood and city. In order to have a maximum impact, this kind of research needs to be embedded in AFC initiatives from the start, with the municipality as a committed and proactive partner. Buffel [17] describes how working with older co-researchers on age-friendly communities in Manchester (UK) was embedded in a partnership between the Manchester City Council, the University of Manchester, various community organizations, and older people, committed to the goal of developing "age-friendly communities." The aspiration for the dissemination of results and acting upon suggestions has to be a product of co-creation between researchers and stakeholders, like a city council. Co-creation can be seen as a practice of interactions between older adults, public professionals, students, researchers, and community stakeholders who jointly define needs and choices, as well as design and implement services and support [31]. Co-creation is when people relate to each other and interact in defining, designing, and implementing a particular service, product, or practice [32]. In the literature, a distinction can be made between three types of involvement: (1) Citizens as co-implementer of public policy, (2) citizens as co-designer, and (3) citizens as co-initiator [32]. The first level is represented most frequently, which involves the citizen as co-implementer of the public service. Here, citizen involvement has already been defined by the public service. The second level approaches the citizen as co-designer of how the product or service should be delivered. In most cases, the initiative for the co-creation lies with the public institution, but citizens decide how the service is being delivered. The third level represents the citizen as initiator and the government as supporting actor. In our video projects, the role of the municipalities was different.

In The Hague, the municipality was setting up a platform "Age-Friendly City." The municipality launched a multitude of new projects, but it was unclear how the results could be embedded.

No arrangements were made to evaluate and discuss the results of the video research. In the final phase of the research, a dialogue between participants, stakeholders, and the municipality would have benefited the follow up [19]. This would have provided an opportunity for improvements and could have fostered empowerment of older people.

In Leiden, not the City council, but the Regional Advisory Board of Older People was co-designer of the research and participated in the research process. Their main aim was to communicate the preferences and needs of older people to policy-makers and stakeholders, like social housing organizations. A short documentary was perceived as more effective than written reports [18]. However, due to Covid-19, we are still in the process of discussing the results of the video research with the municipality, the neighborhood association, and stakeholders. At the neighborhood level, some improvements have already been made. As the neighborhood association is publishing the video research and the improvements for all neighborhood residents in the local newspaper, this may enhance social interaction and feelings of empowerment of the participants. Recently, the municipality has launched a plan to increase age-friendliness of the city, so this provides opportunities to discuss the results and suggestions for improvements on a local level. When we compare the two different approaches, we can conclude that the effect of video research in the context of age-friendly cities is related to the way it is embedded in local policies and agreements with stakeholders on a local level.

Lessons Learned

For future research, it is essential to make some improvements. First, it is important to announce the method in a different way to participants. Instead of focusing on the workshop or video documentaries, participants could be made aware that the results can be used for improvement in an age-friendly city. The focus group could be at the start of the project, discussing the topics more in depth and then focusing on making a documentary on a subtheme. A second focus group could be included to discuss findings and suggestions for stakeholders and the municipality [19]. It is also important to acknowledge that co-creation processes need to address possible barriers both on the organizational level and on the citizen level. On the organizational side, this refers to, for instance, policies that support co-creation, and on the citizen side, this might be the lowering of thresholds for citizens to participate [32]. A prerequisite for co-creation and use of the results is to involve the civil servants from the local municipality and other stakeholders from the start.

Secondly, it is important to discuss with participants the roles and responsibilities, and involve them in the design of the process. For example, instead of editing the films and making a short documentary, more professional assistance in the editing process can be positive for their involvement in the process.

Another important aspect is that participants in both projects in The Hague and Leiden stated that they needed more time for the actual filming. Improvement in a longer period of time, months instead of weeks, may result in more reflection by participants on the theme, the script, and the results, instead of focusing on only learning "something new." It can also enhance the process of filmmaking for the participants. Moreover, it may be beneficial for the involvement of the municipalities and other stakeholders as partners in co-creation and the follow-up process.

These improvements may benefit future video research with older people. In The Hague, one year later, a follow-up project was organized; a new group of participants started with the topic "meaningful ageing". In Leiden, there are also plans for future video research on age-friendliness in another neighborhood.

5. Conclusions

Participatory video research can provide rich data about the age-friendliness of cities and the experiences, preferences, and needs of older people living in these cities and neighborhoods. Older participants showed their own experiences and involved other older people.

The use of participatory video design gives a voice to older people that are interested in a more active approach to research. It also fosters a positive image of older adults as active and motivated persons to improve their living environment. In video research, older people fulfill different roles in the choice of topics, in telling the story, and in directing and editing the videos for a documentary that may lead to improvements. A prerequisite for the follow-up for improvements in age-friendliness is a process of co-creation with relevant stakeholders from the start.

Author Contributions: Conceptualization, M.v.F., Z.T. and S.v.d.P.; methodology, M.v.F., Z.T. and S.v.d.P.; formal analysis, M.v.F., Z.T. and S.v.d.P.; investigation, M.v.F., Z.T. and S.v.d.P.; writing—original draft preparation, M.v.F., Z.T. and S.v.d.P.; writing—review and editing, M.v.F., Z.T. and S.v.d.P.; project administration, S.v.d.P.; funding acquisition, S.v.d.P. All authors have read and agreed to the published version of the manuscript.

Funding: This research was funded by the Dutch Ministry of Health, Welfare and Sport and the Municipality of The Hague.

Acknowledgments: All participants of the video research are thanked for their enthusiastic participation in the studies. We thank Joost van Vliet for his management in the video research in The Hague. We thank Kim Schonewille and Filmhuis Den Haag, as well as Lucas Westerbeek and his assistants of the Bromet Filmstudio/De Frisse Blik for their support in instructing participants, providing iPads, and technical support in editing the films. Karin Krens is acknowledged for her input in the results.

Conflicts of Interest: The authors declare no conflict of interest The funders had no role in the design of the study; in the collection, analyses, or interpretation of data; in the writing of the manuscript, or in the decision to publish the results.

Declaration: Participants of the film projects of the University of Applied Sciences Leiden and The Hague University of Applied Sciences have signed the informed consent, and gave us permission to use the photos taken during the project as illustration in a scientific publication about the film project. The article discusses how film can be used to learn more about the experiences of the elderly and how senior-friendly the city is. The photos are for illustration purposes in the article.

References

1. World Health Organization. *Global Age-Friendly Cities: A Guide*; WHO Press: Geneva, Switzerland, 2007.
2. Van Hoof, J.; Dikken, J.; Buttigieg, S.C.; van den Hoven, R.; Kroon, E.; Martson, H.R. Age-friendly cities in the Netherlands: An explorative study of facilitators and hindrances in the built environment and ageism in design. *Indoor Built Environ.* **2020**, *29*, 417–437. [CrossRef]
3. CBS. Prognose Bevolking; Kerncijfers, 2019–2060. Available online: https://opendata.cbs.nl/statline/#/CBS/nl/dataset/84645NED/table?ts=1594391644164 (accessed on 10 July 2020).
4. Rijksoverheid. Programma Langer Thuis. Available online: https://www.rijksoverheid.nl/documenten/rapporten/2018/06/15/programma-langer-thuis (accessed on 10 July 2020).
5. Rijksoverheid. Pact Voor de Ouderenzorg. Available online: https://www.rijksoverheid.nl/documenten/publicaties/2018/03/08/pact-voor-de-ouderenzorg (accessed on 11 July 2020).
6. Planbureau Voor de Leefomgeving. Regionale Bevolkings- en Huishoudensprognose. Available online: https://themasites.pbl.nl/o/regionale-bevolkingsprognose/ (accessed on 11 July 2020).
7. Cornwall, A.; Jewkes, R. What is participatory research? *Soc. Sci Med.* **1995**, *41*, 1667–1676. [CrossRef]
8. Corrado, A.M.; Benjamin-Thomas, T.E.; McGrath, C.; Hand, C.; Laliberte Rudman, D. Participatory Action Research with Older Adults: A Critical Interpretive Synthesis. *Gerontologist* **2020**, *60*, e413–e427. [CrossRef] [PubMed]
9. Cargo, M.; Mercer, S.L. The Value and Challenges of Participatory Research: Strengthening Its Practice. *Annu. Rev. Public Health* **2008**, *29*, 325–350. [CrossRef] [PubMed]
10. Smaling, A. Participatief onderzoek: Een overzicht. *KWALON* **2009**, *14*, 23–32. (in Dutch).
11. Lake, D.; Wendland, J. Practical, Epistemological, and Ethical Challenges of Participatory Action Research: A Cross-Disciplinary Review of the Literature. *J. High. Educ. Outreach Engagem.* **2018**, *22*, 11. Available online: https://openjournals.libs.uga.edu/jheoe/article/view/1399 (accessed on 12 July 2020).
12. Tangvald-Pedersen, O.; Bongaardt, R. Towards a tinkering participatory research method in mental health. *Scand. J. Disabil. Res.* **2017**, *19*, 7–17. [CrossRef]
13. Fenge, L. Striving towards Inclusive Research: An Example of Participatory Action Research with Older Lesbians and Gay Men. *Brit. J. Soc. Work* **2010**, *40*, 878–894. [CrossRef]

14. Tanner, D. Co-Research with older people with dementia: Experience and reflections. *J. Mental Health* **2012**, *21*, 296–306. [CrossRef]
15. Baur, V.; Abma, T. 'The Taste Buddies': Participation and empowerment in a residential home for older people. *Ageing Soc.* **2012**, *32*, 1055–1078. [CrossRef]
16. Zimmerman, M.A. Empowerment theory. Psychological, organizational and community levels of analysis. In *Handbook of Community Psychology*; Rappaport, J., Seidman, E., Eds.; Kluwer Academic/Plenum Publishers: New York, NY, USA, 2000; pp. 43–64.
17. Buffel, T. Older Coresearchers Exploring Age-Friendly Communities: An "Insider" Perspective on the Benefits and Challenges of Peer-Research. *Gerontologist* **2018**. [CrossRef] [PubMed]
18. Novek, S.; Morris-Oswald, T.; Menec, V. Using photovoice with older adults: Some methodological strengths and issues. *Ageing Soc.* **2012**, *32*, 451–470. [CrossRef]
19. Ronzi, S.; Pope, D.; Orton, L.; Bruce, N. Using photovoice methods to explore older people's perceptions of respect and social inclusion in cities: Opportunities, challenges and solutions. *SSM Popul. Health* **2016**, *2*, 732–744. [CrossRef] [PubMed]
20. Van Hoof, J.; Verhagen, M.M.; Wouters, E.J.M.; Marston, H.R.; Rijnaard, M.D.; Janssen, B.M. Picture Your Nursing Home: Exploring the Sense of Home of Older Residents through Photography. *J. Aging Res.* **2015**. [CrossRef]
21. Pink, S. *Visual Interventions: Applied Visual Anthropology*; Pink, S., Ed.; Berghahn Books: New York, NY, USA, 2007.
22. White, S.A. Participatory Video: A Process that Transforms the Self and the Other. In *Participatory Video: Images that Transform and Empower*; White, S.A., Ed.; SAGE Publications: London, UK, 2003; pp. 63–101.
23. MacDougall, D. (Ed.) *The Corporeal Image: Film, Ethnography, and the Senses*; Princeton University Press: Princeton, NJ, USA, 2006.
24. MacDougall, D. (Ed.) *Transcultural Cinema*; Princeton University Press: Princeton, NJ, USA, 1998.
25. Van Vliet, J.; Ligthart, M.; Boon, M.; van der Pas, S. Leeftijdsvriendelijke stad in beeld. Documentaires maken met ouderen. *Geron* **2018**, *20*, 56–59. (in Dutch). [CrossRef]
26. Van Blijswijk, S.; de Waard, C.S.; van Peet, P.G.; Keizer, D.; von Faber, M.; de Waal, M.; den Elzen, W.; Gussekloo, J.; Blom, J.W. Wishes and needs of community-dwelling older persons concerning general practice: A qualitative study. *PLoS ONE* **2018**, *13*, e0200614. [CrossRef]
27. Mysyuk, Y.; Huisman, M. Photovoice method with older persons: A review. *Ageing Soc.* **2019**, *40*, 1–29. [CrossRef]
28. Blair, T.; Minkler, M. Participatory Action Research with Older Adults: Key Principles in Practice. *Gerontologist* **2009**, *49*, 651–662. [CrossRef]
29. Whiting, R.; Symon, G.; Roby, H.; Chamakiotis, P. Who's Behind the Lens? A Reflexive Analysis of Roles in Participatory Video Research. *Organ. Res. Methods* **2018**, *21*, 316–340. [CrossRef]
30. Gibson, B.E. Co-Producing Video Diaries: The Presence of the "Absent" Researcher. *Int. J. Qual. Methods* **2005**, *4*, 34–43. [CrossRef]
31. Van der Pas, S. Engaging ageing communities as co-creators of social services and support. *Innov. Aging* **2017**, *1*, 1346. [CrossRef]
32. Voorberg, W.H.; Bekkers, W.J.J.M.; Tummers, L.G. A systematic review of co-creation and co-production: Embarking on the social innovation journey. *Public Manag. Rev.* **2015**, *17*, 1333–1357. [CrossRef]

Publisher's Note: MDPI stays neutral with regard to jurisdictional claims in published maps and institutional affiliations.

International Journal of
Environmental Research and Public Health

MDPI

Article

Prioritizing Age-Friendly Domains for Transforming a Mid-Sized American City

Anthony A. Sterns [1,2,3,*], Harvey L. Sterns [4,5] and Ann Walter [6,7]

1 iRxReminder LLC, 1768 E. 25th St., Cleveland, OH 44114, USA
2 Business Administration, School of Professional Studies, City University of New York, New York, NY 10001, USA
3 Management Information Systems, College of Business Administration, Kent State University, Kent, OH 44242, USA
4 Institute for Life-Span Development and Gerontology, Professor Emeritus, Department of Psychology, The University of Akron, Akron, OH 44325, USA; sternsh@uakron.edu
5 Department of Family and Community Medicine, Northeast Ohio Medical University (NEOMED), 4209 St. Rt. 44, P.O. Box 95, Rootstown, OH 44272, USA
6 Consortium of Eastern Ohio Master of Public Health Program, Cleveland State University, 2121 Euclid Ave, Cleveland, OH 44115, USA; a.m.walter@vikes.csuohio.edu
7 Medical Mutual of Ohio, 2060 E 9th Street, Cleveland, OH 44115, USA
* Correspondence: asterns@kent.edu; Tel.: +1-330-606-6675

Received: 30 October 2020; Accepted: 3 December 2020; Published: 6 December 2020

check for updates

Abstract: In May 2019, the city of Akron in the state of Ohio was admitted into AARP's network of age friendly cities and communities. Akron has a long history of aging services initiative that date back to the 1970s. To provide direction for future aging initiatives, an assessment of Akron's current state was conducted in early 2020. A survey designed to capture information on the eight Age-friendly domains was designed and mailed to 3000 randomized individuals in Akron's ten political wards. A total of 656 individuals responded and returned the survey. Akron is rated good to excellent by older Akronites; people want to stay in their neighborhood and in their home. Most Akronites like and use their neighborhood parks, find their streets well-lit, and feel safe walking in their neighborhood. Most respondents rated transportation in Akron as good to very good, but they found sidewalks good to poor. There is a high level of access to social and educational activities and a substantial opportunity to include more people. About two-thirds of respondents participate in faith-based activities, volunteer, and participate in city-sponsored events. Loneliness is not or rarely a problem for three quarters of respondents. Around 56.5% of respondents indicated they disagree they are disconnected from the community. There is high level of access to the Internet and public WiFi in Akron and a substantial opportunity to include more people. Overall, Akron has benefitted from its historical efforts and has the opportunity to impact on more older adults as the older population grows.

Keywords: survey; questionnaire; age-friendly; age-friendly cities; older people; age-friendliness; use of technology

1. Introduction

Beginning in the early 1970s, Akron showed strong leadership and commitment to implementing policies and creating services that benefit older people. The Akron Metropolitan Housing Authority had already developed special housing for older adults. In 1974, the City of Akron created the Senior Citizen Commission to the Mayor and City Council. In addition, United Way took responsibility to oversee the development of the Area Agency on Aging with funding from the Older Americans Act.

These initiatives included establishing a planning process and funding for a three-county area, in which Akron was the largest city with a population approaching 300,000 at that time.

This led to the establishment of services for older adults using existing service providers with other providers added later. This included an information and referral agency, meals-on-wheels and congregate dining, geriatric clinics by the health department, city sponsored senior recreational centers, senior on-demand transportation services, and additional senior cost-supplemented housing. Further, a multi-purpose senior center was established as a cooperative effort between the Akron Metropolitan Housing Authority and the University of Akron with funding from the Area Agency on Aging, United Way and Summit County Welfare Department. The university also launched an AARP Institute of Lifelong Learning and free university-level credit education programming. Another agency created senior job training and job search support. The County of Summit created a response that led to the formation of a cooperative committee that then led to a Robert Wood Johnson Grant to develop a centralized computer allowing for coordinated assessment and services across over 30 agencies.

These services expanded and were maintained in spite of being constrained with a weakening regional economy and the decline in manufacturing for which Akron had become famous as the "rubber capital of the world." Over time, political priorities and a population shrinking toward 200,000 persons led to a loss of the aggressive earlier support. Akron was not in a county that supported an aging services levy and over time United Way and foundations allocated less to aging services. The City of Akron for a number of years did not have an active Senior Citizen Commission. However, in recent years, the Akron Community Foundation has made aging a priority and has funded services planning research and programming.

In 2016, Mayor Daniel Horrigan was elected and supported the reactivation of the Senior Citizen Commission. As the commission assessed needs and wants of older adults, a series of community listening events was conducted. During 2017, there was discussion regarding the possibility of Akron becoming part of the age friendly cities initiative. With encouragement from Ohio AARP, the idea of formally applying was carefully considered. Support from the Director of the Institute for Life-Span Development and Gerontology, who also was chair of the Commission on Aging as well as the Dean of Arts and Sciences and later Interim President of the University of Akron, greatly facilitated moving forward. Direction Home Akron Canton Area Agency on Aging took major leadership responsibility. In February 2019, the application to join the AARP Network of Age Friendly Communities was submitted by Mayor Horrigan.

To focus on aging initiatives and blend them into the general initiatives to enhance the livability of the city of Akron, an effort to guide the next era of development was organized around the AARP network of Age Friendly Cities and Communities [1–3]. The first step in the process was the establishment of a core committee made up of the members of the Commission. The partners in this process include the City of Akron, Direction Home, Akron Canton Area Agency on Aging and Disabilities, the University of Akron, and the City of Akron Senior Citizens Commission to the Mayor and City Council. Members of the Commission on Aging make up the core committee for the Age Friendly Akron initiative. A broader membership of agencies and individuals, the Advisory Committee, was invited to advise the core committee. The development of the assessment involved this group. To guide policy and planning, an assessment of the current state of the City of Akron was planned.

2. Materials and Methods

The study was executed as a randomized cross-sectional study of older residents of the City of Akron. The survey was assembled and mailed through a fulfillment service to ensure the respondents anonymity was maintained. The survey was reviewed and the procedures approved by the University of Akron Institutional Review Board responsible for ethical treatment of human subjects research. Data entry and analysis were conducted by the research team.

2.1. Survey Participants

There were 3000 individuals over the age of 50 randomly selected from all 10 wards in the City of Akron. Surveys were mailed along with prepaid return envelopes. A total of 656 (21.9%) individuals responded and returned the survey. This was comparable to the response rates of Cleveland (n = 283, 28.3% return rate) and Columbus (n = 346, 23.1% return rate). [4,5]

Respondents were predominately female (62.7%), Caucasian (72.4%), and spoke English (87.8%). The age of respondents ranged 50–95 with an average age of 69.3 (s.d. 10) years of age. About two-fifths (40.1%) were married, a quarter divorced (23.9%), one fifth widowed (21.8%), and the remainder never married (14.2%). Respondents most often lived in a home they owned (76%), while others lived in a condominium (7%), a rented apartment (6%), a rented house (5%), a family member's house (2%), subsidized housing (2%), or institutionalized care or community living (2%).

2.2. Instrument

The committee utilized the framework established in the Global Age-friendly Cities Guide by the WHO [1], as well as the conceptual framework and required questions prescribed by the AARP Age-friendly cities and communities' guidebook [6]. The Age Friendly Akron survey looks at the eight proscribed domains of the Age-friendly cities and communities framework: (1) housing and neighborhoods; (2) outdoor spaces and buildings; (3) transportation and walkability; (4) arts, entertainment, and leisure; (5) respect and social inclusion; (6) civic participation and employment; (7) communication and information; and (8) health and wellness. Based on a gerontechnological focus within the committee, additional emphases on technology and health services availability were incorporated into the survey instrument. The importance of additional questions on access and adoption of technology were recently reported by Marston and van Hoof [7].

The Age-friendly Akron survey instrument is shared in Appendix A. The instrument was designed to provide a description of the state of the respondents in each of the eight domains. The core questions drew from the required guidelines of the program survey template [8] as well as drawing on other nearby cities in Ohio including Columbus, the State's capital in the center of the state; Cleveland, just north of Akron on the shores of Lake Erie; and Cincinnati, a city in the south of the state along the Ohio River and the border of the State of Kentucky [4,5,9].

Section 1 of the survey consisted of 12 questions on housing. Some questions had components that consisted of multiple aspects of living situations to consider and on which to report. The overall desire to live in their home, neighborhood, and in the City of Akron were assessed using five-point Likert scale questions.

Section 2 consisted of six multipart questions on outdoor spaces and accessibility. Questions asked respondents to describe the state of city infrastructure including evaluation of street lighting, sidewalk maintenance, walkability, and access to buildings and offices.

Section 3 of the survey consisted of nine questions focused on aspects of transportation and access to various kinds of alternative transportation modalities including walking. Several questions asked respondents to indicate all the transportation modalities they utilize, and the list included various on-demand services including SCAT (on demand paratransit), taxis, Uber/Lyft, and others. Several questions asked about weather's impact on transportation. The City of Akron experiences four distinct seasons; it is hot in the summer and has snow in the winter.

Section 4 of the survey consisted of six multipart questions on arts, leisure, and educational opportunities available to Akron residents. Most questions focused on usage of major facilities (museums, theaters, outdoor venues, and sports facilities) as well as various festival and educational opportunities available throughout the year.

Section 5 of the survey consisted of five questions on respect and social inclusion. These questions asked respondents to indicate the kinds and frequency of interactions they have and to rate the quality of those interactions. One multipart question asked for a rating of the perceived voice older persons have in the community.

Section 6 of the survey consisted of seven questions on civic participation and employment. Questions asked respondents about their employment status, participation in childcare and volunteering, and quantifying access to these opportunities. A question asking about experiences with agism related to employment is also in this section.

Section 7 of the survey consisted of seven questions on access to information and questions about access to and use of communication technologies that include telephony and Internet services. Questions in the section also assessed confidence in knowing how to obtain information on various services and awareness of specific programs designed to support the distribution of information and connect older persons with available services.

Section 8 of the survey consisted of 17 questions on health and wellness. The opening question asked the respondent to rate their overall health. Questions asked about access to grocery stores, medical and pharmacy services, and other health related services such as dentistry. Other questions focused on the use of and frequency of acute challenges related to health, food availability, medical services, and mental health. Several questions focused on loneliness and relationships with others in the respondent's family and in the community. Several questions asked about the use of home modifications required to maintain independence.

A final section of the survey included nine demographic questions including gender, age, income, and marital status.

3. Results

As a first step in the analysis, the internal reliability of the domain-specific questions was examined. Questions with ordinal or quantitative responses in each domain were isolated and a Cronbach's α was calculated for each. The results indicate moderate to high internal consistency within each of the domains (see Table 1). These results, in addition to the consistent approach across the other cities within the WHO and AARP Age-friendly communities provided confidence to examine the individual domains. For a complete list of the questions analyzed, see Appendix B, Table A1.

Table 1. Internal consistency measures of each survey domain.

Domain	Valid n	Cronbach's α
Housing	568	0.672
Outdoor spaces	370	0.685
Transportation	175	0.804
Arts Entertainment and Leisure	627	0.838
Respect and Social Inclusion	569	0.692
Civic participation and employment	562	0.756
Communication	577	0.723
Health	291	0.690

3.1. Housing and Neighborhoods

Respondents rate the city of Akron positively with 88.7% reporting a good or better rating and 34.0% rating it as excellent or very good. Considering the respondents in terms of their average income, there are more favorable views in areas (mailing zip codes) with higher incomes. In the three lower income areas, unfavorable ratings are nearly twice as high (13% vs. 25%), but still a minority (see Figure 1 and Table 2).

Table 2. Ratings of the city of Akron as a place to live based ordered by average income per mailing zip codes. Zip codes are ordered highest income to lowest income and those with less than 8 responses were excluded from this analysis.

	44223	44303	44313	44302	44312	44301	44305	44310	44320	44314	44307	44306	44311	Total
Excellent or Very good	25%	34%	46%	36%	29%	44%	24%	26%	32%	29%	36%	33%	36%	34%
Good	63%	59%	51%	55%	60%	51%	65%	56%	54%	52%	54%	45%	45%	55%
Poor or Very poor	13%	7%	3%	9%	10%	5%	12%	18%	14%	19%	11%	23%	18%	11%
n size	8	29	105	11	58	39	68	57	72	48	28	40	11	574

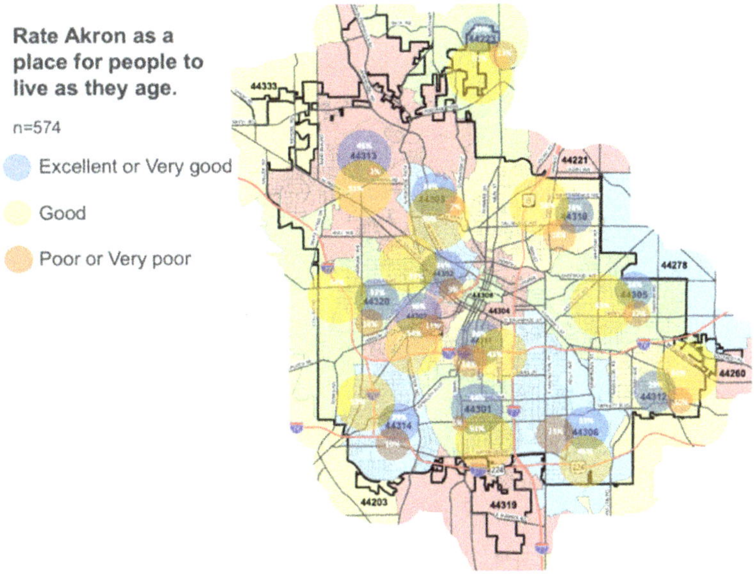

Figure 1. Ratings of the city of Akron as a place to live based on mailing zip codes.

Respondents indicated they most strongly want to remain in their homes and feel slightly less strongly about remaining in their neighborhoods and in the City of Akron. These feelings are stronger for the oldest respondents. (See Figure 2).

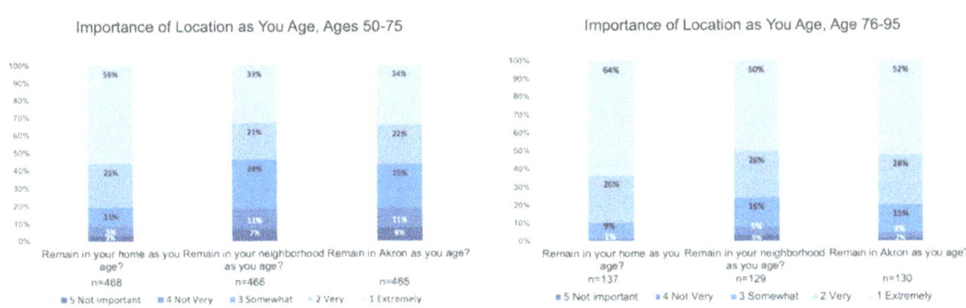

(**a**) (**b**)

Figure 2. Respondents want most to remain in their homes, but they also want to remain in their neighborhoods and in the city of Akron: (**a**) the reported importance of aging in place for respondents aged 50–75; and (**b**) the reported importance of aging in place for respondents aged 76–95.

Several issues in the survey related to housing noted concerns either by absence (e.g., "don't have access") or uncertainty (e.g., "not sure"). These issues included access to affordable housing (29.4% not sure/15.9% no), pedestrian crossing timings (15.9% not sure/24.2% no), access to snow removal services (19.3% not sure/22.7% no), access to lawn services (19.0% not sure/25.5% no), well maintained sidewalks (5.9% not sure/48.8% no), and access to a reliable handyman (23.3% not sure/30.1% no). There were no geographic differences in the acceptability of sidewalks and concerns were citywide.

3.2. Outdoor Spaces and Buildings

Respondents indicated that public parks were extremely (43.0%) or very important (34.7%), and 74.0% of respondents indicated public parks in the neighborhood were good, very good, or excellent. About 9.8% indicated that parks in their neighborhood were poor, and 15.0% indicated they did not have them. Accessibility of outdoor spaces and buildings is summarized in Figure 3.

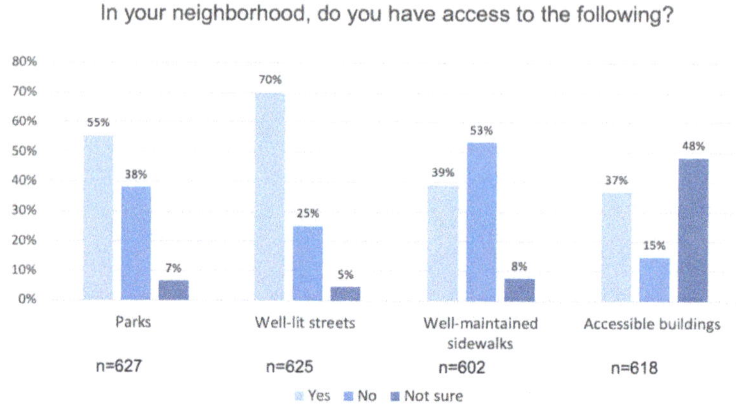

Figure 3. A majority of respondents indicated they have access to parks, well-lit streets, and accessible buildings. In contrast, access to well-maintained sidewalks was a concern.

Access to park benches (86.2%), a park with accessible trails (67.0%), pathways for bikes and people (70.1%), and parks that are maintained in the winter (79.0%) were all generally viewed as available for a majority of respondents.

Buildings were also viewed favorably with accessible front doors (81.4%), having automatic door openers (53.4%), and large enough restrooms (46.6%), all or most of the time.

3.3. Transportation and Walkability

Respondents indicated an overwhelmingly positive view of public transit in the city of Akron with more than half rating the transit system good (57.3%), very good (23.4%), or excellent (6.8%). Regardless of age, driving themselves was the most frequent mode (85.4%) and being driven the next most frequent mode (8.2%). There was a three-fold increase in those respondents reporting being driven for those 50–75 (5.3%) versus those 76–95 (16.5%) years of age (see Figure 4). As driving is the major mode of transit, it is positive that streets signs are perceived as legible (85.7%). Awareness of driver refresher courses, however, is low at only 13.5%.

Akron has both a public fixed route bus system and a dedicated on-demand bus service known as SCAT. Both services are utilized more by those 75 and under and by a very small percentage of older adults (5.2% combined).

The perceptions about public transit are overwhelmingly positive, although there is a substantial number of respondents indicating uncertainty or no opinion. Rating on access to transport for those with disabilities (61.3% yes/3.4% no/35.3% not sure) and access to reliable transit (71.5% yes/7.8% no/20.6% not sure) reflect this trend. Concerns are higher with respect to perceptions of lighting at public transit stops (34.6% all or most/65.4% some, few, or none), public transit stops having seating (25.5% all or most/74.5% some, few, or none), and public transit stops having shelters from the weather (21.5% all or most/79.6% some, few, or none).

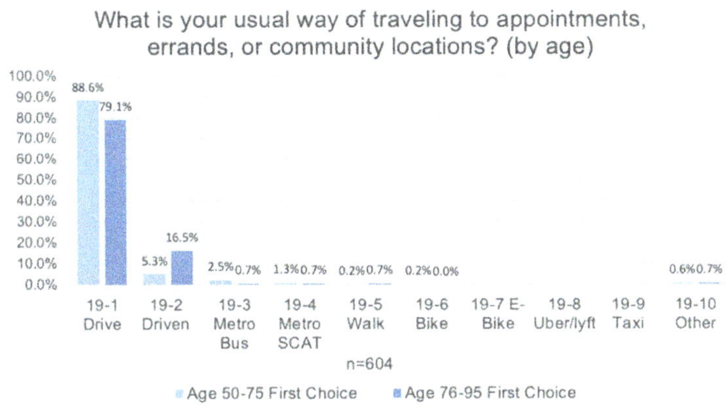

Figure 4. Respondents indicated that a vast majority of travel is done by driving themselves or being driven in a car. This is a low usage of standard public bus (Metro) and public on-demand services (SCAT) as well as walking.

3.4. Arts, Entertainment and Leisure

Akron has historically had a rich cultural environment with the University of Akron as its center with a strong art, dance, and theater program, as well as the Akron Symphony, professional and amateur dance companies, active music scene, numerous live theaters and outdoor concert venues, and a well-respected Museum of Art with a focus on modern works as well as an arts district and monthly art walk. Akron is also home to a downtown baseball stadium for the minor league baseball team as well as stadiums for the University of Akron football, baseball, basketball, and track and field teams. Crisscrossing Akron are the historical locks and canals of the Ohio and Erie Canals and the tow path trail, which connects with walking and bike paths that connect parks and greenspaces throughout the city and along the Cuyahoga River and Summit Lake. Akron is also home to the Akron Zoological Park, Stan Hywett Hall and Gardens, several historical cemeteries, and the Akron Toy Museum as well as many city-sponsored and neighborhood art, cultural, and music festivals throughout the year.

Respondents indicated they have access to social activities (70.3%), educational events (62.7%), and public events (78.9%) (see Figure 5).

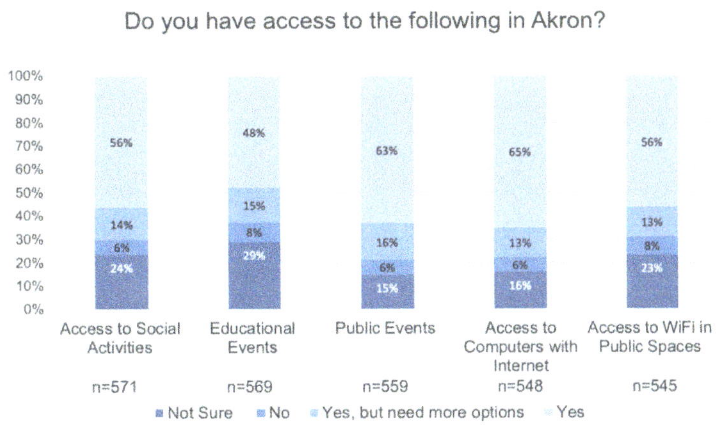

Figure 5. A summary of access social, educational and public events as well as access to computers and WiFi networks.

Questions about participation gauge usage rather than perceptions of access. Respondents were asked how often they participate in events with one quarter (26.6%) participating every other week or more, less than a fifth participating monthly (19.0%), and the remaining majority (54.5%) participating less than monthly (29.6%) or never (25.0%). However, there was an indication that more frequent participation was desired with a third of individuals (32.4%) wanting every other week or more, about a third (30%) wanting monthly event participation, and the remaining quarter interested in less than monthly participation (15.4%), or no participation at all (11.9%).

Respondents were asked if they participate in museums and the zoo. About half (50.2%) indicated yes, while about a sixth (17.3%) indicated they do not but would like too, nearly a quarter (23.8%) indicated they do not but had in the past, and the remainder do not participate and have no interest in doing so (8.6%). A similar pattern was found with live theater, with slightly more participation with city-sponsored events and slightly less participation in sporting events.

Questions were also asked about other activity interests. About half of respondents indicated participation in faith-based activities (50.8% yes/9.1% no but would like too), volunteer activities (34.7% yes/23.3% no, but would like too), and family gatherings (74.4% yes/7.3% no, but would like too).

Leisure activities also include continuing education and physical recreation participation. These appear to offer opportunities for capturing great interest from the community. Only 14.0% of respondents indicated they currently participate in continuing education opportunities, while 34.9% of respondents said they did not participate but would like too. With regard to physical recreation, a larger group (33.4%) indicated they do participate and a similar size group (34.4%) said they do not participate but would like too.

3.5. *Respect and Social Inclusion*

The degree of voice that older persons perceive in the community is an important measure of the respect they feel. Their wellbeing is also connected to the amount of social interaction they experience. These are the focus of the questions related to respect and social inclusion.

3.5.1. Community Interactions

Most (70.7%) older adults interact with friends and family on a daily basis and another 7.1% interact at least monthly. Only 3.1% report highly infrequent contact or have no friends and family. A majority of survey respondents report engaging with other age groups either daily (39.8%), weekly (25.6%), or every other week (8.7%). About one fifth engage with other age groups once per month (9.5%) or less than monthly (8.4%), with 8.4% indicating that they never do so.

About one third (32.0%) of respondents indicated that opinions of older people are valued, while half (50.3%) were not sure, and 17.7% indicated they did not think opinions were valued. Similarly, when respondents were asked if older people were respected by the community: 5.9% strongly agreed, 26.4% agreed, 44.8% were not sure, 20.2% disagreed, and 2.8% strongly disagreed. When respondents were asked if they feel disconnected from the community, a majority strongly disagreed (13.2%) or disagreed (43.3%) with the statement. One quarter (25.1%) of respondents were not sure if they felt disconnected, with 15.4% indicating they agree with feeling disconnected and 3.0% strongly agreeing (see Figure 6).

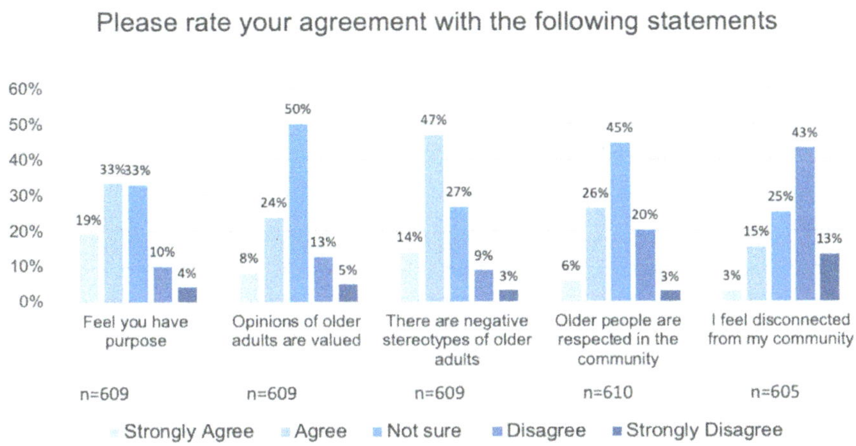

Figure 6. A majority of older adults report having purpose, while a minority indicate their opinions are valued and they are respected in the community. Encountering negative stereotypes of older adults as well as feeling disconnected are reported by a significant minority of respondents.

3.5.2. Purpose and Loneliness

Most respondents strongly agreed or agreed that they feel they have a purpose (52.7%), one third (33.2%) reported not being sure, and 14.1% disagreed or strongly disagreed. Feelings of loneliness are never (44.9%) or rarely (31.1%) experienced by most older adult respondents. However, feelings of loneliness are reported sometimes by about one fifth (21.3%) of respondents. Of most concern are the respondents who report loneliness is experienced most (1.1%) or all of the time (1.6%). Spearman's rho shows a statistically significant correlation between feelings of purpose within a community and feelings of loneliness ($r_s[594] = -2.14$, $p < 0.001$). This correlation is significant but small (see Figure 7).

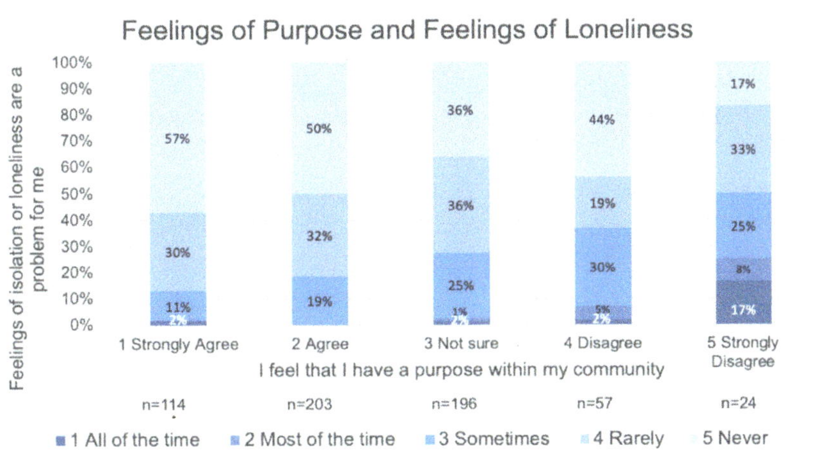

Figure 7. Feelings of purpose and loneliness of negatively related with greater purpose and less loneliness being the most reported state.

3.6. Civic Participation and Employment

About one fifth of respondents reported working full time (19.2%), with 4.8% working part-time, and 1.6% reported themselves as self-employed. When those reporting retired and working (8.2%) are added in, this is about one third of respondents. This is in line with the percentage of 50–67-year-olds who are below the standard retirement age to receive social security. Of those working, 11.0% indicated enjoying working, 9.0% indicated they could not afford to retire, 4.3% were working to maintain healthcare coverage, and 6.7% said they were not yet of retirement age.

There are a groups of respondents who reported themselves as unemployed and seeking work (1.6%), retired and seeking work (6.3%), and underemployed and seeking more work (0.16%). This would be about 50% higher than the unemployment rate for the City of Akron at the time of survey (4.0%) [10]. Some respondents reported providing unpaid childcare (8.2%) and unpaid eldercare (6.6%). Most respondents indicated they had adequate access to volunteer options but less indicated this for job opportunities, see Figure 8.

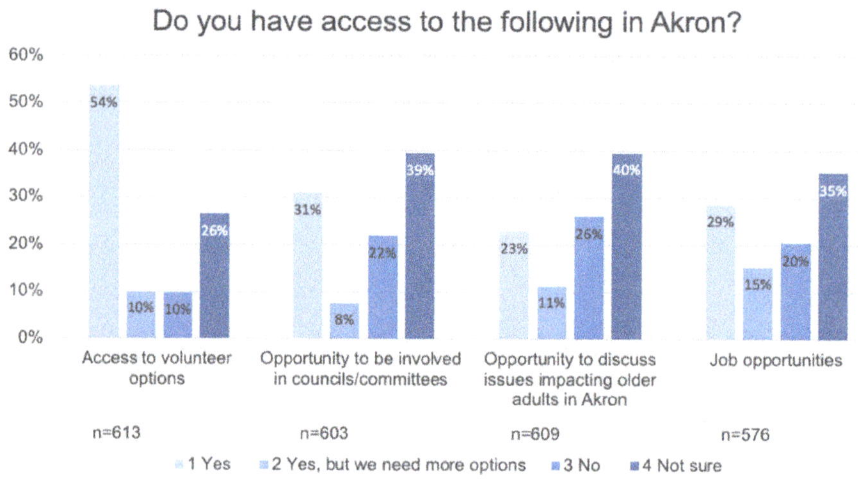

Figure 8. A majority of respondents had access to volunteer opportunities and opportunities to be involved in committees. Many respondents are not sure about various opportunities, which is an opportunity for improving awareness.

The majority of respondents (55.7%) reported being retired and not looking for work. Three quarters (73.3%) of respondents indicated they chose to retire, while the remainder (26.7%) reported they did not choose to retire.

3.7. Communication and Information

Finding information that is needed and being proactive about seeking information are reported by a large majority of respondents. Less than 5.7% of respondents indicated they were rarely or never able to do so and less than 8.1% were rarely or never proactive about doing so. When asked specifically about assistance with housing, 12.5% indicated they were always able to and 34.0% were able to find assistance most of the time. More concerning was that respondents reported they found assistance with housing sometimes (24.1%), rarely (14.0%), or never (15.3%). Similarly, when asked specifically about knowing where to go for assistance with healthcare, 25.2% of respondents always knew where to go and 38.6% knew where to go most of the time. However, 21.1% only knew where to get assistance with healthcare sometimes, 8.1% rarely, and 9.0% never.

For computers, the older the respondent, the less likely they were to have a computer with WiFi, see Figure 9. Respondents indicated most still have a landline, but a greater number have computers, a smartphone, and WiFi at home (see Figure A2 in Appendix C).

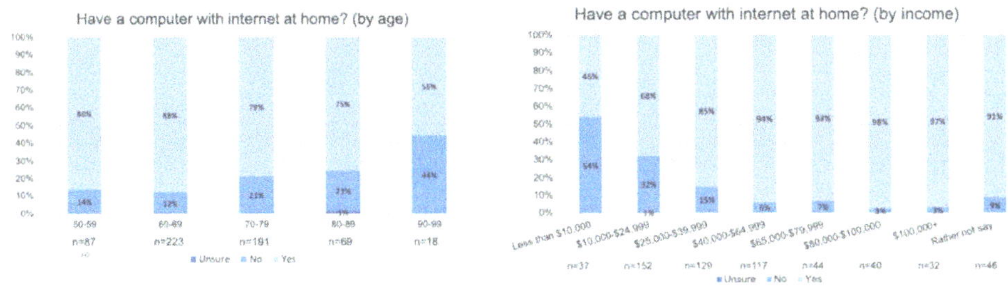

(a) (b)

Figure 9. Respondents generally have computers with Internet in the city of Akron. Having a computer at home with Internet is: (**a**) negatively correlated with age ($r_s[588] = -0.135$, $p < 0.001$); and (**b**) positively correlated with income ($r_s[597] = 0.329$, $p < 0.001$).

3.8. Health and Wellness

The Health and wellness portion of the survey assessed not only respondents' overall health and mental health, but also other factors that contribute to health outcomes such as food security, healthcare affordability, access to healthcare services and providers, and health insurance. Overall, 69.8% of respondents rated their overall health as very good or good, 24.2% responded with fair health, and 6.1% rated their health poor or very poor.

Additional insight into health can be gained by examining location; access to food, pharmacies, and fitness centers, and affordability. A decreasing number of respondents with very good and good health, and an increasing number of those with fair, poor, or very poor health is observed when zip codes are ordered by highest income to lowest income, as seen in Figure 10a. When asked, on average, how often respondents participate in physical activity, the majority of those who reported very good overall health exercise every day to several times per week (73.7%). A gradual decline is observed between frequency of exercise as overall health rating declines as well (see Figures A3 and A4 in Appendix C).

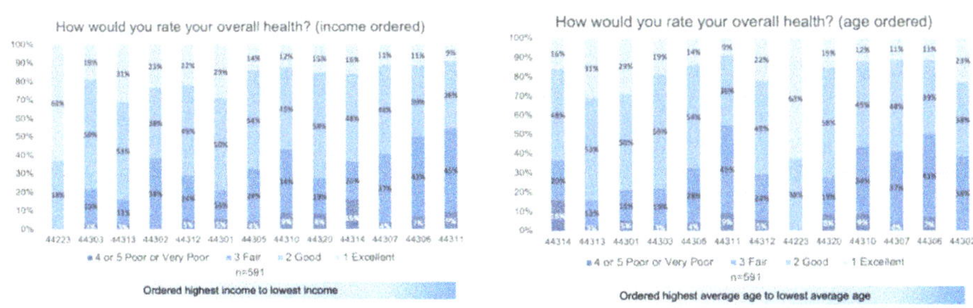

(a) (b)

Figure 10. Respondents rate their overall current health status: (**a**) represents overall health ordered by zip code from highest to lowest incomes of the survey respondents; and (**b**) represents overall health ordered by highest average age to lowest average age of respondents. Zip codes with fewer than eight responses were excluded from this analysis.

Access to a full-service grocery, convenience store, and pharmacy in Akron was indicated by 87.1% or more of respondents in all three categories. The need for more options was highlighted in regard to Healthcare facilities and Urgent care centers (31.8% and 32.7% of respondents, respectively).

Affordability of medications, dentures, glasses/contacts, and hearing aids is considered vital to accessing these items and thereby maintaining low risk of other health issues related to medication adherence, falls, depression, nursing home stays, and dependence on family caregivers [11,12]. Generally, health insurance plans available to older adults including the federally funded Medicare plans for those 65 years and above or disabled do not cover dental, vision, and hearing; these items are often paid for out of pocket.

Seventy-eight percent or more of respondents indicated they can afford regular medications and glasses/contacts always or most of the time (88.2% medications, 77.6% glasses/contacts). Over 52.9% of respondents do not need dentures or hearing aids. Of those that do need these items, approximately 60% reported they could afford them always or most of the time (62.3% dentures, 59.1% hearing aids). See Figure 11.

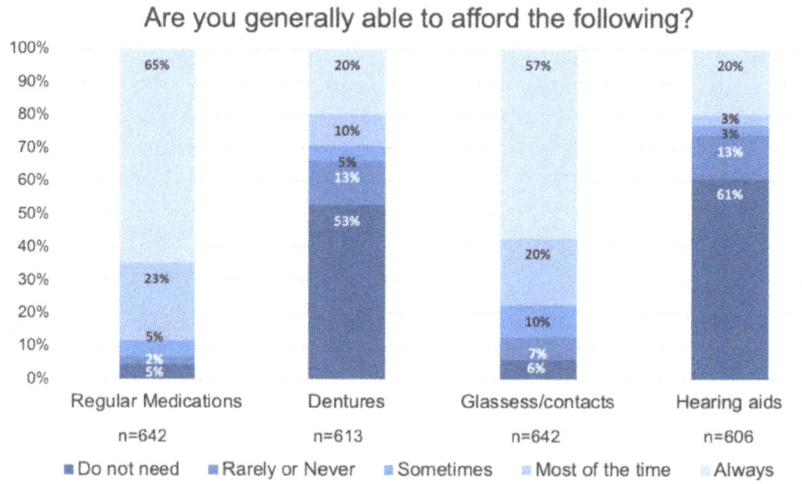

Figure 11. Affordability of regular medications, dentures, glasses/contacts, and hearing aids is reflected in this figure. The majority of respondents can afford regular medications and glasses/contacts always or most of the time. Around 60% of respondents do not need dentures (52.9%) or hearing aids (60.9%) currently.

4. Discussion

Over many years, the planning process of the Area Agency on Aging was the major source of information regarding service needs of older adults. This was an appropriate focus on individuals with greatest needs. In fact, a limitation of this study is that those most frail and living alone may have been the least likely to respond to the survey and may be under-represented. This is limitation is supported by the combined 4% reported to be living in supplemented housing and institutionalized care when we typically expect around 5% in US cities. We also see a comfortingly low level of reported frequent loneliness, although, again, this may be underreported.

However, the focus in not on those in greatest need, but to gather an assessment of the community as a whole from the perspective of the older members of the community. The Age-friendly City approach to looking at a community focusing on the eight domains gives the first multidimensional look at citizens over 50 and their self-reported assessment of the city. This is the first time that the city has been looked at in depth in terms of perceptions of positives and negatives by people ≥50.

The very process of designing and carrying out the survey and the analyses has provided important information for focusing on priorities and possible intervention strategies. This information was collected pre-COVID-19. To take recent experiences into account, focus groups will be conducted in each ward of the city to determine what additional issues need to be considered in planning and priority setting.

One of the key findings was that older adults feel they need to have greater involvement in decision making and their opinions need to be considered by community leadership [13]. This is important as individuals make the transition from work to retirement as evidenced by the survey illustrating a sizeable group participating in work at some level [14]. It also speaks to why the assessment process as a precursor to priority setting is so important. Taking the time to fully explore the results, to understand the heterogeneity of views, and only then engage committees to discuss priorities in each of the eight domains is an important part of the prescribed process [6].

Another key finding is that staying in one's home is a very high priority for Akron residents, higher than the national average for this item, typically 75% in the U.S. [15]. This also leads to a focus on the quality of the neighborhood on many dimensions such as safety, access to grocery shopping, access to health care, and the type of supports such as transportation and home services that are available [13]. Another limitation of the study is that it is apparent that not all areas of the city provide the same experience, and it is possible that those with the least positive experiences were less motivated to respond. However, there are sufficient indications that understanding how to intervein in selected areas with higher dissatisfaction rates will need to be determined.

Most important are the identification of gaps in needed services, need for alternative housing options, and the importance of having access to needed information for services when they become needed [16]. There are disparities that need to be focused on such as key sources of information for needed services. The results show that relatively few individuals were accessing the most helpful information sites and services. However, individuals felt that they were able to find information and felt that they were proactive when it is well known that individuals do not know what they need and only really look for information when there is a problem.

Another important area that was assessed is the quality of the living experience in terms of parks and recreations opportunities, opportunities to attend theater and concerts, attend sports events, engage in educational activities, and ability to have access to jobs and volunteer activities [17]. It becomes very important to carefully explore the areas that need to be addressed first.

To further support older adults in Akron aging in place, several community resources guides have been compiled, notably: the Senior Citizen Information Booklet, produced in Summit County and available online [18]; the Summit County Resource Guide, developed by Getting Wiser and Summit County 2-1-1 [19]; and the Akron Resource Directory, and online resources such as the 2-1-1 Summit County Resource Database.

Many agencies and resources referenced in these guides have found innovative ways to continue their work supporting older adults despite the COVID-19 pandemic. Programs offering minor home repairs at no cost such as Rebuilding Together of Northeast Ohio and Lift Up Ministries continue to provide valuable assistance with repairs around the home including roof/gutters, plumbing, electrical, porch stairs, and furnace. Although many adult day services have been temporarily suspended, organizations such as the Destination Home Akron Area Agency on Aging and Disabilities have been making telephonic wellness calls to residents they support. A plethora of meals programs, albeit with increased safety precautions, have continued their work delivering food to Akronites. In particular, Mobile Meals, Vantage Meals on Wheels, and others have been maintaining vital efforts in meal provision and delivery. As the city pivots to the future, it will be leveraging its strong, growth-ready programmatic infrastructure on which to build.

5. Conclusions

These results represent a summary of the first comprehensive assessment of the key domains of the City of Akron, a typical mid-sized American city, but unique in its history of efforts to provide comprehensive and wide-ranging services to older persons. The reported results document the rationale, tools, and comprehensive nature of the assessments of the Age-friendly cities and communities' domains. They also demonstrate the degree of detail assessed to capture the accessibility and support for functional aging that is the hallmark of the program's current approach.

The commitment to the Age-friendly cities and communities program represents a significant pivot in public policy for the City of Akron and Summit County, Ohio because it demonstrates a return to a unified effort of city government with regional aging services. This is particularly relevant because the City of Akron has a significant history of highly progressive aging services in its past, but a disjointed policy execution over the past two decades.

The analysis provides a comprehensive overview of the current state of each of the domains. It lays the groundwork for a discussion about community priorities. It allows a discussion that not only focuses on the requirements of those with the most need, which is of great importance, but also provides the opportunity to apply resources to improving the livability of the city. Thus, as the population continues growing older, more older adults are positioned to live independently and with greater life satisfaction.

As a summary of the current state of the domains in a typical mid-sized city, the results also provide a point of reference so that future assessments of other cities can make a comparison. Future research should be able to utilize studies such as these to test the accuracy of livability indices that are utilized to compare municipalities throughout the world.

Author Contributions: A.A.S. carried out the coding, labeling, and executed the principal analysis and manuscript generation. H.L.S. as Chair of the City of Akron Commission on Aging and Co-Chair of Age Friendly Akron accepted the role of overseeing the survey research aspects of the project. He contributed to survey design, coordinated research approval, coordinated with project partners, advisory committee and core committee, supervised data encoding, worked with the research team on data analyses and manuscript preparation. A.W. contributed the manuscript, provided a portion of the analysis, as well as developing the graphics and tables for the manuscript. All authors have read and agreed to the published version of the manuscript.

Funding: The survey research was funded by Ohio AARP with a match provided by The University of Akron and carried out by the Institute for Life-Span Development and Gerontology and the Ray C. Bliss Institute of Applied Politics.

Acknowledgments: We want to thank Briana Rummer, M.A. of the Bliss Institute of The University of Akron for her support of the project and for the data coding and input. We also want to thank Douglas Tayek, Associate State Director of Outreach of Ohio AARP for his guidance and support of the work.

Conflicts of Interest: The authors declare no conflict of interest.

Appendix A

AGE-FRIENDLY AKRON

We are conducting a survey of adults ages 50 and over to determine how *Age-Friendly* our Akron community is. Please take a moment to answer the following questions based on the neighborhood where you live. Responses will remain anonymous. If you have questions or need assistance with this survey, please contact Susan Sigmon at (330) 899-5206 or Harvey Sterns at (330) 328-0042

Surveys returned by January 31st will be entered into a drawing to receive a $100 gift card.

Housing and Neighborhoods

1.How many years have you lived in Akron?

____

2. What is your current zip code?

____

3. What Akron neighborhood do you live in?

____

4. What does your current housing situation?

___ Live alone
___ Live with spouse
___ Live with partner
___ Live with family members
___ Live with group

5. Where do you live? *(Check best answer)*

___ Apartment
___ Condo
___ Subsidized housing
___ Owned house
___ Rented house
___ Family member's home
___ Senior living community
    ___ Independent living
    ___ Assisted living
    ___ Nursing home
___ Shared home
Other: _____________________

6. Is your housing restricted to age 55+?

Yes   No

7. How important is it to you to...	**Extremely**	**Very**	**Somewhat**	**Not very**	**Not important**
Remain in your home as you age?					
Remain in your neighborhood as you age?					
Remain in Akron as you age?					

Page **1** of **12**

8. How would you rate Akron as a place for people to live as they age? (Please circle)
excellent very good good poor very poor

9. In your neighborhood, do you have access to the following *(check or circle as appropriate)*:	**Yes**	**Yes, but we need more options**	**No**	**Not sure**
Affordable housing for older adults (active communities, assisted living, etc.)				
Pedestrian crossings with an adequate timed countdown				
Affordable seasonal services like snow removal				
Affordable seasonal services like lawn care				
Well-maintained sidewalks				
Reliable handymen				
Neighborhood watch programs				

10. Do you feel safe walking in your neighborhood? *(Please circle)*
very secure fairly secure unsure some concern very concerned

11. If you were to move, into which housing type would you consider moving?
(Select the five you'd most like; please rank 1 through 5)

___ Apartment
___ Condo
___ Low-income or subsidized housing
___ Owned house
___ Rented house
___ Family member's home
___ Shared home
___ Senior living community
  ___ Independent living
  ___ Assisted living
  ___ Nursing home
___ Shared home
Other: ____________________

12. Is your top housing choice available in your neighborhood?
Yes No Unsure

Outdoor Spaces and Buildings

13. In your neighborhood, do you have access to the following:	**Yes**	**No**	**Not sure**
Well-maintained parks within walking distance of your home			
Well-lit streets			
Well-maintained sidewalks			
Easily accessible buildings for those with disabilities or those who require modifications			

Page **2** of **12**

14. How important do you think it is to have public parks in your community?

___ Extremely important
___ Very important
___ Somewhat important
___ Not very important
___ Not important

15. How do you rate the public parks currently in your neighborhood?

excellent very good good poor very poor don't have

16. If there are parks in your neighborhood do they have…	**Yes**	**Yes, but we need more options**	**No**
Benches?			
Flat surfaces?			
Accessible trails?			
Pathways for bikes and/or pedestrians?			

17. If there are parks in your neighborhood are they well-maintained in the winter from snow and ice?

all the time most of the time sometimes rarely never

18. Do buildings in your neighborhood include the following:	**Always**	**Most of the time**	**Sometimes**	**Rarely**	**Never**
Accessible front doors					
Automatic door openers					
Large enough restrooms					

Transportation and Walkability

19. What is your usual way of running errands, getting to appointments, or attending events? *(Select the three most commonly used; please rank 1 through 3)*

___ I drive myself
___ I am driven by friends or family
___ I take a METRO bus
___ I use METRO SCAT
___ I walk
___ I ride my bike
___ eBike
___ I use Uber/Lyft
___ I use a taxi
Other: _______________

20. How would you rate the public transportation options in Akron?

excellent very good good poor very poor

Page **3** of **12**

21. In your neighborhood do you have access to the following *(check or circle as appropriate):*	**Yes**	**Yes, but we need more options**	**No**	**Not sure**
Special transportation for older adults and/or those with disabilities				
Reliable public transportation				
Legible street signs and street numbers				
Bike lanes for wheelchairs or bikes				

22. Are you aware of any driver education or refresher courses in your neighborhood or community?

Yes No

23. How do you rate the maintenance of the sidewalks in your neighborhood?

excellent very good good poor very poor

24. Do you face any barriers or issues listed below when traveling to an appointment, event, or community location? ***(Select all that apply)***

___ I have no problems getting around
___ I do not drive
___ I do not drive on highways
___ I don't have others willing or able to take me
___ I can't afford a car or car maintenance
___ I don't feel safe walking
___ Do not drive at night
___ I have difficulties with parking
___ I can't afford public transportation
___ There is no METRO bus to take me where I need to go
___ I am unsure how to access or use METRO buses
___ I have problems using METRO SCAT
___ Trouble with medical transportation
___ I need transportation 7 days a week
Other: ____________________

25. Are you aware of travel training by METRO to better navigate public transportation?

Yes No

26. If yes, have you used this service?

Yes No

27. If you use public transportation, do most of the waiting areas at stops for public transportation in Akron include…	**All**	**Most**	**Some**	**Few**	**None**
Safe lighting?					
Seating?					
Shelter from weather?					

Page **4** of **12**

Arts, Entertainment, and Leisure

28. Do you have access to the following in Akron *(circle or check as appropriate)*	**Yes**	**Yes, but we need more options**	**No**	**Not sure**	**Is this free?**
Social activities like book clubs, games, art activities, cultural events, etc					Yes No
Educational events like art classes, gardening classes, or speakers					Yes No
Public events					Yes No
Access to computers with internet access					Yes No
Access to Wi-Fi in public spaces					Yes No

29. Do you participate in the following activities in Akron?	**Yes**	**No but I would like to**	**No and I have no interest**	**No but I have in the past**
Museums (Akron Art Museum, ArtsNow, Akron Zoo, Stan Hywet, etc.)				
Faith-based activities				
Volunteer opportunities				
Live theatre (Akron Civic, E.J. Thomas, Weathervane, etc.)				
City-sponsored events and concerts				
Sporting events (Rubber Ducks, UA sports, local school sports, etc)				
Family gatherings				
Continuing education classes				
Physical recreation (walking groups, yoga, etc)				

30. How often do you engage in social/community events in Akron?

___ Every day to several times a week
___ About once a week
___ About once every other week
___ About once a month
___ Less than once a month
___ Never

31. How often do you <u>want</u> to engage in social or community events in Akron?

___ Every day to several times a week
___ About once a week
___ About once every other week
___ About once a month
___ Less than once a month
___ Never

32. Is transportation a barrier to attending events?

all the time most of the time sometimes rarely never

Page **5** of **12**

33. Are you aware of the different continuing education programs in Akron?

Yes No

Respect and Social Inclusion

34. How often do you interact with friends and family?

___ Every day to several times a week
___ About once a week
___ About once every other week
___ About once a month
___ Less than once a month
___ Never
___ I don't have any friends or family

35. How often do you interact with other age groups?

___ Every day to several times a week
___ About once a week
___ About once every other week
___ About once a month
___ Less than once a month
___ Never

36. Are feelings of isolation or loneliness a problem for you?

all the time most of the time sometimes rarely never

37. Please rate your agreement with the following statements.

	Strongly agree	Agree	Not sure	Disagree	Strongly disagree
I feel that I have a purpose within your community					
Opinions of older adults are valued by decision makers in Akron					
There are negative stereotypes about older adults					
Older people are valued and respected in the community					
I feel disconnected from my community					

38. If you agreed to any of these, why do you feel this way?

____

____

Civic Participation and Employment

39. What is your current employment status?

___ Employed full-time
___ Employed part-time
___ Self-employed
___ Retired and working
___ Retired, not looking for work
___ Retired and seeking work
___ Unemployed, seeking work
___ Underemployed, seeking more work
___ Enrolled in work training program
Other: _________

40. Do you provide unpaid child care?

Yes No

41. Do you provide unpaid eldercare?

Yes No

42. If you are retired, did you choose to retire?

Yes No

43. If you are still working full-time, why? *(Check all that apply)*

___ Enjoy working
___ Cannot afford to retire
___ Maintain healthcare coverage
___ Not yet of retirement age
Other: ____________

44. Have you experienced ageism (discrimination based on a person's age) in the workplace?

definitely yes yes unsure no definitely no

45. Do you have access to the following in Akron?	**Yes**	**Yes, but we need more options**	**No**	**Not Sure**
A range of volunteer options				
Opportunities to be involved in councils and committees				
Opportunities to discuss issues impacting older adults in Akron				
Job opportunities				

Communication and Information

46. In general, are you able to find information on the services you need?

all the time most of the time sometimes rarely never

47. Do you consider yourself proactive in seeking this information?
all the time most of the time sometimes rarely never

48. Do you know where to call to get assistance in choosing service options in areas such as *housing*?
all the time most of the time sometimes rarely never

49. Do you know where to call to get assistance in choosing service options in areas such as *healthcare*?
all the time most of the time sometimes rarely never

50. Do you have any of the following in your home:	Yes	No	Unsure
Landline phone			
Computer with internet			
Smartphone			
Wi-Fi			

51. What do you use to find and access community services?
(Please number the 5 most used; rank 1 through 5)
___Landline telephone
___Mobile phone
___Smartphone
___Internet (websites, email)
___Social media (twitter, facebook, etc)
___Libraries
___TV ads
___Mail
___Radio ads
___Place of worship
___Senior center or other community agency
___Word-of-mouth (friends, family, etc)
___Flyers/bulletin board
___Community newspapers

52. Have you heard of the following information resources?	Yes	No	Use currently
Getting Wiser			
2-1-1			
Direction Home (Area Agency on Aging)			

Health and Wellness

53. How would you currently rate your overall health?
very good good fair poor very poor

54. In your community, do you have access to the following:	**Yes**	**Yes, but we need more options**	**No**	**Not sure**
A full-service grocery store (deli, bakery, produce)				
Farmer's market				
Food pantry / bank				
Convenience store				
A pharmacy				
Home health services				
Fitness programs designed for older adults				
Fully accessible health service facilities		Yes No		
Urgent care		Yes No		

55. Within the past 12 months, have you worried whether food would run out before you could afford to buy more?
Always most of the time sometimes rarely never

56. If you used the food banks and/or pantries in Akron, how often do you have issues getting to them?
Always most of the time sometimes rarely never

57. How often do you experience feelings of sadness or worry?
___ Every day to several times a week
___ About once a week
___ About once every other week
___ About once a month
___ Less than once a month
___ Never

58. Are you aware of mental health services available in Akron?
Yes No Unsure

59. Do you have healthcare providers that accept your insurance	**Yes**	**No**
A primary physician		
A dentist		
An eye doctor		
An audiologist		

60. In general, do you have friends or family you can rely on if you have medical problems?
Always most of the time sometimes rarely never

61. Do you feel that you have access to adequate medical services?
Always most of the time sometimes rarely never

Page **9** of **12**

62. How many medications are you currently prescribed?
0 1 – 7 8+

63. Are you generally able to afford…	**Always**	**Most of the time**	**Sometimes**	**Rarely**	**Never**	**Do not need**
Regular medications?						
Dentures?						
Glasses/contacts?						
Hearing aides?						

64. Are you able to make an appointment with a doctor when you need to?
Always most of the time sometimes rarely never

65. Are you able to make an appointment with a dentist when you need to?
Always most of the time sometimes rarely never

66. On average, how often do you engage in a form of physical exercise?
___ Every day to several times a week
___ About once a week
___ About once every other week
___ About once a month
___ Less than once a month
___ Never

67. How important is it to you to remain physically active for as long as possible?
___ Extremely important
___ Very important
___ Somewhat important
___ Not very important
___ Not important

68. Do you experience difficulties performing these tasks?	**Yes**	**No**	**Unsure**
Preparing meals			
Cleaning your house independently			
Doing errands alone			
Dressing			
Bathing			
Going up or down stairs			

69. Do you think you will need to make the following types of modifications/improvements to your home to enable you to better age in your home?	**Yes**	**No**	**Unsure**	**Already have**

Page **10** of **12**

Handrails on stairs				
Adequate lighting				
Slide resistant floors				
Grab bars and other modifications for bathing/showering				
Easily accessible laundry				
Furniture arrangement to help prevent falls				
No-step entry to the home				

The following questions are for classification purposes only

Age ____________________________
Gender ____________________________
Sexual Orientation ____________________________
Zip Code ____________________________
Native Language ____________________________

Race or ethnicity (please circle)

White/Caucasian
Hispanic or Latino
Black or African American
Native American or American Indian
Asian / Pacific Islander
Other: ______________________

Marital Status (please circle)

Married
Never married
Separated
Divorced
Widowed

Education level (please circle)

Less than a high school diploma
High school degree or equivalent
Some college, no degree
Associate degree
Bachelor's degree
Master's degree
Professional degree
Doctorate

Annual Income (please circle)

Less than $10,000
$10,000 to $24,999
$25,000 to $39,999
$40,000 to $64,999
$65,000 to $79,999
$80,000 to $100,000
$100,000 +
Rather not say

Please give any additional comments on how Akron could become more age-friendly.

____

____

____

____

Page **12** of **12**

Appendix B

Table A1. Variables for each domain of the Cronbach's alpha analysis.

Domain	Questions	Text	Scale	Valid *n*	Cronbach's Alpha	If Item Deleted, Alpha Would be >0.7
Housing	7a	Remain in home	extremely -> not important	568	0.672	
	7b	Remain in neighborhood	extremely -> not important			
	7c	Remain in Akron	extremely -> not important			
	8	Rate Akron for adults as they age	excellent -> very poor			
	10	Feel safe walking in neighborhood	very secure -> very concerned			x
Outdoor spaces	14	How important to have public parks?	Extremely -> not important	370	0.685	x
	17	If parks, are they well maintained in the winter?	All the time -> never			
	18a	Do buildings in your neighborhood include accessible front doors?	Always -> Never			
	18b	automatic door openers	Always -> Never			
	18c	large enough restrooms	Always -> Never			
Transportation	20	Rate public transport in Akron?	Excellent -> very poor	175	0.804	
	23	Rate sidewalk maintenance	Excellent -> very poor			
	27a	If use public transport do the waiting areas have safe lighting?	All -> None			
	27b	seating?	All -> None			
	27c	shelter from weather?	All -> None			
Arts Entertainment and Leisure	30	How often engage in social/community events?	every day -> Never	627	0.838	
	31	How often WANT to engage in social/community events?	Every day -> Never			
Respect and Social Inclusion	36	Feelings of loneliness of isolation a problem?	All the time -> never	569	0.692	
	37a	Feel I have purpose	Strongly agree to disagree			
	37b	opinions of older adults are valued	Strongly agree to disagree			
	37c	negative stereotypes about older adults (recoded)	Strongly agree to disagree			x
	37d	older people are valued and respected in the community	Strongly agree to disagree			
	37e	feel disconnected from my community (recoded)	Strongly agree to disagree			
Civic participation and employment	45a	Do you have access to volunteer options	yes, yes but need more, no, not sure	562	0.756	
	45b	opportunity to be involved in councils or committees	yes, yes but need more, no, not sure			
	45c	discuss issues impacting older adults	yes, yes but need more, no, not sure			
	45d	employment opportunities	yes, yes but need more, no, not sure			
Communication	46	able to find info on services you need?	all the time -> never	577	0.723	
	47	consider yourself proactive?	all the time -> never			
	48	know where to call for housing help?	all the time -> never			
	49	know where to call for healthcare?	all the time -> never			
Health	53	Rate overall health?	very good to very poor	291	0.69	
	55	worried about food in past 12 mos.? (recode)	Always -> Never			
	56	If use foodbanks, see issues? (recode)	always -> Never			
	60	Have friends or family to rely on?	always -> Never			
	61	Access to adequate medical services?	always -> Never			
	64	can make an appt with doc when needed?	always -> Never			
	65	can make appt with dentist when needed?	always -> Never			
	67	how important to remain physically active?	extremely -> not important			x

Appendix C

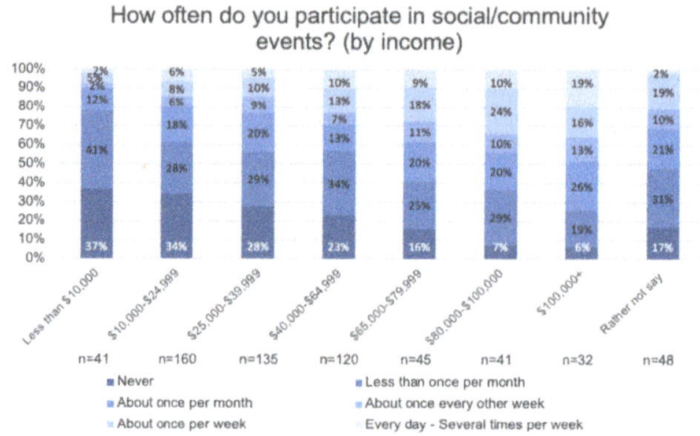

Figure A1. Income is positively related to the amount of activities in which older adults participate.

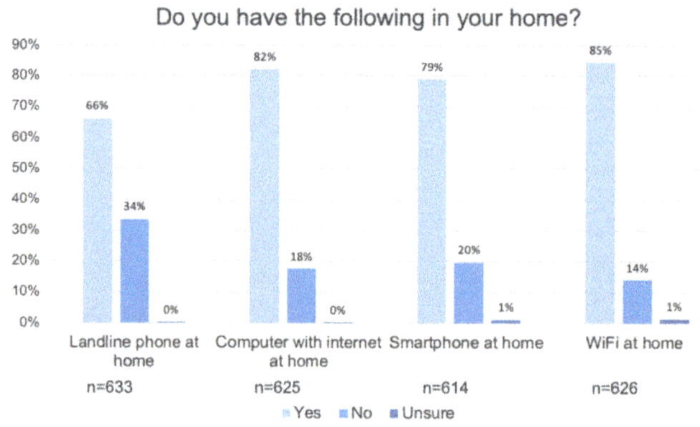

Figure A2. Respondents indicated that 66.9% have a land line telephone, 82.2% have a computer with Internet connection at home, 79.2% have a smartphone, and 84.5% have WiFi service at home.

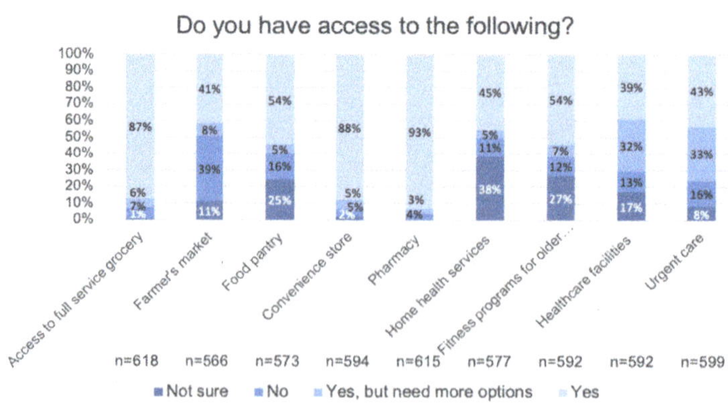

Figure A3. The majority of respondents indicated access to a full-service grocery, convenience store, or pharmacy. This figure represents' ability to access food, fitness, and healthcare centers in the Akron area.

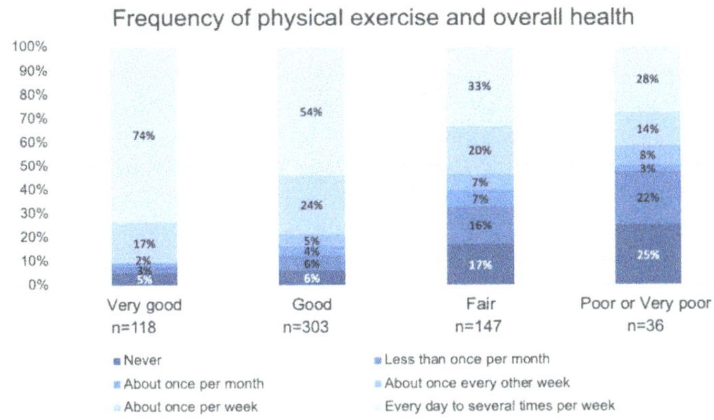

Figure A4. A relation is shown between overall health and frequency of physical exercise. Those respondents who are in very good health exercise the most. A gradual decline is observed in frequency of exercise among those who are in good, fair, poor, and very poor health.

Table A2. Survey population demographic information.

Demographic Characteristic	% (*n*)
Female	62.7% (384)
Male	37.3% (228)
Language:	
English	87.7% (575)
Other	1.8% (12)
Did not respond	10.5% (69)
Race/Ethnicity	
White/Caucasian	72.4% (446)
Hispanic or Latino	0.6% (4)
Black or African American	23.5% (145)
Native American/American Indian	0.8% (5)
Asian/Pacific Islander	0.8% (5)
Other	1.8% (11)
Marital Status	
Married	40.1% (248)
Never Married	14.2% (88)
Separated	0.6% (4)
Divorced	23.3% (144)
Widowed	21.8% (135)
Education level	
Less than high school diploma	4.1% (26)
High school degree or equivalent	23.2% (148)
Some college, no degree	27.8% (177)
Associate degree	9.1% (58)
Bachelor's degree	17.9% (114)
Master's degree	11.1% (71)
Professional degree	3.9% (25)
Doctorate	2.8% (18)
Annual income	
Less than $10,000	6.6% (41)
$10,000 to $24,999	25.7% (160)
$25,000 to $39,999	21.7% (135)
$40,000 to $64,999	19.3% (120)
$65,000 to $79,999	7.2% (45)
$80,000 to $100,000	6.6% (41)
$100,000+	5.1% (32)
Rather not say	7.7% (48)

References

1. World Health Organization. *Global Age-friendly Cities: A Guide*; World Health Organization: Geneva, Switzerland, 2007; ISBN 9789241547307.
2. Greenfield, E.A.; Oberlink, M.; Scharlach, A.E.; Neal, M.B.; Stafford, P.B. Age-friendly community initiatives: Conceptual issues and key questions. *Gerontologist* **2015**, *55*, 191–198. [CrossRef] [PubMed]
3. Plouffe, L.; Kalache, A. Towards global Age-friendly cities: Determining urban features that promote active aging. *J. Urban Health* **2010**, *87*, 33–739. [CrossRef] [PubMed]
4. Center for Community Solutions. *City of Cleveland, Age Friendly Community Assessment*; AARP: Washington, DC, USA, 2016.
5. AgeFriendlyColumbus.org. *Findings Report Age-Friendly Columbus*; AARP: Washington, DC, USA, 2017.
6. AARP. *AARP Roadmap to Livability Collection: Strategies and Solutions that Make a Community Great for People of All Ages*; AARP: Washington, DC, USA, 2018.
7. Marston, H.R.; van Hoof, J. "Who doesn't think about technology when designing urban environments for older people?" A case study approach to a proposed extension of the WHO's Age-friendly cities model. *Int. J. Environ. Res. Public Health* **2019**, *16*, 3525. [CrossRef] [PubMed]
8. AARP. *Age-Friendly Community Survey Template*; AARP: Washington, DC, USA, 2018.
9. City of Cincinnati Aging Office of Aging and Accessibility. *Membership Application to Join the AARP Age-Friendly Communities Program*; AARP: Washington, DC, USA, 2018. Available online: https://www.aarp.org/content/dam/aarp/livable-communities/age-friendly-network/application-letters-resolutions/2018/OH-Cincinnati-Application-2018-Final.pdf (accessed on 29 October 2020).
10. Bureau of Labor Statistics Data. Available online: https://data.bls.gov/timeseries/LAUMT391042000000003?amp%3Bdata_tool=XGtable (accessed on 29 October 2020).
11. Willink, A.; Shoen, C.; Davis, K. How Medicare Could Provide Dental, Vision, and Hearing Care for Beneficiaries. *Commonw. Fund* **2018**, *2018*, 1–12.
12. Neiman, A.B.; Ruppar, T.; Ho, M.; Garber, L.; Weidle, P.J.; Hong, Y.; George, M.G.; Thorpe, P.G. CDC Grand Rounds: Improving Medication Adherence for Chronic Disease Management—Innovations and Opportunities. *MMWR. Morb. Mortal. Wkly. Rep.* **2017**, *66*, 1248–1251. [CrossRef] [PubMed]
13. Morison, R.; Dychtwald, K. *What Retirees Want: A Holistic View of Life's Third Age*; Wiley: Hoboken, NJ, USA, 2020.
14. Sterns, H.L.; Sterns, A.A. Aging and Approaches to Work. In *Handbook of Psychology and Work*; Blustein, D.L., Ed.; Oxford University Press: New York, NY, USA, 2013; pp. 160–184.
15. Binette, J.; Kerri, V. *Home and Community Preferences: A National Survey of Adults Age 18-Plus*; AARP Research: Washington, DC, USA, 2018. [CrossRef]
16. Papalia, D.E.; Sterns, H.L.; Feldman, R.D.; Camp, C.J. *Desarrollo Del Adulto Y Vejez. Spanish Edition*; McGraw Hill: Mexico City, Mexico, 2009.
17. Sterns, H.; McQwoun, C. Age, Work and Retirement. In *Psychology of Aging: A Biopsychosocial Perspective*; Yochim, B.P., Woodhead, E.L., Eds.; Springer Publishing Company: New York, NY, USA, 2017.
18. Senior Citizens Information Booklet. Available online: https://www.akronohio.gov/cms/resource_library/files/a988fcf3c18b645a/senior_handbook.pdf (accessed on 29 October 2020).
19. Getting Wiser Summit County Resource Guide. Available online: https://www.gettingwiser.org/news/getting-wiser-summit-county-resource-guide (accessed on 29 October 2020).

Publisher's Note: MDPI stays neutral with regard to jurisdictional claims in published maps and institutional affiliations.

International Journal of
Environmental Research and Public Health

MDPI

Article

How Can the Lived Environment Support Healthy Ageing? A Spatial Indicators Framework for the Assessment of Age-Friendly Communities

Melanie Davern [1,2,*], Rachel Winterton [3], Kathleen Brasher [4] and Geoff Woolcock [5]

1. Healthy Liveable Cities Group, Centre for Urban Research, RMIT University, Melbourne, VIC 3000, Australia
2. Centre for Health Equity, Melbourne School of Population and Global Health, University of Melbourne, Parkville, VIC 3010, Australia
3. John Richards Centre for Rural Ageing Research, La Trobe Rural Health School, La Trobe University, Bendigo, VIC 3550, Australia; R.Winterton@latrobe.edu.au
4. Age-Friendly Northeast Victoria, Central Hume Primary Care Partnership, Benalla, VIC 3672, Australia; Kathleen.Brasher@centralhumepcp.org
5. Institute for Resilient Regions, University of Southern Queensland, Toowoomba, QLD 4350, Australia; Geoffrey.Woolcock@usq.edu.au

* Correspondence: melanie.davern@rmit.edu.au

Received: 1 September 2020; Accepted: 14 October 2020; Published: 21 October 2020

Abstract: The Age-Friendly Cities and Communities Guide was released by the World Health Organization over a decade ago with the aim of creating environments that support healthy ageing. The comprehensive framework includes the domains of outdoor spaces and buildings, transportation, housing, social participation, respect and inclusion, civic participation and employment, communication and information, and community and health services. A major critique of the age-friendly community movement has argued for a more clearly defined scope of actions, the need to measure or quantify results and increase the connections to policy and funding levers. This paper provides a quantifiable spatial indicators framework to assess local lived environments according to each Age-Friendly Cities and Communities (AFC) domain. The selection of these AFC spatial indicators can be applied within local neighbourhoods, census tracts, suburbs, municipalities, or cities with minimal resource requirements other than applied spatial analysis, which addresses past critiques of the Age-Friendly Community movement. The framework has great potential for applications within local, national, and international policy and planning contexts in the future.

Keywords: age-friendly; health; indicators; planning; tools; spatial; neighbourhoods

1. Introduction

Research has long recognized that environmental factors play a significant role in determining health and wellbeing in older age [1], and there are rising proportions of older people in the populations across the world. Consequently, the recently released United Nations Decade of Healthy Ageing 2020–2030 calls for sustained global action to generate transformative change in four priority areas: addressing ageism; creating age-friendly communities; delivering integrated and person centered care; and providing long-term care [2,3].

Increased urbanization and policy discourses supporting ageing in place add to the urgency to create and plan for age-friendly environments. On a global scale, life expectancy has increased from 47 years in the mid-20th century to an expected 78 years by the mid-21st century [4] and 21% of the world's population is predicted to be aged over 60 years by 2050 [5]. The World Health Organization (WHO) World Report on Ageing and Health [6] documented how age-friendly environments play a significant role in preventing or delaying many of the health changes related to biological ageing and chronic disease. Age-friendly environments can support people to continue to live as independently as possible in their local communities and allow ageing to take place in the social contexts of social and built environments [2].

The social and environmental determinants of healthy ageing are reflected in the eight domains of the WHO Global Age-Friendly Cities and Communities guide [7]. While some local adaption of these domains occur, they are designed as fit for purpose [8] for place-based actions in content areas that are important to later life [9]. Since its inception in 2007, the Age-Friendly Cities and Communities (AFC) movement has evolved into a global movement, with urban and rural communities undertaking action to improve the quality of life for older people in each of these eight domains. Very importantly, AFC supports long term action for ageing in place, which is needed to plan and build cities and towns of the future.

Previous critiques of the AFC movement argued for a narrower scope of actions that are better quantified and connected to policy levers [10]. These suggestions are well justified. Although the movement has brought much attention to planning for ageing, and has been informed by the voice of older people themselves, there has been little: (i) uptake on the community scale [11]; (ii) recognition of AFC in peer-reviewed publications [12]; or (iii) direct application in urban planning [13]. Consequently, this prevents AFC actions being adopted or aligned within existing planning processes, particularly at the municipal level where much AFC policy and planning needs to occur.

In more recent years, the ability to measure age-friendliness across diverse international contexts has also become an important consideration within the age-friendly movement [8,14]. In 2015, the WHO Kobe Centre developed [15] a set of core indicators for age-friendliness to support cities that are part of the WHO Global Network of Age-Friendly Cities and Communities [1]. The WHO report proposed measures relating to wellbeing, equity, and accessible physical and inclusive social environments. In the same year, the Public Health Agency of Canada [16] released an evaluation guide comprising thirty-nine indicators directly relevant to the eight AFC domains. The indicators were selected to provide community-level measures for both quantitative and qualitative outcomes with four indicators to measure longer-term health and social outcomes [17].

In 2018, the WHO Regional Office for Europe synthesized the existing international approach into seven sets of tools to measure and communicate the assessment and monitoring of age-friendly initiatives in Europe [8]. However, there is concern that many of the suggested indicators and measures for the assessment and monitoring of AFC are subjective in nature [14,17] or survey based [12]. These existing approaches are expensive to administer at the community level and beyond the budgets of many local governments who ultimately have the responsibility for local area planning. They are also often tailored to local environments, limiting the ability of state or national governments to have comparative assessments of age-friendly initiatives. New resources are needed to support practitioners and planners seeking to assess, monitor, and promote age-friendliness in the local environments where people live to support healthy ageing in place.

Age-Friendly Communities and the Lived Environment

Age-friendly communities comprise three distinct and interrelated constructs: local liveability; meeting the needs of older people; and ageing as a lifespan developmental process [18]. A set of validated liveability indicators that promote health and wellbeing have been developed for general populations [19]. These provide specific aspects of urban liveability associated with positive health outcomes, including transport [20], walkability [21], public open space [22], housing [23], employment [24], social infrastructure [25], and food environments [26].

This paper builds on these liveability indicators to propose objective spatial indicators to assess the age-friendliness of lived environments. The term "lived environment" is adopted throughout this paper in preference to a built environment to reflect this broader assessment of the key features needed to support healthy ageing. This extends beyond the common conception of the built environment, which often includes transportation systems, land development patterns, and microscale urban design (e.g., footpaths) [27,28]. A lived environment reflects the importance of locality and access to good urban design, as well as human-made and natural environments to support health and wellbeing in the local neighbourhoods where people live. This is consistent with the argument regarding the narrow application of the term "built environment" where both human made and natural worlds are conceived as though there is no separation between them [29].

Spatial indicators provide a quantitative measurement of local lived environments using geocoded data (defined by x and y co-ordinates) developed using Geographic Information Systems (GIS). Data linked to a street address can be mapped using GIS and calculated as spatial indicators, providing aggregated measures across a range of geographic areas, including neighbourhoods or census tracts, suburbs, municipalities, regions, or states. Aggregated geocoded data can be drawn from a range of existing administrative data sources that assess the lived environment and a range of social, economic, and environmental issues. Spatial AFC indicators consequently provide objective and cost-effective assessments of age-friendliness that are easily replicated across large geographic areas using desktop spatial analysis. These indicators can also be made readily accessible to local governments using online digital planning portals and liveability indicator systems for cities, like the Australian Urban Observatory (auo.org.au) [30].

The development of quantifiable spatial indicators of AFC addresses the major critiques of the AFC initiative—that it is too descriptive in approach [31], not measured or monitored by indicators [31], and without a clear understanding of an indicator framework [32]. This paper proposes spatial indicator tools that can be applied for the assessment of AFC in local lived environments using a GIS methodology.

These AFC spatial indicators can also be applied in a variety of international contexts with direct relevance to the Healthy Cities movement [33], the New Urban Agenda, and the 2030 Agenda for Sustainable Development [34]. The 2030 Agenda provides a global framework for sustainable urban development up until 2030 signed by all 193 members states with 169 specific targets. These include Sustainable Development Goals (SDGs) with specific mention of older people in targets for Goal 10 Reduced Inequalities, Goal 11 Sustainable Cities and Communities, and Goal 17 Partnerships for the Goals. In addition, the Decade of Healthy Ageing [3] calls for disaggregated data in twenty-eight indicators across eleven Goals.

Spatial indicators measuring AFC in lived environments are noted by the United Nations as being necessary for the measurement and monitoring of any actions contributing to sustainable development (Goal 17) and multi-stakeholder partnership development and policy and institutional coherence. They have been developed to address segregation or siloed approaches in the current planning approaches and to encourage discussion and action that can promote integrated policy, planning, and practice across urban planning and public health. Often the outcome of AFC remains the sole responsibility of health or social planning with little integration across important portfolios, such as transport or statutory or strategic planning. The implementation of AFC principles must extend beyond practitioners with interest in ageing and should ideally be integrated across policy portfolios with budget and legislative support.

This paper aims to introduce a new set of AFC spatial indicators that can be used to quantify and assess the age-friendliness of local lived environments and monitor changes in age-friendliness over time consistent with the SDGs and 2030 Agenda. These indicators seek to support the Decade of Healthy Ageing, which includes a commitment to action in the development of age-friendly environments and improved measurement, monitoring, and research [8] as well as tools to support planners and practitioners working within government settings. These spatial indicators of AFC also identify the importance of older people and their lived environments in sustainable urban development and the 2030 Agenda.

2. Materials and Methods

Eight interconnected domains are included in AFC (Figure 1). The selection of specific spatial indicators to assess the lived environment of each AFC domain was made following a workshop held with all five authors to identify the most relevant measures for each of these domains. The multidisciplinary experience of the research team spans gerontology, public health, urban planning, psychology, epidemiology, sociology, health geography, health policy, governance, and community development.

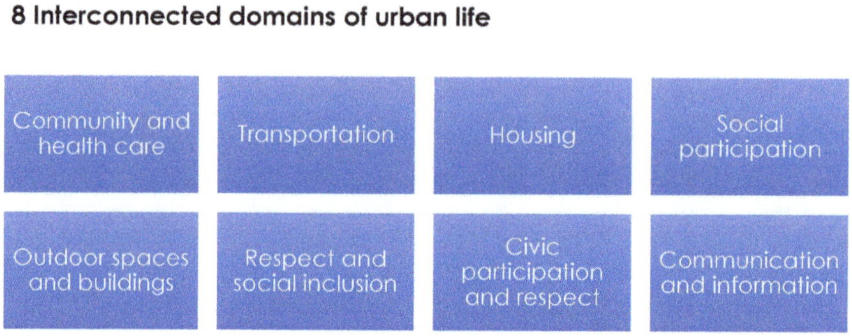

Figure 1. The eight interconnected domains of the Age-Friendly Communities framework [35].

Potential indicators were then judged against the key criteria recommended by the WHO (Box 1) as well as other best practice principles for indicator application [36] including: direct links to policy; connection to theory and existing research; available time series data; connection to budgeting and planning; relevance to most people; and connection to lived reality.

These latter criteria being understood and relevant to most people, particularly older people, are particularly important and informed by previous research in the development of a specific indicator of access to services for older people [37], which included focus groups of older people to determine the local needs and services of highest importance. The selected measures also needed to be relevant to the majority of older people living in a wide range of lived environments, and to measure the most critical requirements for places that support AFC principles.

Box 1. The criteria suggested for defining local AFC indicators [15].

Measurable: Will variations in the indicator be observable over time due to specific actions?
Disaggregation possible: Can the indicator be disaggregated by gender, age group, or across neighbourhoods? There are also other strategies that could be important in the local context, including ethnicity, socioeconomic status, etc.
Aligns with local goals and targets: Does the indicator link to a broader local agenda?
Can be linked to action: Does the indicator provide an understanding of the various actions that might need to be undertaken?
Within local influence: Does the local government or community have the mandate or authority to act on this indicator? For example, a federal insurance scheme is mostly beyond the influence of the municipal government.
Easy to collect: Are the data required to produce the indicator easy to collect in a timely manner?
Socially acceptable: Is the collection of this information acceptable to the communities and individuals concerned?

3. Results

The following section describes each of the selected AFC spatial indicators with research evidence provided to support each indicator (Table 1).

Table 1. Age-Friendly Communities (AFC) domains and suggested spatial indicators.

AFC Domains	Suggested Spatial Indicators for AFC Assessment and Monitoring
1. Outdoor spaces and buildings	• Walkability for transport (with and without footpaths) * • Access to public open space within 400 m * • Intersections serviced with pedestrian crossings • Access to public seating • Access to public toilets (with and without accessibility features) • *Accessible buildings*
2. Transport	• Access to a public transport stop within 400 m * • Access to a public transport stop within 400 m with a regular service every 30 min (7 a.m.–7 p.m.) * • Access to public transport with Disability Standards for Accessible Public Transport • Bus stops with seats/shelters • Disabled car parking access • Community transport measure (if possible)
3. Housing	• Proportion of households in the bottom 40% of incomes spending more than 30% of income on housing costs * • Housing diversity according to eight different housing types • Proportion of government owned dwellings • Access to services for older people [37] *
4. Social Participation	• Access to neighbourhood houses/community centres * • Recreational services catered to older people e.g., a YMCA * • Access to libraries • Access to Universities of the 3rd Age (U3As) • Access to places of worship
5. Respect and social inclusion	• Access to social clubs/senior citizens clubs * • Access to local cafés measured by distance * • Membership of Clubs like Probus and Rotary
6. Civic participation and employment	• Proportion of population aged 60+ years regularly volunteering * • Proportion of population working beyond official retirement age (currently 66 years in Australia) *
7. Communications and information	• Proportion of households with access to the internet * • Proportion of households with mobile phone reception • Access to ABC or national broadcaster radio
8. Community support and health services	• Access to General Practitioners * • Access to Geriatricians • Access to residential aged care accommodation • Access to Commonwealth Support Home Packages (funding supporting ageing in the home if available) *
Additional contextual factors for consideration include: the Estimated Resident Population; proportion of population aged more than 60 years; population age distribution including proportions of older and younger populations in area; ethnicity; education; homeownership; residential density; remoteness e.g., Accessibility/Remoteness Indices or the distance between towns in rural settings; the risk of natural disasters; climatic conditions; and the impact of climate change.	

* Recommended as priority indicators for inclusion.

Selection of Measures

The suggested spatial indicators for each AFC domain are presented in Table 1 with the priority indicators notated with asterisks. This provides flexibility for practitioners in identifying the key spatial indicators of importance to AFC or additional optional indicators where resources are available. Additional information is provided below explaining why these indicators are recommended for each AFC domain with detailed explanations of the supporting research evidence.

The indicators recommended in the following section were identified in accordance with indicators acting as icebergs and highlighting issues of major importance [37]. Only after the major factors have been quantitively assessed should further qualitative assessment be completed, similar to a hierarchy of need. For example, if there are no public open spaces available there is little point in assessing the maintenance, shelter, or facilities available in public open spaces within an area. Additional qualitative assessment could also include local consultation with older residents and relevant stakeholders.

4. Outdoor Spaces and Buildings

The priority indicators identified for this domain are walkability for transport [38,39] and access to public open space within 400 m [22]. These indicators are directly related to walking [40–42], specifically in older people [43], and associated with physical health benefits [44] and mental health benefits [45].

Walkable neighbourhoods are important for older people because, along with the fact that they enable people to reach destinations with commercial and social opportunities [43,46], walking is also associated with maintaining functional independence [47] and better cognitive function [48]. Similarly, public open spaces that are easy to visit with walkable access are important for older people and important in reducing social isolation and increasing physical activity [49].

Data required to create indicators of walkability are commonly available within municipal and planning contexts. Road network analysis (a way to walk), land use mix (destinations to walk to), and housing density (people to service the destinations) are common key components of walkability assessments. Similarly, public open space location data are also regularly held by most municipal governments. Footpaths are an important infrastructure supporting walking in older people [50,51], and walkability can also be refined by superimposing footpath access where spatial data are available. An example of a walkability for transport assessment for the regional city of Launceston in Tasmania, Australia was calculated and is provided in Figure 2 to demonstrate the value of neighbourhood level walkability assessments. The results clearly suggest that the inner neighbourhoods of the city of Launceston have good walkability while the outer neighbourhoods are less supportive of walking for transport, particularly those on the eastern side of town.

Additional spatial indicators for consideration include intersections with visual and auditory signalled pedestrian crossings that allow time for older people to cross over roads, and particularly busy intersections [53,54]. In Australia, many regional towns avoid the use of signalized pedestrian crossings and opt for roundabout intersections, which encourage continual traffic flow and can be frightening for people with reduced mobility.

Access to public seating is also recommended to be available within local public open spaces to encourage rest stops while walking (overlapping with the suggested measure of accessibility to public open space). Clean and safe public toilets are also recommended, including those with accessibility features [51] and should also be included within high quality public open spaces. Accessible buildings are italicised in Table 1 due to the difficulty in sourcing data that measure buildings developed according to universal design principles. If possible, these are recommended, as older people experience difficulties associated with access to public buildings and the lack of handrails, narrow corridors, and steps [51]. Post Occupancy Evaluations are generally more common in sustainability assessments [55] and are time and staff resource intensive but could be considered as an alternative measure if no other data are available to assess buildings.

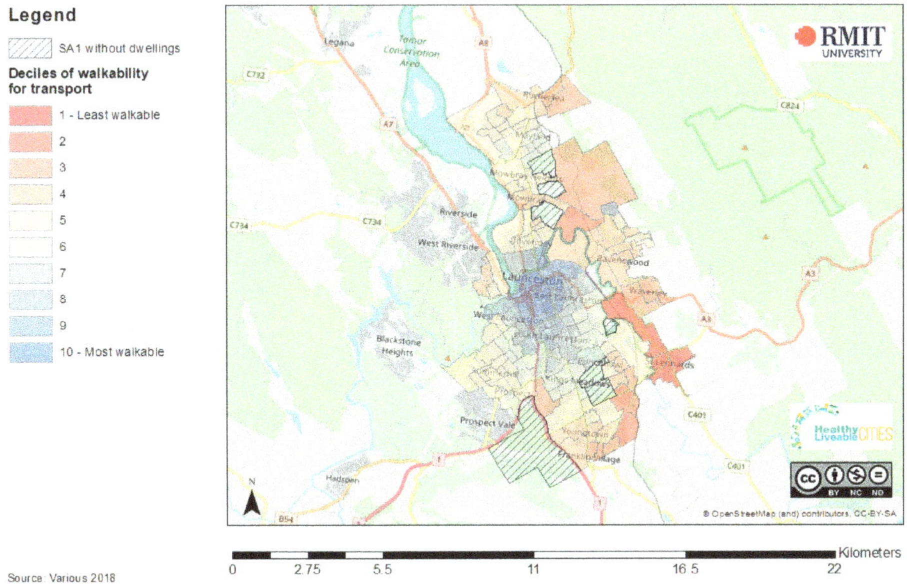

Figure 2. An example of a walkability assessment for the city of Launceston, Tasmania, Australia [52].

There is a growing body of evidence showing a positive association between healthy ageing and blue space [56]. This is worthy of future consideration but is not accessible within all lived environments and, hence, has not been included as a recommended measure within the outdoor space and building domain but could be considered as second tier measures. Blue space is defined as outdoor environments (natural or manmade) that prominently feature water and are accessible proximally (being located in, on, or near water) or distally/virtually (being able to see, hear, or sense water) [57]. Therapeutic design of a built environment using urban green and blue infrastructure was shown to be protective for healthy ageing while supporting those with cognitive decline, or illness [58].

Similarly, a study of largely older people in Hong Kong found that general health was significantly higher in people with a sea view from their home [59], while, in Ireland, older people had a lower risk of depression in those with more sea views [60]. In addition, nature-based solutions, through green and blue space urban management planning, can mitigate the health impacts of climate change while addressing the need for climate resilience in local communities [61]. Future revisions of the AFC principles could consider the inclusion of more detailed measures of green and blue spaces in the domain of outdoor spaces and buildings to address changing climates around the globe. These could include access to local blue spaces, public and private tree canopy coverage, public street tree canopy coverage and the associated shade capability, in combination with the currently recommended measures of walkability and accessibility to public open space. These measures are very worthy of consideration but bring their own challenges in terms of data access and spatial capability making them harder to produce. Consequently, they are suggested as potential expanded, not essential, measures of the AFC lived environment assessment.

5. Transport

Transport is an important determinant of health [62,63] influencing access to local services, engagement in paid and non-paid productive activities (such as employment or volunteering), maintaining and developing social networks and supports, and engaging in social and recreational activities. Public transport has also been identified as a critical influence of liveability in a community [19] and active transport important to older people [64]. Policy-relevant spatial public transport indicators are typically based on 400 m access or a 5-min walk [20,65]. Another important factor that influences the use of public transport is service frequency. Consequently, access to any public transport stop provides a high-level assessment while access to frequent public transport provides a more refined assessment. Similar measures are also included in the Australian Government's National Cities Performance Framework (https://www.bitre.gov.au/national-cities-performance-framework).

For older people, mobility is essential for social participation and wellbeing [66]. Public transport is particularly important for older people who might have a reduced ability to drive. Older people tend to use public transport more frequently if there is easy access to public transport in neighbourhoods at a distance less than 5 min away [67]. This is also consistent with existing research that found that the frequency of public transport and wait time affected older people's willingness to travel [68] and that a high proportion of older people are no longer driving [69].

Data for these indicators can most often be sourced from public access data portals, Open Street Map or General Transit Feed Specification (GTFS) where public transport data are provided by transport agencies into a computer readable format for web developers [70]. Gaining access to more detailed data describing public transport that meets Disability Standards is another very valid indicator and has been associated with increased satisfaction and perceived useability in older people [71]. Similarly, access to a bus stop with an accompanying shelter and seat is also important for older people's mobility, as well as dropped curves, footpaths, and pedestrian signals [54].

6. Housing

Housing is central to living a productive, meaningful, and healthy life, and housing quality is an important influence on self-reported health [72]. Unaffordable housing is detrimental to mental health in low to moderate income households [73]. Unaffordable housing has also been associated with an increased risk of poor self-rated health, hypertension, and arthritis, and renting, rather than owing a home, increases associations between unaffordable housing and self-rated health [74]. Consequently, housing costs and gentrification [75] are particularly important to consider, with housing stress in lower income households being a particularly important indicator for the assessment of age-friendly cities.

Housing needs, sizes, and types can change as people age. Older people might consider downsizing to smaller homes with reduced maintenance needs or to be closer to extended family for support to age in place [76]. In rural and regional areas, older people might need to move from larger farms and back into towns where services are more readily available. Alternatively, frail older residents might require the support of aged care providers to support high care needs. Addressing these issues means that communities need to understand the available housing diversity options (e.g., larger houses, smaller houses, units, and apartments to serve broad community needs) as well as access to services for residents.

AFC supports multiple housing options that are beneficial to all residents with many municipalities thinking primarily about formal aged-care accommodation when addressing housing needs for older people. Even more concerning in Australia, it is common for aged care facilities to be built on the outskirts of cities and towns where there is an abundance of inexpensive and undeveloped land. This isolates older people from the rest of the community, makes it harder for people to access and visit, decreases access to other community services, and decreases intergenerational contact within communities.

The 30/40 housing affordability indicator is recommended and describes the proportion of households in the bottom 40% of household incomes spending more than 30% of their income on housing costs [77]. This measure is also referred to as the Ontario measure where the interest in housing affordability first identified the disproportionate impact of housing costs on lower income households [78,79]. Understanding community demographic profiles, particularly age, in combination with the high incidence of 30/40 housing affordability issues should raise concerns for any community wanting to support age-friendliness. Specifically, older adults on an aged pension within the private rental market will face significant challenges in housing affordability [80].

The indicator of access to services for older people was developed with older people themselves [37] and includes hospitals, General Practitioners, Aged Care Facilities, public transport stops, supermarkets, community centres, libraries, and Universities of the 3rd Age, and could also include places of worship and parks. This indicator also provides a useful assessment for the AFC domain of Community Support and Health Services but is included in the housing domain to reinforce the importance of urban planning that supports the co-locations of services and housing options. The proportion of government owned dwellings could also be investigated as an additional support measure of AFC, particularly in lower income areas.

7. Social Participation

Meaningful social relationships and participation are essential for good health, with health defined as a social phenomenon in the social determinants of health [81]. Social participation has been associated with physical activity [82], mental health [83], reduced psychological distress [84], reduced risk of myocardial infarction [85], and up to a 50% increased likelihood of survival in people with strong social relationships compared to lifestyle risk factors [86].

For older people, social participation provides greater life satisfaction [87], is protective against cognitive decline [88], and contributes to resilience in older people [89], especially in rural communities [90]. Social participation is also being taken seriously internationally, and the United Kingdom appointed a new Minister for Loneliness and a national government action plan on loneliness [91].

The recommended spatial indicators supporting social participation connect to the access to services for older people [92] that are included in the housing domain. Two indicators are recommended: access to community centres and neighbourhood houses; and access to recreational services that cater to the needs of older people. Shared or 'third spaces' such as these are critical social infrastructure [25] and essential in supporting social participation for older adults [93]. Recreational services also support physical and mental health through opportunities for physical activity designed for older people and supporting community connections.

Another indicator recommended for inclusion is access to a local library, which also supports the AFC domains of respect and social isolation, communications and information, and community support and health services. Libraries provide multiple community benefits beyond simply lending books [94,95], including multimedia borrowing, technology training, community classes, lectures, and opportunities for intergenerational and community connections. Libraries also support the need for learning opportunities across the course of life with Universities of the Third Age (U3As) providing social and learning benefits to older people [96,97]. This is associated with better physical health and activity levels [98]. Places of worship are also considered an important facilitator of social connections and social capital [99], particularly in humanitarian arrivals [100] and different cultures [101,102].

8. Respect and Social Inclusion

Respect and social inclusion are essential to ensure social participation for older people. There is much debate on the definition of social inclusion, though most studies refer to an objective participation in society and a more subjective assessment of whether the actual participation meets an individual's preferences [103]. Most definitions of social exclusion emphasise the importance of social activities as a core component [104]. However, the effects of cumulative disadvantage, decreasing social networks, and age discrimination magnify the negative health and wellbeing impacts of social exclusion in later life [105].

A local or lived environment must provide accessible buildings, housing and transport, along with opportunities for social activities to occur if social inclusion and social participation are supported and encouraged. Previous research on the services deemed important for older people has emphasised the importance of local services, such as shops [37,69], and this is supported by the use of new spatial indicators that can access formal and informal places to meet. These include recommended indicators of access to social clubs/senior citizens clubs or participation in international clubs, like Rotary or Probus, that are more formally organised by older people themselves. Alternatively, informal opportunities for social inclusion include an indicator of distance-based access to local cafes that support broader intergenerational social opportunities. Older people need a range of venues to create opportunities for social activities as a foundation for community respect and social inclusion.

9. Civic Participation and Employment

Empowerment, autonomy and control [63,106], and employment conditions [107] were all found to be important influences of actual and self-reported health. Control over one's own destiny has also been proposed [106], consistent with an understanding of health being simultaneously influenced at the individual (micro/personal), place and community context (meso/community) as well as the larger societal context (macro/societal level) [108].

Civic participation and employment are important influences of agency and autonomy in a society. Consequently, it is important to understand how many older people are engaged in paid and unpaid productive activity in the community. This is best measured through the proportion of people who remain employed past the official retirement age (66 years in Australia noting there is no official retirement age and eligibility for the aged pension is currently 66 years increasing to 67 years by 2023) or people aged 60 years or more who are engaged in regular volunteering. These indicators of paid and unpaid productive activity are also important measures of social engagement and civic participation and could be separated into additional age brackets or deciles (e.g., 60–75 years) for more detailed information. It is important to note that employment is also not defined according to hours worked, acknowledging both the civic connections and benefits that come from any level of paid employment and that retirement is not a single event and includes a diverse range of retirement patterns [109].

There has been criticism regarding the dominance of volunteering in measures of collective civic social participation in older people [110] with voting participation argued as a better measure of civic participation [111]. However, voting participation is less relevant in countries like Australia where electoral voting is compulsory and volunteering activities are measured every 4 years. Volunteering is also particularly important in regional areas of Australia where third sector or non-profit organisations rely on older people volunteering [112] with increasing proportions of older people residing in rural locations [113]. In countries where voting is not compulsory (e.g., the USA), then voting participation could be considered as an additional measure of civic engagement.

10. Communications and Information

In 2016, approximately 86% of Australian households had access to the internet [114]. This proportion decreased to 77% in remote areas where it is common to have a high proportion of older people within populations, with entertainment, social networking, and banking the most commonly supported activities supported by internet connection.

Internet access is also becoming more necessary to access information about the government, health, banking, and community services as well as to maintain contact with friends and family. Finding information on services like these is also critical for older people to age in place and is necessary to support independent living and the connection to communities [115]. Th information provision also extends beyond essential services and includes services provided by local libraries, which includes online books, audio, audio-visual, and educational resources that can be made available online for people with physical or geographical mobility restrictions. Online streaming (e.g., Netflix) is another more recent example of recreational activities supporting social connection and information provision. However, all these online resources require household internet access.

Access to a national radio service is another important source of information and becomes particularly important in emergency management, including preparation and recovery from natural disasters, such as floods, droughts, and bushfires, which are becoming increasingly more commonplace in Australia. Emergency SMS messaging systems are also deployed during emergency situations to inform residents of impending safety risks but are worthless without adequate mobile phone reception. Climate change is predicted to increase the likelihood of these emergency situations making telecommunications assessment essential in the support of AFC. It is also necessary for developing technologies, including passive surveillance of movement monitoring within the home, personal alarm devices, and telehealth [116], which have become increasingly accessible and necessary during the 2020 Coronaviruses 2019 (COVID-19) pandemic.

Communication is an important influence on the wellbeing of older people [117], and both household internet and mobile phone reception provide essential telecommunication systems that support both intergenerational communication with family and friends, the communication of essential information [118], and the ongoing adoption of new technologies [119], as well as influence the quality of life [120]. Currently, there is a paucity of references or inclusion of technological solutions offered to support AFC and healthy ageing and technology, and ICTs have recently been suggested as a new smart age-friendly ecosystem framework [118]. Suggestions included in this new framework to assist AFC include: the development of smart housing; the inclusion of ageing in smart cities and engagement with the Internet of Things (IoT); the better use of digital assistants (e.g., Alexa) in the home; the use of digital robots for deliveries; electronic camera enabled doorbells; and motion sensors to detect mobility. Technological features like these require inclusion during new housing development and have benefits across multiple AFC domains beyond communication. They also require a rethink and interdisciplinary collaboration between planners, architects, developers, computer science, industry, and the government. While the opportunities are waiting for action, they also require engagement with older people themselves and their families using qualitative and ethnographic research methods [121]. This is an important area of growth and future development in AFC and requires further research.

11. Community Support and Health Services

Access to primary health support services is essential and necessary for people to age in place. It is also the preferred option for most older people to maximise their health and wellbeing [122]. Within the local community, access to General Practitioners has been identified by older people themselves as essential community support services [36,69,123] and the key access point for primary health care. Consequently, access to General Practitioners was identified as an indicator of primary importance within community support and health services. These practitioners also provide gateway services and referrals to any other medical specialists, including geriatricians, who specialise in treating conditions that affect older people, including dementia.

Additional indicators that should be included relate to housing support either as in-home support packages or residential aged-care accommodation. All of these services are also included within a complete definition of social infrastructure, which has an important influence on subjective wellbeing [25] and are important components of liveability [19].

A Regional Case Study Example

The approaches and spatial measures described above were applied in a case study in a regional context and rural centre in north-eastern Victoria, Australia. The regional town is located over 200 km north-east of the capital city of Melbourne in the centre of the state of Victoria, south-eastern Australia. The major industries are agriculture and manufacturing, with a population of over 9000 people. Both the state government department of health and the local municipality/council were interested in analysing and understanding AFC and broader liveability given an increasingly ageing rural population.

The spatial measures used to assess this included: walkability (with and without footpaths); access to public open space; access to public transport; housing affordability; housing diversity; government owned dwellings (social housing); access to services for older people; libraries; universities of the 3rd Age; places of worship; volunteering; households with internet access; aged care facilities; and access to General Practitioners. The results were presented to the local health department officials, the local municipality, and as a community presentation to residents at the local library.

Many of the challenges and barriers to AFC planning were identified in the spatial measures and were confirmed by the lived experiences of residents from the local community. These included: poor walkability on the outer areas of town; difficulty getting to doctors and medical services located at the regional hospital located on the outer town boundary with limited public transport and poor walkability; disconnection between the older people, families, and younger people in the town due to the location of residential aged care on the town boundary next to the hospital; the importance of cafes and social spaces in the centre of town to support community and social connections; the value of the town's library, art facilities, and public open spaces; and inequity in the disadvantaged areas of the town that had reduced access to public transport and lower levels of household internet connections. The use of mapped spatial measures of AFC was hugely beneficial for inter-agency conversations and planning initiatives as well as community conversations, engagement, and validation of the spatial analyses. The results also highlight the future negative impact of the age-friendliness of the town if future residential aged care development is supported in the outer areas of the town.

12. Discussion

The original WHO Global Age-Friendly Cities Guide was developed in response to the rapid population ageing and urbanisation across the world and was informed by interviews conducted with older people themselves in over 33 different countries [7,15]. The ultimate aim of AFC is to create environments that support healthy ageing. This paper provided detailed, objective, and functional spatial measures of age-friendliness across lived environments that can be used to assess, monitor, evaluate, and communicate age-friendliness refined to the neighbourhood level. Objective spatial measures of the lived environment are critical for the following reasons: to simplify assessments of AFC; to provide a foundation level of knowledge about the age-friendliness of an environment; to assist local and state government planning by informing and monitoring future actions and interventions needed to promote healthy ageing in communities; and to include older people into targets of the 2030 Sustainable Development Goals and the New Urban Agenda.

The movement has previously been criticised for a lack of objective measurements and the need to connect these ideals into functional measures connected to policy, planning, and financial levers [10]. Previous attempts at developing indicators of age-friendliness have been non-specific, non-coordinated, and reliant on survey-based responses (e.g., World Health Organization [15]). Such assessments are also beyond the budget, resources, capabilities, and motivation of local planning agencies and municipalities. The proposed spatial measures of age-friendliness across lived environments is relevant to planners, policymakers, advocacy organisations, governments, architects, industry, citizens and research audiences. The suggested indicators are provided to guide and inform discussions and interventions to promote healthy ageing. The measures can also be adopted and customised to local environments ranging in geographic and population sizes, rurality, climate conditions, and resource limitations.

The proposed spatial indicators of AFC address these issues through the application of GIS technology to produce an objective assessment of the age-friendliness of local lived environments, drawing on indicators from the liveability literature that are specifically relevant to the values, preferences, and needs of older adults. These indicators provide measurement and quantification of AFC domains consistent with the idea that value comes with measurement and leads to knowledge production as argued by Lord Kelvin over 200 hundred years ago [124]. The more simplistic interpretation of this, is that what is measured, is valued, and consequently is done.

12.1. Linking Spatial AFC Indicators to Policy Contexts Outside of Ageing

One of the critical issues raised in the recommended AFC spatial indicators is the connection of all indicators within existing policy and planning contexts [13]. All the recommended indicators can be linked to existing policy and planning environments regardless of whether these have a local/municipal, state, or national focus. The connection of indicators to policy has been long identified within social indicator research [125,126].

These indicators can assist governments in meeting their commitments to the Sustainable Development Goals in a way that is meaningful for a growing segment of their populations. There is also an increasing interest and development in public health digital observatories. For example, relevant liveability indicators for the 21 largest cities of Australia are available in the Australian Urban Observatory (auo.org.au) launched in 2020. There is an opportunity to make spatial indicators available through novel data visualisation and ease of communication providing an influence on the policies required for healthy ageing across communities.

The spatial indicators recommended for assessing AFC domains can all be influenced and improved through policy levers. This includes the indicators suggested for outdoor spaces, transport, housing, social participation, respect and social inclusion, civic participation and employment, communications and information, community support, and health services. The indicator results can be influenced though local and immediate strategies or applied in advocacy with the responsible higher government agencies. This can include reviewing AFC assessments within the context of current policy contexts, existing public health planning, liveability planning, transport planning, strategic planning, land use, and statutory planning

It is also important to acknowledge the limitations of AFC spatial indicators and understanding that these aggregated area-based results effectively act as icebergs of knowledge [35] providing a tip of the iceberg assessment of what is occurring, with additional information required to understand why the result is happening and how it can be addressed. Consequently, the objective AFC spatial indicators should also be combined with additional sources of knowledge. These include consultation and engagement with local older people themselves to expand understanding, prioritise actions, and support the greatest social and economic benefits and returns on investments that support improved health and quality of life for older people.

12.2. Unique Contexts, Regional and Rural Localities

Given the diversity of cities, communities, and places, it is recognised that the achievement of all suggested indicators might not be feasible across all geographic settings. This is particularly relevant to rural and regional locales, which often have a lower population density and reduced levels of physical or social infrastructure. Consultations with older people and combining subjective understandings with more objective AFC spatial indicators will also help to inform the understanding of unique community contexts, including regional and remote areas.

For example, high levels of walkability might not be possible across an entire town in a rural area with a small population. Alternatively, signaled pedestrian crossings might not be necessary. However, a walkability assessment using the recommended walkability indicator could identify walking and transport barriers (e.g., a major road or bridge across a rail line) or identify the best location for new community services. Alternatively, the distances and measures of accessibility listed within indicators may vary across diverse rural and regional settings, but as noted above, these definitions of access within indicators must be determined through consultation with the older adults and communities to a reach consensus on what can be reasonably expected within this locale.

Consequently, in certain settings, these proposed indicators should act as a tool to prompt place-specific discussions around what is important in terms of measurement indicators, and what is achievable (particularly in relation to what should constitute reasonable access). A notable challenge of AFC planning is the absence of the relevant climate change implications in the current AFC principles and domains and inclusion of ICT and new technology. We recommend that future revision of AFC should expand and account for the challenges associated with climate change given the implications on the health and wellbeing of older people [127] and the ultimate AFC goal of healthy ageing. The relationship between older people's physical health and mental health with the environment, urban design, architecture, and AFC could also be considered in the development of future indicators [128].

13. Conclusions

Understanding and expanding AFC spatial indicators for unique contexts and environments is needed in the future and this current foundation of recommended indicators can be applied and tested across a range of different locations. This could include localities with climatic extremes (e.g., heat, cold, and snow), regional and rural locations, international comparisons, and cultural differences to explore how communities differ and what additional indicators should be included. The major aim of this research was to propose a foundational set of objective AFC spatial indicators that can be applied in any location with minimal resources and are directly aligned for policy intervention. This is particularly relevant to planning and policymakers working in government and was neither previously available nor consistently applied within AFC locations. Further research should investigate how this proposed suite of AFC spatial indicators can be added to, refined, or customized to address the needs of many different locations, including the relevant subjective indicators to enhance knowledge. The inclusion of new technology and ICT and addressing climate change are also increasing areas of interest in the future.

Author Contributions: Conceptualization of this paper began with M.D., K.B. and R.W.; Methodology and Analysis was developed by M.D., K.B., R.W. and G.W.; Writing—original draft preparation was led by M.D., R.W. and K.B.; Writing—review and editing was completed by M.D., R.W., K.B. and G.W.; Project Administration and Funding by M.D. All authors have read and agreed to the published version of the manuscript.

Funding: This research was supported by funding from the Clean Air and Urban Landscapes Hub funded by the National Environmental Science Program.

Conflicts of Interest: The authors declare no conflict of interest.

References

1. Rowles, G.D.; Bernard, M.A. *Environmental Gerontology: Making Meaningful Places in Old Age*; Springer Publishing Company: Berlin/Heidelberg, Germany, 2013.
2. Garon, S.; Paris, M. How Healthy Ageing Can Foster Age-Friendly Environment? In *Prevention of Chronic Diseases and Age-Related Disability, Practical Issues in Geriatrics*; Springer: Berlin/Heidelberg, Germany, 2019; pp. 161–167.
3. World Health Organisation. *Decade of Healthy Ageing 2020–2030*; World Health Organisation: Geneva, Switzerland, 2020.
4. Leeson, G.W. The growth, ageing and urbanisation of our world. *J. Popul. Ageing* **2018**, *11*, 107–115. [CrossRef]
5. United Nations. *World Population Prospects: The 2017 Revision, Key Findings and Advance Tables*; United Nations, Department of Economics and Social Affairs: New York, NY, USA, 2017.
6. World Health Organisation. *World Report on Ageing and Health*; World Health Organisation: Geneva, Switzerland, 2015.
7. World Health Organisation. *Global Age-Friendly Cities: A Guide*; World Health Organisation: Geneva, Switzerland, 2007.
8. World Health Organization. *The Global Network for Age-Friendly Cities and Communities: Looking Back Over the Last Decade, Looking Forward to the Next*; World Health Organization: Geneva, Switzerland, 2018.
9. Moulaert, T.; Garon, S. *Age-Friendly Cities and Communities in International Comparison: Political Lessons, Scientific Avenues, and Democratic Issues*; Springer: Berlin/Heidelberg, Germany, 2015.
10. Lawler, K. Age-friendly communities: Go big or go home. *Public Policy Aging Rep.* **2015**, *25*, 30–33. [CrossRef]
11. Park, S.; Lee, S. Age-friendly environments and life satisfaction among South Korean elders: Person-environment fit perspective. *Aging Ment. Health* **2017**, *21*, 693–702. [CrossRef]
12. Dellamora, M.C.; Zecevic, A.A.; Baxter, D.; Cramp, A.; Fitzsimmons, D.; Kloseck, M. Review of assessment tools for baseline and follow-up measurement of age-friendliness. *Ageing Int.* **2015**, *40*, 149–164. [CrossRef]
13. Zhang, X.; Warner, M.E.; Firestone, S. Overcoming Barriers to Livability for All Ages: Inclusivity Is the Key. *Urban Plan.* **2019**, *4*, 31–42. [CrossRef]
14. Kano, M.; Rosenberg, P.E.; Dalton, S.D. A global pilot study of age-friendly city indicators. *Soc. Indic. Res.* **2018**, *138*, 1205–1227. [CrossRef]

15. World Health Organisation. *Measuring the Age-Friendliness of Cities: A Guide to Using Core Indicators*; World Health Organisation: Geneva, Switzerland, 2015.
16. Public Health Agency of Canada. *Age-Friendly Communities Evaluation Guide: Using Indicators to Measure Progress*; Public Health Agency of Canada Ottawa: Ottawa, ON, Canada, 2015.
17. Orpana, H.; Chawla, M.; Gallagher, E.; Escaravage, E. Developing indicators for evaluation of age-friendly communities in Canada: Process and results. *Health Promot. Chronic Dis. Prev. Can. Res. Policy Pract.* **2016**, *36*, 214–223. [CrossRef]
18. Scharlach, A.E. Age-Friendly Cities: For Whom? By Whom? For What Purpose? In *Age-Friendly Cities and Communities in International Comparison*; Moulaert, T., Garon, S., Eds.; Springer: Berlin/Heidelberg, Germany, 2016; pp. 305–329.
19. Badland, H.; Whitzman, C.; Lowe, M.; Davern, M.; Aye, L.; Butterworth, I.; Hes, D.; Giles-Corti, B. Urban liveability: Emerging lessons from Australia for exploring the potential for indicators to measure the social determinants of health. *Soc. Sci. Med.* **2014**, *111*, 64–73. [CrossRef]
20. Badland, H.; Mavoa, S.; Villanueva, K.; Roberts, R.; Davern, M.; Giles-Corti, B. The development of policy-relevant transport indicators to monitor health behaviours and outcomes. *J. Transp. Health* **2015**, *2*, 103–110. [CrossRef]
21. Badland, H.M.; Rachele, J.N.; Roberts, R.; Giles-Corti, B. Creating and applying public transport indicators to test pathways of behaviours and health through an urban transport framework. *J. Transp. Health* **2017**, *4*, 208–215. [CrossRef]
22. Villanueva, K.; Badland, H.; Hooper, P.; Koohsari, M.J.; Mavoa, S.; Davern, M.; Roberts, R.; Goldfeld, S.; Giles-Corti, B. Developing indicators of public open space to promote health and wellbeing in communities. *Appl. Geogr.* **2015**, *57*, 112–119. [CrossRef]
23. Badland, H.; Foster, S.; Bentley, R.; Higgs, C.; Roberts, R.; Pettit, C.; Giles-Corti, B. Examining associations between area-level spatial measures of housing with selected health and wellbeing behaviours and outcomes in an urban context. *Health Place* **2017**, *43*, 17–24. [CrossRef] [PubMed]
24. Badland, H.; Davern, M.T.; Villanueva, K.; Mavoa, S.; Milner, A.; Roberts, R.; Giles-Corti, B. Conceptualising and measuring spatial indicators of employment through a liveability lens. *Soc. Indic. Res.* **2016**, *127*, 565–576. [CrossRef]
25. Davern, M.; Gunn, L.; Whitzman, C.; Higgs, C.; Giles-Corti, B.; Simons, K.; Villanueva, K.; Mavoa, S.; Roberts, R.; Badland, H.M. Using spatial measures to test a conceptual model of social infrastructure that supports health and wellbeing. *Cities Health* **2017**, *1*, 194–209. [CrossRef]
26. Murphy, M.; Badland, H.M.; Koohsari, M.J.; Astell-Burt, T.; Trapp, G.; Villanueva, K.; Mavoa, S.; Davern, M.T.; Giles-Corti, B. Indicators of a health-promoting local food environment: A conceptual framework to inform urban planning policy and practice. *Health Promot. J. Aust. Off. J. Aust. Assoc. Health Promot. Prof.* **2017**, *28*, 82. [CrossRef]
27. Cunningham, G.O.; Michael, Y.L. Concepts guiding the study of the impact of the built environment on physical activity for older adults: A review of the literature. *Am. J. Health Promot.* **2004**, *18*, 435–443. [CrossRef] [PubMed]
28. Frank, L.D.; Engelke, P.O. The built environment and human activity patterns: Exploring the impacts of urban form on public health. *J. Plan. Lit.* **2001**, *16*, 202–218. [CrossRef]
29. Tietz, C. Is it Time to Move Beyond the Limits of 'Built Environment' Thinking? *The Conversation*, 15 October 2018. Available online: https://theconversation.com/is-it-time-to-move-beyond-the-limits-of-built-environment-thinking-102774 (accessed on 18 November 2019).
30. Davern, M.; Both, A.; Higgs, C.; Gunn, L. The Average Regional City Resident Lacks Good Access to Two-Thirds of Community Services, and Liveability Suffers. The Conversation, 2020. Available online: https://theconversation.com/the-average-regional-city-resident-lacks-good-access-to-two-thirds-of-community-services-and-liveability-suffers-131910 (accessed on 18 November 2019).
31. Beard, J.R.; Montawi, B. Age and the Environment: The Global Movement towards Age-Friendly Cities and Communities. *J. Soc. Work Pract.* **2015**, *29*, 5–11. [CrossRef]
32. Steels, S. Key characteristics of age-friendly cities and communities: A review. *Cities* **2015**, *47*, 45–52. [CrossRef]
33. Jackisch, J.; Zamaro, G.; Green, G.; Huber, M. Is a healthy city also an age-friendly city? *Health Promot. Int.* **2015**, *30*, 108–117. [CrossRef]

34. United Nations. *Transforming out World: The 2030 Agenda for Sustainable Development*; United Nations: New York, NY, USA, 2015.
35. World Health Organization. The WHO Age-Friendly Cities Framework. 2019. Available online: https://extranet.who.int/agefriendlyworld/age-friendly-cities-framework/ (accessed on 18 November 2019).
36. Davern, M.T.; Gunn, L.; Giles-Corti, B.; David, S. Best practice principles for community indicator systems and a case study analysis: How community indicators Victoria is creating impact and bridging policy, practice and research. *Soc. Indic. Res.* **2017**, *131*, 567–586. [CrossRef]
37. Lowen, T.; Davern, M.T.; Mavoa, S.; Brasher, K. Age-friendly cities and communities: Access to services for older people. *Aust. Plan.* **2015**, *52*, 255–265. [CrossRef]
38. Giles-Corti, B.; Macaulay, G.; Middleton, N.; Boruff, B.J.; Bull, F.; Butterworth, I.; Badland, H.M.; Mavoa, S.; Roberts, R.; Christian, H. Developing a research and practice tool to measure walkability: A demonstration project. *Health Promot. J. Aust.* **2014**, *25*, 160–166. [CrossRef]
39. Giles-Corti, B. *Transport Walkability Index: Melbourne. McCaughey VicHealth Centre for Community Wellbeing*; The University of Melbourne: Melbourne, Australia, 2014.
40. Boulange, C.; Gunn, L.; Giles-Corti, B.; Mavoa, S.; Pettit, C.; Badland, H. Examining associations between urban design attributes and transport mode choice for walking, cycling, public transport and private motor vehicle trips. *J. Transp. Health* **2017**, *6*, 155–166. [CrossRef]
41. Saelens, B.E.; Handy, S.L. Built environment correlates of walking: A review. *Med. Sci. Sports Exerc.* **2008**, *40*, S550. [CrossRef]
42. Saelens, B.E.; Sallis, J.F.; Black, J.B.; Chen, D. Neighborhood-based differences in physical activity: An environment scale evaluation. *Am. J. Public Health* **2003**, *93*, 1552–1558. [CrossRef] [PubMed]
43. Cerin, E.; Nathan, A.; van Cauwenberg, J.; Barnett, D.W.; Barnett, A.; on Behalf of the Council on Environment and Physical Activity (CEPA)—Older Adults Working Group. The neighbourhood physical environment and active travel in older adults: A systematic review and meta-analysis. *Int. J. Behav. Nutr. Phys. Act.* **2017**, *14*, 15. [CrossRef]
44. Zapata-Diomedi, B.; Boulange, C.; Giles-Corti, B.; Phelan, K.; Washington, S.; Veerman, L.; Gunn, L. Physical activity-related health and economic benefits of building walkable neighbourhoods: A modelled comparison between brownfield and greenfield developments. *Int. J. Behav. Nutr. Phys. Act.* **2019**, *16*, 11. [CrossRef]
45. Davern, M.; Farrar, A.; Kendal, D.; Giles-Corti, B. *Quality Green Space Supporting Health, Wellbeing and Biodiversity: A Literature Review*; Heart Foundation of Australia: Adelaide, Australia, 2017.
46. Winters, M.; Voss, C.; Ashe, M.C.; Gutteridge, K.; McKay, H.; Sims-Gould, J. Where do they go and how do they get there? Older adults' travel behaviour in a highly walkable environment. *Soc. Sci. Med.* **2015**, *133*, 304–312. [CrossRef]
47. Fielding, R.A.; Rejeski, W.J.; Blair, S.; Church, T.; Espeland, M.A.; Gill, T.M.; Guralnik, J.M.; Hsu, F.-C.; Katula, J.; King, A.C.; et al. The lifestyle interventions and independence for elders study: Design and methods. *J. Gerontol. Ser. A Biomed. Sci. Med Sci.* **2011**, *66*, 1226–1237. [CrossRef]
48. Weuve, J.; Kang, J.; Malnson, J. Physical activity, including walking, and cognitive function in older women. *JAMA* **2004**, *292*, 1454–1461. [CrossRef] [PubMed]
49. Aspinall, P.A.; Thompson, C.W.; Alves, S.; Sugiyama, T.; Brice, R.; Vickers, A. Preference and relative importance for environmental attributes of neighbourhood open space in older people. *Environ. Plan. B Plan. Des.* **2010**, *37*, 1022–1039. [CrossRef]
50. Sugiyama, T.; Thompson, C.W.; Alves, S. Associations between neighborhood open space attributes and quality of life for older people in Britain. *Environ. Behav.* **2009**, *41*, 3–21. [CrossRef]
51. Vine, D.; Buys, L.; Aird, R. Experiences of neighbourhood walkability among older Australians living in high density inner-city areas. *Plan. Theory Pract.* **2012**, *13*, 421–444. [CrossRef]
52. Davern, M. *Walkability Factsheet Summary: Assessing Walkability in Brighton, Clarence and Launceston for the Local Government Association of Tasmania*; RMIT University: Melbourne, Australia, 2018.
53. Grant, T.L.; Edwards, N.; Sveistrup, H.; Andrew, C.; Egan, M.Y. Inequitable walking conditions among older people: Examining the interrelationship of neighbourhood socio-economic status and urban form using a comparative case study. *BMC Public Health* **2010**, *10*, 677. [CrossRef]
54. Newton, R.; Ormerod, M.; Burton, E.; Mitchell, L.; Thompson, C.W. Increasing independence for older people through good street design. *J. Integr. Care* **2010**, *18*, 24. [CrossRef]

55. Meir, I.A.; Garb, Y.; Jiao, D.; Cicelsky, A. Post-occupancy evaluation: An inevitable step toward sustainability. *Adv. Build. Energy Res.* **2009**, *3*, 189–219. [CrossRef]
56. White, M.P.; Elliott, L.R.; Gascon, M.; Roberts, B.; Fleming, L.E. Blue space, health and well-being: A narrative overview and synthesis of potential benefits. *Environ. Res.* **2020**, *1*, 110169. [CrossRef]
57. Grellier, J.; White, M.P.; Albin, M.; Bell, S.; Elliott, L.R.; Gascón, M.; Gualdi, S.; Mancini, L.; Nieuwenhuijsen, M.J.; Sarigiannis, D.A.; et al. BlueHealth: A study programme protocol for mapping and quantifying the potential benefits to public health and well-being from Europe's blue spaces. *BMJ Open* **2017**, *7*, e016188. [CrossRef]
58. Andreucci, M.B.; Russo, A.; Olszewska-Guizzo, A. Designing Urban Green Blue Infrastructure for Mental Health and Elderly Wellbeing. *Sustainability* **2019**, *11*, 6425. [CrossRef]
59. Garrett, J.K.; White, M.P.; Huang, J.; Ng, S.; Hui, Z.; Leung, C.; Tse, L.A.; Fung, F.; Elliott, L.R.; Depledge, M.H.; et al. Urban blue space and health and wellbeing in Hong Kong: Results from a survey of older adults. *Health Place* **2019**, *55*, 100–110. [CrossRef] [PubMed]
60. Dempsey, S.; Devine, M.T.; Gillespie, T.; Lyons, S.; Nolan, A. Coastal blue space and depression in older adults. *Health Place* **2018**, *54*, 110–117. [CrossRef]
61. Raymond, C.M.; Breil, M.; Nita, M.R.; Kabisch, N.; de Bel, M. *An Impact Evaluation Framework to Support Planning and Evaluation of Nature-Based Solutions Projects. Report Prepared by the EKLIPSE Expert Working Group on Nature-Based Solutions to Promote Climate Resilience in Urban Areas*; Centre for Ecology and Hydrology: Wallingford, UK, 2017.
62. Delbosc, A. The role of well-being in transport policy. *Transp. Policy* **2012**, *23*, 25–33. [CrossRef]
63. Marmot, M.; Wilkinson, R. *Social Determinants of Health*; OUP Oxford: Oxford, UK, 2005.
64. Klicnik, I.; Dogra, S. Perspectives on Active Transportation in a Mid-Sized Age-Friendly City: "You Stay Home". *Int. J. Environ. Res. Public Health* **2019**, *16*, 4916. [CrossRef] [PubMed]
65. Currie, G. Quantifying spatial gaps in public transport supply based on social needs. *J. Transp. Geogr.* **2010**, *18*, 31–41. [CrossRef]
66. Levasseur, M.; Généreux, M.; Bruneau, J.-F.; Vanasse, A.; Chabot, E.; Beaulac, C.; Bédard, M.-M. Importance of proximity to resources, social support, transportation and neighborhood security for mobility and social participation in older adults: Results from a scoping study. *BMC Public Health* **2015**, *15*, 503. [CrossRef]
67. Truong, L.T.; Somenahalli, S.V. Exploring frequency of public transport use among older adults: A study in Adelaide, Australia. *Travel Behav. Soc.* **2015**, *2*, 148–155. [CrossRef]
68. Wong, R.; Szeto, W.; Yang, L.; Li, Y.; Wong, S. Public transport policy measures for improving elderly mobility. *Transp. Policy* **2018**, *63*, 73–79. [CrossRef]
69. Engels, B.; Liu, G.-J. Ageing in place: The out-of-home travel patterns of seniors in Victoria and its policy implications. *Urban Policy Res.* **2013**, *31*, 168–189. [CrossRef]
70. McHugh, B. Pioneering open data standards: The GTFS Story. *Beyond Transpar. Open Data Future Civ. Innov.* **2013**, *1*, 125–135.
71. Broome, K.; Worrall, L.; Fleming, J.; Boldy, D. Evaluation of age-friendly guidelines for public buses. *Transp. Res. Part A Policy Pract.* **2013**, *53*, 68–80. [CrossRef]
72. Baker, E.; Lester, L.H.; Bentley, R.; Beer, A. Poor housing quality: Prevalence and health effects. *J. Prev. Interv. Community* **2016**, *44*, 219–232. [CrossRef] [PubMed]
73. Bentley, R.; Baker, E.; Mason, M.K.; Subramanian, S.V.; Kavanagh, A.M. Association between Housing Affordability and Mental Health: A Longitudinal Analysis of a Nationally Representative Household Survey in Australia. *Am. J. Epidemiol.* **2011**, *174*, 753–760. [CrossRef] [PubMed]
74. Pollack, C.E.; Griffin, B.A.; Lynch, J. Housing affordability and health among homeowners and renters. *Am. J. Prev. Med.* **2010**, *39*, 515–521. [CrossRef]
75. Versey, H.S.; Murad, S.; Willems, P.; Sanni, M. Beyond Housing: Perceptions of Indirect Displacement, Displacement Risk, and Aging Precarity as Challenges to Aging in Place in Gentrifying Cities. *Int. J. Environ. Res. Public Health* **2019**, *16*, 4633. [CrossRef]
76. Vanleerberghe, P.; De Witte, N.; Claes, C.; Schalock, R.L.; Verté, D. The quality of life of older people aging in place: A literature review. *Qual. Life Res.* **2017**, *26*, 2899–2907. [CrossRef]
77. O'Neill, P. Housing affordability literature review and affordable housing program audit. In *Urban Research Centre*; University of Western Sydney: Sydney, Australia, 2008.

78. Arnold, E.; Skaburskis, A. Measuring Ontario's increasing housing affordability problem. *Soc. Indic. Res.* **1989**, *21*, 501–515. [CrossRef]
79. Senate Select Committee on Housing Affordability in Australia. *A Good Place is Hard to Find: Housing Affordability in Australia*; Australia, C.O., Ed.; Parliament House: Canberra, Australia, 2008.
80. Morris, A. Housing tenure and the health of older Australians dependent on the age pension for their income. *Hous. Stud.* **2018**, *33*, 77–95. [CrossRef]
81. World Health Organisation. *A Conceptual Framework for Action on the Social Determinants of Health: Social Determinants of Health Discussion Paper 2*; World Health Organisation: Geneva, Switzerland, 2010.
82. Kepper, M.M.; Myers, C.A.; Denstel, K.D.; Hunter, R.F.; Guan, W.; Broyles, S.T. The neighborhood social environment and physical activity: A systematic scoping review. *Int. J. Behav. Nutr. Phys. Act.* **2019**, *16*, 14. [CrossRef]
83. Kawachi, I.; Berkman, L.F. Social ties and mental health. *J. Urban Health* **2001**, *78*, 458–467. [CrossRef]
84. Amagasa, S.; Fukushima, N.; Kikuchi, H.; Oka, K.; Takamiya, T.; Odagiri, Y.; Inoue, S. Types of social participation and psychological distress in Japanese older adults: A five-year cohort study. *PLoS ONE* **2017**, *12*, e0175392. [CrossRef]
85. Rosengren, A.; Hawken, S.; Ôunpuu, S.; Sliwa, K.; Zubaid, M.; Almahmeed, W.; Blackett, K.N.; Sitthi-Amorn, C.; Sato, H.; Yusuf, S. Association of psychosocial risk factors with risk of acute myocardial infarction in 11 119 cases and 13 648 controls from 52 countries (the INTERHEART study): Case-control study. *Lancet* **2004**, *364*, 953–962. [CrossRef]
86. Holt-Lunstad, J.; Smith, T.B.; Layton, J.B. Social relationships and mortality risk: A meta-analytic review. *PLoS Med.* **2010**, *7*, e1000316. [CrossRef]
87. Au, A.; Lai, D.W.L.; Yip, H.-M.; Chan, S.; Lai, S.; Chaudhury, H.; Scharlach, A.; Leeson, G. Sense of Community Mediating Between Age-Friendly Characteristics and Life Satisfaction of Community-Dwelling Older Adults. *Front. Psychol.* **2020**, *11*, 86. [CrossRef]
88. Zunzunegui, M.-V.; Alvarado, B.E.; Del Ser, T.; Otero, A. Social networks, social integration, and social engagement determine cognitive decline in community-dwelling Spanish older adults. *J. Gerontol. Ser. B Psychol. Sci. Soc. Sci.* **2003**, *58*, 93–100. [CrossRef]
89. Roth, A.R. Social networks and health in later life: A state of the literature. *Sociol. Health Illn.* **2020**, *42*, 1642–1656. [CrossRef]
90. Neville, S.; Adams, J.; Napier, S.; Shannon, K.; Jackson, D. "Engaging in my rural community": Perceptions of people aged 85 years and over. *Int. J. Qual. Stud. Health Well-Being* **2018**, *13*, 1503908. [CrossRef]
91. Jo Cox Loneliness Commission. *Combatting Loneliness One Conversation at a Time: A Call to Action*; Jo Cox Loneliness Commission: London, UK, 2017.
92. Walker, R.B.; Hiller, J.E. Places and health: A qualitative study to explore how older women living alone perceive the social and physical dimensions of their neighbourhoods. *Soc. Sci. Med.* **2007**, *65*, 1154–1165. [CrossRef]
93. Woolrych, R.; Sixsmith, J.; Fisher, J.; Makita, M.; Lawthom, R.; Murray, M. Constructing and negotiating social participation in old age: Experiences of older adults living in urban environments in the United Kingdom. *Ageing Soc.* **2019**, *2019*, 1–23. [CrossRef]
94. Aabo, V. The role and value of public libraries in the age of digital technologies. *J. Librariansh. Inf. Sci.* **2005**, *37*, 205–211. [CrossRef]
95. Barclay, D.A. Space and the Social Worth of Public Libraries. *Public Libr. Q.* **2017**, *36*, 267–273. [CrossRef]
96. Swindell, R. U3A Online: Building a global learning community of older people. *Australas. J. Ageing* **2009**, *28*, A80.
97. Swindell, R.; Thompson, J. An international perspective on the University-Of-The-3rd-Age. *Educ. Gerontol.* **1995**, *21*, 429–447. [CrossRef]
98. Zajac-Gawlak, I.; Pośpiech, D.; Kroemeke, A.; Mossakowska, M.; Gába, A.; Pelclová, J.; Přidalová, M.; Kłapcińska, B. Physical activity, body composition and general health status of physically active students of the University of the Third Age (U3A). *Arch. Gerontol. Geriatr.* **2016**, *64*, 66–74. [CrossRef]
99. Putnam, R.D. *Bowling Alone: The Collapse and Revival of American Community*; Simon and Schuster: New York, NY, USA, 2000.

100. Chen, W.; Ling, L.; Renzaho, A.M.N. Building a new life in Australia: An analysis of the first wave of the longitudinal study of humanitarian migrants in Australia to assess the association between social integration and self-rated health. *BMJ Open* **2017**, *7*, 11. [CrossRef]
101. Brown, R.K.; Taylor, R.J.; Chatters, L.M. Race/Ethnic and Social-Demographic Correlates of Religious Non-Involvement in America: Findings from Three National Surveys. *J. Black Stud.* **2015**, *46*, 335–362. [CrossRef]
102. Maliepaard, M.; Phalet, K. Social Integration and Religious Identity Expression among Dutch Muslims: The Role of Minority and Majority Group Contact. *Soc. Psychol. Q.* **2012**, *75*, 131–148. [CrossRef]
103. Coombs, T.; Nicholas, A.; Pirkis, J. A review of social inclusion measures. *Aust. N. Z. J. Psychiatry* **2013**, *47*, 906–919. [CrossRef]
104. Morgan, C.; Burns, T.; Fitzpatrick, R.; Pinfold, V.; Priebe, S. Social exclusion and mental health: Conceptual and methodological review. *Br. J. Psychiatry* **2007**, *191*, 477–483. [CrossRef]
105. Walsh, K.; Scharf, T.; Keating, N. Social exclusion of older persons: A scoping review and conceptual framework. *Eur. J. Ageing* **2017**, *14*, 81–98. [CrossRef]
106. Whitehead, M.; Pennington, A.; Orton, L.; Nayak, S.; Petticrew, M.P.; Sowden, A.J.; White, M. How could differences in 'control over destiny' lead to socio-economic inequalities in health? A synthesis of theories and pathways in the living environment. *Health Place* **2016**, *39*, 51–61. [CrossRef] [PubMed]
107. Marmot, M.G.; Stansfeld, S.; Patel, C.; North, F.; Head, J.; White, I.; Brunner, E.; Feeney, A.; Smith, G. Health inequalities among British civil servants: The Whitehall II study. *Lancet* **1991**, *337*, 1387–1393. [CrossRef]
108. Dahlgren, G.; Whitehead, M. *European Strategies for Tackling Social Inequities in Health: Levelling up Part 2. Studies on Social and Economic Determinants of Population Health, No. 3*; World Health Organization Regional Office for Europe Copenhagen: Copenhagen, Denmark, 2007; Volume 89384. Available online: http://www.euro.who.int/__data/assets/pdf_file/0018/103824E (accessed on 18 November 2019).
109. Cahill, K.E.; Giandrea, M.D.; Quinn, J.F. Evolving Patterns of Work and Retirement. In *Handbook of Aging and the Social Sciences*, 8th ed.; George, L.K., Ferraro, K.F., Eds.; Academic Press: San Diego, CA, USA, 2016; pp. 271–291.
110. Serrat, R.; Scharf, T.; Villar, F.; Gómez, C. Fifty-Five Years of Research Into Older People's Civic Participation: Recent Trends, Future Directions. *Gerontologist* **2019**, *60*, e38–e51. [CrossRef]
111. Burr, J.A.; Caro, F.G.; Moorhead, J. Productive aging and civic participation. *J. Aging Stud.* **2002**, *16*, 87–105. [CrossRef]
112. Winterton, R.; Warburton, J. Healthy ageing in Australia's rural places: The contribution of older volunteers. *Volunt. Sect. Rev.* **2014**, *5*, 181–201. [CrossRef]
113. Winterton, R.; Warburton, J. Does place matter? Reviewing the experience of disadvantage for older people in rural Australia. *Rural Soc.* **2011**, *20*, 187–197. [CrossRef]
114. Australian Bureau of Statistics. *Household Use of Information Technology, Australia*; 2016–2017 cat. no. 8146.0 2018; Australian Bureau of Statistics: Canberra, Australia, 2018.
115. Everingham, J.-A.; Petriwskyj, A.; Warburton, J.; Cuthill, M.; Bartlett, H. Information provision for an age-friendly community. *Ageing Int.* **2009**, *34*, 79–98. [CrossRef]
116. Sixsmith, A.; Sixsmith, J. Ageing in place in the United Kingdom. *Ageing Int.* **2008**, *32*, 219–235. [CrossRef]
117. Hummert, M.L.; Wiemann, J.M.; Nussbaum, J.F. *Interpersonal Communication in Older Adulthood*; Sage: Thousand Oaks, CA, USA, 1994.
118. Freeman, S.; Marston, H.R.; Olynick, J.; Musselwhite, C.; Kulczycki, C.; Genoe, M.R.; Xiong, B. Intergenerational Effects on the Impacts of Technology Use in Later Life: Insights from an International, Multi-Site Study. *Int. J. Environ. Res. Public Health* **2020**, *17*, 5711. [CrossRef]
119. Liddle, J.; Pitcher, N.; Montague, K.; Hanratty, B.; Standing, H.; Scharf, T. Connecting at Local Level: Exploring Opportunities for Future Design of Technology to Support Social Connections in Age-Friendly Communities. *Int. J. Environ. Res. Public Health* **2020**, *17*, 5544. [CrossRef]
120. Silvius, H.A.; Tak, E.C.P.M.; Mook-Kanamori, D.O.; Vos, H.M.; Numans, M.E.; Chavannes, N.H. Effects of Technology Use on Ageing in Place: The iZi Pilots. *Int. J. Environ. Res. Public Health* **2020**, *17*, 5052. [CrossRef] [PubMed]
121. Marston, H.R.; van Hoof, J. "Who doesn't think about technology when designing urban environments for older people?" A case study approach to a proposed extension of the WHO's age-friendly cities model. *Int. J. Environ. Res. Public Health* **2019**, *16*, 3525. [CrossRef] [PubMed]

122. Browning, C.; Davis, J.; Thomas, S. Primary Health Care and Older People. In *Ageing in Australia: Challenges and Opportunities*; Oloughlin, K., Browning, C., Kendig, H., Eds.; WHO: Geneva, Switzerland, 2017; pp. 225–237.
123. Van Dijk, H.M.; Cramm, J.M.; Van Exel, J.; Nieboer, A.P. The ideal neighbourhood for ageing in place as perceived by frail and non-frail community-dwelling older people. *Ageing Soc.* **2015**, *35*, 1771–1795. [CrossRef]
124. Ratcliffe, S. *Oxford Essential Quotations*; Oxford University Press: Oxford, UK, 2016.
125. Cobb, C.W.; Rixford, C. *Lessons Learned from the History of Social Indicators*; Redefining Progress: San Francisco, CA, USA, 1998; Volume 1.
126. Innes, J.E. Disappointments and legacies of social indicators. *J. Public Policy* **1989**, *9*, 429–432. [CrossRef]
127. Byrne, C.; Harris, C. Climate Change in an Ageing World. HelpAge International. 2015. Available online: https://reliefweb.int/sites/reliefweb.int/files/resources/COP21_HelpAge_PositionPaper_Final_0.pdf (accessed on 18 November 2019).
128. Dicks, L.; Haddaway, N.; Hernández-Morcillo, M.; Mattsson, B.; Randall, N.; Failler, P.; Ferretti, J.; Livoreil, B.; Saarikoski, H.; Santamaria, L.; et al. *Knowledge Synthesis for Environmental Decisions: An Evaluation of Existing Methods, and Guidance for their Selection, Use and Development: A Report from the EKLIPSE Project*; European Union Funding for Research & Innovation: Brussels, Belgium, 2017.

International Journal of
Environmental Research and Public Health

MDPI

Article

How Older People Experience the Age-Friendliness of Their City: Development of the Age-Friendly Cities and Communities Questionnaire

Jeroen Dikken [1,2], Rudy F.M. van den Hoven [1], Willeke H. van Staalduinen [3], Loes M.T. Hulsebosch-Janssen [4] and Joost van Hoof [1,5,*]

1 Chair of Urban Ageing, Faculty of Social Work & Education, The Hague University of Applied Sciences, Johanna Westerdijkplein 75, 2521 EN Den Haag, The Netherlands; J.Dikken@hhs.nl (J.D.); r.f.m.vandenhoven@hhs.nl (R.F.M.v.d.H.)
2 Faculty of Health, Nutrition & Sport, The Hague University of Applied Sciences, Johanna Westerdijkplein 75, 2521 EN Den Haag, The Netherlands
3 AFEdemy—Academy on age-friendly environments in Europe, Buurtje 2, 2802 BE Gouda, The Netherlands; willeke@afedemy.eu
4 Hulsebosch Advies, Lissenvaart 43, 2724 SJ Zoetermeer, The Netherlands; hulsebosch@hm-advies.nl
5 Institute of Spatial Management, Faculty of Environmental Engineering and Geodesy, Wrocław University of Environmental and Life Sciences, ul. Grunwaldzka 55, 50-357 Wrocław, Poland
* Correspondence: j.vanhoof@hhs.nl; Tel.: +31-6-23381404

Received: 5 September 2020; Accepted: 16 September 2020; Published: 20 September 2020

check for updates

Abstract: The World Health Organization engages cities and communities all over the world in becoming age-friendly. There is a need for assessing the age-friendliness of cities and communities by means of a transparently constructed and validated tool which measures the construct as a whole. The aim of this study was to develop a questionnaire measuring age-friendliness, providing full transparency and reproducibility. The development and validation of the Age Friendly Cities and Communities Questionnaire (AFCCQ) followed the criteria of the COnsensus-based Standards for selection of health Measurement INstruments (COSMIN). Four phases were followed: (1) development of the conceptual model, themes and items; (2) initial (qualitative) validation; (3) psychometric validation, and (4) translating the instrument using the forward-backward translation method. This rigorous process of development and validation resulted in a valid, psychometrically sound, comprehensive 23-item questionnaire. This questionnaire can be used to measure older people's experiences regarding the eight domains of the WHO Age-Friendly Cities model, and an additional financial domain. The AFCCQ allows practitioners and researchers to capture the age-friendliness of a city or community in a numerical fashion, which helps monitor the age-friendliness and the potential impact of policies or social programmes. The AFCCQ was created in Dutch and translated into British-English.

Keywords: survey; questionnaire; validation; age-friendly; age-friendly cities; older people; age-friendliness; AFCCQ

1. Introduction

For over a decade, the World Health Organization (WHO) has been involved in engaging and assisting cities and communities all over the world in becoming "age-friendly" [1–10]. The WHO proposed that policies, services, and structures in an age-friendly city, which are related to the physical and social environment, are designed to support and enable older people to "age actively". A growing number of cities and communities worldwide are striving to better meet the needs of their older residents. The WHO Global Network for Age-Friendly Cities and Communities was established to foster the exchange of experience and mutual learning between cities and communities of different sizes worldwide [11]. According to the WHO, the efforts of these cities and communities to become more age-friendly take place within very diverse cultural and socio-economic contexts. The common ground between these network partners is "the desire and commitment to promote healthy and active ageing and a good quality of life for their older residents". Each member monitors its progress along the age-friendly milestones, and there is a global database of age-friendly practices, as well as a library containing member-uploaded toolkits, publications, research updates and videos [12].

In 2018, the WHO signalled a number of knowledge gaps in terms of age-friendly cities and communities [12]. The largest of these gaps is that the WHO's age-friendly cities approach needs to strengthen its focus on multisectoral action that delivers outcomes in ways that reduce inequities. In the WHO's own words, guidance and tools are needed to support cities and communities to make decisions around which actions are most likely to ensure these outcomes and not leave any groups behind in the process of development [12] (p. 18). According to Buckner et al. [13,14], one of the challenges for the evaluation of age-friendly city initiatives is to identify an evidence-based approach that (i) can be applied in different contexts, (ii) reflects the complexity of the initiatives, (iii) draws on sound data to make assessments of effectiveness, and (iv) presents findings clearly to a mixed audience. The researchers identified ten thematic areas where evidence was required, namely: political support; leadership and governance; financial and human resources; involvement of older people; priorities based on needs assessment; application of existing frameworks for assessing age-friendliness; provision; evidence-based interventions; coordination, collaboration and interlinkages; and monitoring and evaluation.

In short, there is a great need for monitoring, evaluating, measuring and assessing the age-friendliness of cities and communities. The Checklist of Essential Features of Age-Friendly Cities [15] contains a large number of features which are essential to an age-friendly city, and was based on the results of the WHO Global Age-Friendly Cities project consultation in 33 cities in 22 countries. The checklist is a guide for a city's self-assessment and a map for charting progress. This does not mean that all domains are equally relevant in all countries and cities, depending on the status quo in each country that wishes to evaluate. For conducting supportive research, one could also find inspiration in the set of core indicators published by the WHO in 2015 [16], as well as a list of research methodologies, which can be used to investigate the age-friendliness of a city. On top of this, Fulmer et al. [17] called for the creation of an ecosystem, where each of the age-friendly initiatives can create synergies and additional momentum as the population continues to age. Their vision for an age-friendly ecosystem encompasses the lived environment, social determinants of health, the healthcare system, and a prevention-focused public health system. At the same time, Marston and van Hoof [18] argued about the apparent lack of consideration of technology in the existing age-friendly cities literature, which is another direction of investigation that should be included in the assessment of the age-friendliness of cities and communities, and also called for a new ecosystem. To date, despite these noble calls for new ecosystems, the lack of measurability of the age-friendliness of cities and communities is a clear weakness in moving the agenda forward.

Qualitative approaches have tried to measure and assess the age-friendliness of a city, for instance, through photoproduction [19] and photovoice [20] methods, or through citizen science programs of research [21,22]. Various researchers have tried to come up with a more quantitative approach to measure the age-friendliness, often taking the Checklist of Essential Features of Age-Friendly Cities [15] as a basis for their work. Luciano et al. [23] presented a framework for the assessment of the age-appropriateness of housing through a number of metrics that detect and identify physical and non-physical features of a home environment to enable ageing in place. Their study combined data from a systematic literature review expert opinion. A total of 71 metrics were identified and divided into eight main domains to describe the framework. Their study only addressed the age-friendliness of housing, which is just one of the eight domains highlighted by the WHO. In addition, Flores et al. [24]

noted a lack of empirical research exploring the impact of age-friendly cities on older people. Therefore, they evaluated an age-friendly city by analysing its relationship with life satisfaction, taking into account the age cohort variables of older people and whether they live alone or with someone else. They conducted a two-stage study, in which 66 people participated in the qualitative analysis (focus groups) in Stage I and 203 in the quantitative analysis (survey methodology) of Stage II. The regression analysis indicates that for all age cohorts, community support and health services were significantly associated with life satisfaction. Social participation and outdoor spaces and buildings were only significantly associated with life satisfaction for older people who live together. Their research did not produce a validated questionnaire. Zaman and Thornton [25] identified the priority indicators for age-friendly development at the local government level in Unley, South Australia. The study conducted a community perception survey to identify the important indicators, followed by a focus group consultation to identify the priority indicators based on local settings. The study identified 25 indicators as priority indicators for the City of Unley that need to be considered for the development of an age-friendly Unley. Garner and Holland [26] described the development and validation of the Age-Friendly Environment Assessment Tool (AFEAT), assessing whether individual function and frailty impact on perceptions of environmental age-friendliness. The AFEAT was developed using the WHO Age-Friendly Environment Checklist. A total of 132 participants from the United Kingdom, aged 58–96, took part. The AFEAT, which comprises ten items (using a five-point Likert scale system), assesses individual perceptions of the environment. The AFEAT showed the need for an individual-oriented age-friendly environment tool.

All of the instruments described lack transparency of (several phases of) the development and validation process, they do not measure the age-friendliness construct as a whole (covering all eight domains as defined by the WHO) and the methodological rigour in the development process can be questioned, influencing the reliability, validity and usability of these instruments. Therefore, the aim of this study was to develop a questionnaire measuring the age-friendliness of a city or community, in line with state-of-the-art methodology described in the literature, providing full transparency and reproducibility.

2. Materials and Methods

The Age-Friendly Cities and Communities Questionnaire (AFCCQ) for measuring the age-friendliness of a city was developed in a step-by-step approach. For the development and validation of the questionnaire, we based our methods in line with the criteria stated by the COnsensus-based Standards for selection of health Measurement INstruments (COSMIN) [27]. The COSMIN initiative aims to reach consensus about which measurement properties are considered to be important, their most adequate terms and definitions, and how they should be assessed in terms of study design and statistics [28]. The development consisted of the following four phases: (1) development of the conceptual model, themes and items; (2) initial (qualitative) validation; (3) psychometric validation and (4) translating the instrument from Dutch into British English (Figure 1).

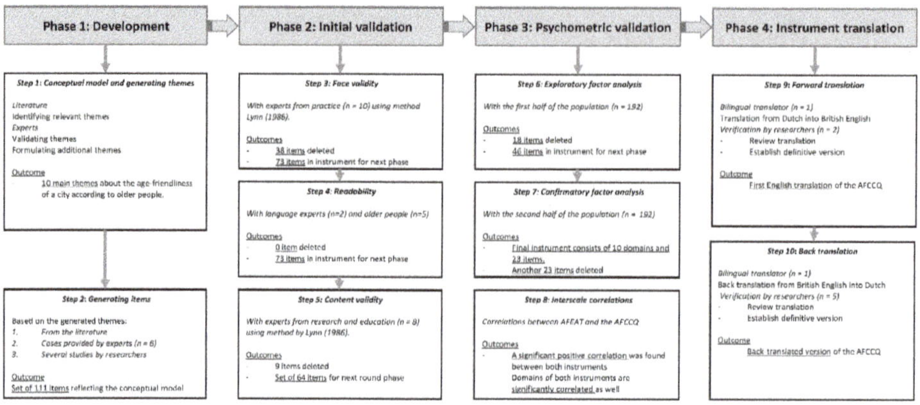

Figure 1. Flowchart representing the phases and steps for developing the Age-Friendly Cities and Communities Questionnaire (AFCCQ).

2.1. Phase 1: Development of the Conceptual Model, Themes and Questions of the AFCCQ (steps 1 and 2)

Within the first step, the goal was to find a theoretical base for the conceptual model of the questionnaire [29] to assess how older people experience the age-friendliness of their city. Models and themes regarding age-friendliness of cities described in international books, guides and scientific articles published after 2007 were identified and discussed by the research team (J.D., R.F.M.v.d.H., W.H.v.S., J.v.H.). This research team was diverse and complementary in each other's respective field of expertise. J.v.H., R.F.M.v.d.H. and W.H.v.S. have a background in housing/technology, social work/andragogy and political sciences, and were responsible for the content of the questionnaire. J.D. has a background in nursing and gerontology and was also responsible for the content of the questionnaire. In addition, he has extensive experience in developing and validating measurement instruments.

Consensus was reached, finding a theoretical basis described in the Global Age-Friendly Cities Guide by WHO [1], as the research team found this guide the best fit with the objective of the study. This guide published a model of age-friendly cities and communities, consisting of eight domains (i.e., themes). These domains are outdoor spaces and buildings; transportation; housing; social participation; respect and social inclusion; civic participation and employment; communication and information; and community support and health services.

Then, the goal was to select and formulate items based on the conceptual model [29], which was the outcome of step 1. The "Checklist of Essential Features of Age-Friendly Cities" published by the WHO [15] was used as a basis. This checklist contains a large number of features which are essential to an age-friendly city and is based on the results of the WHO Global Age-Friendly Cities project consultation in 33 cities in 22 countries. The checklist is a tool for a city's self-assessment and a map for charting progress. The features of this checklist, therefore, formed the foundation of the items for this questionnaire, as well as the WHO documents from 2015 and 2018 [12,16]. The study by Marston and van Hoof [18] on the importance of technology in age-friendly cities (and their age-friendly ecosystem framework), which was further demonstrated for the context of the municipality of The Hague by van Hoof et al. [19], was used as the basis for additional questions on technology in the daily lives of older people. The research report by Bottenheft et al. [30] on The Hague as an age-friendly city was used to come up with additional questions that pertain to the Dutch context of city planning, housing, transport and the system of healthcare. Other efforts, such as the Liveability Index by the American Association of Retired Persons (AARP) [31], which consider many aspects of the (built) environment, were also touched upon. The Hong Kong Special Administrative Region Government stimulates active and healthy ageing by focusing on a multi-dimensional approach. The Hong Kong dimension of financial adequacy [32] was used to produce additional questions related to one's financial situation and skills, as well as feeling financially secure. It also alludes to the notion of equity in health as addressed by WHO, which is defined as the absence of avoidable or remediable differences among groups of people, whether those groups are defined socially, economically, demographically, or geographically [33], and is one of the pillars of the core indicators for age-friendly cities presented by WHO [16].

Items were generated by R.F.M.v.d.H. and J.v.H., which were then provided with multiple rounds of feedback by the other researchers (J.D., W.H.v.S., L.M.T.H.-J.). Next, the items were discussed by the research team until consensus was reached on content and objective. The outcome of this step was a full set of items, which was a depiction of the eight themes as described by the WHO [1] and two additional themes (technology and financial situation).

2.2. *Phase 2: Initial (Qualitative) Validation (Steps 3 to 5)*

The aim of Phase 2 was to assess face validity, readability and content validity and conduct item reduction to establish a definitive selection of items which adequately represent the construct [29].

2.2.1. Step 3: Face Validity—Participants and Measurement

Face validity was assessed using a quantification method [34,35]. A panel from the Dutch Province of South-Holland (n = 14 invited), with a diverse expertise on different domains of the WHO's model of age-friendly cities and communities was contacted for participation. Participants who were willing to participate received an e-mail invitation to rate the relevance of the AFCCQ items regarding construct, study population, and purpose on a four-point Likert scale (1 = not relevant, 2 = somewhat relevant, 3 = quite relevant, 4 = highly relevant). The comprehensiveness was measured by asking the participants whether the items covered the entire construct measured.

2.2.2. Step 4: Readability—Participants and Measurement

The readability was first examined by older people (the target population) (n = 10 invited). They scored all items which were not excluded in the face-validity round (Step 2.1) on language (i.e., difficulty in wording, interpretation of wording and sentences, length of sentences and construction) and understandability of the questions using a ten-point Likert scale (1 = I do not understand the question to 10 = I have no difficulty in understanding the question). Participants were asked to explain a grade below six (i.e., insufficient).

The final questionnaire was examined and improved by "*De Stadskamer*" of the Municipality of The Hague, which specializes in research on how civilians experience the service level of the municipality. This unit did secondary analyses of the wording level (including richness of vocabulary), sentence level (including number of subordinate clauses), and text level (cohesion and structure).

2.2.3. Step 5: Content Validity—Participants and Measurement

The content validity was determined by the same quantification method as used in Step 3 [34,35]. In this round, a Dutch panel of experts in the field of age-friendly cities were contacted for participation (n = 13 invited). All experts were contacted based on holding a doctoral degree and having a track record in the field of gerontology research, specifically in relation to age-friendly cities. Experts were asked by e-mail to independently appraise the relevance of the items with respect to the construct, study population, and purpose on a four-point Likert scale (1 = not relevant, 2 = somewhat relevant, 3 = quite relevant, 4 = highly relevant). Comprehensiveness was again evaluated by asking the experts whether the items comprised the assumed construct and if they missed items or themes.

2.2.4. Statistical Analyses in Phase 2

For the face and content validity of the studies, the Item Content Validity Index (I-CVI) was used, which is defined as the proportion of experts who rate the content as valid (relevance rating of 3 or

4) [34,35]. In both steps, this was calculated for each item. Lynn [34] and Polit et al. [35] found an item to be excellent when the I-CVI value was greater than 0.78.

For the face-validity round (Step 3), items were considered to be excellent when I-CVI ≥ 0.90. These items were retained for the readability (Step 4) and content validity (Step 5) rounds. Items on the threshold (I.CVI = 0.70 to 0.89) were individually assessed by the research team and with consensus were in- or excluded. Items with an I-CVI score of ≤ 0.69 were excluded.

The readability (Step 4) was assessed on a ten-point Likert scale. Individual items with a mean score of < 6 were discussed by the research team and changes in language were made. The readability for the total questionnaire was calculated by averaging all mean grades per item.

In Step 2.3, content validity was assessed, and items were rated excellent when the I-CVI value was greater than 0.78 [34,35]. Items on the threshold (I-CVI = 0.75, having eight raters) were individually assessed by the research team and included or excluded on the basis of consensus. For complete scale validation, all I-CVI values were averaged in order to calculate a Scale Content Validity Index (S-CVIave), for which a value greater than 0.90 is considered excellent [35]. Data of all steps were analysed using SPSS version 25.0 (IBM Corp., Armonk, NY, USA).

2.3. Phase 3: Psychometric Validation (Steps 6 to 8)

The aim of Phase 3 was to statistically assess the validity of the AFCCQ. Exploratory Factor Analysis (EFA) was used to identify the underlying factor structure of the AFCCQ [36]. One of the most important functions of EFA is that it allows for determining how well the items of a scale align with latent factors. In case there is no alignment, or when items are too identical, items can be removed. This improves the overall quality of the instrument. In order to test the factor structure that resulted from the EFA, a Confirmatory Factor Analysis (CFA) was conducted using a second dataset. In CFA, the researchers explicitly test the hypotheses about which items measure which latent factors, and provide more robust validity evidence of the fit of the tested model with the data (i.e., that a scale accurately measures what it purports). In order to investigate the validity of the AFCCQ, the dataset was split randomly in half (n = 192 for each half) and an EFA was conducted using the first half of the data and a CFA on the second half. This approach is used to investigate validity from a single survey administration, especially when the sample is large enough so that resulting subsets represent enough observations to run multiple rounds of factor analyses [36–38].

2.3.1. Data Collection and Participants in Phase 2

For the data collection phase, a sample of community-dwelling older people (65 years and over) were recruited (Table 1). In January 2019, there were 539,040 inhabitants in the municipality of The Hague (https://denhaag.incijfers.nl/jive), of whom 78,073 were aged 65 and over (14.55% of the urban population). A total of 94.6% live independently, or 73,857 inhabitants. With a margin of error of 5% and a confidence level of 95%, this means a total of 383 respondents were needed. The inclusion criteria of the representative sample meant that—ideally—31.3% of the sample had to have a migrant background (according to the definitions of CBS—Statistics Netherlands). The largest group of migrants (47.7%) are migrants from Western countries, followed by people from Suriname (23.0%), as well as Morocco, Turkey, Aruba and the former Netherlands Antilles (Curaçao, Sint Maarten, Bonaire, Sint Eustatius and Saba), and other non-Western countries. The main focus was on recruiting people with a non-Western migration background. The ratio between males and females is 45%–55% in The Hague. Participants came from all boroughs of the city, and older people are not evenly spread across The Hague. A representative distribution across the age cohorts was sought (65–69 (31.0%); 70–74 (27.4%) and 75+ (41.6%)), as well as for the share of the population living in a home that is either rented or owned (58% were owned by the dweller, and 42% rented) [39]. We also recruited people who either lived alone or with a spouse.

Table 1. Demographics of participants (n = 384).

Sex	
Male	n = 188 (49%)
Female	n = 196 (51%)
Age	
Mean (SD)	74.4 (6.36)
60–65	n = 10 (2.6%)
65–69	n = 82 (21.4%)
70–74	n = 118 (30.7%)
75+	n = 156 (40.6%)
Missing values	n = 17 (4.7%)
Born in the European part of the Kingdom of the Netherlands (%) [1]	n = 329 (85.7%)
Educational level	
Primary education only	n= 19 (4.9%)
Secondary school giving entry to intermediate vocational education	n = 101 (26.4%)
Intermediate vocational education	n = 64 (16.7%)
Secondary school giving entry to university (of applied sciences)	n = 35 (9.1%)
University of applied sciences	n = 95 (24.7%)
University	n = 70 (18.2%)
Years living in The Hague	
Mean (SD)	51.3 (22.7)
Type of dwelling	
Owner-occupant	n = 230 (59.9%)
Social housing	n = 110 (28.6%)
Private rent	n = 44 (11.5%)
Living together with a partner (%)	n = 216 (56.3%)
Receiving care (%)	n = 98 (25.5%)
Living with one or more chronic conditions (%)	n = 186 (48.4%)
Using a wheeled walker or wheelchair (%)	n = 56 (14.6%)

[1] Denotes a possible migration background according to Dutch definitions.

The research was carried out by *aha! marktonderzoek en marketingadvies*, Groningen, The Netherlands among members of an existing *Ouderenpanel* database, and additionally recruited older citizens of the municipality of The Hague, between July and September 2020. Participants from the database had consented to their participation by being a part of the panel. Additional participants were asked to sign informed consent forms prior to filling out the questionnaire. Only those aged 65 years or over who lived in their own home and were able to communicate in Dutch were included.

2.3.2. Step 6: Exploratory Factor Analysis

Before running the EFA, the correlations among all items were examined in order to determine if the items that should be related to one another were, in fact, related. Item variance and means were also examined. Ideally, one would like to see relatively high item variance (indicating a wide range of response patterns) and a mean closer to the centre of the scale range [37]. After exploring the data, an EFA was conducted.

Then, the number of latent factors were determined using scree plots, parallel analysis and the conceptual model. The scree plot is a subjective method that allows identification of the number of factors by observing the plot of eigenvalues as a function of the number of factors. The part of the plot with the elbow of the graph indicates the number of factors to be extracted [36]. Then, a parallel analysis was performed which examines eigenvalues in the sample data compared with randomly generated data to determine the number of factors. Triangulation of these sets of information guided decisions about the number of factors to extract.

After determining the number of factors, a maximum likelihood EFA was conducted using the oblimin rotation. Communalities and the loadings of each item were examined to identify those with low or cross-loadings. Specifically, the authors classified any item with a loading of magnitude 0.32 or less as low loading, indicating that less than 10% of the item variance was shared with a latent factor [40], and any item that had loading onto another factor half the magnitude of the main loading as a cross-loading [41]. Low or cross-loading items and items with low communalities (>0.40) were removed one at a time.

2.3.3. Step 7: Confirmatory Factor Analysis

With this CFA, the factor structure resulting from the EFA was tested. First the variance to unity, allowing the factors to co-vary, which is a similar approach to using the promax rotation in the EFA, was set. In order to evaluate the fit of the model, multiple fit indices were considered. First of all, the normed χ^2 was used, which is less sensitive to sample size than the χ^2. Some researchers tolerate values as high as 5 as an adequate model fit [42], while others insist normed χ^2 should be 2 or less, and less than 1.0 is a poor model fit. Shadfar and Malekmohammadi [43] stated that a value below 2 is preferred, but a value between 2 and 5 is considered to be acceptable. Furthermore, the robust Comparative Fit Index (CFI) and Tucker Lewis Index (TLI) were tested, both of which should be 0.9 or greater [44]. The root-mean squared residual (SRMR) should be less than 0.08 for good fit [45]. Finally, the root-mean square error of approximation (RMSEA) was tested, for which MacCallum et al. [46] suggested thresholds of 0.01 or less for excellent fit, 0.05 or less for good fit, and 0.08 for moderate fit, whereas Hu and Bentler [45] described values between 0.05 and 0.1 as a moderate fit. Then, internal consistency of the final model was evaluated using composite reliability which is preferred over Cronbach's alpha with CFA. A composite reliability value of 0.70 was considered appropriate for reliability [47].

2.3.4. Step 8: Interscale Correlation

During data collection, the items of the AFCCQ were supplemented by the ten core questions of the AFEAT (Age-Friendly Environment Assessment Tool) by Garner & Holland [26]. This is a validated questionnaire, and its questions needed to be answered using the same five-point Likert scale as with the AFCCQ (ranging from Strongly Disagree—Disagree—Neither Agree/Disagree—Agree—Strongly Agree). It was hypothesised that sum scores of both scales are highly positively correlated (sig. >0.001), specifically the corresponding latent factors measured by sub-scales of both instruments. The Pearson's correlation coefficient was used to test this hypothesis.

2.4. Phase 4: Instrument Translation (Steps 9 and 10)

The final set of items was translated from Dutch into British English according to the procedure described by Brislin [48] and Maneesriwongul and Dixon [49]. As the first step, the forward translation, a bilingual translator (native Dutch speaker) translated the items into British English. This translation was verified by two bilingual researchers (J.D., J.v.H.), who reviewed the translation and established a definitive version. For the second step, the backward translation, an independent native Dutch speaking translator, who was an English language expert, translated the questions back into the Dutch language. This translator did not have access to the original items written in the Dutch language (i.e., a blind translation). Finally, the original Dutch version of the items were compared with the back-translated version by two researchers (J.D., J.v.H.). If necessary, modifications were made until agreement was reached. The other research team members (R.F.M.v.d.H., W.H.v.S., L.M.T.H.-J.) validated the agreed translated version. This led to the final version of the translation of the instrument.

3. Results

3.1. Phase 1: Development of the Conceptual Model, Themes and Questions of the AFCCQ (Steps 1 and 2)

A total of 111 items were developed for a total of ten domains. The domain Housing consisted of 11 items; social participation of 15 items; respect and social inclusion of 14 items; civic participation and employment of 9 items; communication and information of 8 items; community support and health services of 16 items; outdoor spaces and buildings of 16 items; transportation of 9 items; technology of 7 items; and financial situation of 6 items (see Table S1 for all developed items and reasons for item exclusion in the different steps).

3.2. Phase 2: Initial (Qualitative) Validation

3.2.1. Step 3: Face Validity

A total of 10 respondents scored the AFCCQ on face validity. Respondents were all women and had a mean age of 39.7 (SD = 17.2). Two respondents had a bachelor's degree, seven a master's degree and one a doctoral degree. All had experience (mean 8.1 years, SD = 8.3) working for older people in their current area of practice (policy advisor government, researchers, consultants). Of the total of 111 initially developed items, 38 were excluded from the initial AFCCQ after assessment of face validity scores (Table S1). Multiple items were changed in language following the feedback of this group. Items of the AFCCQ were considered comprehensive and no suggestions for extension were made.

3.2.2. Step 4: Readability

A total of five older people (two men and three women) and two language experts scored the AFCCQ on readability. The older people had a mean age of 74.4 (ranging from 69–81 years old). All respondents had a bachelor's (n = 5) or master's (n = 2) degree and experience with themes regarding age-friendly cities (ranging from 2–50 years). The readability of the AFCCQ was considered excellent with a mean of 8.9. Of the 73 remaining items, seven items (9.6%) scored between 7 and 7.9; 26 items (35.6%) scored between 8.0 and 8.9; and 40 items (54.8%) scored between 9.0 and 10.0. No changes in the AFCCQ were made after this study.

3.2.3. Step 5: Content Validity

In total, eight (international) experts in age-friendly cities participated in this step (six Dutch, two Belgian (Flemish)). Five experts were female and three were male. Their mean age was 42 years (SD = 5.7). All held a doctoral degree and had ample experience within the field. Of the 73 remaining items, nine were excluded in this step after assessment of the content validity (Table S1). The S-CVIave of the remaining 64 items was 0.95 (range 0.88–1.00). Items of the AFCCQ were considered comprehensive, and no suggestions for extension were made.

3.3. Phase 3: Psychometric Validation

3.3.1. Step 6: Exploratory Factor Analysis

The parallel analysis indicated five factors. However, the scree plot was fitting to the number of factors as expected from the conceptual model (10 factors). Therefore, we decided to continue with this number of factors. Then items with low communalities (<0.40) were removed (n = 8). The communality of an item represents how much variation of that item is explained by the latent factors. Although an item's communality should ideally be 0.80 or greater, it is common for communalities to range between 0.40 and 0.70 [50]. Then, items with low (n = 1) or cross-loadings (n = 9) were removed one at a time. This iterative process left a set of 46 items with factor loadings that ranged from 0.35 to 0.88 (Table 2). Ten items loaded on another factor than initially thought when exploring the results, but all could be explained. For example, item 19 *"If necessary, I can get special community transport"* was originally included in the domain "Social participation" but loaded strongly on domain "Community support and health services", which can be explained as the origin of the item can relate to both domains. Items with different factor loadings than originally thought were, therefore, replaced in a further step of the analysis as indicated by the EFA results.

3.3.2. Step 7: Confirmatory Factor Analysis

The next step was to test the fit of the other half of the data with the structure determined by the EFA. This second step is used to confirm that the fit from the EFA is consistent in a more stringent and robust hypothesis-testing model in CFA. The resulting CFA model indicated that the ten-factor model of the AFCCQ did not fit the data well mainly due to low factor loadings. Therefore, we ran several models to maximise model fit with the data (Table 3). First, all items with factor loadings < 0.50 were excluded (model 2), followed by exclusion of all items with loadings < 0.60 (model 3) and excluding all items with loadings < 0.70 (model 4). Finally, items with problematic standardised residual covariances were excluded from the model (model 5). Of the final model, the value of the normed χ^2 was 1.619, which indicates a good fit. Values of the robust CFI and the robust TLI were, respectively, 0.937 and 0.923, both above the 0.9 threshold [44]. The RMSEA was 0.057, which is lower than 0.08 (threshold for moderate fit [46]). The robust SRMR was 0.0569, which is below 0.08. This is considered to be a good fit according to Hu and Bentler [45].

Furthermore, the estimated covariance paths between the factors were all lower than the suggested 0.85 cut-off, indicating discriminant validity. Figure 2 shows the final model. Discriminant validity ensures that the items measure distinct, but perhaps related, factors. Overall, the results of the CFA suggested that the final model resulted from the EFA was (after trimming) a good fit on a second set of data.

Finally, the internal consistency of the model that emerged from the final CFA was examined by calculating the composite reliability per factor (Table 4). All factors demonstrate a value above the threshold for reasonable reliability of > 0.70 that is often reported. The thresholds for composite reliability are up for debate, with different authors offering different threshold suggestions. A lot depends upon how many items there are in the developed scale. Smaller numbers of scale items tend to result in lower reliability levels, while larger numbers of scale items tend to have higher level factors, with five to eight items that should meet a minimum threshold of 0.80 [51]. The results of the present study are in line with these findings.3.3.3. Step 8: Interscale Correlations

Table 5 presents the correlations between the AFCCQ and the AFEAT [26]. The hypothesis that the sum scores of both scales are highly positively correlated ($r = 0.75$, $p < 0.01$) was confirmed (Table 5). Furthermore, the hypothesis that corresponding domains of both instruments were also correlated was confirmed. These results provide evidence for good convergent validity of the AFCCQ.

Table 2. Item Communality and Final Exploratory Factor Analysis Results.

Item	Communality	Factor Loading									
		Housing	Social Participation	Respect and Social Inclusion	Civic Participation and Employment	Communication and Information	Community Support and Health Services	Outdoor Spaces and Buildings	Transportation	Technology	Financial Situation
1	0.702	0.30									**0.67**
3	0.621	**0.51**									
4	0.677	**0.76**									
9	0.628	**0.77**									
10	0.699	**0.41**									
12	0.611		**0.64**								
13	0.611		**0.56**								
16	0.632		**0.67**								
19	0.517						**0.62**				
20	0.505		**0.45**								
21	0.690		0.50						0.38		
22	0.676		**0.66**								
24	0.572										**0.41**
25	0.685		**0.76**								
26	0.639		**0.77**								
27	0.672			**0.74**							
39	0.632			**0.70**							
28	0.538				**0.58**						
36	0.542				**0.51**						
41	0.520				**0.54**						
42	0.495				0.45	0.32					
43	0.566			0.32	0.56						
47	0.625				0.36	0.39					
48	0.564				0.38		0.47				
50	0.506		**0.35**								
54	0.550					**0.54**					
55	0.542					**0.51**					
56	0.578					**0.58**					
57	0.565		0.31			0.51					
59	0.602								**0.49**		
61	0.596						**0.74**				
62	0.554						**0.54**				
64	0.567						**0.58**				
66	0.575						**0.67**				
67	0.637						**0.76**				
69	0.670						**0.54**				
71	0.568						**0.62**				
73	0.533										
74	0.661								**0.53**		

Table 2. *Cont.*

Item	Communality	Factor Loading									
		Housing	Social Participation	Respect and Social Inclusion	Civic Participation and Employment	Communication and Information	Community Support and Health Services	Outdoor Spaces and Buildings	Transportation	Technology	Financial Situation
75	0.695								**0.52**		
76	0.544			**0.51**							
78	0.522		0.30						0.36		
83	0.547							**0.48**			
84	0.562							**0.40**			
85	0.644					0.59					
86	0.654					**0.52**			0.37		
88	0.601							**0.37**			
89	0.652							**0.40**			
90	0.711								**0.76**		
91	0.718								**0.82**		
92	0.663								**0.74**		
93	0.548								**0.40**		
96	0.619					0.35		0.32	0.46		
98	0.564							**0.70**			
106	0.815										**0.87**
107	0.827										**0.88**

Grey cells denote items that demonstrate no loading (item 83) or cross-loadings. bold indicate the included item and the corresponding domain.

Table 3. Models maximising model fit with the data.

Model	Normed χ^2	Comparative Fit Index (CFI)	Tucker Lewis Index (TLI)	Root-Mean Squared Residual (SRMR)	Root-Mean Square Error of Approximation (RMSEA)
Model 1 (45 variables)	2.068	0.757	0.736	0.1041	0.075
Model 2 (35 variables) Exclusion of items with loadings below < 0.50	1.968	0.849	0.829	0.0820	0.071
Model 3 (31 variables) Exclusion of items with loadings < 0.60	1.960	0.878	0.857	0.0796	0.071
Model 4 (27 variables) Exclusion of items with loadings < 0.70	1.752	0.913	0.915	0.0628	0.063
Model 5 (23 variables)	1.619	0.937	0.923	0.0569	0.057

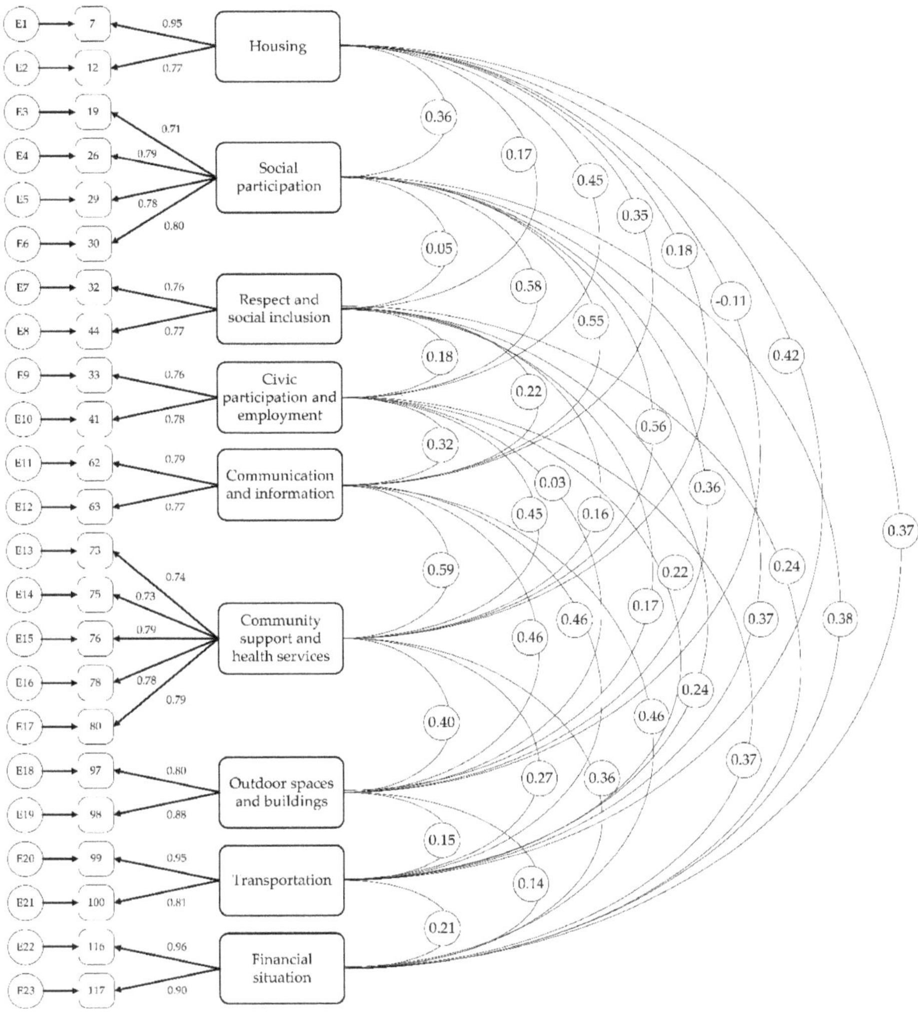

Figure 2. Model of the final confirmatory factor analysis.

Table 4. Reliability per factor of the AFCCQ.

Domain	Housing	Social Participation	Respect and Social Inclusion	Civic Participation and Employment	Communication and Information	Community Support and Health Services	Outdoor Spaces and Buildings	Transportation	Financial Situation
Composite Reliability	0.85	0.85	0.74	0.74	0.76	0.88	0.83	0.88	0.93

Table 5. Interscale correlations (r) between Age-Friendly Environment Assessment Tool (AFEAT) by Garner & Holland [26] and the AFCCQ: total scale and sub-domains (n = 384).

Scales and Domains	AFEAT	AFEAT—Housing	AFEAT—Social Participation	AFEAT—Civic Participation and Employment	AFEAT—Communication and Information	AFEAT—Transportation
AFCCQ total	0.748 **					
AFCCQ—Housing	0.416 **	0.561 **	0.309 **	0.243 **	0.200 **	0.292 **
AFCCQ—Social participation	0.613 **	0.366 **	0.626 **	0.456 **	0.380 **	0.328 **
AFCCQ—Civic participation and employment	0.516 **	0.290 **	0.225 **	0.444	0.356 **	0.306 **
AFCCQ—Communication and information	0.480 **	0.310 **	0.373 **	0.375 **	0.456 **	0.347 **
AFCCQ—transportation	0.507 **	0.532 **	0.298 **	0.261 **	0.251 **	0.551 **

** Correlation is significant at the 0.01 level (2-tailed). Grey cells indicate the expected correlated domains of both scales.

3.4. Phase 4: Instrument Translation (Steps 9 and 10)

Overall, the forward translation was correctly performed by an independent, professional translator. However, some small changes were made by the main researchers to accomplish consequent use of British English (for instance, the word "plenty" was changed to "sufficient" or "enough" and "sick" was changed to "ill"). The end product of the back translation was rather similar to the original items. Occasionally, a loose translation was applied, and some word choices did not fit completely. Consensus was reached that no changes were necessary on the final version of the back translation. Because the aim of this phase was a good translation from Dutch into the British English language, cultural issues were not taken into further consideration. Both the Dutch and British English versions of the AFCCQ can be found in Tables A1 and A2.

3.5. Interpretation and Presentation of Results

The AFCCQ can be used for both research and policy purposes. Total scores range from −46 to +46 points. The number of points per dimension can vary as the number of questions asked per domain varies, too. In order to simplify the interpretation of results and communicate with a larger community of stakeholders, it is advised to use a colour scheme principle (Table 6). As shown, there are several coloured zones. These zones represent how satisfied older people are regarding the city as a whole or a specific domain. Scores in the red zone mean people feel neutral to slightly unsatisfied (−) to very unsatisfied (−−−−). Light green (+) means people feel neutral to slightly satisfied. Scores in the darker green zones mean that people feel satisfied (++) to very satisfied (++++) with their respected city and/or a specific domain. This method allows for a clear and straightforward presentation of findings to a mixed audience, which is in line with the recommendations by Bucker et al. [13,14]. By doing so, policymakers can easily see in which domains they need to act. It can help in prioritising the domains and corresponding interventions for increasing the age-friendliness of their city, as long as the required interventions are a part of the tasks carried out by municipalities or city councils. The colour codes also indicate a sense of urgency. Red scores indicate the need for (immediate or necessary) action. Light green zones indicate that actions may still be needed, and darker green zones mean that there is still room for improvement. Over-time scores can be compared to assess whether policy decisions impacted the age-friendliness of the cities according to research participants. Researchers are advised to use the absolute scores in their analyses. Furthermore, cross-cultural validation may allow researchers to compare between cities within a given country, or between countries.

Table 6. AFCCQ: Interpretation and presentation ($n = 384$).

Scale and Domains of the AFCCQ	Colour Scheme Principle								Mean	SD	Variance	Range
	− − − −	− − −	− −	−	+	++	+++	++++				
AFCCQ Total score	≤−35.1	−23.1–−35.0	−11.5–−23.0	−11.4–0.0	0.1–11.4	11.5–23.0	23.1–35.0	≥35.1	13.3	7.86	61.7	66
Housing	≤−3.1	−2.1–−3.0	−1.1–−2.0	−1.0–0.0	0.1–1.0	1.1–2.0	2.1–3.0	≥3.1	2.3	1.4	1.1	6
Social participation	≤−6.1	−4.1–−6.0	−2.1–−4.0	−2.0–0.0	0.1–2.0	2.1–4.0	4.1–6.0	≥6.1	2.5	1.0	5.8	8
Respect and social inclusion	≤−3.1	−2.1–−3.0	−1.1–−2.0	−1.0–0.0	0.1–1.0	1.1–2.0	2.1–3.0	≥3.1	1.6	1.5	2.5	8
Civic participation and employment	≤−3.1	−2.1–−3.0	−1.1–−2.0	−1.0–0.0	0.1–1.0	1.1–2.0	2.1–3.0	≥3.1	1.4	1.3	1.7	8
Communication and information	≤−3.1	−2.1–−3.0	−1.1–−2.0	−1.0–0.0	0.1–1.0	1.1–2.0	2.1–3.0	≥3.1	1.4	1.3	1.6	8
Community support and health services	≤−7.6	−5.1–−7.5	−2.6–−5.0	−2.5–0.0	0.1–2.5	2.6–5.0	5.1–7.5	≥7.6	2.5	2.9	8.2	20
Outdoor spaces and buildings	≤−3.1	−2.1–−3.0	−1.1–−2.0	−1.0–0.0	0.1–1.0	1.1–2.0	2.1–3.0	≥3.1	0.9	1.4	1.9	8
Transportation	≤−3.1	−2.1–−3.0	−1.1–−2.0	−1.0–0.0	0.1–1.0	1.1–2.0	2.1–3.0	≥3.1	1.7	1.5	2.2	8
Financial situation	≤−3.1	−2.1–3.0	−1.1–−2.0	−1.0–0.0	0.1–1.0	1.1–2.0	2.1–3.0	≥3.1	1.8	1.3	1.6	6

The coloured zones represent how dissatisfied or satisfied older people are regarding the city as a whole or a specific domain. Scores in the red zone mean people are neutral to slightly unsatisfied (−) to very unsatisfied (− − − −). Scores in the green zones mean that people are neutral to slightly satisfied (+) to very satisfied (++++).

Table 6 presents the preliminary results of the sample used in this validation study. These results show how the scores can be presented and interpreted. The AFCCQ presents a relatively high item variance (indicating a wide range of response patterns) and a mean closer to the centre of the scale which is preferred. Furthermore, the results show that most domains score in the light green (++) category, meaning there's room for improvement and actions are wanted. The domains of "Community support and health services" and "Outdoor spaces and buildings" score in the light green zone (+). This means that these two domains may be a priority for policy makers and social programmes or interventions and could be explored in further detail in order to increase the age-friendliness of the city as a whole. Zooming in at the neighbourhood level can further uncover (large) differences in AFCCQ scores and domains and pinpoint where to implement certain interventions.

4. Discussion

The step-by-step rigorous process of development and validation resulted in a valid, psychometrically sound, comprehensive 23-item questionnaire: The Age-Friendly Cities and Communities Questionnaire (AFCCQ) which is reported in full transparency. The AFCCQ can be used to measure the age-friendliness of a city or community. To date, such a validated tool was lacking, and many cities trying to assess their age-friendliness had to resort to a qualitative or mixed methodology approach, which was often based on the Checklist of Essential Features of Age-Friendly Cities [15]. The AFCCQ is the first validated tool that can be used for a quantitative assessment, which still allows for additional qualitative data to be shared with researchers or policy makers. The questions that were not included in the final instrument can nevertheless be used as a source of inspiration for a more in-depth survey per domain. The AFCCQ allows practitioners and researchers to capture the age-friendliness of a city or community in a numerical fashion, which helps to monitor the progress (or decline) of the age-friendliness and the potential impact of policies or social programs.

One of the main questions that needs to be resolved pertains to a cross-cultural validation. Is the current AFCCQ too Dutch in character? The Netherlands have a long-standing tradition of state-organized long-term care, with a nationwide approach to organized nursing home care and district nursing and home, social and domestic care taken care of by the municipalities. This means that for decades, the country has put great effort in improving the well-being of older citizens. This frontrunner position may impact the construct of the questionnaire and its constituting questions. In order to overcome this challenge, two international experts (Belgian nationality) were consulted who had a critical look at items that may have been too Dutch in character. This should have benefits for future cross-cultural validation procedures. Even though a rigorous translation process has been performed as a first step for future cross-cultural research, researchers who want to use the AFCCQ in their respective countries should test the cultural adaptation of the AFCCQ before using it to collect data, especially when cultures are very different from the Dutch/Western Europe culture. One of the most rigorous ways researchers can assess the cross-cultural validity of the AFCCQ is by the assessment of the measurement invariance (MI). MI assesses whether different groups respond in a similar way to a measurement instrument and its items [52,53]. Only when measurement instruments have a certain level of MI can average scores on (sub)scales between different countries/cultures be compared and meaningful interpretations of results be made. One challenge with this analysis is that data from both countries are needed [52].

A more user-friendly approach was presented by Sousa and Rojjanasrirat [54], who described a seven-step guideline from translation (step 1–4) pilot testing (step 5–6) to full psychometric testing (step 7). For the use of the AFCCQ in English-speaking countries, steps 1–4 were already performed in phase 4 of this study. For non-English speaking countries, these steps should be repeated from the translated British-English version into the language of choice.

Some studies from other Western countries have addressed issues concerning national priorities. The study by Zaman and Thornton [25] from Australia identified the priority indicators for age-friendly development at the local government level in South Australia. In their words, the WHO's age-friendly indicators are generalised and overarching and need modification by considering local needs. Garner and Holland [26] did similar important work from a British perspective. Their works show that a meticulous cross-cultural validation may be an important aspect in moving the AFCCQ further. At the same time, the AFCCQ was largely based on the Checklist of Essential Features of Age-Friendly Cities [15], which is also a first indication that most of the factors constituting the questionnaire are international in their origin and applicability.

In addition, Buffel et al. [55]—referring to the Checklist of Essential Features of Age-Friendly Cities [15]—raised the question whether the use of a universal checklist of action items is the most adequate method to deal with the diversity of cities and heterogeneity of their populations. Creating age-friendly communities will require an adjustment of methods and instruments to highly unequal local contexts. This applies not only to the diversity between but also within cities. The question can be asked to what extent instruments such as the AFCCQ survey do justice to the diversity of older people in the city, and whether indicators and items used reflect the different needs, concerns and preferences of particular groups of older people in the city and what they consider to be important aspects of an age-friendly city. This becomes even more important given the growing number of older people with a migration background [52], but also when we take into account existing forms of social inequality and deprivation [3,6]. This applies not only to ethnic or cultural diversity, but also to other factors such as gender, age, socioeconomic position or health status, which influence what people consider important when it comes to the age-friendliness of their living environment. Garner and Holland [26], for example, point to the relation between individual functioning and frailty and perceptions of environmental age-friendliness. When exploring the older people's perception of their neighbourhood, Scharf et al. [56] found that older people's ethnic background has an important influence on people's perceptions. This highlights the importance of paying attention to how dimensions such as gender, ethnicity, income and material deprivation, educational level, household composition and health situation impact on the perception of the age-friendliness of the city and the immediate living environment. This requires that indicators and data can be disaggregated by such dimensions. At the same time, this is also in line with the WHO's plea [16] to disaggregate data—from a perspective of equity—by social stratifications such as gender, age, ethnicity, socioeconomic status and neighbourhood. At the same time, these factors may influence the perceptions different groups have of the age-friendliness of their living environment. The novel AFCCQ provides a tool to move the plethora of smaller qualitative studies towards a more integrative approach of doing research, in which large-scale quantitative studies are supplemented by qualitative approaches. The AFCCQ allows for the inclusion of the abovementioned minority groups, such as people facing social inequalities, and their voices can be analysed separately in a quantitative manner. Quantitative data can help map the magnitude of social inequalities, also between subpopulations. A mixed-methods approach can help study the numerical data in more detail, for instance, when the AFCCQ domains are also studied through qualitative methodologies.

There may be a bias towards the ninth domain of financial situation (as it was taken from Hong Kong SAR (financial adequacy), and because all older people in The Netherlands enjoy a state pension under the 1956 General Old Age Pensions Act). This domain was not part of the original WHO model. Therefore, the panellists did not recognize these elements as age-friendly city indicators or a separate domain. The same can be said for the questions on technology, which correlated with other existing domains, and most questions ($n = 5$) were excluded in the qualitative initial validation rounds. The experts consulted in this study may not have recognized the importance of technology as an integral part of age-friendliness [8,57,58] yet. This may change in the future. At the same time, Marston and van Hoof [18] called for an integrated consideration of technology, and gerontechnology in particular, in all domains of age-friendly cities, instead of technology being a separate novel domain. Future studies could pay particular attention to the role of technology in the structure of the AFCCQ. When doing evaluation studies of age-friendly cities, technology should nevertheless be addressed explicitly, both qualitatively or using an additional instrument addressing the role of gerontechnology.

Local governments and city councils can use the AFCCQ to study the age-friendliness of their respective jurisdictions. The colour scheme approach helps communicate the results of such studies to a larger audience, including older citizens. One of the strengths of the AFCCQ is that it collects data among older people themselves instead of their representatives. Policy makers may even be encouraged to move up in the sequence of colours presented by the colour scheme as a motivator through their social and urban planning policies. Policy makers may also ask for additional research in the fields with low scores. Urban planners and architects could use the outcomes of the AFCCQ as a first indication of satisfaction with aspects of the built environment. At the same time, organisations for the interests of older citizens can use the AFCCQ as well in order to provide a foundation for their actions. Researchers can apply the AFCCQ as a quick scan of a particular city, or to measure age-friendliness in a longitudinal manner, following up on a cohort in a sequence of years. After going through the procedure of cross-cultural validation, cities in various countries (in and between various countries) could be compared as well.

Some considerations regarding this study should be discussed. First, considering the representativity and size of the sample used. The representativeness of the convenient sample of community-dwelling older people (60 years and over) can be questioned as selection bias (the panel used for the study, Dutch speaking older people living in their own home). This may have led to a bias as older people with strong positive or negative experiences/emotions are more likely to participate in such panels. However, for this study, this is acceptable as the primary focus was on the psychometric validation of the AFCCQ and not an exploration of experiences of Dutch older people living in the municipality of The Hague. Regarding the sample size, there is an abundance of recommendations for the appropriate sample size to use when conducting a factor analysis. Suggested minimum sample sizes range from three to 20 times the number of variables, and absolute ranges from 100 to over 1000 participants [59]. Even though this study met the minimum criterion of 1:3 (which means a minimum number of 135 participants), the sample size in this study is on the lower end of the advised number of participants. However, the sample size did not affect the performance of analysis, and over time, multiple studies have demonstrated that rather small sample sizes can be sufficient [60,61]. One strength in this study was the lack of missing data, which maximizes the validity of the item selection during the item reduction process. Now that the AFCCQ is considered psychometrically valid, imputation of data can be performed by researchers in future studies that focus on measuring the experiences and opinions of older people regarding the age-friendliness of their respected localities. Finally, the AFCCQ provided an answer to three of the recommendations made by Buckner et al. [14] regarding the challenges for evaluation of age-friendly city initiatives. The AFCCQ is a validated instrument which (i) can be applied in different contexts, (ii) can make assessments of the effectiveness of an intervention and (iii) presents findings clearly to a mixed audience.

5. Conclusions

The step-by-step rigorous process of development and validation resulted in a valid, psychometrically sound, comprehensive 23-item questionnaire: The Age-Friendly Cities and Communities Questionnaire (AFCCQ), which is reported in full transparency. The AFCCQ was derived through the COnsensus-based Standards for selection of health Measurement INstruments (COSMIN). The AFCCQ covers the eight domains of the WHO Age-Friendly Cities model, and an additional domain of financial situation. The AFCCQ allows practitioners and researchers to capture the age-friendliness of a city or community in a numerical fashion, which helps to monitor the progress (or decline) of the age-friendliness and the potential impact of policies or social programmes. Before the AFCCQ can be used in other countries and cities, it is encouraged to go through the process of cross-cultural validation. In order to facilitate the first steps of such a process, the AFCCQ was translated into British English. Therefore, the AFCCQ is now available in both Dutch and British English.

Supplementary Materials: The following are available online at. Table S1. Reasons for item exclusion in all steps for the Age-Friendly Cities and Communities Questionnaire (AFCCQ).

Author Contributions: Conceptualization, J.v.H. and J.D.; Methodology, J.D.; Validation, J.D. and J.v.H.; Formal Analysis, J.D. and J.v.H.; Investigation, J.D., R.F.M.v.d.H., W.H.v.S., L.M.T.H.-J. and J.v.H.; Writing—original draft preparation, J.D., and J.v.H.; Writing—review and editing, J.D., R.F.M.v.d.H., W.H.v.S., L.M.T.H.-J. and J.v.H.; Visualization, J.D. and J.v.H.; Supervision, J.v.H.; Project administration, L.M.T.H.-J. and J.v.H.; Funding acquisition, J.v.H., L.M.T.H.-J. and W.H.v.S. All authors have read and agreed to the published version of the manuscript.

Funding: This research was funded by the Municipality of The Hague, grant number OCW/2020.1121, and by the Chair of Urban Ageing of The Hague University of Applied Sciences, The Hague, The Netherlands.

Acknowledgments: The participants of the various validation stages are thanked for their contribution and valuable suggestions to improve the questionnaire.

Conflicts of Interest: The authors declare no conflict of interest.

Appendix A

Table A1. The Age-Friendly Cities and Communities Questionnaire (AFCCQ) in Dutch.

	De Age Friendly Cities and Communities Questionnaire (AFCCQ)
	Alle Vragen van de AFCCQ Kunnen Beantwoord Worden op een 5-Punt Likert-Schaal van −2 (Helemaal Oneens); −1 (Oneens); 0 (Noch Mee Eens, Noch Mee Oneens); 1 (Eens); 2 (helemaal Eens).
Item	**Domein**
	Huisvesting
Q1	Mijn woning is toegankelijk voor mij.
Q2	Mijn woning is toegankelijk voor mensen die mij willen bezoeken.
	Sociale participatie
Q3	In mijn buurt zijn voldoende gelegenheden om mensen te ontmoeten.
Q4	Activiteiten en evenementen worden georganiseerd op voor mij bereikbare plaatsen.
Q5	De informatie over activiteiten en evenementen vind ik voldoende en ook geschikt voor mij.
Q6	Ik vind het aanbod van evenementen en activiteiten voldoende afwisselend.
	Sociale inclusie
Q7 *	Ik krijg wel eens vervelende of negatieve opmerkingen vanwege mijn leeftijd.
Q8 *	Ik krijg wel eens te maken met discriminatie vanwege mijn leeftijd.
	Burgerparticipatie en werkgelegenheid
Q9	Ik heb voldoende mogelijkheden om met jongere generaties om te gaan.
Q10	Ik voel mij een gewaardeerd lid van de samenleving.
	Communicatie en informatie
Q11	Gedrukte en digitale informatie van de gemeente en andere maatschappelijke instanties zijn goed leesbaar qua lettertype en grootte.
Q12	Gedrukte en digitale informatie van de gemeente en andere maatschappelijke instanties zijn geschreven in begrijpelijke taal.
	Sociale en gezondheidsvoorzieningen
Q13	Het aanbod van zorg en welzijn in mijn stad is voor mij voldoende.
Q14	Als ik ziek ben, krijg ik de zorg en hulp die ik nodig heb.
Q15	Indien nodig, kan ik zorg en welzijn telefonisch en fysiek gemakkelijk bereiken.
Q16	Ik heb voldoende informatie over zorg en welzijn in mijn buurt.
Q17	Zorg en welzijn werkers in mijn buurt zijn voldoende respectvol.
	Buitenruimte en gebouwen
Q18	Mijn buurt is voldoende toegankelijk voor rollator of rolstoel.
Q19	De winkels in mijn buurt zijn voldoende toegankelijk met rollator of rolstoel.
	Transport
Q20	Ik kan gemakkelijk instappen in de bus of tram in mijn buurt.
Q21	De bus- en tramhaltes in mijn buurt zijn gemakkelijk te bereiken en te gebruiken.
	Financiën
Q22	Mijn inkomen is voldoende om zonder problemen in mijn basisbehoeften te voorzien.
Q23	Ik kan goed rondkomen met mijn inkomen.

Table A1. *Cont.*

De Age Friendly Cities and Communities Questionnaire (AFCCQ)								
Alle Vragen van de AFCCQ Kunnen Beantwoord Worden op een 5-Punt Likert-Schaal van −2 (Helemaal Oneens); −1 (Oneens); 0 (Noch Mee Eens, Noch Mee Oneens); 1 (Eens); 2 (helemaal Eens).								
Item	**Domein**							
	Interpretatie AFCCQ totaalscore en specifieke domeinen							
	− − − −	− − −	− −	−	+	+ +	+ + +	+ + + +
AFCCQ Totaal score	≤−35.1	−23.1—35.	−11.5—23.	−11.4–0.0	0.1–11.4	11.5–23.0	23.1–35.0	≥35.1
Huisvesting	≤−3.1	−2.1—3.0	−1.1—2.0	−1.0–0.0	0.1–1.0	1.1–2.0	2.1–3.0	≥3.1
Sociale participatie	≤−6.1	−4.1—6.0	−2.1—4.0	−2.0–0.0	0.1–2.0	2.1–4.0	4.1–6.0	≥6.1
Sociale inclusie	≤−3.1	−2.1—3.0	−1.1—2.0	−1.0–0.0	0.1–1.0	1.1–2.0	2.1–3.0	≥3.1
Burgerparticipatie en werkgelegenheid	≤−3.1	−2.1—3.0	−1.1—2.0	−1.0–0.0	0.1–1.0	1.1–2.0	2.1–3.0	≥3.1
Communicatie en informatie	≤−3.1	−2.1—3.0	−1.1—2.0	−1.0–0.0	0.1–1.0	1.1–2.0	2.1–3.0	≥3.1
Sociale en geszondheids-voorzieningen	≤−7.6	−5.1—7.5	−2.6—5.0	−2.5–0.0	0.1–2.5	2.6–5.0	5.1–7.5	≥7.6
Buitenruimte en gebouwen	≤−3.1	−2.1—3.0	−1.1—2.0	−1.0–0.0	0.1–1.0	1.1–2.0	2.1–3.0	≥3.1
Transport	≤−3.1	−2.1—3.0	−1.1—2.0	−1.0–0.0	0.1–1.0	1.1–2.0	2.1–3.0	≥3.1
Financiën	≤−3.1	−2.1—3.0	−1.1—2.0	−1.0–0.0	0.1–1.0	1.1–2.0	2.1–3.0	≥3.1

Scoresysteem: Items met een * moeten gehercodeerd worden in tegenovergestelde richting (−2 = 2, −1 = 1, 0 = 0, 1 = −1, 2 = −2). Tel alle scores van de AFCCQ op, om de AFCCQ totaalscore te berekenen. Tel alle scores van de specifieke domeinen op om de domeinspecifieke score te berekenen.

Table A2. The Age-Friendly Cities and Communities Questionnaire (AFCCQ) in English.

The Age Friendly Cities and Communities Questionnaire (AFCCQ)	
All Questions of the AFCCQ Can Be Answered on a 5-Point Likert-Scale Ranging from: −2 (Totally Disagree); −1 (Disagree); 0 (Neutral); 1 (Agree); 2 (Totally Agree).	
Item	**Domain**
	Housing
Q1	My house is accessible to me.
Q2	My house is accessible to the people who come to visit me.
	Social participation
Q3	There are enough opportunities to meet people in my neighbourhood.
Q4	Activities and events are organised in places that are accessible to me.
Q5	The information about activities and events is enough for me and also suitable for me.
Q6	I find the range of events and activities sufficiently varied.
	Respect and Social inclusion
Q7 *	I sometimes get annoying or negative remarks because of my age.
Q8 *	I sometimes face discrimination because of my age.
	Civic participation and employment
Q9	I have enough opportunities to interact with younger generations.
Q10	I feel like a valued member of society.
	Communication and information
Q11	Printed and digital information from the municipality and other social institutions is easy to read in terms of font and size.
Q12	Printed and digital information from the municipality and other social institutions is written in understandable language.
	Community support and health services
Q13	The supply of care and welfare in my city is enough for me.
Q14	When I am ill, I receive the care and help I need.
Q15	If necessary, I can easily reach care and welfare services by telephone and in person.
Q16	I have enough information about care and welfare services in my neighbourhood.
Q17	Care and welfare workers in my neighbourhood are sufficiently respectful.

Table A2. *Cont.*

The Age Friendly Cities and Communities Questionnaire (AFCCQ)	
All Questions of the AFCCQ Can Be Answered on a 5-Point Likert-Scale Ranging from: −2 (Totally Disagree); −1 (Disagree); 0 (Neutral); 1 (Agree); 2 (Totally Agree).	
Item	**Domain**
	Outdoor spaces and buildings
Q18	My neighbourhood is sufficiently accessible for a wheeled walker or wheelchair.
Q19	The shops in my neighbourhood are sufficiently accessible with a wheeled walker or wheelchair.
	Transportation
Q20	I can easily get on the bus or tram in my neighbourhood.
Q21	The bus and tram stops in my neighbourhood are easy to reach and use.
	Financial situation
Q22	My income is sufficient to cover my basic needs without any problems.
Q23	I live well on my income.

Interpretation AFCCQ total score and separate domains.

	− − − −	− − −	− −	−	+	+ +	+ + +	+ + + +
AFCCQ Total score	≤−35.1	−23.1–−35.	−11.5–−23.	−11.4–0.0	0.1–11.4	11.5–23.0	23.1–35.0	≥35.1
Housing	≤−3.1	−2.1–−3.0	−1.1–−2.0	−1.0–0.0	0.1–1.0	1.1–2.0	2.1–3.0	≥3.1
Social participation	≤−6.1	−4.1–−6.0	−2.1–−4.0	−2.0–0.0	0.1–2.0	2.1–4.0	4.1–6.0	≥6.1
Respect and social inclusion	≤−3.1	−2.1–−3.0	−1.1–−2.0	−1.0–0.0	0.1–1.0	1.1–2.0	2.1–3.0	≥3.1
Civic participation and employment	≤−3.1	−2.1–−3.0	−1.1–−2.0	−1.0–0.0	0.1–1.0	1.1–2.0	2.1–3.0	≥3.1
Communication and information	≤−3.1	−2.1–−3.0	−1.1–−2.0	−1.0–0.0	0.1–1.0	1.1–2.0	2.1–3.0	≥3.1
Community support and health services	≤−7.6	−5.1–−7.5	−2.6–−5.0	−2.5–0.0	0.1–2.5	2.6–5.0	5.1–7.5	≥7.6
Outdoor spaces and buildings	≤−3.1	−2.1–−3.0	−1.1–−2.0	−1.0–0.0	0.1–1.0	1.1–2.0	2.1–3.0	≥3.1
Transportation	≤−3.1	−2.1–−3.0	−1.1–−2.0	−1.0–0.0	0.1–1.0	1.1–2.0	2.1–3.0	≥3.1
Financial situation	≤−3.1	−2.1–−3.0	−1.1–−2.0	−1.0–0.0	0.1–1.0	1.1–2.0	2.1–3.0	≥3.1

Scoring system: Items with * should be recorded in the opposite direction (−2 = 2, −1 = 1, 0 = 0, 1 = −1, 2 = −2). Sum all scores of the AFCCQ for the AFCCQ total score. Sum all scores of separate domains for the domain specific score.

References

1. World Health Organization. *Global Age-Friendly Cities: A Guide*; World Health Organization: Geneva, Switzerland, 2007; ISBN 9789241547307.
2. Plouffe, L.; Kalache, A. Towards global age-friendly cities: Determining urban features that promote active aging. *J. Urban Health* **2010**, *87*, 33–739. [CrossRef] [PubMed]
3. Buffel, T.; Phillipson, C.; Rémillard-Boilard, S. Age-friendly cities and communities: New directions for research and policy. In *Encyclopedia of Gerontology and Population Aging*; Gu, D., Dupre, M.E., Eds.; Springer Nature: Cham, Switzerland, 2019. [CrossRef]
4. van Hoof, J.; Kazak, J.K.; Perek-Białas, J.M.; Peek, S.T.M. The challenges of urban ageing: Making cities age-friendly in Europe. *Int. J. Environ. Res. Public Health* **2018**, *15*, 2473. [CrossRef] [PubMed]
5. Chao, T.-Y.S. *Planning for Greying Cities. Age-Friendly City Planning and Design Research and Practice*; Routledge—Taylor & Francis Group: Abingdon, UK, 2018; ISBN 978-0-367-33190-0.
6. Buffel, T.; Handler, S.; Phillipson, C. (Eds.) *Age-friendly Cities and Communities. A Global Perspective*; Policy Press: Bristol, UK, 2019; ISBN 978-1-4473-3134-6.
7. Moulaert, T.; Garon, S. (Eds.) International perspectives on aging. In *Age-Friendly Cities and Communities in International Comparison—Political Lessons, Scientific Avenues, and Democratic Issues*; Springer International Publishing: Cham, Switzerland, 2016; Volume 14, ISBN 978-3-319-24029-9. [CrossRef]
8. Van Hoof, J.; Marston, H.R.; Brittain, K.R.; Barrie, H.R. Creating age-friendly communities: Housing and technology. *Healthcare* **2019**, *7*, 130. [CrossRef] [PubMed]
9. Van Hoof, J.; Kazak, J.K. Urban Ageing. *Indoor Built Env.* **2018**, *27*, 583–586. [CrossRef]
10. Greenfield, E.A.; Oberlink, M.; Scharlach, A.E.; Neal, M.B.; Stafford, P.B. Age-friendly community initiatives: Conceptual issues and key questions. *Gerontologist* **2015**, *55*, 191–198. [CrossRef]

11. World Health Organization. About the Global Network for Age-Friendly Cities and Communities. Available online: https://extranet.who.int/agefriendlyworld/who-network/ (accessed on 30 June 2020).
12. World Health Organization. *The Global Network for Age-Friendly Cities and Communities: Looking Back Over the Last Decade, Looking Forward to the Next*; World Health Organization: Geneva, Switzerland, 2018.
13. Buckner, S.; Mattocks, C.; Rimmer, M.; Lafortune, L. An evaluation tool for Age-Friendly and Dementia Friendly Communities. *Work. Older People* **2018**, *22*, 48–58. [CrossRef]
14. Buckner, S.; Pope, D.; Mattocks, C.; Lafortune, L.; Dherani, M.; Bruce, N. Developing Age-Friendly Cities: An evidence-based evaluation tool. *J. Popul. Ageing* **2019**, *12*, 203–223. [CrossRef]
15. World Health Organization. *Measuring the Age-Friendliness of Cities: A Guide to Using Core Indicators*; World Health Organization: Geneva, Switzerland, 2015; ISBN 9789241509695.
16. World Health Organization. *The Checklist of Essential Features of Age-Friendly Cities*; World Health Organization: Geneva, Switzerland, 2007.
17. Fulmer, T.; Patel, P.; Levy, N.; Mate, K.; Berman, A.; Peloton, L.; Beard, J.; Kalache, A.; Auerbach, J. Moving toward a global age-friendly ecosystem. *J. Am. Ger. Soc.* **2020**, in press. [CrossRef]
18. Marston, H.R.; van Hoof, J. "Who doesn't think about technology when designing urban environments for older people?" A case study approach to a proposed extension of the WHO's age-friendly cities model. *Int. J. Environ. Res. Public Health* **2019**, *16*, 3525. [CrossRef]
19. van Hoof, J.; Dikken, J.; Buttiġieġ, S.C.; van den Hoven, R.F.M.; Kroon, E.; Marston, H.R. Age-friendly cities in the Netherlands: An explorative study of facilitators and hindrances in the built environment and ageism in design. *Indoor Built Environ.* **2020**, *29*, 417–437. [CrossRef]
20. Chan, A.W.; Chan, H.Y.; Chan, I.K.; Cheung, B.Y.; Lee, D.T. An age-friendly living environment as seen by Chinese older adults: A "Photovoice" Study. *Int. J. Environ. Res. Public Health* **2016**, *13*, 913. [CrossRef] [PubMed]
21. King, A.C.; King, D.K.; Banchoff, A.; Solomonov, S.; Ben Natan, O.; Hua, J.; Gardiner, P.; Goldman Rosas, L.; Rodriguez Espinosa, P.; Winter, S.J.; et al. Employing participatory citizen science methods to promote age-friendly environments worldwide. *Int. J. Environ. Res. Public Health* **2020**, *17*, 1541. [CrossRef] [PubMed]
22. Barrie, H.; Soebarto, V.; Lange, J.; McCorry-Breen, F.; Walker, L. Using citizen science to explore neighbourhood influences on ageing well: Pilot project. *Healthcare* **2019**, *7*, 126. [CrossRef] [PubMed]
23. Luciano, A.; Pascale, F.; Polverino, F.; Pooley, A. Measuring age-friendly housing: A framework. *Sustainability* **2020**, *12*, 848. [CrossRef]
24. Flores, R.; Caballer, A.; Alarcón, A. Evaluation of an age-friendly city and its effect on life satisfaction: A two-stage study. *Int. J. Environ. Res. Public Health* **2019**, *16*, 5073. [CrossRef]
25. Zaman, A.U.; Thornton, K. Prioritization of local indicators for the development of an age-friendly city: A community perspective. *Urban Sci.* **2018**, *2*, 51. [CrossRef]
26. Garner, I.W.; Holland, C.A. Age-friendliness of living environments from the older person's viewpoint: Development of the Age-friendly Environment Assessment Tool. *Age Ageing* **2020**, *49*, 193–198. [CrossRef]
27. COSMIN. Consensus-Based Standards for Selection of Health Measurement Instruments. Available online: https://www.cosmin.nl/cosmin-tools/ (accessed on 11 August 2020).
28. Mokkink, L.B.; Terwee, C.B.; Patrick, D.L.; Alonso, J.; Stratford, P.W.; Knol, D.L.; Bouter, L.M.; de Vet, H.C.M. The COSMIN checklist for assessing the methodological quality of studies on measurement properties of health status measurement instruments: An international Delphi study. *Qual. Life Res.* **2010**, *19*, 539–549. [CrossRef]
29. de Vet, H.C.; Terwee, C.B.; Mokkink, L.B.; Knol, D.L. *Measurement in Medicine: A Practical Guide*; Cambridge University Press: Cambridge, UK, 2011. [CrossRef]
30. Bottenheft, C.; van Doleweerd, M.K.; van de Kraats, E.J.; Egter van Wissekerke, N.G.; Engbers, L.H. *TNO-Rapport: TNO 2015 R10311. Wijkdashboard: Age-Friendly City Den Haag*; TNO: The Hague, The Netherlands, 2015. (In Dutch)
31. AARP Public Policy Institute. AARP Livability Index—Great Neighborhoods for All Ages. 2020. Available online: https://livabilityindex.aarp.org/livability-defined (accessed on 23 July 2020).
32. Chief Secretary for Administration's Office. *Active and Healthy Ageing in Hong Kong*; Hong Kong Special Administrative Region Government: Hong Kong, China, 2017.
33. World Health Organization. Equity. Available online: https://www.who.int/healthsystems/topics/equity/en/ (accessed on 1 September 2020).

34. Lynn, M.R. Determination and quantification of content validity. *Nurs. Res.* **1986**, *35*, 382–386. [CrossRef]
35. Polit, D.F.; Beck, C.T.; Owen, S.V. Is the CVI an acceptable indicator of content validity? Appraisal and recommendations. *Res. Nurs. Health* **2007**, *30*, 459–467. [CrossRef]
36. Fabrigar, L.R.; Wegener, D.T.; MacCallum, R.C.; Strahan, E.J. Evaluating the use of exploratory factor analysis in psychological research. *Psychol. Methods* **1999**, *4*, 272. [CrossRef]
37. DeVellis, R.F. *Scale Development: Theory and Applications*; Sage: Los Angeles, CA, USA, 2016; Volume 26, ISBN 9781506341569.
38. Lee, W.C.; Godwin, A. Hermunstad Nave, A.L. Development of the engineering student integration instrument: Rethinking measures of integration. *J. Eng. Educ.* **2018**, *107*, 30–55. [CrossRef]
39. Lijzenga, J.; Gijsbers, V.; Poelen, J.; Tiekstra, C. *Ruimte voor Wonen. De Resultaten van het WoonOnderzoek Nederland 2018*; Ministry of the Interior and Kingdom Relations: The Hague, The Netherlands, 2018; Available online: https://www.woononderzoek.nl/document/Ruimte-voor-wonen--de-resultaten-van-het-WoON2018-(interactief)-/174 (accessed on 22 August 2020).
40. Tabachnick, B.G.; Fidell, L.S.; Ullman, J.B. *Using Multivariate Statistics*; Pearson: Boston, MA, USA, 2007; Volume 5, pp. 481–498. ISBN 9780134790541.
41. Matsunaga, M. How to factor-analyze your data right: Do's, don'ts, and how-to's. *Int. J. Psychol. Res.* **2010**, *3*, 97–110. [CrossRef]
42. Schumacker, R.E.; Lomax, R.G. *A Beginner's Guide to Structural Equation Modeling*, 2nd ed.; Lawrence Erlbaum Associates Publishers: Mahwah, NJ, USA, 2004; ISBN 1-4106-1090-X.
43. Shadfar, S.; Malekmohammadi, I. Application of Structural Equation Modeling (SEM) in restructuring state intervention strategies toward paddy production development. *Int. J. Acad. Res. Bus. Soc. Sci.* **2013**, *3*, 576. [CrossRef]
44. Hu, L.T.; Bentler, P.M. Evaluating model fit. In *Structural Equation Modelling: Concepts, Issues, and Applications*; Hoyle, R.H., Ed.; London Sage: London, UK, 1995; pp. 76–99. ISBN 0803953186.
45. Hu, L.; Bentler, P.M. Cutoff criteria for fit indexes in covariance structure analysis: Conventional criteria versus new alternations. *Struct. Equ. Model.* **1999**, *6*, 1–55. [CrossRef]
46. MacCallum, R.C.; Browne, M.W.; Sugawara, H.M. Power analysis and determination of sample size for covariance structure modeling. *Psychol. Methods* **1996**, *1*, 130–149. [CrossRef]
47. Hair, J.; Hult, C.; Ringle, C.M.; Sarstedt, M. *A Primer on Partial Least Squares Structural Equation Modeling (PLS-SEM)*; Sage: Los Angeles, CA, USA, 2014; ISBN 1452217440.
48. Brislin, R.W. Back-translation for cross-cultural research. *J. Cross Cult. Psychol.* **1970**, *1*, 185–216. [CrossRef]
49. Maneesriwongul, W.; Dixon, J.K. Instrument translation process: A methods review. *J. Adv. Nurs.* **2004**, *48*, 175–186. [CrossRef]
50. Costello, A.B.; Osborne, J.W. Best practices in exploratory factor analysis: Four recommendations for getting the most from your analysis. *Pract. Assess. Res. Eval.* **2005**, *10*, 1–9.
51. Netemeyer, R.G.; Bearden, W.O.; Sharma, S. *Scaling Procedures*; Sage Publications Inc.: Thousand Oaks, CA, USA, 2003. [CrossRef]
52. Van de Schoot, R.; Lugtig, P.; Hox, J. A checklist for testing measurement invariance. *Eur. J. Dev. Psychol.* **2012**, *9*, 486–492. [CrossRef]
53. Dikken, J.; Hoogerduijn, J.G.; Klaassen, S.; Lagerwey, M.D.; Shortridge-Baggett, L.; Schuurmans, M.J. The knowledge-about-older-patients-quiz (KOP-Q) for nurses: Cross-cultural validation between the Netherlands and United States of America. *Nurse Educ. Today* **2017**, *55*, 26–30. [CrossRef] [PubMed]
54. Sousa, V.D.; Rojjanasrirat, W. Translation, adaptation and validation of instruments or scales for use in cross-cultural health care research: A clear and user-friendly guideline. *J. Eval. Clin. Pract.* **2011**, *17*, 268–274. [CrossRef]
55. Buffel, T.; Phillipson, C.; Scharf, T. Ageing in urban environments: Developing 'age-friendly' cities'. *Crit. Soc. Policy* **2012**, *32*, 597–617. [CrossRef]
56. Scharf, T.; Phillipson, C.; Smith, A. Older people's perceptions of the neighbourhood: Evidence from socially deprived urban areas. *Sociol. Res. Online* **2003**, *8*, 153–164. [CrossRef]
57. Baraković, S.; Baraković Husić, J.; van Hoof, J.; Krejcar, O.; Maresova, P.; Akhtar, Z.; Melero, F.J. Quality of life framework for personalised ageing: A systematic review of ICT solutions. *Int. J. Environ. Res. Public Health* **2020**, *17*, 2940. [CrossRef]

58. Verkerk, M.J.; van Hoof, J.; Aarts, S.; de Koning, S.J.M.M.; van der Plaats, J.J. A neurological and philosophical perspective on the design of environments and technology for older people with dementia. *J. Enabling Technol.* **2018**, *12*, 57–75. [CrossRef]
59. Mundform, D.J.; Shaw, D.G.; Ke, T.L. Minimum sample size recommendations for conducting factor analyses. *Int. J. Test.* **2005**, *5*, 159–168. [CrossRef]
60. Wolf, E.J.; Harrington, K.M.; Clark, S.L.; Miller, M.W. Sample size requirements for structural equation models an evaluation of power, bias, and solution propriety. *Educ. Psychol. Meas.* **2013**, *73*, 913–934. [CrossRef]
61. Sideridis, G.; Simos, P.; Papanicolaou, A.; Fletcher, J. Using structural equation modeling to assess functional connectivity in the brain: Power and sample size considerations. *Educ. Psychol. Meas.* **2014**, *74*, 733–758. [CrossRef]

International Journal of
Environmental Research and Public Health

MDPI

Commentary

A Commentary on Blue Zones®: A Critical Review of Age-Friendly Environments in the 21st Century and Beyond

Hannah R. Marston [1,*], Kelly Niles-Yokum [2] and Paula Alexandra Silva [3]

1 Health & Wellbeing Strategic Research Area, School of Health, Wellbeing & Social Care, The Open University, Milton Keynes, Buckinghamshire MK7 6HH, UK
2 Department of Health and Public Management, College of Business & Public Management, University of La Verne, La Verne, CA 91750, USA; kniles-yokum@laverne.edu
3 Centre for Informatics and Systems (CISUC), Department of Informatics Engineering (DEI), University of Coimbra, 3030-290 Coimbra, Portugal; paulasilva@dei.uc.pt
* Correspondence: Hannah.Marston@open.ac.uk

Abstract: This paper explores the intersection of the World Health Organization's (WHO) concepts of age-friendly communities and The Blue Zones® checklists and how the potential of integrating the two frameworks for the development of a contemporary framework can address the current gaps in the literature as well as consider the inclusion of technology and environmental press. The commentary presented here sets out initial thoughts and explorations that have the potential to impact societies on a global scale and provides recommendations for a roadmap to consider new ways to think about the impact of health and wellbeing of older adults and their families. Additionally, this paper highlights both the strengths and the weaknesses of the aforementioned checklists and frameworks by examining the literature including the WHO age-friendly framework, the smart age-friendly ecosystem (SAfE) framework and the Blue Zones® checklists. We argue that gaps exist in the current literature and take a critical approach as a way to be inclusive of technology and the environments in which older adults live. This commentary contributes to the fields of gerontology, gerontechnology, anthropology, and geography, because we are proposing a roadmap which sets out the need for future work which requires multi- and interdisciplinary research to be conducted for the respective checklists to evolve.

Keywords: ageing; age in place; community; Coronavirus; COVID-19; gerontechnology; human centred design; older adults; rural planning; technology; smart ecosystem; smart islands

Citation: Marston, H.R.; Niles-Yokum, K.; Silva, P.A. A Commentary on Blue Zones®: A Critical Review of Age-Friendly Environments in the 21st Century and Beyond. *Int. J. Environ. Res. Public Health* **2021**, *18*, 837. https://doi.org/10.3390/ijerph18020837

Received: 29 November 2020
Accepted: 14 January 2021
Published: 19 January 2021

1. Introduction

There is a growing body of scholarly research [1,2] exploring how urban ageing impacts towns and communities in the Western world while taking an age-friendly approach based on the World Health Organization's (WHO) framework published in 2007 [3]. For nearly twenty years, scholarly research [1,2,4–11] has illustrated how many towns and communities have been working towards ensuring their respective environments include age-friendly features.

At the time of publication (2007), the age-friendly framework proposed by the WHO [3] provided a checklist that offered and afforded academics and policy-makers the opportunity to adapt key facets within their own environments. However, scholarly interest started to grow in the 1990s and at the beginning of the 21st century with regard to technology use by older people [12–28].

Moreover, research from the standpoint of gerontology and age-friendly cities and communities is limited to the domain of Blue Zones®. To date, existing research is taken from the standpoint of epidemiology ranging from dietary [29–35], depression and mental health [36], health, cardiovascular and heart disease [37–42], longevity [43–46], obesity, and physical activity [47] perspectives. Furthermore, while academe has known about

Blue Zones® for approximately 20 years, acknowledging that there is something special about these areas, there is a paucity of scholarly research from the social sciences stance. However, different Blue Zones® characteristics have not been incorporated into the WHO framework published in 2007 [3].

In this commentary, we aim to discuss Blue Zones® and how features of the age-friendly framework posited by the WHO [3] and the smart age-friendly ecosystem (SAfE) framework posited by Marston and van Hoof [48] can be considered for future integration into such environment(s). In particular, we aim to explore and understand how the respective frameworks [3,48] could be integrated in a variety of ways and settings to produce recommendations and notions for future work that could lead to the development of a contemporary framework specifically aimed at incorporating both the Blue Zones® concept and age friendly community principles, offering appropriate interventions and applicable solutions.

The work presented here is significant because it contributes to the fields of gerontology, geography, social sciences, social policy, industry, technology, and health. Furthermore, the work presented in this paper has the potential to impact societies on both national and international scales as it discusses the WHO age-friendly framework, which for 12 years has been used primarily as a marker for towns and cities in the Western world. Moreover, the smart age-friendly ecosystem (SAfE) [48] framework was posited by taking a case study approach using Milton Keynes, United Kingdom, as an exemplar, given the existing notions of a "new town", "smart city". This commentary aims to offer readers a framework as a means of forming an initial basis for future research, case studies and explorations, with a view to enhancing, developing, and improving the blueprint over time.

The content of this commentary is novel in that it bridges the gaps in existing literature from the field of gerontology whereby to date there is a paucity of literature surrounding Blue Zones® and their relationship(s) with the age-friendly cities and communities domain, digital technologies including the relationship(s) and connectors of digital technologies and Blue Zones®.

The outline of this commentary presents an overview of Blue Zones®, and contemporary literature surrounding Western Blue Zones® sites. Furthermore, in Section 3, we present the respective Blue Zones® checklists (Home, Kitchen, Bedroom, and Tribe) and in Section 4 we critically review/analysis of the four checklists. Section 5 discusses the features surrounding the WHO age-friendly and the smart age-friendly ecosystem (SAfE) frameworks. The discussion and conclusion—Section 6—sets out a roadmap for moving this debate forward and proposes recommendations for future steps.

2. Blue Zones®

In this section, we will explore what is meant by Blue Zones® and existing relevant research.

2.1. What Is a Blue Zones®?

The history of the Blue Zones® stems from the founder Dan Buettner, a National Geographic Fellow [49], who has to date discovered five places across the world labelled as Blue Zones®: 1. Okinawa (Japan), 2. Ogliastra Region, Sardinia (Italy), 3. Nicoya Peninsula (Costa Rica), 4. Ikaria (Greece), and Loma Linda (California).

Blue Zones® are places or regions which have a high concentration of centenarians in addition to clusters of people who have reached old age without disease and/or other health conditions such as obesity, cancer, diabetes, and heart problems [49]. Furthermore, Buettner [49] notes how individuals living in these areas or regions not only live longer, but their day-to-day lives are fulfilled with activity, citizens who experience good health, and positive engagements with their families and communities. A Blue Zones® team includes a myriad of team members who are anthropologists, dietitians, demographers, epidemiologists, and medical researchers. However, experts from the field of gerontology do not seem to be included [50].

Buettner and his team identified nine commonalities in four categories and practices across the five Blue Zones® regions and features in the Blue Zones® Solution [49].

These are: move—1. move naturally; right outlook—2. purpose and 3. downshift; eat wisely—4. 80% rule, 5. plant slant, and 6. wine at five; connect—7. right tribe, 8. loved ones first, and 9. belong. These factors are characterized as the Power of 9 and form a triangle, with move naturally at the top, and the notion of belong and the three factors, commonalities or practices forming the base [47,49].

A contemporary piece of research conducted by Riddell [50] puts forth the perspective of urban planning from the standpoint of the USA exploring and identifying correlations between urban planning and design, the physical environment, health, and wellbeing.

Furthermore, there have been additional experiments and explorations across the USA in an attempt to redevelop the areas/regions of Minnesota, California, and Iowa, implementing a Blue Zones® ethos. However, with the exception of Loma Linda—located in California—the other four Blue Zones® were created organically, isolated from their respective mainland regions. Riddell [50] highlights the completed projects across the USA which include: 1. Albert Lea—Minnesota, 2. California Beach Cities—a. Manhattan Beach, b. Hermosa Beach, and c. Redondo Beach, and finally 3. State of Iowa. Furthermore, there are four additional areas which are planned for re-engineering these regions into Blue Zones® and include, 1. Honolulu and Hilo—Hawaii, 2. Wisconsin, 3. Indiana, and 4. Klamath Falls—Oregon [50]. Below, we describe two of the experimental projects to understand how the Blue Zone concept, which was organically created in isolated regions, has been transferred to different regions of the USA.

2.2. *Albert Lea—Minnesota*

Albert Lea was the first region for Buettner [49] sought out for the Blue Zones® experiment, consulting public health officials at the University of Minnesota who in turn requested Buettner to measure and assess each campaign [50]. This town, as Riddell [50] notes, was chosen because it represents a "typical" American city, comprised of ~17.5 K residents [51], which was not too large nor was it too small and therefore could be a model for other regions and cities across the state and the country [50]. Moving forward, the Blue Zones® team chose a 20-mile "life radius" around homes and workplaces because this is where the main activity is conducted during the day [50].

Substantial financial support was provided by the American Association of Retired Persons (AARP), and the University of Minnesota—School of Public Health also joined the pilot project to assist the Blue Zones® team with their assessment of Albert Lea in 2009 [50]. A series of walking groups were formed and met up several times each week to answer whether the environment promoted walking [50]. Such groups, as Riddell [50] notes, are similar to the support groups or *Okinawa's moai* concept which affords physical activity by moving naturally and interacting with the right tribe, coupled with the sense of community. Another creation was developed and included the "walking school bus" which facilitated both parents and children who would usually use the bus to actually walk together to school. Riddell [50] highlights this notion and activity because of its popularity, resulting in older adults volunteering to walk with the "walking school bus". Considering the Power of 9, this approach and implementation engaged several factors, resulting in greater physical activity by all residents, community spirit, and a sense of purpose for the older adults when helping within their own community [49,50].

Both the natural and built environments were analysed, which included grocery stores, schools, restaurants, and included questions relating to the type of food available/displayed, whether the environment was walkable, and whether there were attractive public green spaces being used. Similar approaches have been conducted by van Hoof and colleagues [2] who conducted an assessment based on the age-friendly features in the Dutch municipalities of The Hague and Zoetermeer. By employing a qualitative photoproduction approach based on the Checklist of Essential Features of Age-Friendly cities [3], five neighbourhoods were assessed. Across the two municipalities, large visual representations were identified within five of the eight domains of the WHO age-friendly mode: 1. communication and information; 2. housing; 3. transportation; 4. community support and health services; 5. outdoor spaces and buildings [2,3]. The next area to be explored and assessed by the Blue Zones® team was the built environment which included areas such as grocery stores and their respective layouts. Additionally, the built environment also encompassed policy and budgetary areas which impact on the overall region or city. The Blue Zones® team identified in the grocery stores how healthy food products were not at eye level and instead were placed away from direct eye contact. Yet, unhealthy food products were clearly visible, placed at the checkout areas and on tables [49,50]. Moreover, the Blue Zones® team rearranged the produce throughout the stores, replacing sweets that were visible at the checkout points with fruit and nuts, followed by highlighting sweet potatoes and beans to the consumer with specific "Blue Zones labels" to signify the healthiness of the produce to the consumer [49,50]. Within the school environment, changes to snacks were also introduced and replaced with healthy options in vending machines, replacing crisps, biscuits, and fizzy drinks [49,50]. Buettner [49] highlights that the final stage within this town was working with the residents themselves and at a meeting comprised of 4000 people who pledged to become involved with the project and commenced restocking their own larders and house appliances with healthier food [49,50].

Riddell [50] purports that these changes at various levels of the community from the built environment to the individual ecosystems led to an overall positive change, by employing a three-pronged approach of community, public and private engagement, and partnership. This also included key leadership within the city such as the mayor, presidents of commerce, and educational superintendents, coupled with support and interest from the media, investing various energies into the project for the overall benefit of the town [49,50].

The impact of these changes across various intersections of the community from the home ecosystem, educational environments, and the wider built environments, including community support groups such as the walking groups, as Riddell [50] notes, led to substantial positive health benefits. The impact witnessed a 40% reduction associated with healthcare costs and 12,000 pounds lost (in weight) [49]. Further community and organizational changes were employed in the workplace, although Riddell does not state exactly what changes were made to these restaurants and workplaces.

2.3. State of Iowa

This initiative was rolled out in 2011 to support the State of Iowa to become a healthier state and resulted in the it becoming a demonstrator site. This included twenty towns used to create healthy living environments. One town—Spencer—was comprised of around 11,233 residents [52]. As Riddell [50] notes, this town found the challenge difficult (p. 58) because there was limited leadership and employment positions which resulted in assistance from Alberta Lea and the California beach cities. Riddell [50] notes how the size of this town, coupled with the importance of community engagement, motivation, and spirit, were crucial building blocks to bridge closer relationships [50].

However, between commencing this challenge, over a two-year period, Spencer town was named and granted the first certification for the Blue Zones® community [50] (p. 59) and, as noted in the previous section, included the integration and formed part of the Power of 9 concept [53,54], and fresh fruit and vegetables formed the ethos and activity of the Blue Zones® region. In Spencer town, a total of 36 community plots were created, enabling residents in the community to access fresh produce. These community plots facilitated additional factors within the Power of 9, including moving naturally, plant slant, the right tribe, and a sense of connection and belonging to the community and loved ones first. Riddell [50] also notes how this community created walking moais which facilitated and integrated additional factors surrounding the Blue Zones® ethos of healthy behaviour and happiness within the social and urban environments [53,54]. In the following section, the four Blue Zones® checklists are presented.

2.4. Blue Zones® Checklists

A Blue Zones® checklist is available through membership which offers individuals a tool to understand their home environment, social network, and guidance for improvement [55]. Below is an overview of each of the items of the checklist: 1. Home, 2. Kitchen, 3. Bedroom and 4. Tribe.

2.5. Home Checklist

The *Home* checklist [56] relates to various aspects and activities within the home environment and includes access to weighing scales to enable a person to weigh themselves daily, owning one television, the removal of power tools and instead using hand operated appliances, having the space to grow vegetables, owning a dog for companionship, and conducting physical activity through various and different forms of exercise. Additionally, owning additional transportation such as a bicycle has the potential to encourage regular exercise, as well as owning a variety of sports footwear and equipment (e.g., basketball, baseball, football, golf balls and clubs, inline skates, camping supplies, and running shoes) to motivate additional physical activity. Additionally, it is suggested that growing indoor plants will assist with exercise while maintaining the health of the plants; further space is needed to create a "destination room" which is a popular room in the home, and affords supplementary exercise by climbing the stairs, as well as disconnecting the automatic garage door to encourage a person to get out of their car and open the door. Removing the television remote would enable additional movement when changing the channel, while placing cushions on the floor to facilitate strength training of the thighs, glutes, and lower back.

This 13-item checklist in Table 1 displays a range of questions, answers and points relating to the respective answer(s), enabling a person to gain a maximum of 55 points. Table 1 displays the item checklists, the answer(s), points, and the purpose/additional information that a person can read and learn from.

Table 1. Questions from the "Home" checklist [56].

Checklist Item	Question	Answer(s)	Points	Purpose/Additional Information
1	Place a scale in a prominent spot in your home and weigh yourself daily. *	I do this now Or I don't do this	3 points 0 points	"Why do it: People who weigh themselves every day for two years weigh as much as 17 pounds less after two years than people who never weighed themselves. Daily weight checks take only seconds, and the results can provide powerful reinforcement."
2	Have only one TV in your home. *	I do this now Or I don't do this	5 points 0 points	How to do it: Have only one TV. Put it in a common room, preferably in a cabinet behind doors. The goal here is to nudge you away from screen time that detracts from physical activity and encourages overeating. Why do it: People who watch too much TV are more likely to be overweight. TV-watching actually lowers metabolism, makes us less active, and encourages us to eat junk food via commercials. Kids with a TV in their bedroom are 18 percent more likely to be (or become) obese and have lower grades. The happiest people watch only 30–60 min of TV per day.

Table 1. *Cont.*

Checklist Item	Question	Answer(s)	Points	Purpose/Additional Information
3	Replace power tools with hand tools. *	I do this now Or I don't do this	5 points 0 points	How to do it: Mow your lawn with a push lawn mower, shovel the snow with a hand shovel, and gather the leaves from your lawn with an old-fashioned rake instead of a leaf blower. Why do it: Shoveling, raking, and push-mowing are healthy and productive outdoor workouts. Some burn almost 400 calories an hour. In fact, mowing the lawn or raking leaves burns about the same number of calories as lifting weights.
4	Grown and maintain your own garden. *	I do this now Or I don't do this	3 points 0 points	How to do it: Plant a garden in your yard or take a look through the "how-to projects" from the National Gardening Association website (www.garden.org) and choose a project that's right for you and your space. Start planting and enjoying your delicious produce! Why do it: Gardening is common in all Blue Zones. This activity provides low-intensity range-of-motion exercise, stress reduction, and fresh vegetables. In fact, the CDC points out that you can burn 150 calories by gardening (standing) for approximately 30–45 min.
5	Own a dog. *	I do this now Or I don't do this	3 points 0 points	How to do it: Take a dog home from your local animal shelter or pet store. However, before you do so, visit the American Kennel Club website to determine if you are ready to commit to a dog and learn how to be a responsible dog owner: http://www.akc.org/public_education/responsible_dog_owneo.cfm. Why do it: Pets make for great companions and encourage you to walk or run. Researchers found that if you own a pet, you get over five hours of exercise a week without a lot of added effort. In fact, studies have shown that dog owners have lower rates of health problems compared to those who don't own a dog.
6	Own a bicycle (or clean or repair my current bicycle) and a bicycle helmet. *	I do this now Or I don't do this	5 points 3 points	How to do it: Buy a bike or fix your current bike; then do the same for other family members. Use good quality helmets to prevent injury. Why do it: People who live in Blue Zones areas use active transportation. Not only can you easily incorporate physical activity into your daily life if you own and use a bike, riding at a moderate speed burns approximately 235 calories per half hour. Additionally, wearing a bicycle helmet reduces the risk of serious head injury in crashes by as much as 85% and the risk for brain injury by as much as 88%.

Table 1. *Cont.*

Checklist Item	Question	Answer(s)	Points	Purpose/Additional Information
7	Own at least four of the following: basketball, baseball, football, golf balls and clubs, inline skates, camping supplies, running shoes. *	I do this now Or I don't do this	3 points 0 points	How to do it: Keep sporting equipment nearby to encourage physical activity. Why do it: Owning this equipment makes it easier to practice sports at home. Did you know that inline skating burns more calories than running track and field hurdles and that playing catch for only 30 min burns over 100 calories?
8	Have indoor plants throughout your home. *	I do this now Or I don't do this	3 points 0 points	How to do it: Pick up some pots, potting soil and some of your favorite greenery to place throughout your home. Golden Pothos Vines and Spider Plants are great starter plants and easy to maintain. Why do it: Did you know that watering plants burns the same amount of calories as stretching or walking? Besides their ability to clean the air, indoor plants have been proven to provide health benefits to people who interact with them. If you keep houseplants, then you'll be nudged to nurture them daily.
9	Create a destination room. *	I do this now Or I don't do this	5 points 0 points	How do I do it: Create a room on the top of your home in which you are fully immersed in what you're doing—where it's easy to engage in a hobby, read a book, or do a family activity. Include a large table for family projects, shelves filled with books, and plenty of light. Leave out the clock, TV, computer, or other distracting gadgets. Why do it: A popular room on another level of your home increases stair climbing. Did you know that you burn 10 calories per minute climbing up stairs and four calories per minute climbing down them?
10	Disconnect your garage door opener. *	I do this now Or I don't do this	5 points 0 points	How to do it: Stop using your electric garage door opener. Instead, open the door manually. Why do it: Getting out of the car, raising the door, and returning to the car rather than using a remote control will burn seven calories per minute. Doing this twice a day doesn't take much time, but will burn extra calories!
11	Create an indoor exercise area. *	I do this now Or I don't do this	5 points 0 points	How to do it: Designate a portion of a room in your home for your exercise equipment, stability ball, yoga mat, and/or weight set. Why do it: Exercising is made more convenient when you have a space in your home designated for that specific activity. You are more likely to use the equipment it if is easily accessible and visible. A study at the University of Florida found that women who exercised at home lost 25 pounds in 15 months and maintained that loss.

Table 1. *Cont.*

Checklist Item	Question	Answer(s)	Points	Purpose/Additional Information
12	Get rid of your TV remote. *	I do this now Or I don't do this	5 points 0 points	How to do it: Instead of using your TV remote to change the channel, walk over to your TV and manually switch stations. Why do it: Getting up and changing the channel manually 10 times per day will burn 100 calories.
13	Place cushions on the floor. *	I do this now Or I don't do this	5 points 0 points	How to do it: Instead of sitting on chairs and furniture all the time, sit on cushions on the floor. Why do it: Sitting on the floor works your thighs, glutes, and lower back each time you sit down and stand back up. Supporting yourself without a chair back improves posture and may help you burn up to an additional 130 calories each hour!

* Subscribers to the checklist can enter their email address and receive a copy of their Blue Zones® Home Checklist results.

Upon completion of the checklist the person can calculate their final score and review it to understand where they need to improve (Table 2).

Table 2. Points related to the "Home" checklist [56].

Number of Points	Explanation
55+	Blue Zones Home. You have deconvenienced your living environment in a way that allows you to mindlessly move your way to better health.
30–39	Almost There. You are well on your way to creating an ideal home environment.
15–29	On Your Way. When you begin to pair many of these behaviors together, you'll start engaging in physical activity more often. Which item is first on your list of changes? Get started on that right now.
Below 15	Just Getting Started. Everyone has to start somewhere. Begin the process by prioritizing the changes you want to make and start on them tomorrow.

2.5.1. Kitchen

The Kitchen checklist [57] suggests a person should place snacks into small bags, move the fruit and vegetables to the front of the fridge, while reducing the size of crockery and glassware in a bid to reduce consumption/overeating. Kitchen cupboards (e.g., a specific drawer for junk food) should be organised and all digital devices (e.g., television) should be removed from this environment. While the checklist suggests fruit should be placed at eye level to encourage healthier eating habits, mechanical kitchen appliances should be removed and replaced with hand operated ones. Table 3 displays the 10-item checklists, a range of answers and points relating to the respective answer(s), and the purpose/additional information that a person can read and learn from.

Table 3. Questions from the "Kitchen" checklist [57].

Checklist Item	Question	Answer(s)	Points	Purpose/Additional Information
1	Package your snacks in proportioned, small bags. *	I do this now Or I don't do this	5 points 0 points	How to do it: When you buy snacks like pretzels, portion them into small bags to avoid overeating. Why do it: Re-bagging your snacks will help you eat reasonably sized portions. Additionally, you actually burn more calories by preparing fresh meals and snacks.
2	Dedicate the top shelf of your refrigerator to fruits and vegetables. *	I do this now Or I don't do this	3 points 0 points	How to do it: Get in the habit of keeping your healthy foods on the front of the top shelf of your refrigerator. Why do it: Placing the healthy options at eye level will encourage you to snack mindfully.
3	Only own dinner plates that are 10" or smaller. *	I do this now Or I don't do this	5 points 0 points	How to do it: Replace your oversized plates with smaller 10" plates. Why do it: Eating smaller plates can promote smaller portions. Over the last 20 years, the average U.S. dinner plate has grown to over 12 inches. During the same timeframe we are eating 22 percent more calories. The easiest, mindless way to eat less is to eat off smaller plates.
4	Drink beverages (except for water) out of smaller glasses. *	I do this now Or I don't do this	3 points 0 points	How to do it: Replace your big slurp drinking glasses with smaller glasses. Why do it: Larger glasses may increase consumption.
5	Create a junk food drawer. *	I do this now Or I don't do this	5 points 0 points	How to do it: Put unhealthy snacks and food out of eyes' reach on bottom shelves or behind cabinet doors. Label it "Junk Food." Why do it: Most junk food is consumed because you see it and it looks good. If you're going to have junk food in your house, hiding it from your line of vision will dramatically decrease consumption.
6	Pre-plate your food. *	I do this now Or I don't do this	5 points 3 points	How to do it: Plate your entire meal before sitting down at the table. Avoid eating family style by leaving the serving dishes on the counter. Why do it: Leave the serving dishes on the counter—not on the table—that way, if you really are hungry for seconds, you'll be forced to stand up and walk to the kitchen.
7	Remove the TV from your kitchen and dining room. *	I do this now Or I don't do this	5 points 0 points	How to do it: Remove the TV from your eating environment. Why do it: When other things are going on in your eating environment, you are more likely to pay attention to them rather than the food you are consuming. Avoid multi-tasking while you eat by turning off the TV and radio. Practice this habit while you're at work, too—try not to work while eating. Take some time away from your desk to eat lunch

Table 3. *Cont.*

Checklist Item	Question	Answer(s)	Points	Purpose/Additional Information
8	Put a filled fruit bowl on your countertop. *	I do this now Or I don't do this	3 points 0 points	How to do it: Take a fruit bowl you already have and put it on your countertop in a well-lit, prominent place. Why do it: Placing the healthy options in convenient, eye-level locations will encourage you to snack mindfully. Keeping the fruit bowl filled will also encourage you to buy a variety of fresh produce items.
9	Use hand operated kitchen appliances. *	I do this now Or I don't do this	3 points 0 points	How do I do it: Get rid of your electric can opener and use a hand operated one instead. Also get a potato masher and garlic press, rather than an electric mixer. Why do it: Manual kitchen tasks encourage hand and arm strengthening. Try squeezing fruit juice, mashing potatoes or beans, and opening cans manually.
10	Place a longevity food list on your refrigerator. *	I do this now Or I don't do this	5 points 0 points	How to do it: Create a list with the best longevity foods (nuts, whole grain bread, beans, fruit & vegetables) and the worst junk food (salty snacks, sweetened sugary drinks, processed meats, packaged sweets) and display it on your refrigerator. Why do it: These documents list the best longevity foods to have in your kitchen at all times and the worst junk foods to keep out of your kitchen. They will serve as environmental nudges to help you become more conscious of your consumption.

* Subscribers to the checklist can enter their email address and receive a copy of their Blue Zones® Kitchen Checklist results.

Upon completion, the person can calculate their final score and review it to understand where they need to improve (Table 4), enabling a person to gain a maximum of 40 points.

Table 4. Points related to the "Kitchen" checklist [57].

Number of Points	Explanation
35+	Blue Zones Kitchen. You have set up your eating environment in a way that allows you to eat healthy meals and snacks. Can you get yourself all the way to scoring 40/40 points?
25–34	Mindful Eater. You are well on your way to creating an ideal eating environment. What other changes are you going to make to have a Blue Zones Kitchen?
15–24	On Your Way. When you begin to pair many of these behaviors together, you'll start seeing a healthier environment. Which item is first on your list of changes? Get started on that right now.
Below 15	Just Getting Started. Everyone has to start somewhere. Begin the process by prioritizing the changes you want to make and start on them tomorrow.

2.5.2. Bedroom

The Bedroom checklist [58] relates to one's sleep patterns, and the comfort of the person's bed/mattress and/or pillows, while it is suggested the room temperature should be set to a specific temperature, and the ambience (e.g., lights) should be considered. Individuals should consider removing digital devices (e.g., television, computers, alarm clocks) from this space and to facilitate relaxation a person should consider introducing lavender. Additionally, windows should be larger. This 11-item checklist, presented in Table 5, displays a range of answers and points relating to the respective answer(s), enabling a person to gain a maximum of 45 points, in addition to supplementary information relating to each item.

Table 5. Questions from the "Bedroom" checklist [58].

Checklist Item	Question	Answer(s)	Points	Purpose/Additional Information
1	Know your snore score *.	I do this now Or I want to do this	5 points 0 points	How to do it: Determine your snore score by taking the short assessment below. If you answer "yes" to any of the questions, discuss your symptoms with a medical provider. Why do it: The Snore Score was developed by the American Sleep Apnea Association to help individuals assess their risk of sleep apnea, which is a medical condition that can impair sleep and cause health problems. It is important to identify whether sleep problems are due to a medical condition so the condition can be treated early and appropriately. Are you a loud and/or regular snorer? Have you been observed to gasp or stop breathing during sleep? Do you feel tired or groggy upon awakening, or do you awaken with a headache? Are you often tired or fatigued during the wake time hours? Do you fall asleep sitting, reading, watching TV or driving? Do you often have problems with memory or concentration? If you have one or more of these symptoms you are at higher risk for having obstructive sleep apnea. If you are also overweight, have a large neck, and/or have high blood pressure the risk increases even further. If you or someone close to you answers "yes" to any of the above questions, you should discuss your symptoms with your physician or a sleep specialist. Or ask the American Sleep Apnea Association for more information on the diagnosis and treatment of sleep apnea. Different treatment options exist; which is right for you depends upon the severity of your apnea and other aspects of the disorder. Talk to your doctor about choices. Untreated, obstructive sleep apnea can be extremely serious and cannot be ignored. You may also be interested in attending a meeting of an ASAA A.W.A.K.E. group (A.W.A.K.E. stands for "Alert, Well, And Keeping Energetic," characteristics that are uncommon in people with untreated sleep apnea.) Contact the ASAA for more information about one in your area.

Table 5. *Cont.*

Checklist Item	Question	Answer(s)	Points	Purpose/Additional Information
2	Own a comfortable mattress and comfortable pillows *	I do this now Or I want to do this	3 points 0 points	How to do it: Mattresses should be replaced every 8–10 years. Make sure that your mattress is not sagging or not supporting you comfortably during sleep. When choosing a mattress, spend at least 10 min testing it out before buying. Choose pillows that support your head and neck and are comfortable to you. Why do it: Having a comfortable mattress and comfortable pillows are important to getting a good night's sleep. Getting a good night sleep improves productivity, physical and emotional health, and longevity.
3	Set the temperature in your bedroom to 65 °F at night. *	I do this now Or I want to do this	5 points 0 points	How to do it: Set your thermostat to 65 F at bedtime. If you have a programmable thermostat, program it to automatically adjust to 65 F during sleeping hours. Why do it: Temperatures below 54 F or above 75 F can actually wake you up at night. The ideal temperature for sleep is around 65 F. If it feels a little colder than you'd like, grab a couple of extra blankets.
4	Dim the lights an hour before bed *	I do this now Or I want to do this	3 points 0 points	How to do it: Dim the lights in your home an hour before you go to sleep. Why do it: Practicing good sleep hygiene is the first step to getting the optimal 7–8 h of sleep each night. Dimming the lights before bedtime prepares your body for sleep, allowing you to fall asleep faster and stay asleep longer.
5	Remove digital alarm clocks or turn the clock so it is facing away from the bedside *	I do this now Or I want to do this	3 points 0 points	How to do it: Remove digital alarm clocks from your bedroom or turn your clock away from your bedside so the time is not visible to you. Why do it: The light from digital alarm clocks can disrupt sleep. In addition, hiding your clock from your line of sight will help you avoid clock watching during the night.
6	Hang light blocking window shades in the bedroom *	I do this now Or I want to do this	5 points 3 points	How to do it: Hang dark shades and heavy drapery that can block out all outside light when drawn. Why do it: Light can be disruptive to sleep, even light from a clock or a computer. Make your room as dark as possible for the best sleep.
7	Remove the TV and computer from the bedroom. *	I do this now Or I want to do this	5 points 0 points	How to do it: Remove all screens from your bedroom including televisions, computers and cell phones. Why do it: The bedroom should only be used for sleep and sex. Removing electronic screens from the bedroom helps reinforce the association between the bed and sleep. In addition, artificial light from screens including digital clocks can disrupt sleep.

Table 5. *Cont.*

Checklist Item	Question	Answer(s)	Points	Purpose/Additional Information
8	Remove all phones (including cell phones and land line phones) from your bedroom. *	I do this now Or I want to do this	5 points 0 points	How to do it: Remove all phones from the bedroom. Why do it: Removing phones from the bedroom minimizes interruptions to sleep. The 2011 Sleep in America Poll conducted by the National Sleep Foundation found that cell phones were a sleep disturbance. Twenty percent of generation Y'ers and 18% of generation Z'ers polled said that they are awakened after they go to bed by a phone call, text message or email at least a few nights a week.
9	Put a lavender plant next to the bed *	I do this now Or I want to do this	3 points 0 points	How to do it: Purchase a lavender plant from your local florist or sprinkle a little lavender essential oil on your sheets. Why do it: The smell of lavender is calming, soothing, and helps induce sleep.
10	Install double paned windows in the bedroom *	I do this now Or I want to do this	3 points 0 points	How to do it: Install double paned windows in your bedroom. Why do it: Double paned windows help to block out noise, which can be disruptive to sleep. Another way to block out unwanted sounds is to use earplugs or use "white noise" such as a fan, air cleaner or sound conditioner.
11	Use the bedroom only for sleep and sex *	I do this now Or I want to do this	3 points 0 points	How to do it: Avoid doing work, watching TV, using the computer, or doing anything else that might agitate you in your bedroom. Use your bedroom only for sleep and sex. Why do it: Your bedroom environment should be a comfortable and relaxing place that promotes sleep. Avoiding activities that may lead to stress is one way to ensure the bedroom is a place associated with calm and sleep.

* Subscribers to the checklist can enter their email address and receive a copy of their Blue Zones® Bedroom Checklist results.

Once a person has completed their checklist for the bedroom environment, they can calculate the number of points they have gained and review Table 6 to understand how this specific environment is enriching their health, wellbeing, and lifestyle.

Table 6. Points related to the "Bedroom" checklist [58].

Number of Points	Explanation
35+	Blue Zones Kitchen. You have set up your eating environment in a way that allows you to eat healthy meals and snacks. Can you get yourself all the way to scoring 40/40 points?
25–34	Mindful Eater. You are well on your way to creating an ideal eating environment. What other changes are you going to make to have a Blue Zones Kitchen?
15–24	On Your Way. When you begin to pair many of these behaviors together, you'll start seeing a healthier environment. Which item is first on your list of changes? Get started on that right now.
Below 15	Just Getting Started. Everyone has to start somewhere. Begin the process by prioritizing the changes you want to make and start on them tomorrow.

2.5.3. Tribe

The Tribe checklist [59] relates to a person's lifestyle activities and behaviours, their beliefs, their social networks, their weight, their self-perceived happiness, and feelings of loneliness and social isolation. This 10-item checklist, displayed in Table 7, displays a range of answers and points relating to the respective answer(s) enabling a person to gain a maximum of 65 points. Unlike Tables 1, 3, and 5, there is no explanation to a person about their total score—instead, the person is required to submit their scores online and a person completing this also has the option to include friends who can also answer the same questions.

Table 7. Questions the "Tribe" checklist asks individuals [59].

Checklist Item	Question	Answer(s)	Points
1	In the past month, how many days did you engage in mild or rigorous physical activity (taking stairs, walks, gardening, exercise, etc.)? *	Never Rarely Often	0 points 3 points 5 points
2	During the past month, how often has this person felt sad or depressed? *	Never Rarely Often	5 points 3 points 0 points
3	During the past month, how many days has this person felt lonely? *	Never Rarely Often	5 points 3 points 0 points
4	Does this person smoke? *	No Yes	5 points 0 points
5	Does this person use illegal drugs? *	No Yes	5 points 0 points
6	On average, how many alcoholic drinks does the person have in a typical day? *	None One Two or more	0 points 1 = 3 points 2 or more = 5 points
7	How often does the person participate in social activities? *	Never Once a week More than once a week	0 points 3 points 5 points
8	How often does the person attend religious activities? *	Less than once a week Weekly or more	0 points 5 points
9	Is the person: *	Healthy weight Overweight or obese	5 points 0 points
10	Rate your happiness *	on a scale of 1–10 where 10 represents the best possible life for you and 0 represents the worst possible life for you. What number do you give yourself (or your friends) now?	User inputs their rating into an input box on the website

* Subscribers to the checklist can enter their email address and receive a copy of their Blue Zones® Tribe Checklist results.

It is worth noting that, on the website, there is an option for additional calculations for 1–2 friends, using the same questions above. For the *Tribe* checklist, the person can gain a maximum of 65 points. There is no additional information relating to the total score. However, the person can submit their scores and also print out the related information, enabling the person to look at areas of where they need to improve. In the following section, we provide a critical review of the four checklists presented above.

3. Critical Review

In this section, we provide a critical review/analysis of the four checklists presented in the previous section. To conduct this review/analysis we draw on the work by Munthe-Kaas and colleagues [60] who conducted a systematic mapping of 25 checklists in a bid to assess transferability.

In the respective review, Munthe-Kaas et al. [60] propose nine themes as a way of evaluating content analysis of checklists. In the following sections, we present each of the four Blue Zones® checklists (Home, Kitchen, Bedroom and Tribe) and their viability of transferability against the respective themes: 1. Population, 2. Intervention:, 2a, Intervention characteristics, 2b: Intervention delivery, 3: Implementation Context: 3a. Service providers (individuals), 3b. Implementing organization, 4. Comparison intervention, 5. Outcomes, 6. Environmental context, and 7. Researcher conduct, proposed by Munthe-Kaas et al. [60].

3.1. Overview of Commonalities across Checklists and Analysis

Reviewing all of the checklists against the first theme, *Population*, there is no specific information and/or context presented associated with the respective populations and their characteristics. Munthe-Kaas et al. [60] note that this theme does not only include demographic information but also additional attributes such as health conditions, illness, the acceptability, or reception of the respective checklists by users/subscribers of the checklists, their respective location (e.g., country, state/county, physical space), personnel support, and/or social networks.

3.2. "Home"—Critical Review

In Table 8, the transferability of the "Home" checklist across the 9 themes is limited. Primarily, the items in this checklist are associated with physical activity, weight loss, and tranquillity. However, this checklist and its respective descriptions (Table 1) do not contextualise various populations environments. For example, Item 4—"Grow and maintain your own garden"—aims to facilitate healthy and light physical activities and living. Yet, it assumes that everyone has a garden or at least access to a garden to potentially grow vegetables. This is not the case for many people across the life course, in particular those who live in inner-city housing, who may not even have a balcony, let alone green space (e.g., allotment) to grow their own vegetables.

Item 9, "Create a destination room", assumes that the person will live in a home that affords the luxury of creating a tranquil space. However, for many people, they do not have the space to create a "destination room" and some people choose (or have no other option due to their financial status) to live in a single-story environment (e.g., apartment). Additionally, this checklist does not acknowledge multigenerational living or adults who are ageing without children (AWOC) [61–64]. These two forms of living also impact on the home space and can change quickly—be it through ill health or chaos. Furthermore, this type of societal living arrangement impacts the home environment considerably and, as we move forward into the 21st century, this should be reflected in future iterations of frameworks and domains (e.g., gerontology, gerontechnology, planning, urban design, and social sciences).

Table 8. Critical review of the "Home" checklist based on the systematic mapping by Munthe-Kaas et al. [60].

Blue Zone Checklist	Checklist Item	Mapping of Themes								
		Population	Intervention Characteristics	Intervention Delivery	Individual Service Providers	Implementing Organizations	Comparison Intervention	Outcomes	Environmental Context	Researcher Conduct
Home	Place a scale in a prominent spot in your home and weigh yourself daily	-	-	-		-	-	✓	-	-
	Have only one TV in your home	-	-	-	-	-	-	✓	✓	-
	Replace power tools with hand tools	-	-	-	-	-	-	✓	-	-
	Grown and maintain your own garden	-	-	-	-	-	-	✓	-	-
	Own a dog	-	-	-	-	-	-	✓	-	-
	Own a bicycle (or clean or repair my current bicycle) and a bicycle helmet	-	-	-	-	-	-	✓	-	-
	Own at least four of the following: basketball, baseball, football, golf balls and clubs, inline skates, camping supplies, running shoes.	-	-	-	-	-	-	✓	-	-
	Have indoor plants throughout your home	-	-	-	-	-	-	-	✓	-

Table 8. *Cont.*

Blue Zone Checklist	Checklist Item	Mapping of Themes								
		Population	Intervention Characteristics	Intervention Delivery	Individual Service Providers	Implementing Organizations	Comparison Intervention	Outcomes	Environmental Context	Researcher Conduct
	Create a destination room	-	-	-	-	-	-	-	✓	-
	Disconnect your garage door opener	-	-	-	-	-	-	✓	✓	-
	Create an indoor exercise area	-	-	-	-	-	-	✓	✓	-
	Get rid of your TV remote	-						✓	-	-
	Place cushions on the floor	-	-	-	-	-	-	✓	✓	-

Finally, the "Home" checklist makes some assumptions based on individual and environmental circumstances (Table 8). For example, it assumes that an individual lives in an environment that allows pets, has space for a garden, has a garage, and a separate space for an exercise area. From a physical perspective, not everyone can sit on the floor, or can use hand tools, or practice the sports listed here. As previously noted, information surrounding population characteristics is sparse and does not reflect the respective circumstances of a person's living situation.

3.3. "Kitchen"—Critical Review

In Table 9, the transferability of the "Kitchen" checklist across the 9 themes is limited. Primarily, the items in this checklist are associated with white goods (e.g., fridge), weight loss, and physical space in the living environment. However, this checklist and its respective descriptions (Table 3) do not contextualise various populations environments.

For example, Item 3—"Only own dinner plates that are 10" or smaller"—aims to reduce portion sizes and is set within an American context. There is no information relating to other eating and lifestyle habits surrounding populations living in different continents (e.g., Europe, Asia, etc.). Item 5, "Create a junk food drawer", suggests hiding junk food implying it is more likely to be consumed when visible. However, there is a lack of acknowledgement of prospective multigenerational living circumstances and an assumption that the primary aim is healthier eating/weight loss. Additionally, Item 6—"Pre-plate your food"—aims to reduce and avoid "eating family style by leaving the serving dishes on the counter". As noted in the description (Table 3), if a person is hungry and wants additional servings they can walk to the counter and reduce the temptation to automatically have a second serving. Item 9, "Use hand operated kitchen appliances", assumes that people have the dexterity in their hands to manually use kitchen appliances. However, for some people with chronic illnesses, health conditions and disabilities, using manual appliances is not possible; this is not reflected nor considered in the additional information provided against this item. As previously noted there is no information relating to or associated with population characteristics, suggesting that items such as Item 9 have the potential to alienate many people across the life course from engaging with such a checklist. Item 10, "Place a longevity food list on your refrigerator", has the potential to be adapted for people who may have smart fridges and/or who shop online. For example, while such a list can enable people to remember the good and bad foods to have in their diet, when stocks are getting low, there is the potential to enable Internet of Things (IoT) appliances [65,66] to reorder. Similarly, if a person uses online shopping as their primary method of shopping, then they are able to add such items to their shopping list in preparation for their next delivery.

The "Kitchen" Checklist assumes that an individual lives in an environment whereby they have a kitchen, the person has the space to allow for extra items such as bowls for fruit which in turn can be placed on the countertop. From a physical perspective, not everyone can operate hand appliances or owns appliances, or can reach the top shelf of their refrigerator—if they own one. There are many instances where individuals do not have much choice about the food they have on hand or consume.

3.4. Bedroom Critical Review

As displayed in Table 10, the transferability of the "Bedroom" checklist across the 9 themes is limited. Primarily, the 11 items in this checklist are associated with technology (e.g., TV/computer), physical space and household items (e.g., curtains), temperature, ambience, and bedding.

Table 9. Critical review of the "Kitchen" checklist based on the systematic mapping by Munthe-Kaas et al. [60].

Blue Zone Checklist	Checklist Item	Mapping of Themes									
		Population	Intervention Characteristics	Intervention Delivery	Implementation Context	Individual Service Providers	Implementing Organizations	Comparison Intervention	Outcomes	Environmental Context	Researcher Conduct
Kitchen	Package your snacks in proportioned, small bags	-	-	-	-	-	-	-	✓	-	-
	Dedicate the top shelf of your refrigerator to fruits and vegetables	-	-	-	-	-	-	-	✓	✓	-
	Only own dinner plates that are 10" or smaller	-	-	-	-	-	-	-	✓	-	-
	Drink beverages (except for water) out of smaller glasses	-	-	-	-	-	-	-	✓	-	-
	Create a junk food drawer	-	-	-	-	-	-	-	✓	-	-
	Pre-plate your food	-	-	-	-	-	-	-		-	-
	Remove the TV from your kitchen and dining room	-	-	-	-	-	-	-	✓	✓	-
	Put a filled fruit bowl on your countertop	-	-	-	-	-	-	-	✓	-	-
	Use hand operated kitchen appliances	-	-	-	-	-	-	-	✓	-	-
	Place a longevity food list on your refrigerator	-	-	-	-	-	-	-	✓	-	-

Table 10. Critical review of the "Bedroom" checklist based on the systematic mapping by Munthe-Kaas et al. [60].

Blue Zone Checklist	Checklist Item	Mapping of Themes								
		Population	Intervention Characteristics	Intervention Delivery	Individual Service Providers	Implementing Organizations	Comparison Intervention	Outcomes	Environmental Context	Researcher Conduct
Bedroom	Know your snore score	-	✓	-	-	-	-	✓	-	-
	Own a comfortable mattress and comfortable pillows	-	-	-	-	-	-	✓	-	-
	Set the temperature in your bedroom to 65 °F at night	-	-	-	-	-	-	-	✓	-
	Dim the lights an hour before bed	-	-	-	-	-	-	-	✓	-
	Remove digital alarm clocks or turn the clock so it is facing away from the bedside	-	-	-	-	-	-	-	✓	-
	Hang light blocking window shades in the bedroom	-	-	-	-	-	-	-	✓	-
	Remove the TV and computer from the bedroom	-	-	-	-	-	-	-	✓	-
	Remove all phones (including cell phones and land line phones) from your bedroom.	-	-	-	-	-	-	-	✓	-
	Put a lavender plant next to the bed	-	-	-	-	-	-	-	✓	-
	Install double paned windows in the bedroom	-	-	-	-	-	-	-	✓	-
	Use the bedroom only for sleep and sex	-	-	-	-	-	-	-	✓	-

Item 1, "Know your snore score", relates to one's sleep patterns and habits. In this item, additional information is provided by various sleep associations within the context of America. However, and unfortunately, there is no scholarly work cited to support this item. Furthermore, there are additional questions for people to consider and to follow up, on their own accord (Table 5). Item 2, "Own a comfortable mattress and comfortable pillows" aims to facilitate positive sleep which in turn has the potential to translate into greater productivity and improve overall health and wellbeing. However, purchasing a good mattress is not cheap and this may be beyond many people's financial means. Additionally, while a mattress may or should be replaced nearly every decade, this too can become expensive and wasteful from the standpoint of recycling and sustainability. Item 3, "Set the temperature in your bedroom to 65 °F at night", does not account for various temperature differences found in different continents (e.g., Scandinavia) or the type of materials and age of the housing when built. For some people who live in housing that has been poorly built and insulated, heating would be required during the colder months and may not have the option of setting a specific temperature. For some people who live in housing that is historical, placed in a conservation area and is generally 100–200 years old, heating a room to a certain temperature is not possible because they would need to ensure the temperature is appropriate for them to go to bed, reducing damp and potential health issues resulting from a cold room/living space. However, with recent innovative technologies such as the IoT, there is the option to set individual rooms within the living space to different temperatures that can be set prior to one coming home from work or other outdoor activities [67]. Similarly, this type of technology can also be used for lighting (Item 4) on the Bedroom checklist, and via the various products available on the market, dimming lights can be set for various times of the evening and of the day. For more information relating to IoT devices implemented into real world settings, see Marston and van Hoof [48], and Marston et al. [68–71]. Item 10, "Install double paned windows in the bedroom", assumes users of this checklist own their own home. For people who are renting, which can be more common in European countries and outside of the USA, installing a double paned window may not be possible because of the tenancy agreement and other respective regulations.

Finally, the "Bedroom" checklist assumes that an individual has access to a separate bedroom coupled with the choice of where and how they sleep or rest. Some bedrooms do not have windows and even if they do, not every person can afford to put in new windows. Additionally, a remote control may sometimes be the only option a person has to operate their television and, given the phenomenal rise of smart TVs, the notion of getting up and walking to the television to change a channel may simply not be possible. Furthermore, lighting, temperature, and alarm clocks may not be a matter of personal preference but rather a matter of personal safety, and as noted above, the IoT can afford individuals the opportunity to take control of lighting, temperature, and safety on their own.

3.5. Tribe Critical Review

Table 11 highlights the questions posed in the "Tribe" checklist [59] (Table 7) and analysis of the checklist based on the Munthe-Kaas et al. [60] framework highlights two primary themes: *outcomes* and *environment*. The wording of the items from this checklist is different compared to the other checklists, requiring the individual to self-report or to report on someone else's behalf. Depending on who is completing this checklist, a complete overview may not be ascertained because if a third party is completing the checklist on behalf of someone else, they may not know how many units of alcohol that person drinks, or whether they take part in religious activities, or their level of happiness, or whether they feel lonely, etc.

Table 11. Critical review of the "Tribe" checklist based on the systematic mapping by Munthe-Kaas et al. [60].

Blue Zone Checklist	Check-List Item	Mapping of Themes								
		Population	Intervention Characteristics	Intervention Delivery	Individual Service Providers	Implementing Organizations	Comparison Intervention	Outcomes	Environmental Context	Researcher Conduct
Tribe	In the past month, how many days did you engage in mild or rigorous physical activity (taking stairs, walks, gardening, exercise, etc.)?	-	-	-	-	-	-	✓	-	-
	During the past month, how often has this person felt sad or depressed?	-	-	-	-	-	-	✓	-	-
	During the past month, how many days has this person felt lonely?	-	-	-	-	-	-	✓	✓	-
	Does this person smoke?	-	-	-	-	-	-	✓	-	-
	Does this person use illegal drugs?	-	-	-	-	-	-	✓	-	-
	On average, how many alcoholic drinks does the person have in a typical day?	-	-	-	-	-	-	✓	-	-
	How often does the person participate in social activities?	-	-	-	-	-	-	-	✓	-
	How often does the person attend religious activities?	-	-	-	-	-	-	-	✓	-
	Is the person Healthy weight, overweight or obese	-	-	-	-	-	-	✓	-	-
	Rate your happiness	-	-	-	-	-	-	✓	-	-

The "Tribe" checklist [59] assumes that an individual lives in an environment that allows for physical exercise and can participate in something fitting the definition of exercise; other items included religious activities and social participation, including the number of individuals in one "Tribe" should be viewed from a variety of situational circumstances including preferences. There is a clear distinction to being "lonely" and being "alone".

3.6. Summary

There is little theoretical underpinning associated with the items presented in each of the four checklists in addition to a paucity of research supporting the evaluation of the checklists. As noted in the previous sections, the four checklists seem to be posed in the context of the USA with little consideration for other citizens located in different continents. Furthermore, additional consideration and questioning should be considered when aligning these checklists with the five Blue Zones® and whether there would be similar mapping outcomes. Given the healthy ageing narrative, the concept of incorporating a life course perspective for residents/citizens within the Blue Zones® and who live in other countries and who may be accessing the checklists for their own personal use is needed to fully gauge the understanding and respective situation of a person. Additionally, with this paucity of theoretical underpinning coupled with the notion of implementing a life course perspective, there is the possibility of facilitating actors to capture and complement future data collections, including qualitative data including observations, diaries, and narratives from all citizens not just older people. Access to healthcare, socioeconomic status, age, physical ability, and other factors play important roles in fully understanding one's personal and environmental circumstances.

Our critique of these checklists is intended to widen the perspective of diversity and of the human experience related to older adults and persons with different levels of ability, such as those with chronic health conditions, disabilities, or dementia. Additionally, consideration of the variety of environments in which individuals live is critical for an inclusive approach. In the following section, we explore age-friendly frameworks and approaches that may assist future iterations of Blue Zones® checklists [56–59] and bridge future developments in these two domains.

4. Theoretical Approaches and Frameworks to Age-Friendly Cities and Ecosystems

To date there has been a wealth of research surrounding age-friendly cities and further reading can be found via the works of Marston and van Hoof [48], Marston and Samuels [67], Marston et al. [68], Buffel et al. [7,10,72], and van Hoof et al. [2,6,73], which provide an extensive overview of literature surrounding age-friendly research.

However, the existing work surrounding this framework has been conducted by Buffel et al. [72], Plouffe and Kalache [4], and Rowles [74] who have previously described the historical efforts of the WHO in a bid to positively participate, connect, and support different cities and communities in the remit of the WHO age-friendly initiative in converting respective cities and communities through development processes and following the "Checklist of Essential Features of Age-Friendly Cities" [3] to become more "age-friendly". With this growing body of scholarly work which discusses the WHO age-friendly framework [3] (Figure 1) in conjunction with a recent extended version to this framework proposed by Marston and van Hoof [48] (Figure 2), this contemporary research has identified novel areas for bridging gaps in the literature and working in multi- and cross-disciplinary teams to advance the narrative of this domain.

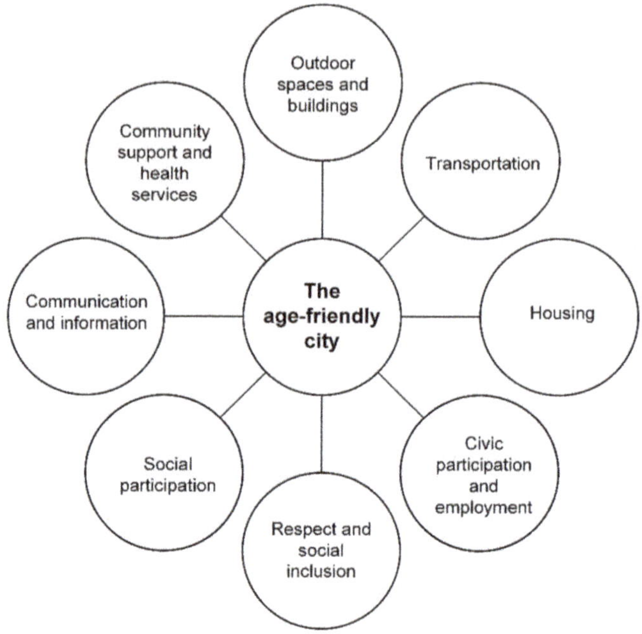

Figure 1. The eight domains of an age-friendly city [3].

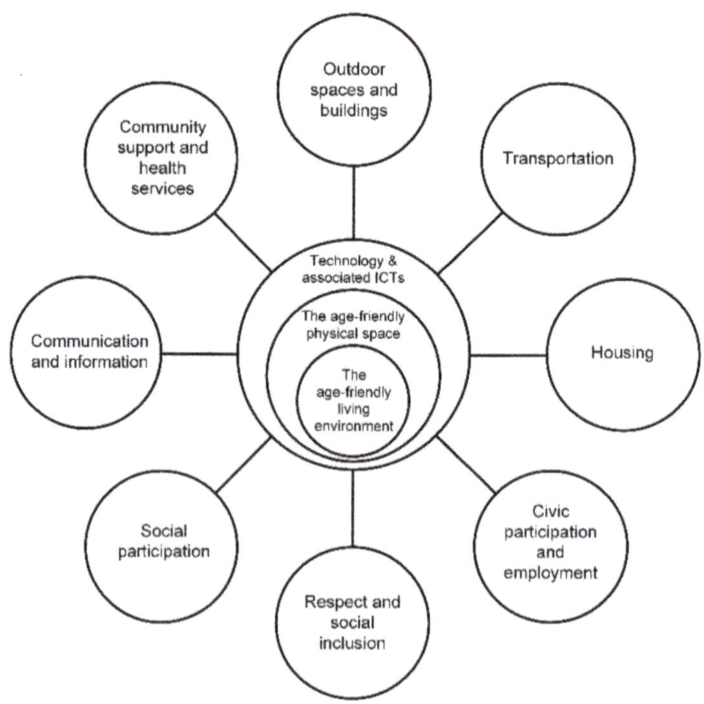

Figure 2. The Smart Age-friendly Ecosystem (SAfE) framework [48]. Permission granted by Drs Marston and van Hoof.

Figure 1 illustrates the eight domains of the framework, making up the original notion of an "age-friendly" environment/community.

However, as noted extensively by Marston and van Hoof in 2019 [48], 13 years after the original framework was published, there has not been any additional iterations coinciding with societal changes such as technology use, deployment, and implementation. This is where the proposed extension—the Smart Age-friendly Ecosystem (SAfE) framework—was created and introduced [48]. Figure 2 illustrates the new framework acknowledging the physical space, technology, and associated ICTs (information communication technology) as described by Marston and van Hoof [48].

The SAfE framework illustrates the relationship technology has with various domains across different segments and interconnections within our respective cities and communities. The physical space, as posited by Marston and van Hoof [48], refers to and acknowledges both the design of urban developments to our towns, cities, and villages—and including a life course perspective [48], the SAfE framework is not solely connected to older adults, but younger people too. Finally, the inner sphere—"The age-friendly living environment"—relates to the physical environments of one's house or apartment, either living on their own or with their families. As noted by Marston and van Hoof [48], this concept has not been previously captured yet. Familial connections and intergenerational relationships are integral to lifestyle, (mental) health and wellbeing, reducing loneliness and social isolation, and enhancing social networks and connectedness.

In the following section, we continue our commentary surrounding age-friendly Blue Zones® frameworks, pulling together a series of recommendations based on the frameworks presented here and offering theoretical insights in an attempt to move the debate and narratives forward.

5. Discussion

In this commentary piece, we have presented contemporary literature surrounding age-friendly cities located in the USA, based on the Blue Zones® checklists. We have provided a critical review of the four Blue Zones® checklists and finally we have presented two age-friendly frameworks: 1. the WHO age-friendly framework [3] and 2. the SAfE framework [48], which present different approaches to contemporary society. The second approach instils a nod to the technological revolution which began at the turn of the 21st century and illustrates how technology can and is being used within the age-friendly domain.

Presently, Blue Zones® have proposed four domains (Home, Bedroom, Kitchen and Tribe) with associated checklists [56–59] comprised of various items and with various motivations. To date, the contemporary literature surrounding Blue Zones® has primarily been from the perspective of health and wellbeing. Yet, there is a paucity of literature surrounding the implementation, use, barriers, enablers, challenges, environmental issues, interventions, and impact surrounding digital technologies in the context of the Blue Zones® checklists and respective regions. Although in the checklists it stipulates that digital technology should kept to a minimum, the 21st century has witnessed and welcomed advances in this area and has not only changed the societal landscape of how we view the use of technology, but also how technology can benefit an individual in all the contexts within these checklists. We have provided examples and suggestions of how technology can be implemented in the home in both the "Kitchen" and "Bedroom" checklists, which may enhance and improve the respective environments should individuals have the financial means to purchase IoT devices and appliances. However, with the implementation of such technological solutions and adaptations, having the digital skillset should also be considered. For many users, old and young, understanding the benefits of purchasing and implementing IoT devices to enhance their living space may not be so evident. While installing the Internet may also be a contentious debate especially if a person is on a low income, this too continues the debate of the digital divide [75]. However, technology and IoT devices cannot be ignored because this area of society has grown phenomenally since the turn of the 21st century and continues to develop and become smarter [48,65–68].

Worldwide, we observe the growing pervasiveness of digital technologies and services in people's everyday living and ecosystems. Yet, while the presence of technology is widely acknowledged [48,68], both the Blue Zones® checklists [56–59] and the WHO age-friendly cities framework [3] devote little attention to this important dimension of societies' current way of living, respective ecosystems, or consideration for future societies. For example, neither the WHO age-friendly cities framework [3] nor the Blue Zones® checklists [56–59] have undergone recent iterations and revisions to reflect the changing world. However, the SAfE framework [48] does reflect contemporary society and provides several recommendations to the academy in a bid to move the narrative forward in this growing domain. Similarly, the work presented by Riddle [50] has attempted to illustrate the transferability of the Blue Zones® concepts into Western society across different locations in the USA. Admittingly, for the specific case of the early studies of Blue Zones®, this was the case because researchers were focusing on the healthy longevity of people rather than technology, which could be less prominent at the time the research took place. However, this appears to be a weakness, if not a gap, in the later developed checklists and area(s) which now deserves greater investigation and understanding. Serving as a tool to "reengineer" particular locations in the USA after the year 2000, to not account for the presence of digital technologies and services is striking, since neglecting such an important aspect may render the application insufficient.

The Power of 9 [53,54] includes nine items organized into four groups: move, right outlook, eat well, and connect. Although the Blue Zones® checklists also propose an equal number of checklists, there seems to be no correspondence between the two. Critical analysis of the checklists, as presented in Section 4, illustrates the primary goal is outcome, followed by environment and Item 1 in the "Bedroom" checklist transfers to "Intervention delivery". There are a number of intended goals of the checklists, including: 1. the promotion of physical activity, 2. the motivation towards eating well, and 3. the encouragement of health promotion. However, these three goals fall short of covering all the dimensions of the Power of 9, specifically the nuances of purpose, downshift, and loved ones first. The Home checklist [56] is almost entirely dedicated to encouraging physical activity, with the exception of Item 8 (see Tables 1 and 7) which seeks to promote air quality, which can also be linked to general health. The Kitchen checklist, [57] is mostly aligned with the eat well dimension, including items that would fall within the three items included in that dimension (the 80% rule, plant slant, and wine at five). Items 4 and 7 of the checklists (see Tables 3 and 9) also extend the move dimension and general health promotion. The Bedroom checklist [58] (see Tables 5 and 10) finds no direct correspondence to the Power of 9. It aims at promoting good quality sleep and, in this way, it aims to promote positive health and wellbeing. The Tribe checklist [59] (see Tables 7 and 11), while designated this way, seems to report on a diverse range of subjects and appears to be an amalgamation of items. This checklist links to general health promotion (Items 4–6, 9) without any direct connection to the Power of 9, physical activity (Item 1), linking to the move dimension of the Power of 9, and an assortment of Items (2, 3, 7–10) could be linked to the right outlook and connect dimensions of the Power of 9. Overall, it is important to underline the underrepresentation of the dimensions: right outlook and connect. As previously noted in earlier sections, population characteristics have not been considered and without this consideration we believe it is difficult to ascertain and fully evaluate the appropriateness of these respective checklists.

Another aspect worth noting is how the Home, Kitchen, and Bedroom checklists [56–58] lack theoretical underpinning and as previously noted, we believe taking a life course perspective would benefit future iterations of these checklists greatly because citizens lives and situations change over a course of years and decades, which in turn may impact one's health and wellbeing. The "Tribe" checklist is subjective and, arguably, difficult to answer and is highly dependent on one's state of mind or quality over the last few days of an individual. This uneven distribution may lead to a skewed application of the checklist, resulting in an added difficulty to replicate the benefits of the Blue Zones®.

The Blue Zones® checklists [56–58] somehow touch upon some of the aspects of the WHO age-friendly cities framework [3]—for example, the inclusion of outdoor spaces and buildings (Home checklist), transport (Home checklist), respect and social inclusion (Tribe checklist), social participation (Tribe checklist), community support, and health services (Bedroom checklist). Aspects such as housing, civic participation and employment, communication and information are neglected and still limited. Furthermore, the critical analysis of the checklists highlights that these elements seem to reflect the reality of populations residing in a wealthy developed Western society, characterised by, for example, houses, gardens, and junk food. This way of living may be found in some parts or regions of wealthy developed countries. However, this is not the case everywhere—for example, parts of the population reside in apartments, or even live-in rooms only or multioccupancy housing environments, with no access to gardens or supplementary spaces to implement the checklist items.

All in all, it appears that in aiming to bring Western societies closer to the Blue Zones® principles, with the notion of offering and pursuing a healthier longevity, the checklists [56–59] have been tailored to a limited segment of society, including individuals and communities who own their own homes, and have few financial worries. This makes the checklists hard to apply in less developed regions or deprived areas of a country, state or county. Future iterations of frameworks should include representative populations from both deprived and affluent areas to gain a complete understanding of how the Power of 9 can increase healthy ageing and longevity.

The various Blue Zones® checklists [56–59] suggest various amendments to the respective three domains (Home, Kitchen and Bedroom) that could be coupled with lifestyle changes and activities in the fourth domain—Tribe. These checklists do not actually take into consideration the domains outlined in the WHO framework (Figure 1); therefore, building on the WHO framework [3] (Figure 1) and the SAfE framework by Marston and van Hoof [48] (Figure 2) would complement both the checklists and the respective age-friendly frameworks [3,48], better representing the intersect of its multiple components within contemporary 21st century society.

The four Blue Zones® checklists [56–59] highlight a dearth of items connecting or even considering the application of technology. From a total of 44 items, only 7 items can be connected to technology and the use of power tools and home appliances. Examples in the checklists include, Home, Items 2, 3, and 11 (see Table 1); Kitchen, Item 7 (see Table 3), and Bedroom, Items 5, 7, and 8 (see Table 5). This lack of acknowledgment of technology may pave the way for the limited use and application of the checklists. With this in mind, the SAfE age-friendly framework [48] could provide actors with a basis to bridge future iterations of the Blue Zones® checklists [56–59] together. Given the SAfE framework [48] illustrates the relationships between the physical space, digital technologies surrounding the living environment and the connections with the respective domains based on the WHO age-friendly framework [3] has the potential to provide a blueprint for this narrative to evolve.

Both the Blue Zones® checklists and the WHO age-friendly cities framework [3] overlook the presence and contribution of technology and associated ICTs. It is hard to imagine a world without technology, even in the Blue Zones® regions where a quick Google search confirms the presence of Internet services and other ICT-related products and services. The important contribution of the environment, physical space, and of technology is stressed in the SAfE framework [48] and offers a good starting point for reflecting on how best to develop an age-friendly physical space and environment in which technology and its associated ICTs can be weaved together, whether it is through assistive devices, smart automation, smart devices, or apps, which act as the connectors between people, physical spaces, and environments in the various Blue Zones®.

Besides offering greater coverage of all the presented items as well as the remaining aspects of the Power of 9, future work should explore how the checklists can potentially evolve, taking guidance from the WHO age-friendly cities framework [3] and the SAfE framework [48]. For example, incorporating the Power of 9 into the framework suggested by Marston and van Hoof [48] may be a way to address the inadequacies of the checklists as they are currently presented and to integrate diversity more fully from a variety of perspectives. This future work should be theoretically underpinned by life course theory [76] and implementing an action research approach [77] to ensure all voices and narratives are considered.

Strengths, Limitations, and Recommendations

This commentary has highlighted an area of social gerontology that has received little attention from scholars who focus on age-friendly and successful age-in-place research. However, given that multi- and cross-disciplinary research is growing, this domain of gerontology—Blue Zones® affords a new area of research for scholars to collaborate and move the narrative forward. This commentary is novel because it highlights gaps in the existing literature and area surrounding the age-friendly domain, Blue Zones® and in this way this innovative piece is a route plan for multi- and cross-disciplinary scholars.

Limitations of this work include the limited evaluation of the checklists [56–59] and frameworks [3,48]. However, in a recent published paper by Dikken and colleagues [78] who present the Age-Friendly Cities and Communities (AFCC) Questionnaire, there are grounds for existing and future evaluations to take place. This in turn forms the basis and groundwork for future iterations of the AFCC.

As a starting point, we propose that the AFCC survey could be complemented by qualitative data collections such as diaries, fieldtrips, first-hand accounts, interviews, and observations, taking an action research approach [77] to ensure a positive impact upon the respective regions as noted by Marston and colleagues [68]. However, it is possible that the AFCC survey [78] may have to be adapted to accommodate the differing facets of the Blue Zones® regions. This would afford various actors interested in age-friendly and Blue Zones® regions the opportunity to specifically create a supplementary iteration of the survey tailored for this domain(s).

Moreover, an alternative approach to measuring Blue Zones® could consider using quantitative measures by building on the work of Davern and colleagues [79], whereby employing a Geographic Information Systems (GIS) to measure spatial indicators associated with Blue Zones® may afford various actors the opportunity to understand the greater importance and associations reflected in the lived environment(s) in an attempt to facilitate and enhance health and wellbeing. In addition to the work published by Davern et al. [79], Jackisch et al. [80] and the United Nations—New Urban Agenda, the 2030 Agenda for Sustainable Development [81] have also employed GIS techniques and approaches as a means of understanding the impact and importance of spatial indicators associated with age-friendly cities and communities.

Previously, we recommended the implementation of a life course perspective [76], an approach that facilitates researchers, policymakers, educators, students, and communities to view solutions through the lens of personal experiences, and historical events that narrate the story of a "personal biography" [76]. In conjunction with participatory action research [77] approaches, and by implementing universal design principles [82], these methodological approaches will afford scholars to capture and complement future qualitative data collection and narratives from all citizens, not just older people.

Indeed, given the existing five various Blue Zones® regions located worldwide, future frameworks and research should account for the differing cultural aspects, and should be represented in future age-friendly frameworks. Instilling, acknowledging, and embedding cultural beliefs, and traditions is integral to prospective positive implementation and adoption of future age-friendly Blue Zones® frameworks within the respective regions. We believe all four checklists [56–59] require substantial revisions supported by published evidence-based research from various fields including gerontechnology, geography, ecology, computer science, and social sciences. Given how the "Tribe" checklist [59] appears to be the less developed checklist, we believe this checklist would benefit from a substantial revision. Such a revision should include contemporary measures associated with loneliness [83], technology use [84,85], and environmental factors (e.g., risk of falling) [85–87].

Extensive fieldwork encompassing a mixed methods approach is needed to achieve these great strides in this domain and as highlighted by Liddle et al. [77], who purports that localised community engagement is needed to fully understand the specific needs, challenges, barriers, and enablers to social connections, using a bottom-up approach.

Reuter and colleagues [88] have taken a participatory action research approach in their respective work in a bid to understand how older adults and stakeholders use technology to provide digital information and communications. Primarily, Reuter and colleagues [88] focus on two domains featured in the WHO age-friendly framework: 1. communication and information, and 2. civic participation. Furthermore, Marston and colleagues [68] propose implementing universal design principles [82] which, if combined with participatory action research [77] while instilling a bottom-up approach, has the potential to understand the needs, perceptions, expectations, requirements, and impacts of incorporating facets from existing age-friendly frameworks [3,48].

6. Conclusions

The aim of this commentary is to outline the initial footprint in a series of future work to bring areas which are limited or lacking in the existing Blue Zones® checklists to the forefront, while also proposing areas for future research within the communities and societies. This is particularly important when we are referring to technology, and globally, we are heading into the third decade of the 21st century.

The authors of this commentary believe this critique is a contribution to the fields of gerontology, gerontechnology, anthropology, geography, and social sciences because, to date, existing research surrounding Blue Zones® regions has primarily focused on the epidemiology and health of citizens, neglecting the opportunity of exploring the social sciences and technological impacts within these regions and looking for an even broader implementation.

We want to open up and welcome further discussions with interested parties, actors, and stakeholders who are interested in age-friendly research, Blue Zones® regions, technology, social sciences, and anthropology, as a way of moving forward with future work, frameworks, and conducting future investigations to advance the knowledge of Blue Zones® regions.

Author Contributions: Conceptualization, all authors; writing—original draft preparation, all authors; writing—review and editing, all authors. All authors have read and agreed to the published version of the manuscript.

Funding: This research received no external funding.

Data Availability Statement: Not applicable.

Conflicts of Interest: The authors declare no conflict of interest.

References

1. Van Hoof, J.; Kazak, J.K.; Perek-Białas, J.M.; Peek, S.T.M. The challenges of urban ageing: Making cities age-friendly in Europe. *Int. J. Environ. Res. Public Health* **2018**, *15*, 2473. [CrossRef] [PubMed]
2. Van Hoof, J.; Boerenfijn, P.; Kolmer, D.B.G.; Marston, H.R.; Kazak, J.K.; Verbeek, H. Chapter 16: Environmental Design for an Ageing Population. In *Changing Horizons in the 21st Century: Perspectives on Ageing*; Phelan, A., O'Shea, D., Eds.; Cambridge Scholars: Cambridge, UK, 2020.
3. World Health Organization. *Global Age-Friendly Cities: A Guide*; World Health Organization: Geneva, Switzerland, 2007; ISBN 9789241547307.

4. Plouffe, L.; Kalache, A. Towards global age-friendly cities: Determining urban features that promote active aging. *J. Urban Health* **2010**, *87*, 733–739. [CrossRef] [PubMed]
5. McDonald, B.; Walsh, K.; Scharf, T. Creating an Age-Friendly County in Ireland: Stakeholders' Perspectives on Implementation. In *Age-Friendly Cities and Communities: A Global Perspective*; Buffel, T., Handler, S., Phillipson, C., Eds.; The Policy Press: Bristol, UK, 2018; pp. 143–166.
6. Van Hoof, J.; Kazak, J.K. Urban ageing. *Indoor Built Environ.* **2018**, *27*, 583–586. [CrossRef]
7. Buffel, T.; Phillipson, C. Can global cities be 'age-friendly cities'? Urban development and ageing populations. *Cities* **2016**, *55*, 94–100. [CrossRef]
8. Dijkstra, L.; Poelman, H. Cities in Europe: The New OECD-EC Definition. Regional Focus A Series of Short Papers on Regional Research and Indicators Produced by the Directorate-General for Regional and Urban Policy RF 01/2012. 2012. Available online: https://ec.europa.eu/regional_policy/sources/docgener/focus/2012_01_city.pdf (accessed on 8 September 2019).
9. Fitzgerald, K.G.; Caro, F.G. An Overview of Age-Friendly Cities and Communities Around the World. *J. Aging Soc. Policy* **2014**, *26*, 1–18. [CrossRef]
10. Buffel, T.; Phillipson, C. Ageing in a Gentrifying Neighbourhood: Experiences of Community Change in Later Life. *Sociology* **2019**, *53*, 987–1004. [CrossRef]
11. Peek, S.T.M.; Wouters, E.J.M.; van Hoof, J.; Luijkx, K.G.; Boeije, H.R.; Vrijhoef, H.J.M. Factors influencing acceptance of technology for aging in place: A systematic review. *Int. J. Med. Inform.* **2014**, *83*, 235–248. [CrossRef]
12. Charness, N.; Czaja, S.; Fisk, A.D.; Rogers, W. Preview Gerontechnology 2002: Creative use of technology for better aging. *Gerontechnology* **2002**, *1*, 198–202. [CrossRef]
13. Tully, C.J. Growing up in technologicalworlds: How modern technologies shape the everyday lives of young people. *Bull. Sci. Technol. Soc.* **2003**, *23*, 444–456. [CrossRef]
14. Adams, R.; Stevenson, M. A Lifetime of Relationships Mediated by Technology. In *Growing Together: Personal Relationships Across the Life Span*; Lang, F., Fingerman, K., Eds.; Cambridge University Press: New York, NY, USA, 2004; pp. 368–393.
15. Barnett, K.; Adkins, B. Computers: Community for aging women in Australia. *Women Environ.* **2001**, *50–51*, 23–25.
16. Becker, S.A. A study of Web usability for older adults seeking online health resources. *ACM Trans. Comput. Hum. Interact.* **2004**, *11*, 387–406. [CrossRef]
17. Blit-Cohen, E.; Litwin, H. Elder participation in cyberspace: A qualitative analysis of Israeli retirees. *J. Aging Stud.* **2004**, *18*, 385–398. [CrossRef]
18. Bradley, N.; Poppen, W. Assistive technology, computers and Internet may decrease sense of isolation for homebound elderly and disabled persons. *Technol. Disabil.* **2003**, *15*, 19–25. [CrossRef]
19. Cody, M.J.; Dunn, D.; Hoppin, S.; Wendt, P. Silver surfers: Training and evaluating Internet use among older adult learners. *Commun. Educ.* **1999**, *48*, 269–286. [CrossRef]
20. Dickinson, A.; Gregor, P. Computer use has no demonstrated impact on the well-being of older adults. *Int. J. Hum. Comput. Stud.* **2006**, *64*, 744–753. [CrossRef]
21. Hargittai, E. Whose space? Differences among users and non-users of social network sites. *J. Comput. Mediat. Commun.* **2007**, *13*, 276–297. [CrossRef]
22. Hargittai, E.; Shafer, S. Differences in actual and perceived online skills: The role of gender. *Soc. Sci. Q.* **2006**, *87*, 432–448. [CrossRef]
23. Kanayama, T. Ethnographic research on the experience of Japanese elderly people online. *New Media Soc.* **2003**, *5*, 267–288. [CrossRef]
24. Kavanaugh, A.L.; Patterson, S.J. The impact of community computer networks on social capital and community involvement. *Am. Behav. Sci.* **2001**, *45*, 496–509. [CrossRef]
25. Laguna, K.; Babcock, R.L. Computer anxiety in young and older adults: Implications for human–computer interactions in older populations. *Comput. Hum. Behav.* **1997**, *13*, 317–326. [CrossRef]
26. McConatha, D.; McConatha, J.T.; Dermigny, R. The use of interactive computer services to enhance the quality of life for long-term care residents. *The Gerontologist* **1994**, *34*, 553–556. [CrossRef] [PubMed]
27. McMellon, C.A.; Schiffman, L.G. Cybersenior empowerment: How some older individuals are taking control of their lives. *J. Appl. Gerontol.* **2002**, *21*, 157–175. [CrossRef]
28. Melenhorst, A.S.; Rogers, W.A.; Bouwhuis, D.G. Older adults' motivated choice for technological innovation: Evidence for benefit-driven selectivity. *Psychol. Aging* **2006**, *21*, 190–195. [CrossRef]
29. Ajala, O.; English, P.; Pinkney, J. Systematic Review and Meta-Analysis of Different Dietary Approaches to the Management of Type 2 Diabetes. *Am. J. Clin. Nutr.* **2013**, 505–516. [CrossRef]
30. Beezhold, B.L.; Johnston, C.S.; Daigle, D.R. Vegetarian Diets Are Associated With Healthy Mood States: A Cross-Sectional Study in Seventh-Day Adventist Adults. *Nutr. J.* **2010**, *9*, 26. [CrossRef]
31. Chrysohoou, C.; Panagiotakos, D.B.; Aggelopoulos, P.; Kastorini, C.M.; Kehagia, I.; Pitsavos, C.; Stefanadis, C. The Mediterranean Diet Contributes to the Preservation of Left Ventricular Systolic Function and to the Long-Term Favorable Prognosis of Patients Who Have Had an Acute Coronary Event. *Am. J. Clin. Nutr.* **2010**, 47–54. [CrossRef] [PubMed]

32. Chrysohoou, C.; Pitsavos, C.; Panagiotakos, D.; Skoumas, J.; Lazaros, G.; Oikonomou, E.; Galiatsatos, N.; Striggou, M.; Xynogala, M.; Stefanadis, C. Long-Term Fish Intake Preserves Kidney Function in Elderly Individuals: The Ikaria Study. *J. Ren. Nutr.* **2013**, e75–e82. [CrossRef]
33. Darmadi-Blackberry, I.; Wahlqvist, M.L.; Kouris-Blazos, A.; Steen, B.; Lukito, W.; Horie, Y.; Horie, K. Legumes: The most important dietary predictor of survival in older people of different ethnicities. *Asia Pac. J. Clin. Nutr.* **2004**, *13*, 217–220. [PubMed]
34. Ford, P.A.; Jaceldo-Siegl, K.; Lee, J.W.; Youngberg, W.; Tonstad, S. Intake of Mediterranean foods associated with positive affect and low negative affect. *J. Psychosom. Res.* **2013**, *74*, 142–148. [CrossRef] [PubMed]
35. Fraser, G.E. Vegetarian diets: What do we know of their effects on common chronic diseases? *Am. J. Clin. Nutr.* **2009**, *89*, 1607S–1612S. [CrossRef]
36. Antonogeorgos, G.; Panagiotakos, D.B.; Pitsavos, C.; Papageorgiou, C.; Chrysohoou, C.; Papadimitriou, G.N.; Stefanadis, C. Understanding the role of depression and anxiety on cardiovascular disease risk, using structural equation modeling; the mediating effect of the Mediterranean diet and physical activity: The ATTICA study. *Ann. Epidemiol.* **2012**, *22*, 630–637. [CrossRef] [PubMed]
37. Bazzano, L.A.; He, J.; Ogden, L.G.; Loria, C.; Vupputuri, S.; Myers, L.; Whelton, P.K. Legume consumption and risk of coronary heart disease in US men and women: NHANES I Epidemiologic Follow-up Study. *Arch. Intern. Med.* **2001**, *161*, 2573–2578. [CrossRef] [PubMed]
38. Bazzano, L.A.; Thompson, A.M.; Tees, M.T.; Nguyen, C.H.; Winham, D.M. Non-soy legume consumption lowers cholesterol levels: A meta-analysis of randomized controlled trials. *Nutr. Metab. Cardiovasc. Dis.* **2011**, *21*, 94–103. [CrossRef] [PubMed]
39. Chrysohoou, C.; Skoumas, J.; Pitsavos, C.; Masoura, C.; Siasos, G.; Galiatsatos, N.; Psaltopoulou, T.; Mylonakis, C.; Margazas, A.; Kyvelou, S.; et al. Long-term adherence to the Mediterranean diet reduces the prevalence of hyperuricaemia in elderly individuals, without known cardiovascular disease: The Ikaria study. *Maturitas* **2011**, *70*, 58–64. [CrossRef] [PubMed]
40. Clarkson, T.B. Soy, Soy Phytoestrogens, and Cardiovascular Disease. *J. Nutr.* **2002**, 566S–569S. [CrossRef]
41. Covas, M.I.; Konstantinidou, V.; Fitó, M. Olive oil and cardiovascular health. *J. Cardiovasc. Pharmacol.* **2009**, *54*, 477–482. [CrossRef]
42. Fontana, L.; Villareal, D.T.; Weiss, E.P.; Racette, S.B.; Steger-May, K.; Klein, S.; Holloszy, J.O.; Washington University School of Medicine CALERIE Group. Calorie restriction or exercise: Effects on coronary heart disease risk factors. A randomized, controlled trial. *Am. J. Physiol. Endocrinol. Metab.* **2007**, *293*, E197–E202. [CrossRef]
43. Carru, C.; Pes, G.M.; Deiana, L.; Baggio, G.; Franceschi, C.; Lio, D.; Balistreri, C.R.; Candore, G.; Colonna-Romano, G.; Caruso, C. Association Between the HFE Mutations and Longevity: A Study in Sardinian Population. *Mech. Ageing Dev.* **2003**, 529–532. [CrossRef]
44. Caselli, G.; Lipsi, R.M. Survival Differences Among the Oldest Old in Sardinia: Who, What, Where, and Why? *Demogr. Res.* **2006**, 267–294. [CrossRef]
45. Caselli, G.; Pozzi, L.; Vaupel, J.W.; Deiana, L.; Pes, G.; Carru, C.; Franceschi, C.; Baggio, G. Family clustering in Sardinian longevity: A genealogical approach. *Exp. Gerontol.* **2006**, *41*, 727–736. [CrossRef]
46. Davinelli, S.; Willcox, D.C.; Scapagnini, G. Extending healthy ageing: Nutrient sensitive pathway and centenarian population. *Immun. Ageing* **2012**, *9*, 9. [CrossRef] [PubMed]
47. Christakis, N.A.; Fowler, J.H. The spread of obesity in a large social network over 32 years. *N. Engl. J. Med.* **2007**, *357*, 370–379. [CrossRef] [PubMed]
48. Marston, H.R.; van Hoof, J. Who Doesn't Think about Technology When Designing Urban Environments for Older People? A Case Study Approach to a Proposed Extension of the WHO's Age-Friendly Cities Model. *Int. J. Environ. Res. Public Health* **2019**, *16*, 3525. [CrossRef] [PubMed]
49. Buettner, D. *The Blue Zones Solution: Eating and Living Like the World's Healthiest People*; National Geographic Books: New York, NY, USA, 2015; Available online: https://www.bluezones.com/about/history/ (accessed on 1 October 2020).
50. Riddell, B. Blue Zones: Rethinking the American Landscape. School of City and Regional Planning, College of Architecture, Georgia Institute of Technology. 2016. Available online: https://smartech.gatech.edu/bitstream/handle/1853/55168/briana_riddell_blue_zones_rethinking_the_american_landscape.pdf (accessed on 1 October 2020).
51. Albert Lea, Minnesota. Wikipedia. Available online: https://en.wikipedia.org/wiki/Albert_Lea,_Minnesota (accessed on 18 October 2020).
52. Spence, Iowa. Wikipedia. Available online: https://en.wikipedia.org/wiki/Spencer,_Iowa (accessed on 18 October 2020).
53. Reverse Engineering Longevity. Available online: https://www.bluezones.com/2016/11/power-9/ (accessed on 27 November 2020).
54. Buettner, D. *Power 9®*; National Geographic Books: New York, NY, USA, 2015.
55. Blue Zones Registration. Available online: https://www.bluezones.com/live-longer-better/checklists/registration/?redirect_to=https%3A%2F%2Fwww.bluezones.com%2Flive-longer-better%2Fchecklists%2F (accessed on 1 October 2020).
56. Home Checklist. Available online: https://www.bluezones.com/live-longer-better/checklists/checklist-home/ (accessed on 1 October 2020).
57. Kitchen Checklist. Available online: https://www.bluezones.com/live-longer-better/checklists/kitchen/ (accessed on 1 October 2020).
58. Bedroom Checklist. Available online: https://www.bluezones.com/live-longer-better/checklists/bedroom/ (accessed on 1 October 2020).

59. Tribe Checklist. Available online: https://www.bluezones.com/live-longer-better/checklists/tribe/ (accessed on 1 October 2020).
60. Munthe-Kaas, H.; Nøkleby, H.; Nguyen, L. Systematic mapping of checklists for assessing transferability. *Syst. Rev.* **2019**, *8*, 22. [CrossRef] [PubMed]
61. Hadley, R.A. Men and Me(n). *Methodol. Innov.* **2020**, *13*. [CrossRef]
62. Hadley, R.A. The Lived Experience of Older Involuntary Childless Men. In *The Annual Journal of the British Sociological Association Study Group on Auto/Biography*; Sparkes, A.C., Ed.; BSA Auto/Biography Group: Durham, UK, 2018; pp. 93–108. ISSN 2040-2996.
63. Hadley, R.A. Ageing Without Children, Gender and Social Justice. In *Ageing, Diversity and Equality: Social Justice Perspectives*; Westwood, S., Ed.; Routledge: Abingdon, UK, 2018; pp. 66–81.
64. Hadley, R.A. Deconstructing Dad. In *The Palgrave Handbook of Male Psychology and Mental Health*; Barry, J., Kingerlee, R., Seager, M., Sullivan, L., Eds.; Springer Nature: Cham, Switzerland, 2019.
65. Smarter. AM. Available online: https://smarter.am/ (accessed on 28 December 2020).
66. Pantri. Available online: https://pantri.net/ (accessed on 28 December 2020).
67. Marston, H.R.; Samuels, J. A Review of Age Friendly Virtual Assistive Technologies and their Effect on Daily Living for Carers and Dependent Adults. *Healthcare* **2019**, *7*, 49. [CrossRef]
68. Marston, H.R.; Shore, L.; White, P.J. How does a (Smart) Age-Friendly Ecosystem Look in a Post-Pandemic Society? *Int. J. Environ. Res. Public Health* **2020**, *17*, 8276. [CrossRef]
69. BBC News. Amazon Echo Trial to Help Elderly and Disabled People. 2018. Available online: https://www.bbc.co.uk/news/av/uk-politics-43869120/amazon-echo-trial-to-help-elderly-and-disabled-people (accessed on 6 March 2019).
70. Hampshire County Council. Hampshire County Council: Pushing the Boundaries by Using Amazon Echo. 2018. Available online: https://www.local.gov.uk/hampshire-county-council-pushing-boundaries-using-amazon-echo (accessed on 6 March 2019).
71. Peskett, J. Virgin Launches New Alexa Initiative to Assist Disabled Passengers. Accessibility Mobility Professional. 2019. Available online: https://www.accessandmobilityprofessional.com/virgin-launches-new-alexa-initiative-to-assist-disabled-passengers/ (accessed on 6 March 2019).
72. Buffel, T.; Phililipson, C.; Rémillard-Boilard, S. Age-Friendly Cities and Communities: New Directions for Research and Policy. In *Encyclopedia of Gerontology and Population Aging*; Gu, D., Dupre, M.E., Eds.; Springer Nature: Cham, Switzerland, 2019.
73. Van Hoof, J.; Dikken, J.; Buttiġieġ, S.C.; van den Hoven, R.F.M.; Kroon, E.; Marston, H.R. Age-friendly cities in The Netherlands: An explorative study of facilitators and hindrances in the built environment and ageism in design. *Indoor Built Environ.* **2020**, *29*, 417–437. [CrossRef]
74. Rowles, G. Place and identity in old age. *J. Exp. Psychol.* **1983**, *3*, 299–313.
75. Marston, H.R. Millennials and ICT—Findings from the Technology 4 Young Adults (T4YA) Project: An Exploratory Study. *Societies* **2019**, *9*, 80. [CrossRef]
76. Elder, G.H., Jr. (Ed.) Perspectives on the Life Course. In *Life Course Dynamics: Trajectories and Transitions, 1968–1980*; Cornell University Press: Ithaca, NY, USA, 1985; Chapter 1; pp. 23–49.
77. Liddle, J.; Pitcher, N.; Montague, K.; Hanratty, B.; Standing, H.; Scharf, T. Connecting at Local Level: Exploring Opportunities for Future Design of Technology to Support Social Connections in Age-friendly Communities. *Int. J. Environ. Res. Public Health* **2020**, *17*, 5544. [CrossRef] [PubMed]
78. Dikken, J.; van den Hoven, R.F.; van Staalduinen, W.H.; Hulsebosch-Janssen, L.M.; van Hoof, J. How Older People Experience the Age-Friendliness of Their City: Development of the Age-Friendly Cities and Communities Questionnaire. *Int. J. Environ. Res. Public Health* **2020**, *17*, 6867. [CrossRef]
79. Davern, M.; Winterton, R.; Brasher, K.; Woolcock, G. How Can the Lived Environment Support Healthy Ageing? A Spatial Indicators Framework for the Assessment of Age-Friendly Communities. *Int. J. Environ. Res. Public Health* **2020**, *17*, 7685. [CrossRef] [PubMed]
80. Jackisch, J.; Zamaro, G.; Green, G.; Huber, M. Is a healthy city also an age-friendly city? *Health Promot. Int.* **2015**, *30*, 108–117. [CrossRef] [PubMed]
81. United Nations. *Transforming out World: The 2030 Agenda for Sustainable Development*; United Nations: New York, NY, USA, 2015.
82. NSAI. EN 17161:2019 Design for All. Accessibility Following a Design for all Approach in Products, Goods and Services. Extending the Range of Users. In Dublin, Ireland: National Standards Authority of Ireland. 2019. Available online: https://www.nsai.ie/about/news/a-design-standard-that-works-for-all/ (accessed on 28 October 2020).
83. De Jong Gierveld, J.; Van Tilburg, T. A 6-Item Scale for Overall, Emotional, and Social Loneliness: Confirmatory Tests on Survey Data. *Res. Aging* **2006**, *28*, 582–598. [CrossRef]
84. Marston, H.R.; Genoe, R.; Freeman, S.; Kulczycki, C.; Musselwhite, C. Older Adults' Perceptions of ICT: Main Findings from the Technology in Later Life (TILL) Study. *Healthcare* **2019**, *7*, 86. [CrossRef]
85. Vaziri, D.D.; Aal, K.; Ogonowski, C.; Von Rekowski, T.; Kroll, M.; Marston, H.R.; Poveda, R.; Gschwind, Y.J.; Delbaere, K.; Wieching, R.; et al. Exploring user experience and technology acceptance for a fall prevention system: Results from a randomized clinical trial and a living lab. *Eur. Rev. Aging Phys. Act.* **2016**, *13*. [CrossRef]
86. Marston, H.R.; Woodbury, A.; Gschwind, Y.J.; Kroll, M.; Fink, D.; Eichberg, S.; Kreiner, K.; Ejupi, A.; Annegarn, J.; de Rosario, H.; et al. The design of a purpose-built exergame for fall prediction and prevention for older people. *Eur. Rev. Aging Phys. Act.* **2015**, *12*, 13. [CrossRef]

87. Delbaere, K.; Smith, S.T.; Lord, S.R. Development and initial validation of the Iconographical Falls Efficacy Scale. *J. Gerontol. Ser. A* **2011**, *66*, 674–680. [CrossRef]
88. Reuter, A.; Liddle, J.; Scharf, T. Digitalising the Age-Friendly City: Insights from Participatory Action Research. *Int. J. Environ. Res. Public Health* **2020**, *17*, 8281. [CrossRef]

International Journal of
Environmental Research and Public Health

MDPI

Article

Developing Age-Friendly Cities and Communities: Eleven Case Studies from around the World

Samuèle Rémillard-Boilard [1,*], Tine Buffel [2] and Chris Phillipson [2]

1 Research Centre on Aging, CIUSSS de l'Estrie—CHUS, Université de Sherbrooke, Sherbrooke, QC J1K 2R1, Canada
2 School of Social Sciences, Manchester Institute for Collaborative Research on Ageing (MICRA), The University of Manchester, Manchester M13 9PR, UK; tine.buffel@manchester.ac.uk (T.B.); christopher.phillipson@manchester.ac.uk (C.P.)
* Correspondence: samuele.remillard-boilard@usherbrooke.ca

Abstract: Developing age-friendly cities and communities has become a key part of policies aimed at improving the quality of life of older people in urban areas. The World Health Organization has been especially important in driving the 'age-friendly' agenda, notably through its Global Network of Age-Friendly Cities and Communities, connecting 1114 (2020 figure) cities and communities worldwide. Despite the expansion and achievements of the Network over the last decade, little is known about the progress made by cities developing this work around the world. This article addresses this research gap by comparing the experience of eleven cities located in eleven countries. Using a multiple case study approach, the study explores the key goals, achievements, and challenges faced by local age-friendly programs and identifies four priorities the age-friendly movement should consider to further its development: (1) changing the perception of older age; (2) involving key actors in age-friendly efforts; (3) responding to the (diverse) needs of older people; and (4) improving the planning and delivery of age-friendly programs. The article concludes by discussing the research and policy implications of these findings for the age-friendly movement.

Keywords: age-friendly cities; ageing; policy; case studies; Global Network of Age-Friendly Cities and Communities; World Health Organization

Citation: Rémillard-Boilard, S.; Buffel, T.; Phillipson, C. Developing Age-Friendly Cities and Communities: Eleven Case Studies from around the World. *Int. J. Environ. Res. Public Health* **2021**, *18*, 133. https://dx.doi.org/10.3390/ijerph18010133

Received: 30 November 2020
Accepted: 24 December 2020
Published: 27 December 2020

1. Introduction

Population ageing is taking place across all countries of the world, raising major issues for the direction of health and social policy. By 2030, two-thirds of the world's population will be residing in cities, with many urban areas in the developed world having 25 per cent or more of their populations aged 60 and over [1]. The period from the mid-2000s saw a substantial growth in interest in age-friendly issues, with a particular focus on problems facing older people in different types of urban areas [2]. This initial period of development recorded a variety of achievements that stimulated new approaches in areas such as housing, social inclusion, and neighborhood design [3]. However, a combination of widening inequalities within urban environments, together with the impact of austerity on local and municipal government budgets, has raised questions about future progress in age-friendly and related activities. Cities produce many advantages for older people in the form of access to medical services, provision of cultural and leisure facilities, and necessities for daily living. At the same time, they may also create feelings of vulnerability and insecurity arising from high levels of population turnover, environmental problems, and reduced availability of low-cost or affordable housing [4].

This article contributes to the debate on age-friendly cities and communities by, first, reviewing the background to the program of 'age-friendly cities and communities' developed by the World Health Organization (WHO); second, reporting on a survey of members of the WHO Global Network of Age-Friendly Cities and Communities; and, third, outlining priorities for the future planning of age-friendly programs.

Developing Age-Friendly Cities and Communities

The 'age-friendly' perspective was first developed by the World Health Organization (WHO) [5–7] through a project examining the experiences of older people living in urban environments. The result of this work was a guide identifying the key characteristics of an age-friendly community in terms of service provision (e.g., health services, transportation), the built environment (e.g., housing, outdoor spaces, and buildings), and social aspects (e.g., civic and social participation) [5]. This guide has since become one of the most frequently used tools to assess the age-friendliness of cities and communities [8]. To encourage dissemination of its work, the WHO launched in 2010 the Global Network of Age-Friendly Cities and Communities (GNAFCC), which by the end of 2020 had reached a membership of around 1114 cities and communities in 44 countries.

Any city or community can join the GNAFCC as long as they make a formal commitment to increase their level of age-friendliness. As the WHO [7] (p. 5) indicates, 'membership of the Network is not a designation but a commitment to making progress on the journey to becoming more age-friendly'. In order to be admitted to the Network participating cities must: (1) agree to share and promote the values and principles of the GNAFCC; (2) commit to developing their work following a 4-step process (i.e., engage and understand, plan, act, measure); and (3) actively participate in the GNAFCC [9].

The Network seeks to support members to become more age-friendly through 'connecting cities and communities worldwide (via its website, www.agefriendlyworld.com) to facilitate the exchange of information, knowledge and experiences'; 'inspiring change by showing what can be done and how it can be done'; and 'supporting cities and communities to find appropriate innovative and evidence-based solutions' [9] (p. 1). Members of the GNAFCC include communities, cities or other sub-national levels of government located in WHO Member States. In addition to the 1114 participating cities and communities in 44 countries, the Network also has 15 affiliates from 11 countries that play a key role in supporting the Network's mission. These affiliated programs advocate the work of the Network and advance knowledge and action on age-friendly environments [7].

Figure 1 identifies three phases in the growth of the Network: first, the *emergence phase*, characterized by relatively slow initial growth; second, the *consolidation phase* from 2014 to 2016, showing a gradual increase in membership; and third, the *expansion* phase, reflecting a marked acceleration in growth from 2017 to date. Membership of the GNAFCC increased four-fold between 2015 and 2018, with an expansion in the number of affiliates. This is a remarkable finding given continued pressures arising from the impact of economic austerity in many countries around the world. The vulnerability of age-friendly programs, faced with economic austerity, has been further compounded by pressures associated with urban change affecting global as well as de-industrializing cities [10]. Such limitations raise important concerns about the effectiveness and sustainability of age-friendly programs, and whether their growth is likely to continue over the next 10 years.

Research on Age-Friendly Issues

The age-friendly movement has begun to attract significant research interest, with groups, for example, in Belgium [11]; Canada [12]; Hong Kong [13]; the UK [14] and the US [15], exploring questions around developing communities responsive to the needs of people as they age. Research in this area has contributed significant knowledge about the ways in which cities are responding to population ageing and building age-friendly communities. Studies have, for example, explored the different steps associated with the age-friendly process, including the planning [16], implementation [17], and evaluation [18] of programs. Researchers have also examined the development of age-friendly initiatives in different contexts, both rural [19] and urban [20], as well as in different countries [21].

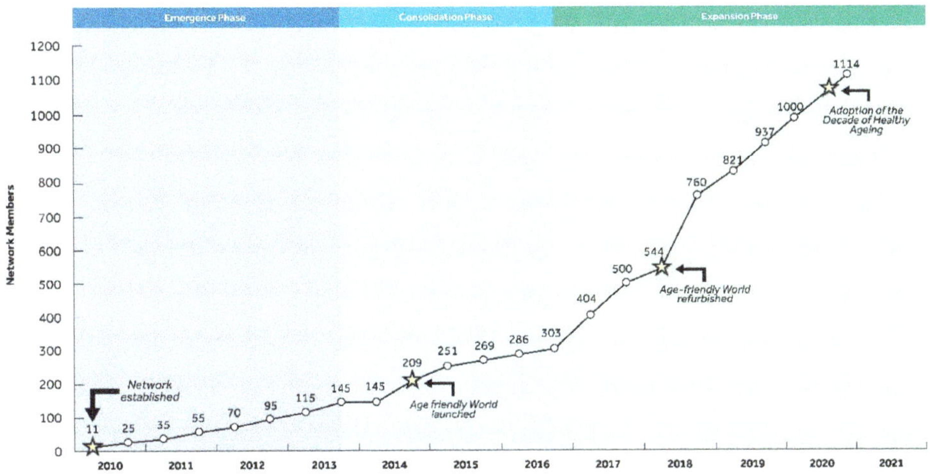

Figure 1. Growth of the Global Network of Age-Friendly Cities and Communities (GNAFCC) (adapted from [7]).

Despite these advances in knowledge, few studies have focused on the type of programs developed by partners in the GNAFCC. Ten years after the launch of the WHO network, little is known about the progress of the movement and the experience of cities developing this work around the world. The need to gain more knowledge of age-friendly initiatives has been highlighted by a number of researchers and has been identified by the WHO as a priority for the future of the age-friendly movement [7]. This interest is reflected in the increasing number of tools published to monitor and evaluate the success of programs. For example, the WHO published a guide in 2015 to help cities select the most appropriate indicators for measuring their level of age-friendliness. This document identified a list of 'core and supplementary indicators' which cities could choose from and adapt when conducting their own evaluations [22]. Similar tools have also emerged in the age-friendly literature focusing on specific national or local settings (see, for example, [18,23,24]).

The research initiatives identified have yet to provide detailed information on the different types of programs within the GNAFCC. This gap in knowledge reflects a range of methodological challenges linked to the integration of interdisciplinary perspectives, cross-national comparison, measurement, and evaluation [21]. Much of the literature published on the development of age-friendly programs and policies has either been based on a review of the literature or a single case study (of a city or a region). To address some of the limitations of existing work, this paper reports on a multiple case study of eleven members of the WHO Global Network of Age-Friendly Cities and Communities, and addresses the following research questions:

(1) What have been the key goals, achievements and challenges faced by local age-friendly programs since joining the GNAFCC?
(2) What are the key priorities to address to improve the development of age-friendly programs in the future?

2. Methodology

The study used a multiple case study approach, one which allows for 'in depth, multi-faceted explorations of complex issues in their real-life settings' [25] to compare the experience of eleven members of the GNAFCC. This approach lends itself to capturing information on more exploratory *'how'*, *'what'* and *'why'* questions, and has shown to be particularly instrumental in comparing the development of age-friendly programs and policies across different cities [20,26].

A purposeful sampling strategy was used to identify the eleven cases, with five criteria guiding the selection process [27]. The aim was to select cities that: (1) had an age-friendly program in place at the time of conducting the study; (2) were members of the Global Network of Age-Friendly Cities and Communities; (3) had been involved in the Network either from the beginning or from a relatively early phase of its development; (4) varied in size; (5) were located in different countries. Representatives from the WHO's Department of Ageing and Life Course assisted in the identification of cases by providing researchers with a list of cities that met the above criteria. The researchers made the final decision and selected the eleven cities presented in Figure 2.

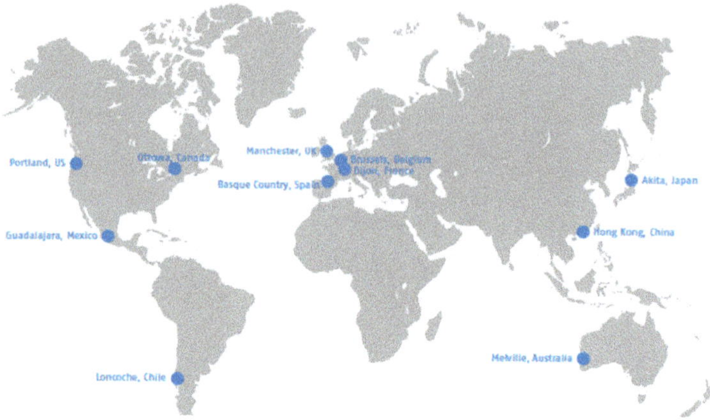

Figure 2. Map of selected cities.

Table 1 summarizes information about the cities which comprised 5 metropolitan areas, 2 medium-size urban areas, 3 small urban areas, and 1 urban cluster [28]. The eleven cities had in most cases joined the GNAFCC in its emergence phase (2010–2013), with the exception of Guadalajara and Loncoche which were admitted to the Network in 2014 and 2016. The percentage of the population aged 65 years and older showed considerable variation, ranging from 9.29% in Manchester to 30% in Akita.

The study was conducted between March 2018 and August 2018. The World Health Organization's Department of Ageing and Life Course was responsible for inviting selected cities to participate in the study, whilst a research team from the University of Manchester took the lead in collecting data. Three data collection tools were used to document the reality of the eleven cases: questionnaires (n = 11), document analysis, and interviews (n = 5).

Program representatives who agreed to take part in the study were invited to complete a questionnaire comprising 20 open-ended questions. The questionnaire explored a variety of themes related to the development of age-friendly programs. Participants were asked, for example, to describe the social and demographic contexts in which their program was developed, to identify some of the key objectives and achievements of their program, to identify the key barriers and enablers to developing age-friendly initiatives, and to share their views on the future of their program and the age-friendly movement. They were invited to complete the questionnaire in the language of their choice (English, French or Spanish) and asked to provide as much information as possible on their program and experience, thus allowing substantial amounts of data to be collected on each case.

Table 1. Key characteristics of the eleven cases.

	City (or Region)	Country	Population	GNAFCC Admission	% of People Aged 65 and Over
Metropolitan areas	Hong Kong	China	7.3 million	2010	14.7
	Basque Country	Spain	2.2 million	2013	22
	Guadalajara	Mexico	1.5 million	2014	10.5 *
	Ottawa	Canada	934,243	2011	15.4
	Portland	USA	647,805	2010	11.6
Medium-size urban areas	Manchester	UK	541,300	2010	9.29
	Akita	Japan	310,407	2011	30
Small urban areas	Brussels	Belgium	179,277	2010	11.1
	Dijon	France	155,114	2010	22.1 *
	Melville	Australia	102,252	2010	18.6
Urban cluster	Loncoche	Chile	23,612	2016	14

* % of people aged 60 and over.

Eleven questionnaires were completed in total. Each member of the research team was responsible for collecting and analyzing the data related to up to three cities in order to allow them to develop a more in-depth understanding of each case and facilitate communications with participating cities. The researchers contacted participants following the questionnaire completion when any clarifications were required. Five follow-up telephone interviews were also conducted with experts in cities to collect additional information. These interviews were audio-recorded, transcribed verbatim and, where necessary, translated into English.

Finally, a review of the key scientific and grey literature on each program was conducted to enrich the case descriptions. Participants were invited to share any document that would help the researchers develop a better understanding of their program and the context in which it was developed. Additional documents (e.g., baseline assessments, action plans, progress reports) were also drawn from the WHO's database of age-friendly programs. The content of these documents was not analyzed, per se, but carefully read and used to further our understanding of each case.

The researchers analyzed data relating to the individual cities first, before making comparisons across cases. The questionnaires served as the main source of information for the analysis. Each questionnaire was carefully read and compared with the interviews and the document analysis to clarify certain information, capture the specificities of each program, understand them in their context, and enrich the case descriptions. The results of this phase of analysis were used to write eleven case study reports, each presenting the reality of one age-friendly program. Whilst these reports were written by researchers, the data were mainly drawn from the questionnaires and reflected the views of local representatives. A similar structure was adopted to write the eleven case studies to facilitate cross-case comparisons. Each report provided a detailed description of one case, covering the five following themes: 'description of the context', 'development of the age-friendly program', 'impact and evaluation', 'opportunities and barriers', and 'future of the age-friendly movement'.

A second phase of analysis was conducted to compare the content of the reports and identify common themes across the eleven cases. Each individual report was carefully read and coded line by line using a thematic analysis approach and the qualitative analysis software NVivo. Two questions were used to focus and guide the analysis: (1) What have been the key goals, achievements and challenges faced by local age-friendly programs since joining the GNAFCC? (2) What are the key priorities to address to improve the development of age-friendly programs in the future? This second phase of analysis led the researchers to identify four priorities the age-friendly movement should consider in order to further its development. The next section of this paper reports on the results of the analysis of the 11 age-friendly programs.

3. Findings

Four main areas were identified as common across the work of the various age-friendly cities and communities: (1) changing the perception of older age; (2) involving key actors in age-friendly efforts; (3) responding to the (diverse) needs of older people; and (4) improving the planning and delivery of age-friendly programs. Each of these is presented and discussed in more detail in the following sections.

3.1. Changing the Perception of Older Age

All participants highlighted the importance of age-friendly programs *challenging the negative image and portrayal of ageing*. The need to shift perception, change mindsets and promote a more positive vision of ageing was identified as a key priority across the eleven cases. Representatives from Akita, for example, considered it important to 'create a society where people consider the 100-year life as a positive opportunity'; representatives from Dijon to 'remind people that living longer lives is a chance'; and representatives from Manchester to 'change the narrative to one that celebrates the valuable role and contribution of older people'. A variety of projects have been developed in participating cities to promote a more positive vision of ageing. One popular way to achieve this goal has been to encourage the development of communication campaigns that use more realistic and non-stereotypical images of ageing, a more positive language, and paint a more diverse portrait of the older population. Cities had also developed communications tools, such as logos, symbols, charters, and slogans to promote age-friendly initiatives and challenge the negative image of ageing. The city of Portland, for example, applied the slogan 'nothing about them, without them' in its communications to describe the city's age-friendly approach and promote the civic engagement of older people.

Promoting the social participation of older people was also seen as a way to challenge ageism, by making this group more visible 'and [making older people] seen as active and essential members of the community' (Loncoche). Participating cities worked toward this goal in two main ways: first, by providing older people with more opportunities to take part in social activities; and second, by involving them more directly in age-friendly interventions. A variety of activities, projects and services aimed at increasing the social participation of older people were created in the eleven cities following their admission to the GNAFCC. One of the key achievements of the age-friendly program in Brussels, for example, has been the opening of seven social meeting spaces for older people across the city. Called 'Spaces S' (for seniors), these offer leisure activities, information, sports, and training sessions for older people that are delivered directly at the neighborhood-level. Similar places have also been created in Dijon and Loncoche and are considered as key resources for the community. Another popular way to promote the participation of older people has been through the formation of representative bodies of different kinds. Various initiatives (e.g., activities, consultations, studies) and mechanisms (e.g., committees, boards, roundtables) have been established in order to give older people a more central role in age-friendly developments. Whilst older people's levels of participation may have differed from one city to another, the need for their expertise to shape the development of age-friendly programs was recognized and considered as a key priority in all cities.

The age-friendly program was also used *to raise awareness of key issues and concerns facing older people*. This was viewed as a way of promoting both a vision of older age and improving the treatment of older people. Participating cities had adopted various strategies to achieve this goal. The city of Guadalajara, for example, had developed training courses for the public sector to help employees become more aware and sensitive towards the specific needs of older people. The cities of Portland and Manchester worked closely with university researchers and held conferences to report on current research and practices on ageing which could feedback to work within the local community. Intergenerational initiatives had also been developed as another approach to raising awareness. Encouraging younger and older people to interact on a more regular basis was seen as way to 'promote the exchange of knowledge' (Guadalajara); 'tackle negative stereotyping of older people' (Guadalajara); and 'increase respect for older generations' (Loncoche).

Responses from the survey suggested that age-friendly initiatives have helped challenge negative perceptions of ageing, with awareness of the existence of these often a driving force behind the development of programs. When asked to describe the impact of their program, a majority of participants reported that this work had contributed to making older people more visible in their city and raised awareness of their views and needs amongst both the population and service providers. The representative from Loncoche, for example, mentioned that the 'perception of older age was changing' in their city; Guadalajara commented that local actors were now 'more aware of the issues surrounding ageing'; and the representative from Ottawa that their program had 'increased awareness of older people's needs and realities'. Despite this progress, changing the perception of older age remained a key concern of respondents. Combating ageism was described not only as an important priority to address to improve the quality of life of older people, but also the delivery of age-friendly programs.

Ageism—and more specifically the lack of interest relating ageing issues—was identified as one of the key *barriers* to developing age-friendly work. Representatives from Dijon went so far as to describe ageism as a '*blockage*' and as '*the principal obstacle the city had to face*'. The difficulty to get traction for ageing issues can be an important barrier to the development of age-friendly initiatives given the wide variety of demands on municipal budgets—not least given new pressures such as those associated with COVID-19. Raising awareness of the needs of older people amongst service providers will be essential to secure more support for developing age-friendly activities.

3.2. Involving Key Actors in Age-Friendly Efforts

The second major theme to emerge from the research was the need to involve key actors in age-friendly projects. When asked to comment on the progress of their work, participants often referred to the development of new partnerships and collaborations as a key goal for the future of their programs. Establishing links with a wide range of actors (e.g., local councils, community organizations, businesses, universities, older people), working in a variety of domains (e.g., housing, transport, health, urban planning, social work, environment), was identified as a key success factor for the development of age-friendly initiatives. The research showed that the cities were able to secure the support of a variety of stakeholders and develop innovative partnerships as part of their work. Akita and Melville, for example, were especially successful in gaining the involvement of businesses. At the time of conducting the research, 88 organizations from the private sector were registered as 'Age-Friendly Partners' and involved in making the city of Akita more age-friendly. Guadalajara, Manchester, Ottawa, and Portland had worked closely with universities and researchers throughout the development of their programs. Portland State University played a leading role in developing age-friendly work in the city, assuming both co-ordination and leadership roles.

Cities had developed a variety of mechanisms to facilitate these collaborations. Dijon, for example, created an innovative platform called '*l'Observatoire de l'Âge*'. This participatory mechanism brings together 83 members (2018 figures) from various groups (i.e., 10 elected officials; 39 local residents; 9 neighborhood representatives; 6 retiree representatives; 4 institutional partners; 10 professional experts; and 5 researchers), divided into work committees. Each committee is allocated a specific theme and asked to develop concrete propositions and projects to improve an ageing issue during the year. As Dijon's representatives explained, this way of working was considered beneficial for the program because it 'encourages stakeholders to compromise and prioritize'. At the time of conducting the study, the cities of Brussels, Manchester and Ottawa were respectively working in close collaboration with a 'Senior Advisory Council', an 'Older People's board' and a 'Senior Roundtable' all comprised of older residents, to shape the development of their program.

The research also highlighted the need to involve actors working at different levels in age-friendly programs. As the movement progresses, scaling up projects and establishing collaborations with actors working at the local, regional, and national level emerged as a growing concern for participating cities. This appeared especially important for large metropolitan areas such as the Basque Country, Hong Kong, and Manchester, which were developing their work at the regional level. More than 50 municipalities had joined the age-friendly movement in the Basque Country, with support from the Department of Employment and Social Policies, and the Matia Gerontological Institute. Melville identified work with the Government of Western Australia as one of the key achievements of its program, whilst the cities of Brussels and Dijon expressed an interest in collaborating with organizations working at the regional and national level to conduct projects on specific themes (e.g., social exclusion and social isolation).

A large majority of participants referred to the development of new collaborations—and the strengthening of existing partnerships—as two of the key achievements of their program. Respondents considered that these collaborations brought important benefits to their work, including the possibility for their program to 'benefit from the expertise of a variety of actors' (Portland); to 'develop a wider range of initiatives' (Manchester); to 'involve the voices of different groups' (Melville); to 'look at ageing issues from different angles' (Dijon); to make a variety of actors 'see the importance of becoming age-friendly' (Akita); and to 'improve the dialogue between the city council and citizens' (Basque Country). Despite this progress, involving key actors in age-friendly efforts was seen as a challenge and considered as an important priority to address for the future of the age-friendly movement. The research found that certain actors remained difficult to involve in age-friendly efforts, especially given budgetary pressures, and competing economic and social priorities [2]. Participants believed they could achieve more with their program if more actors considered their work through 'an ageing lens' and expressed their wish 'for the age-friendly approach to become an automatic consideration in all plans and work' (Manchester) of their city in the future. The lack of interest of certain actors for ageing issues was, however, seen as an obstacle to achieving this goal, reinforcing the idea that raising awareness and challenging the negative perception of older age amongst service providers would be essential for the age-friendly movement to achieve its full potential.

3.3. *Responding to the (Diverse) Needs of Older People*

The third priority to emerge from the research was the need to respond to the (diverse) needs of older people. The research highlighted the need for age-friendly programs to address a variety of themes and domains in order to achieve this goal. Projects aiming to improve the social environments had been especially popular across the eleven cities. Cities had worked on a wide range of issues since launching their programs, ranging from attempts to increase the level of employment in the older working population, to projects aimed at widening participation in arts and cultural activities. Manchester launched a program called 'the Age-Friendly Manchester Culture Program' which brought together 19 cultural organizations (e.g., museums, orchestras, theatres) from across the city with the aim of making arts and culture more accessible to older people. In 2018, more than 150 older volunteers were involved in one of its flagship projects (the 'Culture Champions' scheme), acting as cultural ambassadors in their community.

Another priority for action amongst the cities has been in the area of health promotion. A variety of initiatives have been developed to promote healthy and active ageing, as well as sports and physical activity in older age. Guadalajara developed a program called 'Taking Control of your Health' which sought to encourage healthier eating, physical activity, and healthy cognitive function amongst the older population. The project set a target of reaching 2400 people by the end of 2018. Improving the built environment also emerged as an important area of concerns, with transport and mobility being amongst the themes most frequently addressed. Since joining the GNAFCC, cities have, for example, installed more seating, benches, and lighting in public spaces, and improved pavements and roads to make them safer for older people. They have also developed projects to increase the accessibility of transport systems, public buildings, and specific areas in their city. Dijon, for example, has worked on increasing the age-friendliness of its city center for older people, going as far as to pedestrianize certain areas to increase their accessibility.

Respondents to the survey reported that these projects had had a positive impact on their older population. When asked to describe the key benefits of their programs, participants explained that this work: had allowed them to 'reach a large number of older people' (Guadalajara); had contributed to 'making the community a better place in which to age physically, socially, and economically' (Portland); had 'led to concrete changes in municipal operations, policies and communications' (Ottawa); and had 'increased the accessibility and affordability of programs and services' for older people in their city (Ottawa). Whilst age-friendly programs had undoubtedly led to the development of important and innovative initiatives, participants expressed the wish to raise the ambition of their program in the coming years, albeit aware for constraints on budgets given a climate of economic austerity.

Meeting the needs of diverse groups within the older population was also highlighted by a number of respondents. Representatives from Brussels, for example, highlighted the importance (and difficulty) for the age-friendly program to respond to the needs of different age groups within the older population: 'the 55–65 years old, the 65–80 years old and the 80 and over'. Representatives from Hong Kong and Akita—recognized for the rapid ageing of their populations—expressed a similar concern and stressed the importance of developing initiatives to support the 'oldest-old'. Dijon highlighted the need for age-friendly initiatives to support vulnerable groups, and 'the groups the most at risk of being isolated, such as people with disabilities'; Melville highlighted the need to develop more initiatives for people living with dementia; and the cities of Manchester and Ottawa—considered as ethnically diverse cities—the importance of projects that recognized older people's diverse cultural backgrounds. Manchester, for example, had developed a substantial program of work tackling issues relating to social isolation, linking with a range of organizations representing older people from Black, Asian, and Minority Ethnic (BAME) groups.

These findings illustrate both the importance and complexity of meeting the needs of a rapidly ageing population. In order to increase the age-friendliness of their cities, age-friendly programs must not only address a variety of themes but also address the needs of different groups of older people. Achieving this goal is complex, and even more challenging that age-friendly programs are developed with limited resources. The lack of resources was identified as one of the key barriers to developing age-friendly initiatives. The research found that age-friendly programs were often developed in a context of financial restraint and cuts to public services, with insufficient budget and limited staff, forcing age-friendly programs to prioritize between a wide range of issues and limiting the scope of their work. Securing more resources for age-friendly initiatives will be essential to raise the ambition of age-friendly programs and meet the needs of a wider group of older people. As representatives from Loncoche explained, whilst age-friendly programs 'can be successful with limited resources [...] some projects require more substantial investments in order to achieve their aims'.

3.4. Improving the Planning and Delivery of Age-Friendly Programs

A fourth major theme to emerge from the research was the need to improve the planning and delivery of age-friendly programs. When asked to comment on the progress of their program, a majority of participants referred to the organizational dimension of their work and reflected on ways to improve its development. Cities highlighted the need for age-friendly programs to inform their planning by identifying the key priorities to address in their city. Conducting a baseline assessment and collecting data to better understand 'what communities need and want' (Melville) was often considered as the first step of the planning process. A variety of initiatives were developed across the cities to achieve this goal. The city of Hong Kong, for example, conducted focus groups with 96 participants drawn from a wide range of stakeholders to orient the development of its program, whilst the city of Brussels chose to take part in a research project called 'the Belgian Ageing Studies' to collect data on the needs of their older population and inform its decision-making [29]. Cities have also shown an interest in documenting the needs of a wide range of groups within their older population. The city of Ottawa, for example, conducted 24 public consultation sessions with older people to inform the development of its first age-friendly action plan. Of this number, nine targeted the general population but took place in different locations (allowing urban, rural, francophone and anglophone older residents to be represented) and 15 were designed for older adults with unique needs (e.g., aboriginal elders, natural caregivers, isolated older adults, LGBTQ+ community). Participants highlighted the importance for age-friendly programs to be informed by knowledge and their wish to collect more data to inform their decision-making in the future. The lack of resources was, however, often seen as an obstacle to achieving this goal.

Selecting the type of project to implement also emerged as a key step of the planning process. The research suggested that participating cities had addressed age-friendly issues in different ways since joining the GNAFCC. First, cities had developed new projects and services to increase their level of age-friendliness. These varied in scope and addressed different themes, ranging from promoting the social participation of older people to making public spaces safer and more accessible. Second, cities had developed new ways of working, established innovative partnerships, and created new platforms and mechanisms to facilitate these collaborations. Third, cities had worked on influencing policy and making long-term changes in certain domains. Portland's approach, for example, had been especially focused on shaping policy for the future. As program representatives explained, this choice was made 'intentionally to create sustainable, long-term change that will benefit both current and future generations'. Their efforts allowed for a set of age-friendly policies to be incorporated into Portland's 2035 Comprehensive Plan, a key document which took effect in 2018.

The research indicated that sharing best practices could help cities identify the most beneficial projects to develop in their city. Local representatives saw positively the possibility to take part in knowledge exchange activities. Participants highlighted the need for cities and organizations 'to share best practices' (Ottawa); 'to learn both from failures and successes' (Akita); 'to identify barriers to implementation and develop solutions' (Guadalajara); and 'to showcase their innovations and experimentations' (Dijon) as the age-friendly movement develops. The GNAFCC was seen as a key platform for achieving this goal. When asked to reflect on the future of the age-friendly movement, participants highlighted the important role the Network played in connecting participating cities. The possibility to interact with other cities was considered particularly helpful for communities less advanced in their efforts to become more age-friendly and seen as a way to encourage more cities to join the age-friendly movement.

Securing more political support was also seen as a way to improve the planning and delivery of age-friendly programs. The possibility to rely on strong political support was identified as a key success factor for the development of age-friendly initiatives. Manchester representatives, for example, identified the 'political support and advocacy from the City's leadership' and 'the commitment from services and organizations' as two of the key success factors for developing their program. Ottawa's representatives shared similar views and explained that the strong support they received from political leaders in their city 'provided strength, momentum, credibility and enabled staff buy-in' for their program. As their programs continue to expand, several cities expressed a wish to secure more support for developing this work and involve more city departments in their age-friendly efforts.

Evaluating the success of age-friendly programs finally emerged as a priority for the future of the age-friendly movement. Participants all recognized the importance of evaluating their work. A large majority of them were reflecting on ways to assess the impact of their program at the time of conducting the study. The city of Ottawa, for example, was working on the development of an Age-Friendly Evaluation Framework and had analyzed 'baseline data for 66 indicators covering medium and longer-term outcomes and impacts across the 8 areas of an age-friendly community'. The city of Manchester was developing 'a set of statistical indicators to measure the progress and impact of its work', working in close collaboration with a national foundation on ageing. Despite this progress, the research found that limited evaluation had been carried out in participating cities, but that demonstrating the impact of age-friendly work will be important to raise the ambition of age-friendly programs and ensure their sustainability. As Portland representatives explained, collecting more data could be beneficial for age-friendly initiatives and help 'provide the impetus for the work and support for continuation'.

4. Discussion

This article set out to reflect on the progress of the age-friendly movement by comparing the experience of eleven participating cities in eleven countries. More specifically, it aimed to explore the key goals, achievements, and challenges of age-friendly programs and some of the key cross-cutting themes. The paper identified four priorities to further the development of the age-friendly movement. First, it highlighted the continuing need to change the perception of older age amongst service providers. Despite the progress made by cities, the article showed that promoting ageing remained a challenge for several years after the launch of age-friendly programs. It also showed that tackling ageism was not only important in improving the quality of life of older people, but also in enabling the delivery of age-friendly programs themselves. Gaining prominence for ageing issues can be challenging when there are competing priorities for limited resources. Raising awareness of the needs of older people will be important for age-friendly issues to remain on the political agenda of their city and to ensure the sustainability of local age-friendly programs on the long term.

Second, it highlighted the need to involve key actors in age-friendly projects. The study showed that, on the one hand, mainstreaming ageing was essential to increase the age-friendliness of cities; on the other hand, that certain stakeholders resist direct involvement in age-friendly initiatives. Reflecting on ways to convince actors from different domains and working at different levels to take part in age-friendly efforts will be essential to address the diverse needs of older people. Whilst the importance of developing cross-sectoral collaborations has been acknowledged by a number of researchers in the age-friendly literature, little is known about the key enablers and barriers to establishing these partnerships and the most effective mechanisms to facilitate collaborations. As it continues to expand, the age-friendly movement would benefit from reflecting and conducting more research on these topics.

Third, the survey confirmed the need for age-friendly programs to respond to the (diverse) needs of older people. As this study illustrates, increasing the age-friendliness of cities requires responses to the varied needs of different groups of older people. Whilst they have made significant progress, participating cities all expressed a wish to develop more ambitious projects and reach new groups within the older population in the future, for example those from minority communities, and those living in areas of multiple deprivation. This raises the issue of the extent to which age-friendly programs can tackle wider economic and social inequalities within society, these having become more prominent over the past 10 years [2,10]. In this regard, if success is to be achieved for the kind of initiatives described in this paper—partnerships will be needed with a range of movements seeking to improve the lives of marginalized and excluded groups within cities. This challenge raises important concerns regarding the capacity of cities to achieve this goal with what are often limited resources. Finding ways to secure additional support will be important for the age-friendly movement to achieve its full potential. Linking age-friendly issues to other priorities (or age groups) within cities, for example, might help local actors get more traction for the age-friendly agenda. Establishing partnerships with other social movements might also have benefits, notably around areas such as climate change, and campaigns around rights to the city. Collecting more data and conducting more evaluation might also help demonstrate the benefits of developing this work and help secure the support of influential stakeholders.

Fourth, the survey highlighted the need to improve the planning and delivery of age-friendly programs. Given the large number of needs to address and the limited resources allocated to develop this work, cities are forced to prioritize between a wide range of issues. Identifying the most important challenges to address in their city and deciding how to tackle them requires careful planning. This study suggests that offering programs representatives more opportunities to take part in knowledge exchange activities and share best practices could support their planning and help them select the most optimal projects to develop in their city. As the movement continues to expand, participating cities might also benefit from having access to more tools and information on how to best organize and structure the development of their program. Platforms such as the GNAFCC, or its affiliated programs, can play an important role in this respect by connecting cities and facilitating the sharing of information [7].

Finally, the study suggests that these four priorities overlap and influence each other. Raising awareness of the needs of older people, for example, can help convince more actors to invest in age-friendly efforts, which can, in turn, improve the delivery of age-friendly programs and allow age-friendly initiatives to be more ambitious and better respond to the diverse needs of their population.

Limitations of the Research

Although the study identifies important priorities to address to further the development of the age-friendly movement, the research also has limitations. First, selected cases may not be representative of the whole age-friendly movement. The choice to select more experienced cities was made to allow for a more in-depth reflection on their progress. Whilst their achievements may not represent those of less advanced cities, the challenges and priorities discussed in this paper are likely to speak to any city or community involved in developing this work. There is to date limited information on age-friendly initiatives within low-income countries, and the specific challenges which they face. A research initiative to review issues relating to the scope, implementation, and barriers faced by age-friendly work in this context, is urgently needed. Second, the analysis drew mainly on questionnaires completed by local representatives, and therefore, strongly reflected their perception of their program. Whilst these participants were considered better able to comment on the development of their program and identify the key success factors and challenges to developing age-friendly initiatives, their views may not represent that of other actors in their city. Interviewing a variety of actors, and including the voice of older people in particular, would have allowed the research to paint a more nuanced portrait of each program and develop a more in-depth understanding of each case. Despite these limitations, this exploratory study makes an important contribution to the age-friendly literature by comparing the experience of eleven local age-friendly programs in eleven countries. To our knowledge, this study is the first to compare the experience of that many cities as part of a single research project. This study highlights the need to conduct more empirical, comparative, and cross-national studies on age-friendly initiatives. It also demonstrates the potential of such studies to provide pointers for future research and policy developments on age-friendly issues.

5. Conclusions

This article makes a contribution to the age-friendly literature by identifying four priorities the age-friendly movement should consider to further its development: first, challenging the negative perception of older age and raising awareness of the needs of older people; second, involving key actors in age-friendly programs; third, responding to the (diverse) needs of older people; and fourth, improving the planning and delivery of age-friendly programs. The study also highlighted the benefits of conducting more empirical, comparative, and cross-national studies to better understand the development of the age-friendly movement. As it continues to expand, measuring the progress of the age-friendly movement—and documenting the experience of participating cities—will be essential to demonstrate the benefits of the age-friendly approach, and directions for future policy and practice. Such activity will be especially important in a context of increasing pressure on local authority and municipal budgets given a combination of cuts to the funding of social programs and the impact of the COVID-19 pandemic in amplifying social inequalities [30]. However, it is precisely in this situation that the benefits of adopting an age-friendly approach may become apparent. In particular, in helping to ensure that support for older people is maintained and that the voices of those growing old continue to be heard and acted upon.

Author Contributions: Conceptualization, S.R.-B., T.B. and C.P.; methodology, S.R.-B., T.B. and C.P.; validation, C.P.; formal analysis, S.R.-B.; investigation, S.R.-B. and T.B.; writing—original draft preparation, S.R.-B. and T.B.; writing—review and editing, S.R.-B., T.B. and C.P.; supervision, T.B. and C.P.; project administration, T.B.; funding acquisition, T.B. All authors have read and agreed to the published version of the manuscript.

Funding: This research was supported by funding from the Public Health Agency of Canada and the Government of New Zealand. This work was also supported by the Social Sciences and Humanities Research Council of Canada (SSHRC) through a Doctoral Fellowship at the University of Manchester and the Economic and Social Research Council (ESRC) under the Future Research Leaders scheme (PI, Tine Buffel). Project Reference: ES/N002180/1. The views expressed in this paper are those of the authors and not necessarily those of the WHO.

Institutional Review Board Statement: The study did not require ethical approval.

Informed Consent Statement: Informed consent was obtained from all subjects involved in the study.

Data Availability Statement: Restrictions apply to the availability of these data. Data was obtained through the Word Health Organization (Department of Ageing and Life-Course) and are available from the authors with the permission of the World Health Organisation (Department of Ageing and Life-Course).

Acknowledgments: We would like to thank all participants who agreed to take part in this research. Our appreciation also goes to Alana Officer and Diane Wu for facilitating the research and Natalie Cotterell for her participation to the data collection and the redaction of the case studies.

Conflicts of Interest: The authors declare no conflict of interest.

References

1. Organisation for Economic Co-operation and Development. *Ageing in Cities*; OECD Publishing: Paris, France, 2015.
2. Buffel, T.; Phillipson, C. Can global cities be 'age-friendly' cities? Urban development and ageing populations. *Cities* **2016**, *55*, 94–100. [CrossRef]
3. White, S.; Hammond, M. From representation to active ageing in a Manchester neighbourhood: Designing the age-friendly city. In *Age-Friendly Cities and Communities: A Global Perspective*; Buffel, T., Handler, S., Phillipson, C., Eds.; Policy Press: Bristol, UK, 2018; pp. 193–210.
4. Hertz, N. *The Lonely Century: Coming together in a World that's Pulling Apart*; Sceptre: London, UK, 2020.
5. World Health Organization. *Global Age-Friendly Cities: A Guide*; WHO: Geneva, Switzerland, 2007.
6. World Health Organization. *World Report on Ageing and Health*; WHO: Geneva, Switzerland, 2015.
7. World Health Organization. *The Global Network for Age-Friendly Cities and Communities: Looking Back over the Last Decade, Looking Forward to the Next*; WHO: Geneva, Switzerland, 2018.
8. Plouffe, L.; Kalache, A.; Voelcker, I. A critical review of the WHO age-friendly cities methodology and its implementation. In *Age-Friendly Cities and Communities in International Comparison. Political Lessons, Scientific Avenues, and Democratic Issues*; Moulaert, T., Garon, S., Eds.; Springer International Publishing: Cham, Switzerland, 2016; pp. 19–36.
9. World Health Organization. Membership in the Global Network of Age-friendly Cities and Communities (GNAFCC). Available online: https://www.who.int/ageing/age-friendly-environments/GNAFCC-membership-en.pdf (accessed on 13 November 2020).
10. Buffel, T.; Phillipson, C. A manifesto for the age-friendly movement: Developing a new urban agenda. *J. Aging Soc. Policy* **2018**, *30*, 173–192. [CrossRef] [PubMed]

11. Moulaert, T.; Houioux, G. A Belgian case study: Lack of age-friendly cities and communities knowledge and social participation practices in Wallonia. In *Age-Friendly Cities and Communities in International Comparison. Political Lessons, Scientific Avenues, and Democratic Issues*; Moulaert, T., Garon, S., Eds.; Springer International Publishing: Cham, Switzerland, 2016; pp. 213–228.
12. Garon, S.; Veil, A.; Paris, M.; Rémillard-Boilard, S. How can a research program enhance a policy? AFC-Quebec governance and evaluation opportunities. In *Age-Friendly Cities and Communities in International Comparison. Political Lessons, Scientific Avenues, and Democratic Issues*; Moulaert, T., Garon, S., Eds.; Springer International Publishing: Cham, Switzerland, 2016; pp. 99–120.
13. Phillips, D.R.; Woo, J.; Cheung, F.; Wong, M.; Chau, P.H. Exploring the age friendliness of Hong Kong: Opportunities, initiatives and challenges in an ageing Asian city. In *Age-Friendly Cities and Communities: A Global Perspective*; Buffel, T., Handler, S., Phillipson, C., Eds.; Policy Press: Bristol, UK, 2018; pp. 119–142.
14. Buffel, T.; Handler, S.; Phillipson, C. Age-friendly cities and communities: A manifesto for change. In *Age-Friendly Cities and Communities: A Global Perspective*; Buffel, T., Handler, S., Phillipson, C., Eds.; Policy Press: Bristol, UK, 2018; pp. 273–288.
15. Greenfield, E.A.; Oberlink, M.; Scharlach, A.E.; Neal, M.B.; Stafford, P.B. Age-friendly community initiatives: Conceptual issues and key questions. *Gerontologist* **2015**, *55*, 191–198. [CrossRef] [PubMed]
16. Greenfield. E.A. Getting started: An empirically derived logic model for age-friendly community initiatives in the early planning phase. *J. Gerontol. Soc. Work* **2018**, *61*, 295–312. [CrossRef] [PubMed]
17. McDonald, B.; Scharf, T.; Walsh, K. Creating an age-friendly county in Ireland: Stakeholders' perspectives on implementation. In *Age-Friendly Cities and Communities: A Global Perspective*; Buffel, T., Handler, S., Phillipson, C., Eds.; Policy Press: Bristol, UK, 2018; pp. 143–166.
18. Buckner, S.; Pope, D.; Mattocks, C.; Lafortune, L.; Dherani, M.; Bruce, N. Developing age-friendly cities: An evidence-based evaluation tool. *J. Popul. Ageing* **2017**, *12*, 203–223. [CrossRef]
19. Menec, V.; Bell, S.; Novek, S.; Minnigaleeva, G.A.; Morales, E.; Ouma, T.; Parodi, J.F.; Winterton, R. Making rural and remote communities more age-friendly: Experts' perspectives on issues, challenges, and priorities. *J. Aging Soc. Policy* **2015**, *27*, 173–191. [CrossRef] [PubMed]
20. Buffel, T.; Rémillard-Boilard, S.; Walsh, K.; McDonald, B.; Smetcoren, A.-S.; De Donder, L. Age-friendly approaches and old-age exclusion: A cross-city analysis. *Int. J. Ageing Later Life* **2020**. [CrossRef]
21. Moulaert, T.; Garon, S. (Eds.) *Age-Friendly Cities and Communities in International Comparison. Political Lessons, Scientific Avenues, and Democratic Issues*; Springer International Publishing: Cham, Switzerland, 2016.
22. World Health Organization. *Measuring the Age-Friendliness of Cities: A Guide to Using Core Indicators*; WHO: Geneva, Switzerland, 2015.
23. Chapon, P.-M.; Lefebvre, P.-O.; Philipona, A.; Finot, F. Measuring the impact of an "age-friendly city" approach on a territory by setting up cross-cutting indicators. *Gériatrie Psychol. Neuropsychiatr. Vieil.* **2015**, *13*, 169–175. [CrossRef] [PubMed]
24. Dikken, J.; van den Hoven, R.F.M.; van Staalduinen, W.H.; Hulsebosch-Janssen, L.M.T.; van Hoof, J. How older people experience the age-friendliness of their city: Development of the Age-Friendly Cities and Communities Questionnaire. *Int. J. Environ. Res. Public Health* **2020**, *17*, 6867. [CrossRef] [PubMed]
25. Crowe, S.; Cresswell, K.; Roberston, A.; Huby, G.; Avery, A.; Sheikh, A. The case study approach. *BMC Med. Res. Methodol.* **2011**, *11*, 100. [CrossRef]
26. Rémillard-Boilard, S. Developing Age-Friendly Cities: A Public Policy Perspective. Doctoral Thesis, The University of Manchester, Manchester, UK, 2019.
27. Patton, M.Q. *Qualitative Research & Evaluation Methods: Integrating Theory and Practice*, 4th ed.; SAGE Publications: Thousand Oaks, CA, USA, 2015.
28. Organisation for Economic Co-operation and Development. *Redefining "Urban": A New Way to Measure Metropolitan Areas*; OECD Publishing: Paris, France, 2012.
29. De Donder, L.; De Witte, N.; Verté, D.; Drury, S.; Buffel, T.; Smetcoren, A.S.; Brosens, D.; Verté, E. *Developing Evidence-Based Age-Friendly Policies: A Participatory Research Project*; SAGE Publications: London, UK, 2014. [CrossRef]
30. Buffel, T.; Doran, P.; Goff, M.; Lang, L.; Lewis, C.; Phillipson, C.; Yarker, S. Covid-19 and inequality: Developing an age-friendly strategy for low-income communities. *Qual. Ageing Older Adults* **2020**, *21*, 271–279. [CrossRef]

International Journal of
Environmental Research and Public Health

MDPI

Article

Towards Responsible Rebellion: How Founders Deal with Challenges in Establishing and Governing Innovative Living Arrangements for Older People

Katja M. Rusinovic [1,*], Marianne E. van Bochove [2], Suzanna Koops-Boelaars [2], Zsuzsu K.C.T. Tavy [3] and Joost van Hoof [4,5]

1 Urban Social Development, Faculty of Public Management, Law & Safety, The Hague University of Applied Sciences, Johanna Westerdijkplein 75, 2521 EN Den Haag, The Netherlands
2 Department of Health Care Governance, Erasmus School of Health Policy & Management, Erasmus University Rotterdam, Burgemeester Oudlaan 50, 3000 DR Rotterdam, The Netherlands; vanbochove@eshpm.eur.nl (M.E.v.B.); koops@eshpm.eur.nl (S.K.-B.)
3 Faculty of Health, Nutrition & Sport, The Hague University of Applied Sciences, Johanna Westerdijkplein 75, 2521 EN Den Haag, The Netherlands; z.k.c.t.tavy@hhs.nl
4 Faculty of Social Work & Education, The Hague University of Applied Sciences, Johanna Westerdijkplein 75, 2521 EN Den Haag, The Netherlands; j.vanhoof@hhs.nl
5 Institute of Spatial Management, Faculty of Environmental Engineering and Geodesy, Wrocław University of Environmental and Life Sciences, ul. Grunwaldzka 55, 50-357 Wrocław, Poland
* Correspondence: k.m.rusinovic@hhs.nl; Tel.: +31-6-86-86-52-04

Received: 29 June 2020; Accepted: 16 August 2020; Published: 27 August 2020

check for updates

Abstract: In the Netherlands, there is an increasing need for collective forms of housing for older people. Such housing bridges the gap between the extremes of living in an institutionalised setting and remaining in their own house. The demand is related to the closure of many residential care homes and the need for social engagement with other residents. This study focuses on housing initiatives that offer innovative and alternative forms of independent living, which deviate from mainstream housing arrangements. It draws on recent literature on healthcare 'rebels' and further develops the concept of 'rebellion' in the context of housing. The main research question is how founders dealt with challenges of establishing and governing 'rebellious' innovative living arrangements for older people in the highly regulated context of housing and care in the Netherlands. Qualitative in-depth interviews with 17 founders (social entrepreneurs, directors and supervisory board members) were conducted. Founders encountered various obstacles that are often related to governmental and sectoral rules and regulations. Their stories demonstrate the opportunities and constraints of innovative entrepreneurship at the intersection of housing and care. The study concludes with the notion of 'responsible rebellion' and practical lessons about dealing with rules and regulations and creating supportive contexts.

Keywords: housing; older people; elderly; assisted living facilities; seniors; homes; group living; dwellings; regulations; rebellion; governance; law

1. Introduction

All over the world, people live longer and are generally in better health than previous generations of their age. Age-friendly cities and communities can help improve the quality of life of older citizens. An age-friendly city or community is a place where older people are actively involved, valued, and supported with infrastructure and services that effectively accommodate their needs [1–3]. Housing is one of the key domains of establishing age-friendly cities. Creating appropriate housing for older people is one of the major challenges facing Western countries [2,4,5]. Ever-increasing numbers of older people live independently and remain part of the society at large, also referred to as ageing-in-place. This trend is not just related to the preferences or wishes of older people themselves. Government measures, such as reforms in long-term care, also play an important role [6]. When taking a closer look at the Netherlands, there are several challenges related to housing for older people and the housing career of this cohort [7]. In recent years, for instance, many residential care homes, which bridged the gap between one's own home and a nursing home, have been closed. Some of these vacant premises have been innovatively converted into facilities for independent living [8]. Given the changes in policies, a significant group of older people in need for collectivity are in danger of getting left out. In addition, there are many older people who do not need continuous care and support, but who are nevertheless seeking the safety and jointness of a collective form of housing (sometimes referred to as senior co-housing communities) [9]. A collective form of housing is a type of residence inside a larger building that has housing as its main function. It consists of several residential units, and a minimum of two households voluntarily share at least one living space, and each have at least one private living space. Residents of co-housing communities live in their own apartments but undertake activities together and support one another. There is an administrative separation between the need for housing on the one hand, and the need for care on the other. This is reflected in a lease contract for the home and a separate contract for the provision of care, only if needed by the older tenant. Some of these types of age-friendly housing bridge the gap between the need for ageing-in-place and living in institutional care facilities, as was the case with the former residential care facilities [7].

The Dutch government expects that municipalities, social housing associations and market parties take more action in the coming years, and that more innovative forms of housing that bridge the gap between ageing-in-place and institutional care facilities are developed [10], p. 40. In particular, the current supply of intermediate forms of housing for older people with low and middle incomes is limited in terms of capacity and insufficiently innovative [10], p. 39. However, this does not mean that innovative in-between solutions for lower and middle-income groups are absent. In recent years, various promising initiatives have been launched by directors of established social housing associations and by social entrepreneurs. A social enterprise delivers a product or service just like any other enterprise and has a revenue model, but earning money is a means of achieving a societal mission. For instance, in the case of a social housing association, revenues are re-invested in the quality, affordability and availability of social housing. Founders of innovative initiatives, both directors and social entrepreneurs, often present themselves in catchy one-liners as contrary pioneers, who go against the prevailing views and practices [11]. They emphasise the differences between their own initiatives, presented as innovative and positioned outside traditional frameworks, and the procedures and products of other parties, which they depict as old-fashioned and rigid. When establishing innovative collective housing concepts, directors of social housing associations and social entrepreneurs are faced with a multitude of challenges, such as the large number of national directives which need to be adhered to, and the involvement of numerous stakeholders in concepting and decision making [12]. How founders deal with challenges of establishing and governing innovative new living arrangements is a new field of study. Van Straaten et al. [13] studied the barriers, lessons learnt and pathways towards solutions among founders of new housing arrangements for older people in the Netherlands. The founders experienced a variety of challenges in working together with municipalities, as every municipality has its own methods and procedures. Founders with a track record find it easier to work with municipalities. This can be explained by their experience with dealing with all sorts of organisations as well as their rules and regulations.

In studying how founders deal with internal and external regulations, one can draw on the literature from the healthcare domain, where 'positive deviance', 'tempered radicals' and 'rebellion' have recently received attention [14–17]. In this study, we use the concept of 'rebellion' to refer to those actors who identify with and are committed to their organisations and possess the reflexivity and innovativeness to act otherwise and to find different institutional solutions to do better. This definition is based on central elements of both the concepts of 'tempered radicals' as well as 'positive deviants' [16,17]. The existing literature focused on individuals or teams within traditional care organisations, such as hospitals and nursing homes, who dare to do things differently with the aim of providing a better quality of care. Although this article studies rebellion in a different context, three findings from the existing literature are particularly relevant.

First, *rebels use and create space for doing things differently*. In the Dutch public and political debate, it is often argued that governmental rules and regulations cause the regulatory pressure that many healthcare professionals experience. However, research conducted in Dutch nursing homes showed that—although some of the rules, which were experienced as unnecessary, were indeed formulated by external parties such as ministries or inspectorates—many rules were actually formulated by the care organisations themselves [15]. Instead of complaining about such rules, or blindly obeying them, 'rebellious' directors, middle managers and care professionals working in the nursing homes tried to trace the origin and function of burdensome rules and to bend, change or work around them. Following this strategy enabled some (subunits of) organisations to increase the quality of care by doing things differently in a reflexive, well-considered way.

Second, *rebels shake up organisations, but do not intend to harm or leave them*. Rebels are able to bring about meaningful change by bending or ignoring certain rules [18]. The actions of these rebels can be referred to as 'positive deviance' in the sense that their behaviour deviates from the norm in such a manner that it effectively addresses certain problems [16]. However, this does not mean that they oppose rules in general. Wallenburg and colleagues, who focused on rebels in hospital settings, argue that 'positive deviants (...) tend to shake up the organization, but do not intend to harm or leave the organisation, rather seeking to care for the organization and its purposes' [14], p. 871. In other words, these rebels change the system from within, rather than as complete outsiders.

Third, *rebellion is not only a characteristic of individuals but also of networks*. Related to the previous point, the literature shows that rebels need allies. While rebellion is sometimes studied on an individual level [17], recent studies showed that rebellious behaviour is often displayed in teams [14,15]. Team members discuss which rules are vital to obey, which ones can be changed, and which ones can be ignored. Rebellious individuals, thus, need rebellious teams, which not only include 'deviants' but also 'guardians'. Such guardians ensure the continuity of the operation, reduce the chance for potential risk or damage to the organisation and avoid potential disasters [19]. Rebellious teams, in turn, need organisational contexts that enable them to achieve their goals [14].

The above-discussed findings are relevant for the present study, which aims to research how founders deal with challenges of establishing and governing innovative new living arrangements in the highly regulated context of the Netherlands. In studying how founders deal with regulatory challenges in the establishment and governance of their initiatives, attention will be paid to how founders perceive rules, and what founders do when they come across burdensome rules that do not seem to be related to good quality services. Moreover, it is investigated how the founders relate to other relevant actors, such as various stakeholders within their initiatives, partner organisations and external regulatory bodies. Although this study builds on the findings of earlier studies, it differs from the existing literature on rebellion and innovative housing arrangements in three important ways. While earlier studies focused on rebellious individuals or teams within 'traditional' organisations, this study deals with the initiatives of social entrepreneurs who have established 'rebellious' organisations. Building networks and finding allies might be even more important—and more difficult—for them than for actors who work in established organisations. A second difference from earlier studies on rebellion is that this study includes initiatives on the cutting edge of housing and care, which likely makes dealing with regulatory pressure and knowing how to create room to manoeuvre even more important. Third, this study adds to earlier studies on 'innovative models for ageing-in-place' [20], which mainly focused on the characteristics of various types of arrangements [21]. This study does not aim to generate a typology of new living arrangements, but rather to provide insight into the perceptions and practices of the founders in establishing and governing such arrangements. By combining a focus on rebellion and innovative living arrangements, this study contributes to both fields of the literature.

In the following sections, the selection of 'rebellious' initiatives and important aspects of our qualitative research design are outlined. Thereafter, research findings are presented. In the discussion, the term 'responsible rebellion' is introduced. This is followed by a reflection on the implications of 'responsible rebellion' for theory and practice.

2. Methodology

In order to obtain a closer understanding of the challenges experienced by founders in setting up group living arrangements for older people, a qualitative study was conducted. Data acquisition took place through qualitative (face-to-face) interviews. The decision-making processes in innovative collective housing projects were examined based on the experiences of the founders involved and (un-)successful cases. In addition, the challenges that actors have to deal with regarding (1) internal and external regulations, and (2) establishing (in)formal partnerships and (3) how this is governed by the directors and the supervisory board, were identified.

2.1. Participants, Settings and Interviewing

A total of 17 key figures from the domain of housing for older people were interviewed, among which were social entrepreneurs, directors and members of the supervisory board (Table 1). These founders were recruited through the personal and professional networks of our consortium partners, including small and medium-sized enterprises, knowledge institutes, and stakeholder associations (VTW (Vereniging van Toezichthouders in Woningcorporaties. English: Association of Supervisors of Social Housing Associations), NVTZ (Nederlandse Vereniging van Toezichthouders in Zorg en Welzijn. English: Dutch Association of Supervisors in Care and Welfare) and Aedes (Aedes—Vereniging van Woningcorporaties. English: Aedes—Dutch Association of Social Housing Organisations. Together, Aedes members manage 2.4 million dwellings, constituting 32% of the total housing stock in the Netherlands)), which all have an extensive network in the field of senior co-housing. Purposeful sampling was applied as a technique in selecting the cases. This technique is widely used in qualitative research for the identification and selection of information-rich cases [22]. It involves identifying and selecting participants who are knowledgeable about or experienced with a phenomenon of interest [22]. Participants were selected because they were mentioned by our consortium partners or other participants as someone known as 'rebellious', as someone who works differently, or who possesses the reflexivity and innovativeness to act otherwise.

The initiatives of the founders are all examples of living arrangements positioned on the housing continuum in-between ageing-in-place and institutionalised housing and built for low and middle-income households. In a few cases, the living arrangement is aimed at a specific group of older people, such as people with dementia or older people of ethnic minority groups. Three examples are provided to show the diversity of initiatives included, and to illustrate that the innovation of such housing concepts lies in an innovative approach to both the architectural aspects and the organisation of—and interaction with—care and welfare services.

In one of the housing initiatives older people and students live together. Here, a large social housing association transformed the existing real estate—a former residential care home—into an intergenerational living community. This happened in close collaboration with the local community. The social housing association formed a partnership with a local care partner that provides care for the residents if needed. The housing association leads similar innovative transformation processes in other municipalities in the Netherlands.

Table 1. Overview of the participants.

Participant	Age-Range [Years]	Sex	Position
01	40–49	female	social entrepreneur
02	50–59	male	director
03	≥60	male	director
04	30–39	male	director
05	50–59	female	director
06	50–59	male	director
07	50–59	male	director
08	50–59	male	director
09	≥60	male	member supervisory board
10	≥60	male	social entrepreneur
11	≥60	male	social entrepreneur
12	≥60	male	director
13	50–59	female	member supervisory board
14	40–49	female	director
15	≥60	male	social entrepreneur
16	≥60	male	social entrepreneur
17	50–59	male	social entrepreneur

A second example is a social enterprise that establishes small living communities for more or less self-reliant middle-income seniors. Founded in 2012, the concept originally consisted of a courtyard community, in which multiple smaller housing units make use of an inner courtyard. Here, according to the concept, older people can live independently and age-in-place, as people can help and accompany each other if wanted or needed. The social enterprise works with collective private commissioning, which means a group of private investors, or future residents, is formed in order to finance and further shape the development of the housing facility. Various similar communities were established throughout the country.

A third example is a social enterprise that offers short-term stay in guesthouses where informal care is provided. Older people, who have undergone treatment in a hospital or rehabilitation centre and no longer receive a formal health assessment entitling them to publicly funded 'care with residence' can stay in a guesthouse located in their own neighbourhood. Whenever they need formal care, their familiar professional carers stop by.

There is a large diversity in the sample of participants. The majority (n = 9) of the participants is a director, followed by social entrepreneurs (n = 6). Two members of a supervisory board of a living arrangement were interviewed as well, as these supervisors were involved in the planning and supervision of innovative housing projects. The research strategy to include participants with different positions in the sample, added richness to the data, as it gives different stakeholder perspectives. The sample included 13 males and 4 females. Of the 17 participants, three were members of ethnic minority groups, but for reasons of privacy and potential identification, these data are not shown in Table 1. The large number of participants were aged between 50 and 60 years old (n = 7). Only three were younger than 50 years of age.

The interviews took place at the offices of the participants or at an agreed-on convenient venue between July 2019 and January 2020. All interviews were conducted face-to-face, recorded and transcribed verbatim. The interviews lasted for approximately one hour.

2.2. Topic Lists

Interviews were conducted based on a topic list. The themes of the topic lists were derived from a literature study, including the work by Meyerson [17] and Wallenburg et al. [14] and included dealing with rules and legislation, forming partnerships and networks, and the term rebellion. The topic list was discussed with a number of consortium partners, who are experienced in the field of governance of (collective) housing and adjusted accordingly. The topic list was divided into a structured and a semi-structured section. There were three topics lists, one for social entrepreneurs, one for directors, and one for members of a supervisory board, based on different roles that these positions bring (Supplementary Materials). First, background information, including questions on date of birth, and level of education was collected in order to gain insight into variation within the study population. The topic list contained topics grouped around a number of main themes: (i) the collective living arrangement, (ii) the concept of rebellion, (iii) dealing with rules and regulation and (iv) accountability. The topic list allowed us to gain insight into the participants' experiences, motives, actions and (in)formal partnerships. The focus during the interviews differed, depending on the participants' position, knowledge and expertise.

2.3. Data Analysis

The interviews were anonymised, elaborated and thematically analysed. For the thematic analysis, a qualitative analysis software package (Atlas.ti) was used.

In line with the 'abductive analysis' approach developed by Tavory and Timmermans [23], the analysis consisted of an iterative process of working with the empirical materials in relationship with the literature on rebellion and innovative living arrangements. This approach includes both deductive and inductive reasoning. Based on the existing literature, codes were used, such as 'rules', 'regulations' and 'context', but some codes were generated inductively (for instance, the different ideas respondents had about the term 'rebellion'). During the coding process, three central themes emerged: four central elements of what it means to act 'rebellious'; dealing with the institutional context, consisting of rules and regulations; and creating supportive (external and internal) contexts.

The quotations were translated into English by the authors for the purpose of this article. Contextual information (including names of Dutch public bodies) has been simplified for a better understandability by an international audience.

2.4. Ethics

Since the data and selected cases contain many sensitivities, maintaining participant confidentiality and privacy are of the utmost importance. Confidentiality was addressed during the data collection, data cleaning and dissemination of the research results [24]. This confidentiality is also reflected in the limited case description of the chosen living arrangements. Prior to the phase of data collection, informed consent was obtained from the participants. Participants were asked to read and sign the informed consent statement at the beginning of the interview. After the data were collected, a 'clean' data set was created, one which does not contain information that identifies the participants, such as names or address details. The participants' and organisations' names were replaced with pseudonyms. Finally, in presenting the findings by using specific quotations and examples, it was explicitly considered if this could lead to the identification of a participant via deductive disclosure. If so, we removed additional details in the quotations. The quotations included in this article can only be traced by the researchers, based on the participant code.

3. Results

The following themes are described in the sections below: (1) Four central elements of rebellion: keeping the higher goal in mind; taking action; learning by trial-and-error; and thinking critically. (2) Institutional context: dealing with rules and regulations. (3) Creating supportive external and internal contexts.

3.1. Rebellion: Four Central Elements

The founders were asked what they thought of the term rebellion and whether or not they identified themselves or their initiatives as being rebellious. About half of the participants were positive about the term. Some of them said that they identified themselves as a rebel, and/or their initiatives as rebellious, while others said that they found it difficult to label themselves as rebels.

According to them, that is for others to judge. About a third of the participants had negative associations towards the term rebel. For instance, they related it to warfare or earning success at the expense of others. The remainder of the participants had neither positive nor negative thoughts about the term. Whether or not they liked the term, various participants said that they preferred other terms, such as 'radical' (in the sense of breaking with the past), 'entrepreneur' (who takes risks) and 'pacesetter' (who involves other people and tries to enthuse them).

Despite their different opinions about the terms rebel and rebellious, all participants said that they and their initiatives dare to do things differently. In their explanations of their innovative approach, four central elements could be identified: keeping the higher goal in mind; taking action; learning by trial-and-error; and thinking critically instead of blindly following rules.

The founders talked passionately about the reasons for starting their initiatives and the societal values they pursued. Various founders shared personal stories about their parents who were the reason for starting the initiative: when their parents became older and in need of care, the founders were not satisfied with traditional care services and decided to create an alternative. One founder (Participant 3) said that, in setting-up his initiative, he always kept his mother in the back of his mind. Another founder (Participant 2) said that *'providing older people a safe and sociable home'* is the main objective and he tries to go *'as far as possible'* in achieving that. Others, for instance, describe the quality (Participant 8) and the continuity (Participant 4) of care as the main objectives. According to the participants, rebellion is a means to an end and should never become a goal in itself.

> *"I would not describe it as kicking against something, because that has a negative association; the kicking becomes a goal in itself. For me, it is continuously thinking about what I am doing and trying to do it in different ways."* (Participant 6)

> *"It should not be about the rebellion itself. That you want to be in the spotlights for a moment. It should really be about a specific need or question. Something you want to find a solution for."* (Participant 1)

The personal stories of various founders showed that they were frustrated and sometimes even angry about how housing for older people was organised in the Netherlands. What makes them stand out from many other people who expressed their opinion, was that they decided to take action to change the status quo. Taking action, or in the words of various participants, 'just start doing it', is a central element of rebellion. Rather than endless thinking, talking and planning, they tried to put their idea into practice right away.

> *"I would define rebellion as taking initiative or setting up something and continue doing that, even if it doesn't fit existing frameworks. That is rebellion for me: We are just going to do it. The developer says it doesn't fit, or the municipality says it doesn't fit the way they financially organised care. Despite all this, you say: 'We are just going to do it. The idea is good, so we are doing it'."* (Participant 1)

> *"What makes it rebellious is that we said: 'We are just going to do it. We will see how it turns out'."* (Participant 5)

According to various founders, an action-directed mentality implies learning by doing. Because their initiatives were innovative and broke with existing traditions, there was no existing pathway founders could—or wanted to—follow. By experimentation and trial-and-error, they found out what worked and what did not.

> *"It is about searching how you can do things differently. You try different things and sometimes you don't succeed."* (Participant 6)

Learning by trial-and-error asks for certain personal and organisational characteristics, such as being persistent and daring to take risks.

> *"An entrepreneur sometimes takes risks, that is part of being an entrepreneur. When you say: 'I believe in it', then we believe in it and we go for it and we also take risks. That is also something that I will always do."* (Participant 7)

One final often-mentioned element of rebellion was thinking critically instead of blindly following existing rules or traditions.

> *"When organisations literally do what is prescribed by the rules, I find them so unimaginative."* (Participant 9)

> *"I always call it 'healthy rebellion'. You need people who try colour outside the lines and who see what happens next."* (Participant 13)

The participant quoted above called the critical thinking 'healthy rebellion', another participant said his behaviour was 'friendly rebellious' towards more traditional stakeholders in the field of housing and care (Participant 16). With these specifications, founders tried to make it clear that they did not want to rebel in an aggressive or irresponsible way. In the next section, their critical but responsible stance towards existing rules and regulations is discussed in further detail.

3.2. Institutional Context: Dealing with Rules and Regulations

Although founders mentioned that it is important to 'just start' and take the initiative, they experienced all sorts of limitations and barriers, especially with regard to the institutional context. Founders indicated that the amount of legislation and regulations can be an important barrier in setting up new housing initiatives. The realisation of such new housing initiatives is often complex. Many times, local regulations and procedures are simply not attuned to initiatives that deviate from the 'ordinary'. One of the participants, who was in the process of setting up a new housing initiative, shared the following:

> *"Municipalities are very bureaucratic organisations. I need to fill out an application form, and thereafter, someone from the municipality has to agree on it, and then someone else needs to find a budget for it. These steps take a lot of time."* (Participant 1)

Founders also ran into the organisation and internal procedures of municipalities. Housing initiatives for older people are often seen within the indivisible scope of 'housing and care', such as in the case of nursing homes in which both the provision of shelter and care services are taken care of by a single organisation. At the municipal level—especially in larger municipalities—housing and care are usually two different policy fields, whereby cooperation and coordination between these departments is not always self-evident. As a result, decisions are made slowly because the decision-making process has to flow through the right channels:

> *"Each department has its own set of rules [...] Everything is formally written down. The civil servant in question is certainly not at risk. No one dares to take any risks. One is afraid to operate beyond the existing frameworks."* (Participant 17)

Another barrier experienced by founders, related to the procedures mentioned above, is that the number of rules and regulations result in a rigid institutional system with few opportunities to conduct experiments:

> *"The main problem is that due to all the regulations everything is tied down in rules and budgets. As such, there is no opportunity to experiment in a certain area or neighbourhood."* (Participant 1)

One of the research questions was how 'rebellious' founders found ways to manoeuvre within the boundaries set by the institutional context and if these founders were able to bend, work around or change certain rules and regulations. First of all, almost all founders emphasised the importance of adhering to the existing laws, rules and regulations, especially as the participants are directors of social housing associations or social entrepreneurs, which means that their aim is not only to make a profit that can be reinvested in the organisation, but also to achieve a societal mission. They found it important to operate in a responsible way:

> *"What is very important to me personally, is that we do business in a socially responsible manner. We use public funds and we want to use these funds in the best possible way. If you have other moral standards, I don't think you are suitable to work in this domain. [...] The social responsibility we have is very important to us."* (Participant 7)

Although the founders mentioned the importance of playing by the rules and the importance to manoeuvre within the existing institutional framework, they also felt a responsibility to challenge and sometimes ignore certain rules, as the rules are not always infallible.

> *"We interpret [a certain] law differently so we have had an endless discussion with the Dutch Authority for Social Housing Associations <Dutch: Autoriteit Woningcorporaties>. But in the end, they said: 'OK, we will tolerate [the difference in interpretation]'. That's what it comes down to."* (Participant 2)

The participants were well aware of the opportunities that can be created within the existing legal framework by interpreting the rules and regulations differently:

> *"A creative interpretation of the rules is often regarded as something negative. But the legislation offers an opportunity to act and interpret the rules and regulations differently. It is just more like acting in the spirit of the rules than simply [strictly] following the existing rules."* (Participant 5)

As this quote illustrates, some participants considered it morally legitimate or even morally required to assess existing rules and regulations critically and to challenge them when this seemed justified. For some founders challenging existing rules and acting differently was part of being rebellious. At the same time, they took accountability for their actions and behaviours:

> *"I think I am the one within the organisation who encourages people to do that [colour outside the lines] every now and then. Of course, [you do it] in a responsible way: you always need to take accountability for your actions and explain to others what you have done and how you have done it."* (Participant 13)

Some founders challenged the existing institutional frameworks and also tried to change existing rules or laws, for instance, by lobbying and/or taking action at the local and national levels:

> *"In general, people prefer to follow the rules, otherwise there will be a hassle. However, we are prosecuting against the state about the new Housing Act. The government is convinced about a certain interpretation of the Act. We disagree on this, as it is not written down in the Act."* (Participant 2)

In conclusion, by challenging, bending and sometimes ignoring certain rules or regulations, 'rebellious' founders took certain risks. The reputation of a director or social entrepreneur can be put at risk, especially when there is little support inside or outside the organisation for positive deviance. The following quote stems from an interview with a former director, who had been removed from office by resolution of his supervisory board. As a result, the participant was not able to find a new position in the past few years:

> *"I am [over 60] years old, but I'm already [living of] my retirement savings. In the first years after I was given the sack, I was still asked to give a presentation or a lecture. But at a certain point of time, people in the field don't know you anymore and then there are no more assignments. Therefore, I had to apply for pre-pension."* (Participant 3)

> *"So being a rebel does not always pay off?"* (Researcher)

> *"No. No. Definitely not."* (Participant 3)

In order to limit the abovementioned risks, rebellious founders tried to create support both within and outside the organisation. This is further elaborated in the following section.

3.3. Creating Supportive Contexts

In order to organise support and legitimate their different way(s) of acting, rebellious founders created supportive contexts, both outside and within their organisation. In order to create a supportive context and to minimise risks of acting differently, it was important for founders to take accountability. Founders took accountability to explain and justify their conduct. First of all, explanations and justifications were made towards the health care inspectorate. This involved providing the inspectorate with information, and, in addition, some founders also tried to discuss their differences in interpretation and how and why they questioned certain rules or regulations. Often, the inspection systems were perceived as rigid. Yet, different founders stated that when communication between founders and inspectors took place, inspection systems proved to be more flexible than often thought:

> *"It is assumed that they [the health care inspectorate] need to tick all the boxes. However, if you talk with people from the inspectorate, it becomes slightly different and it appears to be more nuanced."* (Participant 3)

Founders stressed the importance to formalise the agreements made with the inspectors, especially when certain well-considered risks stemming from acting differently were involved. This applied in particular to founders within the health care sector. They challenged rules and regulations that might impact the quality of life of the residents of the collective housing initiative in a negative manner.

> *"We spoke with the inspector before and during the start. [...] It is also important for the inspection to discuss the risks with all parties involved and to record what is discussed and include the outcome in the health care plan."* (Participant 11)

Second, as one founder stated (Participant 11) *'being rebellious starts with communication'*. Communication, transparency and accountability were not only of importance towards the inspectorate, but also in creating wider supportive contexts outside the own organisation. This included the broader political context, as the following quote illustrates:

> *"Well then we invite a few MPs, or a mayor or a top official. We always invite the new General Secretary: 'Come and join us for a day.' And the director of [an inspectorate] did a one-day internship here. Just to understand what and how we are working here."* (Participant 2)

In creating a wider supportive context founders sometimes used the media and the press strategically:

> *"If I am working on something of which I am convinced that it should go in that direction, I use Twitter or LinkedIn to gain support. Often, I receive support from all sides. So, I do approach and use social media to reinforce this."* (Participant 13)

The illustration given above does not mean founders were always open and transparent and/or used the media to create support. Sometimes, they decided to stay under the radar. Founders strategically chose when, how and with whom they created a supportive context.

Third, some founders took accountability or strategically communicated with external parties, and also tried to create coalitions of like-minded parties and/or people:

> *"How do you organise change? I made a list of healthcare organisations, social housing associations and municipalities that are also focused on change. I try to create a coalition of the willing with them."* (Participant 12)

The purpose of moving from an individual actor to a member of a collective force was to bring people together. By creating a collective force through media attention and/or through coalitions of like-minded people, rebellious founders hoped to be better able to exercise influence and achieve desired and sustainable change.

Yet, founders tried to create supportive contexts both outside the organisation and within. Within the organisation, founders tried to nurture relationships with the supervisory board and employees in order to create supportive contexts. In creating support, several founders tried to keep the supervisory board and their employees inspired and emphasised working towards achieving the same higher goal. One founder (Participant 6) talked about sending their employees to visit an innovative housing facility abroad to inspire them and work accordingly. Founders also looked for allies within the organisation with whom they could share their ideas and thoughts. This worked both ways. One founder stressed the importance for employees to discuss cases and dilemmas in which rules or regulations might be challenged or ignored. Therefore, trust within the organisation and between employees was considered important:

> *"Within the organisation employees need to know whether or not they have the support from the board to act differently. You need to feel safe, to know you are supported by the organisation, even if you make a mistake."* (Participant 5)

As the quote above illustrates, transparency and communication were not only important to create a supportive context externally, but internally, within the organisation, as well.

Second, founders mentioned that a supportive context within the organisation consisted of more than just the employees who are more rebellious:

> *"I could always rely on [name of a trusted person]. He kept me with both feet on the ground. Sometimes you might lose sight of reality a little bit. That's something [this person] was always good at: 'You may want this, but there are other factors at play here too'."* (Participant 3)

As the above quotation illustrates, a balance was needed between more rebellious allies or employees and those who could be seen as 'guardians', who were able to challenge the founder and discuss potential risks to the organisation.

4. Discussion

The study on rebellion in the domain of collective housing for older people revealed three central themes. First, the concept of rebellion was discussed, which, according to the participants, contains four elements: keeping the higher goal in mind; taking action; learning by trial-and-error; and thinking critically instead of blindly following rules. Next, the institutional context was discussed and how responsible rebels sometimes work around, bend or change existing rules and regulations. The final theme concerned the creation of supportive contexts, both within and outside the organisation.

The study contributes to existing literature on 'positive deviants', 'radicals' and 'rebels' in three ways. First of all, while earlier research focused on rebellious teams within 'traditional' organisations [14], this study was about founders of rebellious initiatives, who not only have to create supportive contexts within their organisation, but also have to create coalitions of the willing with external stakeholders.

Second, the founders operate on the intersection of two domains, namely housing on the one hand and care on the other. In order to be successful, they have to know the rules of the game of both worlds. As van Straaten et al. [13] showed, experienced founders know how to communicate with municipalities, which are an important player in the Netherlands in both domains. This study adds that founders use various strategies to legitimise their initiative to different stakeholders. Based on their trial-and-error learning style—which they described as central to the innovative character of their initiatives—they know what works under what circumstances. For instance, which rules should be adhered to and which ones can be circumvented or ignored, or when to seek publicity and when staying under the radar seems to be more effective.

Third, the study showed that the terms 'rebel' and 'rebellious' are embraced by some but not all founders of innovative living arrangements. Earlier studies used terms such as 'rebels' and 'radicals' without questioning whether the participants actually identified themselves with these terms. This study shows that the 'rebellious' founders studied had different opinions on the term. Some were very positive about it and even said that the use of the term in the project title was the reason for them to participate in the research. Some others did not have strong positive or negative feelings about it. A third group did not identify with the term, because for them, it had a negative connotation, for instance, because the term suggested that they were fighting others, while in reality, they tried to create alliances.

Based on the above-described contributions, the findings of this study suggest that the rebellious founders are not just rebellious, but also responsible. They find it important to challenge existing formal and informal rules, both within and outside their organisations, but they want to do this in a responsible manner. We coin this 'responsible rebellion', which means that the founders stress the importance of playing by the rules and to manoeuvre within the existing institutional framework on the one hand, but on the other hand also challenge and sometimes ignore certain rules. Founders communicate with and take accountability for explaining and justifying their conduct to external and internal stakeholders. As such, being a 'responsible rebel' can lead to innovative forms of group housing for older people, which less 'rebellious' organisations fail to deliver. Additionally, although they take some risks, the participants are all highly committed to their organisations. Being a responsible rebel implies 'walking the tightrope', as these rebels 'make sure not to harm their organisation and they nurture relationships' but at the same time they sometimes disobey certain rules 'to stay close to their ideas and convictions' [14], p. 879.

There are clear connections between the results of the present study, and previous findings on how to create so-called age-friendly cities. If you consider the foundation of new housing initiatives from the perspective of age-friendly cities and the domain of housing, one needs to look at key characteristics of such age-friendly cities which were reviewed by Steels [25]. Steels found a fruitful collaboration between the different stakeholders, including local and national governments concerning financial and political support, and the involvement and social inclusion of older people themselves, to be important factors. These findings overlap with the perceived barriers of the research participants, who often deal with the boundaries set by the government, a good collaboration with various stakeholders, and the facilitation of participation and having a say of older people.

In addition, the development, design and construction of a new collective housing initiative is a process that can last for many years, and which follows a long administrative process and private and public consultation with a large number of parties. Such initiatives have a mixed level of success [26]. In an administrative landscape, which is the result of previous excesses in the domain of public housing, social entrepreneurs often refer to public administrations as organisations that pose barriers to their initiatives. Internal regulations, the required collaboration and interaction with other stakeholders, can contribute to further delays and barriers for social entrepreneurs when they engage in the development of housing initiatives for older people. Social entrepreneurs want to enjoy a degree of freedom to develop a new concept and bring its services to the marketplace, but supervisory board members are often critical about the quality, durability and sustainability of such initiatives.

Therefore, to set up innovative housing for older people, responsible rebels are needed. For future research, the role of supervisory boards and external inspectorates in how they deal with responsible rebellion among directors within their organisation needs attention. What supervisory styles do they use and when? Do they hinder or stimulate responsible rebellion within their organisation and why? And how do they want their directors to be accountable? Lessons might be learned from the health care sector in which a programme was designed to find new ways of accountability. This 'narrative accountability' is based on a more 'story conscious' way of engaging with the realities of life and care [27]. Moreover, a critical assessment is needed of what the added value of rebellion is for the quality of housing and care. What do rebellious initiatives yield in output compared to 'traditional' initiatives? Are they able to fulfill their ambitions [13]? Furthermore, future research should focus on the participation of older people in decision making concerning new housing concepts. In this study, the focus was on the importance of creating supportive contexts, by nurturing relationships internally, as well as externally [14]. Yet, how are the residents of the collective housing initiatives involved? Are the 'rebellious' initiatives age friendly according to the (future) residents [28,29]? Does the housing initiative contribute to the quality of life of its residents and does the housing initiative fulfil their needs and wishes?

Another important aspect that is of interest for further study is the role financing plays in relationship to the level of rebelliousness. For instance, social housing associations in the Netherlands are bound to an extensive set of financial schemes and regulations, which help protect the financial integrity of the system. Social entrepreneurs who are not bound by these rules have more freedom in seeking and securing a loan from the capital market. The degree of having to adhere to a prescribed system of checks and balances as a founder may impact the level of freedom that founders perceive in their operation. Moreover, housing has a maximum asking price in terms of rent, if a tenant was to stay eligible for rental allowance from the state. Higher rents can be asked but will attract a different group of more affluent tenants. These tenants often own a home and are less prone to sell their house and start renting. Such financial contexts are specific to the Netherlands and impact the applicability of the current findings in an international context. Each country in the European Union has its own cultural and governance contexts when it comes to housing and care for older people, as these two domains are still the responsibility of national governments.

5. Conclusions

The establishment of collective forms of housing for older people in the Netherlands goes together with social entrepreneurship that—when successful—often deviates from the mainstream housing arrangements. The ways that founders dealt with challenges in establishing and governing such initiatives were studied in relation to the concept of 'rebellion'. Rebellion, in the words of the participants, revolves around four elements: keeping the higher goal in mind; taking action; learning by trial-and-error; and thinking critically instead of blindly following rules. The in-depth interviews with founders showed that they encountered various obstacles. Such obstacles are often related to governmental and sectoral rules and regulations, which are specific for each of the domains of housing and care, and which may intersect in the domain of housing for older people. Knowing how to work around them and deal with existing rules and regulations is critical to being successful in the field. In order to succeed in realising plans, one needs to create supportive contexts, both within their own organisations and—no less important—with external stakeholders. Being a 'responsible rebel' can indeed lead to innovative forms of group housing for older people, which less 'rebellious' organisations fail to deliver. Being a 'responsible rebel' is, however, not entirely without risks. If the behaviours displayed and choices made are too challenging, and boundaries are crossed on a continuous basis, irresponsible behaviours may bring a project (or even a career) to a halt. First and foremost, being a responsible rebel is about knowing how to walk the tightrope within the context of the country in which one works.

Supplementary Materials: The following are available online at http://www.mdpi.com/1660-4601/17/17/6235/s1.

Author Contributions: Conceptualisation, K.M.R., M.E.v.B. and J.v.H.; methodology, K.M.R., M.E.v.B. and J.v.H.; formal analysis, K.M.R., M.E.v.B., S.K.-B. and Z.K.C.T.T.; investigation, K.M.R., M.v.B. and S.K.-B.; writing—original draft preparation, K.M.R., M.v.B. and J.v.H.; writing—review and editing, K.M.R., M.v.B., S.K.-B., Z.K.C.T.T. and J.v.H.; project administration, J.v.H.; funding acquisition, K.M.R., M.v.B. and J.v.H. All authors have read and agreed to the published version of the manuscript.

Funding: This research was funded by the Regional Attention and Action for Knowledge Circulation (RAAK) scheme (MKB-3-37), which is managed by the Taskforce for Applied Research (Nationaal Regieorgaan Praktijkgericht Onderzoek SIA). This research was a deliverable of the project *Naar Verantwoorde Rebellie: Governance en Inspraak bij Collectieve Woonvormen voor Ouderen* [Towards Responsible Rebellion: Governance of and Participation in Collective Living Arrangements for Older People] (SIA project number RAAK.MKB09.002). The consortium is made up of The Hague University of Applied Sciences, Erasmus University Rotterdam (Erasmus School of Health Policy & Management (ESHPM)), Rotterdam University of Applied Sciences, Leiden University of Applied Sciences, CareBNB, Stichting Ouderenhuisvesting Rotterdam, Vastgoed Zorgsector, BureauVijftig, Woonz.nl, D'article Enterprise and ProGoDo, and partner organisations Vereniging van Toezichthouders in Woningcorporaties, Nederlandse Vereniging van Toezichthouders in Zorg en Welzijn, Grey Valley, Marjo Visser Advies en Interimmanagement, Atelier Rijksbouwmeester, and Aedes.

Acknowledgments: All participants of the interviews are thanked for their willingness to participate in the study. Marjo Visser (Marjo Visser Advies en Interimmanagement) and Katja van Vliet (Rotterdam University of Applied Sciences) are acknowledged for their constructive feedback on the methodology. We would like to thank Henno Theisens (The Hague University of Applied Sciences) for his input on the discussion.

Conflicts of Interest: The authors declare no conflict of interest. The funders had no role in the design of the study; in the collection, analyses, or interpretation of data; in the writing of the manuscript, or in the decision to publish the results.

References

1. van Hoof, J.; Kazak, J.K. Urban ageing. *Indoor Built Environ.* **2018**, *27*, 583–586. [CrossRef]
2. van Hoof, J.; Kazak, J.K.; Perek-Białas, J.M.; Peek, S. The challenges of urban ageing: Making cities age-friendly in Europe. *Int. J. Environ. Res. Public Health* **2018**, *15*, 2473. [CrossRef] [PubMed]
3. van Dijk, H.M. *Neighbourhoods for Ageing in Place;* Erasmus University Rotterdam: Rotterdam, The Netherlands, 2015.
4. Doekhie, K.D.; de Veer, A.J.E.; Rademakers, J.J.D.J.M.; Schellevis, F.G.; Francke, A.L. Ouderen van de toekomst. In *Verschillen in de Wensen en Mogelijkheden Voor Wonen, Welzijn en Zorg: Overzichtstudies;* Nivel: Utrecht, The Netherlands, 2014; ISBN 978-94-6122-239-8. (In Dutch)
5. Fabian, C.; Janett, S.; Bischoff, T.; Pardani, R.; Leitner, J.; Knöpfel, C. The development of 'age appropriate' living environments: Analysis of two case studies from a social work perspective. *Urban Plan.* **2019**, *4*, 123–133. [CrossRef]
6. Kazak, J.; van Hoof, J.; Świąder, M.; Szewrański, S. Real estate for the ageing society—The perspective of a new market. *Real Estate Manag. Valuat.* **2017**, *25*, 13–24. [CrossRef]
7. van Hoof, J.; Kort, H.S.M.; van Waarde, H. Housing and care for older adults with dementia. A European perspective. *J. Hous. Built Environ.* **2009**, *24*, 369–390. [CrossRef]
8. van Hoof, J.; Boerenfijn, P. Re-inventing existing real estate of social housing for older people: Building a new De Benring in Voorst, The Netherlands. *Buildings* **2018**, *8*, 89. [CrossRef]
9. Rusinovic, K.M.; van Bochove, M.E.; van de Sande, J. Senior co-housing in the Netherlands: Benefits and drawbacks for its residents. *Int. J. Environ. Res. Public Health* **2019**, *16*, 3776. [CrossRef] [PubMed]
10. Ministry of Health, Welfare and Sport. *Programma Langer Thuis;* Ministry of Health, Welfare and Sport: The Hague, The Netherlands, 2018. (In Dutch)
11. Aedes-Actiz. ZorgButler: Wonen in een Verzorgingshuis Nieuwe Stijl. 2018. Available online: https://www.kcwz.nl/doc/woonvariaties/Zorgbutler-wonen-in-een-verzorgingshuis-nieuwe-stijl-2018.pdf (accessed on 15 June 2020).
12. van Hoof, J.; Rusinovic, K.M.; Tavy, Z.K.C.T.; van den Hoven, R.F.M.; Dikken, J.; van der Pas, S.; Kruize, H.; de Bruin, S.R.; van Bochove, M. The participation of older people in concepting and designing new housing facilities in The Netherlands. In *The Age-Friendly Lens;* Gardiner, C., Ed.; Routlegde: Abingdon, UK, 2021. (In Press)
13. van Straaten, B.; van Triest, N.; van Eeden, L. *Woonvarianten Voor Senioren: Hoe Krijg je ze van de Grond? Lessen van Tien Initiatiefnemers;* Platform31: The Hague, The Netherlands, 2020. (In Dutch)
14. Wallenburg, I.; Weggelaar, A.M.; Bal, R. Walking the tightrope: How rebels "do" quality of care in healthcare organizations. *J. Health Org. Manag.* **2019**, *33*, 869–883. [CrossRef]
15. van de Bovenkamp, H.; Stoopendaal, A.; van Bochove, M.; Bal, R. Regeldruk: Van Regelreflex Naar Spiegelreflex. *Qruxx* **2019**. Available online: https://www.qruxx.com/regeldruk-van-regelreflex-naar-spiegelreflex/ (accessed on 22 June 2020).
16. Singhal, A.; Bjurström, E. Reframing the practice of social research: Solving complex problems by valuing positive deviations. *Int. J. Commun. Soc. Res.* **2015**, *3*, 1–12. Available online: http://ijcsr.info/wp/wp-content/uploads/issue%204-1.pdf (accessed on 28 May 2020).

17. Meyerson, D.E. *Rocking the Boat: How Tempered Radicals Effect Change Without Making Trouble*; Harvard Business Press: Boston, MA, USA, 2008.
18. Bevan, H.; Fairman, S. The New Era of Thinking and Practice in Change Transformation: A Call to Action for Leaders of Health and Care, NHSIQ (NHS Improving Quality). 2014. Available online: http://media.nhsiq.nhs.uk/whitepaper/html5/index.html?page=1 (accessed on 25 June 2020).
19. Coleman, A.; Segar, J.; Checkland, K.; McDermott, I.; Harrison, S.; Peckham, S. Leadership for health commissioning in the new NHS: Exploring the early development of clinical commissioning groups in England. *J. Health Org. Manag.* **2015**, *29*, 75–91. [CrossRef] [PubMed]
20. Bookman, A. Innovative models of aging in place: Transforming our communities for an aging population. *Community Work Fam.* **2008**, *11*, 419–438. [CrossRef]
21. Lehning, A.J.; Scharlach, A.E.; Davitt, J.K. Variations on the Village model: An emerging typology of a consumer-driven community-based initiative for older adults. *J. Appl. Gerontol.* **2017**, *36*, 234–246. [CrossRef] [PubMed]
22. Palinkas, L.A.; Korwitz, S.M.; Green, C.A.; Wisdom, J.P.; Duan, N.; Hoagwood, K. Purposeful sampling for qualitative data collection and analysis in mixed method implementation research. *Adm. Policy Ment. Health* **2015**, *42*, 533–544. [CrossRef] [PubMed]
23. Tavory, I.; Timmermans, S. *Abductive Analysis: Theorizing Qualitative Research*; University of Chicago Press: Chicago, IL, USA, 2014.
24. Kaiser, K. Protecting respondent confidentiality in qualitative research. *Qual. Health Res.* **2009**, *19*, 1632–1641. [CrossRef] [PubMed]
25. Steels, S. Key characteristics of age-friendly cities and communities: A review. *Cities* **2015**, *47*, 45–52. [CrossRef]
26. Companen. *Nieuwe Woonvormen Voor de Ouderwordende Samenleving*; Companen: Arnhem, The Netherlands, 2016; Available online: https://www.companen.nl/sites/all/files/downloads/nieuwe_woonvormen_voor_de_ouderwordende_samenleving_companen.pdf (accessed on 12 May 2020).
27. Ubels, G.M. Narrative accountability and quality awareness: Learning about (re)presenting. *J. Aging Stud.* **2015**, *34*, 190–198. [CrossRef] [PubMed]
28. van Hoof, J.; Dikken, J.; Buttiġieġ, S.C.; van den Hoven, R.F.M.; Kroon, E.; Marston, H.R. Age-friendly cities in the Netherlands: An explorative study of facilitators and hindrances in the built environment and ageism in design. *Indoor Built Environ.* **2020**, *29*, 417–437. [CrossRef]
29. Marston, H.R.; van Hoof, J. "Who doesn't think about technology when designing urban environments for older people?" A case study approach to a proposed extension of the WHO's age-friendly cities model. *Int. J. Environ. Res. Public Health* **2019**, *16*, 3525. [CrossRef] [PubMed]

International Journal of
Environmental Research and Public Health

MDPI

Article

Thermal Personalities of Older People in South Australia: A Personas-Based Approach to Develop Thermal Comfort Guidelines

Helen Bennetts [1,*], Larissa Arakawa Martins [1], Joost van Hoof [2,3] and Veronica Soebarto [1]

1 School of Architecture and the Built Environment, The University of Adelaide, North Terrace, Adelaide, SA 5005, Australia; larissa.arakawamartins@adelaide.edu.au (L.A.M.); veronica.soebarto@adelaide.edu.au (V.S.)

2 Faculty of Social Work & Education, The Hague University of Applied Sciences, Johanna Westerdijkplein 75, 2521 EN Den Haag, The Netherlands; j.vanhoof@hhs.nl

3 Institute of Spatial Management, Faculty of Environmental Engineering and Geodesy, Wrocław University of Environmental and Life Sciences, ul. Grunwaldzka 55, 50-357 Wrocław, Poland

* Correspondence: helen.bennetts@adelaide.edu.au; Tel.: +61-8-313-5836

Received: 10 October 2020; Accepted: 10 November 2020; Published: 13 November 2020

check for updates

Abstract: An important consideration for future age-friendly cities is that older people are able to live in housing appropriate for their needs. While thermal comfort in the home is vital for the health and well-being of older people, there are currently few guidelines about how to achieve this. This study is part of a research project that aims to improve the thermal environment of housing for older Australians by investigating the thermal comfort of older people living independently in South Australia and developing thermal comfort guidelines for people ageing-in-place. This paper describes the approach fundamental for developing the guidelines, using data from the study participants' and the concept of personas to develop a number of discrete "thermal personalities". Hierarchical Cluster Analysis (HCA) was implemented to analyse the features of research participants, resulting in six distinct clusters. Quantitative and qualitative data from earlier stages of the project were then used to develop the thermal personalities of each cluster. The thermal personalities represent different approaches to achieving thermal comfort, taking into account a wide range of factors including personal characteristics, ideas, beliefs and knowledge, house type, and location. Basing the guidelines on thermal personalities highlights the heterogeneity of older people and the context-dependent nature of thermal comfort in the home and will make the guidelines more user-friendly and useful.

Keywords: housing; cluster analysis; thermal comfort; design guidelines; heating; cooling

1. Introduction

The ability to stay in one's community and age-in-place is the preferred strategy for most people, including the majority of older Australians [1]. For some people, this may mean moving to a smaller or more manageable dwelling as they approach older age. For others, it may mean making adjustments to their existing homes. The World Health Organization's (WHO, Geneva, Switzerland) Checklist of Essential features of Age-friendly Cities notes that appropriate accommodation is important for the independence and quality of life of older people and that the accommodation should be "appropriately equipped to meet the ambient environmental conditions" [2] (p. 31). This could refer to the design of the house itself and the way it can respond to the environment, or to the heating and cooling equipment installed to assist with the thermal comfort of the occupants. Either approach requires an understanding of local conditions: the climate, housing, and the thermal preferences and behaviours of older people in their homes.

The majority of thermal comfort studies have been conducted with younger people and in non-residential settings such as offices or climate chambers [3]. Studies exploring whether the thermal comfort requirements of older people differ from those of younger people are inconclusive. One review of both climate chamber studies and field studies concluded that there were no significant differences between the comfort temperatures of young and older people once clothing, metabolic, and anthropometric differences were taken into account [4]. Other studies reported that older people preferred higher temperature [3,5,6], or lower [7,8], that their comfort range was narrower [9] or wider [10]. Despite differences in individual studies, both physiological changes (for example, changes to the metabolic rate and cardiovascular system) and behavioural changes (for example, decline in activity, more time spent at home) suggest older people have increased vulnerability to prolonged periods of both high and cold temperatures [11].

While there are a number of design guidelines that provide information about modifying an existing home or building a new one to suit ageing-in-place (for example, Livable Housing Australia [12]), thermal comfort is rarely referred to. The focus is mainly on improving accessibility, supporting self-care, and preventing falls and injury [13]. On the other hand, guidelines and standards for thermal comfort [14–16] rarely address older people or thermal comfort in the home. This is despite knowledge about the impact of ageing on people's thermoregulation [17–22], about the connection between the thermal conditions in the home and older people's health and well-being [23], as well as about the problems of rising energy prices and increasing energy poverty amongst older people [24]. It appears many older people themselves are not aware of these issues. In a recent survey of older people in South Australia, 85% said they had not heard, seen, or received information about how hot and cold weather could affect their health, while 90% said they had not heard, seen, or received information about how to improve their thermal comfort [25].

The research, *Improving the thermal environment of housing for older Australians* (ARC DP180102019), investigates the thermal comfort and thermal behaviours of people aged 65 and over who live independently in South Australia. Data have been collected via telephone survey of 250 respondents [25], focus group discussions with 49 participants about their heating and cooling behaviour [26], and indoor environmental monitoring and occupant surveys in 57 households involving 71 older occupants to capture their attitudes, behaviours, and approaches to achieving thermal comfort [27,28]. The previous stages of this research project revealed the inter-individual differences in the research participants as well as their housing conditions, thermal preferences, (environmental) attitudes and concerns, and heating and cooling practices. In total, 340 people, aged 65 or older who were living independently, participated in the project. The participants exhibited the diversity evident in older people in terms of demographics, with ages from 65 to over 93, and various levels of income, education, health, and well-being. Their thermal behaviours and thermal preferences varied greatly along with the location and thermal performance of their dwellings [29,30].

An important outcome of the project will be thermal comfort guidelines for older people who wish to age-in-place in South Australia. Based on the research data, the guidelines are intended to raise awareness of the links between older people's well-being and thermal comfort in the home and to provide information about keeping cool in hot weather and warm in cold weather. Rather than focusing only on specifying a range of temperatures that are suitable for older people, the guidelines will describe a variety of strategies for achieving thermal comfort, taking into consideration people's personal factors, housing conditions, and knowledge, as well as the actions that older people prefer to take.

Focus groups with older people undertaken earlier in the research project revealed that the strategies employed by individuals to keep cool in hot weather and warm in cold weather were complex, inter-related, and influenced by a range of issues including personal factors and preferences, people's beliefs and experiences, the design and location of the dwelling, the type of heating and cooling equipment, as well as their financial concerns [26]. Some people discussed that their thermal behaviours were mainly influenced by the cost of heating and cooling, while others indicated that they were affected by concern over the impact of the thermal environment on their health and well-being. Recognising these different motivations will be an important aspect of the design guidelines.

Analysis of the data derived from focus group discussions identified four key concepts influencing thermal behaviour: personal factors, doing, knowing, and feeling [26]. The four key concepts highlight the importance of aspects of the housing and lead to important domains and subdomains (Figure 1).

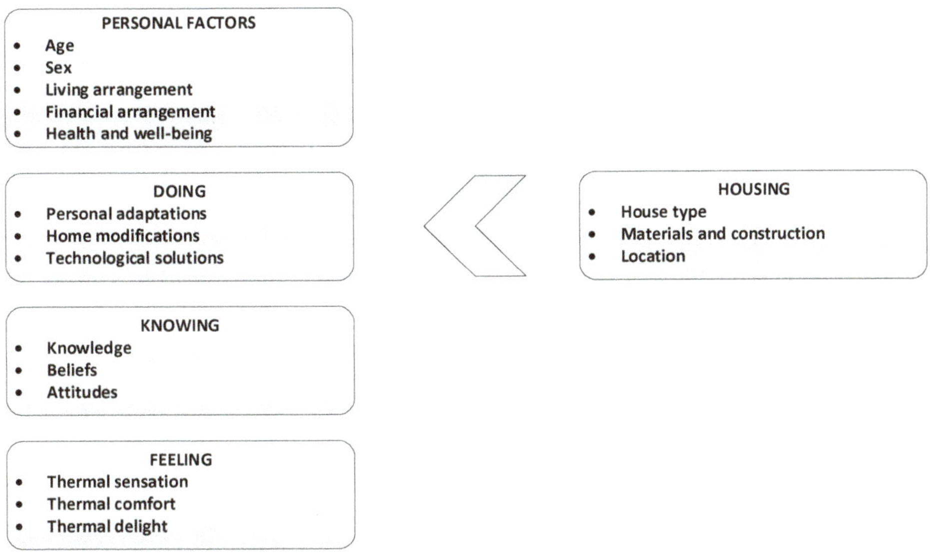

Figure 1. Factors important for understanding heating and cooling behaviours. Adapted from van Hoof et al. [26].

This paper describes the method used to develop the organisation and content of the guidelines. Based on the concept of personas, a number of discrete "thermal personalities" were developed through cluster analysis of quantitative data (for example, personal factors, doing, and housing) from the survey and the monitoring questionnaires, supplemented with qualitative information (for example, about knowing and feeling) from the interviews with the participants of the monitoring and thermal comfort survey and from the focus group discussions.

Personas are "fictitious, specific and concrete representations of target users" [31]. Originally proposed by software developer Alan Cooper [32] as a way to represent the goals and motivations of different types of prospective software users, personas are typically developed from both quantitative and qualitative data and are presented as fictional characters with a name, appropriate image, and a narrative. Personas can be used to summarise and communicate research about people [33], to link such research with design ideas [34], and can stimulate empathy or understanding of user perspectives, particularly where these perspectives are different from those of the designer's [35].

The thermal personalities developed in this study reflect strategies that older people currently use to achieve thermal comfort in the South Australian context and highlight where additional information will be beneficial. Basing the design guidelines on a number of different thermal personalities derived from the experiences and opinions of the participants themselves highlights the different approaches that people have to thermal comfort.

2. Methodology

In order to develop the thermal personalities, cluster analysis was used to identify groups amongst the study participants. In cluster analysis, similar objects are grouped into clusters such that the clusters are distinct from each other, while the members within the cluster are broadly similar to each other [36]. The clustering was based on data from 250 participants of the telephone survey [25] and 71 participants of the indoor environmental monitoring/occupant survey [27–30]. Note that only a small number of the 49 participants of the focus group were included in the cluster analysis, as the rest did not participate in either the telephone survey or the monitoring, where the detailed questionnaire was administered. Further, a number of people participated in all three—the telephone survey, focus group discussions, and indoor monitoring—hence, they were only counted once. This resulted in 303 total participants for the clustering.

After carefully going through all the questions used in the telephone survey and occupant survey, a set of 18 questions were identified as relevant features with which to judge the similarity between each participant in the clustering analysis. Some adjustments on how the data were analysed are explained below.

As the data collection stages—i.e., the telephone survey and indoor environmental monitoring—covered different combinations of questionnaires, the first step of the process involved sorting and separating only the questions that were repeated in both stages and, where possible, combining questions. For example, people were asked to rate their concern about the cost of heating as well as their concern about the cost of cooling on a five-point scale from 1 = not at all concerned, 2 = somewhat concerned, 3 = concerned, 4 = very concerned, to 5 = extremely concerned. As more than 90% of people responded in the same way to both questions, the categories were combined to depict their *Concern about the cost of heating and cooling*. The scale was reduced to a three-point scale, i.e., 1 = not at all concerned, 2 = concerned (covering the previous votes 2 and 3), 3 = very concerned (corresponding to the previous votes 4 and 5). Where the original responses differed for heating and cooling, they were checked. In some cases, the respondent did not use either heating or cooling, so the response for the one they had was recorded to represent the concern over the cost of energy. Otherwise, any responses that included 4 or 5 in the old scale were recoded as 3 (very concerned) in the new scale. Other cases were recorded as the lower value.

During the survey, many respondents had chosen "Declined to answer" when asked about the annual household income, although all had provided the source of income (i.e., either working full or part-time, part or full government-funded aged pension, or self-funded retiree). Note that a self-funded retiree is someone whose retirement income is derived from a contribution-based benefit known as superannuation in Australia or from other sources such as investments or savings. For cases where household income was not given, an amount was calculated based on the source of income that was provided with amounts based on the current means-tested aged pension in Australia for either a single person (AUD 24,000/year) or couple (AUD 36,000/year). Thus, the first category for *Annual household income* (<AUD 30,000) corresponds to a person who lives alone and receives the aged pension. The middle category equates to a single person on part-pension with additional income (for instance, working part-time or investments) or for a couple receiving either the full government pension or a part-pension supplemented by other income. The category for >AUD 50,000 applies for people who do not qualify for the pension as their income from other sources (for instance, superannuation or savings) is too high. The validity of this approach was checked against the cases where both household income and the source of income had been provided.

Both the survey and monitoring questionnaire included separate questions about whether specific health symptoms had been diagnosed by a doctor in either hot or cold weather. While some symptoms were particular to either hot or cold weather (for instance, heat stroke, dehydration, pneumonia), most symptoms occurred in both hot and cold weather (for instance, asthma, bronchitis, renal or kidney condition, heart condition). Thus, these were only counted once per person but combined in the feature 'Weather-affected health symptoms'.

The EQ-5D-5L is a health-related quality of life questionnaire about mobility (the ability to walk about), self-care (washing and dressing oneself), usual activities (work, housework, family or leisure activities), pain or discomfort, and anxiety or depression [37]. Respondents were asked to rate their problems in each category on a scale from 1 (no problems) to 5 (extreme problems or unable to do).

Both the survey and monitoring questionnaire included the question, "When it's very hot, what is the first thing you do to cool down?". Individual responses were grouped for the feature 'First action to keep cool' into personal (i.e., drink water, wear light clothes, reduce activities, stay inside, take cool showers, go for a swim); household (i.e., pull down blinds, shut curtains, keep windows and doors shut during the day or open them up when it cools down); and technology (i.e., turn on fan or air conditioning). Similarly, responses to 'First action to keep warm' were grouped as personal (i.e., hot drinks or hot food, wear warm clothes, keep active, stay in bed longer, use knee rugs, take hot showers); household (i.e., open curtains during day, close them at night, shut doors between rooms); and technology (i.e., turn on heater).

Table 1 shows the 18 features, their data types, and the scales or categories used. The data included different data types: ordinal (such as age group) and nominal (such as sex and living arrangement).

Table 1. Features used for development of the thermal personalities.

Feature		Scale or Categories	Data Type
Age group		1 = 65–74 2 = 75–84 3 = 85+	Ordinal
Sex		0 = female 1 = male	Nominal
Living arrangement		0 = alone 1 = with partner/others	Nominal
Annual household income		1 = less than AUD 30,000 2 = between AUD 30,000 and AUD 50,000 3 = more than AUD 50,000	Nominal
Concern re heating and cooling cost		0 = not concerned 1 = concerned 2 = very concerned	Ordinal
EQ-5D-5L dimensions health-related well-being	Mobility	1 = no problems with walking about 2 = slight problems with walking about 3 = moderate problems with walking about 4 = severe problems with walking about 5 = unable to walk about	Ordinal
	Self-care	1 = no problems washing or dressing myself 2 = slight problems washing or dressing myself 3 = moderate problems washing or dressing myself 4 = severe problems washing or dressing myself 5 = unable to wash or dress myself	Ordinal
	Usual activities	1 = no problems doing my usual activities 2 = slight problems doing my usual activities 3 = moderate problems doing my usual activities 4 = severe problems doing my usual activities 5 = unable to doing my usual activities	Ordinal
	Pain/discomfort	1 = no pain or discomfort 2 = slight pain or discomfort 3 = moderate pain or discomfort 4 = severe pain or discomfort 5 = extreme pain or discomfort	Ordinal
	Anxiety/depression	1 = not anxious or depressed 2 = slightly anxious or depressed 3 = moderately anxious or depressed 4 = severely anxious or depressed 5 = extremely anxious or depressed	Ordinal

Table 1. *Cont.*

Feature	Scale or Categories	Data Type
Number of weather-affected health symptoms	0 = none 1 = 1 2 = 2 3 = 3	Ordinal
First action to keep cool	1 = personal, such as changing clothing level 2 = household, such as close/open doors, windows, curtains, or blinds 3 = technology, such as turning on cooling or fans	Nominal
First action to keep warm	1 = personal such as changing clothing level 2 = household such as close/open doors, windows, curtains, or blinds 3 = technology such as turning on heating	Nominal
Location	1 = Iron Triangle—semi arid (Bsk) 2 = Adelaide metropolitan area—warm temperate (Csa) 3 = Fleurieu Peninsula or Adelaide Hills—mild temperate (Csb)	Nominal
Age of house (years)	1 = less than 10 years 2 = 10–20 years 3 = more than 20 years	Ordinal
In a retirement village?	0 = no 1 = yes	Nominal
Type of cooler	1 = none 2 = ducted reverse cycle (RC) * 3 = split system reverse cycle (RC) 4 = ducted evaporative cooling 5 = portable cooler	Nominal
Type of heater	1 = none 2 = ducted reverse cycle (RC) 3 = split system reverse cycle (RC) 4 = electric panel or portable heater 5 = gas heater 6 = combustion or open wood fire 7 = underfloor heating	Nominal

* RC—reverse cycle air conditioner. In some countries, this is called a heat pump.

The clustering algorithm used was an agglomerative (bottom up) hierarchical cluster analysis (HCA) performed using Anaconda v2019.3 [38], Python v3.7, NumPy, and SciPy libraries. HCA was chosen as there was initially a large number of variables and this approach is considered appropriate for high dimensional and low sample size (HDLSS) data. [39,40]. Additionally, unlike techniques such as k-means, it does not assume or determine the number of clusters (k) in advance but rather, produces a dendrogram diagram that represents the similarity or distance between clusters.

As there were mixed data types used for the clustering analysis (i.e., nominal and ordinal data), each feature required a different distance measure to calculate the similarity between each person. The Gower dissimilarity measure [41] is able to deal with mixed type data types and, therefore, was chosen for this procedure.

The HCA started with all 303 people as separate individual clusters and progressively merged them according to a pre-determined linkage criterion. This criterion determines which distance measure to use between data points. For this study, three linkage criteria, namely weighted, average, and complete [42], were tested in parallel to each other, in order to help choose the best performing cluster merging strategy. The silhouette score [43] was calculated for the different numbers of clusters ranging from 2 to 13. The silhouette score (from −1.0 to +1.0) shows how similar an object is to its designated cluster compared to all the other clusters, with +1.0 representing the best results and negative values representing bad clustering outputs. On consideration, the results for 4–7 clusters were examined in more detail as these appeared the most appropriate number of clusters for the guidelines, while providing enough variation to highlight the difference amongst the participants. For these,

Pearson's Chi-squared (X^2) tests were performed to calculate the significance of the differences between clusters considering each feature.

Once the cluster analysis was finalised, the thermal personalities were developed based on the salient features of each cluster. These were determined by examining the percentage breakdown in each category of each feature. Where the percentage was 75–99%, it was deemed that the category was "highly likely" for that cluster; between 51 and 74%, it was deemed "likely". Where no category exceeded 50%, it was either deemed not salient for that feature or, if appropriate, categories were combined. The thermal personality narratives were further developed with quotes from the focus groups about qualitative aspects of thermal comfort. Information from the monitoring participants not included in the questionnaires (for example, about house design and construction and the way heaters and coolers are operated) was also used to enrich the narratives.

3. Results

3.1. Cluster Analysis Results

The cluster analysis identified that with six clusters, the silhouette score was greater than 0.0 (0.1), and the clusters were considered significantly different in all 18 features tested through Pearson's X^2 tests ($p < 0.05$) (Table 2).

Table 2. Results of Pearson's X^2 test for features used in cluster analysis.

Feature	Pearson's X^2 Significance
Age	0.000
Sex	0.000
Living Arrangement	0.000
Annual household income	0.000
Concern re heating and cooling cost	0.000
Mobility	0.001
Self-care	0.000
Usual Activities	0.000
Pain/discomfort	0.000
Anxiety/depression	0.000
Number of weather-affected health symptoms	0.046
First action to keep cool	0.000
First action to keep warm	0.000
Location	0.000
Age of house	0.014
In a retirement village?	0.000
Type of cooler	0.000
Type of heater	0.000

Figure 2 shows the dendrogram that resulted from the clustering process, truncated to improve visualisation. The dashed horizontal line indicates the height at which the final six clusters, using all 18 features and complete linkage criteria, can be identified. The *y*-axis of this dendrogram reflects the distance between different clusters, from 0 to 1.0. The height (y) at which any two clusters are joined represents how similar they are. Two clusters that are joined at a low y-level are more similar to each other than the ones joined at higher levels.

The results of the cluster analysis are shown in the Supplementary Materials and the description of the salient characteristics of the clusters is shown in Table 3.

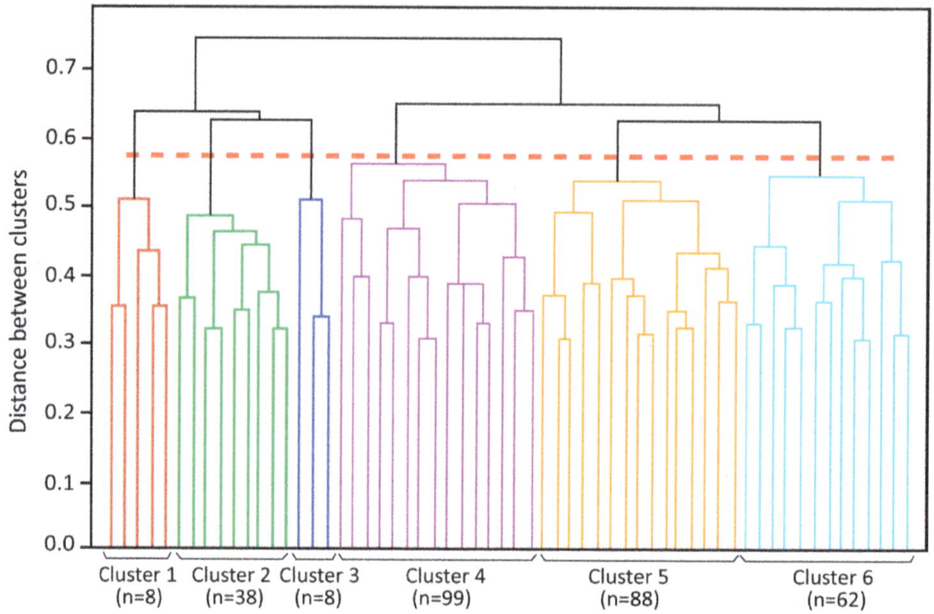

Figure 2. Clustering dendrogram.

3.2. Thermal Personalities

Based on the salient characteristics of each cluster, the narratives for the thermal personalities were developed, as shown in Table 4. A name was assigned for each personality (not a real participant's name) plus, where appropriate, other aspects of personal factors, doing, knowing, feeling, and housing were incorporated to emphasise the identity and indicate specific thermal behaviours. The transcripts of the focus group discussions and the audio recordings of the monitoring participants were examined for quotations to enrich the narratives, particularly in relation to the qualitative aspects of thermal behaviour. These appear in italics in the text of Table 4.

3.3. Development of Thermal Comfort Guidelines

The narratives of each cluster were then used to identify the thermal comfort guidelines that could be relevant for that cluster. The design guidelines are intended to improve people's knowledge (i.e., knowing), particularly about home modifications and technological solutions (i.e., doing), as well as aspects of housing that can affect thermal comfort and energy use.

Table 5 presents the important points for the guidelines of each cluster. Note that the details of the actual guidelines are outside the scope of this paper and will be reported elsewhere.

Table 3. Salient characteristics of clusters.

	Cluster 1	Cluster 2	Cluster 3	Cluster 4	Cluster 5	Cluster 6
Age	Highly likely ** aged 65–74	*	Highly likely aged 85+	*	*	*
Sex	Highly likely female	Highly likely female	Highly likely female	Likely female	Highly likely female	Highly likely male
Live alone/with partner	Lives alone	Highly likely lives alone	Highly likely lives alone	Highly likely lives with other	Likely lives with other	Likely lives with other
Annual household income	Likely > AUD 50,000	Likely < AUD 30,000	Likely < AUD 30,000	Likely > AUD 50,000	*	Likely AUD 30,000–50,000
Mobility	Has problems with mobility	Likely has no problems with mobility	Likely has problems with mobility	Likely has no problems with mobility.	Likely has no problems with mobility.	Likely has no problems with mobility.
Self-care	Highly likely has no problems with self-care	Highly likely has no problems with self-care	Highly likely has no problems with self-care	Highly likely has no problems with self-care	Highly likely has no problems with self-care	Highly likely has no problems with self-care
Undertaking usual activities	Highly likely has problems undertaking usual activities	Likely has no problems undertaking usual activities	Likely has problems undertaking usual activities	Likely has no problems undertaking usual activities	Likely has no problems undertaking usual activities	Likely has no problems undertaking usual activities
Pain and discomfort	Highly likely has moderate to severe pain or discomfort	Highly likely has some pain or discomfort	Likely has some pain or discomfort	Likely has some pain or discomfort	Likely has some pain or discomfort	Likely has some pain or discomfort
Anxiety and depression	Likely has some anxiety or depression	Likely has no anxiety and depression	Likely has no anxiety and depression	Highly likely has no anxiety or depression	Likely has some anxiety or depression	Highly likely has no anxiety or depression
Weather-affected health symptoms	Likely has 1 or more	Likely has none	Likely has 1 or more	Likely has none	Likely has none	Highly likely has none
First thing to keep cool	Highly likely use household strategies	*	Likely use technology	*	Likely use household strategies	Likely use technology

Table 3. *Cont.*

	Cluster 1	Cluster 2	Cluster 3	Cluster 4	Cluster 5	Cluster 6
First thing to keep warm	Likely use technology	Likely use personal strategies	Likely use personal strategies	Likely use personal strategies	Likely use personal strategies	Likely use technology
Concern about cost of heating and/or cooling	Highly likely very concerned	Likely concerned ***	Likely not concerned	Highly likely concerned	Highly likely concerned	Likely concerned
Location	Likely lives in Iron Triangle or Adelaide metropolitan area.	Live in all climate zones.	Highly likely live in Adelaide metropolitan area.	Highly likely live in Adelaide metropolitan area.	Likely live in Adelaide Hills or Fleurieu Peninsula	Likely live in Adelaide Hills or Fleurieu Peninsula
Age of house	Highly likely house > 20 years old	Highly likely house > 20 years old	Likely house > 20 years old	Likely house > 20 years old	Likely house > 20 years old	Highly likely house > 20 years old
Heating	*	*	Highly likely split system reverse cycle	Highly likely ducted reverse cycle	Highly likely split system reverse cycle	Highly likely split system reverse cycle
Cooling	Likely has ducted evaporative cooling.	*	Highly likely has split system reverse cycle	Highly likely ducted reverse cycle	Highly likely split system reverse cycle	Likely split system reverse cycle
In retirement village?	Does not live in a retirement village	Highly likely does not live in a retirement village	Does live in a retirement village	Highly likely does not live in a retirement village	Highly likely does not live in a retirement village	Highly likely does not live in a retirement village

* No salience. ** Highly likely = 75–99% of participants in the cluster; Likely = 51–74%; No salience = Less than 50%. *** combines categories Concerned and Very concerned.

Table 4. Thermal personalities.

	1. Tina, 66, lives alone in Whyalla and is about to renovate her existing house *I was probably much more mobile, in fact I know I was a lot more mobile even a year ago, and I am conscious that I spend a lot of time just sitting now.*	**2. Liz has a low income, lives alone, and wants to reduce her heating and cooling costs** *Oh yes, I care about the bills, when you're on a pension you have to.*	**3. Elsie, 86, lives alone in an independent living unit (ILU) of a retirement village and would like some ideas for improving her comfort** *I am conscious of the power bill because it is expensive and it's scary, but I won't freeze now, I won't freeze with my health and age.*
Personal factors	Recently retired, Tina sometimes has problems walking and often has pain that restricts her activities. She feels that her health is worse in cold weather and often gets colds and flu. In summer, her main problem is that she finds it hard to sleep. She has income from her superannuation.	Liz is often worried about money. She feels she is healthy but has occasional problems with pain in cold weather. *Feeling very, very cold. My limbs aren't as flexible; difficulty in walking; and difficulty in staying warm.*	Elsie receives a government pension. She has a number of ailments and has to use a walking frame. Her eyesight is poor and she also finds she is getting rather forgetful. Elsie has help with shopping and visits the community centre once a week.
Doing	In cold weather, the first thing Tina does to keep warm is turn the heater on. She has electric portable heaters, which she uses in the living room and the bedroom. For cooling, Tina has ducted evaporative cooling. She uses this mostly at night, preferring to shut the house up on a hot day and stay inside.	Although Liz has a split system reverse cycle air conditioner in the living room and a portable heater in the bedroom, she prefers to keep warm by dressing appropriately and working in the garden. Liz only uses cooling during prolonged hot spells.	Elsie has a split system air conditioner in the living room. The first thing she does when she is feeling too warm, is to turn the air conditioner on. In cold weather, she prefers to wait until late afternoon before turning the heating on. She makes sure she is dressed warmly and will often use a knee rug when sitting.
Knowing	Tina has lived in Whyalla for a long time and is familiar with the climate. She is very concerned that her declining health will make it harder to remain in her own home and wants to make adjustments to the house while she can.	Liz is very concerned about the cost of heating and cooling and often finds it difficult to pay her electricity bills. *You pay an electricity account but you go without something else.*	Elsie had the air conditioner installed a few years ago but no one explained how to use it. *I'm never sure that I've got the thing set correctly, whether I've got the wrong instruction book. I always have difficulty, and I don't really know where to go for assistance.*
Feeling	Tina finds her mood lightens on a sunny day. She particularly likes sitting in the sun on a cold day. For Tina, this is pure thermal delight.	Liz prefers hot weather. *I used to love the cold weather and not enjoy the heat so much but my bones love the heat, they don't enjoy the cold.*	Elsie was born in England and she thinks this is why she has never liked the heat. *I certainly get grumpier. It affects my mood and my attitude in the hot weather.*
Housing	Tina lives in a house that was built 30 years ago. It is cavity brick with concrete-slab-on-ground and a corrugated metal roof. Tina thinks it has insulation in the ceiling.	Liz's 100-year-old cottage has sandstone walls and timber floors. The kitchen and living area, added 20 years ago, has brick veneer walls with concrete slab on ground.	Elsie lives in a semi-detached unit built in the 1970s with cavity brick walls, timber floors, and a tiled roof. She thinks there is insulation in the ceiling.

Table 4. *Cont.*

	4. Sophia lives with her husband in Adelaide and is about to renovate her house *I'd just like to be able to do something about it rather than just push a button when it's going to get hot or cold.*	**5. Peggy and her partner are planning to downsize to a township in the Adelaide Hills and want information about sustainable heating and cooling** *If I had a wish in life it would be to live in a home that was environmentally really good, faced the sun and did everything.*	**6. Joe lives with his wife in a seaside town on the Fleurieu Peninsula and is interested in upgrading his air conditioning** *I would say that my heating and cooling is an absolute priority, I'd rather eat mince if you know what I mean and still be warm or cool.*
Personal factors	Sophia and her husband have income from investments and their superannuation. They are healthy and active, regularly going to the gym, travelling, and entertaining family and friends. Sophia has few weather-related illnesses beyond the occasional winter cold.	Since retiring, Peggy has increased her involvement with community and environment groups. Although generally healthy and active, she feels she is slowing down and often becomes anxious both about her future and the state of the world.	Joe is a retired engineer who keeps himself fit and healthy. He has a part-pension that supplements his income from other sources.
Doing	Sophia's house has ducted reverse cycle air conditioning, but Sophia and her husband prefer not to use this as a first response to hot and cold weather. Instead, they make sure they are dressed appropriately for the weather and that they keep active, particularly in cold weather. *Go outside, do something outside. Come back inside and you'll feel warm, work in the garden.*	Peggy has an old split system reverse cycle air conditioner in the living room but rarely uses it. She prefers to dress warmly and keep active in cold weather and to use blinds and curtains to keep the sun out in hot weather. *I very rarely put on the air conditioner because I'm a terrible greenie, and I don't like that air that blows on me.*	Joe's first action if he feels too warm or cold is to turn the air conditioner on. He has one split system reverse cycle air conditioner in the living room and an old window unit in the bedroom but is considering upgrading these along with installing solar panels. *As I get older I must admit... I just flick a switch and it sorts my problems.*
Knowing	Sophia is concerned that the cost of heating and cooling is increasing. She hopes to continue living in the family home but realises they need to make some changes. She is interested in passive design and would like to incorporate some of these principles when they renovate.	Peggy is concerned about climate change and the links between energy use and global warming. While she is very concerned about the financial cost of heating and cooling, she is also concerned about the environmental cost.	Joe is very comfortable with technology. He keeps his own records of the weather and also records his energy use. He likes the sense of control that this knowledge gives him.
Feeling	Sophia likes the idea of having alternatives to the air conditioner to provide comfort. *I'd just like to be able to do something about it rather than just push a button when it's going to get hot or cold.*	Peggy feels much healthier when she is connected to natural elements such as the sun and the wind. *Utilise nature, work with nature and appreciate nature.*	Joe loves living where he does because he finds the salty air healthy and he has a wonderful view of the ocean.
Housing	Sophia and her husband have lived in their bungalow for more than 10 years. It has brick walls, timber floors, and a tiled roof. They are planning to upgrade their house.	Peggy and her partner have lived in their current house for many years, but they are looking to move to a smaller house in an Adelaide Hills town.	Joe's house is elevated lightweight construction with timber floors.

Table 5. Important points to be addressed in the thermal comfort guidelines.

CLUSTER 1—Emphasis: Health and Well-Being	CLUSTER 2—Emphasis: Cost	CLUSTER 3—Emphasis: Comfort and Cost (Retirement Unit)
This cluster will benefit from guidelines consisting of information about: • How hot and cold weather can affect medical conditions in older people (K); • The benefits of simple modifications to the house, (D) for example: ○ improving ceiling insulation; ○ adding window and door seals; • Options for operable windows that are easy to operate (K); • Passive design principles to be incorporated in renovation, particularly to allow sun to come into the living area (K/D/F); • Energy-efficient heating and cooling systems and temperature set points that would be conducive to maintaining good health (D).	This cluster will benefit from guidelines consisting of information about: • How hot and cold weather can affect medical conditions in older people (K); • Low cost household strategies to reduce the running cost of heating and cooling, (D), for example: ○ Installing reversible ceiling fans; ○ Using curtains or blinds to help reduce unwanted heat gain and heat loss; ○ Reducing the volume of rooms to be heated or cooled, for instance, by shutting doors or adding partitions; • Energy-efficient heating and cooling systems (D).	This cluster will benefit from guidelines consisting of information about: • How hot and cold weather can affect medical conditions in older people (K); • Household strategies to improve comfort and reduce the need for heating and cooling (D), for example: ○ Using curtains or blinds to help reduce unwanted heat loss and heat gain; ○ Reducing draughts by improving the sealant around the windows and doors. • Personal heating and cooling devices such as electric rugs or personal fans (D); • How to operate a split system reverse cycle air conditioner efficiently, including thermostat settings, and when to turn it on and off (D); • Easy-to-use remote controls for the air-conditioning system (D).

Table 5. *Cont.*

CLUSTER 4—Emphasis: Comfort and Cost (Own House)	CLUSTER 5—Emphasis: Cost and Environment	CLUSTER 6—Emphasis: Comfort and Technology
This cluster will benefit from guidelines consisting of information about: • How hot and cold weather can affect medical conditions in older people (K); • Passive design principles for house renovation (K). • Household modifications suitable for an old house (D), for example: ○ Summer shading including using deciduous plants; ○ Improving/adding sealant around the windows and doors; ○ Replacing existing glass in windows with better performance glazing, and/or; ○ Replacing existing fixed windows with operable ones; ○ Adding roof vents to the roof space; ○ Checking the insulation on the ceiling and, if needed, replacing/adding new insulation. • Alternatives to the ducted system reverse-cycle air-conditioner for heating and cooling (K/D), for example: ○ Individual/split system so they only need to run the system in the room they occupy; • Solar panels: size, type, payback (K).	This cluster will benefit from guidelines consisting of information about: • How hot and cold weather can affect medical conditions in older people (K); • Passive design principles for building or buying a new house (K), for example: ○ Living areas that face the sun (F); ○ Walls and ceiling are well-insulated; ○ Windows can be opened easily but safely (D/F); ○ Window, door frames, all cracks and joints are well-sealed; ○ Roof eaves and other shading that will block direct sun in summer but allow it to enter the spaces in winter; ○ Large spaces can be divided into small spaces to reduce heating and cooling (D); ○ Using natural materials for building construction, as much as possible, to minimise environmental impact and provide "warm" feeling (F); • Solar panels: size, type, payback (K).	This cluster will benefit from guidelines consisting of information about: • How hot and cold weather can affect medical conditions in older people (K); • Benefits of using energy-efficient heating and cooling systems (i.e., replacing the old window unit) (K/D); • Solar photovoltaic panels, size, cost, and payback (K); • Smart air-conditioning control and application (K/D); • Smart metering system (K); • Benefits of insulation to be installed under the elevated timber floors to reduce heat loss, thus reducing the need for heating (K).

K = Knowing; D = Doing; F = Feeling.

4. Discussion

Based on the concept of personas, this study has identified thermal personalities of older people living independently in South Australia as a basis for producing thermal comfort guidelines for people ageing-in-place in this region. Personas have been used widely in software development, marketing, and product design [44]. In recent decades, the rise of person-centred policies along with an increasing computerisation of information has seen the use of personas spreading. For example, in the health sector, personas have been used when developing public health messages and eHealth platforms for patients [45–47], during the design of medical equipment [48–50], and when developing health policy [51]. Personas of older people have been incorporated in health informatics [52–54]. A project in Europe has developed 30 basic senior personas as a tool for software developers using data derived from the longitudinal survey SHARE (Survey of Health Ageing and Retirement in Europe) [55]. Taşoz and Afacan developed three personas of older people that were used to explore simulated ageing and the effect on basic activities of daily life [56].

In the area of building design and thermal comfort, Jais et al. [57] and McCracken et al. [58] developed personas of people living with dementia to inform architects and designers. Goldstein et al. [59] used inferred and invented personas to develop occupant behaviour models for thermal simulation, while Haines and Mitchell [60] drew on evidence collected from a 4-year study of energy-saving technologies for owner-occupiers to develop personas of different approaches to domestic energy retrofitting. A similar approach was adopted by Ortiz and Bluyssen, who developed five archetypes of residential energy users and suggested that the archetypes will be useful for refining building simulation models and also for building designers wishing to develop building features for specific energy-using archetypes [61].

For this study, the thermal personalities were developed by analysing the characteristics of 303 research participants, and their responses to a range of questions related to how they deal with the weather and how they operate their homes. These characteristics and responses are referred to as features. Using cluster analysis, participants with similar features were grouped together. Whilst the analysis resulted in six distinct clusters, there were a number of challenges in the process. First, data were imbalanced. For example, initially, the participants were grouped into five age groups (65–69, 70–74, 75–79, 80–84, and 85 and over) but upon looking into the data more closely, there were very few participants aged 65–69; thus, a decision was made to reduce the age groups to three (65–74, 75–84, 85 and over). Reducing to three age groups also provided clearer distinctions in terms of age-related thermal behaviour, housing decisions, and health and well-being.

The second challenge was about the number of features included in the cluster analysis. Initially, more than 30 features were considered for the analysis. Many were rejected as the data were incomplete or were consistently evenly distributed (for instance, preference for either hot or cold weather did not show any difference). Indeed, many of the participants had similar characteristics. For example, in line with the general Australian population, the vast majority lived in a separate house built of brick veneer. While using fewer features resulted in a higher silhouette score, indicating that the clusters were distinctive from each other, the results were not comprehensive enough to be useful as a basis for the design guidelines. The process of identifying the features involved constant trying out, considering the outcome.

After a number of iterations, using the 18 features resulted in six distinctive clusters. These features are related to thermal comfort in complex and inter-related ways. For example, thermal comfort requirements and actions are likely to be different for the different age groups. People in the age group 85 years and over are likely to have lower income, more health and well-being issues, and are more likely to live alone than those aged 65–74 [62]. Some chronic health conditions that are common in the older population can be affected by either hot or cold weather. This may cause discomfort or changes to daily routines at one level but, in extreme cases, may lead to hospitalisation or mortality during heat waves or prolonged cold [63–66].

In addition, there may be age-related changes to housing. The majority of people downsizing and moving to a retirement home in South Australia are in the age group of 65–74 [67]. Age may also affect decisions about modifications to the house. During the focus group discussions, it emerged that a person's age was one consideration they took into account when assessing whether it was "worth" doing something, such as installing solar panels to reduce energy costs in light of "how much time is left" (to live). Similarly, the type of housing may determine what modifications are possible. Compared to an owner-occupied home, in a retirement home, the ability to make changes to the fabric of the house (such as adding external shading) is severely constrained.

Along with age, numerous studies have identified living arrangement as a risk factor for heat-related morbidity and mortality, with older people who live alone particularly vulnerable during heat waves [68,69]. In terms of thermal comfort, households with more than one person may have occupants with different thermal requirements (for example, for medical reasons) or different thermal preferences. On the other hand, a household with more than one person is likely to have financial advantages with a higher household income plus a lower energy use and cost per person.

The household income may constrain what is possible in terms of capital changes to a house, the sort of heating and cooling technology that is affordable, and the attitudes to energy usage for heating and cooling. The level of concern that people have about heating and cooling costs is likely to be a driver of thermal comfort behaviour. The costs may not be simply financial costs. A few people indicated that they were "not concerned" about the cost of heating or cooling because they felt the financial cost was less important than the potential cost to their health of being too hot or too cold, while some people were "very concerned" about the environmental cost of heating and cooling energy use rather than the financial cost.

The approach described in this paper of using different thermal personalities as the basis for the guidelines evolved in response to the previous stages of the research, where it became apparent that older people had a range of approaches to thermal comfort depending on their particular circumstances. Complex issues are at play, including the local context (climate, house type, heating and cooling equipment) and the individual's personal situation, habits, beliefs, and preferences. One person may eschew air-conditioning for cooling because of their environmental beliefs, while another may use energy-intensive whole-house heating for many months of the year finding it alleviates their arthritis. In both cases, appropriate (but different) information may help them reduce energy costs and improve their health and well-being.

These design guidelines will differ from existing guidelines and traditional thermal comfort standards, such as ASHRAE Standard 55 [14], ISO 7730 [15], and ISO/TS 14415 [16]. Thermal comfort research has been dominated by building science and quantitative analysis, often with a view to defining or developing standards of optimal environmental conditions. For example, the WHO recommends temperatures between 18 and 24 °C to be the "safe" temperature range where "there is no demonstrable risk to human health of healthy sedentary people" [70]. However, the WHO recommends a minimum temperature higher than 18 °C for older people. On the other extreme, temperature between 25 and 32 °C is recommended by WHO as acceptable maximum temperatures [71]. While recent studies conducted both in environmental chambers [6,72,73] and in dwellings [9,74] have started to make distinctions between thermal comfort for younger and older people, most did not consider people's behaviour in their own home and solely focussed on one's thermal responses. Adopting both quantitative and qualitative approaches, this study, on the other hand, has considered the older people in the true context of their home. This includes their personal factors (i.e., age, sex, living arrangement, financial situation, and health and well-being status), their knowledge, belief, and attitudes, their feeling and sensation about their surroundings, their behaviours and adaptive practices, as well as the interactions with their home environment. It is expected that the guidelines that will be developed from this approach will be more useful in addressing the heterogeneity of older people.

The study, however, has a number of limitations. Firstly, people volunteered to take part in the study and this introduced a bias in terms of people who were interested in research and willing to commit for a long time-frame study. Most were in (relatively) good health. Thus, although the study participants were still heterogeneous, there were some groups who were under-represented in the study including those in poor health, renters, people from non-English speaking backgrounds, and people living in different house types.

Secondly, while the focus group discussions [26] provided qualitative information useful to enrich the understanding from the results of the initial survey [25], the questions posed to the participants during the focus group discussions were not all the same as those used in the survey due to the flow of the discussions at the time. There could have been greater standardisation of questions asked at the different stages of the research and better integration of the non-quantitative aspects.

Thirdly, as there are only three climate zones in South Australia (BSk, Csa, and Csb climate zones according to the Köppen–Geiger climate classification [75]), the results of the study are particularly relevant only to these climates. Similar research in other climate zones is likely to reveal different thermal behaviours and this, in turn, may lead to the identification of different thermal personalities. For instance, someone in northwest Europe living in a Cfb climate may not have to consider the extreme heat that sometimes occurs in South Australia but would have to deal with much lower temperatures. In other words, the thermal behaviours and thermal comfort requirements seen in the participants of this study may be quite different from those living in climates other than the BSk, Csa, and Csb climate zones.

Along with the climate, there are many aspects of thermal comfort that are particular to the local context such as housing tenure and construction methods, heating and cooling equipment, and energy costs. Nevertheless, while the focus of this study is on older people in the particular context of South Australia, the approach can be adopted in other contexts and for other groups in society. One approach could be to conduct a process that is close to the cross-cultural validation of instruments and scales [76]. Such a validation would account for cultural differences, for instance, for older people who arrived in Australia as migrants, or for older people in other countries, or when accounting for existing forms of social inequality and deprivation [77]. This applies not only to ethnic or cultural diversity, but also to other factors such as sex, age, socioeconomic position, or health status, which influence what people consider important when it comes to the age-friendliness of their living environment [78], including the thermal environment of their houses. In addition, for older people in different climate zones, a "cross-climatic validation" could also be conducted, as different climatic conditions may impact behaviours, practices, and beliefs [79]. The circumstances in which societies adapt their cultural values and practices to cold, temperate, and hot climates include the availability of money to cope with the climate [79]. Countries like Australia, which cover various climate zones, could be compared to countries which are located in just one climate zone, such as the United Kingdom, or countries which have a similar diversity in climates (such as the United States of America), and which hold similar cultural practices and share a common language. Conducting a similar study in a climatically and culturally diverse country as India, where many people also speak English, could yield different outcomes in thermal personalities.

5. Conclusions

The research, *Improving the thermal environment of housing for older Australians* (ARC DP180102019), investigates the thermal comfort and thermal behaviours of people aged 65 and over who wish to age-in-place. It adds to our knowledge about the variety of strategies taken by older South Australians to achieve thermal comfort. This paper describes one aspect of the method used to translate the research into information about thermal comfort that is approachable and relevant for a wide audience. The concept of personas was used to develop thermal personalities that reflect personal factors, housing conditions, and knowledge as well as the actions that older people prefer to take to keep warm in cold weather and cool in hot weather. The current study has identified six thermal personalities, which will be developed in more depth for the actual guidelines. Aspects particular to the personality (for instance, preferred strategy for keeping warm or cool, house type, and location) will be incorporated in building simulations to assess the impact on comfort, cost, or energy use of design strategies for each thermal personality. This novel approach to thermal comfort research—based on personas—in turn, will lead to personalised guidelines to achieve thermal comfort in housing for older people.

Supplementary Materials: The following are available online at http://www.mdpi.com/1660-4601/17/22/8402/s1, Table S1. Results of cluster analysis.

Author Contributions: Conceptualization, H.B., L.A.M., J.v.H. and V.S.; funding acquisition, V.S.; methodology, H.B., L.A.M., J.v.H. and V.S.; writing—original draft, H.B., L.A.M. and J.v.H.; writing—review and editing, H.B., L.A.M., J.v.H. and V.S. All authors have read and agreed to the published version of the manuscript.

Funding: This study is funded by the Australian Research Council through the ARC Discovery grant scheme, project number DP180102019. The project has approval from The University of Adelaide Human Research Ethics Committee (approval number H-2018-042).

Acknowledgments: The authors would like to thank all the study participants for their time and insights. Input from researchers Dino Pisaniello, Alana Hansen, Terence Williamson, Renuka Visvanathan and Jian Zuo is acknowledged. The assistance from George Stamatescu with the cluster analysis is also acknowledged.

Conflicts of Interest: The authors declare no conflict of interest. The funders had no role in the design of the study; in the collection, analyses, or interpretation of data; in the writing of the manuscript, or in the decision to publish the results.

References

1. Judd, B.; Liu, E.; Easthope, H.; Davy, L.; Bridge, C. *Downsizing Amongst Older Australians, AHURI Final Report No. 214*; Australian Housing and Urban Research Institute: Melbourne, Australia, 2014.
2. World Health Organization. *Global Age-Friendly Cities: A Guide*; World Health Organization: Geneva, Switzerland, 2007; ISBN 978-92-4-154730-7.
3. Rupp, R.F.; Vásquez, N.G.; Lamberts, R. A review of human thermal comfort in the built environment. *Energy Build.* **2015**, *105*, 178–205. [CrossRef]
4. Wang, Z.; De Dear, R.; Luo, M.; Lin, B.; He, Y.; Ghahramani, A.; Zhu, Y. Individual difference in thermal comfort: A literature review. *Build. Environ.* **2018**, *138*, 181–193. [CrossRef]
5. van Hoof, J.; Hensen, J.L.M. Thermal comfort and older adults. *Gerontechnology* **2006**, *4*, 223–228. [CrossRef]
6. Schellen, L.; van Marken Lichtenbelt, W.; Loomans, M.G.L.C.; Toftum, J.; de Wit, M.H. Differences between young adults and elderly in thermal comfort, productivity, and thermal physiology in response to a moderate temperature drift and a steady-state condition. *Indoor Air* **2010**, *20*, 273–283. [CrossRef]
7. Bills, R. Cold comfort: Thermal sensation in people over 65 and the consequences for an ageing population. In Proceedings of the 9th Windsor Conference: Making Comfort Relevant, Cumberland Lodge, Windsor, UK, 7–10 April 2016; pp. 156–167.
8. Tartarini, F.; Cooper, P.; Fleming, R. Thermal environment and thermal sensations of occupants of nursing homes: A field study. In Proceedings of the International High-Performance Built Environment Conference—A Sustainable Built Environment Conference, Sydney, Australia, 17–18 November 2016.
9. Hwang, R.-L.; Chen, C.-P. Field study on behaviors and adaptation of elderly people and their thermal comfort requirements in residential environments. *Indoor Air* **2010**, *20*, 235–245. [CrossRef]
10. Yang, J.; Nam, I.; Sohn, J.-R. The influence of seasonal characteristics in elderly thermal comfort in Korea. *Energy Build.* **2016**, *128*, 583–591. [CrossRef]
11. Gasparrini, A.; Guo, Y.; Hashizume, M.; Lavigne, E.; Zanobetti, A.; Schwartz, J.; Tobias, A.; Tong, S.; Rocklöv, J.; Forsberg, B.; et al. Mortality risk attributable to high and low ambient temperature: A multicountry observational study. *Lancet* **2015**, *386*, 369–375. [CrossRef]
12. Livable Housing Australia. *Livable Housing Design Guidelines*, 4th ed.; Livable Housing Australia: Forest Lodge, Australia, 2017. Available online: http://www.livablehousingaustralia.org.au/library/SLLHA_GuidelinesJuly2017FINAL4.pdf (accessed on 11 November 2020).
13. Carnemolla, P.; Bridge, C. A scoping review of home modification interventions—Mapping the evidence base. *Indoor Built Environ.* **2018**, *29*, 299–310. [CrossRef]

14. ASHRAE. *Thermal Environmental Conditions for Human Occupancy (ANSI/ASHRAE 55-2017)*; American Society of Heating, Refrigeration and Air-conditioning Engineers: Atlanta, GA, USA, 2017. Available online: https://www.ashrae.org/technical-resources/bookstore/standard-55-thermal-environmental-conditions-for-human-occupancy (accessed on 11 November 2020).
15. ISO. *Ergonomics of the Thermal Environment—Analytical Determination and Interpretation of Thermal Comfort Using Calculation of the PMV and PPD Indices and Local Thermal Comfort Criteria*; ISO 7730:2005; International Organization for Standardization: Geneva, Switzerland, 2005. Available online: https://www.iso.org/standard/39155.html (accessed on 11 November 2020).
16. ISO. *Ergonomics of the Thermal Environment—Application of International Standards to People with Special Requirements, Technical Specification (ISO/TS 14415)*; International Organization for Standardization: Geneva, Switzerland, 2005. Available online: https://www.iso.org/standard/39870.html (accessed on 11 November 2020).
17. Cheshire, W.P. Thermoregulatory disorders and illness related to heat and cold stress. *Auton. Neurosci.* **2016**, *196*, 91–104. [CrossRef]
18. Blatteis, C.M. Age-Dependent Changes in Temperature Regulation—A Mini Review. *Gerontology* **2012**, *58*, 289–295. [CrossRef]
19. Havenith, G. Temperature regulation and technology. *Gerontechnology* **2001**, *1*, 41–49. [CrossRef]
20. Schlader, Z.J.; Coleman, G.L.; Sackett, J.R.; Sarker, S.; Chapman, C.L.; Hostler, D.; Johnson, B.D. Behavioral thermoregulation in older adults with cardiovascular co-morbidities. *Temperature* **2018**, *5*, 70–85. [CrossRef] [PubMed]
21. van Hoof, J.; Kort, H.S.M.; Hensen, J.L.M.; Duijnstee, M.S.H.; Rutten, P.G.S. Thermal comfort and the integrated design of homes for older people with dementia. *Build. Environ.* **2010**, *45*, 358–370. [CrossRef]
22. van Hoof, J.; Schellen, L.; Soebarto, V.; Wong, J.K.W.; Kazak, J.K. Ten questions concerning thermal comfort and ageing. *Build. Environ.* **2017**, *120*, 123–133. [CrossRef]
23. Miller, W.; Vine, D.; Amin, Z. Energy efficiency of housing for older citizens: Does it matter? *Energy Policy* **2017**, *101*, 216–224. [CrossRef]
24. Willand, N.; Horne, R. "They are grinding us into the ground"—The lived experience of (in)energy justice amongst low-income older households. *Appl. Energy* **2018**, *226*, 61–70. [CrossRef]
25. Soebarto, V.; Bennetts, H.; Hansen, A.; Zuo, J.; Williamson, T.; Pisaniello, D.; van Hoof, J.; Visvanathan, R. Living environment, heating-cooling behaviours and well-being: Survey of older South Australians. *Build. Environ.* **2019**, *157*, 215–226. [CrossRef]
26. van Hoof, J.; Bennetts, H.; Hansen, A.; Kazak, J.K.; Soebarto, V. The Living Environment and Thermal Behaviours of Older South Australians: A Multi-Focus Group Study. *Int. J. Environ. Res. Public Health* **2019**, *16*, 935. [CrossRef]
27. Soebarto, V.; Williamson, T.; Bennetts, H.; Arakawa Martins, L.; Pisaniello, D.; Hansen, A.; Visvanathan, R.; Carre, A. Development of an integrated data acquisition system for thermal comfort studies of older people. In Proceedings of the 11th Windsor Conference: Resilient Comfort, Windsor, UK, 16–19 April 2020; pp. 155–170.
28. Soebarto, V.; Williamson, T.; Carre, A.; Martins, L.A. Understanding indoor environmental conditions and occupant's responses in houses of older people. *IOP Conf. Ser. Mater. Sci. Eng.* **2019**, *609*, 042096. [CrossRef]
29. Williamson, T.; Soebarto, V.; Bennetts, H.; Arakawa Martins, L.; Pisaniello, D. Thermal comfort, well-being and health of older residents in South Australia. In Proceedings of the 11th Windsor Conference: Resilient Comfort, Windsor, UK, 16–19 April 2020; pp. 171–186.
30. Arakawa Martins, L.; Williamson, T.T.; Bennetts, H.; Zuo, J.; Visvanathan, R.; Hansen, A.; Pisaniello, D.; van Hoof, J.; Soebarto, V. Individualising thermal comfort models for older people: The effects of personal characteristics on comfort and wellbeing. In Proceedings of the 11th Windsor Conference: Resilient Comfort, Windsor, UK, 16–19 April 2020; pp. 187–199.
31. Adlin, T.; Pruitt, J. *The Essential Persona Lifecycle: Your Guide to Building and Using Personas*; Morgan Kaufmann Publishers: San Francisco, CA, USA, 2010.
32. Cooper, A. *The Inmates are Running the Asylum: Why High Tech Products Drive us Crazy and How to Restore the Sanity*, 2nd ed.; Pearson Education: Indianapolis, IN, USA, 2004; ISBN 9780672326141.
33. Goltz, S. A Closer Look at Personas: What They Are and How They Work Part 1. *Smash. Magaz.* **2014**. Available online: https://www.smashingmagazine.com/2014/08/a-closer-look-at-personas-part-1/ (accessed on 8 July 2020).

34. Tvedebrink, T.D.O.; Jelić, A. Getting under the(ir) skin: Applying personas and scenarios with body-environment research for improved understanding of users' perspective in architectural design. *Pers. Stud.* **2018**, *4*, 5–24. [CrossRef]
35. Van der Linden, V.; Dong, H.; Heylighen, A. Building Empathy: Opportunities for Introducing Future Users' Perspectives in Architectural Design. In Proceedings of the Engineering for Society 2016: Raising Awareness for the Societal Role of Engineering, Leuven, Belgium, 15–16 September 2016; Engineering for Society/KU Leuven/Thomas More: Leuven, Belgium, 2016; pp. 49–53.
36. Bratchell, N. Cluster analysis. *Chemom. Intell. Lab. Syst.* **1989**, *6*, 105–125. [CrossRef]
37. EuroQol. *EQ-5D-5L User Guide*; EuroQoL Research Foundation: Rotterdam, The Netherlands, 2019. Available online: https://euroqol.org/publications/user-guides (accessed on 11 November 2020).
38. Anaconda. Anaconda Software Distribution. Computer Software. March 2019. Available online: Anaconda.com (accessed on 11 November 2020).
39. Steinbach, M.; Ertöz, L.; Kumar, V. The Challenges of Clustering High Dimensional Data. In *New Directions in Statistical Physics*; Springer Science and Business Media LLC: Berlin/Heidelberg, Germany, 2004; pp. 273–309.
40. Holden, R.J.; Kulanthaivel, A.; Purkayastha, S.; Goggins, K.M.; Kripalani, S. Know thy eHealth user: Development of biopsychosocial personas from a study of older adults with heart failure. *Int. J. Med. Inform.* **2017**, *108*, 158–167. [CrossRef] [PubMed]
41. Gower, J.C. Similarity, Dissimilarity, and Distance Measure. In *Encyclopedia of Biostatistics*; Wiley: Hoboken, NJ, USA, 2005.
42. Müllner, D. Modern hierarchical, agglomerative clustering algorithms. *arXiv* **2011**, arXiv:1109.2378. Available online: https://arxiv.org/abs/1109.2378 (accessed on 8 July 2020).
43. Rousseeuw, P.J. Silhouettes: A graphical aid to the interpretation and validation of cluster analysis. *J. Comput. Appl. Math.* **1987**, *20*, 53–65. [CrossRef]
44. Floyd, I.R.; Jones, M.C.; Twidale, M.B. Resolving Incommensurable Debates: A Preliminary Identification of Persona Kinds, Attributes, and Characteristics. *Artifact* **2008**, *2*, 12–26. [CrossRef]
45. Vosbergen, S.; Mulder-Wiggers, J.M.R.; Lacroix, J.P.; Kemps, H.M.C.; Kraaijenhagen, R.A.; Jaspers, M.W.M.; Peek, N. Using personas to tailor educational messages to the preferences of coronary heart disease patients. *J. Biomed. Inform.* **2015**, *53*, 100–112. [CrossRef]
46. Huh, J.; Kwon, B.C.; Kim, S.-H.; Lee, S.; Choo, J.; Kim, J.; Choi, M.-J.; Yi, J.S. Personas in online health communities. *J. Biomed. Inform.* **2016**, *63*, 212–225. [CrossRef]
47. Haldane, V.; Koh, J.J.K.; Srivastava, A.; Teo, K.W.Q.; Tan, Y.G.; Cheng, R.X.; Yap, Y.C.; Ong, P.S.; Van Dam, R.M.; Foo, J.M.; et al. User Preferences and Persona Design for an mHealth Intervention to Support Adherence to Cardiovascular Disease Medication in Singapore: A Multi-Method Study. *JMIR mHealth uHealth* **2019**, *7*, e10465. [CrossRef]
48. Lerouge, C.; Ma, J.; Sneha, S.; Tolle, K. User profiles and personas in the design and development of consumer health technologies. *Int. J. Med. Inform.* **2013**, *82*, e251–e268. [CrossRef]
49. Vincent, C.; Blandford, A. The challenges of delivering validated personas for medical equipment design. *Appl. Ergon.* **2014**, *45*, 1097–1105. [CrossRef]
50. van Hoof, J.; Wetzels, M.H.; Dooremalen, A.M.C.; Overdiep, R.A.; Nieboer, M.E.; Eyck, A.M.E.; van Gorkom, P.J.L.M.; Zwerts-Verhelst, E.L.M.; Aarts, S.; Vissers-Luijcks, C.; et al. Exploring Innovative Solutions for Quality of Life and Care of Bed-Ridden Nursing Home Residents through Codesign Sessions. *J. Aging Res.* **2015**, *2015*, 1–14. [CrossRef] [PubMed]
51. Gonzalez de Heredia, A.; Goodman-Deane, J.; Waller, S.; Clarkson, P.J.; Justel, D.; Iriarte, I.; Hernández, J. Personas for policy-making and health-care design. In Proceedings of the DESIGN 2018 15th International Design Conference, Dubrovnik, Croatia, 21–24 May 2018; pp. 2645–2656.
52. Zhu, H.; Wang, H.; Carroll, J.M. Creating Persona Skeletons from Imbalanced Datasets—A Case Study using U.S. Older Adults' Health Data. In Proceedings of the DIS'19 Designing Interactive Systems conference, San Diego, CA, USA, 23–28 June 2019; pp. 61–70. [CrossRef]
53. Schäfer, K.; Rasche, P.; Bröhl, C.; Theis, S.; Barton, L.; Brandl, C.; Wille, M.; Nitsch, V.; Mertens, A. Survey-based personas for a target-group-specific consideration of elderly end users of information and communication systems in the German health-care sector. *Int. J. Med. Inform.* **2019**, *132*, 103924. [CrossRef] [PubMed]
54. Wildenbos, G.A.; Jaspers, M.; Schijven, M.; Peute, L.D. Mobile health for older adult patients: Using an aging barriers framework to classify usability problems. *Int. J. Med. Inform.* **2019**, *124*, 68–77. [CrossRef] [PubMed]

55. Wöckl, B.; Yildizoglu, U.; Buber, I.; Diaz, B.A.; Kruijff, E.; Tscheligi, M. Basic senior personas. In Proceedings of the 14th International ACM SIGACCESS Conference on Computers and Accessibility—ASSETS' 12, Boulder, CO, USA, 22–24 October 2012; Association for Computing Machinery (ACM): New York, NY, USA, 2012; p. 25.
56. Taşoz, Ş.M.; Afacan, Y. Simulated physical ageing: A prioritized persona-based model for accessible interiors in senior housing environments. *Indoor Built Environ.* **2020**. [CrossRef]
57. Jais, C.; Hignett, S.; Estupinan, Z.; Hogervorst, E. Evidence based dementia personas: Human factors design for people living with dementia. In *Ergonomics for People with Disabilities*; Polak-Sopinska, A., Krolikowski, J., Eds.; Sciendo. De Gruyter Open Ltd.: Warsaw, Poland, 2018; pp. 215–226. [CrossRef]
58. McCracken, I.; de la Harpeand, R.; Ruvo, M.D. Developing dementia personas for user centered architectural design considerations in non-specialized contexts. In Proceedings of the Dementia Lab Conference, Eindhoven, The Netherlands, 21–22 October 2019; Springer International Publishing: Cham, Switzerland, 2019; pp. 48–61. [CrossRef]
59. Goldstein, R.; Tessier, A.; Khan, A. Customizing the behavior of interacting occupants using personas. In Proceedings of the SimBuild 2010: Fourth National Conference of IBPSA-USA, New York, NY, USA, 11–13 August 2010.
60. Haines, V.; Mitchell, V. A persona-based approach to domestic energy retrofit. *Build. Res. Inf.* **2014**, *42*, 462–476. [CrossRef]
61. Ortiz, M.; Bluyssen, P.M. Developing home occupant archetypes: First results of mixed-methods study to understand occupant comfort behaviours and energy use in homes. *Build. Environ.* **2019**, *163*, 106331. [CrossRef]
62. McDougall, K.; Barrie, H. *South Australian Retirement Village Survey 2016*; Prepared for S.A. Health, Office for the Ageing: Adelaide, Australia, 2017.
63. Hansen, A.; Bi, P.; Ryan, P.; Nitschke, M.; Pisaniello, D.; Tucker, G. The effect of heat waves on hospital admissions for renal disease in a temperate city of Australia. *Int. J. Epidemiol.* **2008**, *37*, 1359–1365. [CrossRef]
64. Stewart, S.; Keates, A.K.; Redfern, A.; McMurray, J.J.V. Seasonal variations in cardiovascular disease. *Nat. Rev. Cardiol.* **2017**, *14*, 654–664. [CrossRef]
65. Timmermans, E.J.; van der Pas, S.; Dennison, E.M.; Maggi, S.; Peter, R.; Castell, M.V.; Pedersen, N.L.; Denkinger, M.D.; Edwards, M.H.; Limongi, F.; et al. The Influence of Weather Conditions on Outdoor Physical Activity among Older People With and Without Osteoarthritis in 6 European Countries. *J. Phys. Act. Health* **2016**, *13*, 1385–1395. [CrossRef]
66. Zhang, Y.; Nitschke, M.; Bi, P. Risk factors for direct heat-related hospitalization during the 2009 Adelaide heatwave: A case crossover study. *Sci. Total. Environ.* **2013**, *442*, 1–5. [CrossRef]
67. AIHW. *Older Australia at a Glance*; Australian Institute of Health and Welfare: Canberra, Australia, 2017. Available online: https://www.aihw.gov.au/reports/older-people/older-australia-at-a-glance/report-editions (accessed on 8 July 2020).
68. Vandentorren, S.; Bretin, P.; Zeghnoun, A.; Mandereau-Bruno, L.; Croisier, A.; Cochet, C.; Ribéron, J.; Siberan, I.; Declercq, B.; Ledrans, M. Heat-related mortality—August 2003 Heat Wave in France: Risk Factors for Death of Elderly People Living at Home. *Eur. J. Public Health* **2006**, *16*, 583–591. [CrossRef] [PubMed]
69. Vaidyanathan, A.; Malilay, J.; Schramm, P.; Saha, S. Heat-Related Deaths—United States, 2004–2018. *MMWR. Morb. Mortal. Wkly. Rep.* **2020**, *69*, 729–734. [CrossRef] [PubMed]
70. World Health Organization. *Health Impact of Low Indoor Temperatures: Report from a WHO Meeting, Copenhagen, 11–14 November 1985*; World Health Organization, Regional Office for Europe: Copenhagen, Denmark, 1987.
71. World Health Organization. *Housing and Health Guidelines*; World Health Organization: Geneva, Switzerland, 2018; Licence: CC BY-NC-SA 3.0 IGO.
72. Tsuzuki, K.; Ohfuku, T. Thermal sensation and thermoregulation in elderly compared to young people in Japanese winter season. In Proceedings of the 9th International Conference on Indoor Air Quality and Climate, Monterey, CA, USA, 30 June–5 July 2002; pp. 659–664.
73. Soebarto, V.; Zhang, H.; Schiavon, S. A thermal comfort environmental chamber study of older and younger people. *Build. Environ.* **2019**, *155*, 1–14. [CrossRef]
74. Wang, Z.; Yu, H.; Jiao, Y.; Wei, Q.; Chu, X. A field study of thermal sensation and neutrality in free-running aged-care homes in Shanghai. *Energy Build.* **2018**, *158*, 1523–1532. [CrossRef]

75. Beck, H.E.; Zimmermann, N.E.; McVicar, T.R.; Vergopolan, N.; Berg, A.; Wood, E.F. Present and future Köppen-Geiger climate classification maps at 1-km resolution. *Sci. Data* **2018**, *5*, 180214. [CrossRef]
76. Sousa, V.D.; Rojjanasrirat, W. Translation, adaptation and validation of instruments or scales for use in cross-cultural health care research: A clear and user-friendly guideline. *J. Eval. Clin. Pract.* **2010**, *17*, 268–274. [CrossRef]
77. Buffel, T.; Phillipson, C.; Rémillard-Boilard, S. Age-friendly cities and communities: New directions for research and policy. In *Encyclopedia of Gerontology and Population Aging*; Gu, D., Dupre, M.E., Eds.; Springer Nature: Cham, Switzerland, 2019. [CrossRef]
78. Dikken, J.; van den Hoven, R.F.M.; van Staalduinen, W.H.; Hulsebosch-Janssen, L.M.T.; van Hoof, J. How Older People Experience the Age-Friendliness of Their City: Development of the Age-Friendly Cities and Communities Questionnaire. *Int. J. Environ. Res. Public Health* **2020**, *17*, 6867. [CrossRef]
79. van de Vliert, E. Climates Create Cultures. *Soc. Pers. Psychol. Compass* **2007**, *1*, 53–67. [CrossRef]

International Journal of
Environmental Research and Public Health

MDPI

Article

Innovation Pathways for Age-Friendly Homes in Europe

Frans Sengers [1,*] and Alexander Peine [2]

[1] Athena Institute, Vrije Universiteit Amsterdam, de Boelelaan 1085, 1081 HV Amsterdam, The Netherlands
[2] Copernicus Institute of Sustainable Development, Utrecht University, Princetonlaan 8a, 3584 CB Utrecht, The Netherlands; a.peine@uu.nl
* Correspondence: f.sengers@vu.nl

Abstract: A variety of innovative pilot projects are being implemented to improve the life-course resilience of existing and newly built home environments. We refer to these projects as "socio-technical experiments" that embody different kinds of promising futures and provide direction to current developments in the emerging domain of age-friendly homes. To take stock of this diversity within Europe; this paper provides an overview of 53 ongoing socio-technical experiments that are being conducted in the Netherlands, France, Ireland and Poland. We find that, besides the variation between European countries, there is a more important type variation in terms of the character of the experiments themselves and the differences in development direction that they propose. Our findings suggest that most of the innovations tested in these experiments are not primarily material or technical but primarily social or conceptual in character (i.e., new organizational modes or everyday practices that re-arrange social relations or new housing concepts that bridge the divide between ageing in place individually and a nursing home). This variety of innovations tested in the experiments can be categorized into seven distinct innovation pathways: (1) Showcasing Technology, (2) Innovation Ecosystem, (3) Sheltered Elite, (4) Specific Community, (5) Conscious Retrofitting, (6) Home Sharing and (7) Retrovation Challenge.

Keywords: age-friendly homes; innovation; experiments

Citation: Sengers, F.; Peine, A. Innovation Pathways for Age-Friendly Homes in Europe. *Int. J. Environ. Res. Public Health* **2021**, *18*, 1139. https://doi.org/10.3390/ijerph18031139

Academic Editors: Pauline Van den Berg and Joost van Hoof

Received: 8 December 2020
Accepted: 22 January 2021
Published: 28 January 2021

1. Introduction: Experimenting with Age-Friendly Homes

The ever-increasing life expectancy of Europe's urban population is generally considered to be "a great achievement of modern society" [1], p. 2472, and "the culmination of successful human development" [2], p. 733. But the advent of an ageing society also comes with great challenges for the future. One key challenge is that most present-day home environments are not adapted to permit to older adults to age in place. Large parts of the existing building stock are currently not fit for purpose to enable Europeans to lead healthy, active and meaningful lives at home [3]. At the same time, the home is also a site where digital technologies and other novelties are being introduced at an increasing pace and where a wide gamut of innovations meet the muddled realities of the everyday lives of older adults [4]. Therefore, it is crucial to ensure that our homes are suitable and adaptable to our needs and preferences as we age and that they are conducive to integration of promising innovations. In our view, this should be a key part of the response to the demographics of ageing in European cities.

Whilst most of the articles in this special issue deal with the age-friendly *city*, this contribution provides center stage to the smaller scale of the *home*. The first thing that should be noted is that a home is more than a house, apartment or any other physical shell that harbors a domestic living environment. Philosophers, geographers and architects have a long tradition of engaging with the broad concept of home [5–8]. The notion of home is open to interpretation, sometimes used in a metaphorical way. It is closely related to concepts such as house and dwelling, but it carries with it a set of social and emotional attachments. Home is a "material and an affective space, shaped by everyday practices, lived experiences, social relations, memories and emotions" [8], p. 506, and it is inextricably linked to ideas about "identity, family, nation, a sense of place, and to a sense of responsibility towards who shares this place" [9] and it is a place that offers "security, familiarity and nurture" [6], p. 164. In practical terms for our analysis of innovative activities in the home, this means two things. First, it allows us to focus on social and emotional aspects of a home. These aspects, along with physical elements, together are essential components of what it means to live independently and maintain a good quality life at home [10]. Second, it allows us to look beyond the physical walls of the apartment or house by also including the immediate indoor and outdoor surroundings. Whilst these are not inside the house, they can be included in the wider notion of home. This allows for a focus on a broader set of innovations, not only physical novelties but also social and conceptual novelties—i.e., innovations that do not feature new technology but that feature new ways of organizing social processes or new conceptual housing categories that fill the void between conventional single household apartments and traditional retirement/nursing homes.

Our main concern is thus with the home as a site of *innovation*. Various kinds of organizationally and geographically distinct spaces can be seen as important sites for the concentration and development of particular innovations. These innovative spaces have led to the emergence of new infrastructures, products, activities, services, and industries as well as new sets of user patterns and identities. These spaces include cities, ports, factories, hospitals, offices, but also households or homes. From our perspective as Science and Technology Studies scholars interested in innovation, the home is best described as an "innovation junction". An innovation junction can be defined as "a space in which different sets of heterogeneous technologies are mobilized in support of social and economic activities and in which, as a result of their co-location, interactions and exchanges among these technologies occur" [11], p. 51. In this context "heterogeneous technologies" refers to a broader conceptualization of technology beyond technical elements and material artefacts; instead, it points to the entire network of technical and social relations [12]. These innovations include not only material novelties (technological innovations) but also novelties in stakeholder roles and social relations (social innovations) and conceptually new ways of doing and organizing (conceptual innovations). An important element of an innovation junction is the co-location of innovation, which encourages certain groups of stakeholders to develop mechanisms and arrangements to coordinate the interaction of these innovations, sometimes through the development of so-called mediating technologies that facilitate and stimulate the interaction between various artefacts and innovative practices. For our purposes, we want to stress that many different kinds of stakeholders are introducing innovations into the homes of older adults. The interactions between the innovations and the coordination attempts between diverse stakeholders are crucial to understand how the material composition, social organization and associated identities of what is considered an "age-friendly home", are taking shape.

This paper starts from the observation that an increasing number of innovative designs and visionary ideas to improve the life course resilience of existing and newly built home environments are currently being tested in concrete initiatives throughout Europe. We take these initiatives as our starting point and reveal that they represent something more profound. Our aim is to provide an empirical overview and synthesis of these initiatives. As Science and Technology Studies scholars interested in innovation, we have distinct take on these matters, and we hope that the perspective sketched out in this paper provides a meaningful contribution to this special issue. We begin by introducing some key concepts (Section 2). We conceptualize these newly emerging age-friendly homes initiatives as "socio-technical experiments", and we argue that these experiments are a promising starting point that can lead to wider outcomes in achieving a transition towards age-friendly homes. Next, we present the methodological approach taken to identify and analyze a large set of these experiments (Section 3). We then present the main empirical findings with regard to experimenting for age-friendly housing in different European countries as well as a synthesis (Section 4). A general overview is provided and the specific situation of experimental activity on the ground in four European countries (Poland, France, Ireland and the Netherlands) is sketched out. We also identify a number of general patterns that emerge when we consider this comprehensive set of experiments. Finally, in an effort to synthesize, we articulate a set of "innovation pathways" in order to come to terms with possible futures or potential ways forward. Finally, a reflection is provided on the collection of experiment and the identified innovation pathways, followed by a discussion on the wider support and upscaling dynamics of experiments (Section 5). The paper ends with a brief conclusion (Section 6).

2. Theory: Socio-Technical Experiments and Innovation Pathways

We believe that the notion of a "socio-technical experiment" is a promising concept for discussing the relevance of the recent groundswell of age-friendly housing pilot projects. This concept did not originate from the fields of ageing studies or gerontology but from the field of Sustainability Transitions [13]. The Sustainability Transitions literature argues that contemporary environmental problems, such as climate change, present formidable societal challenges. Addressing these problems requires deep structural changes in the systems that provide transport, energy, healthcare, housing and other societal functions [14]. These are called "socio-technical systems" because they entail an array of social and technological elements, including technological artefacts, infrastructures, policies, markets, consumer practices, cultural meanings and scientific knowledge [15]. Changing the structure of an incumbent socio-technical system (called a "socio-technical regime") requires reconfiguration of the alignment between these elements, and this process starts by experimenting with alternative configurations in a conducive environment that affords a degree of protection from mainstream market selection (called a "socio-technical niche") [16].

It is important to note that a socio-technical experiment is not the same as a scientific experiment carried out by psychologists or physicists. The laboratory—either as a distinct physical space or as a more general metaphor—sets scientific experiments apart from socio-technical experiments. Scientific experiments are practices that take place in the confines of a laboratory or an otherwise strictly controlled environment in order to find hard objective truths about human nature or material reality. Socio-technical experimentation, on the other hand, implies a more engaged and social constructivist position: society is itself a laboratory and a variety of real-world actors commit to the messy experimental processes tied up with the introduction of alternative technologies and practices in order to purposively re-shape social and material realities [17–19].

Socio-technical experiments are thus seen as early expressions of promising new ideas that harbor the seeds of novelty that can contribute to wider socio-technical systems change. Frontrunners or actors who are considered outsiders for incumbent socio-technical systems are often the initiators of these experiments eventually drawing in a broad coalition of actors—from governments and large companies to civil society and grassroots networks of activists. The goal is not simply to establish experimental initiatives as such but to learn about this form of action in the broad sense and find out if the experimental solutions are desirable and effective [16,20]. As the experiment reshapes its institutional environment, fertile ground is created for further chains of experiments and a constituency is built around the alternative socio-technical configuration to form the basis for a new socio-technical system [21]. Formulated in a different way, a socio-technical experiment gives substance to a distinct vision for the future and acts out this future in a small-scale real-life setting. A pilot project with cutting edge smart camera systems and fall detectors in an existing retirement home represents a different possible future as compared to a future represented by a project that demonstrates the feasibility a new form of intergenerational co-housing and formulates this as a challenge to the legitimacy of a traditional retirement home. Since these two very different socio-technical experiments embody distinct future trajectories, they can be said to represent diverging "innovation pathways" for the development of the age-friendly housing niche.

More analytically precise, a socio-technical experiment has been defined by Sengers et al. (2019) as an "inclusive, challenge-led and practice-based initiative designed to promote system innovation through social learning under conditions of uncertainty and ambiguity" [19], p. 161. Let us pick each of the elements of this definition apart. To qualify, an initiative should be *inclusive* in the sense that it is a collective endeavor carried out by a coalition of diverse actors. The *challenge-led* character implies that the initiative is framed as a response to a societal challenge (in our case often related to the pressing need to update the housing with fitting options for older adults). The initiative should be *practice-based* and thus feature a "hands-on" attempt at innovation applied in a real-world setting instead of a laboratory (though sometimes the distinction is not so clear, as in the multitude of "living laboratories" that are now appearing throughout Europe, such as ENoLL, the European Network of Living Labs). The initiative is not simply innovative but should be seen in the context of wider *system innovation,* thus recognizing the material, institutional and cognitive obduracy of the status quo and geared to change key elements of the current way socio-technical systems are configured (in our case systems of housing, care and ICT and their interaction in shaping age-friendly homes). The idea of an initiative promoting *social learning* refers to the way in which stakeholders learn in practice through observation and imitation (important if the experiment is to be followed up) and that they learn in a broad sense; an experiment should allow stakeholders to learn not only about the performance of the innovation itself but also to learn about the wider societal implications of the innovation [21]. The *conditions of uncertainty and ambiguity* in the definition refer to a final feature of these initiatives, namely, that it is unclear to what extent the initiative will attract a wider following in the future (uncertainty), and it is an open question what the desirable and undesirable long-term effects of the intervention will be (ambiguity).

Other scholars have argued for the importance of additional features to characterize a socio-technical experiment. For instance, Vergragt and Brown (2007) talk about "bounded socio-technical experiments" to stress that these initiatives are "bounded" in space and time—i.e., confined within a certain area or community and with a limited duration [22]. The experiments discussed in this paper are bounded by space (the home in the broad sense and experimental site; often territorial boundaries are clear, but sometimes they are more ambiguous), community (older adults or specific sub-groups—e.g., older adults with dementia—are the target audience) and time (sometimes the time during which a new device is being implemented that turns and an existing home into an experimental homes; sometimes the funding duration of a project stipulates the duration, and sometimes there is no clear end for an experiment).

It is important to note that a socio-technical experiment gives substance to a highly distinct vision for the future. Different experiments can be seen as steppingstones toward different futures, which are supported by different values, technologies and institutional arrangements. In other words, experiments can be seen as integral parts of different (competing or complementary) "innovation pathways". Innovation pathways are journeys that involve key drivers, decision-making junctures, agents and opportunities which combine to facilitate the eventual mainstreaming of a particular socio-technical configuration [23]. Identifying a large number of prominent experiments and articulating a set of corresponding innovation pathways for age-friendly homes might help researchers and practitioner in the domain of age-friendly homes to see the bigger picture and develop a more comprehensive understanding of the innovative activities that they encounter or contribute to.

3. Methodological Approach

Our investigation is based on an explorative analysis of socio-technical experiments throughout Europe. Because we set out to collect data about a large number of experiments (our main unit of analysis) within various countries, our research design can be best described as an embedded multiple-case study [24]. Inspired by qualitative methodological approaches for geographers [25], we employ process theory as an explanatory narrative style [26,27]. The approach used for our investigation can be broken down into three separate steps: (1) Scoping, (2) Inquiry and (3) Synthesis.

Our first step of Scoping started with the creation of a database that provides an overview of relevant socio-technical experiments in Europe in the domain of age-friendly homes. To do so we have collected information about projects that pilot test various kinds of innovations related to age-friendly housing. Because we are dealing with socio-technical experiments, we have included not only initiatives that feature technological innovations but also initiatives that feature other kinds of social and conceptual innovations. The experiments that we considered related to age-friendly homes in different ways and brought together elements from multiple logics, rules and institutions ("socio-technical regimes") that structure the systems of physical housing, healthcare and ICT solutions. Various sources were used to collect experiments. For a start, existing repositories that feature good practices throughout Europe were consulted. When looking for information about the experiments within these digital repositories, more weblinks could be found to other potentially interesting experiments, which were then further explored online through online desk research. Table 1 provides an overview of the repositories initially consulted.

Table 1. Overview of repositories of good and innovative practices related to age-friendly homes (1 August 2020).

WHO Global Database of Age-friendly Practices	55 practices worldwide in the category housing, many of which in Europe [28]
EIP AHA repository	26 practices when searched for the term "home" [29]
EIP AHA refence sites	74 European regions as reference sites, which is more about regional innovation ecosystems rather than concrete experiments [30]
AFE-Innovnet repository	55 initiatives within EU countries, with 12 focusing on housing [31]
European Covenant on Demographic Change repository	showcases a number of initiatives within EU countries, including on housing [32]
PROGRESSIVE project examples of good practices	4 interesting age-friendly housing/environment initiatives across Europe [33]
Ireland's Age Friendly Cities and Counties catalogue of age-friendly practices	31 projects and organizations in the domain of "housing" in Ireland, as well as other projects and organizations in the domains of "community support and health services" and "communication and information" [34]
Government of Ireland report on Housing Options for Our Ageing Population	12 comprehensive good practices on housing in Ireland [35]
Aedes-Actiz overview of Dutch smart homes for the future	23 smart homes with a care component within the Netherlands [36]

In addition, we contacted several experts from different European countries with a variety of backgrounds (e.g., university, construction, architecture, policy, civil society) who were in a good position to provide additional suggestions for interesting experiments (e.g., university professors specialized in urban ageing, NGOs promoting age-friendly environments, policy network organizations lobbying for the interests of older adults, etc.) When approaching these experts, a clear idea was formulated in terms of the requirements for an experiment to be added to our database. It was communicated to interviewees that we are looking for pilot projects or novel practices, which feature concrete interventions in a specified living environment/home and embody an approach that is considered promising for the future and to an extent innovative (i.e., the projects should contain an element of novelty in terms of either technological/material novelty, such as the introduction of new building materials or supportive ICT devices, or a conceptual/social novelty, such as new busines model for living together or for integrating care into the home environment).

The second step of Inquiry was geared to investigate the experiments and their context in more detail. This required more in-depth information about the realities on the ground in different European countries. Because Europe is diverse, it would be impossible within the scope of this research to obtain a contextualized overview of experiments in each European country. Therefore, the choice was made not to consider the entirety of Europe but instead to zoom in on the following four countries: The Netherlands, France, Ireland and Poland. These four countries were selected for further inquiry in order to take Europe's diversity into account as much as possible and as a way to compare the situation in different parts of Europe where traditions in their approach to ageing, family structures, care provision as well as the role of the state vary. More specifically, according to Anttonen and Sipilä (1996) each of these four countries represents a distinct "model of social care provision in case of old age" [37]. The Netherlands can be categorized as a part of a "central European subsidiary model" of social care provision in case of old age. In this model the primary responsibility for the care of older adults lies in principle with the family, but the state also plays an important role as steward [37,38]. France can be categorized in terms of a "southern European care model", which puts even more emphasis on family care [37]. Ireland has been categorized a more "Anglo-Saxon" oriented model of care, which features a smaller role for the state and puts more of an emphasis on means-tested service entitlements [37]. Poland does not feature in the categories devised by Anttonen and Sipilä, and neither does any other Central European country. Whilst far less research has been conducted on this region, we believe it is important to include a country such as Poland in our investigation because it emerged from behind the iron curtain with a different set of institutions related to ageing, care and housing as compared to countries in western and southern parts of Europe.

In each of these four countries, one-week field trip was organized and several socio-technical experiments per country were selected for further inquiry through purposive sampling. The choice for these particular experiments was made because they represent different directions for the future of age-friendly homes and because they were considered pioneering and relevant by interviewed "overview experts" (experts who were in key positions in these countries to provide an overview of important innovative projects; this group includes university professors specialized in urban ageing, NGOs promoting age-friendly environments, policy network organizations lobbying for the interests of older adults, etc.) "Pilot stakeholders" (stakeholders who instigated or were centrally involved in the implementation of the selected socio-technical experiments; this group includes architects, policymakers, founders of NGOs and older adults themselves who are living the experimental realities created by the socio-technical experiments) were also visited and interviewed during the field trips. The questions in the interviews with the pilot stakeholders related to the set-up of the experiment itself (the origin story, milestones, vision behind it, stakeholders involved, what was learned, links to other experiments), the upscaling potential (the kinds of mechanisms that might enable the wider impact of the experiment) and the context and support structures (supportive regulation and other conducive structural elements in a country or region, relations between regimes of housing, care and ICT). A total of 34 in-depth interviews (lasting between 1 and 2.5 h) were conducted with overview experts and plot stakeholders during the field trips. Additionally, seven guided site tours were conducted, which included a guided walk through a pilot apartment building or housing scheme by one of the stakeholders involved in the experiments there.

The third step of Synthesis consisted of a deliberate reflective analysis on the database and country findings in order to compare countries and experiments and to distil patterns and innovation pathways. Patterns here refer to recurring ideas about certain innovations and widely shared reflections that can be found in the stakeholders' testimonies, and innovation pathways refer to distinct innovation categories into which most of the experiments in each of the four countries can be said to fit. Each category embodies a different promising direction for future development of age-friendly homes in Europe. It is important to note that it is beyond the scope of this paper to provide an account of how the innovation journeys for each of the individual experiments in the database unfolded. But given our efforts, it is within our scope to reflect upon the kinds of future directions that is being constructed as numerous experiments are being carried out. Therefore, our aim in this final step was to provide a synthesis of directions for future development towards which these innovative activities within experiments seem to point and to categorize the innovation activities into a set of distinct innovation pathways. We should note up front that this will not generate the definitive account of innovation pathways for age-friendly housing but rather a first explorative attempt based on the extensive but incomplete information and based on our personal scholarly interpretation.

4. Findings: General Overview, National Comparisons, Recurring Patterns and Innovation Pathways

The initial stocktaking exercise resulted in the creation of a preliminary database that contains a large but non-exhaustive collection of relevant experiments related to age-friendly homes Europe. This database was complemented with additional entries during the interviews conducted in the Netherlands, France, Ireland, Poland as the four countries that we analyzed in more detail. To illustrate this, Table 2 below presents several (2 per country) of the 53 innovative socio-technical experiments with age-friendly homes in the four countries. For a full overview of each of the 53 experiments, see Table A1 in Appendix A. The '#' symbol in front of each of the experiment names in Tables 2 and A1 provides a shorthand identification number. This # number is used in the findings to quickly refer to a specific experiment (e.g. experiment #1 refers to Knarrenhof (Aahof) experiment).

Table 2. Overview of 8 key age-friendly home experiments in the Netherlands, France, Ireland and Poland (see Table A1 in Appendix A for the complete overview of 53 experiments).

	Experiment Name	Location	Description
# 1	Knarrenhof (Aahof)	Zwolle 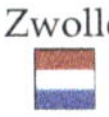	Knarrenhof is an innovative form of housing that actively involves new resident in home making and community support. It is directed at "young older adults" and "old older adults" who want to help each other out and to live independently as long as possible. The attitude and affinity with the neighbors are considered very important, and notions of good neighborship are central. Often those who want to reside here are socially engaged and active (doing voluntary work rather than the stereotype of "bridge clubs and passively sitting at home") and presented as "social people who can in principle be called upon" by their neighbors. The name "Knarrenhof" consists of two parts. The first part, "knarren" takes it from characters of a popular Dutch TV show from the 1980s (van Kooten en de Bie's krasse knarren) who are presented as "hardy old geezers" as a way to stress the agency and vitality of older adults (the logo presents an old man showing off his muscles). The second part "hof" can be translated as "courtyard" and refers to the type of picturesque, secluded set of houses facing each other as part urban planning layout conducive for community building. Because this urban form of the courtyard stems from the Middle Ages in Dutch cities and because notions of good neighborship stem from an earlier age, the ideas are presented as "sprung from the past (but) also a project for the future".

Table 2. *Cont.*

	Experiment Name	Location	Description
# 2	Hogeweyk	Weesp	The Hogeweyk a pioneering care facility/community for older adults with dementia. Compared to traditional nursing homes the residents with dementia are more active and live a more "normal" life. Professionally and inhouse trained staff wear regular clothes instead of a uniform and provide the 169 residents the necessary 24-h support in care, living and wellbeing. The "residents, NOT patients" live in one of several housing types that fit their lifestyle (traditional, urban, cosmopolitan and formal—it used to include Indonesian, but this will stop soon because the cohort of older adults from the former colony is getting smaller). The houses of each type are equipped with a shared living room and bedrooms for several (6–7) residents and they are located in a gated neighborhood setting complete with general store, restaurant and theatre (hence the idea of a dementia "village"). The walls are permeable to an extent and people from society outside are encouraged to come in as a way to eventually create a kind of "reverse emancipation" so that society at large becomes more dementia friendly (bringing the outside world in vs bringing the inside world out; social inclusion is a major objective). The underlying vision is to get away from the large-scale medicalized institutionalized model of care home to small-scale normalized social relational model of care.
# 21	27Delvalle	Nice	A center on connected health and healthy ageing, which includes a model apartment that is designed as a showcase and a testing platform for technologies supporting independent living and autonomy. The Habitat platform of 27Delvalle is a space dedicated to health and autonomy and facilitates cooperation between a variety of regional stakeholders (Overarching network includes FRANCE SILVER ÉCO, Nice Côte d'Azur Metropolis incubator, CIU Santé, PAILLON2020 and more). It relies in particular on the ecosystem of services dedicated to the loss of autonomy. It prepares the return and promotes the home support of vulnerable people and/or people with disabilities around their personal life project. The "demonstration, simulation and experimentation apartment" is equipped with various digital technologies and innovative devices and is set up to provide advice and solutions to users, their families, caregivers and health professionals. In addition, researchers and industry meet to develop innovative technologies. The objectives are to (1) inform, raise awareness and test; (2) facilitate home return and home support; (3) train medical professionals in new technologies; (4) innovate with research by connecting users, professionals, researchers and industry to be a market access facilitator for businesses.
# 22	La Maison des Babayagas	Paris	La Maison Des Babayagas is a feminist cohabitation project that started in Montreuil, in the surroundings of Paris in 2013 (Babayagas is a Slavic term for witch). A group of dynamic women have devised a new kind of communal living for older women based on shared values of feminism and activism. La Maison Des Babayagas is a self-managed social housing project composed of 21 apartments for women over 60 and 4 apartments for young adults below 30; the dwellings are still owned by a social housing landlord. Based on four pillars (self-management, solidarity, citizenship and ecology), this "anti-retirement home" aims to facilitate contacts and mutual care between the community members. One of the main motivations for creating the Babayagas house was battling social isolation and many community projects and social activities are organized both by the inhabitants and with the surrounding community, the two rooms on the ground floor of the building being two municipal rooms.

Table 2. *Cont.*

	Experiment Name	Location	Description
# 23	Great Northern Haven	Dundalk	The Great Northern Haven is a new housing project operational for several years now. It features 16 apartments (including one showroom and testing apartment) built to support "life-time adaptability" and Active Assisted Living for older adults. Each apartment is equipped with sensors and interactive technology to support telecare. To an extent, the experiment has been used as a way to convince developers to adopt universal design by making them "walk in the shoes of a frailer older person". All interviewees in Ireland are familiar with this pioneering high-profile experiment, but according to some of them, the features seem overly hospital-like and heavily reliant on technology. Some of the wiring is now obsolete since smart Wi-Fi solutions were not as prevalent when it was initially designed.
# 24	the Abhaile Project (AVA pilot house)	Dublin	AVA housing offers a solution in the domain of "home sharing", which offers an alternative to older homeowners whereby their homes are adapted to their future needs whist also creating a rental capacity within their home. This provides financial benefits and a sense of security and community for homeowners. The innovative part is the total package of guidance, support and expertise to the homeowner through the process of retrofitting and sharing arrangements. This particular pilot project put these home sharing into practice in a three-bedroom semi-detached house. The severe housing crisis in Ireland is part of the reason why these kinds of home sharing innovations are gaining momentum.
# 52	Mimo Wieku apartment	Warsaw	The U Siebie Mimo Wieku ("at home despite the age") showroom apartment presents a comprehensive set of solutions how to enable older adults to have an active and independent life in their own home. It is the first apartment of this kind in Poland and designed according to best practices regarding accessibility, health, wellbeing and equipped with modern devices to assist older adults and person with disabilities. On about 50 square meters, a well-designed space has been created for a single person or a couple. It is free of physical barriers and ready for upgrades with regard to equipment and amenities. The well thought spatial and physical arrangement, designed by specialized architects, includes solutions with regard to the main aspects of comfort, ergonomics, daylight, illumination and views, indoor air quality, temperature, humidity and air movement and acoustics. The entire array of specially designed building features and smart products make this "larger than the sum of its parts". Another goal aimed at is to get companies in Poland to see older adults as a relevant market for products and services.
# 53	Stalowa-29	Warsaw	The Stalowa-29 intergenerational apartment building is one of the first cohousing solutions in Poland to be inhabited by people from various age groups. It is a retrofit of an older building (renovation is ongoing at this time) and the idea is that it serves as a model for modern, sustainable and well-designed housing modernization under the Integrated Revitalization Program in the Praga district (it is mostly paid for by city of Warsaw). It is also geared to counter negative effects of gentrification and to encourage residents to help one another. On the last two floors, there will be a care and educational institution for youths. On each of the other floors, 4 apartments are planned (12 in total). On the ground floor a space for the local community will be created in the form of a café or other meeting place (how exactly is yet to be determined). Intergenerational design, countering negative effects of gentrification and encouraging residents to help one another are key elements. According to some interviewees, these kinds of projects are difficult to implement in practice because they feature social housing, and legal requirements stipulate that the next person on the waiting list would qualify for the apartment. Selecting people deliberately based on age and skipping others in line might be hard to justify.

The findings per country in Table 2 allow us to compare a set of experiments for one of the four countries with the other three countries. Combined with additional data collected within these countries, this allows to say something broader about the experimental profile of each country in comparative perspective.

Compared to the other countries studied, the Netherlands features a high percentage of social housing, and the overall quality of the housing stock is high. Certain building design requirements that were considered innovative in some of the other countries are standard practice. In the Netherlands, there are many highly innovative experiments at an operational stage. Some of these are not only new to the country but new to the world. Consequently, a few of these experiments have been widely publicized in international media (for instance, experiment #2 Hogeweyk dementia village and experiment #4 Humanitas intergenerational project) and others are considered curious and interesting by non-Dutch interviewees (for instance experiment #1 Knarrenhof). Some interviewees (both Dutch and foreign) consider the Netherlands a frontrunner in terms of age-friendly housing innovation.

France also shows a wide array of age-friendly home experiments. The broadness of this pallet of activities is exemplified by radically different focus of the two experiments of 27Delvalle (experiment #21) and Maison Babayagas (experiment #22)—the first one is technologically innovative, medicalized and entrepreneurial and the second one conceptually innovative, intentional and community oriented without a focus on new technology or economic development. Many projects could be found in France in the same vein as the 27Delvalle project, building on the synergy between the development of new technologies and associated promises of economic activity. The idea of fostering technological innovation as a starting point for more age-friendly homes and the build-up of an "innovation eco-system" with tech start-ups, larger companies, medical professionals and governments agencies that want to boost this form of economic activity might be a promising approach when it becomes a shared agenda by a relatively powerful groups of stakeholders. In Southern France, there is a longer history of setting up experimental home-like environment setting for medical professionals to conduct experiments that feature advanced technology. There is also a wider palette of projects and initiatives to build up innovation ecosystems as a way to boost local high-value economic activity.

Ireland offers a particularly interesting support context since age-friendly housing and the wider agenda of moving towards an age-friendly society have clearly gained momentum there. This is evident in the large amount of national and local support programmes in line with WHO guidelines, and the attention for Universal Design criteria in many planned projects. Age-friendly housing has been successfully positioned on the political agenda and innovative experiments have emerged as a consequence of this, but the experiments have also contributed to bringing actors together to articulate and empower this agenda in the first place. One thing that plays in the background is the ongoing housing crisis, which has resulted in ideas about freeing up larger family homes and relocating older adults to smaller suitable apartments that have to be built first. Besides many small-scale projects designed with Universal Design criteria, there are also several very innovative experiments such as experiment #23 the Great Northern Haven (technologically innovative) and experiments #24 and #25 on new ways of facilitating home-sharing (conceptually innovative). Overall, in Ireland there is a wide array of different innovative experiments and a willing coalition of housing and government agencies that offer support.

The interviewees in Poland argued that their country is not a frontrunner in terms of age-friendly housing provision and innovation compared to some other European countries. Many of the innovative activities mentioned by the interviewees were considered new to Poland but not new to the world at large. In many cases the interviewees referred to activities in Germany that inspired them or at the difficulties to convince Polish companies that older adults present a growing and viable market for them. Nevertheless, our investigation indicates that in Poland a range of innovative activities are currently gaining momentum, including new intergenerational housing projects and a general push for more apartments dedicated to seniors. Furthermore, the unique experiment #52 Mimo Wieku demonstrator apartment (a seemingly isolated initiative within the Polish age-friendly housing landscape) might be ranked amongst the best designed, high-quality and technologically advanced apartments that were observed during all fieldwork site visits.

If we look at the findings per country, we find differences in innovative practices and in levels of policy support. But the palette of innovative activities for each of the countries is broad and we cannot clearly distinguish France, Poland, Ireland and the Netherlands in terms of ideological pre-occupations. In other words, we do not find clearly distinguishable national-level projections or "socio-technical imaginaries" [39] that specify the nature of innovation agendas and set each country apart in terms of how older adults are portrayed as subjects and in terms of distinct national-level visions for what the future of age-friendly homes should look like. Looking more closely at the "where" of the entire set of 53 experiments—so, not just at the level of the country but at the location of the experiments within each country—we find a dispersed rather than a clustered pattern. This is important because many studies about the geography of innovation and experimentation point to a particular clustering of innovation sites; often around science parks or vibrant larger cities that are home to the "creative class" [40–42]. In contrast, if the locations of our 53 experiments would be pinpointed on map for each of the four countries, then a more dispersed pattern would be observed. So, in identifying additional innovative age-friendly home experiments, we should focus our attention not only on booming cities but also on more peripheral towns and villages.

Now let us put national boundaries and locations of experiments aside and consider the focus and directions of the 53 experiments. If the focus of this collection of experiments is in any way representative for the entire array of promising new directions for the future development of age-friendly homes in Europe, then it would seem that most of the associated innovations are not primarily material or technical, but rather social or conceptual in character. These forms of social and conceptual innovation include new organizational modes or everyday practices that re-arrange social relations or new housing concepts that bridge the divide between ageing in place individually and a nursing home. Compared to some of the highly touted technical experiments with smart devices and automated control systems, many of the more radical conceptual innovations with new modes of living together were only identified at a somewhat later stage of the research. The lack of support by powerful business and government coalitions might be a reason why some these conceptual innovations remain under the radar.

For a deeper analysis of innovation activities in experiments, it is crucial to assess the micro processes—or "innovation journeys"—and broader directions—or "innovation pathways" [43]. It is beyond the scope of this paper to provide an account of how the innovation journeys for each of the experiments in the database unfolded (for such an attempt see [44]). But given our efforts, it is within our scope to reflect upon the kinds of future directions that is being constructed as numerous experiments are being carried out. Our aim therefore is to provide a synthesis of directions for future development towards which these innovative activities within experiments seem to point and to categorize the innovation activities into a set of distinct "innovation pathways". The following seven overarching innovation pathways can be identified:

(1) *Showcasing Technology:* The database of 53 experiments includes many smart home pilots with a high degree of focus on technology. Most of these projects are tangible and clearly defined around solving a problem (though in some cases technology seems to feature as a solution looking for a problem rather than the other way around). These experiments are part of this cluster that provides center stage to new (digital) technology, and they share the idea that better technology makes a better home. Often, technology is showcased in a demonstration home rather than an actual home with a permanent resident. Elements of housing, care and new consumer devices feature in these experiments. In some of these experiments, the demonstration of smart products is more clearly emphasized (e.g., experiment #52 Mimo Wieku, experiment #14 het Slimste huis), and in others, the care component is more dominant (e.g., experiment #23 The great Northern Haven, experiment #12 Belevingswoning Schoneveld)

(2) *Innovation Ecosystem*: Related to the Showcasing Technology pathway above, some of the demonstration homes are also part of a larger agenda to build a regional

innovation eco-system around smart home or eldercare technology as their primary goal. In those projects, the demonstration home is not really a home as such since there is no intention of it becoming permanently inhabited by people who can come to call it their place. Examples of experiments in this category include experiment #21 the 27Delvalle and experiment #10 Zorg Innovatie Huis (this is different from the Showcasing Technology pathway above because those apartments are intended to become permanently inhabited by people who will call it their home). Rather than demonstrating to older adults themselves what a future home environment might look like for them, these home-like environments demonstrate technological prowess to investors, healthcare professionals and (to a lesser extent) informal carers. In this case, a building (which might or might not include a home-like demonstrator environment) assumes the role of physical hub to facilitate cooperation between regional stakeholders (such as technology companies, local start-ups, government agencies) and to generate interest amongst other stakeholders that might become enrolled with the eventual goal of strengthening the competitive economic position of the region based on the idea of older adults as a growing market (i.e., a Silver Economy agenda).

(3) *Sheltered Elite*: Also true to the idea of the above Innovation Ecosystem pathway that older adults constitute a lucrative market is the Sheltered Elite pathway. This includes building luxury, high-end sheltered homes designed for older adults who want (and can afford) to live independently with certain well-organized communal facilities and emergency care. It is important to note that this type of housing is not innovative as such, but the reason it is conceptualized here as an innovation pathway is because some of the projects mentioned by interviewees from Poland and to a lesser extent in the other countries included these kinds of housing options when asked about innovative age-friendly housing experiments (e.g., experiment #49 Osiedle Senioralne, experiment #50 Angel Care). Part of the reason for this might be that Poland has a relatively young population that is ageing at a very rapid rate and that still relatively few see this as a potential growth market that is worthy of investment. Apart from issues of growing inequality and whether this would be a desirable pathway in the first place, there is another reason why Sheltered Elite is of interest from an innovation perspective. Compared to more mainstream housing environments, these elite spaces offer an alternative selection environment—or "protective space" [45]—for the development and testing of certain niche innovations.

(4) *Specific Community*: The Sheltered Elite pathway above caters specifically to relatively wealthy older adults, but there are many other examples of experiments directed at other specific sub-groups. Some of experiments feature so-called "intentional communities", which are deliberately founded for members who hold a common social, political or religious vision and follow an alternative lifestyle. The most well-known of these are religious communities and eco-villages, but the experiment Maison Babayagas for older women with shared feminist principles would certainly also qualify. Interestingly, the international Foundation for Intentional Community views these kinds of collective homemaking arrangements as "pathways towards a more sustainable and just world" [46], to which we might ad that our focus highlights pathways towards an age-friendly world. Whilst specific communities' highlights similarities amongst residents and the choice to live in a particular way, other interesting experiments highlight different social groups living together sometimes out of necessity rather than choice. Such projects aim to bridge the divides between these groups and deliberately address certain societal problems. A good example is the array of intergenerational housing experiments (a relatively large category in the database of experiments, and examples include experiment #4 Humanitas Deventer, experiment #53 Stalowa-29, experiment #39 Wólczańska-168 and many others).

(5) *Conscious Retrofitting*: Some of the intergenerational housing experiments mentioned above—as well as a large part of the experiments in the database—are located in

older buildings with heritage characteristics (e.g., experiment #53 Stalowa-29 and experiment #39 Wólczańska-168). Especially buildings with monument or heritage characteristics exemplify the retrofitting challenges that are associated with making a building as age-friendly as possible on the one hand and retaining features of the original built environment on the other hand. This trade-off has to be made in a deliberate manner, conscious of which criteria are valued over others (hence Conscious Retrofitting). Considerations have to made about how "deep" the retrofit should be and to what extent features full accessibility or renewable energy generation (e.g., experiment #34 Rochestown House) will be taken into account. Finding creative solutions when confronted with an earlier design, choosing which features to retain and which to change presents a very different challenge than building new homes on a greenfield site.

(6) *Home Sharing*: Another interesting conceptually innovative solution that involves deep retrofitting is "home-sharing". The idea of an older adult living alone renting out a spare room to a student is not new, but what is new is the way that this can now be organized and facilitated (at least that is how many interviewed stakeholders in Ireland perceived the ideas behind experiment #24 Abhaile Project and associated activities by AVA housing). The idea is that a home is adapted to the future needs of the older homeowner and at the same time create rental capacity within this home, which provides financial benefits and a sense of security and community for homeowner and a way to fund the age-friendly retrofit. This process could be outsourced to an intermediary who coordinates and arranges a builder for the physical retrofit, gains access to funding, and selects potential tenants. It might not be a coincidence that this has received more attention in Ireland because of its severe housing crisis, especially in Dublin. Ideas about "rightsizing" (i.e., downsizing) larger homes now inhabited by a single older adult are a point of focus considered both promising and controversial.

(7) *Retrovation Challenge*: A number of experiments have as their main aim to achieve a paradigm shift by fundamentally challenging incumbent institutions and dominant ways of thinking. Other contributors to this special issue have demonstrated how the "responsible rebels" who initiate such experiments have a difficult time navigating an environment with unfavorable selection pressures [47]. What we would like to add is that some of these institutional challengers argue for innovative alternative models that rehabilitate elements from the past in new way. A few new projects challenge the model of institutionalized care whereby older adults become patients instead of citizens (i.e., they are seen as patients dependent of care rather than individuals with their own values, opinions, needs and wants). In the view of these innovators this represents a loss of control and dignity. There is often an explicit agenda to counter stereotypes about older adults as frail and dependent. Some of these projects feature very innovative ideas about rehabilitating arrangements from the past, for example in terms of livable neighborhood design and good neighborship. This recombination of older ideas in a new form that draw inspiration from an imagined past we could call "retrovation". Interestingly, many retrovation projects are also challengers and vice versa; therefore, these project types have been classified together in name into this "retrovation challenger" category of very innovative conceptual experiments (e.g., experiment #1 Knarrenhof, experiment #2 Hogeweyk, experiment #7 Oudenhuis).

5. Discussion

Since our findings are based on a large collection of socio-technical experiments with age-friendly homes, further reflection is required on what this collection of experiments can be said to represent. First of all, it should be noted that even the very notion of the experiment as our main unit of analysis can be scrutinized and that selecting and delineating experiments is not always straightforward. Sometimes it is unclear how an experiment should be delineated exactly and where its borders should be drawn (e.g., experiment #19 is labeled "Andromède intergenerational district & Modu-Lab" because it is not straightforward what should be considered the innovative focal point of the experiment—should it be the life-stage adaptable houses and appartement that make up the larger Andromède intergenerational district, or should it be the specific collective building called Modu-Lab?) Sometimes it is difficult to tie an experiment to a single location or site (e.g., experiment #25 introduces an innovative home sharing platform nationwide; experiment #15 rolls out "pilots sleep-over care" in 10 locations at once; experiment #1 will be replicated in several other locations). Sometimes there are clear cross-links between experiments, even across national borders (e.g., the creation of experiment #17 Alzheimer Village Landais in France was inspired by experiment #2 Hogeweyk dementia village in the Netherlands and lessons between the stakeholders involved were exchanged). Moreover, not all experiments in our database are created equal. A criterion for an experiment to end up in our collection is that it is considered innovative by key stakeholders in within the context of their respective countries. This means that some of the experiments which were considered to be innovative by experts on the ground in some countries might not be considered innovative in other countries (e.g., some of the social housing schemes that were considered innovative in Poland or Ireland would not be considered innovative in the Netherlands).

Second, the procedure for selecting the experiments for the database also deserves further explanation. Our goal has been to engage with innovative experiments throughout Europe, and to do so, we limited our attention to four countries from different parts of Europe with distinct care and housing traditions. This meant, for instance, that we have not looked into the situation in Nordic countries with potentially highly advanced and innovative experiments. The omission of potentially very interesting projects is an inherent risk of our methodological approach, even within the countries where we conducted fieldwork. After all, the existing databases of innovative good practices (such as those of the WHO and various others) yielded a limited number of results and the interviewed helicopters (people in overview positions) and interviewed frontrunners (people who initiate experiments) will have limited knowledge of what kind the innovative activities are being conducted in their countries. Therefore, we cannot claim that the set of experiments that we distilled from this are in any way exhaustive or even representative of the situation. Similarly, the eight pathways that we distilled—based on our own categorization after carefully considering the results from our desktop research, site visits and interviews—are open to interpretation and not definitive as such. Many of the experiments within the database can be considered part of multiple pathways (for instance, there are several housing experiments in Poland which aim to facilitate inter-generational cohousing solutions for people from various age groups, which points to a Specific Community pathway, within old building with heritage characteristics that force the initiators to develop innovative retrofitting approaches to maximized accessibility, which points to a Conscious Retrofitting pathway). Nevertheless, we do believe that our systematic approach has yielded an extensive and comprehensive overview that will be valued by innovators and policymakers throughout Europe who want to learn about innovative practices and concrete initiatives around age-friendly housing.

A key question that we have not addressed in this paper, which is also relevant for innovators and policymakers, is how these experiments can be "scaled up" and contribute to a larger transition to age-friendly home environments. The notion of "scaling-up" is very popular concept amongst policymakers and practitioners who are propagating the uptake of a particular innovation. However, it is also a term that is very analytically imprecise and open to many different meanings [48–52]. Therefore, it might be better to instead speak about the "embedding" of experiments as a way to come to terms with the impact and their wider outcomes. Peine and Arenthorst [3,4] also use the term embedding to highlight wider outcomes of experimentation with age-friendly housing innovations. For them embedding is about mainstreaming innovations through a process by which the innovation becomes internalized into "dominant cultures, structures and practices of everyday life" [4], p. 1325. In our view, the term embedding also entails a reciprocal process as a journey of accumulating changes in relation to cumulatively more ordered and stable socio-technical configurations which experimental outputs come to have an influence. Our notion of embedding thus characterizes the overall process by which outputs of experiments may come to generate wider influence beyond their initial conception and setting, which can happen through a diverse set of mechanisms [53]. This is not limited to the mechanisms providing economic incentives and fostering the creation market for age-friendly homes (as propagated in the Silver Economy narrative). Instead, other activities are crucial as well, such as lesson drawing and reflexive learning around experiments, building a constituency of stakeholders for deeper long-term support, organizing study tours or developing other modes of knowledge exchange to inspire actors elsewhere to set up a similar experiment. For innovation policy, this means that a broader perspective is needed and that a much wider range of activities need to be considered besides financially supporting marketable technologies. This should include finding meaningful ways to support the embedding of the large number of promising experiments with social and conceptual innovations.

If we consider the socio-technical experiment and its wider outcomes as our entry point for achieving a wider transition toward age-friendly housing, then we should acknowledge the relevance of wider "support structures". By a support structure we mean a more overarching organizational element that is geared to support concrete experimental activities on the ground. In the literature on transitions and socio-technical experiments, a distinction is made between a "local niche" as collection of individual experiments and a "global niche" as distinct networks of actors "who have some distance to the project, but are related through providing resources, such as finance, political support, technical specifications, that generate a space in which local actors can work" [54], p. 378. Examples of support structures include government subsidy programs, new intermediary organizations around a particular agenda, newly developed standards to promote practices that are not yet mainstream. Consider for instance the case of Ireland, where many interesting experiments are taking place, for which fertile ground has been created by nation-wide initiatives (e.g., National Positive Ageing Strategy aligned with the WHO Active Ageing policy framework and the intermediary organization around the Age-friendly Ireland Programme [55]), various county level initiatives (e.g., the Cúltaca initiative and Older People's Councils). Vice versa, the experiments themselves also create fertile ground for new and extended support structures. In Ireland, for instance, the Great Northern Haven experiment was important in bringing various stakeholders together in set up some of the above support structures in the first place. Another interesting example of a different kind of support structure is the European Homes4Life project, which has set out to create a Europe wide certification scheme for innovative age-friendly housing solutions [56]. The idea behind this project is that such a new certificate will stimulate investment and eventually make age-friendliness a mainstream criterion to be considered in housing projects (similar to the green building certificates and energy labels that have become mainstreamed over the last years). The process of developing and testing this certification scheme had other effects as well; for instance, initiators of key experiments learned about other experiments elsewhere, and they reflected and re-evaluated some of the features in their experiments.

6. Conclusions

Throughout Europe, a variety of innovative socio-technical experiments are being implemented to improve the life-course resilience of existing and newly built home environments. These experiments reflect the distinct socio-economic context of their locations and, more importantly, they provide a glance into potential future directions for the development of age-friendly homes. This paper provided an overview of 53 ongoing experiments in the domain of age-friendly housing in the Netherlands, Poland, Ireland and France as countries that represent different parts of Europe with distinct approaches to housing and care for older adults. Overall, we find that, besides the variation between these countries, there is a more important type variation in terms of differences in the character of these experiments and the directions proposed by these experiments. Most of the associated innovations tested in age-friendly home experiments are not primarily material or technical but primarily social or conceptual in character (i.e., new organizational or everyday practices that re-arrange social relations or new housing concepts that bridge the divide between ageing in place individually and a nursing home). This variety of innovations tested in the experiments has been categorized into seven distinct innovation pathways (Showcasing Technology, Innovation Ecosystem, Sheltered Elite, Specific Community, Conscious Retrofitting, Home Sharing and Retrovation Challenge). We hope that our overview, interpretation and reflection on innovative practices for age-friendly housing and its future directions are a valuable contribution for scholars and practitioners alike.

Author Contributions: Conceptualization, F.S. and A.P.; methodology, F.S.; formal analysis, F.S. and A.P.; investigation, F.S.; resources, F.S. and A.P.; data curation, F.S.; writing—original draft preparation, F.S.; writing—review and editing, F.S. and A.P.; visualization, F.S.; supervision, A.P.; project administration, A.P.; funding acquisition, A.P. All authors have read and agreed to the published version of the manuscript.

Funding: The research presented in this article is part of a project that has received funding from the European Union's Horizon 2020 research and innovation programme under agreement No 826295.

Institutional Review Board Statement: Not applicable.

Informed Consent Statement: Not applicable.

Data Availability Statement: The first part of the data supporting reported results can be found on publicly available websites and databases (hyperlinks have been provided in the text). The second part of the data supporting reported results are interviews and field visits (interview transcripts, photographs and field visit notes are not publicly available, but can be can be provided by the corresponding author upon request).

Conflicts of Interest: The authors declare no conflict of interest.

Appendix A

Table A1. Full overview of 53 age-friendly home experiments in the Netherlands, France, Ireland and Poland.

	Experiment Name	Location	Description
# 1	Knarrenhof (Aahof)	Zwolle	Knarrenhof is an innovative form of housing that actively involves new resident in home making and community support. It is directed at "young older adults" and "old older adults" who want to help each other out and to live independently as long as possible. The attitude and affinity with the neighbors are considered very important and notions of good neighborship are central. Often, those who want to reside here are socially engaged and active (doing voluntary work rather than the stereotype of "bridge clubs and passively sitting at home") and presented as "social people who can in principle be called upon" by their neighbors. The name "Knarrenhof" consists of two parts. The first part, "knarren" takes it from characters of a popular Dutch TV show from the 1980's (van Kooten en de Bie's krasse knarren) who are presented as "hardy old geezers" as a way to stress the agency and vitality of older adults (the logo presents an old man showing off his muscles). The second part "hof" can be translated as "courtyard" and refers to the type of picturesque secluded set of houses facing each other as part urban planning layout conducive for community building. Because this urban form of the courtyard stems from the Middle Ages in Dutch cities and because notions of good neighborship stem from an earlier age, the ideas are presented as "sprung from the past ... (but) also a project for the future". Aside from the Aahof in Zwolle, there are plans to create more Knarrenhof locations in several other Dutch municipalities.

Table A1. *Cont.*

	Experiment Name	Location	Description
# 2	Hogeweyk	Weesp	The Hogeweyk a pioneering care facility/community for older adults with dementia. Compared to traditional nursing homes the residents with dementia are more active and live a more "normal" life. Professionally and inhouse trained staff wear regular clothes instead of a uniform and provide the 169 residents the necessary 24-h support in care, living and wellbeing. The "residents, NOT patients" live in one of several housing types that fit their lifestyle (traditional, urban, cosmopolitan and formal—it used to include Indonesian, but this will stop soon because the cohort of older adults from the former colony is getting smaller). The houses of each type are equipped with a shared living room and bedrooms for several (6–7) residents and they are located in a gated neighborhood setting complete with general store, restaurant and theatre (hence the idea of a dementia "village"). The walls are permeable to an extent and people from society outside are encouraged to come in as a way to eventually create a kind of "reverse emancipation" so that society at large becomes more dementia friendly (bringing the outside world in vs bringing the inside world out; social inclusion is a major objective). The underlying vision is to get away from the large-scale medicalized institutionalized model of care home to small-scale normalized social relational model of care.
# 3	Empatisch Wonen	Roermond	59 social housing apartments in a former care home give substance to the vision of "empathic living" (Empathisch Wonen). The main idea behind emphatic living is that a building can be easily transformed to adapt to changing needs of resident groups (i.e., because it is adaptable it "lives with" older adults during their life course, but also for next cohorts of residents such younger people or families). The concept is still relatively open, currently being substantiated. The approach features elements of co-creation and is loosely related to work by visionary Dutch architects from the 1970s. On a secondary level, the emphatic living concept as used in Roermond implies certain features, such as soft walls between one-bedroom apartments (modularity to facilitate future reshuffling of rooms), storage space close to the apartment (for a scoot mobile, but generally useful), a common room (to foster community), broad common hallways (for the scoot mobile and to foster community), lighting solutions for common hallways (daylight to foster experience or solutions with floors that indicate direction) placemaking (has to do with identity and atmosphere and the experience of living), new temperature management, fiber optic internet cabled through a technical room located on the same places on every floor to enable easy access and future smart solutions (to make the home "domotics-ready"), green on balconies (for livability). Aside from Roermond, there are two other locations that will serve as a test site for the Empatisch Wonen concept.
# 4	Humanitas woonstu-denten	Deventer	An innovative intergenerational housing arrangement in the Netherlands as an example of how a local long-term older people care practice evolved in response to a national agenda to close down nursing homes in the Netherlands. From 2012 to 2020, there will be 6 students ("woonstudenten") living amongst the older residents. For a minimum of 30 h a month they are tasked to be a "good neighbor", for instance by serving bread at the common restaurant.
# 5	Selficient Huis	Utrecht	A self-sufficient modular age-friendly house. Selficient is the name for a housing concept created by a new start-up, and they have a demonstration house in Utrecht, which is portrayed as "the house of the future". The idea of the Selficient company is to change traditional building practices. Their concept house can be built in a short time through standardized practice. The house is presented as "circular" because sustainable materials are used, can be broken down and rebuilt, and it generates its own energy. Moreover, the house is presented as "modular" because it can be adjusted to "live with you" across the life course. Two specific elements are mentioned as a way to give substance to modularity: future-proof (living as long as possible in the house by adjustments into account in the building process) and life course resilience (house "lives along with you" through the life course since it can be made bigger and smaller with adjustable rooms).

Table A1. *Cont.*

	Experiment Name	Location	Description
# 6	Woon service zone	Haarlemmer-meer	An innovative home care concept and funding model. A Cristian healthcare foundation and a consultancy and construction management company are developing an affordable "home service zone" (woonservicezone) for various groups in Haarlemmermeer. Such a home service zone is a residential area for 5000 to 20,000 people with many care service facilities and adapted homes. Housing and spatial planning are presented as the "glue" that makes sure that affordable home care is possible. Another interesting associated financial innovation is the idea of an Investment Memorandum as a tool to coordinate investments amongst various kinds of care and construction domain stakeholders involved.
# 7	Ouden Huis	Bodegraven	These 22 apartments provide an alternative for a care home targeted at older adults with or without special care needs. According to the founders "the (traditional) care home strips away your strength and sense of dignity". the Oudenhuis concept relies on a few key principles related to independence (living on your own and finding company when you want it), aspects of co-living (independent living but aspects of co-living—e.g., shared meals—"so that you know you are not in it alone"), affordability (to include less affluent households), inhouse professional care (through carers in the house, including palliative care), couples stick together (sense of control). Aside from Bodegraven, there are also plans for an Ouden Huis in Woerden and Waddinxveen
# 8	Tuindorp Oost	Utrecht	Since 2016 youth lived alongside older adults in this innovative care home. A stop was introduced which resulted in too many vacant rooms and younger adults looking for housing were allowed to move in. In 2018, it was announced that both younger and older adults had to vacate the place by the end of that year. They were angry about this and did not understand why, especially since this was perceived as a successful experiment. As a result, the younger and older adults banded together to draft a manifesto for better care for older adults. In the manifesto, the younger adults say: "we have a unique perspective on the life of older adults because we have lived amongst them for two years. That is, until [the housing organization] decided to pull us apart too early". The manifesto is called "give older adults back their voice".
# 9	De Benring	Voorst	A residential complex with 72 apartments. It was the site of an innovative transformation project which shows how social and technological innovations can be integrated through retrofitting existing real estate for older adults. The built environment is used flexibly, which makes the building "system- and customer preference proof". De Benring traditional care home was marked for demolition in 2013, but 400 members of the local community spoke out against it and challenged the government. After co-creation workshops they took full responsibility for future functionalities of the building and its prospective future residents. This resulted physically in a refurbished complex (new floor plans and refurbished apartments) with an intergenerational character (10% of the residents being viral youngsters of max 22 years old and 90% older adults of over 55 years old, who learn from each other and help each other out; the youngsters have to take a test to see if they fit and possibly buddy up with an older resident). Various types of home care are also provided, more than possible under normal legal conditions, which effectively safeguards the project against changes in government policy.
# 10	Zorg Innovatie Huis	Baarn	A life course resilient house where older adults, informal carers, healthcare professionals, product and service providers and education stakeholders strive for innovative personalized care. The house provides an inspiring location that collects innovation and new technology for home care and makes it tangible. These smart solutions are tested and learned from in a real world setting with the goal to improve them and to share best practices. The innovations are sub-divided into four groups: (1) physical support, (2) care at a distance, (3) motion, interaction and activation, (4) autonomy and well-being. Examples include smart rollator walkers, smart beds and many robots shaped as small companions or of stuffed animals for cuddling (e.g., Dino Dirk, Maatje, flowerpot Tessa, etc.)

Table A1. *Cont.*

	Experiment Name	Location	Description
# 11	Het Zorg(T)huis	Winschoten	Project about showcasing technology and giving information; it integrates ideas on smart homes and on care.
# 12	Belevingswoning Schoneveld	Doetinchem	An "experience" apartment showcasing how older adults can live longer at home.
# 13	Huis van Zelfredza-amheid	Enschede	Project about showcasing technology and giving information; it integrates ideas on smart homes and on care.
# 14	Het slimste huis	Alkmaar	Project about showcasing technology and giving information; it integrates ideas on smart homes and on care.
# 15	Pilots logeerzorg	Zeist	The "pilots sleep-over care" are a way to temporarily lift the burden from the shoulder of informal carers. For 10 pilot municipalities the option is given for older adults with high care needs or dementia to temporarily move to a care institution to give some space to informal carers. The programme runs until 2020 and the 10 municipalities are Westland, Capelle a/d IJssel, Dordrecht, Hoeksche Waard, Zeist, Nieuwegein, Helmond, Ede, Heerde and Assen.
# 16	Vivre aux Vignes	Grenoble	A communal living facility that amounts to a novel housing formula with pooled services and care. It is conceptually in between an individual a home and a nursing home and also aimed at older adults with a modest budget.
# 17	Alzheimer Village Landais	Dax	An Alzheimer village in the Southwest of France, inspired by the Dutch project, the Hogeweyk (see above in this table).
# 18	La Note Bleue	Limonest	A residence complex to support ageing in place through adapted housing with 23 units of which 17 are equipped to accommodate people with loss of autonomy.
# 19	Andromede intergenera-tional district & Modulab	Blagnac	20 houses and 80 apartments are of part of the Andromède intergenerational district, located in Blagnac. The latter is made up of evolving housing that can be adapted to the various stages of life and especially to the loss of autonomy. On this site is also collective building called the Modu-Lab.
# 20	Bailleur social	Lille	Small experiment implementing a modular housing system.
# 21	27Delvalle	Nice	A center on connected health and healthy ageing, which includes a model apartment that is designed as a showcase and a testing platform for technologies supporting independent living and autonomy. The Habitat platform of 27Delvalle is a space dedicated to health and autonomy and facilitates cooperation between a variety of regional stakeholders (Overarching network includes FRANCE SILVER ÉCO, Nice Côte d'Azur Metropolis incubator, CIU Santé, PAILLON2020 and more). It relies in particular on the ecosystem of services dedicated to the loss of autonomy. It prepares the return and promotes the home support of vulnerable people and/or people with disabilities around their personal life project. The "demonstration, simulation and experimentation apartment" is equipped with various digital technologies and innovative devices and is set up to provide advice and solutions to users, their families, caregivers and health professionals. In addition, researchers and industry meet to develop innovative technologies. The objectives are to (1) inform, raise awareness and test; (2) facilitate home return and home support; (3) train medical professionals in new technologies; (4) innovate with research by connecting users, professionals, researchers and industry to be a market access facilitator for businesses.

Table A1. *Cont.*

	Experiment Name	Location	Description
# 22	La Maison Des Babayagas	Paris	La Maison Des Babayagas is a feminist cohabitation project that started in Montreuil, in the surroundings of Paris in 2013 (Babayagas is a Slavic term for witch). A group of dynamic women have devised a new kind of communal living for older women based on shared values of feminism and activism. La Maison Des Babayagas is a self-managed social housing project composed of 21 apartments for women over 60, and 4 apartments for young adults below 30; the dwellings are still owned by a social housing landlord. Based on four pillars (self-management, solidarity, citizenship and ecology), this "anti-retirement home" aims to facilitate contacts and mutual care between the community members. One of the main motivations for creating the Babayagas house was battling social isolation and many community projects and social activities are organized both by the inhabitants and with the surrounding community, the two rooms on the ground floor of the building being two municipal rooms.
# 23	Great Northern Haven	Dundalk	The Great Northern Haven is a new housing project operational for several years now. It features 16 apartments (including one showroom and testing apartment) built to support "life-time adaptability" and Active Assisted Living for older adults. Each apartment is equipped with sensors and interactive technology to support telecare. To an extent, the experiment has been used as a way to convince developers to adopt universal design by making them "walk in the shoes of a frailer older person". All interviewees in Ireland are familiar with this pioneering high-profile experiment, but according to some of them, the features seem overly hospital-like and heavily reliant on technology. Some of the wiring is now obsolete since smart Wi-Fi solutions were not as prevalent when it was initially designed.
# 24	the Abhaile Project (AVA pilot house)	Dublin	AVA housing offers a solution in the domain of "home sharing", which offers an alternative to older homeowners whereby their homes are adapted to their future needs whist also creating a rental capacity within their home. This provides financial benefits and a sense of security and community for homeowners. The innovative part is the total package of guidance, support and expertise to the homeowner through the process of retrofitting and sharing arrangements. This particular pilot project put these home sharing into practice in a three-bedroom semi-detached house. The severe housing crisis in Ireland is part of the reason why these kinds of home sharing innovations are gaining momentum.
# 25	Elder Home Share	nation-wide	New platform that allows older homeowners to continue to live at home with a greater degree of security at night, companionship and help with practical tasks such as light housework and shopping. The other side of the match is a responsible and caring (younger) person who wants an affordable living situation in exchange for sleeping in the house 5 to 6 nights a week and providing 8 h a week companionship and support. The severe housing crisis in Ireland is part of the reason why these kinds of home sharing innovations are gaining momentum.
# 26	Inchicore Housing with Supports	Dublin	Planned housing project with 52 apartments to develop a new model of "housing with supports" for older adults, featuring a physical environment adapted according to universal design principles and appropriate care and supports provided on site, integrated within the local community.
# 27	Broome Lodge	Dublin	43 new apartments built according to Universal Design criteria and rented out social housing by an approved housing body.
# 28	Proudstown	Navan	4 new apartments built on a previously derelict site. Small-scale development that also features renewable energy innovations.
# 29	McAuley Place	Naas	a non-medical, intergenerational and not-for-profit housing association with 53 apartments for social and private housing.
# 30	Colivet Court	Southill	35 apartments designed to be a catalyst in both the social and physical regeneration of the area, generating a sense of pride, empowerment, ownership and mutual respect.

Table A1. *Cont.*

	Experiment Name	Location	Description
# 31	Leighlinbridge Housing	Leighlinbridge	15 apartments on the grounds of an old presbytery building, providing for security and passive-surveillance and a sense of community.
# 32	Father Lemass Court	Dublin	32 apartments with the goal to create a community through the provision of al central courtyard with an adjoining community room and a communal roof garden, all designed so as to provide passive supervision and social contact.
# 33	SVP Malahide	Dublin	37 apartments devised over wo ranges of housing along opposing sides of the site. This makes the enclosed garden the central focal point, which provides a secure ambience that maximizes passive surveillance and generates an environment of communal engagement.
# 34	Rochestown House	Dublin	34 apartments from the 1970s undergoing a deep energy retrofit to counter fuel poverty and geared to maximize the number of units on this site, which is close to existing services and public transport (this way underused larger council owned houses become available for larger families).
# 35	Glór Na Srútha	Cloncara	12 apartments in a rural village setting and incorporating Age Friendly Design guidelines and universal design principles. Lifetime adaptability, efficiency of technology, and integration with the existing community were all key components (the design responded to site contours and poor ground conditions, and the traditional styles of clustered communities in the locality. The overall design creates a sense of community enclosure through the slow curve of the design whilst retaining its connectivity with adjoining housing scheme through a pedestrian link).
# 36	Cuan an Chláir	Ennis	12 houses and communal facilities. Funding was received from a mix of government funding and other sources based on donations, local fundraising and land allocated by the church.
# 37	Ballygall	Dublin	39 apartments from the 1970s, remodeled, refurbished and energy retrofitted and fully accessible.
# 38	Annamore Court	Dublin	70 newly built social apartments in an existing derelict 1960s social housing scheme with a higher density development (this way underused larger council owned houses become available for larger families). Additional supports and services are provided on site with the aim of supporting independent living in the community for as long as possible. This was the first social housing new-build to benefit from funding provided by the Housing Finance Agency and the European Investment Bank.
# 39	Wólczańska-168	Lodz	This integrational house was partly Inspired by the Warsaw Stalowa-29 exemplar but is now actually at a further stage. This project is about converting an 1883 villa to fit with senior apartments. The project was initiated by seniors from the Forum for the Fatherland Association, who in 2013 submitted their project "Multi-generational House" to the Citizens' Budget competition where it gained interest among members of the City Council, who in the next year indicated the property at Wólczańska-168 for the Multi-generational House. The funds were secured for a thorough renovation with the adaptation of flats to the needs of the older people, with disabilities (handles in bathrooms, floor showers, no architectural barriers). In 2016, an interdisciplinary team was established within the office, responsible for the development of the Multi-generational House operation program, the work of which in 2018 was supported by the expert team of the Laboratory Foundation for Architecture 60+ as part of a pilot project of revitalization (carried out on behalf of the Ministry of Investment and Development from European funds). The developed model is currently being implemented. Soon the first residents should move in (in accordance with the recommended social mix), an NGO has been running the Neighborhood Club—a place for meetings and integration of future tenants and neighborhood—on the site.

Table A1. *Cont.*

	Experiment Name	Location	Description
# 40	Inter-generational tenement house Szczecin	Szczecin	A multi-generational house actually in operation. It seems to be a project with senior apartment linked to an orphanage to foster the multi-generation exchange of support (though not much information could be found about this).
# 41	Sheltered housing tenants are waiting for	Ostrów Wielkopolski	14 sheltered apartments were created as part of a larger program in response to the needs of a growing number of seniors and the lack of flats currently dedicated to people 60+ in Ostrów Wielkopolski. Common problems faced by seniors include stairs, no elevator, and a lack of help. This project aims to solve these issues. It is divided into 2 tasks: Sheltered housing Municipal housing Ostrów decided to implement the 1st sheltered flat in order to offer support to seniors who require assistance in everyday functioning but do not have support from their family and do not need service 24/7. It is an alternative to a Social Welfare Home. The Apartments are built in 2 buildings and are adapted to the needs of seniors (lift, wide corridors). They are in the town center, close to a church and a bus stop. The 14 apartments are geared to find out more about the needs of needs older adults (a needs-assessment is conducted).
# 42	Orpea Polska Mieszkania dla seniorów	Wrocław	Housing investment dedicated to older people and independent apartments dedicated to older people with or without assistant needs.
# 43	Orpea stoya rest home	Warsaw	Like the Orpea Polska Mieszkania dla seniorów example above, also a type of alternative nursing home by Orpea.
# 44	Dom dla seniora Szczecin	Szczecin	Dom dla seniora (translated Senior Citizen's Home) features 15 well-designed apartments (12 one-room units and 3 two-room units). They are located in a building located in the city center of Szczecin, which is equipped with an elevator and designed with older adults in mind, i.e., without architectural barriers.
# 45	Assisted living flats Szczecin	Szczecin	38 assisted living flats for older adults funded local government (though not much information could be found about this).
# 46	Assisted living in Stargard	Stargard Szczeciński	Social housing for older adults with the help of ICT systems and volunteers, the first of this type in Poland. Further search of a WHO database suggests that there are 24 apartments and that this is part of the "house needed" program and the "not alone" program (though not much information could be found about this).
# 47	Mieszkania dla seniorow	Poznan	141 apartments designed exclusively for seniors are located in three buildings. These apartments are intended for older people who have applied for housing in the past but have not received them due to the lack of such a possibility. The apartments became available due to signed collaborations between the city of Poznan and a TBS (a TBS is an institution for a particulate category of semi-social housing).
# 48	Dom Seniora Opole	Opole	102 rental apartments for rent in the TBS Senior system, with 3 buildings of 34 apartments in each. In each building there is a room for shared use by residents (a common room) and facilities for those with mobility impairments.
# 49	Osiedle senioralne	Warsaw	Presented as the First Senior Housing Estate in Poland, which provides an alternative to a nursing home. It is suggested that people feel guilty when they put their parents in a nursing home, but that they should not feel guilty if their parents move to this type of living arrangement. There are 1-bedroom and 2-bedroom apartments available and there is a rehabilitation program to various conditions.

Table A1. *Cont.*

	Experiment Name	Location	Description
# 50	Angel Care centrum seniora	Wrocław	Angel Care is a nursing home with high-quality nursing support and high-level facilities. This "best nursing home" consist of 48 fully furnished and safe apartments designed for one or two people. In addition. The complex will offer its permanent residents individually designed facilities and tailor-made entertainment and room for their own hobbies. In addition, 24-h nursing, physiotherapy and medical support and specialized beds for medical care are provided. There is a library, common space and workplaces.
# 51	Senioral Apart Hotel Zarabia	Bielsko-Biała	Apartments for older adults on with proximity of mountains and rivers or ski resorts. Their unique selling point is the excellent geographical location.
# 52	Mimo Wieku apartment	Warsaw	The U Siebie Mimo Wieku ("at home despite the age") showroom apartment presents a comprehensive set of solutions how to enable older adults to have an active and independent life in their own home. It is the first apartment of this kind in Poland and designed according to best practices regarding accessibility, health, wellbeing and equipped with modern devices to assist older adults and person with disabilities. On about 50 square meters a well-designed space has been created for a single person or a couple. It is free of physical barriers and ready for upgrades with regard to equipment and amenities. The well thought spatial and physical arrangement, designed by specialized architects, includes solutions with regard to the main aspects of comfort, ergonomics, daylight, illumination and views, indoor air quality, temperature, humidity and air movement and acoustics. The entire array of specially designed building features and smart products make this "larger than the sum of its parts". Another goal aimed at is to get companies in Poland to see older adults as a relevant market for products and services.
# 53	Stalowa-29	Warsaw	The Stalowa-29 intergenerational apartment building is one of the first cohousing solutions in Poland to be inhabited by people from various age groups. It is a retrofit of an older building (renovation is ongoing at this time), and the idea is that it serves as a model for a modern, sustainable and well-designed housing modernization under the Integrated Revitalization Program in the Praga district (it is mostly paid for by city of Warsaw). It is also geared to counter negative effects of gentrification and to encourage residents to help one another. On the last two floors, there will be a care and educational institution for youths. On each of the other floors, 4 apartments are planned (12 in total). On the ground floor a space for the local community will be created in the form of a café or other meeting place (how exactly is yet to be determined). Intergenerational design, countering negative effects of gentrification and encouraging residents to help one another are key elements. According to some interviewees, these kinds of projects are difficult to implement in practice because they feature social housing and legal requirements stipulate that the next person on the waiting list would qualify for the apartment. Selecting people deliberately based on age and skipping others in line might be hard to justify.

References

1. Van Hoof, J.; Kazak, J.; Perek-Białas, J.; Peek, S. The Challenges of Urban Ageing: Making Cities Age-Friendly in Europe. *Int. J. Environ. Res. Public Health* **2018**, *15*, 2473. [CrossRef]
2. Plouffe, L.; Kalache, A. Towards Global Age-Friendly Cities: Determining Urban Features that Promote Active Aging. *J. Urban Health Bull. N. Y. Acad. Med.* **2010**, *87*, 733–739. [CrossRef] [PubMed]
3. Peine, A.; Arenthorst, M. Towards a European Reference Framework for Age-Friendly Housing 2016. Available online: http://ec.europa.eu/newsroom/document.cfm?doc_id=43991 (accessed on 3 September 2020).
4. Arentshorst, M.; Peine, A. From niche level innovations to age-friendly homes and neighbourhoods: A multi-level analysis of challenges, barriers and solutions. *Technol. Anal. Strateg. Manag.* **2018**, *30*, 1325–1337. [CrossRef]
5. Heidegger, M. Building dwelling thinking. In *Poetry, Language, Thought*; Heidegger, M., Ed.; Harper & Row: New York, NY, USA, 1971; pp. 145–161.
6. Tuan, Y.F. Home. In *Patterned Ground: The Entanglements of Nature and Cuture*; Pile, S., Thrift, N., Harrison, S., Eds.; Reaktion Books: London, UK, 2004; pp. 164–165.

7. De Visscher, J. Wonen: De nabijheid van de ander in de bezieling van de dingen. In *Wonen: Architectuur in Het Denkenvan Heidegger*; de Visscher, J., de Saeger, R., Eds.; SUN: Nijmegen, The Netherlands, 1991; pp. 117–146.
8. Blunt, A. Cultural geography: Cultural geographies of home. *Prog. Humran Geogragphy* **2005**, *29*, 505–515. [CrossRef]
9. Duncan, J.; Lambert, D. Landscapes of home. In *A Companion to Cultural Geography*; Duncan, J.S., Johnson, N.C., Schein, R.H., Eds.; Blackwell: Oxford, UK, 2003; pp. 382–403.
10. Homes4Life. KPI Framework for Smart Age Friendly Living Environments. 2019. Available online: http://www.homes4life.eu/wp-content/uploads/2020/04/Homes4Life_D2.4_D3.1.pdf (accessed on 1 September 2020).
11. De Wit, O.; Van Den Ende, J.; Schot, J.; Van Oost, E. Innovative Junctions: Office Technologies in the Netherlands, 1880–1980. *Technol. Cult.* **2002**, *43*, 50–72. [CrossRef]
12. Law, J. Technology and heterogeneous engineering. In *The Social Construction of Technological Systems*; Bijker, W.E., Hughes, T.P., Pinch, T.J., Eds.; MIT Press: Cambridge, MA, USA, 1987; pp. 111–134.
13. Markard, J.; Raven, R.; Truffer, B. Sustainability transitions: An emerging field of research and its prospects. *Res. Policy* **2012**, *41*, 955–967. [CrossRef]
14. Grin, J.; Rotmans, J.; Schot, J.; Geels, F.; Loorbach, D. *Transitions to Sustainable Development: New Directions in the Study of Long Term Transformative Change*; Routledge: New York, NY, USA, 2010.
15. Geels, F. Technological Transitions as Evolutionary Reconfiguration Processes: A Multi-level Analysis and A Case Study. *Res. Policy* **2002**, *31*, 1257–1274. [CrossRef]
16. Kemp, R.; Schot, J.; Hoogma, R. Regime shifts to sustainability through processes of niche formation: The approach of strategic niche management. *Technol. Anal. Strateg. Manag.* **1998**, *10*, 175–198. [CrossRef]
17. Latour, B. Which Protocol for the New Collective Experiments? In *Kultur Im Experiment*; Schmindgen, H., Geimerand, P., Dierig, S., Eds.; Kadmos Verlag: Berlin, Germany, 2004; pp. 17–36.
18. Karvonen, A.; Van Heur, B. Urban laboratories: Experiments in reworking cities. *Int. J. Urban Reg. Res.* **2014**, *38*, 379–392. [CrossRef]
19. Sengers, F.; Wieczorek, A.; Raven, R. Experimenting for Sustainability Transitions: A Systematic Literature Review. *Technol. Forecast. Soc. Chang.* **2019**, *145*, 153–164. [CrossRef]
20. Hoogma, R.; Kemp, R.; Schot, J.; Truffer, B. *Experimenting for Sustainable Transport: The Approach of Strategic Niche Management*; Spon Press: London, UK, 2002.
21. Schot, J.; Geels, F. Strategic niche management and sustainable innovation journeys: Theory, findings, research agenda and policy. *Technol. Anal. Strateg. Manag.* **2008**, *20*, 537–554. [CrossRef]
22. Vergragt, P.J.; Brown, H.S. Sustainable mobility: From technological innovation to societal learning. *J. Clean. Prod.* **2007**, *15*, 1104–1115. [CrossRef]
23. Naturevation. Navigating Innovation Pathways. 2020. Available online: https://naturvation.eu/action/navigating-innovation-pathways (accessed on 1 September 2020).
24. Yin, R. *Case Study Research: Design and Methods*, 5th ed.; Sage: Thousand Oaks, CA, USA, 2004.
25. Limb, M.; Dwyer, C. *Qualitative Methods for Geographers*; Arnold: London, UK, 2001.
26. Van de Ven, A.; Poole, M. Explaining development and change in organizations. *Acad. Manag. Rev.* **1995**, *20*, 510–540. [CrossRef]
27. Pettigrew, A. What is processual analysis? *Scand. J. Manag.* **1997**, *13*, 337–348. [CrossRef]
28. WHO. Global Database of Age-friendly Practices. 2019. Available online: https://extranet.who.int/agefriendlyworld/afp/ (accessed on 1 August 2020).
29. EIP AHA. General Repository. 2019. Available online: https://ec.europa.eu/eip/ageing/repository (accessed on 1 August 2020).
30. EIP AHA. Reference Sites. 2019. Available online: https://ec.europa.eu/eip/ageing/reference-sites_en (accessed on 1 August 2020).
31. AFE-Innovnet. Repository. 2020. Available online: http://www.afeinnovnet.eu/repository/ (accessed on 1 August 2020).
32. European Covenant on Demographic Change. Repository. 2019. Available online: https://www.agefriendlyeurope.org/repository (accessed on 1 August 2020).
33. PROGRESSIVE. Examples of Good Practices. 2019. Available online: https://progressivestandards.org/examples-of-good-practices/ (accessed on 1 August 2020).
34. Age-friendly Ireland. Ireland Age Friendly Cities and Counties catalogue. 2016. Available online: http://agefriendlyireland.ie/wp-content/uploads/2016/07/WHO-compendium-4.pdf (accessed on 1 August 2020).
35. Government of Ireland. Housing Options for Our Ageing Population. 2019. Available online: ttps://assets.gov.ie/9398/ca553fa753b64f14b20e4a8dcf9a46ab.pdf (accessed on 1 August 2020).
36. Aedes-Actiz. Mapped Examples of Dutch Smart Homes for the Future. 2020. Available online: https://www.kcwz.nl/thema/woonzorgtechnologie/slim-wonen-in-de-toekomst-voorbeeldwoningen-op-de-kaart (accessed on 1 August 2020).
37. Anttonen, A.; Sipilä, J. European social care services. Is it possible to identify models? *J. Eur. Soc. Policy* **1996**, *6*, 87–100. [CrossRef]
38. Bettio, F.; Plantega, J. Comparing care regimes in Europe. *Fem. Econ.* **2004**, *10*, 85–113. [CrossRef]
39. Jasanoff, S.; Kim, S. Containing the atom: Socio-technical imaginaries and nuclear power in the United States and South Korea. *Minerva* **2009**, *47*, 119–146. [CrossRef]
40. Porter, M. *Clusters and the New Economics of Competition*; Harvard Business Review: Boston, MA, USA, 1998.

41. Breschi, S.; Malerba, F. The Geography of Innovation and Economic Clustering: Some Introductory Notes. *Ind. Corp. Chang.* **2001**, *10*, 817–833. [CrossRef]
42. Florida, R. *The Rise of the Creative Class: And How It's Transforming Work, Leisure, Community and Everyday Life*; Basic Books: New York, NY, USA, 2002.
43. Van de Ven, A.; Polley, D.; Garud, R.; Venkataraman, S. *The Innovation Journey*; Oxford University Press: New York, NY, USA, 1999.
44. Enninga, T. *Armchair Travelling the Innovation Journey: Building a Narrative Repertoire of the Experiences of Innovation Project Leaders*; Delft University Press: Delft, The Netherlands, 2018.
45. Smith, A.; Raven, R. What is protective space? Reconsidering niches in transitions to sustainability. *Res. Policy* **2012**, *41*, 1025–1036. [CrossRef]
46. Foundation for Intentional Community. Our Mission. 2020. Available online: https://www.ic.org (accessed on 1 August 2020).
47. Rusinovic, K.; van Bochove, M.; Koops-Boelaars, S.; Tavy, Z.; van Hoof, J. Towards Responsible Rebellion: How Founders Deal with Challenges in Establishing and Governing Innovative Living Arrangements for Older People. *Int. J. Environ. Res. Public Health* **2020**, *17*, 6235. [CrossRef]
48. Douthwaite, B.; Kuby, T.; Van de Fliert, E.; Schulz, S. Impact pathway evaluation: An approach for achieving and attributing impact in complex systems. *Agric. Syst.* **2003**, *78*, 243–265. [CrossRef]
49. Dees, J.; Anderson, B.; Wei-Skillern, J. Scaling social impact: Strategies for spreading social innovations. *Stanf. Soc. Innov. Rev.* **2004**, *1*, 24–32.
50. Van den Bosch, S.; Rotmans, J. *Deepening, Broadening and Scaling Up: A Framework for Steering Transition Experiments*; Knowledge Centre for Sustainable System Innovations and Transitions: Rotterdam, The Netherlands, 2008.
51. Smith, B.; Stevens, C. Different types of social entrepreneurship: The role of geography and embeddedness on the measurement and scaling of social value. *Entrep. Reg. Dev. Int. J.* **2010**, *22*, 575–598. [CrossRef]
52. Westley, F.; Antadze, N.; Riddell, D. Five configurations for scaling up social innovation: Case examples of nonprofit organizations from Canada. *J. Behav. Sci.* **2014**, *50*, 234–260. [CrossRef]
53. Sengers, F.; Turnheim, B.; Berkhout, F. Beyond experiments: Embedding outcomes in climate governance. *Environ. Plan. C Politics Space* **2020**, *0*, 1–24. [CrossRef]
54. Geels, F.; Raven, R. Non-linearity and expectations in niche-development trajectories: Ups and downs in Dutch biogas development (1973–2003). *Technol. Anal. Strateg. Manag.* **2006**, *18*, 375–391. [CrossRef]
55. WHO. Global Age-friendly Cities: A Guide. 2007. Available online: https://www.who.int/ageing/publications/Global_age_friendly_cities_Guide_English.pdf (accessed on 1 September 2020).
56. Homes4Life. About Certification for Ageing in Place. 2020. Available online: http://www.homes4life.eu/about/ (accessed on 1 September 2020).

International Journal of
Environmental Research and Public Health

MDPI

Article

Perspectives on Active Transportation in a Mid-Sized Age-Friendly City: "You Stay Home"

Irmina Klicnik [1] and Shilpa Dogra [2,*]

[1] Faculty of Health Sciences (Community Health), University of Ontario Institute of Technology, Oshawa, ON L1G-0C5, Canada; Irmina.Klicnik@ontariotechu.net

[2] Faculty of Health Sciences (Kinesiology), University of Ontario Institute of Technology, Oshawa, ON L1G-0C5, Canada

* Correspondence: Shilpa.Dogra@uoit.ca; Tel.: +1-905-721-8668 (ext. 6240)

Received: 23 October 2019; Accepted: 2 December 2019; Published: 5 December 2019

Abstract: Background: Active transportation is an affordable and accessible form of transportation that facilitates the mobility of older adults in their communities. Age-friendly cities encourage and support physical activity and social participation among older adults; however, they often do not adequately address active transportation. Our goal was to identify and understand the constraints to active transportation that older adults experience in order to inform the development of viable solutions. Methods: Focus group interviews were conducted with community dwelling older adults (n = 52) living in the City of Oshawa in Ontario, Canada; each focus group targeted a specific demographic to ensure a diverse range of perspectives were represented. Data were analyzed to identify themes; sub-group analyses were conducted to understand the experience of those from low socioeconomic status and culturally diverse groups. Results: Themes pertaining to environmental, individual, and task constraints, as well as their interactions, were identified. Of particular novelty, seemingly non-modifiable constraints (e.g., weather and personal health) interacted with modifiable constraints (e.g., urban design). Culturally diverse and lower socioeconomic groups had more favorable perspectives of their neighborhoods. Conclusion: While constraints to active transportation interact to exacerbate one another, there is an opportunity to minimize or remove constraints by implementing age-friendly policies and practices.

Keywords: physical activity; aging; social isolation; cycling; walking

1. Introduction

Active transportation is a mode of transportation in which people get to places using their own power [1]. It is a form of physical activity wherein individuals travel or commute using modes such as walking or cycling. The purpose of the travel is not leisure, but work or task oriented. It is typically used for travel to school or work among children or young adults. Among older adults, active transportation can be used for travel associated with volunteer commitments, daily activities, or medical appointments. This form of transportation contributes significantly to daily physical activity levels and healthy aging [2]. Of utmost importance, it is a form of transportation that is both affordable and accessible.

Encouraging and enabling active transportation in cities may reduce the health burden and social isolation among older adults by facilitating mobility in the community, particularly among older adults who do not have access to a personal vehicle, or in cities where public transportation is suboptimal. However, the design of many communities does not support active transportation, particularly for older adults. The constraints to participating in active transportation are somewhat unique for older adults. For example, research indicates that, unlike young adults, older adults are not comfortable walking on snow-covered sidewalks [3], they require access to public toilets [4], and want benches or rest stops along their route [5]. Thus, the built environment and urban design are critical determinants of active transportation among older adults as it can either serve to limit or promote active transportation.

1.1. Transportation and the Age-Friendly Cities Guideline

To ensure that communities are designed with older adults in mind, the World Health Organization (WHO) put together a guideline on age-friendly cities in 2007 [6]. Many cities around the world have since committed to becoming age-friendly and have developed plans or strategies that have been approved by their municipal government. However, these age-friendly cities still lack significantly in the infrastructure necessary to support active aging and active transportation. Furthermore, active transportation is not directly addressed in the WHO guideline. Much of the emphasis in the *transportation* dimension is on public transportation, while the emphasis of the *outdoor spaces and buildings* dimension is on recreational physical activity. The latter addresses some important issues, however, there is a significant gap in supporting municipalities in creating age-friendly active transportation plans for their older residents.

To inform policies and practices pertaining to the design of age-friendly communities, we must first gather evidence of the issues experienced by older adults in their community. In a review of urban environments and age-friendly cities, Buffell and colleagues [7] cited several constraints that impact the lives of older adults. They suggested that there are many urban hazards that older adults must deal with in order to participate in life or to age in place. Importantly, they argued that older adults must be included in the development and maintenance of age-friendly environments. This may be particularly important in the transportation domain.

According to Shergold and colleagues, the mobility of older adults in their community is compromised by an increasing focus on the car, particularly in rural areas [8]. They also highlighted that many of the activities and services accessed by older adults are within short distances, making active transportation a feasible option. While previous commentaries have noted the need for better active transportation infrastructure [9,10], it is important to highlight again that active transportation is not part of the WHO age-friendly city guideline. As suggested by Lawler (2015), the scale required for transportation infrastructure to support adequate transportation options for older adults is grand, and will require significant investment. Alternatives to the car are needed to support active aging [10]. In fact, alternatives to public transit are also needed. In many cases, older adults cannot afford public transportation, and are thus unable to participate in activities of interest [11].

While some cities have included older adults in understanding transportation related concerns, the focus again has been on public transit [12]. Many cities have some form of public transportation, but some cities are too small to offer door-to-door services. In such cases, transportation becomes multi-modal because older adults may rely on active transportation to get to and from bus stops or train stations. Encouraging use of public transit leads to an increase in time spent in active transportation [13]. However, few plans are available to ensure safe and accessible active transport. We argue that in order for a city to be truly age-friendly, it must increase its focus on active transportation, not just public transit or recreational physical activity.

1.2. Theoretical Model

Work to date has investigated the many environmental constraints [5] as well as the individual constraints, such as fear of falling or health conditions such as arthritis [14], that older adults must negotiate when engaging in active transportation; however, little work has simultaneously assessed a broad array of constraints to understand the interaction between these constraints. This is critical for understanding how we can overcome constraints, and facilitate active transportation in older adults. This gap in knowledge can be addressed using a comprehensive theoretical approach as proposed by Newell [15]. The model is based on the concept that throughout the lifespan, certain constraints have more salience because of developmental stages. Older adulthood is characterized by developmental changes that affect functional independence, thus this model is useful in capturing a crucial stage of development in relation to an individual's environment, and the demands of active transportation. Newell conceptualized optimal behavior and performance as a product of the interaction between three types of constraints: individual, environmental, and task. Individual constraints include structural factors (e.g., height, weight, and fitness) and functional factors (e.g., psychological qualities such as motivation and personality). Environmental constraints include geographical area, the physical environment, sociocultural environment, and policies. Finally, task constraints include the demands of an activity (e.g., ability to balance while performing a specific task) as well as equipment required (e.g., size of wheels on a gait aid such as a walker). The dynamic nature of Newell's [15] model lends itself well to the study of constraints to active transportation because it recognizes that, although some constraints may be more salient for one individual than for another, the lack of one constraint type does not necessarily result in the desired outcome. Rather, it positions the outcome active transportation as a multifaceted problem, which requires multifaceted approaches for development of solutions. Of note, the literature also identifies promotors or facilitators of active aging and active transportation [16,17]. These may limit or counter constraints, but are not necessarily the inverse of constraints.

The purpose of this study was to understand the perspectives of a diverse group of older adults on the individual, environmental, and task constraints to participating in active transportation. While several studies have looked at specific types of constraints, that is, either environmental [4,5] or individual [14], our study is the first, to our knowledge, to investigate task constraints, as well as the interaction between constraints. This is an essential first step in identifying opportunities to properly address constraints. We were interested in speaking to a culturally diverse group of older adults from different socioeconomic environments to ensure that recommendations generated from this work would lead to the development of equitable solutions. Understanding these constraints is an important first step to helping cities support active transportation in older adults.

2. Materials and Methods

Study Design: This qualitative study used phenomenology, a method that is used to understand participant experiences [18]. A qualitative approach was necessary as we wanted to hear the voices of a diverse group of older adults whose voices are not often included in discussions pertaining to active transportation. Qualitative research is particularly important in gerontology as it helps clarify important issues related to the experience of aging [19]. Importantly, a survey of constraints would not provide an understanding of the constraints, nor does a validated or reliable survey of such nature exist. Nine focus groups were conducted with older adults, at separate locations, between October 2018 and January 2019. All methods and communications were approved by the Research Ethics Board at the University of Ontario Institute of Technology.

Participants: Community dwelling older adults (aged 55 years and older) were eligible to participate in this study. That is, older adults in assisted living facilities or long-term care were not included. Recruitment was done using several methods and through several contacts from the local senior's community centers. Specifically, to ensure a representative sample of our city, we targeted "newcomer" social groups (n = 2, groups targeted at older adults who had recently immigrated to the country and/or did not speak English), low-income neighborhoods (n = 2, as per the Region of Durham Building on Health in Priority Neighbourhoods Report), and several different community locations including the library (n = 2), seniors centers (n = 2), and an apartment complex (n = 1). This resulted in a sample of 52 older adults. Participation in the study was voluntary, and all participants provided written informed consent.

Place: The focus groups were conducted with residents who lived in a mid-sized city (City of Oshawa) in southern Ontario, Canada. This city recently completed the consultation process to become an Age-Friendly designated city through the WHO. Approximately 1/3 of the population is over the age of 55 years, and there are five community centers in the city that specifically cater to this age group. The city is experiencing significant growth, and will need to prioritize active transportation to support urban mobility. Of note, there is a strong history of car manufacturing in the city which means much of the City's identity and culture is based in cars. The culture is changing, and there is some political will to encourage active transportation.

Interview Guide: The purpose of these focus groups was to uncover and understand the constraints that older adults experience when engaging in active transportation. The focus group interview guide included an explanation of the research and purposes, a definition of active transportation, as well as questions that specifically probed participants about their current engagement in active transportation or their desire to engage in active transportation; their individual, environmental, and task constraints pertaining to active transportation; and their perception on whether their community supported active transportation. No personal, identifying data were collected from any of the participants; however, all participants met our eligibility criteria.

Research Team: The principal researcher and senior author of this paper has a PhD in kinesiology and health sciences with research expertise in the area of active aging. She and two research students conducted all of the focus groups. In some instances, a staff member was present because the participants were being recruited from a specific program. The first author on this paper was not present for data collection. She has expertise in the area of physical activity constraints, is a therapeutic recreation specialist with a bachelor's degree in psychology, a master's degree in health sciences, and several years of clinical experience working with older adults in hospital. The first and last author were responsible for all data analysis and interpretation.

Data Analysis: Audio tapes were transcribed verbatim and reviewed to ensure accuracy. Field notes were taken during the interview by a research student. Each focus group lasted roughly 30–45 min. Focus group transcripts were reviewed and analyzed by IK and SD.

A consensus approach was taken in the directed content analysis of the data. Directed content analysis was guided by processes described by Hsieh and Shannon [20]. A list of relevant concepts and terms was compiled based on existing literature on active transportation, and used as initial coding categories. Data analysis was completed manually by IK and SD. Codes were extracted independently in relation to each of the major areas outlined by the questions from the interview guide. From there, major themes were identified for each of the interview questions by collapsing codes. The research team discussed major themes and any disagreements were resolved during that time. As suggested by Miles and Huberman [21], major themes and corresponding codes were plotted into a flow chart, which identified relationships. The flow chart reflected themes identified during content analysis and identified underdeveloped areas that can be used to inform future research.

Themes were also compared between groups to better understand the differences between culturally diverse groups and groups of different socioeconomic backgrounds.

3. Results

Several themes arose from the data. These were: constraints (environmental, individual, and task) and the interactions between constraints, neighborhood perception, and promoters. Several subthemes arose during the content analysis of the nine focus group transcriptions. These themes and their respective subthemes are detailed below along with a comparison of the perspectives of those from different cultural and socioeconomic groups.

3.1. Theme 1: Constraints and Interactions

Environmental (Table 1), individual (Table 2), and task (Table 3) constraints that arose were consistent with previous literature. Sub-themes and sample quotes are provided in the respective tables.

Table 1. Environmental Constraints: Subthemes, examples and supporting quotations.

Subthemes	Examples Cited	Sample Quotations
Weather	Ice, humidity, cold, rain, snow, and slippery conditions	Like, uh, some places there's too slippy I think and then one has to sort of be careful.
Sidewalks and Roads	Lack of residential snow clearing Quality and width of sidewalk/roads/bike lanes Lack of curb cuts Increased traffic and construction Lack of bike lanes Lack of cross-walks Insufficient length of pedestrian traffic lights	When you get to the winter time the city relies on every individual...to clear their path... But if you ever try walking down them [sidewalks], you'll find that not everyone does, right? Walking is too dangerous. They'll do a bike lane by painting a line, but that doesn't keep the bicycles and cars separate
Urban Design	Car-centric Lack of bike racks Continuity of bike trails Lack of rest stops/benches Lack of phone booths Lack of washrooms/water fountains Distance to stores/services	Um I was wondering how practical it was to um put out some rest stops, you know perhaps a bench or something like that for people who can walk short distances, but just need to stop and-and you know? I think a lot of it is some drivers, car drivers don't accept bikes on the road. They just...I mean you see them go around and they just cut you off. So, I get to the grocery store, where do I put my bike?
Transit	Accommodation for mobility issues Cleanliness of shelters and stops Lack or benches/shelters Connectivity of routes	What we need and not necessarily a full size bus that uses a lot of gas, but a small bus say coming every hour right outside ABC Street, not upon XYZ Road or anywhere else. We need it outside the door. And like maybe a small bus that would take us to doctors appointments, clinics, hospital for appointments and stuff.
City/regional policies and practices	Cars parked in bike lanes Lack of enforcement (snow removal, construction, driving through cross-walks) Trail maintenance (e.g., garbage, animal control)	And they [buses]- they'll sit there for 20–25 min, and that's right in the bike lane, and those are region buses by the way. And if you have a car coming, done, you're done, you're toast . . . I just talked to an officer. He says-he says unless it specifically states on those streets where you have the bike lanes for bicycle, that is enforceable you know, no parking on the bicycle lanes, they don't enforce it. So this at your own discretion, take your chances you know.

Table 2. Individual Constraints: Subthemes, examples and supporting quotations.

Subthemes	Examples Cited	Sample Quotations
Health	*Previous surgeries* *Cognitive impairment* *Pain* *Arthritis* *Herniated disc*	Arthritis slows you down. As you get older you know, your abilities go down …
Fear of falls/injury	Functional fitness Risk of injury Embarrassment Social Isolation	At this stage you can't afford to have a fall, a fall means a fracture or something … so we have to be very careful. I won't even ride my bike on the road anymore. To me, its just too scary. You stay home.
Perception of Personal Safety	Presence of drugs/illicit activity on trails Lack of security patrols Wild animals Lack of lighting and phone booths Poor signage	Drunks, men [people] that are yelling at the top of their voices they're swearing they're … scary. The trails, um, they might be more comfortable knowing that they were um patrolled if it was a paved trail.
Functional Fitness	Balance Agility Mobility Fatigue Strength	I'm afraid of falling that's … a big one for me. Balance, my balance is bad and a lot of us have the same problem. I can't get my leg over the seat to get on the bicycle...
Financial	Cost of bicycle	What about financial barrier to um cycling? What if I don't have a bike or I don't have...and I have to get that stuff.
Personal Characteristics	Lazy Body Lack of knowledge of bike use/safety	Well I'm active at home, but I am too lazy to walk, so in the summer during the days when its hard to get parking over here... I would walk.

Table 3. Task Constraints: Subthemes, examples and supporting quotations.

Subthemes	Examples Cited	Sample Quotations
Task *Walking related*	Gait aids not optimized for outdoor/all terrain use Difficulty with some tasks	I um sometimes have to use a walker because I have arthritis my knees and in the-in the winter, I live in a residential neighbourhood in ABC and in the winter lots of people don't clear their snow properly its everyone's responsibility, and the people at the corers especially. This is really a problem for a person with a walker. ...going to the grocery store, and you have a couple of bags, well it's, I'd rather take my car because of the strength issue involved there.
Cycling related	Height of bike seat Size of seat Balance required to ride	There's all kinds of places I can learn how to drive a car, where do I learn how to drive a bike.

Participants independently generated several unique interactions between constraints while describing their experience (Figure 1). These arose without explicit priming by focus group facilitators. First, the health or functional fitness related constraints (individual) such as arthritis were exacerbated by poor weather (environmental).

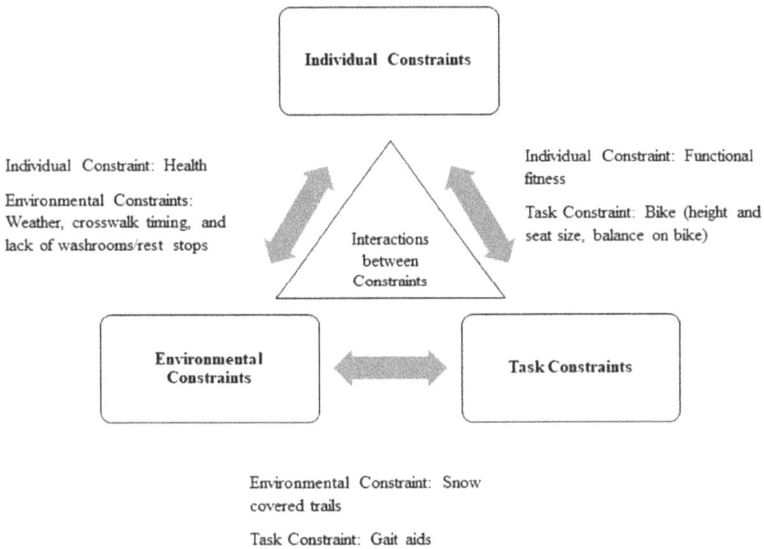

Figure 1. A depiction of the interaction between the constraints to active transportation in older adults.

"In my case I've got a form of cerebral palsy, which I've had all my life and I fall just by looking at a patch of ice, let alone if there's a slight rise in uh sidewalk, I trip if I'm not watching."

Health also interacted with urban design factors such as sidewalks, crosswalk light timing, and lack of washroom facilities, or rest stops. Participants commented on health issues related to aging (e.g., arthritis, pain, and cognitive impairment) with their perception of difficulties navigating their neighborhood.

"So, 15 seconds or 19 seconds or 23 seconds to get from whatever that street is over to the mall is not enough for maybe somebody with a cane or a walker."

Second, navigating bumpy or snow-covered sidewalks with gait aids was also mentioned, suggesting an interaction between environmental and task constraints. The environmental constraint here is two-fold: weather and sidewalk maintenance.

"I sometimes have to use a walker because I have arthritis my knees and in the-in the winter ... lots of people don't clear their snow properly its everyone's responsibility, and the people at the corners especially. This is really a problem for a person with a walker."

This sentiment was echoed by other participants, who also recalled stories of friends or neighbors who experienced similar constraints.

Finally, an interaction between individual and task constraints was mentioned when participants discussed their functional fitness in relationship to the height, seat size, and balance required on a bike. This was in the context of falls among older adults, where one participant noted that:

"At this stage [of life], you can't afford to have a fall ... a fall means a fracture, so we have to be very careful".

The fear of falling was expressed by participants who were not using cycling as a mode of active transportation as well.

3.2. Promoters of Active Transportation

Some constraints raised were subsequently followed up with ways in which participants had negotiated the constraint; thus, participants made positive remarks about factors which facilitated their engagement in active transportation. Participants shared promoters related to the physical and built environment, health benefits, and a number of other factors.

Well maintained trails, the presence of local parks, and city-maintained gardens were all cited as municipality related promoters.

" we are well provided for, but it's just this niggling stuff".

Participants also commented on using active transportation more frequently in the summer or in good weather. Further, some participants mentioned the health benefits of walking.

"If I go for a walk, I'm pain free for hours."

Participants who used public transit spent more time in active transportation due to their walk to and from the bus stop as well as around the destination, and those who had a "buddy system" also engaged in more active transportation. Similarly, a lack of parking spaces forced some older adults to engage in active transportation.

3.3. Neighborhood Perception

Participants identified both positive and negative views of the neighborhood in which they lived. Some participants felt that their neighborhood in the city did not support active transportation and specifically said "we have nothing" or that it was fine for walking but not for cycling. They also mentioned that the infrastructure to support active transportation was not keeping up with urban sprawl and that despite these issues, they did not want to see an increase in their taxes. Those who felt positively about their neighborhood and its ability to support active transportation mentioned that most issues were relatively minor, and that overall the city was doing a good job. The differences in these views may be directly related to socioeconomic status and the neighborhood in which participants reside. For example, sidewalk quality was listed as a constraint in some groups, but others praised the infrastructure in their neighborhood.

3.4. Sub-Group Analysis

Participants in the low SES group generally espoused a more positive neighborhood perception with respect to infrastructure for active transportation, citing easy access to public transit and pride in their neighborhood. In some cases, their perspective was more negative. They cited perception of personal safety and a lack of residential snow clearing more frequently than other groups. Participants shared stories about incidents of crime that they had heard about from acquaintances, in the context of trails and walking paths being unsafe. One participant suggested:

" ... the trails ... [we] might be more comfortable knowing that if they were um patrolled or if it was a paved trail".

Participants in the high SES group shared positive and negative neighborhood perceptions, acknowledging that, although they were generally "well provided for", there were many improvements that needed to be made. Specifically, they cited policy issues as significant constraints to active transportation. These included policies related to infrastructure (wide, paved sidewalks), fines for drivers who fail to stop at a crosswalk or who park vehicles in cycling lanes, and the prospect of having to pay more taxes. As one participant, shared;

" ... there seems to be a lot of inertia in city hall."

Participants recruited from "newcomer" groups shared overall very positive neighborhood perceptions. They judged trails, accessibility (e.g., ramps and accessible entryways to buildings), community gardens and landscaping, and the presence of parks favorably. They frequently cited weather and traffic (secondary to road construction) related constraints, which was similar to other groups.

4. Discussion

Active transportation is an accessible and affordable mode of physical activity that facilitates active ageing. Supporting active transportation in older adults is critical for a city to be truly age-friendly. In fact, our data reveal that lack of support for active transportation prevented older adults from leaving their home, or participating in life. A novel finding of this study was that the constraints that older adults negotiate often interact with one another, exacerbating the primary constraint. It is clear from our data, that, to increase cycling as a mode of active transportation in older adults, several infrastructure investments, policy changes, and supports need to be in place. While walking is associated with fewer constraints, these constraints appear to affect a larger portion of the population. Our data reveal several opportunities for increasing active transportation in age-friendly cities.

Several constraints, such as weather and personal health, could be considered non-modifiable from the perspective of researchers and municipal governments. However, these constraints interacted with *modifiable constraints* such as urban design or skill, which enables development of interventions to increase active transportation. For example, older adults with physical impairments who required gait aids had additional constraints to walking in the winter due to sidewalks being covered in snow or ice. While it would appear that their own physical limitations are the primary constraint, this constraint can be removed or minimized by ensuring that sidewalks are properly maintained throughout the year. This can be dealt with in a number of ways by the municipality: they can make use of novel technologies and implement heated sidewalks, they can change policies and practices so that the onus of winter maintenance is not placed on residents, or they can create covered walking paths. Thus, seemingly non-modifiable constraints may be overcome through appropriate intervention.

This is an important consideration as cities work towards becoming age-friendly. It was clear from our data that urban design and the policies and practices of municipalities are key influencers of engagement in active transportation among older adults. This is in line with previous research that has also found sidewalk characteristics [22], lack of rest stops [23], and timing of lights at cross-walks or intersections [24,25] to be significant constraints to active transportation. A unique urban design constraint that was identified in this work was a lack of public phones. This is interesting in the context of safety. Many youth and adults have personal cellular phones, and thus feel safer when using trails or when out walking or cycling; however, many older adults have not fully adopted this technology, and rely upon pay phones. As cities continue to modernize, such utilities are being removed, and are having unintended consequences. In this case, removal of phones and the safety concerns arising may promote social isolation or reliance of cars [26].

Social isolation was an issue that arose through several focus groups. Participants indicated that fears associated with falling and traffic as well as lack of supportive infrastructure kept them at home. This is problematic as social isolation is a significant concern in our aging population. Estimates suggest that over 20% of older adults are socially isolated, with another 30% at risk [27]. Many age-friendly communities provide programming that encourages social participation of older adults, but are unable to provide appropriate access to active transportation, thus limiting participation. Active transportation, therefore, might be a critical counter measure to social isolation being experienced by older adults.

A novel and interesting aspect of the current work was the sub-analysis of those of lower SES and those who were from culturally diverse backgrounds. Interestingly, participants from newcomer groups were more satisfied with services and urban design compared to other groups. We also found that those in lower socioeconomic groups were more likely to have concerns around safety and urban design issues such as sidewalks, but had more positive overall perceptions of their neighborhood. On the other hand, older adults of higher socioeconomic backgrounds have more concerns with municipal policies and practices. This may be due to a higher level of volunteerism or their own career backgrounds, increasing their awareness and understanding of the importance of municipal workings [28]. The social capital garnered through regular or incidental interactions with neighbors or one's community while engaging in active transportation has also been shown to increase health-promoting behavior [29]. People who live in neighborhoods which promote active transportation have a greater sense of social capital than those who live in car-centric communities [30,31]. Participants in the low socioeconomic groups were the only groups who commented that bus use contributed to their active transportation, which may explain their more positive neighborhood perceptions in the context of social capital gained through this mode.

There are some strengths and weaknesses of this work that should be considered. First, we used a diverse group of older adults from a variety of neighborhoods and formal groups that allowed for important sub-group analyses, and provide a representative sample of our city. Our sample size was also sufficient to reach saturation, and all data were collected over the fall and winter seasons. Some weaknesses of the current study are that we did not include older adults living in assisted living or retirement residences. Isolated older adults living in the community who do not access community centers were also not included. In addition, actual time spent engaging in active transportation was not considered due to the scope of this study, nor was perceived level of loneliness or isolation. Finally, we were unable to include Indigenous Canadians in our study due to the timelines and approval requirements. Future research should consider the experience of older Indigenous Canadians to better understand their experience of active transportation and age-friendly cities.

Implications and Recommendations

This work provides novel insights into active transportation and age-friendly communities. First, based on our findings that constraints to active transportation facilitated social isolation, it is clear that communities aiming to be truly age-friendly must address active transportation in their plans. Second, the interactions identified clearly indicate that many of the non-modifiable constraints to active transportation, such as weather and functional capacity, are exacerbated by policies and practices of local municipalities. Thus, an age-friendly and accessibility lens needs to be applied to all working committees in municipalities. Finally, the differences observed between neighborhoods indicates that there is an inequity in the way municipalities prioritize infrastructure related to active transportation. To ensure accessibility across the diverse range of older adults, more equitable policies and practices need to be put in place.

Based on our work, we would recommend that the WHO Age-Friendly guideline be updated to include active transportation. This would ensure that cities and communities around the world who are interested in the age-friendly designation be required to undertake significant consultation in their communities to better understand the needs of their residents. Given that many cities around the globe are declaring climate emergencies, and there is increasing concern about the health effects of climate change and air pollution [32], an increased emphasis on active transportation is both timely and necessary. We would also recommend that municipalities include active transportation in their master transportation plans, and consult with older adults when working on these plans. According to statistics from major cities, older adults are disproportionally the victims of traffic related fatalities [33], and many cities have unknowingly promoted victim blaming strategies to help older adults in reducing these fatalities. For example, police and municipalities have encouraged pedestrians to wear reflective clothing, remove earphones, and make eye contact with drivers while walking or cycling, instead of putting in appropriate infrastructure that ensures the safety of those engaging in active transportation. This is an indicator of the car-centric culture of cities. Finally, it is clear that urban design is critical for facilitating active transportation. Thus, municipal staff in charge of urban planning need to develop more age-friendly policies. For example, new developments could be required to ensure appropriate multi-use pathways, protected bike lanes, and rest stops and benches. While it requires significant finances to retrofit old neighborhoods, no new car-centric neighborhoods should be created moving forward.

Ultimately, we found that active transportation is central to an age-friendly city, and needs to be more carefully considered by the WHO as well as local municipalities. Future research comparing health and quality of life of older adults living in communities that support active transportation to those who do not is needed to determine the magnitude of the impact of active transportation.

5. Conclusions

Focus group data from a diverse group of older adults indicate that they negotiate several individual, environmental, and task related constraints to participating in active transportation, and, while these constraints interact to exacerbate one another, there is an opportunity to minimize or remove constraints by implementing age-friendly policies and practices. For a city to be truly age-friendly, active transportation must be prioritized.

Author Contributions: S.D. was responsible for conceptualization and data collection. I.K. and S.D. performed data analysis, drafted the manuscript, and approved the final version of the manuscript.

Funding: This research was funded by the Social Sciences and Humanities Research Council, grant number 892-2018-1029, as well as the City of Oshawa's Teaching City fund.

Acknowledgments: We would like to thank the Oshawa Senior Community Centres for their support throughout this work, especially the support of Colleen Zavrel who assisted greatly with recruitment.

Conflicts of Interest: The authors declare no conflict of interest.

Ethics: All procedures were approved by the Research Ethics Board at the University of Ontario Institute of Technology (#15018), and all participants provided written consent prior to participation in the study.

References

1. Government of Canada. Active Transportation. 2014. Available online: https://www.canada.ca/en/public-health/services/being-active/active-transportation.html (accessed on 4 December 2019).
2. Mueller, N.; Rojas-Rueda, D.; Cole-Hunter, T.; De Nazelle, A.; Dons, E.; Gerike, R.; Goetschi, T.; Panis, L.I.; Kahlmeier, S.; Nieuwenhuijsen, M. Health Impact Assessment of Active Transportation: A Systematic Review. *Prev. Med.* **2015**, *76*, 103–114. [CrossRef]
3. Clarke, P.; Hirsch, J.A.; Melendez, R.; Winters, M.; Gould, J.S.; Ashe, M.; Furst, S.; McKay, H. Snow and Rain Modify Neighbourhood Walkability for Older Adults. *Can. J. Aging Rev. Can. Vieil.* **2017**, *36*, 159–169. [CrossRef] [PubMed]
4. Aspinall, P.A.; Thompson, C.W.; Alves, S.; Sugiyama, T.; Brice, R.; Vickers, A. Preference and Relative Importance for Environmental Attributes of Neighbourhood Open Space in Older People. *Environ. Plan. B Plan. Des.* **2010**, *37*, 1022–1039. [CrossRef]
5. Barnett, D.W.; Barnett, A.; Nathan, A.; Van Cauwenberg, J.; Cerin, E. Built Environmental Correlates of Older Adults' Total Physical Activity and Walking: A Systematic Review and Meta-Analysis. *Int. J. Behav. Nutr. Phys. Act.* **2017**, *14*, 103. [CrossRef] [PubMed]
6. World Health Organization. *Global Age-Friendly Cities: A Guide*; World Health Organization: Geneva, Switzerland, 2007.
7. Buffel, T.; Phillipson, C.; Scharf, T. Ageing in Urban Environments: Developing 'Age-Friendly'cities. *Crit. Soc. Policy* **2012**, *32*, 597–617. [CrossRef]
8. Shergold, I.; Graham, P.; Musselwhite, C. Rural Car Dependence: An Emerging Barrier to Community Activity for Older People. *Transp. Plan. Technol.* **2012**, *35*, 69–85. [CrossRef]
9. Fitzgerald, K.G.; Caro, F.G. An Overview of Age-Friendly Cities and Communities around the World. *J. Aging Soc. Policy* **2014**, *26*, 1–18. [CrossRef]
10. Lawler, K. Age-Friendly Communities: Go Big or Go Home. *Public Policy Aging Rep.* **2015**, *25*, 30–33. [CrossRef]
11. Sheila, N.; Menec, V.H. Older Adults' Perceptions of Age-Friendly Communities in Canada: A Photovoice Study. *Ageing Soc.* **2014**, *34*, 1052–1072.
12. Shiau, T.-A.; Huang, W.-K. User Perspective of Age-Friendly Transportation: A Case Study of Taipei City. *Transp. Policy* **2014**, *36*, 184–191. [CrossRef]
13. Coronini-Cronberg, S.; Millett, C.; Laverty, A.A.; Webb, E. The Impact of a Free Older Persons' Bus Pass on Active Travel and Regular Walking in England. *Am. J. Public Health* **2012**, *102*, 2141–2148. [CrossRef] [PubMed]

14. Mertens, L.; Delfien, V.D.; Benedicte, D.; De Bourdeaudhuij, I.; Brondeel, R.; Van Cauwenberg, J. Individual, Social, and Physical Environmental Factors Related to Changes in Walking and Cycling for Transport among Older Adults: A Longitudinal Study. *Health Place* **2019**, *55*, 120–127. [CrossRef] [PubMed]
15. Newell, K. Constraints on the Development of Coordination. In *Motor Development in Children: Aspects of Coordination and Control*; Martinus Nijhoff Publishers: Dordrecht, The Netherlands, 1986.
16. Manson, J.D.; Hala, T.; Baker, J. Barriers and Promoters for Enrollment to a Community-Based Tai Chi Program for Older, Low-Income, and Ethnically Diverse Adults. *J. Appl. Gerontol.* **2017**, *36*, 592–609. [CrossRef] [PubMed]
17. Loitz, C.C.; Spencer-Cavaliere, N. Exploring the Barriers and Facilitators to Children's Active Transportation to and from School from the Perspectives of Practitioners. *J. Phys. Act. Health* **2013**, *10*, 1128–1135. [CrossRef]
18. Creswell, J.W.; Hanson, W.E.; Clark Plano, V.L.; Morales, A. Qualitative Research Designs: Selection and Implementation. *Couns. Psychol.* **2007**, *35*, 236–264. [CrossRef]
19. Phoenix, C. Why Qualitative Research Is Needed in Gerontology and How We Can Do It Better. *J. Gerontol. Ser. B* **2018**, *73*, 81–85. [CrossRef]
20. Hsieh, H.-F.; Shannon, S.E. Three Approaches to Qualitative Content Analysis. *Qual. Health Res.* **2005**, *15*, 1277–1288. [CrossRef]
21. Miles, M.B.; Huberman, A.M. *Qualitative Data Analysis: An Expanded Sourcebook*, 2nd ed.; Sage Publications: London, UK, 1994.
22. Lee, E.; Dean, J. Perceptions of Walkability and Determinants of Walking Behaviour among Urban Seniors in Toronto, Canada. *J. Transp. Health* **2018**, *9*, 309–320. [CrossRef]
23. Mackett, R.L.; Thoreau, R. Transport, Social Exclusion and Health. *J. Transp. Health* **2015**, *2*, 610–617. [CrossRef]
24. Duim, E.; Lebrão, M.L.; Antunes, J.L.F. Walking Speed of Older People and Pedestrian Crossing Time. *J. Transp. Health* **2017**, *5*, 70–76. [CrossRef]
25. Webb, E.A.; Bell, S.; Lacey, R.E.; Abell, J.G. Crossing the Road in Time: Inequalities in Older People's Walking Speeds. *J. Transp. Health* **2017**, *5*, 77–83. [CrossRef] [PubMed]
26. Yen, I.H.; Flood, J.F.; Thompson, H.; Anderson, L.A.; Wong, G. How Design of Places Promotes or Inhibits Mobility of Older Adults: Realist Synthesis of 20 Years of Research. *J. Aging Health* **2014**, *26*, 1340–1372. [CrossRef] [PubMed]
27. Keefe, J.; Andrew, M.; Fancey, P.; Hall, M. *A Profile of Social Isolation in Canada*; Report Submitted to the F/P/T Working Group on Social Isolation; Mount Saint Vincent University: Halifax, NS, Canada, 2006.
28. Tang, F. Socioeconomic Disparities in Voluntary Organization Involvement among Older Adults. *Nonprofit Volunt. Sect. Q.* **2008**, *37*, 57–75. [CrossRef]
29. Giles-Corti, B.S.; Foster, T.S.; Falconer, R. The Co-Benefits for Health of Investing in Active Transportation. *N. S. W. Public Health Bull.* **2010**, *21*, 122–127. [CrossRef]
30. Leyden, K.M. Social Capital and the Built Environment: The Importance of Walkable Neighborhoods. *Am. J. Public Health* **2003**, *93*, 1546–1551. [CrossRef]
31. Lund, H. Pedestrian Environments and Sense of Community. *J. Plan. Educ. Res.* **2002**, *21*, 301–312. [CrossRef]
32. Orru, H.; Ebi, K.L.; Forsberg, B. The Interplay of Climate Change and Air Pollution on Health. *Curr. Environ. Health Rep.* **2017**, *4*, 504–513. [CrossRef]
33. Vanlaar, W.; Hing, M.M.; Brown, S.; McAteer, H.; Crain, J.; McFaull, S. Fatal and Serious Injuries Related to Vulnerable Road Users in Canada. *J. Saf. Res.* **2016**, *58*, 67–77. [CrossRef]

International Journal of
Environmental Research and Public Health

MDPI

Article

The Role of Mobility Digital Ecosystems for Age-Friendly Urban Public Transport: A Narrative Literature Review

Eugène Loos [1,*,†], Maria Sourbati [2,†] and Frauke Behrendt [3,†]

1 Utrecht University School of Governance, Utrecht University, Bijlhouwerstraat 6, 3511 ZC Utrecht, The Netherlands
2 School of Media, University of Brighton, Brighton BN2, UK; M.Sourbati@brighton.ac.uk
3 Department of Industrial Engineering and Innovation Sciences, Eindhoven University of Technology, PO Box 513, 5600 MB Eindhoven, The Netherlands; f.behrendt@tue.nl
* Correspondence: e.f.loos@uu.nl
† Authors contribute equally.

Received: 31 August 2020; Accepted: 6 October 2020; Published: 14 October 2020

check for updates

Abstract: Within the context of the intersection of the global megatrends of urbanisation, ageing societies and digitalisation, this paper explores older people's mobility, with a particular interest in public transport, and a strong consideration of digital/ICT elements. With a focus on (smart) mobility, the paper aims to conceptualise transport, one of the main domains of age-friendly cities as a core element of a smart, age-friendly ecosystem. It also aims to propose a justice-informed perspective for the study of age-friendly smart mobility; to contribute towards a framework for the evaluation of age-friendly smart transport as a core element of the global age-friendly cities programme that comprises mobility practices, digital data, digital networks, material/physical geographies and digital devices and access; and to introduce the term "mobility digital ecosystem" to describe this framework. The paper uses the method of a narrative literature review to weave together a selected range of perspectives from communications, transport, and mobility studies in order to introduce the embeddedness of both communication technology use and mobility practices into their material conditions. Combining insights from communications, mobility and transport and social gerontology with a justice perspective on ICT access and mobility, the paper then develops a framework to study age-friendly smart mobility. What we call a "mobility digital ecosystem" framework comprises five elements—mobility practices, digital data, digital networks, material geographies, digital devices and access to services. The paper contributes a justice-informed perspective that points towards a conceptualisation of age-friendly smart mobility as a core element of the age-friendly cities and communities in the WHO's global age-friendly cities programme.

Keywords: age-friendly cities; age-friendly urban public transport; smart mobility; age-friendly transport; mobility justice; ICT; older people

1. Introduction

"In 2016, there were 512 cities with at least 1 million inhabitants globally. By 2030, a projected 662 cities will have at least 1 million residents." [1].

"Today, more than half of the world's population live in cities, with this proportion set to rise to two-thirds by 2050. The global population is also ageing rapidly, with the numbers of people aged over 60 set to pass the 1 billion mark over the next decade. A significant and growing number of the world's urban residents are older people—more than 500 million." [2].

These statistics clearly show that two trends, urbanisation and population ageing, are occurring rapidly. Living in an urban area has impact on older people's everyday life and, for this reason, reports on age-friendly/urban ageing have been published by the World Health Organisation (WHO) (2007, 2018) and the Organisation for Economic Cooperation and Development (OECD) [3]. An important point enhancing older people's living conditions is to stay mobile because this contributes to their social inclusion. Digitalisation is a third global trend that intersects with urbanisation and ageing societies. Having access to digital elements of and information about transport in urban settings is crucial for older people. The WHO global age-friendly cities programme [4] and the WHO age-friendly environment programme [4] paid attention to age-friendly and inclusive transport attributes, but less so to Information and Communication Technology (ICT).

One can travel in a city by walking, cycling ((e-)bike), motorcycle, mobility scooter, (shared) taxi, (shared/rented/own) car or by using public transport/mass transit (land and water-based). In terms of their broadly similar general mobility patterns, older people travel less than younger people, considering all modes of travel, and often replace driving a private car, after retirement, by walking and the use of public transport, especially buses [5]. Public transport and walking are the most recurring modes of transport among older people, who are less likely to have cars, in cities in Europe [6,7]. Unsuitability or unavailability of service provision in particular areas or for specific destinations [8] can be major barriers to using public transport. The social element of interacting with others on public transport is an important positive element. Musselwhite, Holland and Walker [9] discuss walking, cycling and public transport in relation to health benefits and speculate about the increasing importance of public and community transport for our ageing societies, alongside technological advances that may enable car use later in live (e.g., assisted and autonomous driving). In terms of active transport, there is limited literature that considers walking [10,11] and cycling [12–14] and both modes [15]—in relation to old age. Walking is often a key link to public transport, as many public transport users (of all ages) walk to and/or from their access point to public transport [16]—known as "door to vehicle" or the "last mile" portion of the journey.

Many studies on transport and age focus on driving and driving cessation [17,18]. One of the few papers taking a broader perspective has been published by Musselwhite, Holland and Walker [9], going beyond the car in terms of modes and also including virtual mobilities in their approach.

Flexible transport services include demand-responsive transport [19] (DRT) and community transport. The latter is positively regarded, especially by women and the oldest old, but a lack of awareness and information amongst older people is often reported [8]—which is interesting as it has similarities to the "trendy" Mobility-as-a-Service (MaaS) (https://maas-alliance.eu/). Several studies show that walking and cycling were viable options for short trips in the urban context, pointing at the role of the walkability of the built environment [8]. There appear to be less unfulfilled travel needs in urban areas compared to other geographies. Overall, studies in this field reviewed by Luiu et al. [8] "show that at least one-third of older people report unmet travel needs" with "women and the oldest older (75 years old and above)" and those without car access reporting these needs the most [8].

Despite the importance of urban public transport to older people's mobility in cities—which could be considered as a fundamental right (see Section 3.3)—this area is characterised by a lack of studies [20]. Our paper will critically discuss the intersection of theoretical and empirical studies pertaining to age-friendly urban public transport in developed countries, embedded in what we call a "mobility digital ecosystem", a notion including also all kinds of digital devices and (access to) services playing a crucial role in this regard (see Section 3.4). Thus, we respond to Marston and Van Hoof's [21] call for making technologies and ICT central to the WHO's age-friendly city checklist and to include transport more centrally in their discussions. Their paper reviews a wider range of technology domains such as smart houses, considers technology barriers to use of public transport and the use of delivery robots, alongside a transport-focused case study—all in relation to age.

After having explained the way we have proceeded with our narrative literature review to explore this field in Section 2, we present its results in Sections 3.1–3.4. The insights will be used in Section 4 to propose a framework for a research agenda that combines insights into the ways older adults make sense of their mobility digital ecosystem, focusing on older people's ICT (in)capability in relation to the role of the built urban environment (including technologies and systems of transport/communications) to enhance inclusive mobilities in later life.

In our paper, we will adopt a mobility approach to age, which means that, instead of focusing on functional/utilitarian (economic/engineering) and trip aspects, we will use a broader understanding of mobility that includes social, emotional, embodied and political elements [9,22,23].

2. Method: Narrative Literature Review

We conducted a narrative literature review "in which the findings (...) of relevant studies are outlined and discussed with a view to presenting an argument about the conclusions that can be drawn from the current state of knowledge in a field" [24]. Systematic literature reviews, often used in the field of quantitative evidence-based empirical studies, are not well suited to social science topics that explore new topics, and particularly not for multi-disciplinary areas such as the focus of this paper (see e.g., [25]).

Insights from communications [26–28] and transport technology use [29,30] and transport mobility practices [31,32] will be used in Section 3.1 as a starting point to explore the materialities and digital elements of communications, mobility and transport. Reports from the World Health Organization and publications such as those by Alley, Liebig, Pynoos and Banerjee [33], Buffel, Handler and Phillipson [34] and Steels [35] will be used to get an insight into transport and mobility in age-friendly cities (Section 3.2). In Section 3.3, we will discuss the importance of mobility rights for older people by building on Sheller's concept of *"mobility justice"* [36] comprising differential access to spaces, services and social goods as "not just the result" of racial, gendered, classed, sexed, and, in our study, aged formations, but also "as *productive* of those hierarchical systems of differentiation, through various kinds of enablement and disablement" [36]. The studies by Behrendt, Murray, Hancox, Sourbati and Huber [37] and Sourbati and Behrendt [38] will be used to explore how we can move forward to age-friendly smart mobility in Section 3.4. Then, in Section 4, we will use the insights from Sections 3.1–3.4 as a conceptual framework to understand the dynamics of the use of digital devices and (access to) services as practices in an urban "mobility digital ecosystem".

3. Literature

3.1. Communications, Mobility and Transport as Material and Digital Entanglements

This section weaves together a selected range of perspectives from communications studies, transport studies and mobility studies to introduce the embeddedness of both communication technology use [26,27] and transport mobility practices [31,32] into their material conditions.

Historically, electronic communication technologies and motorised transport have been commonly contextualised in terms of one another [29]. During the interwar period of the 20th century, both new media technologies (radio and moving image) and transportation (the automobile, air travel) were "[c]onsistently paired" in public discourse as the prime agents behind the proliferation of modes of connection and contact between people and places [30,31]. Originating in the early years of communications studies, this perspective on communication as "organized movement and action" [30] has been revisited in the study of more recent developments surrounding mobility and contact as media technology and transportation "remain inextricably linked in ways that are both conceptual and material" [29]. Over the last 10–15 years, transportation, typically understood as a form of organised movement, has embedded digital ICT [39,40]. Research into the ways digital ICTs, in particular the smartphone, have profoundly changed the ways in which transport systems are perceived and used, and mobilities performed, has underlined the contribution of smart apps to the encouragement of sustainable travel [41].

Both communication and transport are entanglements of material and virtual elements, comprising fixed, in-place infrastructures, including roads, railways, pavements, transit stations, bus stops, traffic lights, and Wi-Fi infrastructure; motorised and non-motorised vehicles [5,7,42] communications devices; connectivity, such as mobile internet, street sensors or cameras; systems of licensing and regulation (e.g., governing the provision of telecommunications/network connectivity and the collection, ownership and sharing of digital data [43]), and embodied practices of movement [44]. Moving around the city integrates mediated communication with material forms of movement and action [27,30,45]. Communication can be seen to play an important role in the constitution of socio-spatial territories [28] by combining and integrating the movement of people and information. Thus, mobile media use has profound social consequences as "not only means of communication but increasingly also of generating data" [46] Contextualised in terms of its material surroundings, mobile communications can be likewise seen to "meld with pedestrian urban ecologies" [45]. Within this entanglement, the interaction of walkers, passengers, drivers, riders, etc., combines material infrastructures and mediated or symbolic forms, such as information, data and meanings. Infrastructures, understood as systems that facilitate action in communication [47] and transport [48] are shaped by pre-existing cultural logics that serve to inform, but also "amplify', and "inflect" their adoption and contemporary uses, often producing stratified, mediated connections [28].

Social imaginaries of age [49] are an example of how cultural logics have historically informed the design of infrastructures and technologies in transport systems [31], pedestrian movement and journey planning applications [50] and, more generally, ICT design [51,52], smart mobile telephony [53–55] and Artificial Intelligence (AI) [56].

Within a broader context of wider social changes such as the growing and ageing urban populations that overlay and interact with mobility [5], the needs of older city residents are beginning to receive some acknowledgement across Europe as an area of smart city policy outcomes [57] but these are yet to be addressed by stakeholders. In this socio-economic context, the digital ICT capabilities of older groups and the growing diversity of ageing urban populations constitute an important conversation to be held on the future of urban mobility—and of the city [58]. In Section 3.4, we will focus on the specific role of digital devices for (access to) urban public transport services.

3.2. *Transport and Mobility in Age-Friendly Cities*

The creation of age-friendly environments worldwide has been promoted by the World Health Organization (WHO) [59,60] who define an "age-friendly" city as a city that "optimiz[es] opportunities for health, participation, and security in order to enhance quality of life as people age" [59]. Transportation, including accessible and affordable public transport, is a key theme in the WHO age-friendly city checklist [59]. Alley, Liebig, Pynoos, Banerjee and Choi [33] underline the involvement of older people in age-friendly environments and describe age-friendly cities and communities as "places that actively involve, value, and support older adults, both active and frail, with infrastructure and services that effectively accommodate their changing needs" while Buffel, Handler and Phillipson [34] underline the significance of finding ways older people themselves can be involved in the co-production of age-friendly policies and practices. For more information about the characteristics of age-friendly cities, see also [21,61].

Age-friendly cities and communities (AFCC) [60] have become an important area of work in the field of public policy and ageing, reflecting the importance of the physical and social environment in maintaining the quality of life of older people, given the complexity of demographic change [61] in the context of global "megatrends" [62,63] that also include rapid urbanisation, digital ICT and climate change. The age-friendly agenda has resulted in an increased discussion of problems facing older people living in urban environments as well as of strategies and initiatives which ensure policies, services and products meet the needs of older persons [21,35]. As population aging becomes a widely noted "issue-fied"matter [64] that is granted urgency, significant political motivations are emerging to pursue "age-friendly" community initiatives [65]. This growth in interest in "age-friendly" issues by public policy and stakeholders has stimulated new approaches to the built environment, housing and neighbourhood design that highlight the importance of physical contexts [66]. Information and communication technology (ICT) has been integral to these approaches [5,7,42].

With AFCC debates and initiatives now taking off, social policy and critical gerontology scholars are highlighting the need to integrate research with policy [34] for age-friendly strategies to promote the health and wellbeing of older adults [67]. Applying a more inter-generational perspective, sustainable all age-friendly models [68,69] can create urban spaces and places inclusive of social and emotional aspects of intergenerational belonging and community [58]. From the perspective of mobility (and transport), we understand age-friendly models to embrace social and environmental citizenship in addition to social policy goals, including safe and sustainable travel and connection to other people.

Transport and mobility, both in their traditional forms as well as in "smart" mode, should, therefore, be seen as a core component of age-friendly cities and communities. Transportation has been highlighted by the WHO [59] as a key factor that influences active and healthy aging, and so is "Information and Communication" (see also Figure 1). Smart Transport is arguably situated at the intersection of these two topics—as it refers to the use of digital technologies to improve transport by improving access to information about any aspect of the journey, including destination and pickup points, booking and payment systems, timetable, etc. Smart Transport can enhance age-friendly outcomes, such as the ability to move about the city, which in turn "determines social and civic participation and access to community and health services" [59]. According to Gassmann, Böhm and Palmié [70], smart mobility pursues sustainable, innovative, and secure transportation systems; access to diverse transportation modes; good availability in the entire city; inclusion of nonmotorized transportation; integration of ICT in transportation systems (see also Section 3.4, where the concept of smart mobility will be discussed more in detail). These objectives can promote the "age-friendly" agenda [59,60] based on inclusive ICT: we propose the concept of all age-friendly transport (similar to Murray's [22] argument) where the design and deployment of digital ICT and data are steered towards the creation of tools to support inclusivity, e.g., by widening the participation of excluded older groups who are typically the most excluded in the digital economy (though not the only ones), and sustainability. A focus on transport and mobility can highlight broader areas of impact of the converging trends in digital ICT, datafication, mediatisation, climate and demographic change [38]. Accordingly, we conceptualise age-friendly infrastructures as smart, green, public, inclusive, sustainable, and safe. This approach links the WHO's Age-Friendly Cities and Communities to the UN sustainability goals, specifically the goals "reduced inequalities" and "sustainable cities and communities" [71]; see also Figure 1.

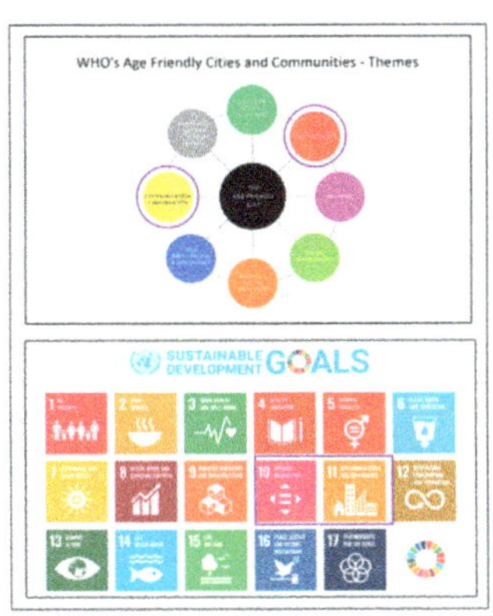

Figure 1. The two key themes of the WHO's Age-Friendly Cities and Communities and of the UN's Sustainable Development Goals (highlighted in purple) most relevant to this paper. Author's illustration, based on illustrations by [72] and by [73].

3.3. Access, Equity and Mobility Justice in the City

If we wish to ensure that older people can continue to participate in our society, then access to services and (digital) information about these services are of prime importance [74]. Van den Hoven [75], referring to Rawls [76,77], goes so far as to refer to accessible information as a "primary good". As all citizens have an equal right to access to information, Bovens [78] and Bovens and Loos [79] even advocate granting citizens information rights, next to the classic (freedom) rights. It is important to refer here to an initiative to guarantee the rights of older people, The Madrid Plan of Action [80], offering "a bold new agenda for handling the issue of ageing in the 21st-century. It focuses on three priority areas: older persons and development; advancing health and well-being into old age; and ensuring enabling and supportive environments." See also the related UN Report of the Second World Assembly on Ageing [81] and the Follow-Up to the Second World Assembly on Ageing [82].

In the context of access to mobility and transport services (and information about them), cultural age-related bias remains a major impediment to age-friendly city initiatives. Older people have been systematically excluded from participation in decision making [34,83] and continue to remain invisible in research and datasets [38,56]. In order to widen the participation of excluded groups such as older (and younger) pedestrians and public transport users in transport and social policy, it is therefore important to focus on age as a social category in its own right while simultaneously recognizing social inequalities within the older adult population [84].

Enhancing the participation of excluded groups and their access to services points towards a conceptualisation of smart mobility as a core element of the age-friendly city that aims to frame smart transport mobility [34,85] as an area for debate and policy intervention based on a better understanding of the mobility activity, transport use and travel patterns [31,86], and mobile media use patterns of a diversity of (older) groups and how these are developing during their life course. While mobility and/or digital connectedness are key to reaching many opportunities, it is important not to conflate mobility (or digital connectedness for that matter) with accessibility.

Attuned to human rights and freedoms perspectives [31], access to ICT connectivity, destinations, and modes of transport foregrounds questions of resource (re)distribution, equity and justice, as captured in evolving discussions of transport and mobility justice [39,87,88]. Mobility is "a prerequisite for citizens to have independence and participate in activities, access services, and form social relations" [31]. Accordingly, differential access to spaces, places, services and social goods through transport systems are "not just the result" of inequality but are "also *productive* of [...] hierarchical systems of differentiation, through various kinds of enablement and disablement" [39].

Fainstein's [89,90] concept of a "just city" and her work to identify approaches to realizing it within the urban context can provide a bridge between justice-oriented perspectives on mobility, transport and the city.

To assess implementation of policy goals, justice-oriented research into mobility [91], transport [92] and ICT [93] has been drawing on the capabilities approach (CA) as developed by Sen [94] and Nussbaum [95]. The concept of capabilities for wellbeing has been applied here to study policy responses to the needs, experiences and practices of diverse groups. Capabilities define the sets of freedoms and opportunities available for individuals to choose and to act to fulfil their basic potential. At a minimum, these comprise rights to life, health, bodily integrity, access to education, and the ability to participate politically and materially in shaping one's environment [94,95]. Conceptualising capabilities as an interface of situated individuals and contextual factors [96] helps to identify areas for policy intervention to address the social basis of capabilities [95,97] and strategies to influence the opportunities and overcome barriers. Since the 1990s, the capabilities approach has provided a well-reasoned case, based on a justice perspective for the promotion of the UN's Millennium Goals [98] and Sustainable Development Goals (SDGs) [99], linked to the WHO's definition of Healthy Ageing [100,101]. In this paper, we take a capability approach to the study of mobility in old age based on a multidimensional understanding of accessibility that acknowledges the diversity of people's needs and constraints [31,91,92]. A "capability approach" offers a strong conceptual framework to assess the implementation of policy goals, including those surrounding age-friendly cities and communities (AFCC) and, more generally, the progress of the Sustainable Development Goals (see also Figure 1). Like the SDGs, the capability approach takes a multi-dimensional perspective, is applicable to all societies, shows concern for "all people, everywhere", and has interconnectedness across dimensions at its core [102].

3.4. Towards Age-Friendly Smart Mobility

The studies by Behrendt, Hancox, Huber, Murray and Sourbati [37] and Sourbati and Behrendt [84] into the role of inclusive public transport address wider societal challenges such as loneliness and isolation, civic participation, connectivity and health and wellbeing in relation to mobility and the physical–environmental context. Here, they are brought into conversation from the perspective of age-friendly, inclusive transport, especially the topic areas of "transportation" and "information and communication" in the WHO Global age-friendly cities programme [5] (https://www.who.int/ageing/projects/age_friendly_cities/en/) to highlight the importance of smart mobility and transport for the social inclusion of ageing urban populations.

Jeekel [102] discusses smart mobility in the context of those who are involuntarily "transport disadvantaged" by having greater efforts in getting to locations that are relevant for their regular activities, either through distance or through "forms of disability", which, for him, include age [103]. Out of the four smart mobility elements he identifies—vehicle technology, intelligent transport systems, data, and mobility as a service—he highlights that the potential of data for public transport is currently not very well realised, while automated driving is likely to serve those older people who are not disadvantaged [103]. Jeekel [102] sees the best potential in mobility as a service. However, he also cautions how this will be financed for the transport disadvantaged, how prices will be set, how subsidies will work, and also how MaaS would be replacing or complementary to public transport [102]. We agree with Jeekel [102] that it is important to be aware that "digital literacy" is required to engage with mobile devices for booking MaaS. Being able to buy and handle user-friendly digital devices for (access to) services for urban public transport is crucial (see also Section 4).

Battarra et al. [103] consider a number of projects to identify seven categories of smart mobility measures for older citizens (improvement of public transport, improvement of public transport comfort, improvement of road network, ITS for private transport, promotion of soft mobility, promotion of shared mobility, implementation of info-mobility services) and analyse Italian cities (across several parameters each for safety, accessibility, ICT). However, while some ICT items measured might be useful for older inhabitants, e.g., electronic bus stop signs, others might instead act as barrier, e.g., electronic travel tickets on mobile devices, and, in that sense, can be considered as enabling constraints [104].

The social element of mobility is also a key consideration in the context of ageing societies. Jeekel [102] calls for creating "a transport system that maximises the possibility to meet, via mobility, all sorts of people, and is basically about the power of joint experiences, dialogue, and creating community via transport and transport services" [102]. This is an issue relevant for both ICT and mobility, but is often forgotten at their intersection.

Just as cycling is often excluded from "smart mobility" industry and policy agendas in favour of a car-centric approach [105] it would be pertinent to analyse if the same is true for older people (in favour of those of "working" age). National policies on transport and mobility need to take an inclusive approach [103], including considerations around (older) age. The same is true for ICT/digital policies. The quickly growing intersection between both—where mobility and smart technologies merge—needs to be high on policy agendas to make inclusivity and age diversity key requirements and features of current and future smart mobility developments, to channel the rapid industry development (in both the digital and transport sector) in these areas towards inclusive, sustainable and just cities and societies.

4. Mobility Digital Ecosystems in Later Life: Framework for a Research and Policy Agenda

The preceding discussion shows the importance of integrating the examination of continuities in media technologies and transport systems, the socio-cultural logics informing their design, and changes made possible by digital connectivity and data in order to understand the affordances of (smart) transport systems in promoting or impeding mobility for older people as well as younger age groups. Drawing on capability analysis, transport and mobility were discussed as person–environment, interactive and resource-dependent practices, highlighting the role of public policy in shaping access to those systems. The policy, the design, the spatial, the personal and the social elements can be understood as interconnected in the provision of opportunities to access transport and mobility capacity.

In this final section, we will use these insights in a framework for developing research and policy that recognises the importance of smart transport as an integral element of smart, age-friendly cities of the future (see also Figure 2). We coin the term "mobility digital ecosystem" for this framework; see also Marston and Van Hoof's [21] concept of a "digital ecosystem", proposed for a critical discussion of the WHO's notion of an "age-friendly city". We put the word "mobility" in front of their "digital ecosystem" to highlight how the cultural, social and political context of public urban transport used by older people increasingly intertwines digital and mobility elements. The mobility digital ecosystem is composed of five elements—mobility practices, digital data, digital networks, material geographies, digital devices and (access to) services—as follows:

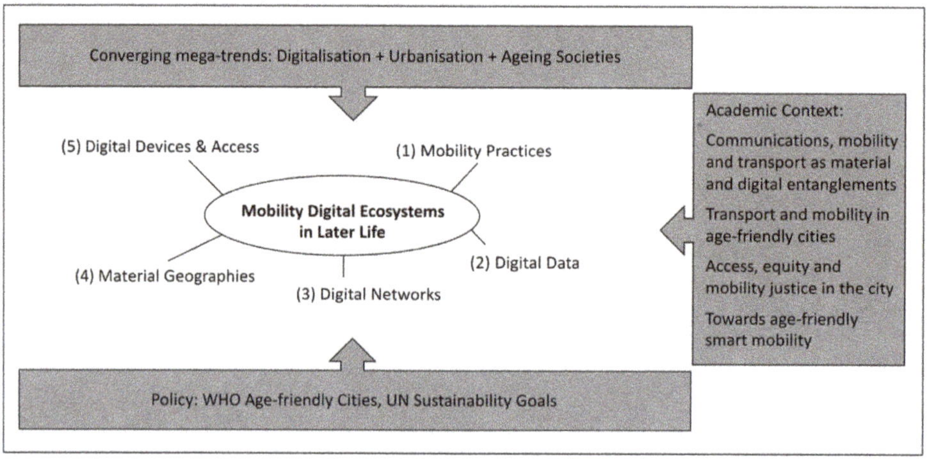

Figure 2. The framework "Mobility Digital Ecosystems in Later Life" and its five elements, within the larger societal (top), policy (bottom) and academic (right) contexts.

(1) Mobility has been broadly defined in relation to the embodied practices of moving around (Merriman and Pearce [44] and the wellbeing of individuals, as the ability to choose where and when to travel and which activities to participate in outside the home in everyday life [91]. Mobility practices integrate personal and environmental components [31] and combine material and digital objects [106]. Digital, mobile ICTs such as the mobile phone not only support social connectivity when their users are in physical motion [107] but also support movement in place, through the production and use of digital data [89]. ICT and data infrastructures are increasingly integrated into an expanding range of mobility including walking, velomobility/cycling [106] and other non-motorised means of transport, as well as electrically assisted modes of transport including bicycles, cargo bicycles and freight vehicles, push scooters, skateboards, trikes and personal mobility devices alongside motorised vehicles such as private cars, car sharing and public transport. All these modes describe complexes of social practice (including working, shopping, leisure, visiting friends and family) which are embedded into their material

conditions [31] and connected to infrastructural arrangements across space and time [108] (e.g., routes, destinations, shelters, data infrastructures) and included or excluded [109] in ways that cannot be controlled by individuals alone. Thus, mobility can usefully be analysed as a "person–environment relationship" (see, e.g., [110]) of transport mobility, comprising the physical/geography of places and the built environment, the social/cultural and the institutional/regulatory systems [111,112]. These practices of mobility and experiences of age shape and influence each other. Older people's mobility patterns are changing but not in a homogenous manner. With mobility widely recognised as an important factor in older people's wellbeing, Levin emphasises the need to consider variations in experiences of age and mobility practice among older groups, including in health and fitness and places of residence, in the application of recurrent concepts of wellbeing and independence. Multi-modal mobility can therefore play a key role in encouraging the use of public transport along more active modes in the transition from automobility, including after the cessation of driving licenses.

(2) Digital data: As the range of digital ICT applications is expected to increase, our cities and transport systems become more instrumental in providing data for digital AI application development [113], combined with data generated through mobile ICT use [38]. Accordingly, both the role of this data and our expectations and use of AI are bound to increase. Age-friendly smart public urban transport requires algorithms that are capable of setting up bias-free training datasets and statistical models capable of incorporating the digital media practices of broader population segments [56].

(3) Smart mobility relies on digital networks, in addition to mobile physical objects and people, while smart mobility involves data collection and analysis on a scale [114]. Smart mobility systems combine physical, digital and data infrastructures. These comprise intelligent transport systems, where networked ICT capability is applied in existing mobility systems, including sensors in public roads and parks, Internet of Things (IoT) solutions built into public and private transportation modes such as buses and cars, and citizens' use of networked ICT (e.g., traffic management), data, and new mobility services [115]. According to Gassmann, Böhm and Palmié [74], smart mobility pursues the core objectives of sustainable, innovative, and secure transportation systems, access to diverse transportation modes, good availability in the entire city, the inclusion of nonmotorized transportation, and the integration of ICT in transportation systems. Expanding the conceptualisations of mobility as a person–environment relationship [115,116] to encompass digital data generation, registration and use, we can develop a socially oriented analysis of smart mobility in urban settings for later life.

(4) Together with material geographies and built environments (such as roads, pavements, parks, city centres, the systems of roads and pavements, traffic lights, Wi-Fi) [7,27], the digital infrastructures of a city have consequences for transport and mobility. Their construction and regulation shapes both the kinds of effects that existing spatial arrangements may have (on transport systems and organised movement) and the new spaces created by smart ICT (see [117]). These also highlight areas of opportunity. Older people are currently underserved by transport systems with physical and digital infrastructures, including the surface of pavements, the provision of benches, seating areas in terminals and bus stops [5], pedestrian crossing lights [117], digital interfaces such as journey planners and maps designed for more able-bodied younger users, and can be seen as discriminatory [5]. Smart transport solutions can make public transport, and community/flexible transport services more accessible by both addressing barriers to access relating to difficulties in getting information about the provision of services, as well as by enabling the signalling of demand for travel services and making viable flexible transport solutions [40] as well as issues relating to security/safety on board [8] In an urban context, promoting opportunities to access mobility entails both physical and social infrastructures of media and transport access.

(5) Digital devices and (access to) services are crucial to enable (e.g., by providing access to transport information) older people's urban mobility. However, we should beware of the fact that, at the same time, digital devices also risk constraining older people—for example, when people are incapable or not willing to use digital devices, e.g., because they are perceived as too complex or

expensive [118,119]. Thus, digital devices can be seen as enabling constraints [104]. It is also important to mention the so called "I-methodology', which is "the reliance on personal experience, whereby the designers consider themselves as representatives of the user" [120] and, without being aware of it, produce user representations that resemble themselves (designers tend to be younger adults). To enable older people to be mobile in an urban setting as much as possible, it is therefore important to give them a voice by involving them in the co-design of user-friendly digital devices (see [121]) and the co-production of age-friendly digital policies and practices (see [33]).

5. Conclusions

Within the context of the intersection of the global megatrends of urbanisation, ageing societies and digitalisation, this paper explores older people's mobility, with a particular interest in public transport, and a strong consideration of digital/ICT elements. It presents a transdisciplinary and a mobilities approach to age that is a "broader navigation of the experiences of ageing and the ways in which people of different ages experience urban spaces" [22]. The approach integrates the examination of continuities in media technologies and transport systems, the socio-cultural logic informing their design, and changes made possible by digital connectivity and data, in that order. This involves understanding the affordances of (smart) transport systems in promoting or impeding mobility for older people as well as younger age groups.

The paper combined insights from the communications, mobility and transport literature (including [26,27,31,32]) and social–gerontology research on transport, mobility, and age-friendly cities (including Alley, Liebig, Pynoos and Banerjee [33], Buffel, Handler and Phillipson [61], Buffel and Phillipson [34] and Steels [35]). Furthermore, it drew on justice perspectives related to media/technology access, equity and mobility (such as Sheller [88]) and on age-friendly smart mobility [38,103]. The paper also drew on the policy literature and initiatives such as the WHO Global age-friendly cities and communities programme and the UN's sustainable development goals. Building on these bodies of academic and grey literature, the paper developed the concept of the "mobility digital ecosystem", which engages with the services and digital information around public urban transport used by older people. This concept forms the backbone of the proposed framework for a research and policy agenda that combines insights into the ways older adults make sense of their mobility digital ecosystem, focusing on older people's ICT (in)capability in relation to the role of the built urban environment (technologies and systems of transport/communications) to enhance inclusive mobilities in later life. The "mobility digital ecosystem" is comprised of five elements—mobility practices, digital data, digital networks, material geographies, digital devices and (access to) services (see also Figure 2).

This interdisciplinary review has highlighted that smart urban public transport for older people is currently under-researched, despite its growing importance in the context of the urbanisation, digitalisation and ageing of societies around the globe. Future research in this area could include empirical work that draws on the literature and concepts identified in this narrative literature review, such as analysing policy documents at transnational, national regional or local levels, and interviews with older people, as well as relevant policy and industry stakeholders. Furthermore, studies on urban mobilities, public transport, old age, and digital society should ideally take into consideration each of these elements, rather than only focusing on one of them. This is also relevant to research on smart cities. Future research should also consider structural differences between countries and areas to understand in more detail how urban mobility and digital literacy differ for older people, for example, between Northern and Southern Europe, but also on a global scale. The research options sketched out here would also contribute to validating (elements) of the framework we developed in this paper.

The review has also shown how important it is that international, national, regional and local policies on both transport/mobility and ICT take an age-inclusive approach. This could translate into a number of practical policy steps. Funding opportunities as policy tools in the areas of mobility and ICT could stipulate the inclusion of older age groups, for example, as participants in pilots or in design/user experience (UX) approaches, such as personas or user journey maps. This could also be extended to commissioned policy reports, tendering and commissioning. It is important for policy agendas to make inclusivity and age diversity a key requirement and feature of current and future smart mobility developments, in order to channel the rapid industry development (in both the digital and transport sector) in these areas towards inclusive, sustainable and just cities and societies. Overall, this paper contributed a justice-informed perspective that points towards the conceptualisation of smart mobility as a core element of an age-friendly city.

Author Contributions: Conceptualization, E.L., M.S.; methodology, E.L.; formal analysis, E.L., M.S., F.B.; resources, E.L., M.S., F.B.; writing—original draft preparation, E.L., M.S., F.B.; writing—review and editing, E.L., M.S., F.B.; visualization, F.B.; funding acquisition, F.B. All authors have read and agreed to the published version of the manuscript.

Funding: The research for this article was partially funded by the Arts and Humanities Research Council (AHRC) under grant AH/S004475/1 "Creative and Industry Approaches to Mobility in the Age of the Internet of Things, Blockchain and Data (CIAM)".

Conflicts of Interest: The authors declare no conflict of interest.

References

1. United Nations Department of Economic and Social Affairs. The World's Cities in 2016: Data Bookelt. *Int. J. Electrochem. Sci.* **2016**. Available online: https://www.un.org/en/development/desa/population/publications/pdf/urbanization/the_worlds_cities_in_2016_data_booklet.pdfURL (accessed on 10 October 2020).
2. *HelpAge International Ageing and the City: Making Urban Spaces Work for Older People*; AGE Platform Europe: Brussels, Belgium, 2016.
3. OECD. *Ageing in Cities*; OECD: Paris, France, 2015.
4. Anon Global Age-Friendly Cities Project. Available online: https://www.who.int/ageing/projects/age_friendly_cities/en/ (accessed on 21 February 2020).
5. Foresight, A. *Time of Unprecedented Change in the Transport System*; Foresight: Palo Alto, CA, USA, 2019.
6. LaPlante, J.; Kaeser, T.P. A History of Pedestrian Signal Walking Speed Assumptions. In Proceedings of the 3rd Urban Street Symposium: Uptown, Downtown, or Small Town: Designing Urban Streets That Work, Seattle, WA, USA, 24–27 June 2007; The National Academies of Sciences, Engineering, and Medicine: Seattle, WA, USA, 2007.
7. Arup. Help Age International; Intel; Systematica Shaping Ageing Cities. 10 European Case Studies. 2015. 102. Available online: https://ifa.ngo/wp-content/uploads/2015/09/Shaping-Ageing-Cities_A4_web-1.pdf (accessed on 10 October 2020).
8. Luiu, C.; Tight, M.; Burrow, M. The unmet travel needs of the older population: A review of the literature. *Transp. Rev.* **2017**, *37*, 488–506. [CrossRef]
9. Musselwhite, C.; Holland, C.; Walker, I. The role of transport and mobility in the health of older people. *J. Transp. Health* **2015**, *2*, 1–4. [CrossRef]
10. Ghani, F.; Rachele, J.N.; Washington, S.; Turrell, G. Gender and age differences in walking for transport and recreation: Are the relationships the same in all neighborhoods? *Prev. Med. Rep.* **2016**, *4*, 75–80. [CrossRef] [PubMed]
11. Pollard, T.M.; Wagnild, J.M. Gender differences in walking (for leisure, transport and in total) across adult life: A systematic review. *BMC Public Health* **2017**, *17*, 1–11. [CrossRef] [PubMed]
12. Winters, M.; Sims-Gould, J.; Franke, T.; McKay, H. "I grew up on a bike": Cycling and older adults. *J. Transp. Health* **2015**, *2*, 58–67. [CrossRef]
13. Van Cauwenberg, J.; Clarys, P.; De Bourdeaudhuij, I.; Ghekiere, A.; de Geus, B.; Owen, N.; Deforche, B. Environmental influences on older adults' transportation cycling experiences: A study using bike-along interviews. *Landsc. Urban Plan.* **2018**, *169*, 37–46. [CrossRef]
14. Van Cauwenberg, J.; de Geus, B.; Deforche, B. Cycling for transport among older adults: Health benefits, prevalence, determinants, injuries and the potential of e-bikes. *Geogr. Transp. Ageing* **2018**, 133–151. [CrossRef]
15. Mertens, L.; Van Dyck, D.; Deforche, B.; De Bourdeaudhuij, I.; Brondeel, R.; Van Cauwenberg, J. Individual, social, and physical environmental factors related to changes in walking and cycling for transport among older adults: A longitudinal study. *Health Place* **2019**, *55*, 120–127. [CrossRef]

16. Daniels, R.; Mulley, C. Explaining walking distance to public transport: The dominance of public transport supply. *J. Transp. Land Use* **2013**, *6*, 5–20. [CrossRef]
17. Musselwhite, C.; Scott, T. Developing a model of mobility capital for an ageing population. *Int. J. Environ. Res. Public Health* **2019**, *16*, 3327. [CrossRef]
18. Davey, J.A. Older people and transport: Coping without a car. *Ageing Soc.* **2007**, *27*, 49–65. [CrossRef]
19. Coutinho, F.M.; van Oort, N.; Christoforou, Z.; Alonso-González, M.J.; Cats, O.; Hoogendoorn, S. Impacts of replacing a fixed public transport line by a demand responsive transport system: Case study of a rural area in Amsterdam. *Res. Transp. Econ.* **2020**. [CrossRef]
20. Haustein, S.; Siren, A. Older People's Mobility: Segments, Factors, Trends. *Transp. Rev.* **2015**, *35*, 466–487. [CrossRef]
21. Marston, H.R.; Van Hoof, J. "Who doesn't think about technology when designing urban environments for older people?" A case study approach to a proposed extension of the who's age-friendly cities model. *Int. J. Environ. Res. Public Health* **2019**, *16*, 3525. [CrossRef]
22. Murray, L. Age-friendly mobilities: A transdisciplinary and intergenerational perspective. *J. Transp. Health* **2015**, *2*, 302–307. [CrossRef]
23. Garrod, J.Z. The Real World of the Decentralized Autonomous Society. *TripleC* **2016**, *14*, 62–77. [CrossRef]
24. Lewis-Beck, M.; Bryman, A.; Liao, T. The SAGE Encyclopedia of Social Science Research Methods 2003. Sage Publications: Thousand Oaks, CA, USA.
25. Papaioannou, D.; Sutton, A.; Carroll, C.; Booth, A.; Wong, R. Literature searching for social science systematic reviews: Consideration of a range of search techniques. *Health Info. Libr. J.* **2010**, *27*, 114–122. [CrossRef]
26. Morley, D. For a Materialist, Non—Media-centric Media Studies. *Telev. New Media* **2009**, *10*, 114–116. [CrossRef]
27. Morley, D. Communications and transport: The mobility of information, people and commodities. *Media Cult. Soc.* **2011**, *33*, 743–759. [CrossRef]
28. Morley, D. *Communications and Mobility: The Migrant, the Mobile Phone, and the Container Box*; Wiley-Blackwell: Hoboken, NJ, USA, 2017; ISBN 978-1-405-19201-9.
29. Popp, R. Machine-Age Communication: Media, Transportation, and Contact in the Interwar United States. *Technol. Cult.* **2011**, *52*, 459–484. [CrossRef]
30. Sterne, J. Transportation and Communication: Together as You've Always Wanted Them. In *Thinking With James Carey: Essays on Communication, Transportation, History*; Jeremy, P., Craig, R., Eds.; Peter Lang: New York, NY, USA, 2006.
31. Levin, L. How may public transport influence the practice of everyday life among younger and older people and how may their practices influence public transport? *Soc. Sci.* **2019**, *8*, 96. [CrossRef]
32. Levin, L. How to Integrate Gender Equality in the Future of "Smart" Mobility: A Matter for a Changing Planning Practice. In *Proceedings of the HCI in Mobility, Transport, and Automotive Systems*; Krömker, H., Ed.; Springer International Publishing: Cham, Germany, 2019; pp. 393–412.
33. Alley, D.; Liebig, P.; Pynoos, J.; Banerjee, T.; Choi, I.H. Creating elder-friendly communities: Preparations for an aging society. *J. Gerontol. Soc. Work* **2007**, *49*, 1–18. [CrossRef]
34. Buffel, T.; Phillipson, C. A Manifesto for the Age-Friendly Movement: Developing a New Urban Agenda. *J. Aging Soc. Policy* **2018**, *30*, 173–192. [CrossRef] [PubMed]
35. Steels, S. Key characteristics of age-friendly cities and communities: A review. *Cities* **2015**, *47*, 45–52. [CrossRef]
36. Sheller, M. Theorising mobility justice. *Tempo Soc.* **2018**, *30*, 17–34. [CrossRef]
37. Behrendt, F.; Murray, L.; Hancox, A.; Sourbati, M.; Huber, J. *Intelligent Transport Solutions for Social Inclusion, Project Report*; ITSSI: Viterbo, Italy, 2017.
38. Sourbati, M.; Behrendt, F. Smart mobility, age and data justice. *New Media Soc.* **2020**, 1–17. [CrossRef]
39. Cohen-Blankshtain, G.; Rotem-Mindali, O. Key research themes on ICT and sustainable urban mobility. *Int. J. Sustain. Transp.* **2016**, *10*, 9–17. [CrossRef]
40. Gössling, S. ICT and transport behavior: A conceptual review. *Int. J. Sustain. Transp.* **2018**, *12*, 153–164. [CrossRef]
41. Banister, D.; Stead, D. Impact of information and communications technology on transport. *Transp. Rev.* **2004**, *24*, 611–632. [CrossRef]

42. Ormerod, M.; Newton, M.R.; Phillips, J.; Musselwhite, A.C.; Mcgee, S.; Russell, R. *How can Transport Provision and Associated Built Environment Infrastructure be Enhanced and Developed to Support the Mobility Needs of Individuals as they Age? Future of an Ageing Population: Evidence Review*; Government Office for Science: London, UK, 2015.
43. Kitchin, R.; Lauriault, T.P.; McArdle, G. (Eds.) Data and the City. In *Data and the City*; Routledge: Milton Park, Abingdon, Oxfordshire, 2017; pp. 1–12.
44. Merriman, P.; Pearce, L. Mobility and the humanities. *Mobilities* **2017**, *12*, 493–508. [CrossRef]
45. Ito, M. Personal Portable Pedestrian: Lessons from Japanese Mobile Phone Use. *Proc. Asia Pac. J.* **2006**, 3.
46. Breiter, A.; Hepp, A. (Eds.) The Complexity of Datafication: Putting Digital Traces in Context. In *Communicative Figurations*; Palgrave Macmillan: Cham, Germany, 2018; pp. 387–405.
47. Star, S.L.; Bowker, G.C. How to Infrastructure. In *Handbook of New Media: Social Shaping and Consequences of ICTs*; Lievrouw Leah, A., Livingstone, S., Eds.; Sage Publications: Thousand Oaks, CA, USA, 2006; pp. 151–162.
48. Cox, P. *Theorising infrastructure: In The Politics of Cycling Infrastructure*; Cox, P., Koglin, T., Eds.; Policy Press: Cambridge, UK, 2020; pp. 15–34.
49. Higgs, P.; Gilleard, C. The ideology of ageism versus the social imaginary of the fourth age: Two differing approaches to the negative contexts of old age. *Ageing Soc.* **2019**, 1–14. [CrossRef]
50. Sourbati, M. Age and the City: The case of smart mobility. In Proceedings of the Human Aspects of IT for the Aged Population: Technology and Society. 6th International Conference, ITAP 2020, Held as Part of the 22nd HCI International Conference, HCII 2020, Copenhagen, Denmark, 19–24 July 2020; Gao, G., Zhou, J., Eds.; Springer International Publishing: Cham, Germany, 2020.
51. Peine, A.; van Cooten, V.; Neven, L. Rejuvenating Design. *Sci. Technol. Hum. Values* **2017**, *42*, 429–459. [CrossRef]
52. Peine, A. Technology and Ageing—Theoretical Propositions from Science and Technology Studies (STS). In *Ageing and Digital Technology*; Springer: Singapore, 2019; pp. 51–64.
53. Comunello, F.; Fernández Ardèvol, M.; Mulargia, S.; Belotti, F. Women, youth and everything else: Age-based and gendered stereotypes in relation to digital technology among elderly Italian mobile phone users. *Media Cult. Soc.* **2017**, *39*, 798–815. [CrossRef]
54. Fernández-Ardèvol, M.; Sawchuk, K.; Grenier, L. Maintaining connections: Octo- and nonagenarians on digital 'use and non-use'. *Nord. Rev.* **2017**, *38*, 39–51. [CrossRef]
55. Rosales, A.; Fernández-Ardèvol, M. Smartphone Usage Diversity among Older People. In *Perspectives on Human-Computer Interaction Research with Older People*; Springer: Cham, Germany, 2019; pp. 51–66.
56. Rosales, A.; Fernández-Ardèvol, M. Structural ageism in big data approaches. *Nord. Rev.* **2019**, *40*, 51–64. [CrossRef]
57. European Commission. Smart Cities Digital Single Market. *Eur. Comm. Strateg.* **2017**, *1*, 1–5.
58. Biggs, S.; Carr, A. Age- and Child-Friendly Cities and the Promise of Intergenerational Space. *J. Soc. Work Pract.* **2015**, *29*, 99–112. [CrossRef]
59. World Health Organisation. *Global Age-friendly Cities: A Guide*; World Health Organisation: Geneva, Switzerland, 2007.
60. World Health Organization. *Measuring The Age-Friendliness of Cities: A Guide To Using Core Indicators*; World Health Organization: Kobe, Japan, 2015; Available online: https://apps.who.int/iris/bitstream/handle/10665/203830/9789241509695_eng.pdf?sequence=1 (accessed on 10 October 2020).
61. Buffel, T.; Handler, S.; Phillipson, C. (Eds.) *Age-Friendly Cities and Communities: A Global Perspective*; Press: Cambridge, UK, 2019; ISBN 9781447331346.
62. Modly, T. *Five Megatrends and Their Implications for Global Defense & Security*; Price Waterhouse Coopers: London, UK, 2016; pp. 1–52. Available online: https://www.pwc.com/gx/en/archive/archive-government-public-services/publications/five-megatrends.html (accessed on 10 October 2020).
63. PwC, Megatrends—Issues—Price Waterhouse Coopers UK. 2015. Available online: https://www.pwc.co.uk/issues/megatrends.html (accessed on 10 October 2020).
64. Rogers, R.; Sánchez-Querubín, N.; Kil, A. *Issue Mapping for an Ageing Europe*; Amsterdam University Press: Amsterdam, The Netherlands, 2015; ISBN 9089647163.
65. Woo, J.M.; Choi, M. Why and How Have Korean Cities Embraced the World Health Organization's Age-Friendly Cities and Communities Model? *J. Aging Soc. Policy* **2020**, 1–18. [CrossRef]

66. Buffel, T.; McGarry, P.; Phillipson, C.; De Donder, L.; Dury, S.; De Witte, N.; Smetcoren, A.S.; Verté, D. Developing Age-Friendly Cities: Case Studies From Brussels and Manchester and Implications for Policy and Practice. *J. Aging Soc. Policy* **2014**, *26*, 52–72. [CrossRef]
67. Lehning, A.J.; Greenfield, E.A. Research on Age-Friendly Community Initiatives: Taking Stock and Moving Forward. *J. Hous. Elderly* **2017**, *31*, 178–192. [CrossRef]
68. Facer, K.; Manchester, H.; Horner, L. *Towards the All-Age-Friendly City Working Paper 1 of the Bristol All-Age-Friendly City Group*; Future Cities Catapult: London and University of Bristol: Bristol, UK, 2014.
69. Facer, K.; Horner, L.; Manchester, H. *A Manifesto for All-Age Friendly Cities*; Future Cities Catapult: London and University of Bristol: Bristol, UK, 2016.
70. Gassmann, O.; Bohm, J.; Palmié, M. *Smart Cities: Introducing Digital Innovation to Cities*; Emerald Publishing: Bradford, UK, 2019.
71. UN Sustainable Development Goals. Available online: https://sustainabledevelopment.un.org/?menu=1300 (accessed on 15 May 2020).
72. Buffel, T.; Phillipson, C.; Rémillard-Boilard, S. Age-Friendly Cities and Communities: New Directions for Research and Policy. In *Encyclopedia of Gerontology and Population Aging*; Gu, D., Dupre, M.E., Eds.; Springer: Cham, Germany, 2019; pp. 1–11.
73. United Nations Communications Materials. Available online: https://www.un.org/sustainabledevelopment/news/communications-material/ (accessed on 26 August 2020).
74. De Jong, J.; Rizvi, G. *The State of Access: Success and Failure of Democracies to Create Equal Opportunities*; Brookings Institution Press: Washington, DC, USA, 2008; ISBN 0815701764.
75. Van den Hoven, M.J. Towards ethical principles for designing politco-administrative information systems. *Informatiz. Public Sect.* **1994**, *3*, 353–373.
76. Rawls, J. *A Theory of Justice*; Belknap Press and Harvard University Press: Cambridge, MA, USA, 1971.
77. Rawls, J. *Political Liberalism*; Columbia University Press: New York, NY, USA, 1993.
78. Bovens, M.A. Information rights. Citizenship in the information society. *J. Polit. Philos.* **2002**, *10*, 317–341. [CrossRef]
79. Bovens, M.A.P.; Loos, E.F. The digital constitutional state: Democracy and law in the information society. *Inf. Polity* **2002**, *7*, 185–197. [CrossRef]
80. Secound World Assembly on Ageing Madrid Political Declaration and International Plan of Action on Ageing 2002. Available online: https://www.un.org/esa/socdev/documents/ageing/MIPAA/political-declaration-en.pdf (accessed on 10 October 2020).
81. United Nations. *Report to the Second World Assembly of Aging*; United Nations: New York, NY, USA, 2002; ISBN 9211302218.
82. United Nations. *Follow-up to the International Year of Older Persons: Second World Assembly on Ageing*; United Nations: New York, NY, USA, 2013.
83. Zukin, S. *Naked City: The Death and Life of Authentic Urban Places*; Oxford University Press: Oxford, UK, 2010; ISBN 9780195382853.
84. Greenfield, E.A. Age-Friendly Initiatives, Social Inequalities, and Spatial Justice. *Hastings Cent. Rep.* **2018**, *48*, S41–S45. [CrossRef]
85. Beard, J.R.; Montawi, B. Age and the Environment: The Global Movement Towards Age-Friendly Cities and Communities. *J. Soc. Work Pract.* **2015**, *29*, 5–11. [CrossRef]
86. Hjorthol, R.J.; Levin, L.; Sirén, A. Mobility in different generations of older persons. The development of daily travel in different cohorts in Denmark, Norway and Sweden. *J. Transp. Geogr.* **2010**, *18*, 624–633. [CrossRef]
87. Verlinghieri, E.; Schwanen, T. Transport and mobility justice: Evolving discussions. *J. Transp. Geogr.* **2020**, *87*, 1–7. [CrossRef]
88. Sheller, M. *Mobility Justice*; Verso: London, UK, 2018.
89. Fainstein, S. *The Just City*; Cornell University Press: Ithaca, NY, USA, 2010.
90. Fainstein, S. The Just City. *Int. J. Urban Sci.* **2014**, *18*, 1–18. [CrossRef]
91. Nordbakke, S. Capabilities for mobility among urban older women: Barriers, strategies and options. *J. Transp. Geogr.* **2013**, *26*, 166–174. [CrossRef]
92. Pereira, R.H.M.; Schwanen, T.; Banister, D. Distributive justice and equity in transportation. *Transp. Rev.* **2017**, *37*, 170–191. [CrossRef]

93. Sourbati, M. Disabling communications? A capabilities perspective on media access, social inclusion and communication policy. *Media Cult. Soc.* **2012**, *34*, 571–587. [CrossRef]
94. Sen, A. *Development as Freedom*; Oxford: Oxford University Press: Oxford, UK, 1999.
95. Nussbaum, M.C. *Women and Human Development*; Cambridge University Press: Cambridge, UK, 2000.
96. Nussbaum, M.C. *Frontiers of Justice: Disability, Nationality, Species Membership*; Harvard University Press: Cambridge, MA, USA, 2005.
97. Hulme, D. *The Making of the Millennium Development Goals: Human Development Meets Results-Based Management In an Imperfect World Creating and Sharing Knowledge to Help end Poverty*; BWPI (Brooks World Poverty Institute): Manchester, UK, 2007.
98. Hummels, H. *The 18th Sustainable Development Goal: Social Entrepreneurship in a Global Society*; U.S.E. Working Paper Series: Uterchaht, The Netherlands, 2018.
99. Stephens, C.; Breheny, M.; Mansvelt, J. Healthy ageing from the perspective of older people: A capability approach to resilience. *Psychol. Health* **2015**, *30*, 715–731. [CrossRef] [PubMed]
100. Stephens, C. From success to capability for healthy ageing: Shifting the lens to include all older people. *Crit. Public Health* **2017**, *27*, 490–498. [CrossRef]
101. Deneulin, S.; Alkire, S. *The Real Wealth of Nations: Sen's Capability Approach and the Sustainable Development Goals*; United Nations: London, UK, 2018.
102. Jeekel, H. *Inclusive Transport: Fighting Involuntary Transport Disadvantages*; Elsevier: Amsterdam, The Netherlands, 2018; ISBN 9780128134535.
103. Battarra, R.; Zucaro, F.; Tremiterra, M.R. Smart Mobility and Elderly People Can Ict Make the City More Accessible for Everybody? *Tema-J. L. Use Mobil. Environ.* **2018**, 23–42. [CrossRef]
104. Giddens, A. *The Constitution of Society: Outline of the Theory of Structuration*; Polity Press: Cambridge, UK, 1984; ISBN 0855207825.
105. Behrendt, F. Cycling the Smart and Sustainable City: Analyzing EC Policy Documents on Internet of Things, Mobility and Transport, and Smart Cities. *Sustainability* **2019**, *11*, 763. [CrossRef]
106. Behrendt, F. Why cycling matters for Smart Cities. Internet of Bicycles for Intelligent Transport. *J. Transp. Geogr.* **2016**, *56*, 157–164. [CrossRef]
107. Campbell, S.W. Mobile media and communication: A new field, or just a new journal? *Mob. Media Commun.* **2013**, *1*, 8–13. [CrossRef]
108. Shove, E.; Watson, M.; Spurling, N. Conceptualizing connections. *Eur. J. Soc. Theory* **2015**, *18*, 274–287. [CrossRef]
109. Springgay, S.; Truman, S. (Eds.) An immanent account of movement in walking methodologies. Re-thinking participation beyond a logic of inclusion. In *Walking Methodologies in a More-than-Human World: WalkingLab*; Routledge: Abingdon, UK, 2019; pp. 66–81.
110. Iwarsson, S.; Ståhl, A. Accessibility, usability and universal design—Positioning and definition of concepts describing person-environment relationships. *Disabil. Rehabil.* **2003**, *25*, 57–66. [CrossRef]
111. Wennberg, H. *Walking in Old Age: A Year-Round Perspective on Accessibility in the Outdoor Environment and Effects of Measures Taken*; Lund University: Lund, Sweden, 2009; Volume 247, ISBN 9789162879259.
112. Batty, M.; Axhausen, K.W.; Giannotti, F. Smart cities of the future. *Eur. Phys. J. Spec. Top.* **2012**, *214*, 481–518. [CrossRef]
113. Abduljabbar, R.; Dia, H.; Liyanage, S.; Bagloee, S.A. Applications of artificial intelligence in transport: An overview. *Sustainability* **2019**, *11*, 189. [CrossRef]
114. Jeekel, H. Social Sustainability and Smart Mobility: Exploring the relationship. In *Proceedings of the Transportation Research Procedia*; Elsevier: Amsterdam, The Netherladns, 2017; Volume 25, pp. 4296–4310.
115. Smith, A.E. *Ageing in Urban Neighbourhoods: Place Attachment and Social Exclusion*; Polity: Bristol, UK, 2009; ISBN 9781847422729.
116. Couldry, N.; McCarthy, A. (Eds.) Introduction. In *Media Space*; Routledge: London, UK, 2004; pp. 1–19.
117. Asher, L.; Aresu, M.; Falaschetti, E.; Mindell, J. Most older pedestrians are unable to cross the road in time: A cross-sectional study. *Age Ageing* **2012**, *41*, 690–694. [CrossRef] [PubMed]
118. Loos, E.F. Senior citizens: Digital immigrants in their own country? *Observatorio* **2012**, *6*, 1–23. [CrossRef]
119. Loos, E.F. *De Oudere: Een Digitale Immigrant in Eigen Land? Een Verkenning Naar Toegankelijke Informatievoorziening*; Older people: Digital Immigrants in their own country? Exploring accessible information delivery; inaugural lecture; Boom Lemma: The Hague, The Netherlands, 2010.

120. Akrich, M. User representations: Practices, methods and sociology. In *Managing Sociology in Society: The Approach of Constructive Technology Assessment*; Rip, A., Misa, T.J., Schot, J., Eds.; Pinter: London, UK, 1995; pp. 167–184.
121. Östlund, B.; Fischer, B.; Marshall, B.; Dalmer, N.; Fernandez-Ardévol, M.; Garcia-Santesmases, A.; Lopez, D.; Loos, E.; Chang, F.; Chen, X.; et al. Using Academic Work Places to Involve Older People in the Design of Digital Applications. Presentation of a Methodological Framework to Advance Co-design in Later Life. In Proceedings of the Human Aspects of IT for the Aged Population. Technologies, Design and User Experience HCII 2020; Gao, Q., Zhou, J., Eds.; Springer International Publishing: Cham, Germany, 2020; pp. 45–58.

Publisher's Note: MDPI stays neutral with regard to jurisdictional claims in published maps and institutional affiliations.

International Journal of
Environmental Research and Public Health

MDPI

Article

Is Consultation-Liaison Psychiatry 'Getting Old'? How Psychiatry Referrals in the General Hospital Have Changed over 20 Years

Silvia Ferrari [1], Giorgio Mattei [1,2], Mattia Marchi [1], Gian Maria Galeazzi [1] and Luca Pingani [1,3,*]

1 Department of Biomedical, Metabolic Sciences and Neurosciences, University of Modena and Reggio Emilia, Via del Pozzo 71, 41124 Modena, Italy; silvia.ferrari@unimore.it (S.F.); giorgio.mattei@unimore.it (G.M.); mattia-marchi@libero.it (M.M.); gianmaria.galeazzi@unimore.it (G.M.G.)

2 Department of Economics "Marco Biagi", University of Modena and Reggio Emilia, Via Jacopo Berengario 51, 41121 Modena, Italy

3 Department of Health Professions, Azienda USL–IRCCS di Reggio Emilia, Via Amendola 2, 42122 Reggio Emilia, Italy

* Correspondence: luca.pingani@unimore.it; Tel.: +39-0522-522077

Received: 29 June 2020; Accepted: 9 October 2020; Published: 10 October 2020

Abstract: There is an ever-growing awareness of the health-related special needs of older patients, and Consultation-Liaison Psychiatry Services (CLPS) are significantly involved in providing such age-friendly hospital care. CLPS perform psychiatric assessment for hospitalized patients with suspected medical-psychiatric comorbidity and support ward teams in a bio-psycho-social oriented care management. Changes in features of the population referred to a CLPS over a 20-year course were analysed and discussed, especially comparing older and younger referred subjects. Epidemiological and clinical data from all first psychiatric consultations carried out at the Modena (North of Italy) University Hospital CLPS in the period 2000–2019 (N = 19,278) were included; two groups of consultations were created according to the age of patients: OV65 (consultations for patients older than 64 years) and NONOV65 (all the rest of consultations). Consultations for OV65 were about 38.9% of the total assessments performed, with an average of approximately 375 per year, vs. the 589 performed for NOV65. The number of referrals for older patients significantly increased over the 20 years. The mean age and the male/female ratio of the sample changed significantly across the years in the whole sample as well as both among OV65 and NOV65. Urgent referrals were more frequent among NOV65 and the rate between urgent/non urgent referrals changed differently in the two subgroups. The analysis outlined recurring patterns that should guide future clinical, training and research activities.

Keywords: consultation-liaison psychiatry; elderly; psycho-geriatrics; general hospital

1. Introduction

Consultation-liaison psychiatry (CLP) is a branch of psychiatry aimed at dealing with the complex interactions of 'multi-morbidity' [1], including its psycho-social causes and effects. Born with a strong operative accent, i.e., how to perform psychiatric consultations on patients admitted to the general hospital (GH) or in other contexts of health care ("consultation"), and how to support and favour communication among health care professionals ("liaison"), it has moved to be the operationalized arm of psychosomatic medicine and of the bio-psycho-social paradigm promoted by George Engel and many other researchers and clinicians over the second half of 20th century [2–4].

CLP everyday activities in the GH most commonly consist in performing diagnostic assessments and activate treatment plans when medical-psychiatry comorbidity may be present, including adjustment disorders, anxiety, self-harm behaviours and suicidality, delirium, medically unexplained physical symptoms, eating disorders, alcohol and substance-related disorders, and so forth. Prevention of work-related stress and burn-out syndrome of health professionals as individuals or teams is another typical target of a CLP Service (CLPS) [3]. Strong interaction with related health and social agencies inside and outside the GH (i.e., general practice or social services) is one of the core principles of CLP, to achieve better integration and coordination of care, rationalization of health care resources and reduction of excessive medical sectorialization [5,6].

Research has confirmed how effective CLP clinical actions may help improving outcome indicators of health care, i.e., long-term prognosis of medical conditions, adherence to care plans, quality of life and disability of patients, length of hospital stay, health direct and indirect costs [7–10].

Older patients represent the vast majority of patients admitted to the GH, especially in western countries, with rates ranging between 40 and 65% [11,12]. Referrals for in-patients aged more than 65 have increased consistently, e.g., raising from 0.7 to 2.89% over a 30-year period in an UK CLPS [13]. Old age is a significant risk factor for many psychiatric conditions that may complicate the course and management of multimorbidity, such as depressive and anxiety disorders and neurocognitive disorders [11,14]: up to 40% of geriatric patients may present concomitant psychiatric complaints [15]. Complex bio-psycho-social health care needs impact massively on health outcomes of older patients [16], but may still be neglected, mostly due to delayed diagnosis, inadequate use of psychotropic medications and other therapeutic tools, fear of stigma and limited integration of care. Referrals for psychiatric consultation is performed less frequently for old age patients than other age ranges [15].

In the "*Global Age-Friendly Cities: A Guide*" published by the WHO, older people from 33 different countries were asked to discuss positive and negative aspects of their living situations; when reporting on health-related issues, disease prevention and health promotion were cited as the most relevant expectations, whereas lack of coordination among services, causing complications and reducing effectiveness, was quoted as a common problem [17]. Indeed, taking care of older patients both inside and outside the hospital setting requires specific attention combined to dedicated skills. For example, the rate and severity of multimorbidity increases with the age of patients, and, consistently, efforts in providing coordinated and integrated care should be made. This is known to improve health performances in terms of prognosis and quality of life, as well as reducing and rationalising health costs [18]. Interestingly, the same topics are among the most important targets of CLP, particularly by means of a close interaction with community health services [19,20]. The solid holistic tradition of psychosomatic medicine inspires all CLP's clinical, training and research actions, aiming at making the statement "the patient at the centre" not just an empty metaphor but a real effort towards autonomy and active involvement of patients in their care action plans [21,22].

Aim of this paper was describing changes of socio-demographic and clinical characteristics in the population referred to a hospital-based CLPS over a 20-year (2000–2019) lag-time. Specifically, the variables were examined as referred to the whole sample of older people (aged 65 or more—OV65) and in comparison, to the rest of the population assessed by the service (aged between 18 and 64—NOV65).

2. Methodology

The Modena GH is a 611-bed university hospital, belonging to the Regional Health System (Regione Emilia-Romagna); it is located in the central city area of Modena, a middle town in the North of Italy, and its catchment area is of about 200 thousand inhabitants. It includes an Accident & Emergency (A&E) unit. The Modena CLPS was instituted in 1989 by Prof. Marco Rigatelli and administratively belongs to an operative unit of Adult Mental Health Care, also including a 12-bed psychiatric rehabilitation residential facility and a community mental health service. The CLPS is staffed by three half-time psychiatrists and three to four full-time residents in psychiatry; residents stay for 12 months at the CLPS, during the intermediate-final stages of residency (moderate-to-high level of clinical autonomy according to Italian regulations for resident training). A varying number of final-year medical students and volunteer medical doctors regularly take part to clinical and research activities. PhD students at pertinent Doctorate Schools of the University of Modena & Reggio Emilia also collaborate to research activities. The CLPS does not staff other professionals than medical doctors (e.g., nurses, clinical psychologists, social workers) [23].

The CLPS provides routine (non-urgent) and urgent psychiatric referrals to all the wards of the GH, excluded the paediatric ward and included the A&E unit. Patients referred are mostly in-patients, but protocols of collaboration with a limited number of out-patient clinics are available. The CLPS is open on working days from 8 am to 3 pm and on Saturdays from 8 am to 1 pm. In the remaining hours and during festivities, only for urgent referrals, the 24/7 on-call general psychiatrist (operating in a different hospital of the town) is contacted.

Request forms for psychiatric consultations are sent electronically through the IT system. The form specifically differs from generic consulting request forms for all other medical specialties and is semi-structured for psychiatric referrals, to help clinicians in the formulation of a more defined clinical question [3,24] and to provide consultants with relevant information; particularly, a list of possible pre-defined reasons for referrals and diagnostic hypotheses is provided. Routine referrals are guaranteed within 48 h but are provided most of the times within 24 h. Urgent referrals may be prompted via phone call and are provided within 1 h. One or two first assessments each day are programmed in due advance for patients attending day-hospitals or out-patient clinics.

At the beginning of the working day, a staff meeting for group reading and distribution of received referrals takes place to organize activities. In the afternoon, collegial discussion of clinical cases and supervision of residents is carried out. Psychiatric consultation letters are then written electronically and sent back to referring wards, accompanied by verbal details by phone when necessary. For urgent referrals, the back-referral system is accelerated and often takes place in the ward, right after visiting the patient. Clinical procedures for psychiatric consultations follow indications from international evidence adapted to local context features. An electronic database was adopted by the CLPS for audit purposes after the involvement of the service in the research studies on CLP promoted in Europe by the ECLW in the late '90s [25–27]. For privacy reasons, it was decided to work on the aggregate data provided by this electronic database (through the request of appropriate "queries"). A complete, homogeneous, and reliable electronic documentation is available from year 2000. In this study, all first psychiatric consultations carried out at the CLPS in the period 2000–2019 (20 years; N = 19,278) were considered and analysed. More in detail, the following clinical and non-clinical variables were considered: number of first consultations per year; age (in years) and gender (male/female) of patients; waiting time (time—in days—from referral to actual performance of the assessment); number of referrals per year received by seven top-referring hospital wards (internal medicine, oncology, gastroenterology, headache centre, transplant surgery, general surgery, nephrology-dialysis); number of the eight most recurring reasons for referral among both sub-populations (abuse of alcohol/drugs/psychotropic drugs; anxiety; delirium; depression; medical unexplained physical symptoms; pre-orthotopic liver transplantation (pre-OLTx); psychomotor agitation; re-evaluation of psychopharmacological therapy); proportion of urgent referrals (defined as to be carried out within three hours from request). Scalar and interval variables were described as means and standard deviations (SD), ordinal and categorical variables as absolute values and percentages. Statistically significant differences between OV65 and NOV65 were searched for by means of the t-test for interval and scalar variables and of the Chi-square test for categorical and ordinal ones. The ANOVA test was performed to evaluate the variation of an interval or scalar variable over the years. This research was approved by local Ethics Committee (Prot. AVEN 886/2020/OSS*/AUSLMO).

3. Results

Table 1 summarizes a complete description of the sample, including results of statistical analysis of comparison between OV65 and NONOV65 over time. Over the 20 years of activity considered, the Modena CLPS carried out 19,278 consultations: 11,783 (61.12%) for NOV65 and 7495 (38.88%) for OV65. The year with the highest number of consultations performed was 2005 (N = 1206; 6.26%), while the one with the lowest was 2001 (704; 3.65%). The total mean annual number of 1st consultations was 963.90 (SD = ±157.93), 589.05 for NOV65 (SD = ±108.06) and 374.65 (SD = ±75.46) for OV65 populations.

Figure 1a,b describe the variation over time in the absolute numbers and proportions of total assessments for OV65 and NONOV65. Both comparison of annual numbers of consultations for OV65 vs. NONOV65 and variation of proportion over time were found statistically significant, with evidence of an increase in the number of referrals for older patients (t = 9.69; df = 19; $p < 0.001$).

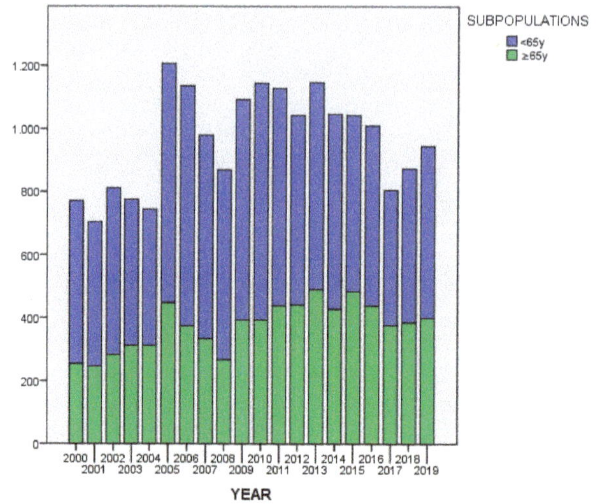

(a)

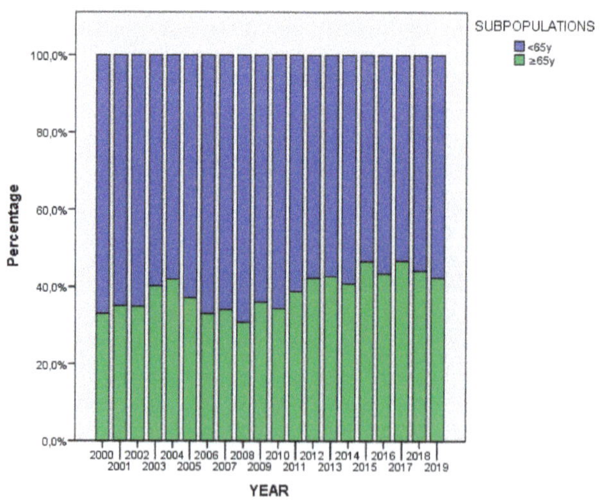

(b)

Figure 1. Consultations carried out from 2000 to 2019, divided into the two subpopulations. (**a**) Absolute value of psychiatric consultations carried out; (**b**) Percentage of psychiatric consultations carried out.

Table 1. Descriptive analysis of the collected clinical and sociodemographic variables.

	Entire Population (N = 19278)		Not Over 65 Subpopulations (NOV65)		Over 65 Subpopulations (OV65)		Not Over 65 (NOV65) vs. Over 65 (OV65) Subpopulations during Years	Variation of Mean/Ratio during Years	
	Mean	DS	Mean	DS	Mean	DS		NOV65	OV65
Number of consultations	963.90	±157.93	589.05	±108.06	374.65	±75.46	t = 9.69; df = 19; $p < 0.001$	t = 24.38; df = 19; $p < 0.001$	t = 22.21; df = 19; $p < 0.001$
Age	57.86	±18.09	45.93	±12.29	75.90	±7.25	Not calculated	F = 15.59; df = 19; $p < 0.001$	F = 4.08; df = 19; $p < 0.001$
Mean waiting time from referral to assessment (days)	1.52	±4.47	1.75	±5.09	1.17	±3.31	t = 7.62; df = 14473; $p < 0.001$	F = 19.86; df = 16; $p < 0.001$	F = 12.47; df = 16; $p < 0.001$
	N	%	*N*	%	*N*	%			
Sex									
Male	8885	46.09%	5394	45.78%	3489	46.55%	X^2 = 134.97; df = 19; $p < 0.001$	X^2 = 84.11; df = 19; $p < 0.001$	X^2 = 62.31; df = 19; $p < 0.001$
Female	10,376	53.82%	6373	54.08%	4001	53.38%			
Missing	17	0.09%	16	0.14%	5	0.07%			
Number of referrals according to ward									
Internal medicine	6749	35.01%	3411	28.95%	3338	44.54%	X^2 = 297.45; df = 19; $p < 0.001$	Not calculated	
Oncology	1840	9.54%	950	8.06%	890	11.87%	X^2 = 43.51; df = 16; $p < 0.001$		
Gastroenterology	1088	5.64%	799	6.78%	288	3.84%	X^2 = 26.38; df = 17; $p = 0.07$		
Headache centre	945	4.90%	870	7.38%	75	1.00%	X^2 = 32.84; df = 19; $p = 0.03$		
Transplant surgery	979	5.08%	798	6.77%	179	2.39%	X^2 = 44.90; df = 11; $p < 0.001$		
Surgery	902	4.68%	508	4.31%	394	5.26%	X^2 = 175.45; df = 19; $p < 0.001$		
Nephrology-dialysis	624	3.24%	265	2.25%	359	4.79%	X^2 = 29.83; df = 19; $p = 0.06$		
Reason for referral									
Abuse of alcohol/drugs/psychotropic drugs	665	3.45%	587	4.48%	78	1.04%	X^2 = 25.50; df = 15; $p = 0.04$	Not calculated	
Anxiety	1414	7.33%	981	8.33%	432	5.76%	X^2 = 23.76; df = 15; $p = 0.07$		
Delirium	449	2.33%	93	0.79%	356	4.75%	X^2 = 16.94; df = 15; $p = 0.32$		
Depression	4591	23.81%	2364	20.06%	2227	29.71%	X^2 = 45.66; df = 15; $p < 0.001$		

Table 1. *Cont.*

	Entire Population (N = 19278)		Not Over 65 Subpopulations (NOV65)		Over 65 Subpopulations (OV65)		Not Over 65 (NOV65) vs. Over 65 (OV65) Subpopulations during Years	Variation of Mean/Ratio during Years	
	Mean	**DS**	**Mean**	**DS**	**Mean**	**DS**		**NOV65**	**OV65**
Medical Unexplained Physical Symptoms	1246	6.46%	93	0.79%	312	4.16%	$X^2 = 33.42$; df = 19; $p = 0.02$		
Pre-OLTx	1160	6.02%	1043	8.85	116	1.55%	$X^2 = 53.82$; df = 14; $p < 0.001$		
Psychomotor agitation	1581	8.02%	512	4.35%	1068	14.25%	$X^2 = 18.29$; df = 15; $p = 0.25$		
Re-evaluation of psychopharmacological therapy	831	4.31%	481	4.08%	350	4.67%	$X^2 = 26.80$; df = 14; $p = 0.02$		
Number of urgent referrals									
Urgent	4689	24.32%	3070	26.05%	1619	21.60%	$X^2 = 428.99$; df = 19; $p < 0.001$	$X^2 = 248.38$; df = 19; $p < 0.001$	
Not urgent	12,210	63.34%	7178	60.92%	5032	67.14%			
Missing information	2379	12.34%	1535	13.03%	844	11.26%			

The mean age of the entire sample was 57.86 (SD = ±18.09): the variations over years of the mean age of NOV65 (45.93; SD = ±12.29) and OV65 (75.90; SD = ±7.25) were statistically significant ($F = 15.59$; $df = 19$; $p < 0.001$ and $F = 4.08$; $df = 19$; $p < 0.001$, respectively), though that observed among OV65 was more marked (Figure 2).

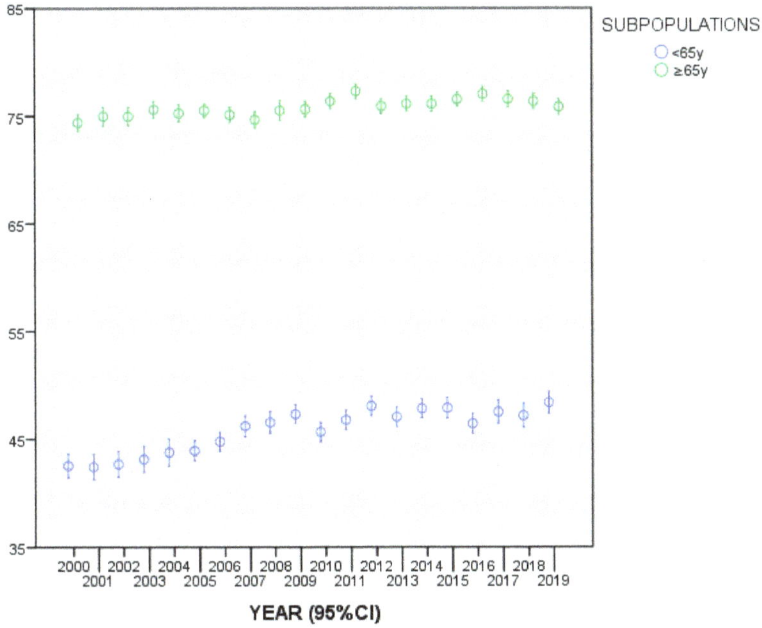

(a)

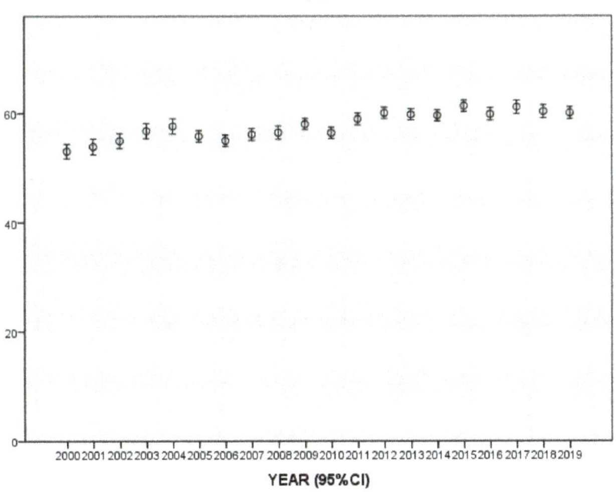

(b)

Figure 2. (**a**) Mean age of the two subpopulations (NOV65 and OV65). (**b**) Mean age of the entire sample.

Females were most frequent than males in the general sample (*N* = 10,376; 53.82%) as well as among both the NOV65 subpopulation (*N* = 6373; 54.09%) and the OV65 (4001; 53.38%). The variation of the male/female ratio over the years was statistically significant ($X^2 = 134.97$; df = 19; $p < 0.001$) (Figure 3), and the same was found among both the subpopulations (NOV65 population: $X^2 = 84.11$; df = 19; $p < 0.001$ and OV65 population $X^2 = 62.31$; df = 19; $p < 0.001$).

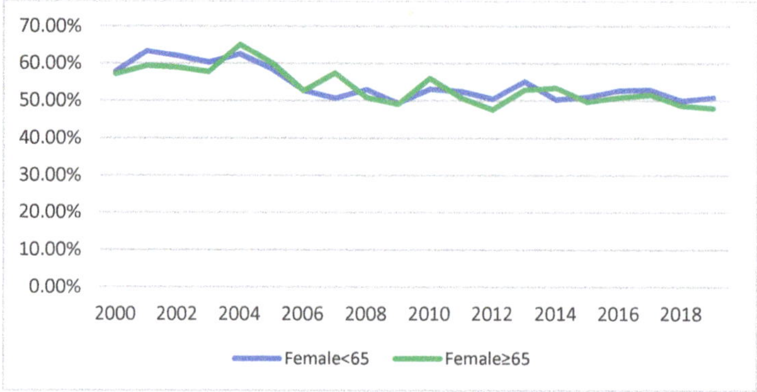

Figure 3. Percentage of consultations, per year, made to female patients.

The mean waiting time for a consultation was 1.52 days (SD = ±4.47) in the total sample, 1.75 (SD = ±5.09) for NOV65 and 1.17 (SD = ±3.31) for OV65. The variation across the years of the waiting time in the two subpopulations was statistically significant (t = 7.62; df = 14,473; $p < 0.001$) (Figure 4), as well as for each individual sub-population (NOV65: F = 19.86; df = 16; $p < 0.001$ and OV65: F = 12.47; df = 16; $p < 0.001$).

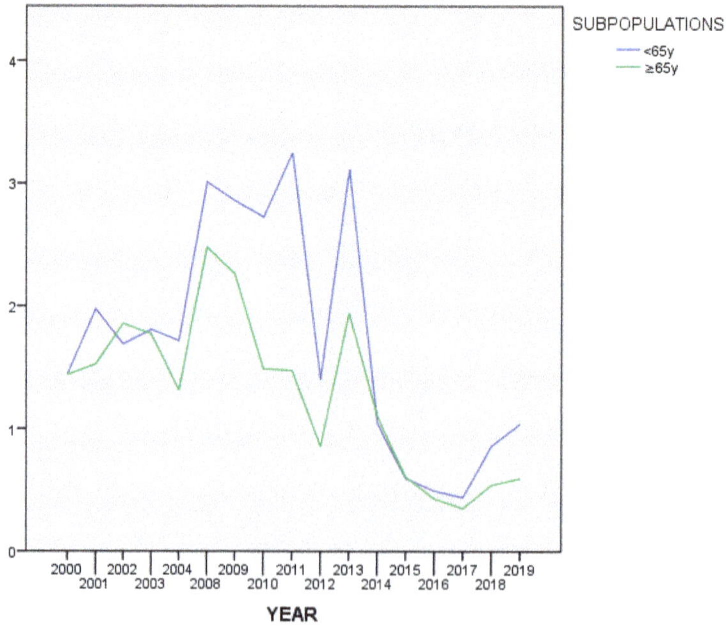

Figure 4. Mean waiting time from referral to assessment (days).

A peculiar feature of this trend, for both populations, should also be noticed: mean waiting times increased considerably in 2008 and then dropped to values even lower than before from 2013 onwards.

This finding is chronologically related to the increase, from 2007, in the collaboration of the CLPS with the outpatient clinic of the liver transplant unit. At first, this required an adjustment process of organization, since patients came from different parts of the national territory and it was more difficult to synchronize all different diagnostic procedures, including the mandatory psychiatric evaluation. The organization gradually improved over time, resulting in mean waiting times even lower than before in more recent years.

The ward that requested the highest number of consultations was internal medicine, both in the whole sample (N = 6749; 35.01%) and in the two age-subpopulations, though the rate of referrals from this ward decreased constantly over the 20 years for both adults (aged between 18 and 64 years) and older people (aged 65 years and more). On the contrary, the rate of referrals from the transplant unit and gastroenterology increased over the years. This is the expression of the establishment of a liver transplantation assessment circuit that, as mentioned before, took place in the Modena Hospital in 2007, being these two the wards where potential candidates for liver transplantation are admitted and referred for mandatory psychiatric consultation, according to the clinical protocol. Figure 4 (from (a) to (g)) illustrates trends over time of proportions of referrals from the different wards in the two age groups. The comparison between proportions of referrals in the two age groups across time was statistically significant in all wards but gastroenterology (X^2 = 26.38; df = 17; p = 0.07) and nephrology-dialysis (X^2 = 29.83; df = 19; p = 0.06).

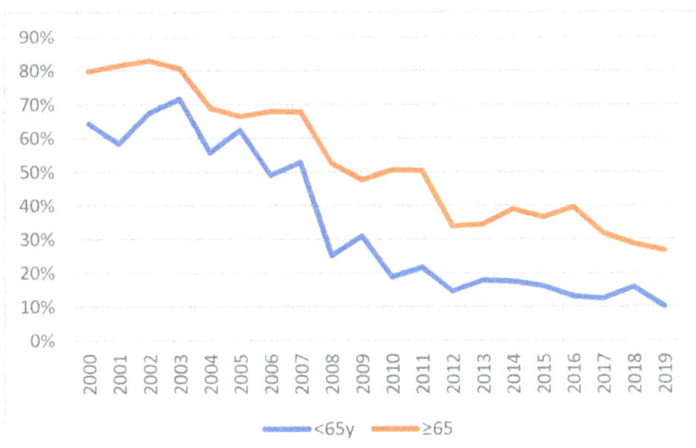

(a)

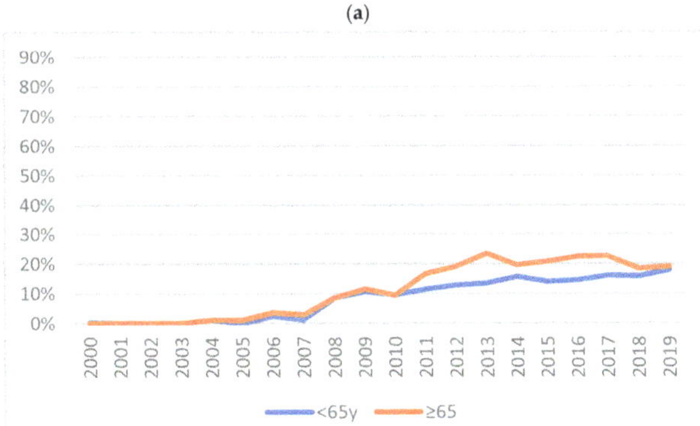

(b)

Figure 4. *Cont.*

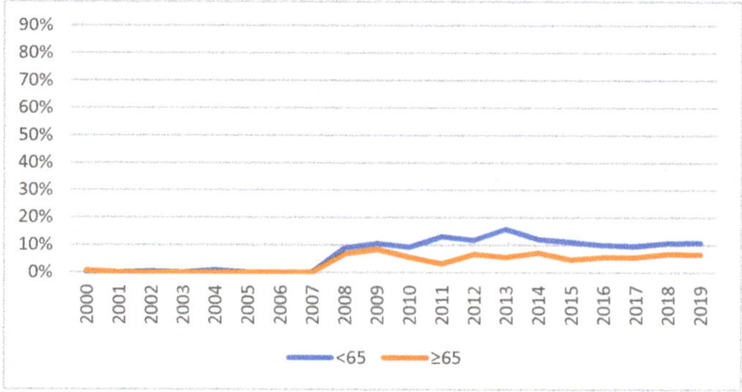

(c)

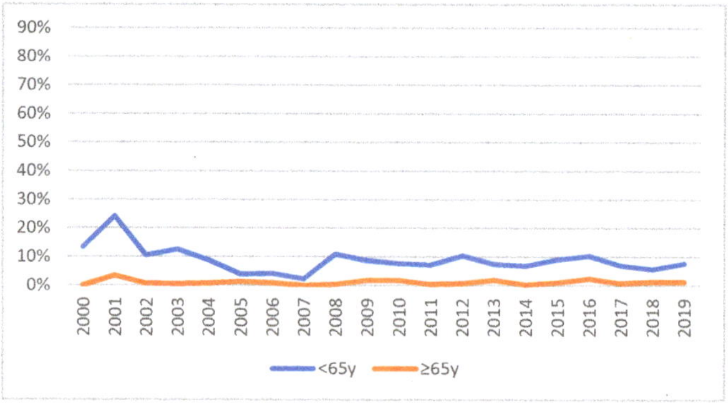

(d)

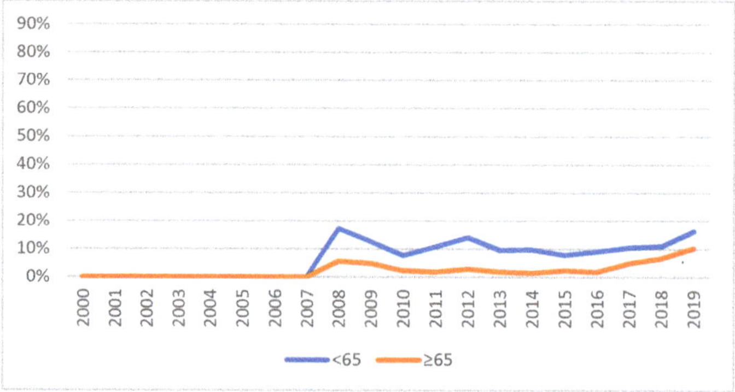

(e)

Figure 4. *Cont.*

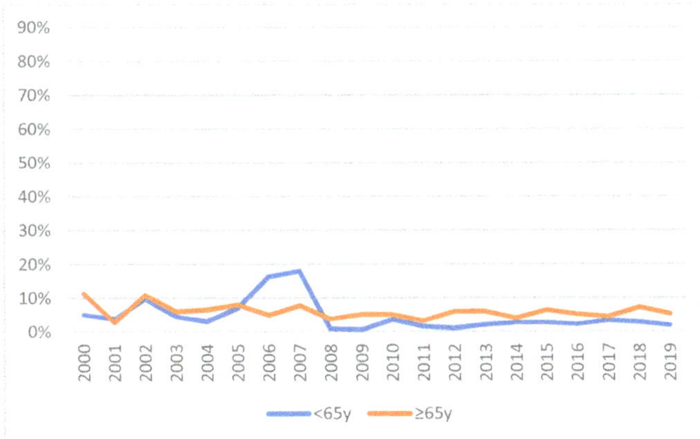

(f)

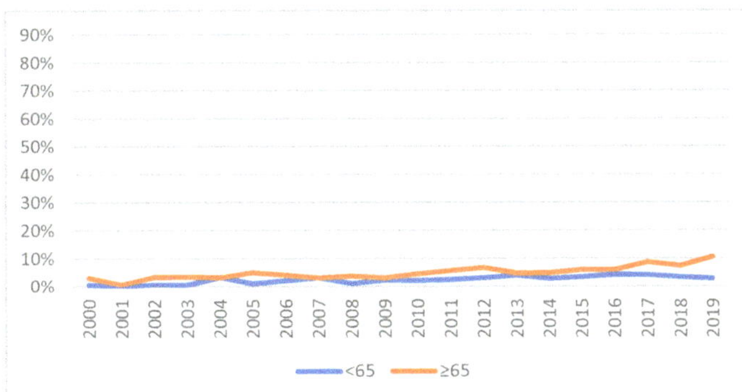

(g)

Figure 4. Trends over time of percentage of referrals from wards for the subgroups NOV65 and OV65. (**a**) Internal medicine; (**b**) Oncology; (**c**) Gastroenterology; (**d**) Headache centre; (**e**) Transplant surgery; (**f**) Surgery; (**g**) Nephrology-dialysis.

The most common reason for referral was clinical suspicion of depression both in the entire sample (N = 4591; 23.81%) and in the two age subpopulations, though this was more evident among the OV65 (N = 2227; 29.71% vs. N = 2364; 20.06%), with a statistically significant difference ($X^2 = 45.66$; df = 15; $p < 0.001$). Trends over time in the two age subgroups were different in a statistically significant way also when the reasons for referral was clinical suspicion of alcohol/substance/psychotropic drug abuse ($X^2 = 25.50$; df = 15; $p = 0.04$), medically unexplained physical symptoms (MUPS) ($X^2 = 33.42$; df = 19; $p = 0.02$), pre-OLTx ($X^2 = 53.82$; df = 14; $p < 0.001$) and rehearsal of on-going psychotropic medications ($X^2 = 26.80$; df = 14; $p = 0.02$), but not for delirium, psychomotor agitation and anxiety. Figure 5 (from (a) to (h)) illustrates the trends over time of such proportions.

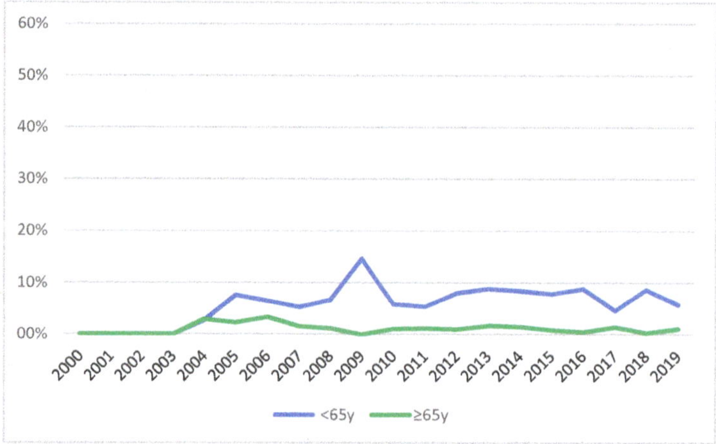

(a)

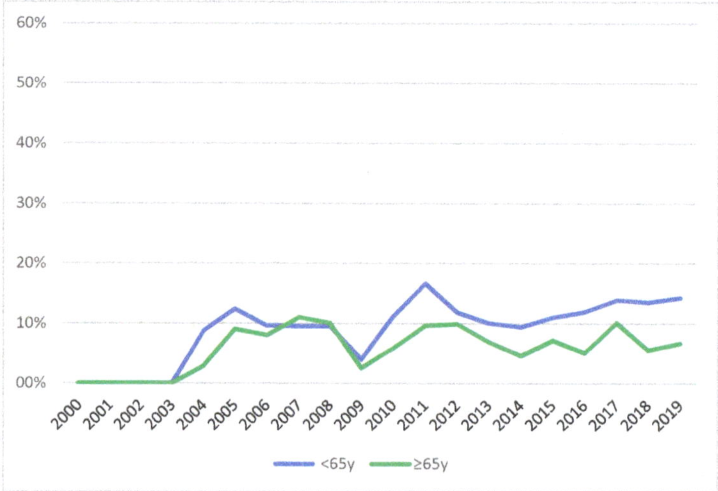

(b)

Figure 4. *Cont.*

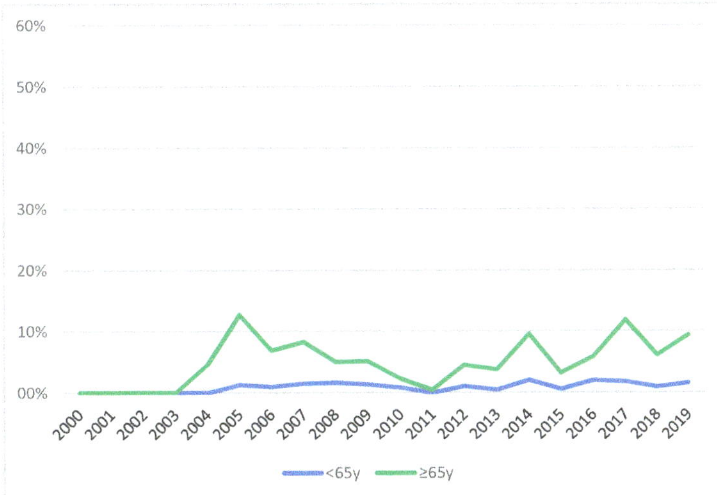

(c)

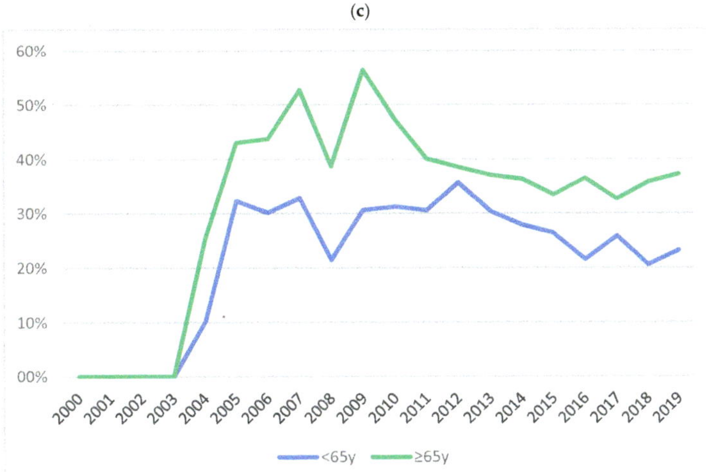

(d)

Figure 4. *Cont.*

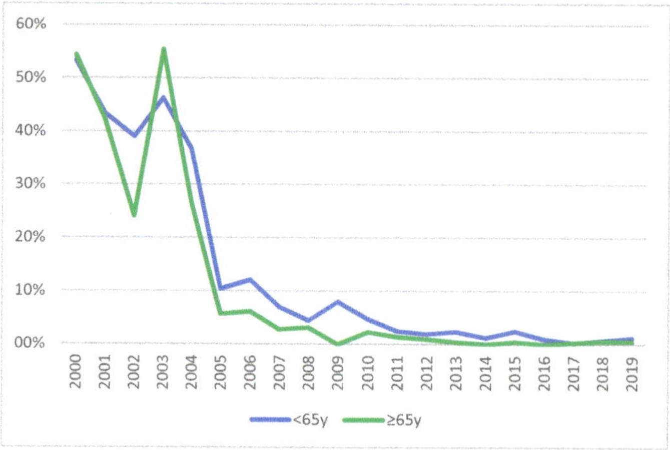

(e)

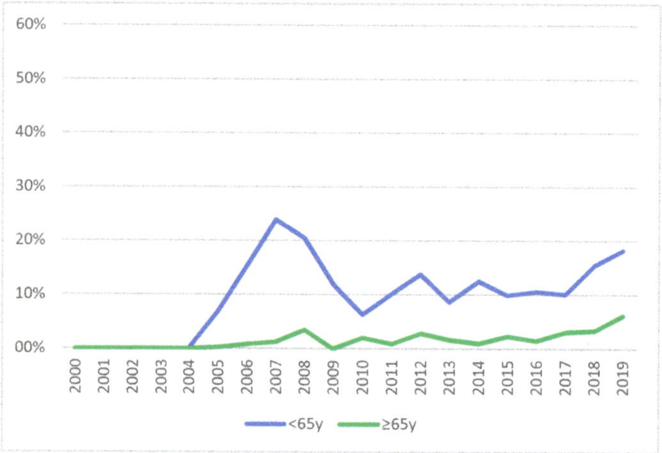

(f)

Figure 4. *Cont.*

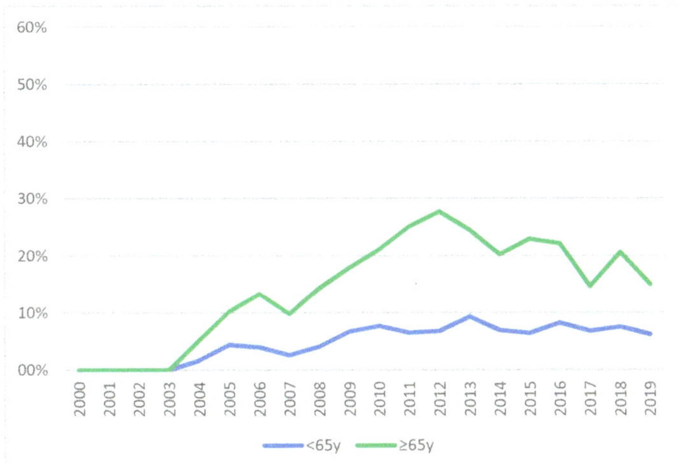

(**g**)

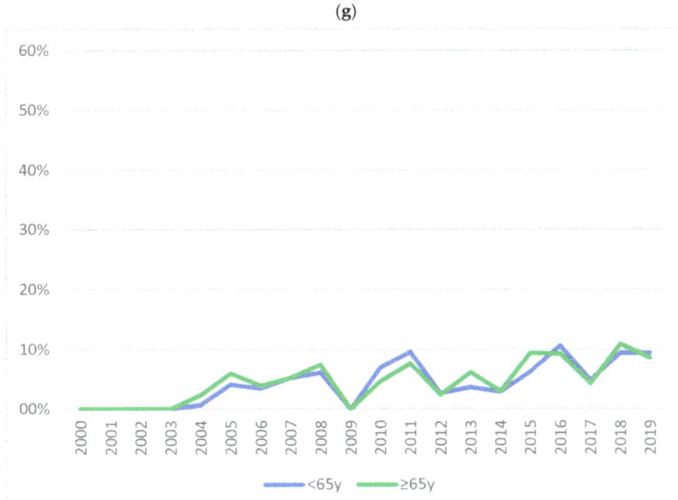

(**h**)

Figure 5. Trends over time of percentage of reasons for referrals for the subgroups NOV65 and OV65. (**a**) Abuse of alcohol/drugs/psychotropic drugs; (**b**) Anxiety; (**c**) Delirium; (**d**) Depression; (**e**) Medical Unexplained Physical Symptoms; (**f**) Pre-OLTx; (**g**) Psychomotor agitation; (**h**) Re-evaluation of psychopharmacological therapy.

Urgent referrals were more frequent among NOV65 (N = 3070; 26.05%) than in the OV65 subpopulation (N = 1619; 21.60%). The trend over time in the proportion of urgent vs. non-urgent referrals was found to be different with statistical significance between the two age groups ($X^2 = 428.99$; df = 19; $p < 0.001$). Figure 6 illustrates such trend.

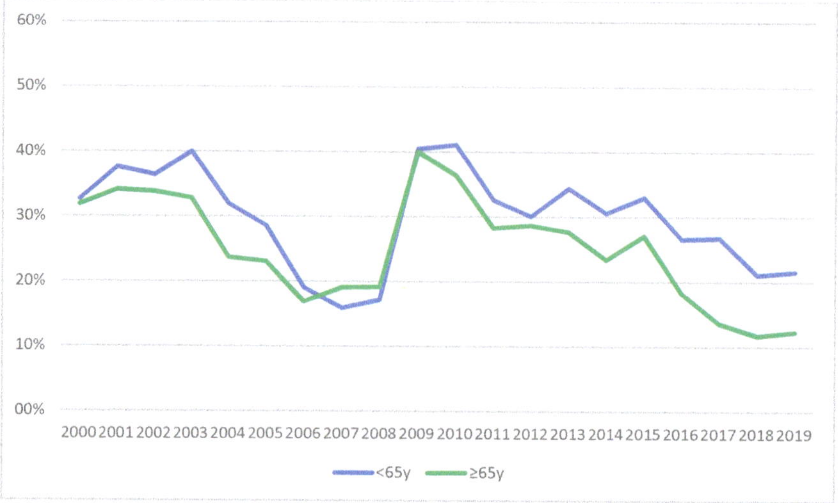

Figure 6. Percentage of urgent requests over time.

4. Discussion

The clinical activities of a northern Italy hospital-based CLPS were analysed over a period of 20 years, with the aim to recognize and discuss relevant features and changes related to the population referred for psychiatric consultations, with specific attention to comparison of different features related to age. Such an analysis was felt relevant, and confirmed to be, to provide helpful hints to improve the performances of the CLPS. For example, it could suggest improvements in organizational aspects (e.g., dedicated pathways to care), or training activities (e.g., on psychogeriatric topics), or further research initiatives.

Activities dedicated to the older population represent a significant amount of the whole of clinical responsibilities of the CLPS, an average of about 40%. Moreover, this amount progressively increased over the 20 years considered, and the variation of mean age was more evident among older patients. All these findings are consistent with the phenomenon of aging of both general and hospital populations [13,20,28] and confirms the relevance to study these patterns of utilization. Both consultees and consultants should be aware of specific needs of their geriatric patients in terms of mental health when they refer and assess them, respectively: these needs are known to be different than those of younger patients [14,16,29], and require specific knowledge and skills (i.e., the ability to perform a differential diagnosis between depression and hypoactive delirium, or a safe and appropriate management of psychotropic medications).

This was also clearly outlined by results related to most common reasons for referrals: depression, the most common reason for psychiatric referral both in the total sample and in the two age-groups, was particularly frequent in the over-65 patients.

Depression in older patients is easily missed and mismanaged, due for example to multimorbidity and difficulties in appropriate interpretation of somatic symptoms or to uneasiness of clinicians in using antidepressants for fear of side effects or interactions [30,31], but also to a more implicit conceptual reason, that is the tendency to feel that it is normal or inevitable to be depressed when old [30,32]. The increase here reported may be a positive sign, meaning that clinicians are more aware of the need to properly address and treat depression among their older patients. No statistically significant change in the proportion of diagnoses of delirium in the two age groups was found, this being also a confirmation not only of the epidemiology of this condition, but also of the good reliability of physicians in diagnosing it.

The amount of referrals received changed significantly in the two subpopulations for other diagnostic categories: abuse of alcohol, substances or medications was more common but also much more variable among younger patients. Referrals for pre-transplant assessments were also more common among patients with less than 65 years, as expected, being age a significant parameter that influences the choice of candidates by surgeons, though the number of referrals with this indication evidently increased in both age groups in recent years, consistently with the growing importance as surgical hub for transplantation of the Modena centre [33]. Generic referrals for psychomotor agitation, increasing particularly for older patients until 2012, have become less common in more recent years: this may also reflect an improvement in the diagnostic skills of consultees, who are able to use more detailed diagnostic frameworks such as that of delirium, as already commented. The observation of such changes, allowed by the long-time of activity here considered, is also an indirect evidence that day-by-day work on liaison and more formal training initiatives promoted by the CLPS are effective in the long run and help a better use of resources [34]. Another relevant change observed over the 20 years in both age-groups was the drop in the referrals due to MUPS: this finding is maybe the expression of a conceptual twist in the nosography of somatisation and the so-called functional disorders, variously addressed in the scientific literature [35].

Female patients referred to the CLPS were more common both among older and among younger patients, but also their proportion progressively decreased along the years in both subpopulations. This change, though, was more marked in the older research participants. One possible way to interpret this finding is the increased amount of patients referred for pre-OLTx, who are mostly male [36]. Gender-related issues in geriatric patients are very relevant, considering the higher proportion of more severe forms of some disorders in male patients, e.g., depression [37]: awareness on the consequent increased risk of self-harm behaviours should be an important priority in the organization of the CLPS as well as in the definition of training activities.

The Modena CLPS confirms to perform well in terms of waiting times for back-referral, with an average of 1 day and half. This time is even less for older patients, who may be felt as a priority in the scheduling of the activities of the day by the consultants. Urgent referrals, though, were more common for younger subjects, but decreased considerably in both groups over the 20 years, as a possible sign that consultees have learnt to "trust" the CLPS in providing prompt reaction when needed. With reference to changes in the trend of waiting times, moreover, a significant increase was noticed, in both populations, around 2008, followed by a big drop in 2013. This trend is related to the history of the Modena CLPS, which, in 2008, increased significantly its regular collaboration with the outpatient clinic of the Liver Transplant Unit, resulting, for some years, in more difficult and timely organization of appointments. This finding is a clear example of how useful the regular recording of clinical activities is in understanding trends and changes that reflect internal and external events [3].

The study has some limitations that must be clarified to understand the discussion of the results: (1) the professionals who collected the data were different over the years. Each professional was given a short introductory course however this may not have prevented some errors in entering data; (2) data collection was done following privacy regulations but not through a dedicated software. Using a spreadsheet did not allow to avoid errors in data entry; (3) for the majority of hospital wards, requests for psychiatric consultation were not defined by a protocol or a criteria check-lists: medical doctors decided in total autonomy when to request a consultation for their hospitalized patient. This subjectivity may have characterized the distribution of requests in the different wards; (4) some wards (for example transplant surgery) had a very strong collaboration with the CLPS, using its support in their protocols. This strong synergy has certainly influenced the number of requests from that wards; (5) the database does not collect variables measuring level of dependence, activities of daily living, social support or even degree of frailty, whose possible interesting changes over time we were therefore not able to document.

5. Conclusions

One major goal of CLPSs operating in the GH should be the acquisition of an attitude more strongly focused on prevention and health promotion. The epidemiologic approach to clinical data achieved by this study, together with its wide time-span (20 years of activity), supports the recognition of obstacles, opportunities and other needs in the organization of the CLPS, in order to improve its effectiveness in dealing with medical-psychiatric comorbidity of older patients.

Consultations for older patients accounted for a large amount, more than one third, of the whole activities of the CLPS, and a significant increasing trend was evident. Depression was by far the most common diagnosis not only in the general population assessed by the CLPS, but in the older age group particularly. Changes in mean lag-times between referral and assessment as well as in proportion of urgent/routine referrals were evident.

These findings suggest that along with the phenomenon of progressive ageing in hospital populations, there is an increased need for hospital-based CLPS to potentiate their skills in managing old-age specific psychopathology and tailor their organization, training, and research activities accordingly. The present study provides support to a better tuning to the needs of older people by identifying high-risk disease patterns or promoting dedicated clinical processes (i.e., detection of mild cognitive impairment, coordination with primary care or social services, prevention of delirium).

Author Contributions: Conceptualization, S.F. and G.M.G.; methodology, L.P. and G.M.; data curation, L.P. and M.M.; writing—original draft preparation, S.F.; writing—review and editing, S.F., G.M., M.M., G.M.G. and L.P.; supervision, G.M.G. All authors have read and agreed to the published version of the manuscript.

Funding: This research received no external funding.

Conflicts of Interest: The authors declare no conflict of interest.

References

1. Smith, G.C. From Consultation–Liaison Psychiatry to Integrated Care for Multiple and Complex Needs. *Aust. N. Z. J. Psychiatry* **2009**, *43*, 1–12. [CrossRef] [PubMed]
2. Ferrari, S.; Blum, J.; Kelly, P. How to collaborate with other specialities. In *How to Succeed in Psychiatry: A Guide to Training and Practice*; Fiorillo, A., Calliess, I.T., Sass, H., Eds.; J. Wiley & Sons: Chichester, West Sussex, UK, 2012; pp. 211–235, ISBN 978-1-119-99866-2.
3. Ferrari, S.; Dreher, A.; Mattei, G.; Diefenbacher, A. Liaison psychiatry—Is it possible? In *Psychiatry in Practice*; Fiorillo, A., Volpe, U., Bhugra, D., Eds.; Oxford University Press: Oxford, UK, 2016; pp. 389–408, ISBN 978-0-19-872364-6.
4. Engel, G. The need for a new medical model: A challenge for biomedicine. *Science* **1977**, *196*, 129–136. [CrossRef] [PubMed]
5. Meller, W.; Specker, S.; Schultz, P.; Kishi, Y.; Thurber, S.; Kathol, R. Using the INTERMED complexity instrument for a retrospective analysis of patients presenting with medical illness, substance use disorder, and other psychiatric illnesses. *Ann. Clin. Psychiatry* **2015**, *27*, 38–43.
6. de Jonge, P.; Huyse, F.J.; Slaets, J.P.J.; Söllner, W.; Stiefel, F.C. Operationalization of Biopsychosocial Case Complexity in General Health Care: The INTERMED Project. *Aust. N. Z. J. Psychiatry* **2005**, *39*, 795–799. [CrossRef]
7. Oldham, M.A.; Chahal, K.; Lee, H.B. A systematic review of proactive psychiatric consultation on hospital length of stay. *Gen. Hosp. Psychiatry* **2019**, *60*, 120–126. [CrossRef]
8. Kishi, Y.; Meller, W.H.; Kathol, R.G.; Swigart, S.E. Factors Affecting the Relationship between the Timing of Psychiatric Consultation and General Hospital Length of Stay. *Psychosomatics* **2004**, *45*, 470–476. [CrossRef]
9. Udo, I.; Odeyale, F.; Gash, A.; Fossey, M. The rise of liaison psychiatry: Challenges and implications for sustainability. *Br. J. Hosp. Med.* **2016**, *77*, 523–528. [CrossRef]
10. Yrondi, A.; Petiot, D.; Arbus, C.; Schmitt, L. Economic impact of consultation-liaison psychiatry in a French University Hospital Centre. *Encephale* **2016**, *42*, 112–115. [CrossRef] [PubMed]
11. Nogueira, V.; Lagarto, L.; Cerejeira, J.; Renca, S.; Firmino, H. Improving quality of care: Focus on liaison old age psychiatry. *Ment. Health Fam. Med.* **2013**, *10*, 153–158.

12. National Center for Health Statistics. *Percent Distribution, Rate, Days of Care with Average Length of Stay, and Standard Error of Discharges from Short-Stay Hospitals, by Sex and Age 2010*; National Center for Health Statistics: Hyattsville, MD, USA.
13. Anderson, D.; Nortcliffe, M.; Dechenne, S.; Wilson, K. The rising demand for consultation-liaison psychiatry for older people: Comparisons within Liverpool and the literature across time. *Int. J. Geriatr. Psychiatry* **2011**, *26*, 1231–1235. [CrossRef]
14. Ferrari, S.; Signorelli, M.S.; Cerrato, F.; Pingani, L.; Massimino, M.; Valente, S.; Forlani, M.; Bonasegla, P.; Arcidiacono, E.; De Ronchi, D.; et al. Never too late to be anxious: Validation of the geriatric anxiety inventory, Italian version. *Clin. Ter.* **2017**, *168*, 120–127. [CrossRef]
15. Schellhorn, S.E.; Barnhill, J.W.; Raiteri, V.; Faso, V.L.; Ferrando, S.J. A comparison of psychiatric consultation between geriatric and non-geriatric medical inpatients. *Int. J. Geriatr. Psychiatry* **2009**, *24*, 1054–1061. [CrossRef] [PubMed]
16. Wild, B.; Heider, D.; Maatouk, I.; Slaets, J.; König, H.-H.; Niehoff, D.; Saum, K.-U.; Brenner, H.; Söllner, W.; Herzog, W. Significance and costs of complex biopsychosocial health care needs in elderly people: Results of a population-based study. *Psychosom. Med.* **2014**, *76*, 497–502. [CrossRef] [PubMed]
17. World Health Organization (Ed.) *Global Age-Friendly Cities: A Guide*; World Health Organization: Geneva, Switzerland, 2007; ISBN 978-92-4-154730-7.
18. Stiefel, F.C.; Huyse, F.J.; Söllner, W.; Slaets, J.P.J.; Lyons, J.S.; Latour, C.H.M.; van der Wal, N.; de Jonge, P. Operationalizing Integrated Care on a Clinical Level: The INTERMED Project. *Med. Clin. N. Am.* **2006**, *90*, 713–758. [CrossRef]
19. Wild, B.; Herzog, W.; Schellberg, D.; Böhlen, F.; Brenner, H.; Saum, K.; Maatouk, I. A short intervention targeting psychosomatic care in older adults with complex health care needs—Results of a randomized controlled trial. *Int. J. Geriatr. Psychiatry* **2019**, *34*, 272–279. [CrossRef]
20. Glass, O.M.; Hermida, A.P.; Hershenberg, R.; Schwartz, A.C. Considerations and Current Trends in the Management of the Geriatric Patient on a Consultation–Liaison Service. *Curr. Psychiatry Rep.* **2020**, *22*, 21. [CrossRef]
21. Smith, G.C. From Consultation—Liaison Psychiatry to Psychosocial Advocacy: Maintaining Psychiatry's Scope. *Aust. N. Z. J. Psychiatry* **1998**, *32*, 753–761. [CrossRef]
22. Wild, B.; Heider, D.; Schellberg, D.; Böhlen, F.; Schöttker, B.; Muhlack, D.C.; König, H.-H.; Slaets, J. Caring for the elderly: A person-centered segmentation approach for exploring the association between health care needs, mental health care use, and costs in Germany. *PLoS ONE* **2019**, *14*, e0226510. [CrossRef]
23. Pingani, L.; Fiorillo, A.; Luciano, M.; Catellani, S.; Vinci, V.; Ferrari, S.; Rigatelli, M. Who cares for it? How to provide psychosocial interventions in the community. *Int. J. Soc. Psychiatry* **2013**, *59*, 701–705. [CrossRef]
24. Rigatelli, M.; Ferrari, S. The Modena Consultation–Liaison Psychiatry Service, Italy. *Br. J. Psychiatry* **2004**, *184*, 268–269. [CrossRef]
25. Huyse, F.J.; Herzog, T.; Lobo, A.; Malt, U.F.; Opmeer, B.C.; Stein, B.; Creed, F.; Crespo, M.D.; Gardoso, G.; Guimaraes-Lopes, R.; et al. European Consultation-LiaisonPsychiatric Services:the ECLW Collaborative Study. *Acta Psychiatr. Scand.* **2000**, *101*, 360–366. [CrossRef] [PubMed]
26. Huyse, F.J.; Herzog, T.; Lobo, A.; Malt, U.F.; Opmeer, B.C.; Stein, B.; de Jonge, P.; van Dijck, R.; Creed, F.; Crespo, M.D.; et al. Consultation-Liaison psychiatric service delivery: Results from a European study. *Gen. Hosp. Psychiatry* **2001**, *23*, 124–132. [CrossRef]
27. Gala, C.; Rigatelli, M.; De Bertolini, C.; Rupolo, G.; Gabrielli, F.; Grassi, L. A multicenter investigation of consultation-liaison psychiatry in Italy. *Gen. Hosp. Psychiatry* **1999**, *21*, 310–317. [CrossRef]
28. De Giorgio, G.; Quartesan, R.; Sciarma, T.; Giulietti, M.; Piazzoli, A.; Scarponi, L.; Ferrari, S.; Ferranti, L.; Moretti, P.; Piselli, M. Consultation-Liaison Psychiatry—From theory to clinical practice: An observational study in a general hospital. *BMC Res. Notes* **2015**, *8*, 475. [CrossRef]
29. Kastenschmidt, E.K.; Kennedy, G.J. Depression and Anxiety in Late Life: Diagnostic Insights and Therapeutic Options. *Mt. Sinai J. Med.* **2011**, *78*, 527–545. [CrossRef]
30. Alexopoulos, G.S.; Bruce, M.L.; Hull, J.; Sirey, J.A.; Kakuma, T. Clinical Determinants of Suicidal Ideation and Behavior in Geriatric Depression. *Arch. Gen. Psychiatry* **1999**, *56*, 1048. [CrossRef]
31. Neviani, F.; Belvederi Murri, M.; Mussi, C.; Triolo, F.; Toni, G.; Simoncini, E.; Tripi, F.; Menchetti, M.; Ferrari, S.; Ceresini, G.; et al. Physical exercise for late life depression: Effects on cognition and disability. *Int. Psychogeriatr.* **2017**, *29*, 1105–1112. [CrossRef]

32. Stanners, M.N.; Barton, C.A.; Shakib, S.; Winefield, H.R. Depression diagnosis and treatment amongst multimorbid patients: A thematic analysis. *BMC Fam. Pract.* **2014**, *15*, 124. [CrossRef]
33. Olivieri, T.; Magistri, P.; Guidetti, C.; Baroni, S.; Rinaldi, S.; Assirati, G.; Catellani, B.; Chierego, G.; Cantaroni, C.; Bondi, F.; et al. University of Modena Experience with Liver Grafts From Donation after Circulatory Death: What Really Matters in Organ Selection? *Transplant. Proc.* **2019**, *51*, 2967–2970. [CrossRef]
34. Rigatelli, M.; Ferrari, S.; Uguzzoni, U.; Natali, A. Teaching and Training in the Psychiatric-Psychosomatic Consultation-Liaison Setting. *Psychother. Psychosom.* **2000**, *69*, 221–228. [CrossRef]
35. Ferrari, S.; Poloni, N.; Diefenbacher, A.; Barbosa, A.; Cosci, F. From hysteria to somatic symptom disorders: Searching for a common psychopathological ground. *J. Psychopathol.* **2015**, *21*, 372–379.
36. Mattei, G.; Laghi, A.; Balduzzi, S.; Moscara, M.; Piemonte, C.; Reggianini, C.; Rigatelli, M.; Ferrari, S.; Pingani, L.; Galeazzi, G.M. Indicators of Complex Care During the Consultation-Liaison Psychiatry Activity at the Transplant Center of the Policlinico Hospital, Modena. *Transpl. Proc.* **2017**, *49*, 2105–2109. [CrossRef] [PubMed]
37. Craig Nelson, J. Management of Late-Life Depression. In *Antidepressants*; Macaluso, M., Preskorn, S.H., Eds.; Handbook of Experimental Pharmacology; Springer International Publishing: Cham, Switzerland, 2018; Volume 250, pp. 389–413, ISBN 978-3-030-10948-6.

International Journal of
Environmental Research and Public Health

MDPI

Article

Smart and Age-Friendly Cities in Russia: An Exploratory Study of Attitudes, Perceptions, Quality of Life and Health Information Needs

Liliya Eugenevna Ziganshina [1,2,3,4,*], Ekaterina V. Yudina [5], Liliya I. Talipova [1], Guzel N. Sharafutdinova [1] and Rustem N. Khairullin [1]

1 Interregional Clinical Diagnostic Centre (ICDC), The Ministry of Health of the Republic of Tatarstan, 12A Karbysheva Street, 420101 Kazan, Russia; tli13@mail.ru (L.I.T.); guzel_792@mail.ru (G.N.S.); icdc@icdc.ru (R.N.K.)

2 Federal State Budgetary Educational Institution of Continuing Professional Education "Russian Medical Academy of Continuing Professional Education", The Ministry of Health of the Russian Federation (RMANPO), 2/1, Barrikadnaya Street, 123995 Moscow, Russia

3 Department of Pharmacology, Kazan State Medical University (KSMU), The Ministry of Health of the Russian Federation, 49 Butlerov Street, 420012 Kazan, Russia

4 Department of Medicinal Chemistry, Kazan Federal University (KFU), The Ministry of Science and Higher Education of the Russian Federation, 18 Kremlevskaya Street, 420008 Kazan, Russia

5 Children's Hospital N 1 of the City of Kazan, 125a Dekabristov Street, 420034 Kazan, Russia; ekaterina.v.yudina@mail.ru

* Correspondence: lezign@gmail.com; Tel.: +7-987-296-8496

Received: 28 October 2020; Accepted: 8 December 2020; Published: 9 December 2020

Abstract: In Russia, initiatives for healthy ageing have been growing over the last two decades; however, none use an evidence-based (EB) approach. It is proposed that Kazan, a city with a population of over a million in the European part of Russia, has good chances of moving towards age-friendliness and contributing to raising awareness about healthy ageing through Cochrane evidence. One of the eight essential features of age-friendly cities by the World Health Organisation (WHO) directly points to health services. This exploratory study assesses the health information needs of the ageing population of Kazan and the challenges people face in improving their health and longevity. Survey data were used from 134 participants, patients, caregivers and healthcare providers of the Interregional Clinical Diagnostic Centre (ICDC), aged from 30 to over 80 years, and potential associations of the studied parameters with age, gender, quality of life and other characteristics were analysed. Older people (60+) were less positive about their quality of life, took medicines more often on a daily basis (10/16 compared to 29/117 of people under 60), encountered problems with ageing (9/16 compared to 21/117 of people under 60) and rated their quality of life as unsatisfactory (4/14 compared to 9/107 of people under 60). Awareness of EB approaches and Cochrane was higher within health professions (evidence-based medicine: 42/86 vs. 13/48; Cochrane: 32/86 vs. 2/48), and health information needs did not differ between age or gender groups or people with a satisfactory and unsatisfactory quality of life. The minority (10%—13/134) were aware of ageism without age or gender differences. The low awareness calls for the need of Cochrane intervention both for consumers and those in the health profession to raise awareness to contribute to Kazan moving towards an age-friendly city.

Keywords: Kazan; Russia; health information; quality of life; ageing; ageism; Cochrane; evidence-based; medicines; consumers; awareness; age-friendly cities

1. Introduction

The strive for healthy ageing is universal. Healthy ageing is defined by the WHO as *"maintaining the functional ability that allows you to do the things you value"*, *"preserving physical and mental capacity"* in an accessible and supportive environment for older people. It is not surprising that one of the eight essential domains of age-friendly cities by the WHO deals with health services. Raising evidence-based awareness campaigns about ageing is the most important action, mandated by the WHO, in order to ensure that societies become more just and fairer with institutions becoming stronger to benefit the ageing population [1]. Further development of the WHO's age-friendly framework was proposed recently with the focus on the role of technology in a modern urban environment [2].

In Russia, the proportion of the population over the working age reached one-quarter of its population in 2018, according to the Federal State Statistics Service [3]. At that time, the working age was declared as over 60 years for men and over 55 years for women until 2019 when the retirement age was raised. This demographic shift caused tensions and strains in health and welfare systems [3,4].

Most countries in the world have declared the chronological age of 65 as older age. Currently, there is no United Nations standard numerical criterion; however, the UN agreed that the cut-off age value for the older population is 60+ [5].

The Republic of Tatarstan (RT) is one of the most vibrantly developing regions of the Russian Federation with a population of 3.9 million people living in a territory of 67,836 square kilometres and has experienced, over the last three years, a 0.5% population growth. There has also been an increase in the ageing population, both in cities and the countryside, among men and women [4,6]. Therefore, the issues of healthy ageing are relevant for Russia and RT. Kazan is the capital of the Republic of Tatarstan, an ancient city with more than 1000 years of history, located on the left bank of the Volga River (https://www.kzn.ru/o-kazani/) with a current population of 1,257,391 people as of 1 January 2020 (the fifth location in Russia) [7,8]. Kazan is a vibrant city of sustainable economic growth and opportunities, comfortable for everyday life for its citizens, with a safe urban environment and age-friendly city [9].

Recently, an impressive number of initiatives, targeted at healthy lifestyle promotion, have been established and implemented in the Russian Federation and Tatarstan. However, there is a scarcity of published reports in the public domain. From our detailed searches of PubMed and eLIBRARY, the Russian database, we learnt that research on the ageing population, primarily of Moscow and Saint Petersburg, has been conducted since the 1990s using mostly the survey methodology [10,11]. The most extensive and recent monitoring of Moscow's ageing population was performed in a framework of a longitudinal monitoring study over five years (2011–2015) by the centre for monitoring studies, with special emphasis on the indicators of the level and quality of life and attention to the changing needs of the ageing Muscovites [12]. Researchers have looked mostly at social and economic factors, emotions and quality of life of the older people. Over the last five years, Russian research attention has turned to information and training needs of older adults as a factor contributing to healthy ageing [13,14].

However, none of the published studies addressed or used the concept of an evidence-based approach to healthy ageing. We did not find any studies performed in Kazan, showing that there is an urgent need for raising evidence-based awareness amongst the ageing population of Kazan (Tatarstan, Russia). This might enable Kazan to join the European movement of transforming age-friendly cities to become age-inclusive cities [15].

Cochrane is an international organisation, a registered charity in the UK that has contributed to world health by pioneering and implementing the concept of organising medical research findings in a unique form of Cochrane systematic reviews. Cochrane systematic reviews facilitate informed decisions about treatment and other health interventions for better health. Over the last 25 years, Cochrane has gained international recognition for providing the benchmark of high-quality, unbiased and independent trusted evidence for better health [16,17]. Cochrane Russia was formed in Kazan 2015 to empower the Russian health system and Russian people with the best-synthesised research evidence.

From our practical work at Cochrane Russia, we recognise that the majority of current initiatives for healthy lifestyle promotion in Kazan and Tatarstan have been delivered by newly formed nongovernmental or private organisations utilising governmental funds run by young entrepreneurs who are unaware of research evidence, such as Cochrane, as witnessed by the results of our one-question survey at the meetings of health-promotion entrepreneurs. In our capacity of Cochrane Russia, we developed an Evidence School project for the ageing population of Tatarstan to improve health and longevity through Cochrane Knowledge Translation in the framework of the Cochrane consumers initiative Geographic Groups Consumer Engagement and Involvement Challenge Fund and were successful in our application. Here, we report the findings of the baseline survey.

Direct involvement of consumers in health care with shared decision making has evolved as a new approach or concept in health care over recent decades [18–21]. The language to define the new concepts and approaches in research and practice have evolved and require special attention to terminology that has not yet been fully unified [21]. The implementation of shared decision making should rely on knowledge and skills in evidence-based medicine, not only of health professionals but also of patients or consumers for quality and transparency of decision making [20]. Research in consumer training potential has emerged recently. It was shown that training in evidence-based medicine (EBM) was feasible [18,19] and better, and long-term implementation and further research are needed [18].

The aim of this study was to explore the health information needs of the ageing population of Kazan and the challenges people face in improving their health and longevity based on their attitudes, perceptions and assessment of their quality of life to ultimately raise evidence-based awareness about ageing. It is the most important action, mandated by the WHO, in order to ensure that societies become more just and fairer and institutions stronger to benefit the ageing population.

2. Materials and Methods

For this exploratory project, we performed a descriptive study among patients, caregivers and health care workers of the Interregional Clinical Diagnostic Centre (ICDC, Kazan, Republic of Tatarstan, Russian Federation), using the simple survey methodology. The Interregional Clinical Diagnostic Centre (ICDC) is one of the largest clinical hospitals of the Republic of Tatarstan, Kazan. It deals with the major burden of disease, disability and mortality of the Tatarstan population and cardiovascular diseases. The majority of regular ICDC patients belong to the older age groups. We planned to use the survey results as the basis for the Cochrane Evidence School development to enable targeting the most pertinent local health environment issues of the ageing population.

The survey consisted of 25 questions grouped into 3 sections: "Participant Portrait," "Awareness Level" and "Exploring Ageing/Health Problems" and were a mixture of closed-ended and open-ended formats (the English translation of the survey questionnaire is presented in Supplementary Material S1).

The original plan was to focus on the ageing population only; however, at the time of the study, which coincided with the time of the expansion of the COVID-19 pandemic in Kazan, due to the scarcity of in-patients, we decided not to use any specific cut-off age value to include as many participants into our study as possible. All patients, caregivers and staff members of the ICDC, who agreed to participate in the study at that point of time, were included. This approach allowed us to determine whether there were any differences amongst various age groups in knowledge needs, perceptions, attitudes, quality of life, contentment with current position and challenges people face in maintaining and improving their health with ageing. Every participant gave their informed consent to participate in the study and anonymise the processing of personal demographic information (for an English translation of the Informed Consent Form, please see Supplementary Material S2 and the Ethics Approval section) before taking part in the survey. They received a printed hard copy of the questionnaire at the ICDC and filled it in themselves or with the assistance of a caregiver over a period of 2 weeks in (10–25) April 2020.

Ethics Approval: the study obtained ethics approval from the Ethics Committee of the ICDC, numbered 259 dated 30th of March 2020. All the participants gave their informed consent before taking part in the survey. The English translation of the Informed Consent form is in Supplementary Material S2.

A total of 134 people participated in the study.

The survey results were combined in an Excel spreadsheet by the calculating absolute and relative numerical measurements for which we used the numbers of participants of various categories (age, gender, health profession, etc.) as the measurements. The results of open-ended questions were used in a descriptive way. Various subgroups of participants were compared to explore the potential associations of the studied parameters (answers to survey questions) with age, gender, representing health profession or not and other participant characteristics (but not a participant status with the ICDC (employee/patient/caregiver) using Fisher's exact test [22]. The predefined significance threshold was $p < 0.05$ for a two-tailed test.

3. Results

Of a total of 134 people, who participated in the survey, there were: 44 patients of ICDC, 2 caregivers (family members) of the ICDC patients and 88 ICDC staff members.

3.1. General Characteristics of the Survey Participants, Their Lifestyle, Health Problems, Income, Quality of Life and Satisfaction

The distribution of participants by their general characteristics (gender, age, professional affiliation, etc.) is presented in Table 1. In total, 87 women (65%) and 47 men (35%) participated in the survey, and the majority of participants were under 60 years old (117/134; 87%). More than half of the participants had higher or secondary specialised medical/pharmaceutical education (73/134; 54%) and were healthcare workers (86/134; 64%).

Table 1. General characteristics of the survey participants.

Age	*N* (%)	**Gender**	*N* (%)
Under 60 years	117 (87%)	Women	87 (65%)
60+ years	16 (12%)	Men	47 (35%)
Unknown	1 (1%)		
Total (%)	134 (100%)	Total (%)	134 (100%)
Education	*N* (%)	**Occupation**	*N*(%)
Higher or secondary specialised medical/pharmaceutical education	73 (54%)	Health care providers	86 (64%)
Higher/secondary specialised education (excl. med/pharm)	53 (40%)	Non-health-care workers	23 (17%)
Secondary education	8 (6%)	Retired	25 (19%)
Total (%)	134 (100%)	Total (%)	134 (100%)
Unhealthy Lifestyle (Including Smoking, Alcohol Consumption, Etc.)	*N* (%)	**Chronic Diseases (Long-Term Health Conditions)**	*N*(%)
Yes	92 (69%)	Yes	115 (86%)
No	19 (14%)	No	19 (14%)
Unknown (no answer)	23 (17%)		
Total (%)	134 (100%)	Total (%)	134 (100%)
Income Level Per Month			
Under 8000 RUB (88 Euro)			3 (2%)
8000–12,000 RUB (88–133 Euro)			9 (7%)
12,000–20,000 RUB (133–221 Euro)			29 (21%)
20,000–30,000 RUB (221–332 Euro)			39 (29%)
30,000–60,000 RUB (332–663 Euro)			43 (32%)

Table 1. *Cont.*

Income Level Per Month	
60,000–90,000 RUB (663–995 Euro)	8 (6%)
>90,000 RUB (995 Euro)	2 (2%)
Unknown	1 (1%)
Total (%)	134 (100%)

N–number, %–percentage of total number.

Most participants (115/134; 86%) indicated that they had various chronic diseases or long-term health conditions, and many of them had more than one health problem. Among the most frequently mentioned were cardiovascular diseases (37/134; 28%), gastrointestinal diseases (31/134; 23%), bone and joint diseases (25/134; 19%), neurological diseases (22/134; 16%) and respiratory diseases (13/134; 10%).

The majority of participants considered their lifestyle to be unhealthy (92/134; 69%), including having a sedentary lifestyle (33/134; 25%), a lack of attention to their health (28/134; 21%), an unhealthy diet (26/134; 19%), smoking (21/134; 16%) and excess alcohol consumption (3/134; 2%).

The income level of the participants ranged from under 8 thousand rubles per month to over 90 thousand rubles per month, and the median income level among all participants was 20–30 thousand rubles per month. For the majority of participants (>80%), the income level ranged from 12 to 60 thousand rubles. The income level of participants over 60 years old (16 people) also ranged from under 7–8 thousand rubles to over 90 thousand rubles per month, and almost half of the participants (7 out 16 people) had an income level within 12–20 thousand rubles.

Regarding the frequency of medicine use, 52 out 134 people (38%) responded that they rarely took medicines, 39 people (29%) took medicines every day, 29 people (22%) took medicines periodically, 13 people (10%) answered never and 1 person did not answer this question. However, when comparing the frequency of taking medicines in the age groups of our interest (60+ vs. <60), it was found that more people aged 60+ (10 out 16 people) took medicines every day whereas more people under 60 years of age (49 out 132 people) took medicines rarely (Table 2).

Table 2. Frequency of medicine use among the participants by age.

Frequency of Medicine Use	Number of Participants Aged Under 60	Number of Participants Aged 60+	Total Number of Participants
Daily	29 *	10 *	39 (29%)
Periodically	26	3	29 (22%)
Rarely	49	2	51 (38%)
Never	12	1	13 (10%)
No answer	1		1 (1%)
In total	117	16	133 (100%)

* $p = 0.006$ (Fisher's exact test).

When comparing the answer "daily use" with all other answers combined among people aged under 60 and aged 60+, it was found that more of the older participants took medicines on a daily basis: 10 out of 16 compared to 29 out of 117 of people under 60 ($p = 0.006$, Fisher's exact test).

There were also differences in medicine use between men and women: half of the male participants answered that they took medicines every day whereas fewer than one-fifth of women responded that they took medicines every day (Table 3). Most of the female participants responded that they took medicines rarely (38 out 87 women; 44%) or periodically (25 out 87 women; 29%).

Table 3. Frequency of medicine use among the participants by gender.

Frequency of Medicine Use	Number of Men	Number of Women	Total Number of Participants
Daily	23 *	16 *	39 (29%)
Periodically	4	25	29 (22%)
Rarely	14	38	52 (38%)
Never	5	8	13 (10%)
No answer	1		1 (1%)
In total	47	87	134 (100%)

* $p = 0.0003$ (Fisher's exact test).

When comparing the answer "daily use" with all other answers combined among men and women, it was found that more of the men than women took medicines on a daily basis ($p = 0.0003$, Fisher's exact test).

Thus, medicine use was heavier in the older participants (aged 60+) and men.

All participants were asked to rate their quality of life on a 10-point scale. We attributed a score of 1–4 points to low quality of life, 5–7 points to moderate quality of life and 8–10 points to high quality of life.

Out of 134 participants, 131 assessed the quality of their life, but since 1 of them did not indicate her age (woman with low quality of life), we were able to compare the quality of life among 130 participants with a known age. The results of assessing the quality of life of survey participants by age (under 60 years vs. 60+ years) are presented in Table 4.

Table 4. Participants' quality of life (self-reported) by age.

Participants' Quality of Life	Number of Participants Aged under 60	Number of Participants Aged 60+	Total Number of Participants
High (8–10 points)	65	4	69 (52%)
Moderate (5–7 points)	42	6	48 (36%)
Low (1–4 points)	9	4	13 (10%)
Unknown	1	2	3 (2%)
Total	117	16	133 (100%)

Many participants rated their quality of life high enough: more than half of the participants (69/133; 52%) considered their quality of life to be high, and 48 out 133 participants (36%) considered their quality of life to be moderate.

We combined participants with high and moderate quality of life together as participants with satisfactory quality of life and compared the quality of life (satisfactory vs. unsatisfactory) among participants aged under 60 years and 60+ years (Table 5). Low quality of life was considered unsatisfactory. Four participants were excluded from this assessment because three of them did not assess their quality of life and one did not indicate her age.

Table 5. Satisfactory and unsatisfactory quality of life (self-reported) by age.

Participants' Quality of Life	Number of Participants Aged under 60	Number of Participants Aged 60+	Total Number of Participants
Satisfactory (5–10 points)	107 *	10 *	117 (90%)
Unsatisfactory (1–4 points)	9 *	4 *	13 (10%)
Total	116	14	130 (100%)

* $p = 0.03$ (Fisher's exact test).

The proportion of the participants with unsatisfactory quality of life was higher among participants aged 60+ compared to the participants aged under 60. However, the number of participants over 60 was small. With the use of Fisher's exact test to assess the significance of differences between compared groups, the probability of such a result was found to be approximately 0.03. This means that we can refute the null hypothesis that there are no differences between groups, and the quality of life of participants aged 60+ is worse compared to participants aged under 60.

It was important to determine if the quality of life of the participants changed with age in their opinion and, if changed, what the changes were. For the question "Has the quality of life changed with age?" 52 out of 134 people (39%) answered "yes" (9 people aged 60+, 42 people aged under 60 and 1 person with unknown age). Twelve out of these 52 people answered that their quality of life improved with age (1 person aged 60+ and 11 people aged under 60). However, 22 out of 52 people answered that their quality of life worsened with age (4 people aged 60+ and 18 people aged under 60).

The analysis of the responses regarding participants' satisfaction with their current situation and their life in general showed that more than half of the participants (73/134; 55%) answered that they were satisfied with their current situation, 39 out 134 participants (29%) answered that they were unsatisfied, 21 out 134 participants (16%) answered that they had difficulties with this question and 1 participant did not answer at all.

When comparing participants' satisfaction with their current situation between the two age groups (60+ vs. under 60), there were no significant differences after using Fisher's exact test (Table 6). Two participants were excluded from this assessment because one of them did not assess her quality of life (woman >80 years) and one participant (unsatisfied) did not indicate her age. Thus, slightly more than half of the participants, regardless of age, were satisfied with their current situation.

Table 6. Participants' satisfaction with their current situation.

Participants' Satisfaction	Number of Participants Aged under 60	Number of Participants Aged 60+	Total Number of Participants
Satisfied	65	8	73 (55%)
Unsatisfied	32	6	38 (29%)
Difficult to answer	20	1	21 (16%)
Total	117	15	132 (100%)

The participants who were unsatisfied with their current situation were asked to answer what they would like to change. Twenty-two people out of 38 answered. Many participants responded they would welcome positive changes in their wellbeing, health and lifestyle (nine people), in their financial situation (nine people) and some of them would like changes in professional development (career), health care, family support and personal life.

3.2. *Age-Related Problems, Awareness about Ageism and Participation in Antiaging Programmes*

Since at the inception of the study it was planned to include mostly older people to participate in our survey, one of the questions of our questionnaire asked if people experienced age-related problems. Thirty-one out 134 participants (23%) answered that they had encountered problems related to their age (21 people aged under 60, 9 people aged 60+ and 1 person with unknown age).

When comparing the proportion of participants who had encountered age-related problems or not within the two age groups (60+ vs. under 60), it was found that older participants (60+) reported age-related problems more frequently (Table 7).

Table 7. Experience of age-related problems by age.

Have You Encountered Any Problems Related to Your Age?	Number of Participants Aged under 60	Number of Participants Aged 60+	Total Number of Participants
Encountered	21 *	9 *	30 (22%)
Not encountered	84	6	90 (68%)
Difficult to answer	12	0	12 (9%)
No answer	0	1	1 (1%)
Total	117	16	133 (100%)

* $p = 0.002$ (Fisher's exact test).

When using Fisher's exact test to assess the association of reporting on age-related problems with age, it was found that the probability of the association was there with the value of approximately $p = 0.002$. Unsurprisingly, the participants aged 60+ encountered more age-related problems.

However, one cannot be sure that the participants reported about their personal experiences of age-related problems, particularly those of the younger participants. It cannot be ruled out that they meant not only their personal experience but also the experience of their relatives or friends.

The majority of participants (17 out 30 people; 12 people aged from under 30 to 60, 4 people aged 60+ and 1 person with unknown age) described these problems as health-related problems (diseases, impairment of vision and hearing, memory and endurance, as well as overweight, decreased alertness and reaction, and fatigue). Some participants (3 people aged 50–70) reported social problems (deprivation of work, decrease in income (salary), lack of funds for living) and one participant (aged 40–50) noted problems associated with appearance (wrinkles).

It was important to know if our participants had heard about ageism and, if yes, what it was in their opinion. According to Wikipedia, ageism is determined as "stereotyping and/or discrimination against individuals or groups on the basis of their age" [23]. According to the WHO, ageism is defined as "*stereotypes, prejudice, and discrimination against older people on the basis of their chronological or perceived age.*" it is widespread and has harmful effects on the health of older adults, their social life, employment and other aspects of life [1].

It was found that only 13 out of 134 participants (10%; 7 men and 6 women) previously heard about ageism (Table 8), including 11 people aged under 60 and 2 people aged 60+. Nearly all of them were health care providers (12 people). There were no differences in the awareness about ageism between the two age groups (60+ vs. under 60).

Table 8. Participants' awareness of ageism.

Awareness about Ageism	Number of Participants Aged under 60	Number of Participants Aged 60+	Total Number of Participants
Aware (previously heard) about ageism	11	2	13 (10%)
Unaware (not previously heard) about ageism	60	14	74 (55%)
Difficult to answer	5	0	5 (4%)
No answer	41	0	41 (31%)
Total	117	16	133 (100%)

Only nine participants were able to correctly explain what ageism was. It could be suggested that the low awareness about ageism among our survey participants may be due to insufficient use of this English-language-originating term in Russia and the absence of a Russian-language analogue of this term. Since the number of participants was small, further research with more people is needed to study the awareness of the phenomenon of ageism.

Regarding participation in antiaging programmes, only 2 out of 134 people answered that they had previously participated in antiaging programmes. Two men aged 40–50 and 60+, both health care providers, with an income level of 60–90 thousand rubles per month, who rated their quality of life as high and were satisfied with their current situation, had never heard about ageism before. One of them thought that participation in antiageing programmes was beneficial for him to facilitate quitting bad habits, and the other considered it to aid in improving his wellbeing.

It could be assumed that not all of the participants understood what antiaging programmes were since there was no explanation in the question and it was the English term "antiaging" that was used in the questionnaire (Supplementary Material S1). Perhaps additional clarifications to this question and the use of the Russian-language analogue of the name of antiaging programmes would lead to different results of the answer to this question.

3.3. *Awareness about Evidence-Based Medicine, Cochrane and Health Information Needs*

The specially designed series of questions asked about awareness of evidence-based medicine (EBM), Cochrane and the needs for health information or knowledge (willingness to participate in the Evidence School).

Fifty-five out 134 participants (41%) had previously heard about evidence-based medicine (50 people aged 60+ and 4 people aged under 60; 25 men and 30 women; 42 health care providers, 9 non-health-care providers and 4 people retired (unemployed)). There were no significant differences in awareness about evidence-based medicine between the two age groups (60+ vs. under 60) after using Fisher's exact test. Only a weak tendency to the potential association that awareness was higher in participants aged under 60 ($p = 0.2$) could be suggested. It was noteworthy that EBM-awareness was higher among men than women ($p = 0.04$).

Assuming that EBM-awareness should be higher among health care providers, we compared the proportion of participants who had previously heard about EBM among health care providers and non-health-care workers, combined with retired (and unemployed) participants (Table 9).

Table 9. Participants' awareness of evidence-based medicine (EBM).

Awareness about (EBM)	Number of Health Care Providers	Number of Non-Health-Care Workers	Number of Retired Participants	Total Number of Participants
Aware about EBM	42 *	9 *	4 *	55 (41%)
Unaware about EBM	31	4	13	48 (36%)
Difficult to answer	13	9	9	31 (23%)
Total	86	22	26	134 (100%)

* $p = 0.01$ (Fisher's exact test).

EBM-awareness was higher among health care providers compared to non-health-care workers combined with nonworking participants (Fisher's exact test, $p = 0.01$).

The survey asked about participants' awareness of Cochrane and Cochrane evidence and contribution as Cochrane is the leading international organisation for evidence synthesis, knowledge translation, and independent quality research advocacy.

It was found that the majority of participants (93 out of 134 people; 70%) had not heard about Cochrane. Out of 134 people, 34 (25%) answered that they were aware of Cochrane and Cochrane work, and 7 out 134 people (5%) could not answer this question.

When comparing Cochrane awareness between the two age groups of the participants (60+ vs. under 60), no differences were found.

When comparing the numbers of aware and unaware (in relation to Cochrane) participants between health care providers and non-health-care workers, it was found that Cochrane awareness was associated with health care professionals both when compared to unaware people ($p = 0.001$) and when compared to the combined group of unaware and people experiencing difficulties to answer ($p = 0.000008$) (Table 10).

Table 10. Participants' awareness of Cochrane and Cochrane work.

Awareness about Cochrane	Number of Health Care Providers	Number of Non-Health-Care Workers	Number of Retired Participants	Total Number of Participants
Aware of Cochrane	32	1	1	34 (25%)
Unaware of Cochrane	50	20	23	93 (70%)
Difficult to answer	4	2	1	7 (5%)
Total	86	23	25	134 (100%)

Thus, our survey confirmed that awareness about evidence-based medicine and Cochrane was higher within the healthcare profession than all others. However, it turned out that more than one-third of health care providers had never heard about EBM (31 out 86 health care workers; 36%) and more than half had never heard about Cochrane (50 out 86 health care providers; 58%).

In the framework of our project of Evidence School for the ageing population of Tatarstan aimed at improving health and longevity, it was planned to explore the needs in the knowledge of EBM and Cochrane for further designing the Evidence School project. Forty-six out of 134 people answered that they were interested in learning (34%), 34 people (25%) answered that they were not interested, 44 people (33%) could not answer and 10 people (8%) did not answer.

When comparing the need for knowledge about EBM and Cochrane between the two age groups (60+ vs. under 60), as well as between men and women, participants with satisfactory or unsatisfactory quality of life, no significant differences were found. Initially, assuming that the knowledge needs are possibly higher in health care workers compared to other workers or nonworking people, it was important to check if there are differences in knowledge needs between them (Table 11).

Table 11. Need for knowledge about evidence-based medicine (EBM) and Cochrane.

Need for Knowledge about EBM And Cochrane	Number of Health Care Providers	Number of Non-Health-Care Workers	Number of Retired Participants	Total Number of Participants
Interested in gaining knowledge (learning)	38	3	5	46 (34%)
Not interested in gaining knowledge (learning)	16	10	8	34 (25%)
Difficult to answer	27	7	10	44 (33%)
No answer	5	3	2	10 (8%)
Total	86	23	25	134 (100%)

The need for knowledge about EBM and Cochrane was higher among health care providers in the following comparisons:

(1) "Interested in gaining knowledge (learning)" vs. "not interested" amongst health care providers and non-health-care workers ($p = 0.003$);
(2) "Interested in gaining knowledge (learning)" combined with "difficult to answer" vs. "not interested" amongst health care providers and non-health-care workers ($p = 0.009$);
(3) "Interested in gaining knowledge (learning)" vs. "not interested" amongst health care providers and non-health-care workers combined with retired (not working) participants ($p = 0.001$);
(4) "Interested in gaining knowledge (learning)" combined with "difficult to answer" vs. "not interested" amongst health care providers and non-health-care workers combined retired (not working) participants ($p = 0.01$).

4. Discussion

A descriptive study (survey) was performed among patients, caregivers and health care providers of the Interregional Clinical Diagnostic Centre (Kazan, Republic of Tatarstan, Russian Federation), using the simple survey methodology for this exploratory project. The age of the participants ranged from under 30 to over 80 years. The majority of the participants were people under 60 years old, women, healthcare providers with medical or pharmaceutical education, with long-term health conditions and an unhealthy lifestyle. This age disposition of participants is not representative of the current population of Tatarstan because, in 2016, Tatarstan moved to the very high level of demographic old age, with people aged 60+ comprising 18% of the population and more [4]. However, it is characteristic of the pandemic situation at the ICDC and loosely reflects the age disposition of in-patients in Russia [4,10]. The majority of the participants rarely took medicines, but there were more participants taking medicines more often (daily) among people aged 60+ and men, which is, again, in line with the findings of Belokon on the importance of medicines and reliance on them within the retired Russian population [10].

Most participants positively assessed their quality of life: half noted high quality of life, and over one-third of participants noted moderate quality of life. Ageing contributed to the lower perception of quality of life. The proportion of participants who rated their quality of life as unsatisfactory was higher among participants aged 60+. This is in line with the findings of the large-scale (about 700 respondents) survey in six territories of Russia in the vicinity of Moscow, reporting low quality of life of older adults. The survey showed that the low quality of life was due to low (below the subsistence level) pensions, but was not limited to this financial aspect only, demonstrating that the older people perceived their quality of life low because of the lack of respect for their personality [10].

Most participants in our study noted that their quality of life has changed with age negatively primarily due to health problems. Very few participants included financial problems to their characteristics of poor quality of life; however, some participants noted a positive change in their quality of life with age, describing more emerging opportunities, freedom and becoming smarter. More than half of the participants were satisfied with their current situation without any age differences. These findings suggest that, indeed, the ageing population of Kazan may be in a better situation compared to the rest of the country. Though this assumption needs to be confirmed in larger-scale studies, it could be suggested that Kazan is closer to age-friendly cities than others in the country.

It could be assumed that the significance of the different components of quality of life varies among different people, and this is probably a rather subjective assessment. Although some participants who reported an improvement in the quality of their life with age noted that they became smarter with more opportunities and more freedom, the participants who reported worsening of their quality of life with age noted an increase in health problems. Thus, the participants assessed the quality of life from different perspectives, both from social situations, interactions and health conditions, depending on what affected and worried them most. This is in line with the findings of a large community survey of retired citizens of Saint Petersburg (1500 people), which identified social components of the quality of life of older adults with mainly the worsening of financial status and becoming less satisfied with their current situation and more reliant on their children in taking responsibility for their wellbeing [11]. Certainly, it could be assumed that the age of participants in our study might have affected their perception of the change in quality of life with age, though we could not assess this factor quantitatively. For instance, participants aged 60+ more often encountered age-related problems, primarily perceiving them as health-related problems, commented less often on financial or work-related problems. This perception could be one of the potential reasons for the low awareness of ageism among our participants. However, there may be simply a lack of familiarity with the term per se. Noteworthy is the fact that none of the identified publications on ageing problems in Russia used this term, though studied components of what constitutes ageism [10].

The awareness of evidence-based medicine and its approaches was low. Less than half of participants were aware of EBM and only a quarter were aware of Cochrane. Health professionals were more informed about EBM and Cochrane, and age did not contribute to better or poorer awareness. This is our pioneering finding, and though it needs verification and confirmation in larger studies, we will use the data from this survey to design and conduct the Cochrane Evidence School at the ICDC. This will actively involve both patients and healthcare providers in the design and production of Cochrane Knowledge Translation products for their personal use and use by their peers. We will survey participants of the School at its first-round completion and report or new findings. We think that this work will help us to plan further research in this area and design a more informed plan of action for better Cochrane Knowledge Translation specifically tailored to the needs of the ageing population of Kazan.

We hope to bring closer the times of Kazan becoming not only a smart but truly age-friendly [24] and even an age-involved city when society will get to the position of being able to celebrate the current increases in longevity and life expectancy. Our project will empower the ageing population of Kazan and further raise awareness of the need for evidence and "action to ensure good health in older ages" following the Cochrane Campbell Global Ageing Partnership and its Wikipedia Project [25]. We hope that our findings and future development of the project will contribute to the expanding area of research on the proposed extension of the WHO's age-friendly cities model by following its recommendations on including citizens from all sectors of society, consultations and data collection, including a qualitative approach to measure attitudes and perceptions [2].

Finally, about a third of the surveyed people were interested in new knowledge and learning (participating in Cochrane Evidence School). Unsurprisingly, the need for knowledge was higher among healthcare providers, but otherwise, there were no differences between participants aged 60+ or under 60, men and women, participants with satisfactory or unsatisfactory quality of life and other characteristics. This is in line with the findings of the survey study in Saratov Day-Care Centre for Social Services the Population of Saratov (for retired people), which looked at the mechanisms and drivers of social activity of older citizens [14]. The author identified internal resources of the older people for voluntary work, namely spare time, experience, knowledge, the desire to contribute and components of motivation: "the need for communication and the desire to be socially useful to other people; the need for new knowledge and, accordingly, in new social roles. Retirement leisure in the social service forms an active position (physical, educational activity). The results of the research showed the presence of interest and the desire to take the initiative in organising social events" [14].

These findings together with the results of our exploratory study provide a good background for the implementation of Cochrane Evidence School and later hopefully scaling up the experience and the impact to contribute to the vision for an age-friendly ecosystem and prevention-focused public health system [26].

Strength and Limitations

This study is the first to explore the concept of an evidence-based approach and specifically Cochrane for healthy ageing and to address a number of factors contributing to the challenges of ageing in Kazan, Tatarstan, Russia. Data were collected with the same standardised questionnaire in all participants and analysed the data quantitatively and qualitatively.

When planning the study, we aimed to survey 50 people but did not limit the target number in case more people volunteered to participate, ending up with nearly three times the initial target.

All patients of the ICDC (at the time of the survey (end of March–beginning of April 2020), Russia was under a strict lockdown period, and only emergency patients were at the ICDC) were included as well as their family members who agreed to participate. This allowed us to subgroup participants by age to determine if there were any differences amongst various age groups in knowledge, perceptions, attitudes and challenges people face in maintaining and improving their health with ageing. Involving health care providers allowed for a new dimension of the study and comparison of answers from consumers to the answers from within the health profession.

However, the findings of this exploratory study should be interpreted with caution and need to be confirmed in a larger-scale research project owing to the number of limitations: small numbers of survey participants from a single health care setting, small and unequal numbers of participants in compared subgroups; substantial representation of health professionals and people under 60 years of age. The possibility that some of the questions were not clear enough to all the participants could not be ruled out, although there is hope that participants answered the questions with full sincerity.

Although the sample is small, despite having over 130 participants, this is the first exploratory study in a region of Russia that has a diverse community (Tatar/Russian), and this work forms a basis to progress this domain in Russia across rural and urban environments.

5. Conclusions

This exploratory study provides data on the health information needs of the ageing and middle-aged population of Kazan by documenting that less than half of the survey participants were aware of evidence-based medicine and only a quarter of them were aware of Cochrane and Cochrane work. EBM-awareness was higher within the healthcare profession than others and among men than women, with a weak tendency to be higher in participants under 60 years of age than in people of 60+ years old. Cochrane awareness was also higher within the healthcare profession. The need for EBM and Cochrane knowledge was also higher within the health profession without age or gender differences or between participants with satisfactory and unsatisfactory quality of life.

Most of the survey participants were generally positive in assessing their quality of life despite the fact that many have long-term health conditions and unhealthy lifestyles. A few reported improvements in quality of life with age.

Older participants were less positive about their quality of life. More participants aged 60+ took medicines on a daily basis than people under 60 years of age.

Ageing was the challenge in improving health and longevity with more participants aged 60+ rating their quality of life as unsatisfactory than participants under 60 years old, and encountering more age-related problems. Only 10% of participants were aware of ageism without age or gender differences.

Low awareness of EBM, Cochrane, ageing problems and ageism, together with the scarcity of independent, accessible, quality information about the effectiveness and safety of therapeutic and diagnostic interventions, nondrug treatment and prevention measures, present a case for the urgent need for raising awareness of ageing problems, ageism and evidence-based approach to tackling the problems of the ageing population of Kazan, which strives to be an age-friendly city.

Cochrane Evidence Schools designed not only for patients and consumers but also for health care providers might become a beneficial instrument both for raising awareness and advancing knowledge and attitudes of the citizens of Kazan as a pilot city with the potential of scaling up.

The hope is that this exploratory study would contribute to Kazan becoming not only a fully age-friendly city but moving towards age-inclusiveness.

Supplementary Materials: The following are available online at http://www.mdpi.com/1660-4601/17/24/9212/s1. Supplementary Material S1: English translation of the survey questionnaire "Health evidence for consumers". Supplementary Material S2: English translation of the informed consent form.

Author Contributions: Conceptualization, L.E.Z. and E.V.Y.; methodology, L.E.Z.; software, L.E.Z; validation, R.N.K., L.I.T. and G.N.S.; formal analysis, G.N.S. and E.V.Y.; investigation, E.V.Y. and L.E.Z.; resources, R.N.K. and L.I.T.; data curation, G.N.S. and E.V.Y.; writing—original draft preparation, E.V.Y. and L.E.Z.; writing—review and editing, L.E.Z.; visualization, E.V.Y.; supervision, L.E.Z.; project administration, L.I.T. and R.N.K.; funding acquisition, L.E.Z. and R.N.K. All authors have read and agreed to the published version of the manuscript.

Funding: This research will receive funding from the Cochrane Geographic Groups and Consumers Challenge Fund: https://community.cochrane.org/news/call-proposals-cochrane-geographic-groups-consumer-engagement-and-involvement-challenge-fund#:~:text=As%20part%20of%20the%20Cochrane,consumers%20and%20sharing%20examples%20of.

Acknowledgments: We would like to acknowledge Cochrane Consumer Network and Cochrane Central Executive for administrative and logistical support and the leadership of ICDC for in-kind support.

Conflicts of Interest: The authors declare no conflict of interest. The funders had no role in the design of the study; in the collection, analyses, or interpretation of data; in the writing of the manuscript, or in the decision to publish the results.

References

1. WHO. Ageing and Life-Course. Healthy Ageing and the Sustainable Development Goals. 2020. Available online: https://www.who.int/ageing/sdgs/en/ (accessed on 9 December 2020).
2. Marston, H.R.; Van Hoof, J. "Who Doesn't Think about Technology When Designing Urban Environments for Older People?" A Case Study Approach to a Proposed Extension of the WHO's Age-Friendly Cities Model. *Int. J. Environ. Res. Public Health* **2019**, *16*, 3525. [CrossRef] [PubMed]
3. Rosstat1. The Older Generation. 2020. Available online: https://rosstat.gov.ru/folder/13877 (accessed on 7 October 2020). (In Russian)
4. Fakhrutdinova, E.V.; Yagudin, R.K.; Rybkin, L.I. Problems of the adult population of the Republic of Tatarstan: Medical and demographic aspect. In *Economic and Legal Issues*; Limited Liability Company "Economic Sciences": Moscow, Russia, 2016; pp. 64–68.
5. WHO. Health Situation and Trend Assessment. Elderly Population. 2020. Available online: http://origin.searo.who.int/entity/health_situation_trends/data/chi/elderly-population/en/#:~{}:text=Trends%20in%20proportion%20of%20older%20persons%20(60%2B)&text=The%20UN%20agreed%20cutoff%20is,110%2B)%20are%20also%20made (accessed on 9 December 2020).
6. Russia Today, R. Rating of Regions by Demography. 2020. Available online: https://riarating.ru/infografika/20200421/630168368.html (accessed on 7 October 2020).
7. Rosstat2. Population of the Russian Federation by Municipalities. 2020. Available online: https://rosstat.gov.ru/compendium/document/13282 (accessed on 7 October 2020). (In Russian)
8. Wikipedia. Population of Kazan. In Wikipedia. 2020. Available online: https://ru.wikipedia.org/wiki/%D0%9D%D0%B0%D1%81%D0%B5%D0%BB%D0%B5%D0%BD%D0%B8%D0%B5_%D0%9A%D0%B0%D0%B7%D0%B0%D0%BD%D0%B8#cite_note-1 (accessed on 7 October 2020).
9. Duma, K.C. *On the Strategy of Socio-Economic Development of the Municipal Formation of Kazan until 2030*; Duma, K.S., Ed.; 2020; Volume 14, p. 103. Available online: https://www.kzn.ru/upload/about-kazan/strategiya-kazani-2030/%D1%81%D1%82%D1%80%D0%B0%D1%82%D0%B5%D0%B3%D0%B8%D1%8F.doc (accessed on 7 October 2020).
10. Belokon, O.V. Modern problems of the quality of life of the elderly in Russia (results of surveys). *Adv. Gerontol.* **2005**, *17*, 87–101.
11. Shmeleva, E.V. Elderly Petersburgers today: Factors of quality of life. *J. Sociol. Soc. Anthropol.* **2005**, *8*, 146–156.
12. Kornilova, M.V. Sociological monitoring of the level and quality of life of elderly Muscovites: New methodological and organisational approaches. *Sci. Result Ser. Sociol. Manag.* **2016**, *2*, 12–19.
13. Grokhotova, E.V. Teaching the basics of computer literacy for people of the third age: Problems and solutions. *Bull. Sib. State Univ. Railw. Humanit. Res.* **2018**, *8*, 42–48.
14. Grigorieva, S.A. Formation of conditions for social activity of older citizens. *Soc. Humanit. Knowl.* **2018**, *4*, 164–172.
15. Van Hoof, J.; Marston, H.R.; Brittain, K.; Barrie, H. Creating Age-Friendly Communities: Housing and Technology. *Healthcare* **2019**, *7*, 130. [CrossRef] [PubMed]
16. Useem, J.; Brennan, A.; LaValley, M.; Vickery, M.; Ameli, O.; Reinen, N.; Gill, C.J. Systematic Differences between Cochrane and Non-Cochrane Meta-Analyses on the Same Topic: A Matched Pair Analysis. *PLoS ONE* **2015**, *10*, e0144980. [CrossRef] [PubMed]
17. Koletsi, D.; Fleming, P.S.; Michelaki, I.; Pandis, N. Heterogeneity in Cochrane and non-Cochrane meta-analyses in orthodontics. *J. Dent.* **2018**, *74*, 90–94. [CrossRef] [PubMed]
18. Berger, B.; Gerlach, A.; Groth, S.; Sladek, U.; Ebner, K.; Mühlhauser, I.; Steckelberg, A. Competence training in evidence-based medicine for patients, patient counsellors, consumer representatives and health care professionals in Austria: A feasibility study. *Zeitschrift für Evidenz Fortbildung und Qualität im Gesundheitswesen* **2013**, *107*, 44–52. [CrossRef] [PubMed]

19. Berger, B.; Steckelberg, A.; Meyer, G.; Kasper, J.; Mühlhauser, I. Training of patient and consumer representatives in the basic competencies of evidence-based medicine: A feasibility study. *BMC Med. Educ.* **2010**, *10*, 16. [CrossRef] [PubMed]
20. Gibson, A.; Boddy, K.; Maguire, K.; Britten, N. Exploring the impact of providing evidence-based medicine training to service users. *Res. Involv. Engagem.* **2015**, *1*, 10. [CrossRef] [PubMed]
21. Sarrami-Foroushani, P.; Travaglia, J.; Debono, D.; Braithwaite, J. Key concepts in consumer and community engagement: A scoping meta-review. *BMC Health Serv. Res.* **2014**, *14*, 250. [CrossRef] [PubMed]
22. Fisher, R. On the Interpretation of $\chi 2$ from Contingency Tables, and the Calculation of P. *J. R. Stat. Soc.* **1922**, *85*, 87. [CrossRef]
23. Wikipedia. Ageism. Available online: https://en.wikipedia.org/wiki/Ageism#:~{}:text=Ageism%2C%20also%20spelled%20agism%2C%20is,patterned%20on%20sexism%20and%20racism (accessed on 9 December 2020).
24. Ivan, L.; Beu, D.; van Hoof, J. Smart and Age-Friendly Cities in Romania: An Overview of Public Policy and Practice. *Int. J. Environ. Res. Public Health* **2020**, *17*, 5202. [CrossRef] [PubMed]
25. Cochrane Campbell Global Ageing Partnership Wikipedia Project. Available online: https://globalageing.cochrane.org/cochrane-campbell-global-ageing-partnership-wikipedia-project#:~{}:text=Cochrane%20Campbell%20Global%20Ageing%20Partnership%20Wikipedia%20Project,-Welcome%20to%20our&text=The%20CCGAP%20wikipedia%20project%20was,ageing%20in%20the%2021st%20century (accessed on 18 October 2020).
26. Fulmer, T.; Patel, P.; Levy, N.; Mate, K.; Berman, A.; Pelton, L.; Beard, J.; Kalache, A.; Auerbach, J. Moving Toward a Global Age-Friendly Ecosystem. *J. Am. Geriatr. Soc.* **2020**, *68*, 1936–1940. [CrossRef]

Publisher's Note: MDPI stays neutral with regard to jurisdictional claims in published maps and institutional affiliations.

International Journal of
Environmental Research and Public Health

MDPI

Perspective

The Academic Collaborative Center Older Adults: A Description of Co-Creation between Science, Care Practice and Education with the Aim to Contribute to Person-Centered Care for Older Adults

Katrien Luijkx *, Leonieke van Boekel, Meriam Janssen, Marjolein Verbiest and Annerieke Stoop

Department Tranzo, Tilburg School of Social and Behavioral Sciences, Tilburg University, P.O. Box 90153, 5000 LE Tilburg, The Netherlands; L.vanBoekel@tilburguniversity.edu (L.v.B.); M.Janssen4@tilburguniversity.edu (M.J.); M.E.A.Verbiest@tilburguniversity.edu (M.V.); H.J.Stoop@tilburguniversity.edu (A.S.)

* Correspondence: K.G.Luijkx@tilburguniversity.edu; Tel.: +31-13-466-2895

Received: 16 October 2020; Accepted: 27 November 2020; Published: 3 December 2020

check for updates

Abstract: Long-term care for older adults is in transition. Organizations offering long-term care for older adults are expected to provide person-centered care (PCC) in a complex context, with older adults aging in place and participating in society for as long as possible, staff shortages and the slow adoption of technological solutions. To address these challenges, these organizations increasingly use scientific knowledge to evaluate and innovate long-term care. This paper describes how co-creation, in the sense of close, intensive, and equivalent collaboration between science, care practice, and education, is a key factor in the success of improving long-term care for older adults. Such co-creation is central in the Academic Collaborative Center (ACC) Older Adults of Tilburg University. In this ACC, Tilburg University has joined forces with ten organizations that provide care for older adults and CZ zorgkantoor to create both scientific knowledge and societal impact in order to improve the quality of person-centered care for older adults. In the Netherlands, a "zorgkantoor" arranges long-term (residential) care on behalf of the national government. A zorgkantoor makes agreements on cost and quality with care providers and helps people that are in need of care to decide what the best possible option in their situation is. The CZ zorgkantoor arranges the long-term (residential) care in the south and southwest of the Netherlands. This paper describes how we create scientific knowledge to contribute to the knowledge base of PCC for older adults by conducting social scientific research in which the perspectives of older adults are central. Subsequently, we show how we create societal impact by facilitating and stimulating the use of our scientific knowledge in daily care practice. In the closing section, our ambitions for the future are discussed.

Keywords: person-centered care; older adults; co-creation; perspective of older adults; quality improvement

1. Introduction

Due to demographic changes and economic constraints, healthcare in general as well as long-term care for older adults are in transition. People prefer to participate in society and to live at home for as long as possible. Governments are pursuing agendas that seek to enable older adults to do so [1,2]. Enabling autonomy and community support and health services that are tuned to the needs and possibilities of older adults are key domains for the World Health Organization (WHO) in their aim to create age-friendly communities [3]. Due to ageing of the population and a presumed unattractiveness of the profession, shortages in caregiving staff in long-term care for older adults are already a fact [4,5]. To date, the large-scale implementation of technological solutions that aim to support older adults to lead the life they desire is rather an ideal than reality [6–9]. Moreover, over the last decades, the care for older adults, especially within nursing homes, has been shifting from the biomedical care model towards a person-centered care (PCC) model [10,11]. PCC is suitable for age-friendly communities, because both stress the importance of older adults to be valued, actively involved and supported when needed [12–14]. Nursing homes providing PCC would be excellent age-friendly living environments, according to the new smart age-friendly ecosystem framework [12]. PCC refers to the recognition and appreciation of the individuality of both care receivers (i.e., older adults) and caregivers. PCC aims to enable older adults with complex care needs to continue to live their lives as they prefer despite an increasing dependency on others [10,11,15–17]. To provide tailored care and support for older adults, sensitivity regarding their individual needs, wishes and possibilities is essential, but challenging for care professionals. There is an implementation gap; although care organizations embrace PCC, they struggle to bring it into practice [18].

In order to address the aforementioned challenges, organizations providing long-term care for older adults increasingly use scientific knowledge to evaluate and innovate long-term care [19–22]. The use of scientific knowledge to improve the quality of PCC for older adults incorporates the stimulation and facilitation of care professionals to reflect on and creatively and critically think about the care they provide. The education of current and future care professionals is one of the ways this can be achieved. Close, intensive and equivalent collaboration between science, care practice and education in the development of innovative, evidence-based knowledge—also called co-creation—is key in the success of improving long-term PCC for older adults by using scientific knowledge [19–22].

Such co-creation is central in the Academic Collaborative Center (ACC) Older Adults of Tilburg University in the Netherlands. This ACC is a long-term structural partnership of ten organizations providing long-term care for older adults, CZ zorgkantoor and Tilburg University (see Box 1 for the organizational embedding of the ACC Older Adults and Table 1 for an overview of the stakeholders involved). In the Netherlands, a "zorgkantoor" arranges long-term (residential) care on behalf of the national government. A zorgkantoor makes agreements on cost and quality with care providers and helps people that are in need of care to decide what the best possible option in their situation is. The CZ zorgkantoor arranges the long-term (residential) care in the south and southwest of the Netherlands. The ACC Older Adults chose a social scientific perspective for two reasons. First, the shift from the biomedical care model towards a PCC model underlines the fact that compared to medical care, living is at least equally important to nursing home residents. Second, Tilburg University has no medical school and therefore no medical expertise. Our slogan "science in practice to contribute to PCC for older adults" summarizes our ambitions:

1. Creating scientific knowledge by contributing to the knowledge base on PCC for older adults by conducting social scientific research in which the perspectives of older adults are central;
2. Creating societal impact by facilitating and stimulating the use of our scientific knowledge in daily care practice to enhance PCC.

This paper aims to describe how we are joining forces in the ACC Older Adults to realize our ambitions. Although the first ambition is mainly scientific and the second mainly societal, they are strongly interwoven. Co-creation is the key approach for realizing both ambitions and includes intensive and equal collaboration between various stakeholders operating on different levels, ranging from older adults, caregivers, nurses, psychologists, managers, teachers, policymakers, and scientists. The next section starts with a description of how we create scientific knowledge, because this is the starting point for all our activities. We elaborate on how we are co-creating with various stakeholders in order to ensure that our scientific results are relevant and usable for daily care practice. The following section subsequently elaborates on how we are creating societal impact based on our scientific results and insights.

Table 1. Stakeholders involved in the ACC Older adults.

Stakeholders Involved	Employed by	Number in the ACC Older Adults (November 2020)	Background and/or Expertise	Main Tasks
Professor	Tilburg University	1	PhD degree in social sciences	Supervision of research projects and projects creating societal impact, chairing the ACC, strategy
Senior researcher/research broker	Tilburg University	4	PhD degree in social or health sciences, or psychology	Supervision of research projects and fostering collaboration and knowledge exchange between science and care practice and strategy
Communication expert	Tilburg University	1	Expertise in marketing and communication	Creating communication strategy and communication materials
Education expert	Tilburg University	1	Expertise in education, teaching	Fostering collaboration with education institution and making knowledge accessible in training and current curricula
Implementation expert	Tilburg University	1	Expertise in management and quality improvement	Supervising and monitoring implementation of our knowledge
Regular PhD student	Tilburg University	3	Various backgrounds	Conducting PhD research in collaboration with care practice and older adults
Science practitioner	Care organization and Tilburg University	7	Various backgrounds	Conducting research in collaboration with care practice and older adults
Science-to-practice project researcher	Tilburg University	1	Various backgrounds	Conducting research in collaboration with care practice and older adults
Post doc researcher	Tilburg University	3	Various backgrounds	Conducting research in collaboration with care practice and older adults
Care professionals	Care organization	Depending on the projects		Learning of and providing feedback to our studies, co-creating products, and providing feedback on our approach
Older adults	Not applicable	Depending on the projects		Provide their feedback about our knowledge development and spreading, being a respondent in our studies, and teaching us what is important in old age
Teachers	Educational organization	Depending on the projects		Co-creating education and using our scientific insights in teaching their students

Box 1. Organizational embedding of the Academic Collaborative Center (ACC) Older Adults.

ACC Older Adults

The ACC Older Adults is a long-term structural partnership of ten organizations that care for older adults (Azora, BrabantZorg, De Riethorst Stromenland, De Wever, Groenhuysen, Schakelring, Surplus, SVRZ, Volckaert and Zorggroep West- en Midden-Brabant (Thebe)), CZ Zorgkantoor and Tilburg University. All partners invest both in-kind and financially in the ACC. Since 2018, the Dutch Ministry of Health, Welfare and Sport has structurally funded the ACC Older Adults to further develop and strengthen the knowledge infrastructure, i.e., improve and expand the collaboration and knowledge transfer between science and care practice in our ACC.

Tranzo, Tilburg University

The ACC Older Adults is embedded within Tranzo, which is one of the departments of Tilburg University in the Netherlands. Tranzo aims to bridge the gap between science and practice in different domains of care and welfare. In addition to the ACC Older Adults, Tranzo consists of ten other ACCs with different areas of interest, such as mental health care and people with an intellectual disability.

National Embedding

In addition to the ACC Older Adults in Tilburg, five comparable ACCs in the field of Care for Older Adults exist across the Netherlands. The other ACCs are affiliated with Maastricht University, Radboud University Medical Center Nijmegen, Leiden University Medical Center, Amsterdam University Medical Center—location VUmc and University Medical Center Groningen. Each ACC has its own specific expertise, ambition, approach and research focus in the field of care for older adults. On a national level, however, joined forces across the six ACCs add value to obtaining the shared goal of improving overall quality of care for older adults in agenda setting of the national government. For example, during the current COVID-19 outbreak, the six ACCs are cooperating in various corona-related studies in order to inform policymakers on a national level [23–25]. All six ACCs receive structural funds from the Dutch Ministry of Health, Welfare and Sport to strengthen the knowledge infrastructure.

2. Creating Scientific Knowledge

PCC is taking shape in the care relationship between older adults and care professionals. Therefore, when aiming to contribute to the knowledge base on PCC for older adults, it is important to address research topics that are of importance to older adults and care professionals and especially to discover the perspectives on these topics of older adults themselves. To ensure that we develop relevant and applicable knowledge, we are creating knowledge via co-creation in which older adults, care professionals, and researchers are involved. In the following sections, we elaborate on the specific themes of our studies, and on the stakeholders involved.

2.1. Themes of Research

Research projects in the ACC Older Adults—of which the majority are PhD studies—all relate to PCC and revolve around the following four themes: 1. autonomy; 2. technology; 3. social needs and social networks; 4. quality improvement.

Researchers, care professionals, and older adults together determine research topics, questions and designs for specific PhD studies, thus ensuring our research themes are of relevance for daily care practice. Partnership organizations facilitate data collection within their organization. Our PhD studies are financed in two ways, the first being competitive external research funding. Proposals for these PhD studies are always written in collaboration between researchers, care professionals of our partnership organizations, and older adults or their representatives. Research topics are determined based on gaps in scientific knowledge in combination with experiences of older adults and care professionals in care practice. These research projects are executed by full-time PhD students motivated to advance care practice with their scientific knowledge.

The second way PhD studies are financed is via funding by partnership organizations of one of their employees as a science practitioner. Science practitioners combine their PhD study with their current work as a care practitioner, for example, as a nurse, a psychologist, a manager, or a policy maker in a care organization. Their research topics relate to problems or questions they come across in their daily work, such as access to care [26–28], love, intimacy, and sexuality of nursing home residents with dementia [29–32], or autonomy [33,34]. Within their care organization, science practitioners are seen as experts in their field of research, and they also motivate their colleagues to use scientific knowledge. Moreover, care organizations explicitly connect to science by providing their science practitioner with the opportunity to conduct their PhD study, and they stress the importance of knowledge about the studied topic.

2.2. Stakeholders Involved

PhD students, both science practitioners and full-time PhD students, are supervised by the professor and one of the four senior researchers of the ACC. These senior researchers are employed by Tilburg University and hold a PhD degree. We aim to involve both scientific and societal expertise in our supervising teams. Therefore, if possible, an employee with a PhD degree of the care organization where the science practitioner is employed is involved as co-supervisor. This strengthens the collaboration between Tilburg University and the care organization. In addition to supervising PhD students, the four senior researchers of the ACC together with the professor further develop and expand the ACC Older Adults, prepare competitive research grant proposals, and also work partly as so-called "research brokers" within the partnership organizations to foster the collaboration and knowledge exchange between science and care practice. Each of them is responsible for the collaboration with two or three of the partnership organizations. In these organizations, the research brokers ensure that care practice and university are connected in various ways and at different levels. They meet and collaborate with people who are relevant for the use of scientific knowledge in daily care practice, they participate in relevant committees, and they know when and how to showcase the knowledge that is available in the ACC. The close connection that research brokers have with daily practice contributes to a detailed understanding of the struggles and interests of care professionals and older adults. This is essential for conducting science that is relevant and useful for daily practice.

Moreover, for each PhD study, we install an expert group of care professionals, managers and older adults. We regularly share and discuss our (preliminary) study findings and future study directions with this group to stimulate and facilitate care professionals in using our study findings in their daily work. Such an expert group ensures that insights from the study immediately are translated into daily care practice on a small scale. Additionally, due to the feedback of care professionals and older adults on the ongoing study, the study may be adapted to remain relevant and applicable for daily care practice.

2.3. Perspective of Older Adults

In order to be able to improve PCC by conducting scientific research and achieving its translation to care practice, it is essential to understand the perspectives of older adults. In our research, we always study the perspective of older adults on a specific topic, such as access to long-term care [26,35], technology acceptance [36–40], love, intimacy and sexuality [31,32], and social needs and networks [41–44]. Although physical or cognitive limitations—including dementia—may complicate this, we showed that it is possible and worthwhile [45]. The scarce number of studies that compare the perspective of older adults with that of proxies, such as loved ones or care professionals, shows that these perspectives differ [46–49]. These (sometimes nuanced) differences in perspective may affect the older adult's experience of being respected as a unique individual and the genuine experience of PCC. To maximize the impact of understanding the perspective of older adults, we study it in the first empirical study of most research projects. Because older adults are a heterogeneous group regarding their capacities, limitations, goals, preferences, and habits, qualitative methods of data gathering are the most helpful for understanding the perspectives of older adults.

To clarify the value of studying the perspective of older adults, we give two examples. Repeated interviews with community dwelling older adults revealed that emotional attachment, need compatibility, cues to use, proficiency to use, input of resources, and support together influence the frequency of technology use. The interplay between these factors can be modified by factors, such as social influence, alternative means, and changing personal needs, which can cause changes in the frequency of technology use [39]. Interviews with older adults living with dementia in a nursing home and their spouses revealed that love, intimacy and sexuality are still important in their relationship despite the dementia and the move to a nursing home. However, the nursing home is not always conducive to satisfactory experiences regarding love, intimacy, and sexuality due to practical, emotional, and communicational problems and limitations [31].

To contribute to PCC, we aim to create an ACC with, for, and by older adults. Therefore, older adults need to be involved in the ACC on other levels as well. The research brokers aim to meet annually with the central client council of the partnership organizations to learn what is important to older adults and which topics we need to study, as well as to ask for feedback on our ambitions, research and products. Moreover, we are currently developing an expert panel of older adults to incorporate their perspectives structurally in the ACC. For instance, we invite older adults to share their opinions and perspectives on a certain topic during our symposia or events. These older adults like to share their story and to talk in public. In addition, we have a group of client representatives or members of special-interest organizations for older adults who are consulted in research proposals for funding opportunities and in ongoing research projects. These client representatives often have experience with a specific area such as policy, management or informal caregiving, depending on the topic of the project or research we invite them to collaborate on. Finally, we strive to set up a test panel of older adults from the general public who can pilot test our products and materials and provide us with feedback on this.

3. Creating Societal Impact

We aim to create societal impact by facilitating and stimulating the use of scientific knowledge in daily care practice to enhance PCC. Therefore, our study findings need to be translated in such a way that care professionals whom they concern can easily find, understand, and work with them. Moreover, with our scientific knowledge, we want to stimulate them to critically reflect on their care giving approaches and to inspire them to change these according to the study findings. Although dissemination is an important first step, it is also important to translate study insights into education and into practical tools that are ready to be implemented and used in daily care practice.

Our "science-to-practice team", consisting of a communication expert, an education expert, and an implementation expert, plays a crucial role in creating societal impact and is complete as from the beginning of 2020. These team members work from their respective expertise in communication, education and care practice, and although they are not scientific staff, they understand and embrace the value of science to further improve care. Their mutual collaboration is close, and they collaborate closely with the researchers and other stakeholders in the ACC as well. These experts often notice other or earlier opportunities than our scientists to communicate or share research findings. Hence, working in such a multidisciplinary team with scientists as well as communication, education, and implementation experts is essential in creating both scientific knowledge and societal impact in order to strengthen PCC for older adults.

Moreover, care professionals are important stakeholders in creating societal impact because PCC needs to be realized in the care relationship between older adults and care professionals. Therefore, we incorporate the perspective of care professionals structurally in the ACC by having an expert team of care professionals. This expert team is consulted, for example, regarding the topics that need to be studied, the tools we develop based on the findings of our PhD studies, and the resources they use to find information. Furthermore, they may act as ambassadors for the ACC and help us to further disseminate and implement our knowledge among relevant stakeholders, such as their co-workers.

The following section shows how we translate our scientific knowledge into daily care practice in so-called "science-to-practice projects". Subsequently, we elaborate on communication, education and implementation.

3.1. Science-to-Practice Projects

In so-called "science-to-practice projects", in co-creation between researchers, older adults, care professionals, and teachers, we translate relevant scientific knowledge into daily care practice and education. Within these projects, based on our research findings, we develop tools and educational programs that can directly be applied in daily care practice, in vocational education, or for training on the job purposes. In general, these tools aim to help care professionals to analyze and evaluate their daily care giving practice and to pay attention to perspectives of older adults, which contributes to more PCC. An example of a "science-to-practice project" is the practical evaluation tool which is useful for care practice to evaluate and improve geriatric rehabilitation care [50]. This evaluation tool has been developed based on our previous scientific insights about evaluation of integrated care interventions and is described in detail elsewhere [51]. Another example is the Gerontechnologies Matchmaking (GTM) tool (see Figure 1) [52] that is based on our scientific insights about why older adults use or do not use digital technology [38]. The GTM tool was co-created with technology consultants and aims to help professionals to match the most appropriate technology at the right time with the needs of the older adult. Moreover, it structurally involves the perspective of informal caregivers, because they are important in the lives of older adults in general and regarding technology acceptance. The common boxes in Figure 1 depict objective information that is the same for the older adult and the informal caregiver, while the doubled boxes represent the topics in which the attitude and experience of both parties might differ. In the development of the GTM tool, we used our scientific insights about origins and consequences of technology acquirement by older adults and we observed the matchmaking dialogues between technology consultants and older adults. Together, these scientific and practical insights and observations were combined in the first version of the tool and thereafter drafted, tested and adapted. The approach has been described in detail elsewhere [52].

In some cases, the science-to-practice projects reveal undiscovered research areas and are the start of a new PhD study. For example, the PhD study on love, intimacy, and sexuality [29–32,45] revealed the perspective of residents and their loved ones on how nursing home residents with dementia, and possibly their partners, can be best supported in their wishes and needs with regard to intimacy and sexuality [53]. To translate the knowledge of this PhD study into daily care practice, the science-to-practice project started with semi-structured interviews with various nursing home professionals to discover their perspective. These interviews revealed that these care professionals usually perceive expressions of sexuality as problematic behavior and find it difficult to address the wishes and needs of residents with dementia with regard to love, intimacy and sexuality. To address the need of a training program to help care professionals to cope with all kinds of expressions of intimacy and sexuality, and to provide PCC with regard to such a sensitive topic, we started a new PhD study. In this PhD study, based on an understanding of the perspectives of both nursing home residents and care professionals, we aim to develop, implement and evaluate a comprehensive program to help care professionals cope with problematic behavior and to address needs and wishes regarding love, intimacy, and sexuality as well.

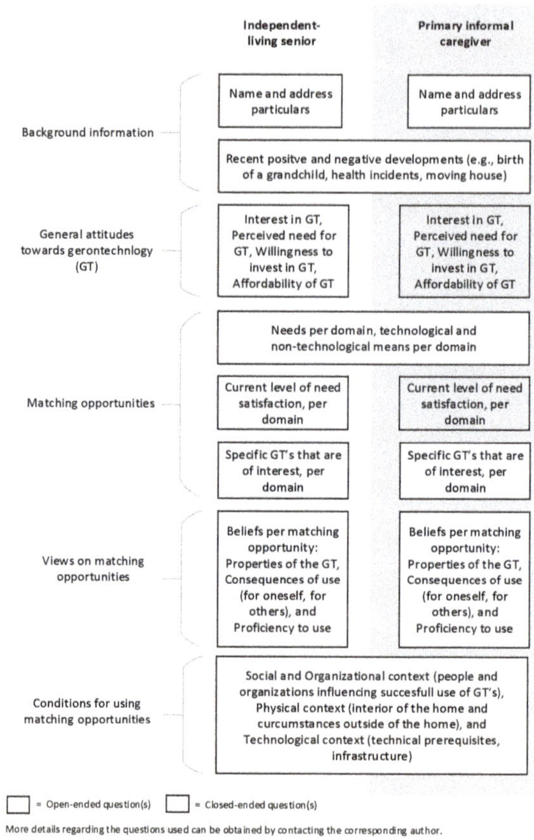

Figure 1. Gerontechnologies Matchmaking (GTM) tool [52].

3.2. Communication

Communication is essential when aiming for societal impact, and it is interwoven in all activities to create societal impact. Our communication expert, who is employed by Tilburg University, with a background in marketing and communication, developed a marketing and communication strategy, including a recognizable corporate identity that is attractive to care professionals. Moreover, she formulated a slogan that summarizes our ambitions concisely and helps us focus: "science in practice to contribute to PCC for older adults". We study our communication target group, professionals working in care for older adults, to understand how we can best reach them. In an attempt to overcome the implementation gap, we develop attractive and easy to understand personalized communication materials to inform care professionals about our study results and tools and to help them to change daily care practice according to our scientific knowledge.

The research brokers, the education expert, and the implementation expert use the communication materials as an aid to translate our scientific knowledge towards daily care practice. Moreover, our communication expert facilitates all our researchers in communicating in an attractive and accessible manner for an audience of care professionals. Furthermore, our meetings are interactive with the use of creative work forms, based on to the assumption that knowledge is more easily incorporated when offered through various approaches [54].

3.3. Education

The majority of professional caregivers in daily care for older adults do not have many years of education and is low or moderately skilled. Because educating current and future care professionals is an excellent means of translating scientific knowledge into daily care practice, middle and high vocational teachers as well as education experts of our partnership organizations have been involved in our ACC in recent years. Based on our research findings, our education expert, who is employed by Tilburg University and is an experienced teacher at both vocational levels, designs and tests education in co-creation with these stakeholders. For example, she designed, in close collaboration with a teacher from middle vocational education, a three-piece workshop based on the findings of our PhD study on love, intimacy and sexuality among nursing home residents [29–32,45]. The workshops have already been used in a number of classes, and we are now searching for opportunities to disseminate the tested and improved workshop "intimacy and sexuality" among teachers of vocational education on a national level.

We aim for education to be used by teachers and education experts themselves and aim for our scientific knowledge to be incorporated in the current curricula because we are convinced that this is most sustainable. Furthermore, we aim to spread our knowledge in care organizations and educational institutions across the Netherlands, without providing education by people employed by university. This ambition does not fit with the ambitions of a university department, in which research and educating academic students are rewarded, while teaching future and current caregivers and nurses is not. Moreover, other parties are experts in this, with whom we collaborate to realize our societal ambitions. We are convinced that this will lead to more sustainable results with which we can reach many more stakeholders.

Furthermore, in line with our ambitions, we organized a national inspiration day (see Figure 2) exclusively for (student) nurses and caregivers about love, intimacy and sexuality among nursing home residents. Together with teachers of higher vocational education, we designed and facilitated this day. We offered 100 (student) nurses and caregivers the opportunity to be actively involved and to learn about the topic. We invited them to design innovations for facilitating intimacy and sexuality in the nursing home in a person-centered way. All innovations were presented in an exposition. Visitors of the exposition selected the two most promising innovations: a board game (see Figure 3) and a leaflet. Both innovations are currently further fine-tuned, prototyped, and tested in care practice. This is conducted in co-creation between the ACC, the involved institution for higher vocational education, and the involved current and student professional caregivers. The board game aims to stimulate and facilitate conversation among team members regarding intimacy and sexuality in the nursing home. The leaflet aims to inform older adults who are going to live in a nursing home that not living together does not have to mean not being together—it is an invitation to bring this subject to the table. These products will become available for our partnership organizations, but also for other nursing homes in the Netherlands.

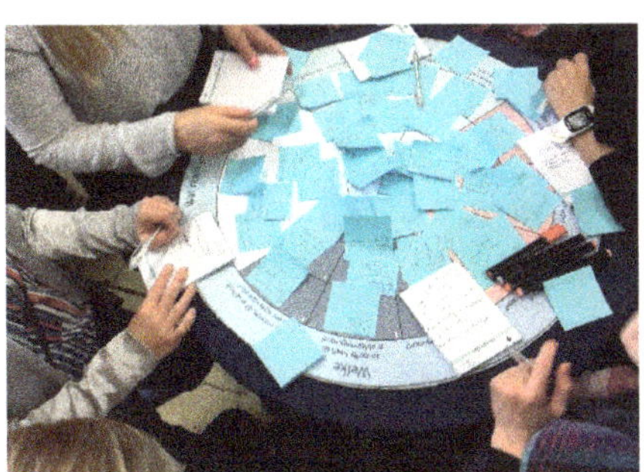

Figure 2. National inspiration day 2019.

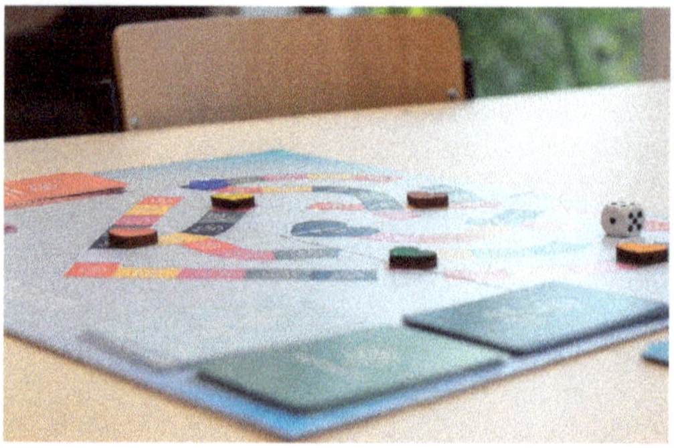

Figure 3. Board game to stimulate and facilitate conversation among team members regarding intimacy and sexuality in the nursing home.

3.4. Implementation

Despite the aforementioned efforts and practical tools resulting from our science-to-practice projects, the utilization of these tools is not always obvious and easy from the care organization perspective. Therefore, we need to stimulate and facilitate implementation of our tools in daily care practice. To this end, our implementation expert, who is employed by Tilburg University as from the beginning of 2020, works on the cutting edge of care practice and science. With a background in management and quality improvement within care for older adults, she is familiar with the setting and challenges of adopting innovations. She offers our tools to our partnership organizations based on their demand within the organization. Moreover, she verifies whether an organization or a specific team is ready to use the tool, i.e., not hindered by daily chores, such as severe staff shortages, reorganization, or other organizational factors.

Although we aim for all Dutch nursing homes to use our tools, we do not introduce our tools in all nursing homes. In order to serve as much stakeholders as possible, our implementation expert trains self-employed professionals or nursing home professionals on how to implement our tools. To ensure the implementation of our tools is of high quality and performed as intended, she supervises and monitors the implementation process.

4. Future

The current state of the ACC Older Adults as described in this paper is characterized by a long-term, structural equal collaboration between various stakeholders, in which everyone's expertise is respected and valued and mistakes are seen as opportunities to learn from. A clear focus and aim of the ACC and the research, which adheres to the mission and interests of stakeholders involved, is essential. Moreover, collaboration within multidisciplinary teams is important to address research topics that are relevant for care practice. It takes time over the years and every day to collaborate successfully on different levels and between different people and thus investments of all parties involved.

The ACC Older Adults was founded in 2003 as the ACC Chronic Care and made a focus shift towards PCC for older adults in 2013. It has always been our ambition to develop usable scientific knowledge, to translate this knowledge to daily care practice, and to facilitate its use. Structural funds of the Dutch Ministry of Health, Welfare and Sport to expand the knowledge infrastructure as from 2018 have provided us with the opportunity to enlarge the activities described above in recent years and will continue to do so in the future. We aim for our knowledge and tools to be translated and implemented into care practice. Co-creation is key in our approach. Combining the expertise of all stakeholders involved leads to the best possible outcomes for both science and care practice, and, thus, for PCC for older adults. For now, we focus on our partnership organizations, but we ultimately strive to reach all Dutch organizations providing long-term care for older adults and all institutions that educate professional caregivers in care for older adults. Therefore, we aim to use existing roads to disseminate our scientific knowledge, research findings, and tools, for example, by collaborating with institutes that share applicable knowledge or institutes that provide educational materials on a national level. We do not guide the implementation or education because we are convinced that it is more sustainable when we collaborate with other parties who are experts in implementation or education and are eventually able to serve all stakeholders across the Netherlands. Moreover, both implementing tools in care practice and vocational education do not fit the ambitions of a university department.

To date, our focus has mainly been on the development of scientific knowledge and evidence-based tools to implement in daily care practice and of education. In the future, when a tool has been implemented in different teams and organizations, we intend to evaluate the implementation processes and the impact on daily care practice and especially client outcomes. In this manner, we strive to strengthen our expertise in developing relevant scientific knowledge and in translating this knowledge into care practice to improve caregiving and especially to contribute to PCC and age-friendly communities.

Author Contributions: Conceptualization, K.L., L.v.B., M.J., M.V. and A.S.; writing—original draft preparation, K.L.; writing—review and editing, L.v.B., M.J., M.V. and A.S.; supervision, K.L., L.v.B., M.J., M.V. and A.S.; project administration, K.L., L.v.B., M.J.; funding acquisition, K.L., L.v.B., M.J. All authors have read and agreed to the published version of the manuscript.

Funding: The ACC Older Adults is funded by our partnership organizations: Azora, BrabantZorg, De Riethorst Stromenland, De Wever, Groenhuysen, Schakelring, Surplus, SVRZ, Volckaert and Zorggroep West-en Midden-Brabant (Thebe), CZ Zorgkantoor. The Dutch Ministry of Health, Welfare and Sport structurally funds the expansion of the knowledge infrastructure in nursing home care.

Acknowledgments: We thank the employees and older adults of our partnership organizations and teachers of various educations institutions for collaborating with us in the ACC Older Adults.

Conflicts of Interest: The authors declare no conflict of interest.

References

1. Hsu, H.C. Exploring elderly people's perspectives on successful ageing in Taiwan. *Ageing Soc.* **2007**, *27*, 87–102. [CrossRef]
2. Thanakwang, K.; Soonthorndhada, K.; Mongkolprasoet, J. Perspectives on healthy aging among Thai elderly: A qualitative study. *Nurs. Health Sci.* **2012**, *14*, 472–479. [CrossRef]
3. WHO. Age-Friendly Cities and Communities. Available online: https://www.who.int/ageing/projects/age-friendly-cities-communities/en/ (accessed on 13 November 2020).
4. Leensen, R.; Poulssen, R.; Weststrate, E. *Barometer Nederlandse Gezondheidszorg 2019. Rating en Rendement Dalen Door Toegenomen Verzuim en Verloop*; Ernst & Young: London, UK, 2019.
5. Tooren, M.V.D.; Hooftman, W.; Hulsegge, G.; Bouwens, L.; Rosenkrantz, N. *Arbeidsmarktproblematiek in de sector Zorg en Welzijn*; in opdracht van het onderzoekprogramma Arbeidsmarkt Zorg en Welzijn; TNO: Leiden, The Netherlands, 2019.
6. Balta-Ozkan, N.; Davidson, R.; Bicket, M.; Whitmarsh, L. Social barriers to the adoption of smart homes. *Energy Policy* **2013**, *63*, 363–374. [CrossRef]
7. Lazar, A.; Demiris, G.; Thompson, H.J. Evaluation of a multifunctional technology system in a memory care unit: Opportunities for innovation in dementia care. *Inform. Health Soc. Care* **2016**, *41*, 373–386. [CrossRef]
8. Schulz, R.; Wahl, H.W.; Matthews, J.T.; De Vito Dabbs, A.; Beach, S.R.; Czaja, S.J. Advancing the Aging and Technology Agenda in Gerontology. *Gerontologist* **2015**, *55*, 724–734. [CrossRef]
9. Wigg, J.M. Liberating the wanderers: Using technology to unlock doors for those living with dementia. *Sociol. Health Illn.* **2010**, *32*, 288–303. [CrossRef]
10. Koren, M.J. Person-Centered Care For Nursing Home Residents: The Culture-Change Movement. *Health Aff.* **2010**, *29*, 1–6. [CrossRef]
11. White-Chu, E.F.; Graves, W.J.; Godfrey, S.M.; Bonner, A.; Sloane, P. Beyond the medical model: The culture change revolution in long-term care. *J. Am. Med Dir. Assoc.* **2009**, *10*, 370–378. [CrossRef]

12. Marston, H.R.; van Hoof, J. "Who Doesn't Think about Technology When Designing Urban Environments for Older People?" A Case Study Approach to a Proposed Extension of the WHO's Age-Friendly Cities Model. *Int. J. Environ. Res. Public Health* **2019**, *16*, 3525. [CrossRef]
13. Van Hoof, J.; Kazak, J.K. Urban ageing. *Indoor Built Environ.* **2018**, *27*, 583–586. [CrossRef]
14. Van Hoof, J.; Kazak, J.K.; Perek-Białas, J.M.; Peek, S.T.M. The Challenges of Urban Ageing: Making Cities Age-Friendly in Europe. *Int. J. Environ. Res. Public Health* **2018**, *15*, 2473. [CrossRef] [PubMed]
15. Donnelly, L.; MacEntee, M.I. Care Perceptions among Residents of LTC Facilities Purporting to Offer Person-Centred Care. *Can. J. Aging* **2016**, *35*, 149–160. [CrossRef] [PubMed]
16. McCormack, B. Person-centredness in gerontological nursing: An overview of the literature. *J. Clin. Nurs.* **2004**, *13*, 31–38. [CrossRef] [PubMed]
17. McCormack, B.; McCance, T.V. Development of a framework for person-centred nursing. *J. Adv. Nurs.* **2006**, *56*, 472–479. [CrossRef] [PubMed]
18. Stoop, A.; Lette, M.; Ambugo, E.; Gadsby, E.; Goodwin, N.; MacInnes, J.; Minkman, M.; Wistow, G.; Zonneveld, N.; Nijpels, G.; et al. Improving Person-Centredness in Integrated Care for Older People: Experiences from Thirteen Integrated Care Sites in Europe. *Int. J. Integr. Care* **2020**, *20*. [CrossRef] [PubMed]
19. Garretsen, H.F.L.; Bongers, I.M.B.; de Roo, A.A.; van de Goor, I.A.M. Bridging the Gap between Science and Practice: Do Applied Academic Centres Contribute to a Solution? A Plea for International Comparative Research. *J. Comp. Soc. Welf.* **2007**, *23*, 49–59. [CrossRef]
20. Koopmans, R.T.; Lavrijsen, J.C.; Hoek, F. Concrete steps toward academic medicine in long term care. *J. Am. Med Dir. Assoc.* **2013**, *14*, 781–783. [CrossRef]
21. Verbeek, H.; Zwakhalen, S.M.; Schols, J.M.; Hamers, J.P. Keys to successfully embedding scientific research in nursing homes: A win-win perspective. *J. Am. Med Dir. Assoc.* **2013**, *14*, 855–857. [CrossRef]
22. Verbeek, H.; Zwakhalen, S.M.G.; Schols, J.M.G.A.; Kempen, G.I.J.M.; Hamers, J.P.H. The Living Lab in Ageing and Long-Term Care: A Sustainable Model for Translational Research Improving Quality of Life, Quality of Care and Quality of Work. *J. Nutr. Health Aging* **2020**, *24*, 43–47. [CrossRef]
23. Hamers, J.; Koopmans, R.; Gerritsen, D.; Verbeek, H. *"Intens Gelukkig dat ze weer Bezoek Mocht Ontvangen". Ervaringen met de Verruiming van de Bezoekregeling in Verpleeghuizen*; Tweede Kamer der Staten-Generaal: The Hague, The Netherlands, 2020.
24. Koopmans, R.; Gerritsen, D.; Luijkx, K.; Zuidema, S.; Hertogh, C.; Verbeek, H.; Hamers, J. *Verruiming van de Bezoekregeling in Verpleeghuizen: Bevindingen van de Diepte-Monitoring na 3 Weken; Factsheet*; Ukon: Nijmegen, The Netherlands, 2020.
25. Van Loon, A.; Rutten, J.; Buul, L.V.; Van Kooten, J.; Joling, K.; Smalbrugge, M.; Hertogh, C. *COVID-19 bij Verpleeghuisbewoners. Factsheet 2: Patiëntkenmerken en Risicofactoren*; Universitair Netwerk Ouderenzorg, Amsterdam UMC; VUmc (UNO-VUmc): Amsterdam, The Netherlands, 2020.
26. Schipper, L.; Luijkx, K.; Meijboom, B.; Schalk, R.; Schols, J. Access to long-term care: Perceptions and experiences of older Dutch people. *Qual. Ageing Older Adults* **2015**, *16*, 83–93. [CrossRef]
27. Schipper, L.; Luijkx, K.; Meijboom, B.; Schols, J. The 3 A's of the access process to long-term care for elderly: Providers experiences in a multiple case study in the The Netherlands. *Health Policy* **2015**, *119*, 17–25. [CrossRef] [PubMed]
28. Schipper, L.; Meijboom, B.; Luijkx, K.; Schols, J. Front/back office considerations in the operational access to long-term care for older people: Findings of a multiple case study. *Int. J. Healthc. Manag.* **2013**, *6*, 252–262. [CrossRef]
29. Roelofs, T.; Luijkx, K.; Embregts, P. The attitudes of residential care staff towards the sexuality of residents with dementia: Organizational factors. *Innov. Aging* **2018**, *2*, 340. [CrossRef]
30. Roelofs, T.S.; Luijkx, K.G.; Embregts, P.J. Intimacy and sexuality of nursing home residents with dementia: A systematic review. *Int. Psychogeriatr.* **2015**, *27*, 367. [CrossRef]
31. Roelofs, T.S.; Luijkx, K.G.; Embregts, P.J. Love, Intimacy and Sexuality in Residential Dementia Care: A Spousal Perspective. *Dementia* **2019**, *18*, 936–950. [CrossRef]
32. Roelofs, T.S.; Luijkx, K.G.; Embregts, P.J. Love, intimacy and sexuality in residential dementia care: A client perspective. *Clin. Gerontol.* **2019**, 1–11. [CrossRef]
33. Boumans, J.; van Boekel, L.C.; Baan, C.A.; Luijkx, K.G. How Can Autonomy Be Maintained and Informal Care Improved for People With Dementia Living in Residential Care Facilities: A Systematic Literature Review. *Gerontologist* **2019**, *59*, e709–e730. [CrossRef]

34. Van Loon, J.; Luijkx, K.; Janssen, M.; de Rooij, I.; Janssen, B. Facilitators and barriers to autonomy: A systematic literature review for older adults with physical impairments, living in residential care facilities. *Ageing Soc.* **2019**, 1–30. [CrossRef]
35. Schipper, L.; Luijkx, K.G.; Meijboom, B.R.; Schols, J.M.G.A. 'It is a completely new world you step into.' How older clients and their representatives experience the operational access to Dutch long-term institutional care. *J. Aging Stud.* **2015**, *35*, 211–220. [CrossRef]
36. Luijkx, K.; Peek, S.; Wouters, E. "Grandma, you should do it—It's cool" Older Adults and the Role of Family Members in Their Acceptance of Technology. *Int. J. Environ. Res. Public Health* **2015**, *12*, 15470–15485. [CrossRef]
37. Peek, S.; Luijkx, K.; Rijnaard, M.; Nieboer, M.; van der Voort, C.; Aarts, S.; van Hoof, J.; Vrijhoef, H.; Wouters, E. Older Adults' Reasons for Using Technology while Aging in Place. *Gerontology* **2016**, *62*, 226–237. [CrossRef] [PubMed]
38. Peek, S.T.M.; Luijkx, K.G.; Vrijhoef, H.J.M.; Nieboer, M.E.; Aarts, S.; van der Voort, C.S.; Rijnaard, M.D.; Wouters, E.J.M. Origins and consequences of technology acquirement by independent-living seniors: Towards an integrative model. *BMC Geriatr.* **2017**, *17*, 189. [CrossRef] [PubMed]
39. Peek, S.T.M.; Luijkx, K.G.; Vrijhoef, H.J.M.; Nieboer, M.E.; Aarts, S.; van der Voort, C.S.; Rijnaard, M.D.; Wouters, E.J.M. Understanding changes and stability in the long-term use of technologies by seniors who are aging in place: A dynamical framework. *BMC Geriatr.* **2019**, *19*, 236. [CrossRef] [PubMed]
40. Peek, S.T.M.; Wouters, E.J.M.; Luijkx, K.G.; Vrijhoef, H.J.M. What it Takes to Successfully Implement Technology for Aging in Place: Focus Groups With Stakeholders. *J. Med. Internet. Res.* **2016**, *18*, e98. [CrossRef] [PubMed]
41. Ten Bruggencate, T.; Luijkx, K.; Sturm, J. When your world gets smaller: How older people try to meet their social needs, including the role of social technology. *Ageing Soc.* **2019**, *39*, 1826–1852. [CrossRef]
42. Ten Bruggencate, T.; Luijkx, K.; Sturm, J. How to fulfil social needs of older people: Exploring design opportunities for technological interventions. *Gerontechnology* **2019**, *18*, 156–167. [CrossRef]
43. Ten Bruggencate, T.; Luijkx, K.G.; Sturm, J. Friends or frenemies? The role of social technology in the lives of older people. *Int. J. Environ. Res. Public Health* **2019**, *16*, 4969. [CrossRef]
44. Vos, W.H.; van Boekel, L.C.; Janssen, M.M.; Leenders, R.T.; Luijkx, K.G. Exploring the impact of social network change: Experiences of older adults ageing in place. *Health Soc. Care Community* **2020**, *28*, 116–126. [CrossRef]
45. Roelofs, T.; Embregts, P.; Luijkx, K. A person-centered approach to study intimacy and sexuality in residential care facility (RCF) clients with dementia: Methodological considerations and a guide to study design. *Neuropsychol. Rehabil.* **2017**, *41*, 359–373. [CrossRef]
46. Dröes, R.; Boelens-Van Der Knoop, E.C.C.; Bos, J.; Meihuizen, L.; Ettema, T.P.; Gerritsen, D.L.; Hoogeveen, F.; De Lange, J.; SchöLzel-Dorenbos, C.J.M. Quality of life in dementia in perspective: An explorative study of variations in opinions among people with dementia and their professional caregivers, and in literature. *Dementia* **2006**, *5*, 533–558. [CrossRef]
47. Gerritsen, D.L.; Ettema, T.P.; Boelens, E.; Bos, J.; Hoogeveen, F.; Lange, J.d.; Meihuizen, L.; Scholzel-Dorenbos, C.J.; Droes, R.M. Quality of life in dementia: Do professional caregivers focus on the significant domains? *Am. J. Alzheimer Dis. Other Dement.* **2007**, *22*, 176–183. [CrossRef] [PubMed]
48. Kane, R.A.; Caplan, A.L.; Urv-Wong, E.K.; Freeman, I.C.; Aroskar, M.A.; Finch, M. Everyday matters in the lives of nursing home residents: Wish for and perception of choice and control. *J. Am. Geriatr. Soc.* **1997**, *45*, 1086–1093. [CrossRef] [PubMed]
49. Larsson, H.; Edberg, A.-K.; Bolmsjö, I.; Rämgård, M. Contrasts in older persons' experiences and significant others' perceptions of existential loneliness. *Nurs. Ethics* **2019**, *26*, 1623–1637. [CrossRef] [PubMed]
50. Janssen, M.M.; Vos, W.; Luijkx, K.G. Development of an evaluation tool for geriatric rehabilitation care. *BMC Geriatr.* **2019**, *19*, 206. [CrossRef]
51. Busetto, L.; Luijkx, K.; Vrijhoef, H.J.M. Development of the COMIC Model for the comprehensive evaluation of integrated care interventions. *Int. J. Care Coord.* **2016**, *19*, 47–58. [CrossRef]
52. Haufe, M.; Peek, S.T.M.; Luijkx, K.G. Matching gerontechnologies to independent-living seniors' individual needs: Development of the GTM tool. *BMC Health Serv. Res.* **2019**, *19*, 26. [CrossRef]

53. Roelofs, T. *Love, Intimacy and Sexuality in Nursing Home Residents with Dementia: An Exploration from Multiple Perspectives*; Tilburg University: Tilburg, The Netherlands, 2018.
54. Birnbaum, M.S.; Kornell, N.; Bjork, E.L.; Bjork, R.A. Why interleaving enhances inductive learning: The roles of discrimination and retrieval. *Mem. Cogn.* **2013**, *41*, 392–402. [CrossRef]

Publisher's Note: MDPI stays neutral with regard to jurisdictional claims in published maps and institutional affiliations.

International Journal of
Environmental Research and Public Health

MDPI

Article

The Homestead: Developing a Conceptual Framework through Co-Creation for Innovating Long-Term Dementia Care Environments

Bram de Boer [1,2,*], Belkis Bozdemir [2,3], Jack Jansen [2,3], Monique Hermans [2,3], Jan P. H. Hamers [1,2] and Hilde Verbeek [1,2,*]

1 Department of Health Services Research, Care and Public Health Research Institute, Maastricht University, 6229 GT Maastricht, The Netherlands; jph.hamers@maastrichtuniversity.nl
2 Living Lab in Ageing and Long-Term Care, 6229 GT Maastricht, The Netherlands; BelkisBozdemir@mgzl.nl (B.B.); JackJansen@mgzl.nl (J.J.); moniquehermans@mgzl.nl (M.H.)
3 MeanderGroep Zuid Limburg, 6372 PP Landgraaf, The Netherlands
* Correspondence: b.deboer@maastrichtuniversity.nl (B.d.B.); h.verbeek@maastrichtuniversity.nl (H.V.)

Abstract: Alternative care environments for regular nursing homes are highly warranted to promote health and well-being of residents with dementia that are part of an age-friendly and dementia-friendly city and society. Insight is lacking on how to translate evidence-based knowledge from theory into a congruent conceptual model for innovation in current practice. This study reports on the co-creation of an alternative nursing home model in the Netherlands. A participatory research approach was used to co-create a conceptual framework with researchers, practitioners and older people following an iterative process. Results indicate that achieving positive outcomes for people with dementia, (in)formal caregivers, and the community is dependent on how well the physical, social and organizational environment are congruently designed. The theoretical underpinnings of the conceptual model have been translated into "the homestead," which is conceptualized around three main pillars: activation, freedom and relationships. The Homestead Care Model is an illustrative example of how residential care facilities can support the development of age-friendly communities that take into consideration the needs and requirements of older citizens. However, challenges remain to implement radical changes within residential care. More research is needed into the actual implementation of the Homestead Care Model.

Keywords: long-term care; dementia; physical environment; social environment; organizational environment; environmental design

Citation: de Boer, B.; Bozdemir, B.; Jansen, J.; Hermans, M.; Hamers, J.P.H.; Verbeek, H. The Homestead: Developing a Conceptual Framework through Co-Creation for Innovating Long-Term Dementia Care Environments. *Int. J. Environ. Res. Public Health* **2021**, *18*, 57. https://dx.doi.org/10.3390/ijerph18010057

Received: 16 November 2020
Accepted: 19 December 2020
Published: 23 December 2020

1. Introduction

The care environment plays a crucial role to support people with dementia in their daily functioning and well-being. It can be seen as an active part of care and service delivery, especially when the disease progresses and 24-hour care is required. Traditionally, nursing homes for people with dementia are confining, closed environments which are separated from communities [1]. Routines can be rigid and structured with little affordances for residents [1–3]. Current evidence suggests that traditional nursing homes are not effective in supporting everyday functioning. For example, nursing home residents are often inactive [4,5], display high levels of neuropsychiatric symptoms such as agitation and depression [6,7], and are restricted in their autonomy as physical and chemical restraints are often used [8,9]. As a result, a cultural change movement has been employed in nursing homes [10–12]. The focus is to let people with dementia live their lives as they want to, in a self-determined manner.

Alternative care environments are highly warranted to promote health and well-being of residents with dementia and are part of an age-friendly and dementia-friendly city and society. Design should facilitate human rights and dignity of people with dementia [13,14]. Radical changes in the physical, social and organizational environment are necessary to provide a care setting that enables people with dementia to be part of society. The physical design of the buildings and surroundings of innovative residential care facilities aims to follow the most recent design principles focusing on optimizing helpful stimulation, supporting movement and engagement, creating a familiar place and designing according to a clear model on the way of life at the facility [14]. An effective design of the physical environment enables people with dementia to better find their way, reduces challenging behavior such as agitation and improves independence in activities of daily living [15–18]. Furthermore, the physical environment and architectural design help to support care and activities, as well as the approach through which staff are able to maintain and reinforce the capabilities of people with dementia. Studies have suggested that higher quality of life is associated with buildings that facilitate engagement with a variety of activities both inside and outside, are familiar, provide a variety of private and community spaces, and provide opportunities to take part in domestic activities [14,19,20]. Therefore, a large variety of different types of innovative residential care facilities are developing in many countries, including the Netherlands. A recent report illustrates the variety of concepts by reporting on 84 case studies from 27 countries [21]. These include various types of small-scale homelike care models, including 24 h green care farms.

Green care farms that are 24 h have been developed as an alternative to traditional nursing homes, putting a congruent physical, social and organizational environment into practice [22]. Originating outside the healthcare sector, green care farms combine agriculture with care activities and aim to enable independence and participation in people with dementia for as long as possible. The rationale of green care farms is that people should be able to participate in daily activities as much as possible and care service delivery is integrated in daily life [23]. Furthermore, the physical environment (including animals, plants, natural elements) offers many opportunities to incorporate these activities into normal daily care practices. Residents can move more freely than in existing nursing homes as they have the opportunity to participate in outdoor, domestic, work-related, and other activities incorporated into normal daily life [22,24]. Farmers transfer their care philosophy to their staff by acting as a role model. Staff is selected based on competencies that support the individual green care farm vision and are continuously guided in providing care according to this philosophy [25,26]. Although there is large variety between green care farms (e.g., some have a degree of commercial farming such as crops, livestock, and woodland, while others do not), early evidence on outcomes for residents with dementia living at green care farms are promising. Green care farms appear to have a direct impact on the daily lives of residents. Residents living at green care farms were found to be more active, socially engaged and came outside more often [27]. This is important, as being outside was correlated with a positive mood [28]. Furthermore, the self-reported quality of life by residents was higher in green care farms compared with regular nursing homes [29]. Similar findings were found for day care services at green care farms [23,30]. Although various types of small-scale homelike care models exist, there is a lack of theoretical frameworks underpinning components and possible working mechanisms. There is an increased interest in concepts such as green houses, care villages and green care farms [10,27,31]. However, a clear theoretical framework describing the underlying principles on alternative nursing home care for people with dementia is currently lacking. Such a theoretical framework can increase our understanding of possible working mechanisms and can guide future hypothesis testing. Therefore, the novelty of the current study lies in the provision of insight into how to translate evidence-based knowledge from theory into a congruent care model.

An important facilitator of translating scientific evidence into practice is co-creation between researchers, professionals of care organizations and end-users (residents and family members) [32–36]. In the development of innovative dementia care settings, staff and family members have rarely reported to be involved [37]. Previous research indicates that studies that address the outcomes of co-creation processes are scarce [32]. This is problematic, given the increased focus on client-centered services within care practice, and the importance of true partnership between formal and informal care. Within care, co-creation is more than simple collaboration between stakeholders. It is the joint creation of vital goals for patients through the process of sharing knowledge and values [32,33]. This resonates with marketing concepts related to balanced centricity and stakeholder theory, which call for a situation where the interests of all actors in a network are secured [34]. Furthermore, existing collaboration initiatives within long-term care suggest that close, intensive collaboration between science and care practice is key to success of improving long-term care for older adults [35,36].

At the moment, many residential care facilities in the Netherlands are being redesigned and there is a high need for new care models. This article reports on the co-creation of an alternative nursing home model called the Homestead (in Dutch it is called de Hoeve). It presents the results of a co-creation process in which the underlying principles of green care farms have been translated into a new care model. Older people, their families and representatives, long-term care staff, management, architects and design staff have worked with researchers to put scientific knowledge on how to design the physical, social and organizational environment in everyday care into practice.

2. Materials and Methods

2.1. Design

A case study design was used studying the development of a new nursing home model called the Homestead. An existing farm-like building was acquired by the care organization, and plans were made to purposefully redesign the building in order to facilitate care provision according to the new care model, based on principles of green care farms and other innovative residential care models (e.g., putting a congruent physical, social and organizational environment in practice, and aiming to enable independence and participation in people with dementia for as long as possible). A participatory research approach was used in which researchers and practice co-created the new care model and planned for the redesign of the facility. The current study reports on a co-creation process of two years, starting August 2018 and ending in August 2020.

2.2. Case and Context Description

The research was conducted within a care organization in the southern part of the Netherlands. The care organization provides care across the full long-term care spectrum, including home care services, rehabilitation, palliative care and residential care in nursing homes to a wide variety of target groups. It has 17 nursing home locations, with approximately 1160 residents in total. It is a large organization with over 5000 staff members (covering home care, domestic services, nursing home care, palliative care and other staff). The care organization is part of the Living Lab in Ageing and Long-term Care, which is a formal interdisciplinary collaboration between research, education and care organizations in the southern part of the Netherlands [36].

The Homestead will be realized in a small village with approximately 5500 inhabitants. The village used to have a traditional large scale nursing home that needed to be renovated. However, the care organization chose to buy a different building that would be more fitting to implement and support the new care model.

2.3. Participants

The care model was developed with both practice and research in mind. Due the participatory research approach, participants of the current study included all stakeholders involved during the development of the care model (including older people, their families and representatives, long-term care staff, management, architects and design staff). The following groups were structured to guide the development process:

The core development group ($n = 7$) led the development process and managed the co-creation by deciding on the overall planning, making first drafts based on scientific literature and lessons learned in practice, and deciding on which topics to discuss in other working groups or with external experts. Furthermore, they discussed the final decisions regarding the care model. The core development group consisted of the project leader, the board of directors of the care organization, the director within the care organization, the nursing home manager, and two researchers from the university. Members of this core development group also participated in other working groups and brought information discussed in the other working groups together. Furthermore, this group was responsible for communication with the municipality (relevant civil servants and councilors) and the general practice of the region.

The project group ($n = 13$) consisted of the project leader, director within the care organization, nursing home manager, architect, client representative, janitor, care staff (both vocationally trained and higher educated nursing staff, $n = 4$), catering manager, employee from resident administration and a researcher from the university. Furthermore other (medical) staff such as medical doctors, psychologists, GPs, physiotherapists and occupational therapists gave input to the working group on relevant topics. This working group discussed everything related to the new residential care model with a specific focus on the elaboration of the most important pillars of the care model including the physical redesign of the building, possible competencies for staff and community engagement. A small portion the project group also focused on visiting many innovative care practices in the country in order to identify possible successful elements that could fit the developed care model. The following working groups were set up on specific themes to advice the project group.

- Resident, family and community engagement working groups: these working groups focused on engaging residents, family and people or organizations in the community in the development of the care model. Again, these took different forms ranging from large meetings with over 50 clubs and organizations from the local community, to smaller gatherings with family members and possible future residents. Besides standard gatherings, this working group also organized an official opening of the Homestead, informing the local community about the planning and concept of the Homestead. This opening was attended by more than 500 residents from the village. This working group also informed the community by sending multiple information letters regarding the state of affairs.
- Staff working groups: these working groups took several different forms during the development process ranging from brainstorm sessions with large groups of care staff (e.g., all staff of the original traditional nursing home of the village), and smaller gatherings of care staff focusing on e.g., describing what a day of a resident should look like in the Homestead, how to incorporate the outside areas more, etc. Thus, these groups varied from 3 to 30 staff members (including direct care staff, registered nurses from home-care teams, social workers and case manager).
- Technology working group ($n = 6$): this working group consisted of a nursing home manager, an innovation manager, an information advisor, care staff, ICT staff and a researcher from the university. This working group focused on all relevant technological questions and issues in order to facilitate providing care according to the care model such as home automation, beacon technology, etc.

2.4. Procedure

We used common methodology in co-creation research [32,33]. The co-creation process is an iterative process of identification of needs/aims, sharing knowledge on theory and scientific evidence and balancing this with what is possible in practice. Furthermore, careful reflection on whether the practical application is in line with the intended goals was part of the process. The development of the Homestead Care Model resulted from an iterative process of determining the main pillars of the care model, incorporating recent insights from the scientific literature, having meetings and sessions within the different working groups, working visits to existing facilities and drafting concept documents describing the care model. The core development group coordinated the process and connected the different working groups by exchanging information, feeding intermediate outcomes and results and facilitated discussions. For example, if a staff working group highlighted certain design issues, members from the core development group made sure this was communicated with the architect and other members from the project planning group. Furthermore, a log was kept that showed the overall planning and kept track of all decisions made within all working groups. If decisions were made that led to certain desired actions from other stakeholders within the development process, this was shared via the log. The role of the researchers was to monitor the process, to share scientific evidence with the other stakeholders, encourage out-of-the-box thinking and highlight best-practices. Furthermore, the researchers aided in translating evidence into practice and shared critical reflections on developed ideas. Final decisions regarding the Homestead Care Model were made by the care organization.

2.5. Data Collection and Analyses

Due to the participatory research approach, data collection and data analysis were performed in parallel. Data were collected by the researchers through direct observation and participation of meetings related to the development of the care model. During these meetings, the researchers kept track of a log which covered the date of the meeting, the type of meeting (e.g., workshop, board meeting, staff meeting, etc.), the topic of the meeting (e.g., physical environment, staff selection, care vision), and the participants (their position/function). Furthermore, the log contained information on which decisions/actions were made based on the meetings. In addition, the researchers held separate meetings with the primary involved nursing home manager to discuss the development process. Data analysis was thematic in nature, and dependent on the stage of development, meant that in early stages of development the researchers analyzed which themes were discussed in the meetings and how scientific evidence was used to support first ideas. In later stages of development, the researchers analyzed which main pillars of the care model were identified and how these were translated into practice examples.

Furthermore, archival data was collected. All reporting that was made during the development process was shared with the research team by the involved stakeholders. This archival data contained internal documents made during meetings (e.g., minutes), preliminary care model documents, planning documents, documents created by involved external stakeholders (e.g., architect), and presentations during board meetings. The research team saved all received documents on their university server and analyzed all documents as a whole. Relevant documents were labeled regarding the topic of the document (e.g., minutes project group meeting, action/decision list project group meeting, provisional care model document). Next, documents that were given the same/similar label, where grouped together to be read and analyzed sequentially. The data were abstracted further by summarizing main themes regarding the underlying theoretical principles and practical conceptualization.

3. Results

First, the theoretical principles of how nursing homes ideally support a meaningful daily life of residents with dementia are highlighted. Second, these principles were translated into practice, which is detailed below.

3.1. Theoretical Framework

The underlying theoretical framework that has guided the co-creation process is presented in Figure 1.

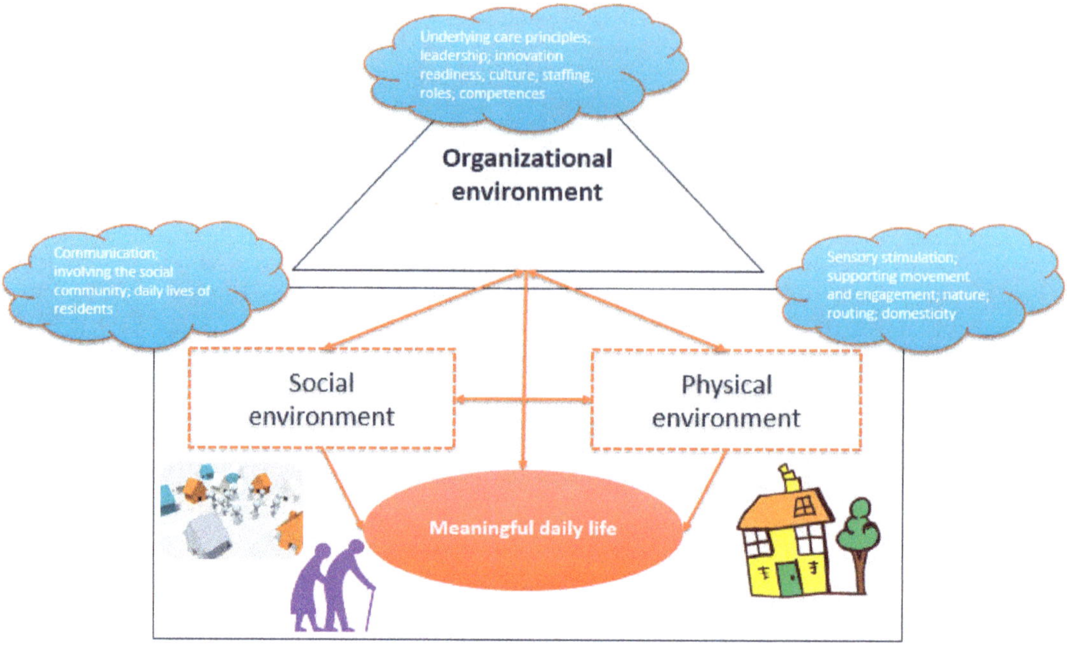

Figure 1. Underlying theoretical framework which integrates the physical, social and organizational environment.

Behavior and everyday functioning are the result of an interaction between the individual and her/his environment, although exact working mechanisms for people with dementia are unknown. Theories from various scientific backgrounds (i.e., psychology, nursing, gerontology, geriatrics) stress that a match is needed between the person's needs, his/her abilities and environmental demands to elicit adequate behavior in people with dementia, also referred to as person–environment fit [3,15,17,38,39]. If environmental demands exceed a persons' ability to cope, they will have more difficulty maintaining adequate behavior.

Within residential dementia care settings, the literature indicates three environmental components that impact everyday life and functioning for residents with dementia (see Figure 1):

- Physical aspects, including interior design, outdoor areas (e.g., gardens), architecture, built environment, lay-out aspects and sensory elements.
- Social aspects, including interactions with others in the environment. This includes resident, staff, family and friends and also the wider community and social context in which a dementia care setting is situated (e.g., local entrepreneurs, societies, and schools).
- Organizational aspects, including the way dementia care is organized and how the organizational culture is being perceived (e.g., values, expectations, attitudes that guide behavior of staff working in the dementia care setting).

The physical and social environment directly impact outcomes for residents with dementia. There is substantial evidence showing that the built environment can positively impact meaningful activities and quality of life for people with dementia [20]. Furthermore, restrictive physical environments can have unintended negative consequences. Therefore, the environment should contain opportunities that encourage activity [40–42]. Various studies show the importance of environmental aspects for people with dementia (e.g., sunlight, sounds, view, spatial layout, nature, orientation, music, privacy, autonomy, windows, comfort, facilities, staff, group size, non-institutional character, and domesticity). These studies show that careful consideration of the physical environment can support person-centered care, social interactions and daily activities of people with dementia [2,14,39,43–48]. For instance, features of the environment such as long corridors and lack of distinction between different areas may cause troubles in wayfinding [49], whereas minimizing long corridors may facilitate the domesticity of the environment [2]. Furthermore, careful consideration of signs, colors and furniture may improve orientation [49,50]. Another important aspect of the physical environment is the sensory stimulation it provides. Sensory stimulation can also be used to facilitate wayfinding and familiarity of the environment [51,52]. Environmental features such as accessibility of activity rooms, the use of artwork, plants and windows can be important factors influencing physical activity [53]. Furthermore, the use of outdoor spaces can be facilitated by incorporating environmental features such as seasonal plants and outdoor seating [54].

Although optimizing the built environment in residential aged care is important to facilitate activities and engagement, it is pivotal that changes in the physical environment are made in conjunction with considerations regarding how care should be provided [14]. Here, social aspects are crucial to consider. For instance, environmental features have been found to be able to create a familiar place for people with dementia, and to provide links to their family and community [14]. However, staff should then allow and facilitate residents to personalize their living space (e.g., by bringing photographs, paintings and pieces of furniture) [55,56]. People with dementia have to deal with the possibility of a declining ability to initiate activities and to communicate with others, showing the importance of support in maintaining social relationships. Activities can still be meaningful for people with dementia if they cause feelings of pleasure, involvement, connection and belonging. Being autonomous and having their own identity is important for people with dementia, therefore it is pivotal that staff ensure that activities are matched with roles, interests, routines and experiences of individual residents [57,58]. Over the last decade, there has been increased focus on providing person-centered care, in which the needs of people with dementia (such as the need for inclusion or identity) are considered. More recent scientific insights suggest that person-centered care insufficiently captures the interdependencies and reciprocities that underpin caring relationships, showing the importance of relationship-centered care and the reciprocity within a caring relationship [1,59–62]. Therefore, the building of relationships should be facilitated during the daily life of residents.

The theoretical model shows that the organizational context conditions any environmental design (both physical and social) and thereby influences everyday life and functioning of residents with dementia. Within long-term care, factors related to organizational culture and leadership to maintain culture are viewed as central aspects of the organizational context that impact outcomes [63–65]. Evidence suggests that shared values and supportive leadership for staff help in setting priorities and improve the delivery of individualized care [66,67]. For example, wards characterized by staff with positive caring climates had significantly less agitated behaviors (restlessness, wandering) compared with negative caring climate wards [66,68]. Furthermore, dementia wards characterized by an organizational culture of shared values and strong cohesion provided better quality of care [69]. The organizational environment, therefore, is an important prerequisite to innovate and directly impacts other environmental aspects. Congruence is needed between the different environmental components (physical, social and organizational), in order to promote well-being and adapted behaviors for residents with dementia and their caregivers.

3.2. Translation into Practice: The Homestead Care Model

The above-mentioned theoretical framework and underlying scientific principles were used in the co-creation process with all stakeholders and translated into three pillars leading to the Homestead Care Model: (1) activation, (2) freedom and (3) relationships.

The activation principle is the first pillar of the care model. Scientific evidence shows that people with dementia wish to be involved in meaningful activities and when they are more involved in these kinds of activities, this can affect their overall well-being and affect fundamental psychological needs [58,70–73]. In addition, it is known that a more active daily life is associated with aspects related to quality of life [73,74]. All stakeholders in the development process emphasized the value and importance of an active, meaningful life for people with dementia. As a result, the core development group decided that activation should be central in all facets of care delivery and in living at the Homestead in general. The project group discussed that the underlying idea is that because people with dementia can be more active during their daily life they will also remain cognitively and physically fit longer. This is in line with the "use it or lose it" principle, which suggests that if people do not use certain functionalities of the brain for a longer period of time, they will get worse at those functionalities (or lose them completely) [75–77]. For instance, if a person with dementia has little or no physical activity for a longer period of time, this will negatively affect his/her physical functioning (hence, he/she is less able to walk independently). The same applies for other functionalities such as communication, reasoning or emotional skills.

The freedom principle is the second pillar of the care model and refers to freedom of movement, freedom of choice and overall autonomy. Within the staff working groups, it was discussed that even though people with dementia experience limitations in daily life, their autonomy can be supported by engaging in true partnership between the residents, their family, and formal caregivers. This is also referred to as relational autonomy, which indicates that people with dementia can still exercise autonomy, regardless of being dependent on others [78–82]. Building on this, the core development group decided that freedom is the second important principle. This indicated that, at the Homestead, the residents should decide how they want their care to be arranged and formal caregivers can support this. When people with dementia live at home, they are in charge. As the Homestead is their new home, they are still in charge. People with dementia sometimes need help and support to express their preferences, which is something that family and formal caregivers can support with. Hence, freedom of choice is paramount in everything including living, eating, exercising, day planning, activities, and care. In the project group, examples put forward by the staff working group were mentioned. For example, the resident can choose where to eat and with whom, he/she can choose to sleep in or not, and he/she can decide to undertake an activity alone, in a group, or not at all. The environment shapes the behavior of residents and should increase personal agency of people with dementia. Agency refers to a persons' capacity to act within his or her environment and is influenced by contextual factors such as whether there is the possibility to act or to make choices independently. This emphasizes the importance of making sure that the physical and social environment of residents encourages them to make optimal use of their living space in the most meaningful way [3,83].

The relationship principle is the third pillar of the care model. A main aspect mentioned (in particular from the resident, family and community engagement working group) was that for people with dementia, it is important that they are supported to build a bond and forge relationships with other residents and formal caregivers. Therefore, the core development decided that relationships is the third important principle. Based on the principles of relationship-centered care, care should be provided to a small group of residents, by a small, permanent team of formal caregivers. Relationship-centered care means that care goes beyond just looking at the resident (as it is in person-centered care). The focus is on optimizing the residents' closest relationship triangle (resident–family–formal caregiver). Quality of care is defined as the perceived quality by residents (based on their expectations with regard to care and the interactions between residents, their loved ones, and their care providers). Making shared decisions about living arrangements, lifestyle, and treatment, and monitoring these decisions to improve care will result in higher experienced quality of care.

The pillars have been translated into choices in practice. Within the core development group, it was decided that all decisions made during the development of the Homestead Care Model should be made based on promoting the three pillars of the care model. This included choices regarding the physical environment (e.g., building, outdoor spaces, furnishing), as well as choices about the social and organizational environment (e.g., staffing, required competencies, involvement of the community). The consequences for the physical and social environment are mainly based on discussion within the project group, which received input from the other working groups. The practical translations are presented below.

3.2.1. The Physical Environment

Within the Homestead Care Model, it is of utmost importance that residents are physically, cognitively and socially activated or can remain active themselves during their life. To implement these principles in practice, the Homestead aims to provide an optimal person–environment fit, tailoring the environment as much as possible to the needs of individual residents, family and staff [17]. The Homestead is an existing building which is a typically rural square farm, built of limestone, with a courtyard that is more than 100 m deep. It was built around the year 1400. It has a chapel attached to the courtyard. The courtyard is accessed through a large gate. The building has a rich history and is well-known by the local community (see Figure 2 for illustrative images).

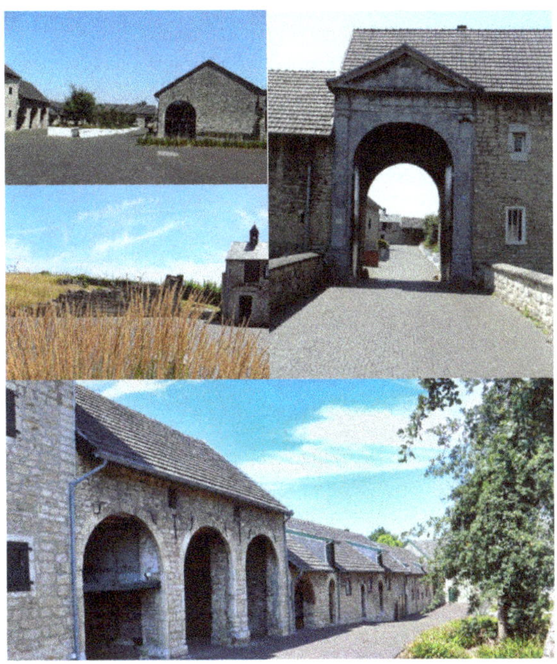

Figure 2. Illustrative images of the building in which the Homestead will be realized.

The Homestead has three floors (ground, first and second), and offers a living environment for 52 people with dementia. Figure 3 shows the floor plan of the first floor. In order to respect the privacy of residents and to facilitate their autonomy in terms of self-care, there are 52 individual rooms for residents with their own sanitary facilities. Furthermore, there are communal kitchens, living rooms and activity areas. To support residents' agency and freedom, all residents have direct access to the outdoors, regardless of where they live in the Homestead. This means that paths, access roads and places are created on all floors that support residents to go outside and seek contact in the general outdoor spaces (garden, courtyard, etc.). A portion of the outdoor space has a raised soil-level so that residents from the first floor can walk outdoors without having to take an elevator or stairs. In addition, lines of sight, walking routes, and familiarity are taken into account in the design of the Homestead to make sure residents are able to find their way independently. Orientation to find their own room, living room, or the outdoors are facilitated. All possible spaces and rooms are used to accommodate activities for residents. Hence, there will be no separate areas for nursing staff (e.g., nurses station).

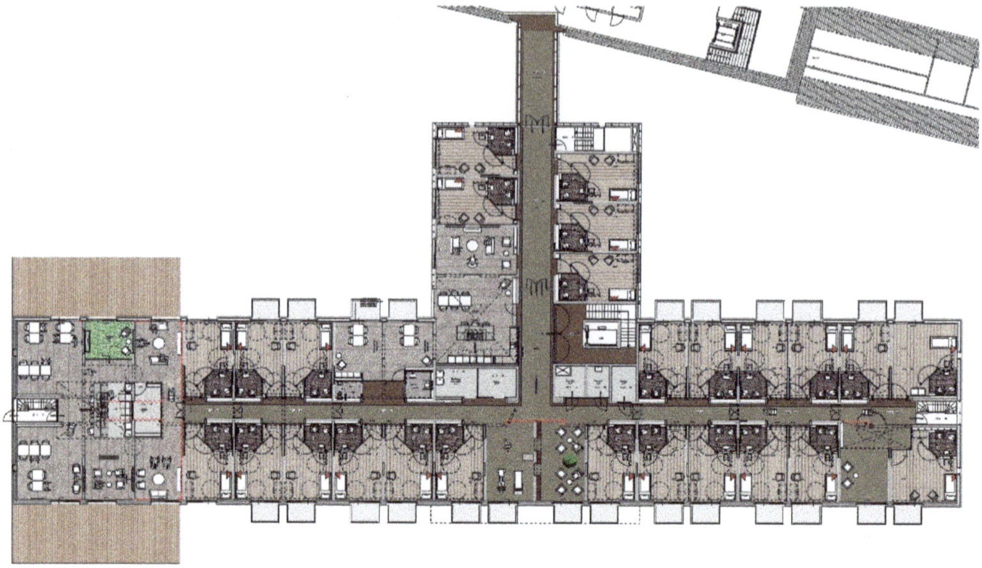

Figure 3. Floor plan of the Homestead (© Reproduced with permission from Widdershoven Architecten bv).

Thus, the building and the outdoor spaces are inviting and inspire residents to be active. There are many options for residents to choose how they want to spend their day. Examples include activities in the garden, working with plants, taking care of animals, or just taking a walk outside. Furthermore, indoor activities such as hobbies, preparing dinner, watching a movie, playing games, or just having a pleasant chat are some of the options. Many of these activities are also organized by or for the local community, which will facilitate the building of relationships. Within the Homestead there is a restaurant for residents and family as well as for the general public. A vibrant, social gathering place for the community is created which will facilitate the social integration of residents. There is a free water tap for passing hikers or cyclists. Furthermore, playing areas for children will facilitate intergenerational interactions.

To give the residents maximum freedom of movement, there is an open door policy, meaning that no doors are locked. Residents can choose when they want to go outside. Opportunities for social interactions as well as privacy are facilitated. Furthermore, both the indoor and outdoor areas are equipped with care communication technology. By using smart technologies, a resident is supported in their freedom (e.g., camera if needed, GPS tracking, etc.). Together with residents, family, and formal caregivers it is decided which optimal degree of freedom is possible.

3.2.2. The Social Environment

Within the project group one of the themes discussed was around what a typical day at the Homestead should look like, in which it was discussed how the pillars of the care model influence daily life of residents, family and staff. Practical applications of the pillars of the care model were summarized in basic principles which were described in a document called Living and Working at the Homestead. One important principle is that the Homestead is the actual house of the resident, meaning that staff are visiting people in their own house and should act accordingly. This is a crucial principle which indicates that staff should always respect residents' privacy, and that there should always be mutual consent in all actions. This is relevant in all aspects of care delivery.

A second important principle is related to an equal partnership between residents, family and staff. People with dementia all have their own story/history, in which they create relationships with others. Their story should not stop when they move to the Homestead. Rather, residents should be able to continue their story as they see fit, and their social environment should facilitate this. Therefore, relationship centered care and social health are important principles at the Homestead [59,84]. There is active family participation and the capacity to fulfil residents' full potential at the center of care practice. Residents should be able to manage their life, regardless of their degree of independence. At the Homestead there is no fixed day program that determines what a resident can do. Instead, together with family, formal caregivers and residents, an equal partnership is used to determine which sources should be used to meet the needs and wishes of residents. The residents are supported to make their own choices, as they would also do in their own home.

Furthermore, the transition process to a residential care facility impacts the experiences quality of care after transition. Therefore, staff at the Homestead visit the residents and family before they actually move to the Homestead in order to familiarize themselves with the home situation, preferences, needs and existing relationships of future residents. Information that is shared by residents and family before moving to the Homestead is used to optimally support the transition process and maintain the life people are used to as much as possible. Aspects that are considered are how an optimal fit can be created with the other residents, the community and how existing habits can be implemented into normal daily care practices. For example, if a resident slept until 11:00 a.m. in their home situation, this is also possible at the Homestead, or if a resident is used to participating in certain activities, they can still do that at the Homestead (even if these activities take place outside of the Homestead).

The Homestead is more than a nursing home—the social context is intensively involved and should be seen as a house of the community. It is a lively center for the neighborhood. The areas for communal activities, outdoor spaces, and the restaurant are arranged in such a way that they can also be made available to the general public. In addition, the Homestead actively seeks connection to the neighborhood by contacting specific organizations (such as the local primary school), clubs or societies in the community (e.g., local sports club, orchestra, choir, band, etc.). With these organizations they form a reciprocal relationship (focusing on what the Homestead can do for the organizations, and what the organizations can do to contribute to a meaningful life for residents). Residents are encouraged to participate as much as possible in the activities that are going on at the Homestead. There is always something to do and residents can choose what they would like to do. By including a larger social context in the Homestead, residents are still part of larger social groups and give a meaningful contribution to the community.

3.2.3. The Organizational Environment

The Homestead can be seen as an innovation platform in which new scientific insights are applied in practice in the form of experiments or pilot studies. A culture is created in which learning, development and innovation, guided by scientific insights, are central to continuously improve the care that is provided to residents. Constant discussion about each other's actions is necessary to implement the care model completely. For instance, it is important that all options for activities are not seen as separate interventions or organized activities. They are part of the normal course of events and are integrated into normal daily life at the Homestead. However, in order to successfully implement them, staff need to be reminded and think about how to do so. It is important that there is coaching staff on all levels in the organization who are constantly coaching the rest of the team. At the

Homestead, this coaching is mostly performed by management and bachelor-educated nursing staff.

At the Homestead, it is important that managers facilitate innovation by creating shared values and setting priorities. Effective management is only one dimension of leadership which also involves, for example, exercising of charisma and demonstrating commitment to innovation. Being a role model for staff is an important part of implementing the care model. The style of leadership at the Homestead is therefore consultative, facilitative and flexible. Ideally, several leaders will be operating simultaneously at multiple organizational levels. Therefore, there are role models in place on all levels of the organizations (board level, director level, management level and direct care staff level). These people are given different roles within the Homestead. They are part of the development of the care model and other staff members know that they can be seen as the voice of the care model.

In line with this, important parts of the organizational environment of the Homestead are the staff roles, the competence based selection and training of staff. The three main pillars of the care model impose adjusted requirements on staff. Staff members are selected on the basis of the care model and are required to let go of traditional ways of working. Staff roles (including living counselor, well-being coach, culinary employee and manager) are formulated. For each role, the required competencies and expertise are elaborated on. These competencies include the ability to switch between the pillars of the care model in order to properly anticipate the needs of residents. Staff is required to oversee many things at the same time and they must be flexible and creative in order to integrate activities into normal daily care practices. Based on relationship centered care, involving the residents and informal caregivers as partners in the care process and the daily life of residents is one of the requested requirements. Other competencies include facilitating residents' autonomy, focusing on remaining capabilities, being respectful and having knowledge on dementia. In order to achieve an environment that successfully implements and maintains the care model, the Homestead uses competence based selection and training for staff. All staff receive an extensive introduction and training program about the care model. The training is aimed at the pillars of the care model and covers how staff should facilitate activation, freedom, autonomy and relationship building. All staff have a trial period of six months. If it turns out that a staff member is not employing the care model correctly, he/she is not hired to work at the Homestead. Furthermore, all staff have a personal development plan which is evaluated periodically.

4. Discussion

This article reports on the Homestead Care Model, which is the result of a co-creation between older people, their families and representatives, long-term care staff, management, architects and design staff and researchers. Scientific knowledge shows that the physical, social and organizational environment should be congruent in order to promote overall well-being and everyday functioning of residents and caregivers in dementia care. These principles were translated into the Homestead Care Model and conceptualized around three main pillars: activation, freedom and relationships. This means that the Homestead is aimed at providing residents with an active, meaningful daily life in which they are enabled to live their lives as they want to, in a self-determined matter. Freedom of movement, freedom of choice, and overall autonomy is facilitated by focusing on remaining capabilities, rather than on limitations of residents. Furthermore, the Homestead aims to be more than a nursing home—it is a lively center for the community that facilitates relationships and enables residents to contribute and be part of society. A crucial underlying principle of the Homestead care model is that the pillars should lead to choices regarding the physical, social and organizational environment. These different facets of the environment are interrelated and achieving the aims of the Homestead Care Model is dependent on how well the physical, social and organizational environment are attuned to each other.

The Homestead Care Model is an illustrative example of how residential care facilities can support the development of age-friendly communities that take into consideration the needs and requirements of older citizens, which is an important aim of the world-wide program by the World Health Organization (WHO) on age-friendly cities and communities [85]. Furthermore, a recent age-friendly framework also highlights the importance of considering actual physical environments that are associated with age-friendly living, which was seen as a relevant addition to the WHO domains of an age-friendly city [86]. We present an example of an innovative residential care model that may facilitate a more positive social attitude towards older people and people with dementia in the community.

As previous studies have indicated, it is challenging to implement radical changes within residential care (e.g., [10]). Besides the redesign of the physical environment, a main possible barrier of successful implementation is the lack of highly qualified staff with the competences necessary to implement the Homestead Care Model. Managers are expected to apply competence-based selection for staff. Given the current workforce challenges and high turnover within residential care, this will be challenging [87]. However, the Homestead aims to facilitate a culture focusing on personal development and innovation, which is suggested to positively impact staff-turnover [88]. Staff making the transition will be trained beforehand. Furthermore, on-the-job coaching and training of this radically new way of working will be an ongoing process before and after the move.

Some limitations of the current study should be considered. First, using a participatory research approach can be considered a strength. However, such an approach requires sensitivity to the relationship between involved stakeholders [89]. In some cases, researchers needed to make deliberate decisions to trade-off their expected outcomes with what the care organization considers to be realistic outcomes. Outcomes of the current study were therefore sometimes the result of a compromise between completely evidence based principles and considerations of the care organization in terms of resources and possibilities. This however illustrates the real world application of research findings. Second, so far the Homestead Care Model is a theoretical concept which is currently being implemented in practice. More research is needed to address the gaps in knowledge regarding which actions deliver actual positive outcomes. Future studies should include outcomes both from a psychophysiological perspective (e.g., functional ability, physical fitness, blood pressure) and a psychosocial perspective (e.g., maintaining relationships, daily life, quality of life). This is in line with the WHO statement that guidance and tools are needed to support communities to make decisions which promote actions that are most likely to ensure these outcomes [90].

5. Conclusions

The Homestead Care Model is a translation of underlying principles that takes into consideration the interrelatedness of the physical, social and organizational environment. It incorporates scientific knowledge which indicates that the physical, social and organizational environment should be congruent in order to promote overall well-being and everyday functioning of residents and caregivers in dementia care. Future studies should focus on the actual implementation and effectiveness of the Homestead Care Model.

Author Contributions: Conceptualization, B.d.B., B.B., J.J., M.H., J.P.H.H. and H.V.; formal analysis, B.d.B.; methodology, B.d.B. and H.V.; supervision, H.V.; visualization, B.d.B. and B.B.; writing—original draft, B.d.B. and H.V.; writing—review & editing, B.d.B., B.B., J.J., M.H., J.P.H.H. and H.V. All authors have read and agreed to the published version of the manuscript.

Funding: This project was funded by Maastricht University.

Acknowledgments: The authors would like to acknowledge the architect that participated in the co-creation of the Homestead care model and provided illustrative images (Widdershoven Architecten bv).

Conflicts of Interest: The authors declare no conflict of interest.

References

1. Wiersma, E.C.; Pedlar, A. The nature of relationships in alternative dementia care environments. *Can. J. Aging* **2008**, *27*, 101–108. [CrossRef] [PubMed]
2. De Boer, B.; Beerens, H.C.L.; Katterbach, M.A.; Viduka, M.; Willemse, B.M.; Verbeek, H. The physical environment of nursing homes for people with dementia: Traditional nursing homes, small-scale living facilities, and green care farms. *Healthcare* **2018**, *6*, 137. [CrossRef] [PubMed]
3. Topo, P.; Kotilainen, H.; Eloniemi-Sulkava, U. Affordances of the care environment for people with dementia—An assessment study. *HERD* **2012**, *5*, 118–138. [CrossRef] [PubMed]
4. den Ouden, M.; Bleijlevens, M.H.C.; Meijers, J.M.M.; Zwakhalen, S.M.G.; Braun, S.M.; Tan, F.E.S.; Hamers, J.P.H. Daily (in) activities of nursing home residents in their wards: An observation study. *J. Am. Med. Dir. Assoc.* **2015**, *16*, 963–968. [CrossRef] [PubMed]
5. Donovan, C.; Donovan, A.; Stewart, C.; McCloskey, R. How residents spend their time in nursing homes. *Can. Nurs. Home* **2014**, *25*, 13–17.
6. Wetzels, R.B.; Zuidema, S.U.; de Jonghe, J.F.M.; Verhey, F.R.J.; Koopmans, R.T.C.M. Course of neuropsychiatric symptoms in residents with dementia in nursing homes over 2-year period. *Am. J. Geriatr. Psychiatry* **2010**, *18*, 1054–1065. [CrossRef] [PubMed]
7. Helvik, A.S.; Selbaek, G.; Saltyte Benth, J.; Roen, I.; Bergh, S. The course of neuropsychiatric symptoms in nursing home residents from admission to 30-month follow-up. *PLoS ONE* **2018**, *13*, e0206147.
8. Lam, K.; Kwan, J.S.; Kwan, C.W.; Chong, A.M.; Lai, C.K.; Lou, V.W.; Leung, A.Y.; Liu, J.Y.; Bai, X.; Chi, I. Factors associated with the trend of physical and chemical restraint use among long-term care facility residents in Hong Kong: Data from an 11-year observational study. *J. Am. Med. Dir. Assoc.* **2017**, *18*, 1043–1048. [CrossRef]
9. Ferreira, A.R.; Simões, M.R.; Moreira, E.; Guedes, J.; Fernandes, L. Modifiable factors associated with neuropsychiatric symptoms in nursing homes: The impact of unmet needs and psychotropic drugs. *Arch. Gerontol. Geriatr.* **2020**, *86*, 103919. [CrossRef]
10. Ausserhofer, D.; Deschodt, M.; De Geest, S.; van Achterberg, T.; Meyer, G.; Verbeek, H.; Sjetne, I.S.; Malinowska-Lipien, I.; Griffiths, P.; Schluter, W.; et al. "There's No Place Like Home": A scoping review on the impact of homelike residential care models on resident-, family-, and staff-related outcomes. *J. Am. Med. Dir. Assoc.* **2016**, *17*, 685–693. [CrossRef]
11. Koren, M.J. Person-centered care for nursing home residents: The culture-change movement. *Health Aff.* **2010**, *29*, 312–317. [CrossRef] [PubMed]
12. Verbeek, H.; Van Rossum, E.; Zwakhalen, S.M.G.; Kempen, G.I.; Hamers, J.P.H. Small, homelike care environments for older people with dementia: A literature review. *Int. Psychogeriatr.* **2009**, *21*, 252–264. [CrossRef]
13. Charras, K.; Eynard, C.; Viatour, G. Use of space and human rights: Planning dementia friendly settings. *J. Gerontol. Soc. Work* **2016**, *59*, 181–204. [CrossRef]
14. Fleming, R.; Zeisel, J.; Bennet, K. *World Alzheimer Report 2020: Design, Dignity, Dementia: Dementia-Related Design and the Built Environment*; Alzheimer's Disease International: London, UK, 2020.
15. Chaudhury, H.; Cooke, H.A.; Cowie, H.; Razaghi, L. The influence of the physical environment on residents with dementia in long-term care settings: A review of the empirical literature. *Gerontologist* **2018**, *58*, e325–e337. [CrossRef] [PubMed]
16. Chaudhury, H.; Cooke, H. Design matters in dementia care: The role of the physical environment in dementia care settings. *Excell. Dement. Care* **2014**, *2*, 144–158.
17. Jao, Y.-L.; Liu, W.; Chaudhury, H.; Parajuli, J.; Holmes, S.; Galik, E. Function-Focused Person-Environment Fit for Long-Term Care Residents with Dementia: Impact on Apathy. *Gerontologist* **2020**. [CrossRef]
18. Wong, C.; Leland, N.E. *Applying the Person-Environment-Occupation Model to Improve Dementia Care*; OT Practice: London, UK, 2018; pp. CE-1–CE-7.
19. Barnes, S. Space, choice and control, and quality of life in care settings for older people. *Environ. Behav.* **2006**, *38*, 589–604. [CrossRef]
20. Fleming, R.; Goodenough, B.; Low, L.-F.; Chenoweth, L.; Brodaty, H. The relationship between the quality of the built environment and the quality of life of people with dementia in residential care. *Dementia* **2016**, *15*, 663–680. [CrossRef]
21. Fleming, R.; Zeisel, J.; Bennet, K. *World Alzheimer Report 2020: Design Dignity Dementia: Dementia-Related Design and the Built Environment Volume 2: Case Studies*; Alzheimer's Disease International: London, UK, 2020.
22. De Bruin, S.R.; Oosting, S.; van der Zijpp, A.; Enders-Slegers, M.-J.; Schols, J. The concept of green care farms for older people with dementia: An integrative framework. *Dementia* **2010**, *9*, 79–128. [CrossRef]
23. De Bruin, S.R.; Stoop, A.; Molema, C.C.; Vaandrager, L.; Hop, P.J.; Baan, C.A. Green care farms: An innovative type of adult day service to stimulate social participation of people with dementia. *Gerontol. Geriatr. Med.* **2015**, *1*, 2333721415607833. [CrossRef]
24. Hassink, J.; Van Dijk, M. *Farming for Health: Green-Care Farming across Europe and the United States of America*; Springer: Berlin/Heidelberg, Germany, 2006.
25. de Bruin, S.R.; de Boer, B.; Beerens, H.C.; Buist, Y.; Verbeek, H. Rethinking dementia care: The value of green care farming. *J. Am. Med. Dir. Assoc.* **2017**, *18*, 200–203. [CrossRef] [PubMed]
26. Buist, Y.; Verbeek, H.; de Boer, B.; de Bruin, S.R. Innovating dementia care; implementing characteristics of green care farms in other long-term care settings. *Int. Psychogeriatr.* **2018**, *30*, 1057–1068. [CrossRef] [PubMed]
27. de Boer, B.; Hamers, J.P.H.; Zwakhalen, S.M.G.; Tan, F.E.S.; Beerens, H.C.; Verbeek, H. Green care farms as innovative nursing homes, promoting activities and social interaction for people with dementia. *J. Am. Med. Dir. Assoc.* **2017**, *18*, 40–46. [CrossRef]

28. Beerens, H.C.; Zwakhalen, S.M.G.; Verbeek, H.; Tan, F.E.S.; Jolani, S.; Downs, M.; de Boer, B.; Ruwaard, D.; Hamers, J.P.H. The relation between mood, activity, and interaction in long-term dementia care. *Aging Ment. Health* **2018**, *22*, 26–32. [CrossRef] [PubMed]
29. de Boer, B.; Hamers, J.P.H.; Zwakhalen, S.M.G.; Tan, F.E.S.; Verbeek, H. Quality of care and quality of life of people with dementia living at green care farms: A cross-sectional study. *BMC Geriatr.* **2017**, *17*, 155. [CrossRef]
30. Ellingsen-Dalskau, L.H.; de Boer, B.; Pedersen, I. Comparing the care environment at farm-based and regular day care for people with dementia in Norway—An observational study. *Health Soc. Care Community* **2020**. [CrossRef]
31. Cohen, L.W.; Zimmerman, S.; Reed, D.; Brown, P.; Bowers, B.J.; Nolet, K.; Sandra Hudak, R.N.; Horn, S.D. The Green House Model of Nursing Home Care in Design and Implementation. *Health Serv. Res.* **2016**, *51*, 352–377. [CrossRef] [PubMed]
32. Voorberg, W.H.; Bekkers, V.J.J.M.; Tummers, L.G. A Systematic Review of Co-Creation and Co-Production: Embarking on the social innovation journey. *Public Manag. Rev.* **2015**, *17*, 1333–1357. [CrossRef]
33. Bergdahl, E.; Ternestedt, B.M.; Bertero, C.; Andershed, B. The theory of a co-creative process in advanced palliative home care nursing encounters: A qualitative deductive approach over time. *Nurs. Open* **2019**, *6*, 175–188. [CrossRef]
34. Verleye, K.; Jaakkola, E.; Hodgkinson, I.R.; Jun, G.T.; Odekerken-Schroder, G.; Quist, J. What causes imbalance in complex service networks? Evidence from a public health service. *J. Serv. Manag.* **2017**, *28*, 34–56. [CrossRef]
35. Luijkx, K.; van Boekel, L.; Janssen, M.; Verbiest, M.; Stoop, A. The Academic Collaborative Center Older Adults: A Description of Co-Creation between Science, Care Practice and Education with the Aim to Contribute to Person-Centered Care for Older Adults. *Int. J. Environ. Res. Public Health* **2020**, *17*, 9014. [CrossRef] [PubMed]
36. Verbeek, H.; Zwakhalen, S.M.G.; Schols, J.M.; Kempen, G.I.; Hamers, J.P.H. The Living Lab in Ageing and Long-Term Care: A Sustainable Model for Translational Research Improving Quality of Life, Quality of Care and Quality of Work. *J. Nutr. Health Aging* **2020**, *24*, 43–47. [CrossRef] [PubMed]
37. Charras, K.; Bébin, C.; Laulier, V.; Mabire, J.-B.; Aquino, J.-P. Designing dementia-friendly gardens: A workshop for landscape architects: Innovative Practice. *Dementia* **2018**, *2018*, 1471301218808609. [CrossRef] [PubMed]
38. Edvardsson, D. Therapeutic environments for older adults: Constituents and meanings. *J. Gerontol. Nurs.* **2008**, *34*, 32–40. [CrossRef] [PubMed]
39. Lawton, M.P.; Nahemow, L. Ecology and the Aging Process. 1973. Available online: https://psycnet.apa.org/record/2004-15428-020 (accessed on 30 September 2020).
40. Low, L.-F.; Draper, B.; Brodaty, H. The relationship between self-destructive behaviour and nursing home environment. *Aging Ment. Health* **2004**, *8*, 29–33. [CrossRef] [PubMed]
41. Torrington, J. What has architecture got to do with dementia care? Explorations of the relationship between quality of life and building design in two EQUAL projects. *Qual. Ageing* **2006**, *7*, 34. [CrossRef]
42. Whear, R.; Coon, J.T.; Bethel, A.; Abbott, R.; Stein, K.; Garside, R. What is the impact of using outdoor spaces such as gardens on the physical and mental well-being of those with dementia? A systematic review of quantitative and qualitative evidence. *J. Am. Med. Dir. Assoc.* **2014**, *15*, 697–705. [CrossRef]
43. Davis, S.; Byers, S.; Nay, R.; Koch, S. Guiding design of dementia friendly environments in residential care settings: Considering the living experiences. *Dementia* **2009**, *8*, 185–203. [CrossRef]
44. Woodbridge, R.; Sullivan, M.; Harding, E.; Crutch, S.; Gilhooly, K.; Gilhooly, M. Use of the physical environment to support everyday activities for people with dementia: A systematic review. *Dementia* **2018**, *17*, 533–572. [CrossRef]
45. Chaudhury, H.; Hung, L.; Badger, M. The role of physical environment in supporting person-centered dining in long-term care: A review of the literature. *Am. J. Alzheimers Dis. Dement.* **2013**, *28*, 491–500. [CrossRef]
46. Fleming, R.; Crookes, P.A.; Sum, S. A Review of the Empirical Literature on the Design of Physical Environments for People with Dementia. 2008. Available online: https://ro.uow.edu.au/cgi/viewcontent.cgi?article=3923&context=hbspapers (accessed on 25 September 2020).
47. Day, K.; Carreon, D.; Stump, C. The therapeutic design of environments for people with dementia: A review of the empirical research. *Gerontologist* **2000**, *40*, 397–416. [CrossRef] [PubMed]
48. Dijkstra, K.; Pieterse, M.; Pruyn, A. Physical environmental stimuli that turn healthcare facilities into healing environments through psychologically mediated effects: Systematic review. *J. Adv. Nurs.* **2006**, *56*, 166–181. [CrossRef] [PubMed]
49. Marquardt, G. Wayfinding for people with dementia: A review of the role of architectural design. *HERD* **2011**, *4*, 75–90. [CrossRef] [PubMed]
50. Davis, R.; Weisbeck, C. Creating a supportive environment using cues for wayfinding in dementia. *J. Gerontol. Nurs.* **2016**, *42*, 36–44. [CrossRef]
51. Chenoweth, L.; Forbes, I.; Fleming, R.; King, M.; Stein-Parbury, J.; Luscombe, G.; Kenny, P.; Jeon, Y.-H.; Haas, M.; Brodaty, H. PerCEN: A Cluster Randomized Controlled Trial of Person-Centered Residential Care and Environment for People with Dementia. 2014. Available online: https://ro.uow.edu.au/cgi/viewcontent.cgi?article=2827&context=smhpapers (accessed on 25 September 2020).
52. Davis, R.; Ohman, J.M.; Weisbeck, C. Salient cues and wayfinding in Alzheimer's disease within a virtual senior residence. *Environ. Behav.* **2017**, *49*, 1038–1065. [CrossRef]
53. Douma, J.G.; Volkers, K.M.; Engels, G.; Sonneveld, M.H.; Goossens, R.H.; Scherder, E.J. Setting-related influences on physical inactivity of older adults in residential care settings: A review. *BMC Geriatr.* **2017**, *17*, 97. [CrossRef] [PubMed]

54. van den Berg, M.E.; Winsal, M.; Dyer, S.M.; Breen, F.; Gresham, M.; Crotty, M. Understanding the Barriers and Enablers to Using Outdoor Spaces in Nursing Homes: A Systematic Review. *Gerontologist* **2020**, *60*, e254–e269. [CrossRef] [PubMed]
55. Charras, K.; Zeisel, J.; Belmin, J.; Drunat, O.; Sebbagh, M.; Gridel, G.; Bahon, F. Effect of personalization of private spaces in special care units on institutionalized elderly with dementia of the Alzheimer type. *Non-Pharmacol. Ther. Dement.* **2010**, *1*, 121–137.
56. Van Hoof, J.; Janssen, M.L.; Heesakkers, C.M.C.; Van Kersbergen, W.; Severijns, L.E.J.; Willems, L.A.G.; Marston, H.R.; Janssen, B.M.; Nieboer, M.E. The importance of personal possessions for the development of a sense of home of nursing home residents. *J. Hous. Elder.* **2016**, *30*, 35–51. [CrossRef]
57. Phinney, A.; Chaudhury, H.; O'connor, D.L. Doing as much as I can do: The meaning of activity for people with dementia. *Aging Ment. Health* **2007**, *11*, 384–393. [CrossRef]
58. Vernooij-Dassen, M. *Meaningful Activities for People with Dementia*; Taylor & Francis: New York, NY, USA, 2007.
59. Adams, T.; Gardiner, P. Communication and interaction within dementia care triads: Developing a theory for relationship-centred care. *Dementia* **2005**, *4*, 185–205. [CrossRef]
60. McCormack, B.; McCance, T.V. Development of a framework for person-centred nursing. *J. Adv. Nurs.* **2006**, *56*, 472–479. [CrossRef] [PubMed]
61. Wilberforce, M.; Batten, E.; Challis, D.; Davies, L.; Kelly, M.P.; Roberts, C. The patient experience in community mental health services for older people: A concept mapping approach to support the development of a new quality measure. *BMC Health Serv. Res.* **2018**, *18*, 461. [CrossRef] [PubMed]
62. Wilberforce, M.; Challis, D.; Davies, L.; Kelly, M.P.; Roberts, C. The preliminary measurement properties of the person-centred community care inventory (PERCCI). *Qual. Life Res.* **2018**, *27*, 2745–2756. [CrossRef]
63. Goodman, C. The organisational culture of nursing staff providing long-term dementia care is related to quality of care. *Evid. Based Nurs.* **2011**, *14*, 88–89. [CrossRef]
64. André, B.; Sjøvold, E.; Rannestad, T.; Ringdal, G.I. The impact of work culture on quality of care in nursing homes—A review study. *Scand. J. Caring Sci.* **2014**, *28*, 449–457. [CrossRef]
65. Etherton-Beer, C.; Venturato, L.; Horner, B. Organisational culture in residential aged care facilities: A cross-sectional observational study. *PLoS ONE* **2013**, *8*, e58002. [CrossRef]
66. Edvardsson, D.; Fetherstonhaugh, D.; McAuliffe, L.; Nay, R.; Chenco, C. Job satisfaction amongst aged care staff: Exploring the influence of person-centered care provision. *Int. Psychogeriatr.* **2011**, *23*, 1205. [CrossRef]
67. Backman, A.; Ahnlund, P.; Sjögren, K.; Lövheim, H.; McGilton, K.S.; Edvardsson, D. Embodying person-centred being and doing: Leading towards person-centred care in nursing homes as narrated by managers. *J. Clin. Nurs.* **2020**, *29*, 172–183. [CrossRef]
68. Edvardsson, D.; Sandman, P.-O.; Nay, R.; Karlsson, S. Associations between the working characteristics of nursing staff and the prevalence of behavioral symptoms in people with dementia in residential care. *Int. Psychogeriatr.* **2008**, *20*, 764. [CrossRef]
69. Van Beek, A.; Gerritsen, D. The relationship between organizational culture of nursing staff and quality of care for residents with dementia: Questionnaire surveys and systematic observations in nursing homes. *Int. J. Nurs. Stud.* **2010**, *47*, 1274–1282. [CrossRef]
70. Jones, C.; Liu, F.; Murfield, J.; Moyle, W. Effects of non-facilitated meaningful activities for people with dementia in long-term care facilities: A systematic review. *Geriatr. Nurs.* **2020**, *41*, 863–871. [CrossRef] [PubMed]
71. Han, A.; Radel, J.; McDowd, J.M.; Sabata, D. Perspectives of people with dementia about meaningful activities: A synthesis. *Am. J. Alzheimers Dis. Dement.* **2016**, *31*, 115–123. [CrossRef] [PubMed]
72. Nyman, S.R.; Szymczynska, P. Meaningful activities for improving the wellbeing of people with dementia: Beyond mere pleasure to meeting fundamental psychological needs. *Perspect. Public Health* **2016**, *136*, 99–107. [CrossRef] [PubMed]
73. Travers, C.; Brooks, D.; Hines, S.; O'Reilly, M.; McMaster, M.; He, W.; MacAndrew, M.; Fielding, E.; Karlsson, L.; Beattie, E. Effectiveness of meaningful occupation interventions for people living with dementia in residential aged care: A systematic review. *JBI Database Syst. Rev. Implement. Rep.* **2016**, *14*, 163–225. [CrossRef] [PubMed]
74. Beerens, H.C.; De Boer, B.; Zwakhalen, S.M.G.; Tan, F.E.S.; Ruwaard, D.; Hamers, J.P.H.; Verbeek, H. The association between aspects of daily life and quality of life of people with dementia living in long-term care facilities: A momentary assessment study. *Int. Psychogeriatr.* **2016**, *28*, 1323–1331. [CrossRef] [PubMed]
75. Mistridis, P.; Mata, J.; Neuner-Jehle, S.; Annoni, J.M.; Biedermann, A.; Bopp-Kistler, I.; Brand, D.; Brioschi Guevara, A.; Decrey-Wick, H.; Démonet, J.F.; et al. Use it or lose it! Cognitive activity as a protec-tive factor for cognitive decline associated with Alzheimer's disease. *Swiss Med. Wkly.* **2017**, *147*, w14407.
76. Fielding, R.A.; Guralnik, J.M.; King, A.C.; Pahor, M.; McDermott, M.M.; Tudor-Locke, C.; Manini, T.M.; Glynn, N.W.; Marsh, A.P.; Axtell, R.S.; et al. Dose of physical activity, physical functioning and disability risk in mobility-limited older adults: Results from the LIFE study randomized trial. *PLoS ONE* **2017**, *12*, e0182155. [CrossRef]
77. Garshol, B.F.; Ellingsen-Dalskau, L.; Pedersen, I. Physical activity in people with dementia attending farm-based dementia day care–a comparative actigraphy study. *BMC Geriatr.* **2020**, *20*, 1–10.
78. Simmons, S.F.; Rahman, A.; Beuscher, L.; Jani, V.; Durkin, D.W.; Schnelle, J.F. Resident-directed long-term care: Staff provision of choice during morning care. *Gerontologist* **2011**, *51*, 867–875. [CrossRef]
79. Verkerk, M.A. The care perspective and autonomy. *Med. Health Care Philos.* **2001**, *4*, 289–294. [CrossRef]
80. McCormack, B. Autonomy and the relationship between nurses and older people. *Ageing Soc.* **2001**, *21*, 417. [CrossRef]

81. Morgan, L.A.; Brazda, M.A. Transferring control to others: Process and meaning for older adults in assisted living. *J. Appl. Gerontol.* **2013**, *32*, 651–668. [CrossRef] [PubMed]
82. Bosisio, F.; Barazzetti, G. Advanced care planning: Promoting autonomy in caring for people with dementia. *Am. J. Bioeth.* **2020**, *20*, 93–95. [CrossRef] [PubMed]
83. Boyle, G. Recognising the agency of people with dementia. *Disabil. Soc.* **2014**, *29*, 1130–1144. [CrossRef]
84. Dröes, R.M.; Chattat, R.; Diaz, A.; Gove, D.; Graff, M.; Murphy, K.; Verbeek, H.; Vernooij-Dassen, M.J.F.J.; Clare, L.; Johannessen, A.; et al. Social health and dementia: A European consensus on the operationalization of the concept and directions for research and practice. *Aging Ment. Health* **2017**, *21*, 4–17. [CrossRef] [PubMed]
85. World Health Organization. *Measuring the Age-Friendliness of Cities: A Guide to Using Core Indicators*; World Health Organization: Geneva, Switzerland, 2015.
86. Marston, H.R.; van Hoof, J. "Who doesn't think about technology when designing urban environments for older people?" A case study approach to a proposed extension of the WHO's age-friendly cities model. *Int. J. Environ. Res. Public Health* **2019**, *16*, 3525. [CrossRef]
87. Gilster, S.D.; Boltz, M.; Dalessandro, J.L. Long-term care workforce issues: Practice principles for quality dementia care. *Gerontologist* **2018**, *58*, S103–S113. [CrossRef]
88. Banaszak-Holl, J.; Castle, N.G.; Lin, M.K.; Shrivastwa, N.; Spreitzer, G. The role of organizational culture in retaining nursing workforce. *Gerontologist* **2015**, *55*, 462–471. [CrossRef]
89. Mackenzie, J.; Tan, P.-L.; Hoverman, S.; Baldwin, C. The value and limitations of participatory action research methodology. *J. Hydrol.* **2012**, *474*, 11–21. [CrossRef]
90. World Health Organization. *The Global Network for Age-Friendly Cities and Communities: Looking Back over the Last Decade, Looking forward to the Next*; World Health Organization: Geneva, Switzerland, 2018.

International Journal of
Environmental Research and Public Health

MDPI

Article

How is Respect and Social Inclusion Conceptualised by Older Adults in an Aspiring Age-Friendly City? A Photovoice Study in the North-West of England

Sara Ronzi [1,2,*], Lois Orton [2,3], Stefanie Buckner [4], Nigel Bruce [2] and Daniel Pope [2]

1 Department of Health Services Research and Policy, Faculty of Public Health and Policy, London School of Hygiene and Tropical Medicine, London WC1H 9SH, UK
2 Department of Public Health, Policy and Systems, University of Liverpool, Liverpool L69 3DT, UK; l.orton@sheffield.ac.uk (L.O.); nigelbruce16@outlook.com (N.B.); danpope@liverpool.ac.uk (D.P.)
3 Department of Sociological Studies, University of Sheffield, Sheffield S10 2TU, UK
4 Cambridge Public Health, University of Cambridge, Cambridge CB2 0SR, UK; sb959@medschl.cam.ac.uk
* Correspondence: sara.ronzi@lshtm.ac.uk

Received: 30 October 2020; Accepted: 7 December 2020; Published: 10 December 2020

check for updates

Abstract: The World Health Organisation (WHO) Global Age-Friendly Cities (AFC) Guide classifies key characteristics of an AFC according to eight domains. Whilst much age-friendly practice and research have focused on domains of the physical environment, those related to the social environment have received less attention. Using a Photovoice methodology within a Community-Based Participatory Research approach, our study draws on photographs, interviews and focus groups among 26 older Liverpool residents (60+ years) to explore how the city promotes respect and social inclusion (a core WHO AFC domain). Being involved in this photovoice study allowed older adults across four contrasting neighbourhoods to communicate their perspectives directly to Liverpool's policymakers, service providers and third sector organisations. This paper provides novel insights into how: (i) respect and social inclusion are shaped by aspects of both physical and social environment, and (ii) the accessibility, affordability and sociability of physical spaces and wider social processes (e.g., neighbourhood fragmentation) contributed to or hindered participants' health, wellbeing, intergenerational relationships and feelings of inclusion and connection. Our findings suggest that respect and social inclusion are relevant across all eight domains of the WHO AFC Guide. It is core to an AFC and should be reflected in both city-based policies and evaluations.

Keywords: Age-Friendly Cities; photovoice; qualitative research; healthy ageing; active ageing; older people; social inclusion; participation; UK

---

1. Introduction

1.1. Age-Friendly Cities Initiatives

Population ageing and urbanisation present unique public health challenges requiring urgent action [1]. Involving older adults in creating social and physical environments that better support healthy ageing is important for public health policy [2]. The past fifteen years have seen a proliferation of efforts across the world to create environments that are 'age-friendly' (see References [2–5]). Many of these endeavours have concentrated on urban environments, although a parallel focus on ageing in rural settings has also emerged [6–9]. In this study, an Age-Friendly City (AFC) or environment is defined as one that "encourages active ageing by optimising opportunities for health, participation and security in order to enhance quality of life as people age" [10] (p. 1), and where "policies, services, settings and structures support and enable people to age actively" (ibid., p. 5). In line with the World

Health Organisation (WHO) [10] definition, we use the term 'older adults' to refer to people aged 60+ years.

The WHO has played a leading role in the development of AFCs, producing a range of products from planning and implementation guidance and outcomes indicators (e.g., References [10–13]). Launched in 2006, the AFC Initiative [10] classified the key characteristics of an AFC according to eight core domains (Figure 1a).

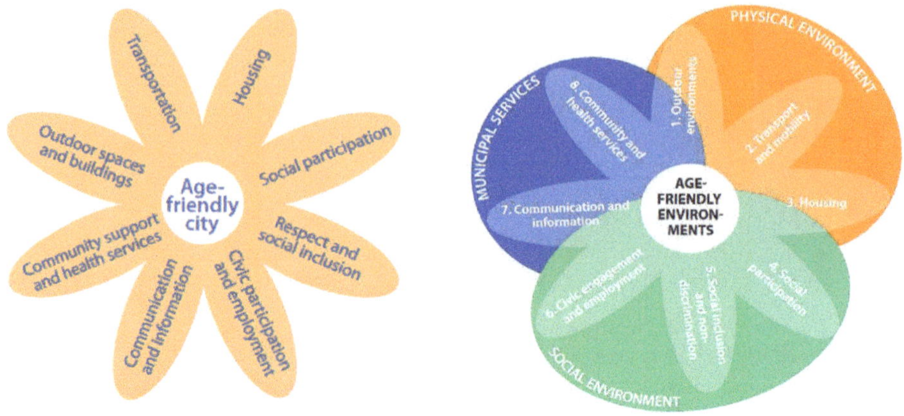

(a) (b)

Figure 1. (**a**) Age-Friendly City (AFC) domains [10]. (**b**) Eight domains for age-friendly action [14].

The WHO AFC guide is based on appraisal of the evidence and global empirical research involving older people and city stakeholders (Vancouver Protocol) [15]. Over time, the AFC domains have evolved (Figure 1b), highlighting three themes that cut across the domains of age-friendly environments—the physical and social environment, and municipal services. The WHO domains aim to represent the multifaceted nature of age-friendliness in complex real-world environments. Although presented as distinct elements, the domains overlap and are interlinked [7]. Treating them as distinct elements, however, provides a useful analytical framework for exploring important elements within each domain and when using the AFC Guide for purposes of evaluation benchmark of AFCs [13].

The AFC Guide has become one of the most commonly employed instruments to evaluate the age-friendliness of cities, and it continues to guide initiatives globally [14,16–19]. Since the publication of the Guide, other age-friendly frameworks and definitions have been developed that reflect the varying approaches to, and organisations participating in, the development of age-friendly environments [16,18,20–22]. Some have focused more on the physical structure of an AFC (e.g., housing, accessible pavements and outdoor spaces), while others have focused on the social aspects of an AFC (e.g., social participation) [23].

1.2. Respect and Social Inclusion

Whilst much age-friendly practice and research have focused on the domains that relate to the physical environment (e.g., housing, outdoor spaces and transportation) [24–28], those related to the social environment (e.g., respect and social inclusion) have received less attention [20,29–31]. This leaves an important gap in knowledge to inform policy and practice on healthy ageing.

Among the studies that have examined social aspects of the urban environment, Woolrych et al. [32] used semi-structured interviews in three cities and nine neighbourhoods in the United Kingdom, which shed light into how older adults constructed and negotiated elements of social participation within their everyday urban environments. In another study [33], qualitative photoproduction conducted by researchers of two municipalities in the Netherlands explored aspects of the built environment that reinforced age-stereotypes and ageism explicitly or implicitly—using the eight WHO AFC domains as an analytical framework. However, an important limitation of the study is that older people were not directly involved in the photo-production process, with photographs taken and disseminated (to health professionals and older adults) by the research team. In evaluating age-friendly programmes in the USA, Scharlach and Lehning [20] highlighted the potential for initiatives to harness communities in promoting the respect and social inclusion of older adults. Buffel et al. [34], through policy document review and secondary qualitative data from interviews with stakeholders, considered the extent to which AFC initiatives in Brussels, Dublin and Manchester were reducing social exclusion in older people. Findings showed that in each city, AFC initiatives had been designed to reduce single or multiple areas of social exclusion (e.g., promoting participation, tackling social isolation and reducing neighbourhood exclusion). Although with some overlaps, their study focused on aspects of social exclusion, rather than on the WHO AFC domain of respect and social inclusion.

With regards to the importance of making older adults feeling valued and respected, persistent disrespectful attitudes, and misconceptions about ageing, have been identified as significant barriers to the development of effective public health policies on healthy ageing [35,36]. These barriers have consequences for the way ageing is perceived and can negatively impact on the health and wellbeing of older adults [37]. According to Swift and Steeden [38], societal attitudes towards older adults can take the form of 'benign indifferences', with ageism tending to manifest indirectly, for instance, as lack of respect. Ageism can be defined as "a combination of how we think about age (stereotypes), how we feel about age (prejudice) and how we behave in relation to age (discrimination)" [39] (p. 2). Research on what makes people feel valued and respected as they age can therefore provide insights that are of value in combating ageism, a strategic objective in the *WHO's Global Strategy and Action Plan on Ageing and Health* [39]. This Action Plan urges a move away from problematising ageing towards a positive respectful and inclusive perspective of older adults that highlights their contributions. It advocates an approach to healthy ageing based on a salutogenic model that focuses on aspects that make people healthy [30,40].

Building on existing literature, our study focused on examining the WHO AFC social domain of respect and social inclusion. We define respect and social inclusion as 'enhancing the opportunities for people of all ages to (i) cultivate social relationships, (ii) have access to resources and support, (iii) feel valued and respected and (iv) feel part of their community' [20]. Urban environments have an important role in fostering respect and social inclusion by being "socially inclusive of all people—regardless of age, gender, social position, health or disability—[ensuring they] are respected and have opportunities to participate and contribute" [14] (p. 69). A specific commitment must be to create interventions that reach those most in need, including those at risk of social exclusion and ill health. Supporting a community to foster respect and social inclusion can have important public health benefits. In a systematic review of qualitative and quantitative studies conducted in high-income countries, Ronzi et al. [41] described positive associations between interventions promoting respect and social inclusion and a variety of health outcomes among older adults aged 60 and over, including a positive impact on wellbeing, subjective health, quality of life and physical and mental health.

1.3. Study Aim

This paper is based on doctoral research by S.R. conducted in Liverpool, UK (2013–2016). It draws on data collected from older residents across four contrasting neighbourhoods in the city. We employed a Photovoice methodology within a Community-Based Participatory Research approach to: (i) explore the extent to which respect and social inclusion were promoted as the city sought to become more age-friendly/an AFC, and (ii) actively involve older adults in the research process and to allow them to directly communicate issues with stakeholders involved in AFC policy.

Previous photovoice studies have explored positive and negative factors for promoting age-friendliness in both rural and urban environments [33,42,43]. These factors have included aspects related to physical activity [44], ability to walk outside [45], access to green spaces [26], perceptions of ageing-in-place [46], places and health [47] and social participation [48]. However, none have focused primarily on respect and social inclusion, as a crucial domain of the WHO AFC Guide.

2. Materials and Methods

2.1. Study Setting

The study took place in Liverpool, North West of England (UK). Over the years, as many cities in the UK, Liverpool has seen a notable increase in its population of older adults. According to latest data (June 2020), the number of people aged 65+ years is approximatively 73,514 [49], with a projected increase to 96,400 by 2035 [50]. This has important implications not only for promoting healthy ageing, but also for the increased urbanisation in Liverpool.

In an ageing population, the years of life gained do not necessarily equate to healthy-life years. Liverpool's residents have worse health than the rest of England, with the city continuing to be ranked among the most deprived local authorities in the UK, according to The English Indices of Deprivation 2019 [51]. Inequalities in health are also clearly seen at a local level, with as much as a 12-year gap in life expectancy at birth between Liverpool's least and most deprived wards [51]. Addressing these health inequalities should therefore be central to AFC policies designed to enable positive ageing experiences.

2.2. Participants

Four groups of older adults aged 60+ years (n = 26) were recruited from four geographical areas with contrasting socioeconomic conditions in Liverpool, to explore potentially different experiences of respect and social inclusion in the city. Criteria for recruitment are described in Table 1.

Table 1. Inclusion criteria of study participants.

1. Being able to consent for themselves.
2. Being an older person aged 60+ years.
3. Being able to speak English fluently.
4. Living in Liverpool.
5. Being British or having lived in the UK for at least 10 years.
6. Being able to manage simple digital cameras and take pictures about the topic under study.
7. Being able to attend and participate in group meetings and an individual interview.

We included anyone who was able to communicate fluently in English. This included those older people of non-British heritage able to speak English fluently. We required fluency in English (criterion 3) as, due to budget constraints, we were not able to have an interpreter. We recruited people who had lived in the UK for at least 10 years, for participants to provide insightful information about respect and social inclusion based on their familiarity with the City. Potential participants who did not meet these criteria were excluded.

Participants were recruited through connections that S.R. developed with gatekeepers working in local grassroots organisations in each of the four geographical areas. Grassroots organisations are typically small and work directly with the community in the surrounding area. Such organisations played an essential role in helping S.R. to recruit a mix of more and less socially included older people, by reaching those who were less actively involved in the community. One organisation, in particular, targeted people of all ages who were less embedded in the community for several reasons (e.g., mental and/or physical disability and/or socio-economic difficulties) and provided transportation to those not able to use public transportation.

Gatekeepers were provided with details of the study inclusion criteria (Table 1) and personally introduced S.R. to prospective participants. They also advised on other aspects of the data collection process (e.g., preferred times and days to conduct focus groups). S.R. spent between four to eight months building a trusting relationship with prospective participants through informal visits during weekly activities at each centre where recruitment of participants was planned. Such relationship building was also important in understanding the context in which older adults were living and to explore and understand the dynamics of the participant group. S.R. explained the purpose of the study to the community centre users and assessed their eligibility using a set of open questions that reflected the inclusion criteria. Those meeting all inclusion criteria were invited to take part in the initial focus group and provided with an information sheet and a consent form. Participants included four people with limited mobility (e.g., use of the stroller and walking sticks). All participants were informed that assistance with taking photographs was available from S.R. if required. Three participants were accompanied to places they wanted to photograph, and they were assisted with setting up the camera.

2.3. Photovoice

One of the key mechanisms necessary to build AFCs and create inclusive environments is the active involvement of older adults in identifying priorities for action and in decision-making processes [2]. Doing so not only helps older adults to express their views, but it also ensures that developments for AFCs respond to their needs [30,52].

An interpretivist phenomenological approach guided our study [53], which focused on identifying meanings and perceptions that older people had of respect and social inclusion in the urban context. We employed a Photovoice methodology within a Community-Based Participatory Research (CBPR) approach, focused on participation, action and collaborative investigation [54,55]. Photovoice, a methodology developed by Wang and Burris [56], involves participants photographing aspects of their lives and communities that are important to them, with group discussions being held to facilitate critical reflection about community strengths and issues [57,58]. Photovoice was used to provide a unique perspective on the issue of respect and social inclusion in the urban context whilst creatively involving participants in the research process.

A modification of Wang and Burris' [56] original methodology was adopted, adding individual semi-structured interviews (SSIs) to the process in addition to focus group discussions (FGDs) that are used for photovoice. The addition of SSIs has previously been reported by, for example, Novek et al. [59]. The SSIs helped to (i) build a relationship with each participant and (ii) examine the individual views of participants in relation to the photographs they had taken in greater depth than could be achieved through FGDs, the latter focusing on stimulating discussions around the photos. Each photovoice project (Phase 1–4, Table 2) lasted about one month and a half and was repeated separately for each group. At the end of the study, each participant received a supermarket voucher (valued £20) as a thank you for their time.

Table 2. Photovoice phases adopted in this study.

Photovoice Phase	Description
Phase 1: Photographic and ethical training session and initial Focus Group Discussion (FGD)	Overview of the project aims. Distribution of the digital cameras to participants with training. FGD explored general perceptions of respect and social inclusion in Liverpool. The FGD was audio recorded with permission. Participants were asked to photograph aspects of their environment that they felt 'enabled or prevented feeling valued and part of the community' and to identify potential solutions to any problems identified. Participants could photograph any object/person/place that referred to their views of respect and social inclusion in the city and neighbourhood. Participants did not receive examples of potential photos that they could take, in order to reduce the researcher's influence over the participants' choice of photographs [60–62]. Photographic and ethical training, including photo ownership and ethical implications of individuals appearing in photos [63,64]. Participants were given the 'rules' on when consent was needed (e.g., when a person or group is 'featured') and when not (where individuals can be considered a crowd). Participants were instructed to inform every person who appeared in the photographs on the study aim and that the photos were to be used as a part of publications and photo-exhibitions [62].
Phase 2: Taking the photographs	Participants took photographs over a period of approximatively a week.
Phase 3: Individual Semi-Structured Interview (SSI)	Each participant was shown their photographs on a laptop and asked to select approximatively six photographs they wanted to discuss at the interview and in the subsequent focus group. Restricting the number to six enabled a more in-depth exploration of each photograph [59]. Participants took part in an SSI (audio-recorded with permission). Questions explored the meanings associated with each photograph and informed by the *SHOWeD* technique [56]. The *SHOWeD* technique consists of different questions that relate to the photograph: 'What do you See here? What's really Happening here? How does this relate to Our lives? Why does this problem, concern, or strength Exist? What can we Do about it?'. Other questions were adapted from reviewing the literature on ageing and AFCs (Appendix A). To explore unrecorded issues of perceived importance, participants were asked to discuss any photograph that they had wanted to take, but for different reasons had been unable to [63,64].
Phase 4: Second FGD	Participants took part in a second FGD, where they collectively interpreted the photographs, including similarities and differences among images [65]. They identified key themes emerging from the discussion of the photographs. They then discussed how they wanted to communicate the findings to policy makers and relevant stakeholders (e.g., through a photo-exhibition event), including preferences for potential venues and plans for the photo-exhibition event. The FGD was audio-recorded with permission.
Phase 5: Summarising photos' texts and checking these with participants	From transcripts, captions were developed by S.R. based on the participant's explanation of each photograph. To guarantee that each caption accurately reflected the correct meanings, each participant reviewed and approved the captions in advance of the photo-exhibition [60]. Participants also reviewed and agreed on the selection of the photographs and accompanying texts to display in the photo-exhibition.
Phase 6: Disseminate the findings and advocacy (e.g., photographic exhibition)	In total, seventy-one people attended a public and stakeholder event, including participants, community members, representatives from Liverpool City Council, services for older people in the city, local TV and radio journalists, and academics. Twenty-three participants (out of 26) presented their photographs and narratives to the attendees of the event. Sixty-one photographs (out of 127) were displayed, with each participant having between two and three photographs and accompanying texts exhibited. The photographic exhibition provided a forum for participants to (i) directly communicate their views to city stakeholders and (ii) stimulate discussion of their priorities for healthy ageing and the way forward for respect and social inclusion in the city.

2.4. Data Analysis

The data presented in this paper come from the photographs (n = 127), FGDs (n = 8) and SSIs (n = 21 individual interviews; n = 2 interviews were conducted in pairs, with a total N = 25 participants being interviewed). SSIs and FGDs were transcribed and anonymised, and imported into NVivo 11 software [66] for analysis.

Techniques from thematic analysis [67] were used and focused on identifying meanings and perceptions that older people had of respect and social inclusion in the urban context. S.R. (i) reviewed the transcripts one-by-one, applying provisional thematic codes, and (ii) incorporated these into emerging sub-themes. L.O. double coded 20% of the transcripts for accuracy. Any discrepancy was resolved by discussing with a third reviewer (D.P./N.B.). S.R. iteratively refined sub-themes and themes as the analysis progressed. Over the course of focused analysis sessions, data were discussed, and themes adapted and agreed with the other members of the research team. Whilst data from the FGD transcripts offered a group view on respect and social inclusion (Phase 1 and Phase 4, Table 2), data from the SSIs provided an individualised and often more intimate view, offering in-depth information about the context, meaning and importance associated with the chosen photographs (Phase 3, Table 2).

According to Wang and Burris [56], the meaning of the images resides in the ways that participants interpret those images. Therefore, photographs and their associated meanings were considered within the context of the corresponding transcripts and not analysed separately. The meanings of each photograph was captured during the SSIs and FGD2, which were guided by the visual images (Phase 2 and Phase 4, Table 2) [25,68]. Further details about the data analysis and the link between transcripts and photos are included in our companion paper [64].

3. Results

The demographic composition of the study sample is shown in Table 3.

Table 3. Study participants. M = male, F = female.

Group	Area	Level of Deprivation	N	Gender	Age Group	Ethnic Background
1	A	High	10	3 M, 7 F	60–64: 2 65–70: 2 70–75: 2 75–80: 1 80–85: 3	5 White British, 2 Asian British, 3 Black African British
2	B	Low	4	2 M, 2 F	60–64: 1 65–70: 2 70–75: 1	4 White British
3	C	Low	6	2 M, 4 F	60–64: 2 75–80: 2 80–85: 1 >85: 1	5 White British, 1 Other White Background
4	D	High	6	6 F	65–70: 1 70–75: 3 75–80: 1 80–85: 1	6 White British

3.1. Overview

Older adults highlighted both contrasting and complimentary aspects of the urban context that fostered or hindered perceived respect and social inclusion, and ways in which some of the barriers identified could be reduced. Overall, the combination of accessibility, affordability and sociability of physical spaces contributed to older adults' mental wellbeing, feelings of inclusion, sense of independence and connection. Participants also identified aspects of the physical (e.g., litter on the streets) and the social environment (e.g., a lack of respect for the older generation and people living in more disadvantaged areas) that contributed to feelings of vulnerability and a sense of exclusion. Wider social processes (e.g., family and neighbourhood fragmentation) were reported to lead to difficulty in cultivating intergenerational relationships.

To facilitate the presentation of the results, we have structured the different sub-themes that emerged from the analysis around the three key dimensions of an AFC, as described by the revised WHO AFC framework (Figure 1b): physical environment, social environment and services.

3.2. Physical Environment

3.2.1. Green and Blue Spaces

Green and blue spaces were the most photographed and talked about places by participants across the four groups. They offered (free) opportunities to do physical activity and provided a space for multi-generational interactions (Figure 2).

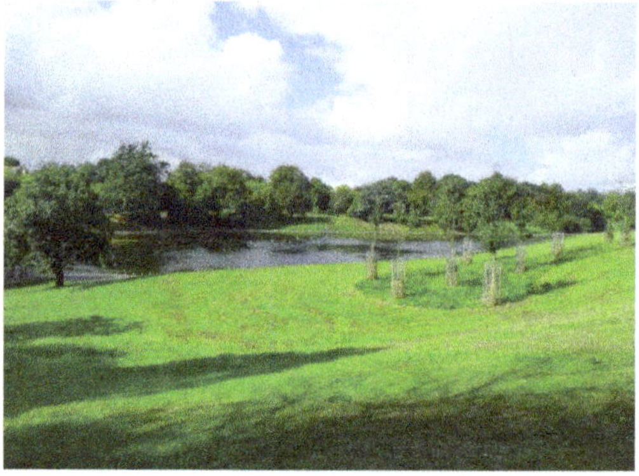

Figure 2. Example of green spaces promoting respect and social inclusion (P1) (Sefton Park, Liverpool).

"We have so many good open spaces with trees and water around the city ... and they're really good for your mental health and wellbeing ... and feeling included, as you mix with everybody in a park! It gives you interest, it gets you out, and it gets you in the open area. Sefton Park is a focal point for life in the city. It is a real bonus that we have. We're lucky!" (P1, M, 65, Group 1) (Figure 2)

Paved, flat and accessible walking paths and parks were believed to be particularly important not only for older people, but for everyone with functional limitations or disabilities (Figure 3).

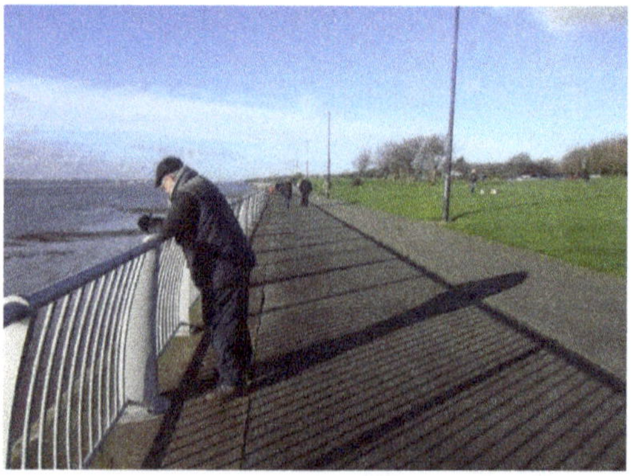

Figure 3. Example of green spaces promoting respect and social inclusion (P17) (Otterspool Promenade, Liverpool).

'This is the Promenade, it's a great facility. [...] it's all on the flat for everyone to go for a walk. There are no hills involved ... and you've got the nice aspect of the river... It's a lovely facility to have and it's used by lots of different age groups.' (P17, F, 64, Group 3) (Figure 3)

As shown by these examples, an important aspect that made these green spaces 'inclusive' was that all age groups could access and use them. The quote below, however, highlights that the geographical location of many green spaces in Liverpool is in the most affluent parts (e.g., the South of Liverpool) and may not be so easily accessible to everyone.

'People of all ages can access it, there's parking, so you can walk down and on a nice summer's day people of all ages are out, [...] ... it's a good place to go and have a good walk and take the fresh air. ... we're lucky in the South end of Liverpool that we have something like this'. (P9, M, 71, Group 2) (Figure 4)

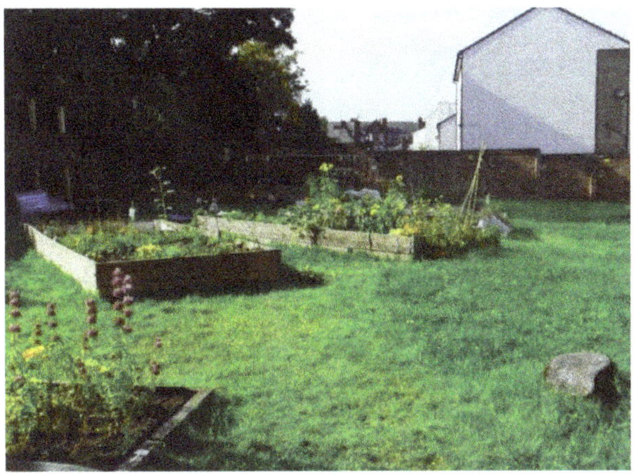

Figure 4. Example of a community garden promoting respect and social inclusion (P3) (Ferngrove community garden, Liverpool).

Alongside parks, allotments and leisure facilities encouraged physical activity, by providing a space for people to walk, exercise and volunteer. They also had an indirect impact on wellbeing due to their sociability—providing a space for people to come together and cultivate hobbies (Figure 4).

'I have one of those plots in the community garden. It's an occupation that I enjoy. [...] It's engaging with others, there're all sort of people involved in this. [...] from my memories ... it was a wasteland, and people used to throw rubbish in there ... and now it's a beautiful oasis in Liverpool 8!' (P3, M, 63, Group 1) (Figure 4)

Another interesting aspect that emerged from this study is the role that blue spaces played in participants' perception of social inclusion (in this case, the River Mersey). Walking along the river not only created a sense of attachment to the aesthetic aspect of the river (Figure 5), but it was perceived as an integral part of participants' sense of identity towards Liverpool.

'I think that's a wonderful idea and a real achievement for Liverpool. It gets me out in the fresh air ... I like to walk anyway, but how pleasant is to walk there along the river? [...] this is about the feel-good factor that's so important in life.' (P20, F, 81, Group 4) (Figure 5)

'The river has always been a part of my life. It just feels Liverpool when you stand by the river [...]'. (P12, M, 68, Group 2)

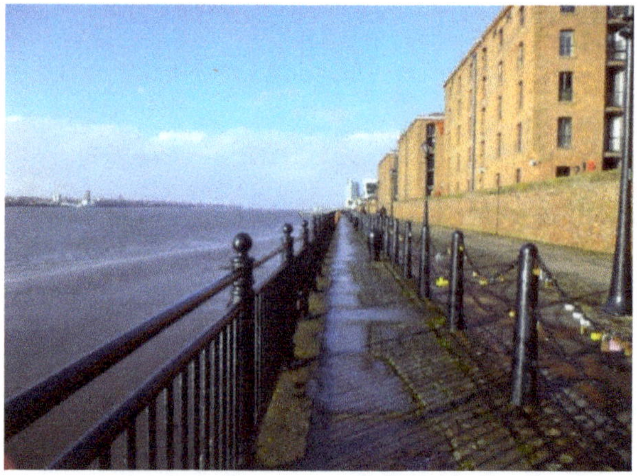

Figure 5. Example of blue spaces promoting respect and social inclusion (P20) (Albert Dock, Liverpool).

The combination of accessibility, affordability and sociability of green and blue spaces contributed to participants' mental wellbeing, feeling of inclusion and sense of connection.

3.2.2. Transportation

Alongside green and blue spaces, public transportation was perceived as a key resource that strengthened participants' sense of inclusion and respect. It was necessary for older people's ability to remain independent, and to participate regularly in community life. Overall, participants felt very satisfied with the public transport system in Liverpool. It was perceived as efficient and accessible, giving them the freedom to reach local places as well as more iconic places in the city centre (Figure 6).

> *'I really appreciate our very good bus and train services. [...] I can come out in the morning and I can get on a bus and go to so many places, and I don't have to wait long for a bus. It gives me freedom: freedom to get out. We are so lucky! Buses and trains are such a vital part in our lives.'* (P20, F, 81, Group 4) (Figure 6)

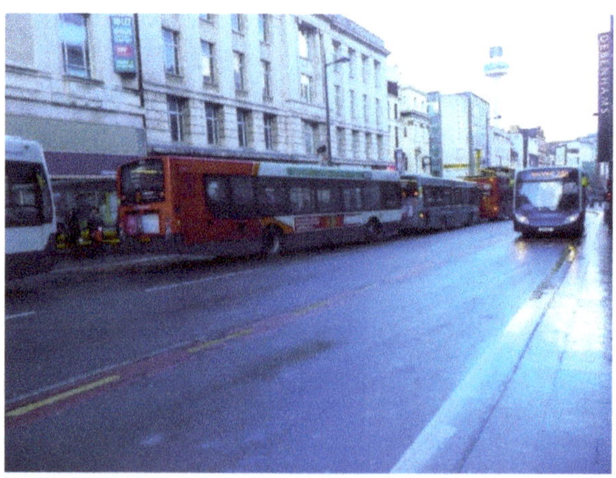

Figure 6. Example of transportation options promoting respect and social inclusion (P20) (Buses in Liverpool city centre).

The affordability of transportation options was essential, particularly for those less willing to drive, with no access to a car, or on a low income.

'The free travel pass helps me to connect with the community that I live in. […] it allows me to travel across Merseyside for free and do things that I would not otherwise be able to do […]' (P3, M, 63, Group 1)

The free travel pass for people aged 60+ covers buses, trains and ferries across the areas surrounding Liverpool (called Merseyside), offering additional opportunities to access places that are not necessarily in the local 'community'.

'In Liverpool, we can use the buses but [also] the trains and the Mersey Ferry, […] … we've got a lot more on offer with our bus pass than people in other parts of the country.' (P17, F, 64, Group 3)

Accessibility was not only perceived in terms of the transportation itself, but also *how* participants accessed it. The quotes and photos below show two contrasting examples of local stations, and how they enabled or hindered participants' sense of respect and social inclusion. The first one provided a safe and warm environment for people waiting for the bus or train (Figure 7). Moreover, the integration of different public transports offered more options and made it easier to travel.

'I am very lucky because I have got all of that near to me, and it gives me access to a lot of options to travel. We've got the trains in and out and the buses in and out … it just makes it so much easier for people to travel. Once you get inside the building, you're protected from the weather and the wind, it is very cosy, convenient, and very accessible. Older people deserve the respect and a good travel experience.' (P1, 65, M, Group 1) (Figure 7)

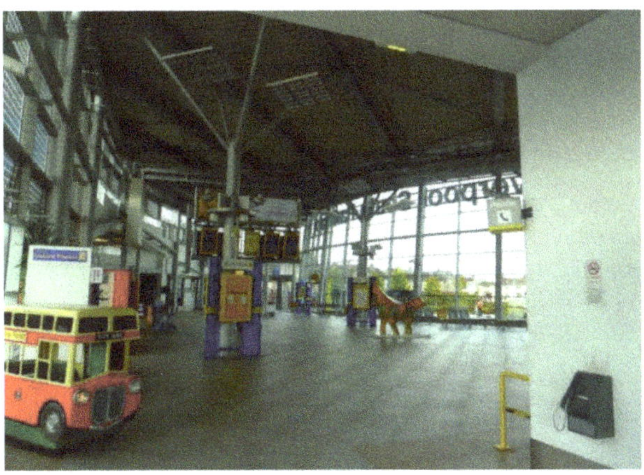

Figure 7. Example of train and bus stations promoting respect and social inclusion (P1) (South Parkway Railway Station, Liverpool).

By contrast, the second bus station (located at the heart of the city) was perceived as very uncomfortable due to lack of protection from the wind, and not particularly safe (Figure 8).

'Growing older is not about changing a lot … or being in a transition … but it's about keeping the opportunities the same for you as they are for everybody else. So, things like this [transportation] become very important. As you can see, Liverpool One bus station is completely open, and the wind can still get in! We should use the learning from South Parkway station [Figure 7], and apply it to this station, so that you're behind closed doors, in comfort, while waiting for a bus.' (P1, 65, M, Group 1) (Figure 8)

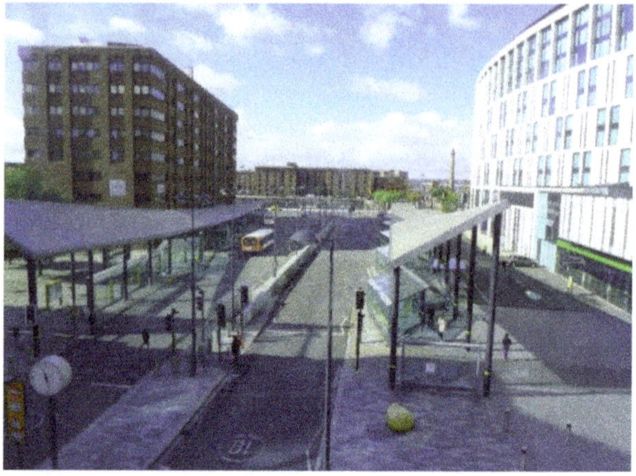

Figure 8. Example of bus stations hindering respect and social inclusion (P1) (Liverpool One bus station).

Both photos were taken by the same participant, who used photographs and their associated meanings to illustrate the concept of accessibility as an important dimension of social inclusion in the urban context.

As shown in the quotes related to Figures 6 and 7 (and already in Figure 3), participants described themselves to 'be lucky'. This seems to indicate a positive outlook for these participants and a strong personal attachment to the city.

3.2.3. Additional Public Facilities: Public Toilets and Pavements

Participants identified other public facilities that shaped their perceptions of accessibility. These included public toilets and pavements. Shortage of toilets, especially in spaces regularly used by the community, was reported as preventing many people from going out, impacting negatively on their ability to feel confident in public spaces (Figure 9).

> *'This toilet's not inviting, it's not accessible ... and I'll be a bit anxious about getting locked in ... It's counterproductive to meeting the needs of older people. Your body is changing and you've different needs ... , but you need immediate access to clean toilets. It's against social inclusion. It's a barrier because not many older people will be confident to go to the city centre if there're not enough accessible public toilets.'* (P1, 65, M, Group 1) (Figure 9)

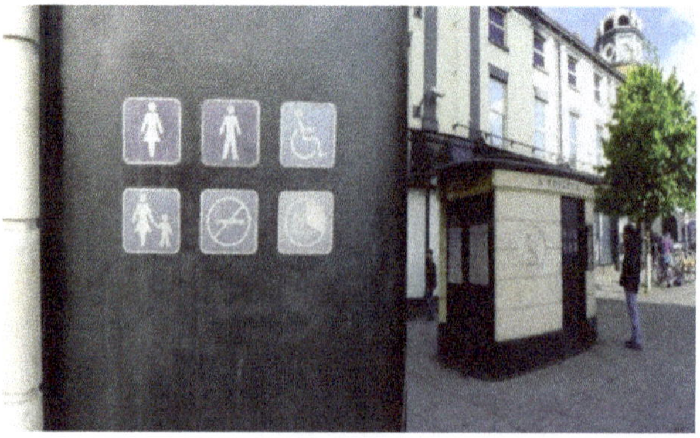

Figure 9. Example of public toilets hindering respect and social inclusion (P1) (Bold Street, Liverpool).

The same participant who took the photo in Figure 9. Suggested that premises in the city centre (e.g., cafes and restaurants) could allow older people provided with the free travel pass to use their toilets:

> *'[...] the city council could have a scheme whereby if you are an older person with a bus pass, or if you have disabilities and you have your car badge, they should negotiate with all the restaurants and cafes, and pubs that people won't be stopped from accessing those toilets.'* (P1, 65, M, Group 1)

Tactile paving at the end of the sidewalks was identified as particularly important not only for older adults, but for everyone with lower levels of mobility and/or disability. Being able to walk safely in the neighbourhood was perceived as having a positive impact on social participation, as people could get out more often (Figure 10).

> *'These little bumps ensure safety when there's bad weather. For some people, just stepping off the side is not much, but when you've got bad legs, it is awful; so, if you have these bumps to help you getting around, then it helps you in the community; you can actually get out more, and you can socialise a bit more [...]'.* (P23, F, 70, Group 4) (Figure 10)

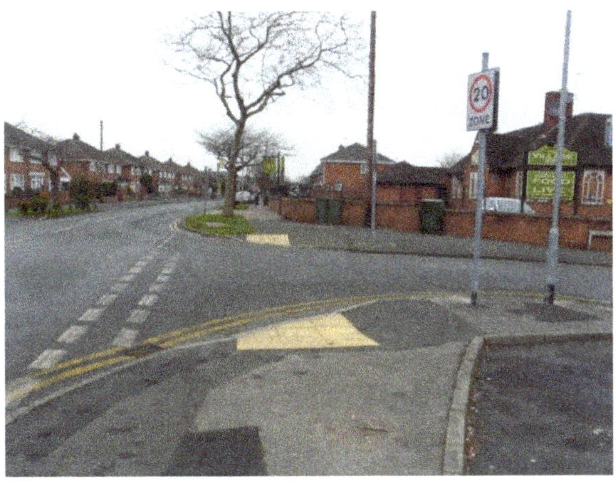

Figure 10. Example of sidewalks promoting respect and social inclusion (P23) (Road, Liverpool).

3.2.4. Disrespectful Environmental Attitudes and Sense of Disregard and Alienation towards the Community

Whilst many aspects of the urban space helped participants feel valued and part of their community, poorly maintained environments (uncleanliness, litter on the streets and general decline of the neighbourhood) contributed to feelings of vulnerability and a sense of exclusion. It is interesting to note that all the photographs and quotes relating to negative perceptions of the physical environment originated from participants living in more disadvantaged areas (Table 3). This may suggest that participants living in more affluent areas did not identify or perceive similar issues in their neighbourhoods. In fact, they reported positive perspectives of their neighbourhoods.

According to some participants, the uncleanliness of the streets was mainly to do with lack of respectful attitudes of some people towards their local community and failure of the Council to address this. The litter in the street was not only seen to lower the tone of the neighbourhood. It was perceived as a bad example for young people, meaning they did not learn how to be respectful towards their community and, by implication, its residents, including older adults (Figure 11).

'This lowers the tone of the neighbourhood. I think I live in a quite nice neighbourhood [...] the bin man's just been ... but that mess is still there. [It] does not engender any respect in the young. The young see that and think "well, everyone else is throwing away their rubbish". [...] The people who live there should be aware of it [...] There's no respect for yourself or for anyone else with that around.' (P20, F, 81, Group 4) (Figure 11)

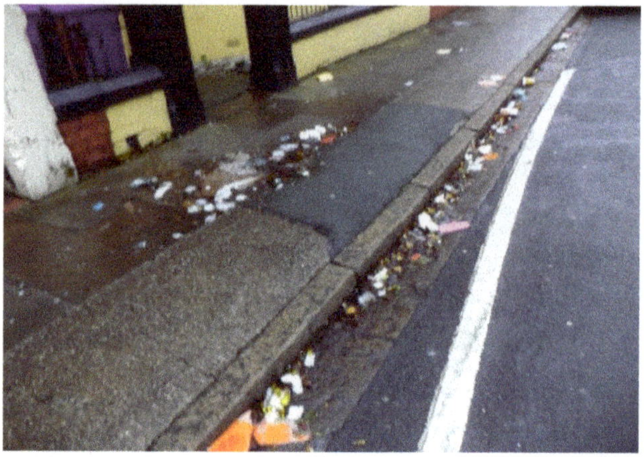

Figure 11. Example of litter in the street hindering respect and social inclusion (P20) (Road, Liverpool).

The following quotes show a close interlink between aspects of the physical environment (e.g., litter on the streets) and the social environment (e.g., a lack of respect for the older generation) that contributed to feelings of vulnerability and a sense of exclusion. At times, participants' efforts to address disrespectful attitudes led to a more direct experience of disrespect, as shown in this quote:

*'The other day a young woman was eating a package of crisps. She finished the crisps and threw the package on the floor. Five yards away there was a rubbish bin. I said to her: "why you don't put the package on the rubbish bin?" And she told me to f**k off. So, I said ok, bye! It's a very disappointing aspect, but ... never mind.'* (P3, M, 63, Group 1)

On other occasions, some participants reported that people living in more affluent areas often displayed stigmatising attitudes towards the more disadvantaged areas (where some study participants lived). Such episodes contributed to a perceived sense of exclusion and frustration, given that many felt unable to change the situation, for instance, by going to live in a nicer neighbourhood:

'[...] I have been on the bus sometimes and I have been hearing people [from a particular affluent area] saying: "How do people live here? [...] sometimes there are troubles and gangs". I would like to hear people saying there're good people here as well, and a lot of us have no choice to live anywhere else and move out.' (P21, F, 75, Group 4)

Living in a deprived neighbourhood not only adversely affected the attachment that participants felt towards these spaces, but in some instances, caused a feeling of alienation.

'I feel alienated by the community when I see rubbish in the streets.' (P3, M, 63, Group 1)

Participants used their photos and narratives to raise awareness of some issues that they felt were not currently addressed by the Council and/or were the responsibility of residents.

3.3. Social Environment

As reported earlier on, participants identified a close connection between the physical and social dimensions of their living environment, with aspect of the physical environment (e.g., parks) contributing to many social aspects of their lives (e.g., meeting people).

3.3.1. Places to Cultivate Learning, Art and Culture

Places to cultivate learning, art and culture were the second most photographed and talked about aspect by participants. With only one exception (Section 3.4), participants took photographs of libraries located in their area of residence, suggesting that libraries tend to be facilities mainly used by people who live locally. In a similar way to green spaces, libraries were free and accessible facilities to cultivate interests, as well as meeting places to open to everyone. Furthermore, this example shows how the aesthetic of the library contributed to the sense of attachment perceived towards Liverpool Figure 11.

> *'This is the library. I like books and inside it's absolutely beautiful ... we have such a lovely facility here [...] it's lovely to have a look and see whatever you want to see ... it's open for anyone in Liverpool to go in, so it's not local community but it's for the community of Liverpool'.* (P15, F, 64, Group 3) (Figure 12)

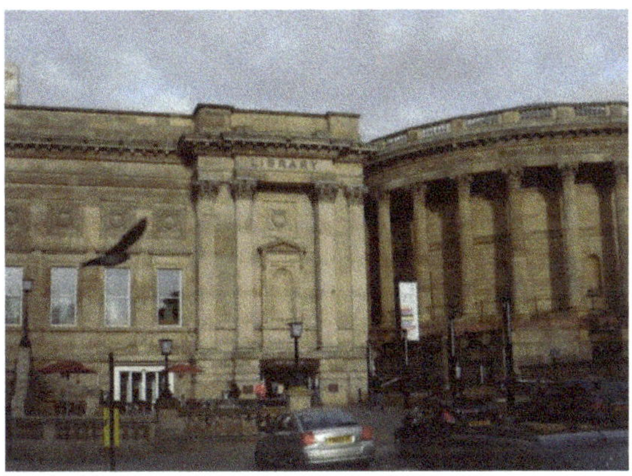

Figure 12. Example of libraries promoting respect and social inclusion (P15) (Central Library, Liverpool).

Alongside libraries, museums were identified as very valuable assets in the city. In these examples, a participant identified three main aspects that facilitated ease of access and frequency of use: (i) accessibility and affordability of museums (Figure 13) and (ii) the aspect of proximity to the local community (Figure 14).

> *'This is Liverpool Museum ... it's just a lovely facility. All the museums that we have in Liverpool ... they're all free.'* (P17, F, 64, Group 3) (Figure 13)

> *'This is Sudley House. It's been kept as a 19th century house; it has also very nice art inside. [...] They also do Shakespeare's plays in there in the summer. I use it because it's a local facility for me, and I can walk there.'* (P15, F, 64, Group 3) (Figure 14)

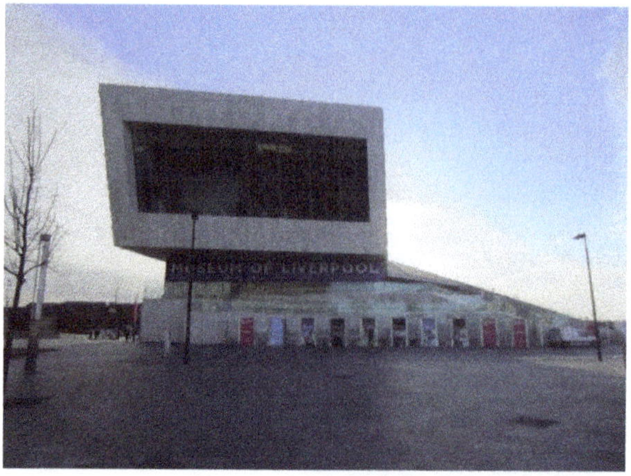

Figure 13. Example of museums promoting respect and social inclusion (P15) (Museum of Liverpool).

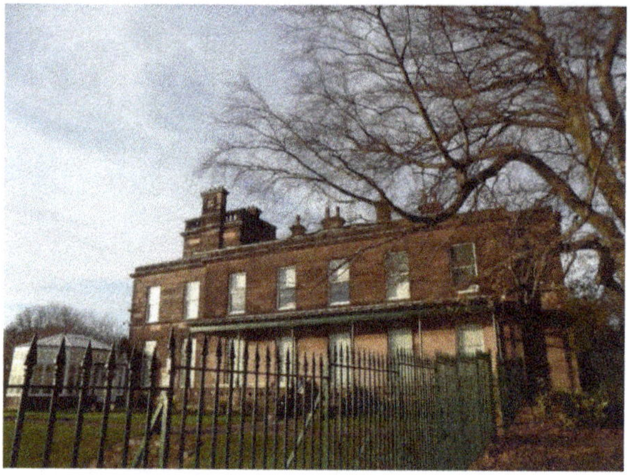

Figure 14. Example of museums promoting respect and social inclusion (P15) (Sudley House, Liverpool).

3.3.2. Places to Cultivate Informal and Formal Relationships

When reflecting about spaces to cultivate informal and formal relationships, participants stressed the value of community centres. Community centres were often described as an inclusive space for social interaction, which contributed to a sense of wellbeing and feeling valued.

> *'[...] It gives me something to live for, something to look forward to. It gets you out and it's another reason to get up in the morning. It makes you feel good because we're all nice people, and we all talk and have ideas together. We help each other.'* (P22, F,67, Group 4) (Figure 15)

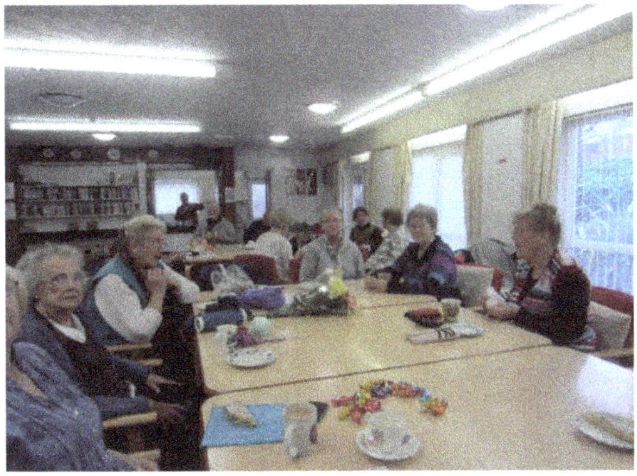

Figure 15. Example of a community group promoting respect and social inclusion (P22) (community group, Liverpool).

Soup kitchens, instead, were considered a good alternative for those who were not interested in joining a club:

> *'I go there [to the Soup Kitchen] every week [...] it makes people who wouldn't normally come out to meet up with people. Lots of people don't want to join a club ... this is a nice way to have a bowl of soup, and some nice crusty bread, [...] and you can just talk to the people of your table [...]!'* (P20, F, 81, Group 4)

In terms of public spaces, benches at the bus stops or in green spaces were key places for informal socialisation, where people could rest and have a chat with others.

> *'This is the new bus shelter and [the council] provided seating again. [...] that is very good because [...] you can rest while you're waiting for the bus, you can get chatting to people, and you also are covered from the wind. [...] it's part of the community because you get to be more sociable if you're sitting down, and you will talk to people'.* (P23, F, 70, Group 4) (Figure 16)

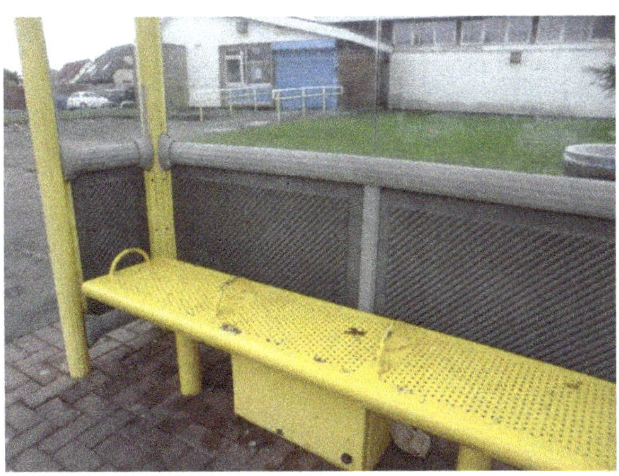

Figure 16. Example of a bus bench promoting respect and social inclusion (P23) (Bus stop, Liverpool).

3.3.3. Negative Age Perceptions and Disrespectful Attitudes towards Older Adults and Ageing as a Barrier

Despite that many aspects made participants feel valued and included, disrespectful attitudes towards older adults contributed to feelings of vulnerability in the community and a sense of exclusion.

> *'More respect for older people. I think that's where we are lacking now.'* (P21, F, 75, Group 4)

Some participants reported instances that they felt intensified negative perceptions of ageing in society. The quote below shows how the language used to refer to older adults was perceived as disrespectful:

> *'A lot of it it's about feeling valued. I really don't like being called an old, aged pensioner [...] I like the phrase elder. In Australia, we call older people 'elder' because we respect them, and I really think that's missing in English society'.* (P3, M, 63, Group 1)

In fact, although older adults made useful contributions to society (e.g., voluntary work), it was perceived that Liverpool and society in general tended to consider people to have a value only in terms of working life (economic value):

> *'Not just in Liverpool, within Western culture, we don't value older people. It's almost like that you retire, and you don't work anymore for money, so you have no value in society, while we have a great deal of resources up here. [...] we have a great deal of knowledge and wisdom that we could pass on young people if they want to listen to us.'* (P3, M, 63, Group 1)

However, participants did challenge these negative perceptions through photographs and associated narratives. For instance, some facilities (e.g., allotments) were supporting people with lower mobility or forms of disabilities to carry out daily hobbies and activities in the community (Figure 17).

> *'This [photograph] shows that people can still do outdoor activities and grow for themselves vegetables ... and disability or immobility is not gonna stop them doing it! [...] they are raised beds: if you're old and you can't get down, you can sit next to the beds and it makes it much easier [...].'* (P9, M, 71, Group 2) (Figure 17)

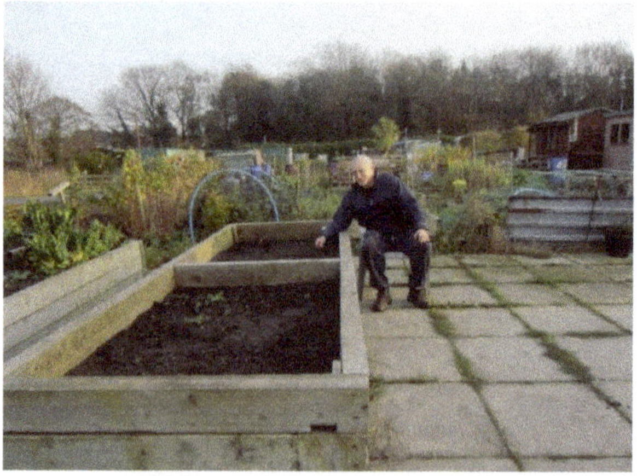

Figure 17. Example of allotments promoting respect and social inclusion (P9) (Allotment in Mersey Road, Liverpool).

There were fewer photos portraying negative social aspects such as disrespectful attitudes towards older adults, although these were reported extensively during the SSIs and FGDs. Participants reported that they found it more difficult to take photographs of negative social concepts (e.g., social isolation) compared with negative physical aspects (e.g., rubbish in the street) or positive social concepts (e.g., social participation) (findings presented in our companion paper) [65].

3.3.4. Neighbourhood Fragmentation and Lack of Social and Intergenerational Interactions as a Barrier

Wider social processes (e.g., family and neighbourhood fragmentation) were reported to lead to difficulty in cultivating intergenerational relationships, as families increasingly lived away from each other. Lack of knowledge exchange between generations was linked to negative age perceptions and disrespect, which participants believed could be addressed by encouraging contact between different age groups:

> *'Young children can go and get to know older people, because there's a lot of them that don't talk to older people. If their own grandparents have died, they don't get used to know older people...they just see old people as being old and miserable. But when they get to know them, they'd realise that they're not. It's like old people thinking young boys with hoods on are all bad children, but they're not.'* (P23, F, 70, Group 4)

Linked to this, participants highlighted that in the past people used to know their neighbours more than today, and they used to mix with each other. The sense of community was perceived as getting lost. People were constantly moving houses and out of communities, and this made it difficult to cultivate trusting relationships with neighbours and a community in which older people could feel embedded.

> *'[...] what we lost is possibly the community aspect where people in the road looked after other people.'* (P15, F, 64, Group 3)

> *'[...] because families lived very close to each other, there was a very close community. I have just found out the name of the lady opposite to me! And I have been in that house for 17 years ... .'* (P20, F, 81, Group 4)

This included reduced opportunities for older adults to informally meet young people in the neighbourhood. The problem was seen to be exacerbated by more people using cars for their transport and children now typically playing inside.

> *'I used to walk to school, and you met people; but people come out of their house now, get into a car and go [...].'* (P11, F, 64, Group 2)

> *'I have lived in the same street now for 36 years, and I knew everyone. I knew all the kids, but now the kids are all indoors, you don't see them, so it's a ghost town.'* (P21, F, 75, Group 4)

This concern was not echoed by all participants. Some of those from a more affluent area stressed that there was a sense of strong community in their streets with good neighbourhood relations leading to a feeling of inclusion:

> *'Our road is very neighbourly; people are around all the time. We know all our neighbours, we say hello to them, it may be not much more than that but [...] we do see them, and our next door is actually one of our friends, [...] so I think that depends on the road.'* (P10, F, 67, Group 2)

3.4. *Services*

Communication and Access to Information

Access to the Internet (IT) and computing skills was an important aspect of participants' perceptions of social and digital inclusion. IT was the most common means of accessing information by the study participants. IT was perceived as particularly important not only to access information more easily, but also to counteract some practical challenges such as not being able do shopping due to health issues:

'When you have difficulties, as I did, I have done the online shopping and it was a great help to me. When I am fit enough to go out, I will go out shopping ... but when you know how to use Internet, it makes you independent.' (P22, F, 67, Group 4)

IT training was often facilitated by community organisations (Figure 18) and libraries (Figure 19), which created a supportive environment in which older people felt encouraged to learn.

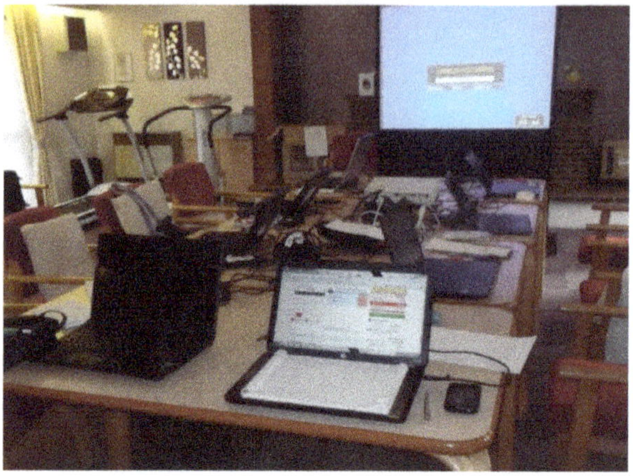

Figure 18. Example of a computing classes promoting respect and social inclusion (P21) (St. Luke's court, Liverpool).

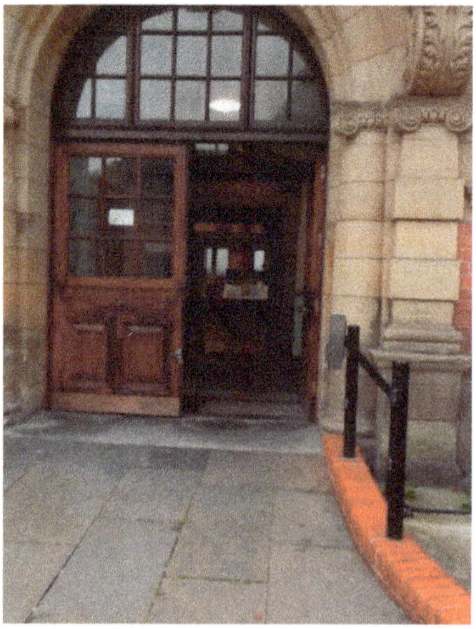

Figure 19. Example of libraries promoting respect and social inclusion (P2) (Toxteth Library, Liverpool).

'Going to this computer class with the other girls, they're all the same age as me and I do not feel embarrassed. It's very helpful, particularly shopping online. I was very ill last year, and I could not get out; people had to do my shopping, but it would have been easier if I could have done the shopping online.' (P21, F, 75, Group 4) (Figure 18)

'This is our library, and anybody can go there and read the books ... if you want to learn computers ... they can teach you. It's nice and quiet, and it's a mixed community that goes in there. It's a place to meet up with each other and discuss things, and you can make new friends in there!' (P2, F, 64, Group 1) (Figure 19)

However, a lack of computing or IT skills stood in the way to participation in the community, as access to information was limited.

'It's about knowing what's going on even in the neighbourhood down the road or across the park ... it's still a problem if you have missed out on the technology thing.' (P1, M, 65, Group 1)

'We live in a society which just uses computers all the time [...] so if you haven't got a computer, or if you aren't computer literate in my age group, it's a barrier'. (P17, F, 64, Group 3)

Despite IT being commonly used to access information, local leaflets and free newspapers held value for older adults in increasing their awareness of activities in their local area and city. To make access to information more inclusive for those who were not using IT, and to increase social inclusion through engagement with activities, participants suggested that organisations could put some leaflets and/or small display boards in the bus stops, post offices and supermarkets to advertise weekly events and activities. In fact, these amenities were accessed daily by most people.

'They should advertise [events] more: in the papers, in the supermarkets, because [...] everybody goes in the supermarkets [...].' (P4, F, 70, Group 1)

'[...] all the local shops could have just little weekly or monthly summary on what's going on in the immediate neighbourhood in the next few weeks. So, if you go to the post office in the area, or you're going to the local shop, or supermarket, you are going to be able to see it in the notice board.' (P1, M, 65, Group 1)

4. Discussion

To our knowledge, this is the first photovoice study to actively engage community members in exploring their perceptions of factors influencing their respect and social inclusion in a city seeking to become more age-friendly/an AFC. This study provides novel insights into how respect and social inclusion are shaped by aspects of the physical and social environment, and the role that accessibility, affordability and sociability of physical spaces had on older adults' wellbeing, feelings of inclusion, sense of independence and connection. Participants also identified some aspects of the physical (e.g., litter on the streets) and social environment (e.g., age-stereotypes) that contributed to feelings of vulnerability and a sense of exclusion. Wider social processes (e.g., family and neighbourhood fragmentation) also contributed to difficulties in cultivating intergenerational relationships.

In line with what others [20,22] have reported, our findings suggest that rather than a discrete entity, respect and social inclusion is highly interconnected with the other AFC domains, including social participation, communication and information, outdoor spaces, transportation and housing [20,42]. As such, it should be considered a guiding principle for cities aspiring to become more age-friendly. Cities need to ensure that respect and social inclusion is reflected in city-based policies, including local strategies for older adults as well as services in the community [16].

For example, our findings showed that parks and iconic places (e.g., museums) in the city provided an accessible (and free) space for multi-generational interactions, and for which older people felt a strong sense of connection. The sense of identity and inclusion expressed by participants was often connected with the participant's aesthetic experience, particularly concerning outdoor spaces and architecture. This result is consistent with previous research [24,45,46], which highlights an interaction with the different aspects of the environment (e.g., green spaces, iconic buildings) fostering a sense of community connection and identity. Moreover, our study clearly showed that older adults accept that they themselves have a responsibility for their own wellbeing and a big role to play in ensuring they remain included. For example, by going out, joining a club, meeting people, practicing physical activity, doing volunteering, or learning something new. However, to be truly 'age-friendly', a city must provide an environment where older adults feel both respected and included, and support them in overcoming physical and social barriers that can limit their involvement in their communities [34].

In our study, older adults saw IT as important in improving their access and sense of connection with the communities and wider social networks. The provision of free IT training classes equipped them with the skills needed to negotiate opportunities within their city (e.g., being digitally connected, doing online shopping,). Accordingly, IT can play a critical role in increasing awareness of existing activities and promoting social inclusion [69]. Connectivity beyond IT was still valued by participants and highlights the need for wider communication and knowledge sharing. Our results are consistent with other studies that have stressed the importance of sharing local information through the use of leaflets or notice boards displayed in places regularly used by older adults (e.g., supermarkets, bus stops and post offices) [22,70].

Accessibility and affordability emerged as key features of inclusive environments. Affordable transportation and accessible stations enabled older adults to use and access places in the city and remain independent. From our findings, the free travel pass in Liverpool was highly valued and provided an opportunity for *all* people aged 60+ to reach key destinations in the city. An AFC should include provision of affordable and accessible transportation options in related policy to ensure that older adults maintain participation in social life [27,70,71]. Responding to the different transport needs of the population can also have important benefits on equity, which is key to create inclusive environments [71]. A primary challenge for many older adults is, in fact, to maintain mobility, regardless of their physical limitations or disabilities associated with advancing age [15,44]. A city with paved, flat, accessible pathways, sidewalks and transportation options enables older adults to be mobile and to participate in the community, as our findings illustrate.

Our findings showed some differences in perceptions among participants living in affluent or more disadvantaged areas (Table 3). For instance, those living in more disadvantaged areas generally reported feeling disappointed with the appearance of, and people's attitudes in, their local area. This included disappointment in how clean the community was kept and a general decline of the neighbourhood. These reports created a sense of exclusion and frustration, which was exacerbated when people living in more affluent areas displayed stigmatising attitudes towards areas where some of the study participants lived. These findings have important implications when considering people's perceptions of age-friendly environments and in the development of AFCs. They highlight the importance of paying attention to the diversity not only between cities, but also within cities. This does include the social exclusion experienced by many older adults living in disadvantaged areas [16,34]. Conversely, in our study, all participants living in more affluent areas reported positive perceptions and feelings of inclusion towards their local area.

In addition to the feeling of social exclusion that older people who reside in disadvantaged and/ or stigmatised neighbourhoods might feel, such environments can have negative impacts on health and quality of life [72,73], even from an early age [74]. With advancing age, people are likely to become more emotionally attached to their local community and homes. Therefore, if older adults live in an environment they feel is supportive, they are more likely to experience a sense of belonging, and this can improve their wellbeing [24]. If, instead, they live in an environment perceived as neglected, and poorly maintained, they are more likely to experience a sense of exclusion and a negative influence on their wellbeing. This can also reduce their social participation within and outside the community [74,75].

Cities committed to developing AFCs need to consider policies that respond to the unequal contexts and disadvantages experienced by older adults [76]. Taking an equity lens in developing AFCs and addressing social, gender, ethnic and other forms of inequalities will not only benefit older adults but all age groups, especially those most at risk of experiencing social exclusion and disadvantage [77].

4.1. Implications for Research, Policy and Practice

Recognising respect and social inclusion as fundamental principles for age-friendliness has implications for both policy and practice. Research in the related field of dementia friendliness provides relevant insights [3]. Buswell et al. [78] highlight raising awareness (in this case, of dementia) and, thus, generating understanding in the community as the necessary starting point for creating an environment that enables people affected by dementia to live well. In the context of AFCs, awareness raising relates closely to the strategic objective of combating ageism in the *WHO's Global strategy and action plan on ageing and health* [39]. This entails, for instance, tackling misconceptions and negative attitudes on ageing and drawing attention to the contributions made by older adults.

In our study, participants reflected to what extent the city made them feel respected as older adults. A perceived decline in respect accompanied by negative perceptions of ageing in society were negatively impacting how some participants viewed themselves and the activities they thought they could engage with. Participants reported that to challenge macro-societal barriers such as negative perceptions of ageing, change needed to happen beyond the local level (e.g., improving the terminology used to refer to older people in the media). This finding highlights that AFCs do not operate in a vacuum, but there needs to be a match between what they are working towards and efforts at the national level and across many sectors. At the macro level, what is critical to this is addressing ageism and tackling the discourses that promote the persistence of age-stereotypes and a negative view of ageing [38]. Awareness raising to foster respect and social inclusion can thus be advocated as a foundational activity for aspiring AFCs. In practice, this might take the form of intergenerational projects and spaces that promote a cohesive community and public information campaigns that promote the contribution of older people in a city, coupled with advertising of the city's AFC initiative [70].

Another fundamental aspect for the successful development of an AFC is to ensure that respect and social inclusion are reflected in older adults' experiences of their city/community. This can be achieved through an active involvement of older adults in decision-making processes, including working in partnership with community members and multiple stakeholders (local policy makers, public, private and third sector). The cities of Manchester (UK), Brussels (Belgium) and Quebec (Canada) represent some exemplars where collaborative partnerships were key to the successful implementation of AFC models [16,79]. For instance, Manchester (UK) has used a co-productive approach to engage older people as co-researchers in exploring features of age-friendliness in their city, and findings have provided evidence to assist in development of their AFC initiative.

However, significant challenges stand in the way of those aspiring to create equitable AFCs, most notably competing priorities in relation to allocation of resources within the local authorities [16]. In times of austerity with limited budgets, interventions needed to achieve an AFC may be given a low priority. Liverpool, together with several cities in the UK and globally, have experienced significant reductions in funding allocated to services for older adults [34,80].

Liverpool's AFC history dates from 2012, when its Mayor signed a pledge committing the city to become an AFC, in accordance with the WHO AFC initiative. In 2014, Liverpool joined the WHO's Global Network of Age-Friendly Cities and Communities. Despite the initial commitment, in a context of budget reductions, the AFC initiative in Liverpool got off to a slower start than many had anticipated. In 2019, Liverpool's AFC initiative has regained momentum with the appointment of an AFC Lead and with the Deputy Mayor reaffirming the pledge to become an AFC [81]. Supported by a steering group with representation from older residents and from sectors across the city (transportation, art and culture, health), work to enhance Liverpool's age-friendliness has progressed in different ways. The AFC coordinator has indicated that our study findings are still relevant for Liverpool, and city developments are very much in line with our results [80].

For instance, many study participants highlighted the need to foster intergenerational relationships in the city. Recently commissioned projects in Liverpool include intergenerational initiatives bringing together socially isolated older adults and allow them to teach their life skills to parents and children in their community [82]. At the Liverpool City Region level, there are plans to display AFC window stickers in premises [83]. Inspired by Nottingham City Council's work [84] (UK), premises displaying the AFC window sticker aim to provide a free seat, make toilet facilities available and offer tea, coffee, or a glass of water to older residents. This initiative will address lack of accessible public toilets in Liverpool city centre: a barrier to respect and social inclusion identified by our study participants.

Our study has also highlighted the need to incorporate older residents' views in AFC plans and promote partnership work across sectors. According to the AFC lead, one of the notable changes has been Liverpool City Council's approach to work, which is now more focused on considering older residents' needs and working closely with third sector organisations [80]. Recently, Liverpool City Council has been working with an independent organisation, Health Watch, to identify residents' views on priorities that need addressing. Engagement is happening through a wide range of methods, including face to face and telephone interviews, and surveys [80]. A current challenge in Liverpool, is, however, finding other ways to routinely engage with a wider range of older residents, particularly those most at risk of experiencing social exclusion and disadvantage [80]. This highlights a common challenge for other cities developing AFC (or related) approaches: the need to find more effective ways of engaging with older adults. Our study has demonstrated the appropriateness of taking a CBPR approach in accessing older people to elucidate their views on respect and social inclusion in the city. We believe that the periodic use of photovoice methods should be considered by policy makers and public health practitioners as a tool to maintain engagement with older people in identifying priorities for action and ensuring that their views are included in decision-making processes for their city.

4.2. Strengths and Limitations

Photovoice, with the combination of FGDs, SSIs and photos, brought to the surface older people's views about what was most important for their respect and social inclusion in an aspiring AFC, providing us with a unique angle to the issue, whilst engaging participants throughout the research [57,64].

A potential limitation of this study relates to the gender imbalance in the sample (males: 7; females: 19). The guiding principle for recruiting participants was to have a mix of included and less included participants, rather than focusing on gender differences. Moreover, we realised that (i) our strategy to recruit participants from grassroots organisations in order to include a mix of more or less socially included older adults and (ii) our requirement for participants to physically attend the sessions and being able to walk (even if for short distances only) to take photographs, meant that we did not reach some of the most excluded older people. However, our sample included a mix of affluent and less affluent participants from a range of locations in the city, as well as different age ranges and a mixture of ethnic and cultural groups. Finally, whilst our study was not designed to produce generalisable findings (e.g., to other contexts in the UK or elsewhere), some aspects identified by older adults in Liverpool are potentially applicable to other contexts (e.g., age-friendly non-urban communities). Our study therefore offers an opportunity to apply the same or similar research methods to explore perceptions of respect and social inclusion among older residents living in smaller and rural age-friendly communities.

5. Conclusions

This study has provided novel insights into how respect and social inclusion are shaped by aspects of the physical and social environment, and the role that accessibility, affordability and sociability of physical spaces contributed to older adults' mental wellbeing, feelings of inclusion, sense of independence and connection.

This research has shown that respect and social inclusion is a key domain of an AFC, and one that cuts across most—if not all—other domains identified in the original WHO framework for AFCs. As such, it should be a guiding principle for cities and communities aspiring to become more age-friendly. AFCs need to ensure that respect and social inclusion are appropriately reflected in city-based policies, including local strategies for older adults as well as services in the community. Our study has also shown the importance of perspectives about ageing and deprivation held more widely across society. The AFC movement could make a collaborative effort nationally and internationally to help society as a whole to evolve in these regards.

Cities and communities developing AFC (or related) approaches need to find better ways of engaging with older adults, including those most at risk of experiencing social exclusion and disadvantage. The periodic use of photovoice methods should be considered by policy makers and public health practitioners as a tool to maintain engagement with older adults in identifying priorities for action and ensuring that their views are included in decision-making processes for their city.

Author Contributions: Conceptualization, S.R., D.P., L.O. and N.B.; Data curation, S.R.; Formal analysis, S.R., L.O., S.B., D.P. and N.B.; Funding acquisition, D.P. and N.B.; Investigation, S.R.; Methodology, S.R., D.P., L.O. and N.B.; Project administration, N.B.; Resources, S.R.; Supervision, D.P., L.O. and N.B.; Visualization, S.R. and S.B.; Writing—original draft, S.R. and S.B.; Writing—review and editing, S.R., L.O., S.B., D.P. and N.B. All authors have read and agreed to the published version of the manuscript.

Funding: This doctoral research was supported by the National Institute for Health Research School for Public Health Research. Since April 2020, Sara Ronzi has been supported by the National Institute for Health Research School for Public Health Research Fellowship, Grant Reference Number PD-SPH-2015. The views expressed are those of the author(s) and not necessarily those of the NIHR or the Department of Health and Social Care.

Acknowledgments: The authors would like to thank the participants of the research for their generosity in sharing their time and experiences; Joe Monoghan and Sue Donald (Liverpool Citizen Advocacy), Joan Davies (St. Mary's Church, Grassendale) and Jackie Connolly (Plus Dane Group), who provided access to participants, and space to conduct our interviews and focus groups; the Museum of Liverpool, particularly Carol Rogers and Dawn Caroll, who kindly provided the space and help for the photo-exhibition. Thank you to the Age-Friendly City Lead Gemma Black, for her input in this research and information provided about the development of the Age-Friendly City Initiative in Liverpool. We are also grateful to other members of the NIHR SPHR, particularly Margaret Whitehead, Rory McGill, Cherie McCracken, Emma Halliday and Jennie Popay, for their valuable input in this research.

Conflicts of Interest: The authors declare no conflict of interest. The funders had no role in the design of the study; in the collection, analyses, or interpretation of data; in the writing of the manuscript, or in the decision to publish the results.

Appendix A

Main questions asked at the interview

- Tell me why you took this photograph.
- Why do you want to share this photograph?
- Why is it important for you?
- How, in what way does this photograph (name of the building/place in the photograph) make you feel valued and/or part of your community?

The SHOWeD technique [56,84]:

- ○ What do you *See* here?
- ○ What is really *Happening* here?
- ○ How does this relate to *Our* lives?
- ○ Why does this problem, concern, or strength *Exist*?
- ○ What can we *Do* about it?

- What does this photograph represent in terms of positive and negative aspects which support or do not support you to feel valued and part of your community?
- How do you think that this photograph/aspect you portrayed may be helping to support other elder people to age healthily and feel valued and/or part of their community?
- Think of two challenges within your neighbourhood/local community/Liverpool that you face every day which constitute a barrier for you to make you feel valued and/or part of the community.
- Think of two aspects within your neighbourhood/local community/Liverpool that support you to make you feel valued and/or part of the community.

- Think of services/aspects/activities of Liverpool that are inclusive of elder people. Can you give me some examples of this? What type of services would you like to see/do you think that can be inclusive of elder people in the community?
- Imagine that there was the possibility to make your neighbourhood/local community/Liverpool a better place for elder people to feel valued and part of their community. In this, imagine that you have all the resources to make it possible. What would you do?
- How would like to communicate what is meaningful to you and the results of the project to people who work in the council and representatives of services for elder people in the city?

Exploring photographs not taken:

- Are there any photographs that you might have wanted to take but you did not? If yes, can you tell me more about that? [63].

References

1. World Health Organization. *The World Report on Ageing and Health*; WHO Press: Luxembourg, 2015.
2. World Health Organization. *The Global Network for Age-Friendly Cities and Communities: Looking Back over the Last Decade, Looking Forward to the Next*; WHO Press: Geneva, Switzerland, 2018.
3. Buckner, S.; Pope, D.; Mattocks, C.; LaFortune, L.; Dherani, M.; Bruce, N. Developing Age-Friendly Cities: An Evidence-Based Evaluation Tool. *J. Popul. Ageing* **2019**, *12*, 203–223. [CrossRef]
4. Gonyea, J.G.; Burnes, K. Aging Well at Home: Evaluation of a Neighborhood-based Pilot Project to 'Put Connection Back into Community. *J. Hous. Elder.* **2013**, *27*, 333–347. [CrossRef]
5. Lehning, A.J.; Greenfield, E.A. Research on Age-Friendly Community Initiatives: Taking Stock and Moving Forward. *J. Hous. Elder.* **2017**, *31*, 178–192. [CrossRef]
6. Keating, N.; Eales, J.; Phillips, J.E. Age-Friendly Rural Communities: Conceptualizing 'Best-Fit'. *Can. J. Ageing* **2013**, *32*, 319–332. [CrossRef]
7. Menec, V.H.; Novek, S.; Veselyuk, D.; McArthur, J. Lessons Learned from a Canadian Province-Wide, Age-Friendly Initiative: The Age-Friendly Manitoba Initiative. *J. Aging Soc. Policy* **2013**, *26*, 37–41. [CrossRef]
8. Spina, J.; Menec, V.H. What Community Characteristics Help or Hinder Rural Communities in Becoming Age-Friendly? Perspectives From a Canadian Prairie Province. *J. Appl. Gerontol.* **2015**, *34*, 444–464. [CrossRef]
9. Walsh, K.; O'shea, E.; Scharf, T.; Shucksmith, M. Exploring the impact of informal practices on social exclusion and age-friendliness for older people in rural communities. *J. Community Appl. Soc. Psychol.* **2014**, *24*, 37–49. [CrossRef]
10. World Health Organization. *Global Age-Friendly Cities: A Guide*; WHO Press: Geneva, Switzerland, 2007.
11. World Health Organization. *Measuring the Age-Friendliness of Cities: A guide to Using Core Indicators*; WHO Press: Geneva, Switzerland, 2015.
12. Rosenberg, M.; Rosenberg, P.E.; Dalton, S.D. A Global Pilot Study of Age-Friendly City Indicators. *Soc. Indic. Res.* **2017**, *138*, 1205–1227. [CrossRef]
13. Dikken, J.; Hoven, R.F.V.D.; Van Staalduinen, W.H.; Hulsebosch-Janssen, L.M.; Van Hoof, J. How Older People Experience the Age-Friendliness of Their City: Development of the Age-Friendly Cities and Communities Questionnaire. *Int. J. Environ. Res. Public Health* **2020**, *17*, 6867. [CrossRef]
14. World Health Organization. *Age-Friendly Environments in Europe: Indicators, Monitoring and Assessments*; WHO Press: Geneva, Switzerland, 2018.
15. Plouffe, L.; Kalache, A. Towards global age-friendly cities: Determining urban features that promote active aging. *J. Urban. Health* **2010**, *87*, 733–739. [CrossRef]
16. Buffel, T.; Phillipson, C. A Manifesto for the Age-Friendly Movement: Developing a New Urban Agenda. *J. Aging Soc. Policy* **2018**, *30*, 173–192. [CrossRef] [PubMed]
17. Moulaert, T.; Garon, S. *Age-Friendly Cities and Communities in International Comparison*; Springer International Publishing: Basel, Switzerland, 2016.
18. Steels, S. Key characteristics of age-friendly cities and communities: A review. *Cities* **2015**, *47*, 45–52. [CrossRef]

19. Plouffe, L.; Kalache, A.; Voelcker, I. A Critical Review of the WHO Age-Friendly Cities Methodology and Its Implementation. In *Age-Friendly Cities and Communities in International Comparison*; Moulaert, T., Garon, S., Eds.; Springer International Publishing: Basel, Switzerland, 2016; pp. 19–36.
20. Scharlach, A.E.; Lehning, A.J. Ageing-friendly communities and social inclusion in the United States of America. *Ageing Soc.* **2012**, *33*, 110–136. [CrossRef]
21. Handler, S. *A Research & Evaluation Framework for Age-Friendly Cities A Research & Evaluation Framework for Age-Friendly Cities*; Urban Ageing Consortium: Manchester, UK, 2014.
22. Menec, V.H.; Means, R.; Keating, N.; Parkhurst, G.; Eales, J. Conceptualizing age-friendly communities. *Can. J. Aging* **2011**, *30*, 479–493. [CrossRef]
23. Lui, C.-W.; Everingham, J.-A.; Warburton, J.; Cuthill, M.; Bartlett, H. What makes a community age-friendly: A review of international literature. *Australas. J. Ageing* **2009**, *28*, 116–121. [CrossRef]
24. Finlay, J.; Franke, T.; McKay, H.A.; Sims-Gould, J. Therapeutic landscapes and wellbeing in later life: Impacts of blue and green spaces for older adults. *Health Place* **2015**, *34*, 97–106. [CrossRef]
25. Belon, A.P.; Nieuwendyk, L.M.; Vallianatos, H.; Nykiforuk, C.I.J. How community environment shapes physical activity: Perceptions revealed through the PhotoVoice method. *Soc. Sci. Med.* **2014**, *116*, 10–21. [CrossRef]
26. Plane, J.; Klodawsky, F. Neighbourhood amenities and health: Examining the significance of a local park. *Soc. Sci. Med.* **2013**, *99*, 1–8. [CrossRef]
27. Broome, K.; Worrall, L.; Fleming, J.; Boldy, D. Evaluation of age-friendly guidelines for public buses. *Transp. Res. Part. A Policy Pr.* **2013**, *53*, 68–80. [CrossRef]
28. Wigglesworth, S.; Barnes, S.; Tait, M.; Crookes, L.; Park, A. Designing for Wellbeing in Environments for Later Life Project (DWELL) 2016. Available online: http://dwell.group.shef.ac.uk/ (accessed on 20 September 2016).
29. Domínguez-Párraga, L. Neighborhood influence: A qualitative study in Cáceres, an aspiring age-friendly city. *Soc. Sci.* **2019**, *8*, 195. [CrossRef]
30. Rémillard-Boilard, S.; Buffel, T.; Phillipson, C. Involving Older Residents in Age-Friendly Developments: From Information to Coproduction Mechanisms. *J. Hous. Elderly* **2017**, *31*, 146–159. [CrossRef]
31. Greenfield, E.A.; Oberlink, M.; Scharlach, A.E.; Neal, M.B.; Stafford, P.B. Age-friendly community initiatives: Conceptual issues and key questions. *Gerontologist* **2015**, *55*, 191–198. [CrossRef]
32. Woolrych, R.; Sixsmith, J.; Fisher, J.; Makita, M.; Lawthom, R.; Murray, M. Constructing and negotiating social participation in old age: Experiences of older adults living in urban environments in the United Kingdom. *Ageing Soc.* **2019**, 1–23. [CrossRef]
33. Van Hoof, J.; Dikken, J.; Buttiġieġ, S.C.; van den Hoven, R.F.M.; Kroon, E.; Marston, H.R. Age-friendly cities in the Netherlands: An explorative study of facilitators and hindrances in the built environment and ageism in design. *Indoor Built Environ.* **2019**, *29*, 417–437. [CrossRef]
34. Buffel, T.; Rémillard-Boilard, S.; Walsh, K.; McDonald, B.; Smetcoren, A.-S.; De Donder, L. Age-Friendly Approaches and Old-Age Exclusion: A Cross-City Analysis. *Int. J. Ageing Later Life* **2020**, 1–29. [CrossRef]
35. Officer, A.; Schneiders, M.L.; Wu, D.; Nash, P.; Thiyagarajan, J.A.; Beard, J.R. Valuing older people: Time for a global campaign to combat ageism. *Bull. World Health Organ.* **2016**, *94*, 710–710A. [CrossRef] [PubMed]
36. Swift, H.; Steeden, B. Exploring Representations of Old Age and Ageing. Literature Review. 2020. Available online: https://www.ageing-better.org.uk/sites/default/files/2020-03/Exploring-representations-of-old-age.pdf (accessed on 20 September 2020).
37. Chang, E.-S.; Kannoth, S.; Levy, S.; Wang, S.-Y.; Lee, J.E.; Levy, B.R.E.S. Global reach of ageism on older persons' health: A systematic review. *PLoS ONE* **2020**, *15*, e0220857. [CrossRef] [PubMed]
38. Swift, H.; Steeden, B. Doddery but Dear? Examining Age-Related Stereotypes. 2020. Available online: https://www.ageing-better.org.uk/sites/default/files/2020-03/Doddery-but-dear.pdf (accessed on 20 September 2020).
39. World Health Organisation. *Global Strategy and Action Plan on Ageing and Health (2016–2020)*; WHO Press: Geneva, Switzerland, 2017.
40. Vaandrager, L.; Kennedy, L. The Application of Salutogenesis in Communities and Neighborhoods. In *The Handbook of Salutogenesis*; Mittelmark, M.B., Sagy, S., Eriksson, M., Bauer, G.F., Pelikan, J.M., Lindström, B., Espnes, G.A., Eds.; Springer Science and Business Media LLC: Cham, Switzerland, 2016; pp. 159–170.
41. Ronzi, S.; Orton, L.; Pope, D.; Valtorta, N.K.; Bruce, N.G. What is the impact on health and wellbeing of interventions that foster respect and social inclusion in community-residing older adults? A systematic review of quantitative and qualitative studies. *Syst. Rev.* **2018**, *7*, 26. [CrossRef]

42. Novek, S.; Menec, V.H. Older adults' perceptions of age-friendly communities in Canada: A photovoice study. *Ageing Soc.* **2014**, *34*, 1052–1072. [CrossRef]
43. Torku, A.; Chan, A.P.C.; Yung, E.H.K. Age-friendly cities and communities: A review and future directions. *Ageing Soc.* **2020**, 1–38. [CrossRef]
44. Mahmood, A.; Chaudhury, H.; Michael, Y.L.; Campo, M.; Hay, K.; Sarte, A. A photovoice documentation of the role of neighborhood physical and social environments in older adults' physical activity in two metropolitan areas in North America. *Soc. Sci. Med.* **2012**, *74*, 1180–1192. [CrossRef] [PubMed]
45. Mitra, R.; Siva, H.; Kehler, M. Walk-friendly suburbs for older adults? Exploring the enablers and barriers to walking in a large suburban municipality in Canada. *J. Aging Stud.* **2015**, *35*, 10–19. [CrossRef] [PubMed]
46. Van Hees, S.; Horstman, K.; Jansen, M.; Ruwaard, D. Photovoicing the neighbourhood: Understanding the situated meaning of intangible places for ageing-in-place. *Heal. Place* **2017**, *48*, 11–19. [CrossRef] [PubMed]
47. Petteway, R.J. Intergenerational photovoice perspectives of place and health in public housing: Participatory coding, theming, and mapping in/of the 'structure struggle. *Heal. Place* **2019**, *60*, 102229. [CrossRef]
48. Andonian, L.; MacRae, A. Well older adults within an urban context: Strategies to create and maintain social participation. *Br. J. Occup. Ther.* **2011**, *74*, 2–11. [CrossRef]
49. Liverpool City Council. Liverpool: Population. 2020. Available online: https://liverpool.gov.uk/council/key-statistics-and-data/data/population/ (accessed on 26 October 2020).
50. Public Health England. Local Authority Health Profiles: Liverpool. 2020. Available online: https://fingertips.phe.org.uk/profile/health-profiles/data#page/12/gid/1938132696/pat/6/par/E12000002/ati/202/are/E08000012/cid/4 (accessed on 26 October 2020).
51. Ministry of Housing Communities and Local Government. The English Indices of Deprivation. 2019. Available online: https://www.gov.uk/government/statistics/english-indices-of-deprivation-2019 (accessed on 20 September 2020).
52. Buffel, T.; McGarry, P.; Phillipson, C.; De Donder, L.; Dury, S.; De Witte, N.; Verté, D. Developing Age-Friendly Cities: Case Studies from Brussels and Manchester and Implications for Policy and Practice. *J. Aging Soc. Policy* **2014**, *26*, 52–72. [CrossRef]
53. Green, J.; Thorogood, N. Analysising qualitative data. In *Qualitative Methods for Health Research*, 2nd ed.; SAGE: Los Angeles, CA, USA, 2009; pp. 195–228.
54. Israel, B.; Coombe, C.M.; Cheezum, R.R.; Schulz, A.J.; McGranaghan, R.J.; Lichtenstein, R.; Reyes, A.G.; Clement, J.; Burris, A. Community-based participatory research: A capacity-building approach for policy advocacy aimed at eliminating health disparities. *Am. J. Public Health* **2010**, *100*, 2094–2102. [CrossRef]
55. Benjamin-Thomas, T.E.; Corrado, A.M.; McGrath, C.; Rudman, D.L.; Hand, C. Working Towards the Promise of Participatory Action Research: Learning From Ageing Research Exemplars. *Int. J. Qual. Methods* **2018**, *17*, 1609406918817953. [CrossRef]
56. Wang, C.C.; Burris, M.A. Photovoice: Concept, Methodology, and Use for Participatory Needs Assessment. *Heal. Educ. Behav.* **1997**, *24*, 369–387. [CrossRef]
57. Carlson, E.D.; Engebretson, J.; Chamberlain, R.M. Photovoice as a social process of critical consciousness. *Qual. Health Res.* **2006**, *16*, 836–852. [CrossRef]
58. Liebenberg, L. Thinking Critically About Photovoice. *Int. J. Qual. Methods* **2018**, *17*, 160940691875763. [CrossRef]
59. Novek, S.; Morris-Oswald, T.; Menec, V. Using photovoice with older adults: Some methodological strengths and issues. *Ageing Soc.* **2012**, *32*, 451–470. [CrossRef]
60. Evans-Agnew, R.A.; Rosemberg, M.-A.S. Questioning Photovoice Research: Whose Voice? *Qual. Health Res.* **2016**, *26*, 1019–1030. [CrossRef] [PubMed]
61. Wang, C.C.; Redwood-Jones, Y.A. Photovoice Ethics: Perspectives from Flint Photovoice. *Heal. Educ. Behav.* **2001**, *28*, 560–572. [CrossRef] [PubMed]
62. Budig, K.; Diez, J.; Conde, P.; Sastre, M.; Hernán, M.; Franco, M. Photovoice and empowerment: Evaluating the transformative potential of a participatory action research project. *BMC Public Health* **2018**, *18*, 1–9. [CrossRef]
63. Hodgetts, D.; Chamberlain, K.; Radley, A. Considering Photographs Never Taken During Photo-production Projects. *Qual. Res. Psychol.* **2007**, *4*, 263–280. [CrossRef]
64. Ronzi, S.; Pope, D.; Orton, L.; Bruce, N. Using photovoice methods to explore older people's perceptions of respect and social inclusion in cities: Opportunities, challenges and solutions. *SSM Popul. Health* **2016**, *2*, 732–745. [CrossRef]

65. Díez, J.; Conde, P.; Sandin, M.; Urtasun, M.; López, R.; Carrero, J.L.; Gittelsohn, J.; Franco, M.J. Health & Place Understanding the local food environment: A participatory photovoice project in a low-income area in Madrid, Spain. *Health Place* **2016**, *43*, 95–103. [CrossRef]
66. QSR International. NVivo 11 2020. Available online: https://www.qsrinternational.com/nvivo-qualitative-data-analysis-software/support-services/nvivo-downloads (accessed on 26 October 2020).
67. Miles, M.B.; Huberman, A.M. Early Steps in Analysis. In *Qualitative Data Analysis*; SAGE Pubblications Ltd.: London, UK, 1994; pp. 50–89.
68. Keats, P.A. Multiple text analysis in narrative research: Visual, written, and spoken stories of experience. *Qual. Res.* **2009**, *9*, 181–195. [CrossRef]
69. World Health Organization. *Age-Friendly Environments in Europe A Handbook of Domains for Policy Action*; WHO Press: Geneva, Switzerland, 2017.
70. Housing Lin. *Place-Making with Older Adults: Towards Age-Friendly Cities and Communities*; Heriot-Watt University Edinburgh: Scotland, UK, 2019.
71. Hallgrimsdottir, B.; Svensson, H.; Ståhl, A. Long term effects of an intervention in the outdoor environment-a comparison of older people's perception in two residential areas, in one of which accessibility improvements were introduced. *J. Transp. Geogr.* **2015**, *42*, 90–97. [CrossRef]
72. Prattley, J.; Buffel, T.; Marshall, A.; Nazroo, J. Area effects on the level and development of social exclusion in later life. *Soc. Sci. Med.* **2020**, *246*, 112722. [CrossRef] [PubMed]
73. Ruff, R.R.; Ng, J.; Jean-Louis, G.; Elbel, B.; Chaix, B.; Duncan, D.T. Neighborhood Stigma and Sleep: Findings from a Pilot Study of Low-Income Housing Residents in New York City. *Behav. Med.* **2018**, *44*, 48–53. [CrossRef] [PubMed]
74. Marmot, M.; Allen, J.; Boyce, T.; Goldblatt, P.; Morrison, J. Health Equity in England: The Marmot Review 10 Years On. *BMJ* **2020**, *368*, m693. [CrossRef]
75. Scharf, T.; Phillipson, C.; Smith, A.E. Social exclusion of older people in deprived urban communities of England. *Eur. J. Ageing* **2005**, *2*, 76–87. [CrossRef]
76. Buffel, T.; Phillipson, C.; Scharf, T. Ageing in urban environments: Developing 'age-friendly' cities. *Crit. Soc. Policy* **2012**, *32*, 597–617. [CrossRef]
77. Buffel, T.; Phillipson, C. Ageing in a Gentrifying Neighbourhood: Experiences of Community Change in Later Life. *Sociology* **2019**, *53*, 987–1004. [CrossRef]
78. Buswell, M.; Goodman, C.; Russell, B.; Bunn, F.; Mayrhofer, A.; Goodman, E. *Community Engagement Evidence Synthesis: A Final Report for Alzheimer's Society*; University of Hertfordshire: Hatfield, UK, 2017. [CrossRef]
79. Garon, S.; Paris, M.; Beaulieu, M.; Veil, A.; Laliberté, A. Collaborative Partnership in Age-Friendly Cities: Two Case Studies From Quebec, Canada Collaborative Partnership in Age-Friendly Cities: Two Case Studies From Quebec, Canada. *J. Aging Soc. Policy* **2014**, *26*, 73–87. [CrossRef] [PubMed]
80. Black, G.; (Centre for Ageing Better, Liverpool, UK). Phone Conversation with the Age-Friendly City Lead in Liverpool. Personal Communication, 2020.
81. Black, G. Reflections on Being an Age-Friendly Community from an Age-Friendly Lead. 2019. Available online: https://www.ageing-better.org.uk/blogs/reflections-being-age-friendly-community-age-friendly-lead (accessed on 26 October 2020).
82. Social Care Institute for Excellence. Practice Examples: Challenges and Solutions of Commissioning During COVID-19. 2020. Available online: https://www.scie.org.uk/care-providers/coronavirus-covid-19/commissioning/challenges-and-solutions/practice-examples (accessed on 26 October 2020).
83. Liverpool City Region. Age Friendly Liverpool City Region. 2020. Available online: https://www.liverpoolcityregion-ca.gov.uk/age-friendly/ (accessed on 26 October 2020).
84. Centre for Ageing Better. Age-Friendly Case Study: Take a Seat Campaign. 2019. Available online: https://www.ageing-better.org.uk/stories/age-friendly-nottingham-take-seat (accessed on 26 October 2020).

International Journal of
Environmental Research and Public Health

MDPI

Article

Prisons, Older People, and Age-Friendly Cities and Communities: Towards an Inclusive Approach

Helen Codd

School of Justice, University of Central Lancashire, Preston PR1 2HE, UK; hlcodd@uclan.ac.uk

Received: 28 October 2020; Accepted: 7 December 2020; Published: 9 December 2020

Abstract: This original and ground-breaking interdisciplinary article brings together perspectives from gerontology, criminology, penology, and social policy to explore critically the nature and consequences of the lack of visibility of prisons, prisoners, and ex-prisoners within global research, policy and practice on age-friendly cities and communities (AFCC), at a time when increasing numbers of people are ageing in prison settings in many countries. In addition, the COVID-19 pandemic continues to pose challenges in the contexts both of older peoples' lives, wellbeing, and health, and also within prison settings, and thus it is timely to reflect on the links between older people, prisons, and cities, at a time of ongoing change. Just as there is an extensive body of ongoing research exploring age-friendly cities and communities, there is extensive published research on older people's experiences of imprisonment, and a growing body of research on ageing in the prison setting. However, these two research and policy fields have evolved largely independently and separately, leading to a lack of visibility of prisons and prisoners within AFCC research and policy and, similarly, the omission of consideration of the relevance of AFCC research and policy to older prisoners and ex-prisoners. Existing checklists and tools for assessing and measuring the age-friendliness of cities and communities may be of limited relevance in the context of prisons and prisoners. This article identifies the potential for integration and for cross-disciplinary research in this context, concluding with recommendations for developing inclusive research, policies, and evaluation frameworks which recognise and include prisons and older prisoners, both during and after incarceration.

Keywords: prisons; prisoners; older offenders; ex-prisoners; age-friendly cities and communities

1. Introduction

1.1. Age-Friendly Cities, Crime, and Criminology

The development of "age-friendly cities and communities" (AFCC) has become a highly significant theme in relation to public policy and ageing that has resulted in a Global Network for Age-Friendly Cities and Communities, launched in 2010, and a panoply of locally-developed age-friendly policies [1]. When engaging with the research literature for the first time, however, an academic working on crime and justice issues is likely to be struck by a vague sense of cognitive dissonance. Age-friendly cities are promoted as spaces, places, and communities where people of all ages are valued, engaged, and facilitated to live active lives. This overarching vision of the age-friendly city portrays a positive image of a harmonious, inter- and multi-generational space, place, and community where all are welcomed and included. However, for criminologists, cities have always been linked to crime, urban deprivation, and a range of social issues including drug use, organised crime, homelessness, "gangs" and high levels of both criminal residence and criminal victimisation.

That is not to say, of course, that criminological research has not identified positive aspects of cities—there is a substantial body of research on community cohesion in cities, and on designing cities to encourage crime prevention—but from the early days of the pioneer researchers of the Chicago

School, who used the city of Chicago as their laboratory for empirical social research, there has been no shortage of research exploring crime, policing and victimisation within urban environments, although a detailed exposition of this vast body of research is beyond the scope of this article [2,3].

Thus, on encountering research and policy documents on age-friendly cities and communities for the first time, a criminologist is very likely to wonder where the crime has gone, and indeed, where all the criminals have gone. Indeed, from a more penological perspective, one could also wonder where the prisons and ex-prisoners have gone, especially when, in the UK and many other countries, prisons situated in urban environments are still common. That is not to say there is no mention of crime at all, as in some of the research there is some mention of policing and older people as victims, for example, but the relative invisibility of prisons, older offenders, older prisoners, and former prisoners is striking. This reflects the relative neglect of older peoples' experiences as offenders, prisoners, and ex-prisoners within gerontology as a whole, although a recent edited collection exploring diversity and difference in experiences of ageing included a chapter on ageing in prison, and this inclusion is to be welcomed [4].

To some extent this is surprising, as the evolution and development of the "age-friendly cities and communities" (AFCC) movement from the early 1980s onwards has been mirrored by a growing recognition of the involvement of older people in the criminal justice process, as victims but also as offenders. This growth in awareness and expansion in the published research literature reflects both demographic shifts, with older people living longer, and also changes in penal policies and practices which have led to high levels of imprisonment in some jurisdictions. This "mass imprisonment epidemic", perhaps most visible in the US but replicated to some extent in other countries including England and Wales, has been characterised by mandatory minimum sentencing, whole life tariffs, and life sentences without the possibility of parole. The abolition of capital punishment in many countries has also meant that individuals are growing old in prison when prior to abolition they would have been executed. In addition, as seen in recent cases in the UK and the US, prosecutions of historical state, war, and sexual crimes which took place in the past are leading to people who are now in older age being tried and sentenced, sometimes with no previous experience of involvement in the criminal justice system. However, these two fields of research have emerged and evolved largely independently of each other and whilst there is a great deal of potential for exchange of good practice at present these two disciplinary approaches seem to constitute primarily separate academic and policy-making spaces.

1.2. The Aims and Structure of This Paper

The aims, objectives, and purposes of this review are to explore the extent to which the needs and experiences of older prisoners and former prisoners are recognised within the extensive and growing literature on age-friendly cities; to assess the relevance of existing measures of age-friendliness in relation to older prisoners and former prisoners, and to identify gaps in the literature and outline directions for future research. This paper is based on a thorough and comprehensive literature review including not only monographs and peer-reviewed articles but also relevant reports by non-governmental organisations (NGOs) and governmental policy guidance documents.

The structure of this paper reflects the potential readership which includes academics and policy-makers with expertise in criminology and also those with expertise in relation to age-friendly cities. Whilst some readers will approach this paper with some knowledge of older prisoners, they may not be familiar with the literature on age-friendly cities, and the converse may also be the case. Recognising this diverse potential readership, Section 2 of the paper outlines key issues identified in the published research into older people and prisons. Section 3 provides a summary of the development of the concept of age-friendly cities and communities (AFCC), including an introduction to the eight WHO themes. Section 4 brings these two research areas together to explore the age-friendliness of cities and communities for older prisoners and ex-prisoners, using the eight WHO themes as a starting point. Section 5 sets out conclusions, including recommendations for future research.

2. Older People and Prisons

2.1. The Rising Number of Older Prisoners

In many countries including the UK, Ireland, the US, Canada, and Australia, older prisoners, make up a significant and growing minority within a penal estate populated primarily by young men [5–8]. Rising numbers of older prisoners have become a matter of concern for policy-makers, practitioners, and researchers in many jurisdictions including the US, the UK, and Japan. Although these numbers are increasing, older prisoners form a minority of the prison population, and within this population older women constitute a minority within a minority [8].

2.2. The Experiences of Older Prisoners

Alongside the "greying" of the prison population, research has flourished and there is now a substantial body of relevant literature, utlilisinga range of quantitative and qualitative methodological approaches, which have served to render older prisoners and their experiences and needs much more visible in criminological and penological contexts. This research includes perspectives from law, psychiatry, psychology, medicine, health and gerontology, sociology, social work, social and penal policy, criminology, corrections, and prison management [6,7,9–24]. There is also an extensive body of research on criminal behaviour by, and against, older people, discussion of which is beyond the scope of this article [10,25].

The term "prison" is used in this article in the usual UK sense, meaning an establishment tasked with the custodial care of those accused of crimes awaiting trial or sentence, and those who have been sentenced to terms of imprisonment (or youth custody for young offenders). This includes a wide range of institutions, including the equivalents of jails and also the equivalents of federal penitentiaries, as exist in the US. Prisons are not homogenous environments, but they all involve compulsory detention and associated restrictions on liberty. They vary not only in terms of their physical environments and facilities, but also their populations: for example, a city-centre Victorian prison such as HMP Preston, is populated mainly by remand prisoners and experiences a high level of prisoner turnover ("churn") and an unstable and ever-changing population, with security appropriate to holding Category B prisoners. This can be contrasted with long-term training prisons and contrasted again with the highest security "dispersal" prisons (such as HMP Long Lartin) and prisons operating under open conditions (such as HMP Kirkham). Some prisons have higher proportionate numbers of older offenders as a reflection of their specialist status as exemplified by HMP Wymott and its high population of sex offenders. All prisons in England and Wales are subject to the same inspection regime but these same inspection reports illuminate differences between establishments.

Prisons fulfil multiple functions for those who live in them due to their sentence. They provide bed, board, and a place to live. They are the source of medical care, of education and training and for some prisoners very low-wage employment. They can provide psychological care, counselling, and spiritual support and opportunities to practise one's faith (or not). The prison can create new friendships but also expose older people to aggression and bullying. Prison can entrench people in offending lifestyles, as reflected in reoffending rates. From the point of view of an older prisoner, the prison fulfils multiples roles, often at the same time. Some of these mirror outside activities and provision. Others make "ordinary" life challenging, such as restrictions on family visits and contact. Access to telephones and the internet may make older people's lives easier in the community, but their use in prison is highly proscribed. The COVID19 pandemic has created a necessity for new forms of communication between prisoners and their friends and family, including approved prison-issued mobile phones and online-based "Purple Visits", but these are tightly regulated and, at the time of writing, subject to technological and infrastructural uncertainties and the challenges of digital poverty.

2.3. The Age-Friendly Prison?

There are ongoing debates about if and how prisons can be age-friendly institutions, especially as a core element of age-friendliness involves maintaining autonomy and choice and it is inherent in the nature of the prison itself that such autonomy and choice is restricted. The most straightforward approach to age-friendliness in prisons is to mirror the "-friendly" suffix from other aspects of prison provision, such as prisons being "family- friendly" or "child-friendly", then applying these ideas to exploring whether prisons respond adequately to the needs of prisoners from diverse age groups, primarily in the context of ageing (and elderly) prisoners. Applying this approach, there is an array of published research which highlights failures to be age-friendly, especially in relation to physical factors such as prison design, medical, and healthcare facilities, and which documents the challenges experienced by older prisoners [6,20,21,26]. To some extent the literature on older prisoners has, until relatively recently, tended to view older people in prison through a medicalised lens. More broadly, older prisoners are also included in research on adult social care in prison settings [26,27].

2.4. Good Practice in Working with Older Prisoners

RECOOP, an organisation which supports older prisoners, has published guides to good practice in working with older prisoners, and also for approved premises [28]. There is no shortage of research literature criticising prison environments for the barriers to participation they create for older offenders, especially those with mobility difficulties, and attention has been drawn to access to educational and dining areas; problems of allocating older people the top bunk of bunk beds; sports and recreation facilities, and the limitations to access and movement inherent in old prison buildings, many of them, such as HMP Dartmoor, built initially in the nineteenth century. Some attention has been drawn to the social needs of older prisoners but much of the research focuses on physical and environmental factors, and issues of provision to respond to the medical, health and welfare needs of older people in prison. This approach focuses on a medicalised, pathological model of ageing and to some extent focuses on micro-environmental factors (grab rails, ramps, and so on) which are relatively low-cost to amend and which do not require major changes to prison regimes, provision of activities, and a whole scale rethinking of prison for older people [6,12,18,21].

There are also several policy reports and guidance documents aimed specifically at prison governors and service commissioners to help them to respond to the needs of the older prisoner population within prisons, as exemplified in HMPPS Model for Operational Delivery: Older Prisoners [29] and the work of the Prisons and Probations Ombudsmen [30]. Similarly, research reports and policy documents from government agencies and NGOs provide information and guidance on specific aspects of the needs and experiences of older prisoners, including health and social care needs [27,31,32] and issues arising from the needs of older people on release [33]. The ageing of the prison population has also prompted discussions around life-limiting illness and end-of-life care, including palliative care, the ethical challenges and issues around assisted suicide and assisted dying, and the impacts of the deaths of loved ones during the period of custody [34–37].

2.5. The Challenges of Defining "Older" in the Prison Setting

Older prisoners are no longer "invisible" in penological research and policy development, nor conversely are older people in prison completely invisible in research on ageing, but in spite of the expansion of academic and practitioner interest in older offenders a number of core questions still vex researchers. From the outset, the definitions of "older people" and "older prisoners" have been contested, and there is no agreed national or international definition, each researcher or policymaker adopting their own definition which sets the threshold somewhere between 45 and over 70 [38]. Although the UN has recognised older prisoners as "special needs prisoners" [39] there is no shared international definition, which makes comparisons difficult, and research tends to use the terms "older" and "elderly" interchangeably [13]. Defining people as older at 45 or 50 may seem very low, but it has been argued that accelerated aging can occur for some prisoners, who are argued to be functionally older than their chronological age [19] as a consequence of previous lifestyle, lack of medical care prior to imprisonment, and the experience of incarceration itself [13–15]. Thus, a prisoner in their fifties may have the health problems and physical appearance of someone living in the community who is at least ten years older [9,10,37]. This view is controversial, however, some commentators arguing that prison healthcare can mitigate the accelerated aging process and that individuals experience aging differently [38].

3. Age-friendly Cities and Communities

3.1. The Development of Age-Friendly Cities (AFCC)

The AFCC movement traces its origins to the United Nations First World Assembly on Ageing, which was convened by the General Assembly of the UN and held in Vienna in 1982 [40–42]. Subsequent to this conference, which led to the first ever international instrument on ageing (the Vienna International Plan of Action on Ageing), the 1986 WHO Ottawa Charter for Health Promotion led to the launch of the Healthy Cities movement. In 2002, twenty years after the First World Assembly, the UN met to review the outcomes of the Vienna International Plan on Ageing. This 2002 event led to the adoption of two major policies which provided the foundation for the AFCC movement (i.e., The Madrid International Plan of Action on Ageing and the WHO Active Ageing Policy Framework. The WHO defined an age-friendly city as one which could promote active ageing, defined as, "the process of optimizing opportunities for health, participation and security in order to enhance quality of life as people age" [42].

The age-friendly city programme, having first been introduced at the World Congress of Gerontology and Geriatrics, was launched in 2006, as the WHO Global Age-Friendly Cities project, which brought together 33 cities around the world in order to identify the core features of an age-friendly city. This research, which focused on the viewpoints of older people, caregivers, and local service providers, identified eight themes in order to increase and maximise the age-friendliness of cities, each including a checklist of key features. This guide and checklist aimed to provide cities with a tool to identify strengths and areas for improvement, to plan change and to monitor progress [43,44].

The WHO is not the first, nor indeed the only, organisation to focus on age-friendly developments, but the WHO has become a highly significant and influential resource for defining AFCCs [45]. Other initiatives have been developed, including the creation of an Action Group by the European Commission, which more recently has created a joint project (Age-Friendly Environments in Europe (AFEE)) with the WHO Regional Office for Europe; the AARP livable communities approach; the AdvantAge Initiative created by the Visiting Nurse Service of New York, the US Environmental Protection Agency's Building Healthy Communities for Active Aging (BHCAA) Award Program, and the "Village Movement", among others. The WHO has facilitated links, support and dialogue between different cities, communities, and regions, via a global network, and the identification of the eight domains has encouraged and enabled an integrated approach to ageing and urbanisation which goes beyond health and social care programmes alone [42]. Beyond urban environments, age-friendliness has been applied to exploring the lived experiences and social exclusion of older people in rural environments [44].

The concept of the "livability" of cities predates research and policies exploring AFCCs [45]. Terms such as livability and "age-friendliness" are used to describe how cities and communities are recognising and responding to the needs of an ageing population, often being used interchangeably. However, these concepts emerged at different times. Livability emerged during the 1980s in relation to cities and can include but is not limited to ageing people within cities. In a significant and useful scoping review, Chonody and Teatra [45] utilise a five-step process to explore the similarities and differences between these approaches, exploring whether they are underpinned by a similar perspective. Their review explores how livable and age-friendly communities are conceptualised in the existing literature, the specific elements that are identified as formulating the concepts, such as frameworks or indices, and the extent to which these frameworks and indices are interrelated and/or independent. Their thorough methodological approach identified 21 studies which met their criteria for inclusion, which were analysed in order to identify the elements of livable and age -friendly communities in each, that were generated through along with the frequency of their occurrence over all the studies included.

Chonody and Teatra's article provides several tables identifying the core terms and themes used within each study to identify livability and age-friendliness. The amount of variation as to how these themes are defined and framed is striking. Overall, however, they find several overlapping and common thematic frameworks, such as health, social engagement/connectivity, opportunities for recreation, and employment or volunteering opportunities. The most frequently included community elements were health, housing, safety and security, social participation, transportation, civic participation, the built environment, recreation and cultural activities, the natural environment, income, and respect or social inclusion. Some of the definitions of livability, those which considered citizens' inclusion, included age-friendliness. Overall, the age-friendly frameworks were more focused on ageing and ageing populations in comparison with the livability frameworks which seemed in some settings to be more directed towards young professionals [46]. As Kashef [47] pointed out, "The cities that tend to rise to the top of the livability rankings are those with relatively small percentages of people living below the poverty line, low birth rates, low percentage of children, and are more hospitable to tourists/business travelers than immigrants." If, however, livability is assessed from the points of view, for example, of those people who are from a lower socioeconomic status, then this highlights gaps in services and structures.

3.2. The Eight WHO Themes of Age-Friendly Cities

The eight WHO themes have become one of the most commonly used tools for evaluating age-friendliness in varied environments around the world [48] following the publication of the WHO guide, "Global age-friendly cities" in 2007 [42]. The eight themes explored in the guide are:

1. Outdoor spaces & buildings
2. Transportation
3. Housing
4. Social Participation
5. Respect and social inclusion
6. Civic participation & employment
7. Communication and Information
8. Community support and health services

Within research and policy documents on age-friendly cities and communities, it is a foundational principle that every community and city will have its own unique challenges and opportunities to address, the WHO encouraging each community and city to implement evidence-based planning and to develop their own mechanisms in order to increase their age-friendliness A number of toolkits, resource packs and guides have been developed so as to provide a basic understanding of age-friendly cities, some providing templates to help cities assess and evaluate the effectiveness of their programmes across each of their domains [48,49]. The challenges of measuring age-friendliness have been recognised by the WHO itself—"age-friendliness is a moving target; thus, it does not easily lend itself to standardization of measurement" [50]. From criticisms that initial frameworks for assessing and evaluating age-friendliness, the WHO has published further core and supplementary AFC indicators, some of which are very specific [49].

The first step as encouraged by the WHO is to conduct a baseline assessment of age-friendliness, such as by consulting with older people, organisations, and other stakeholders via focus groups or more innovative participatory methods such as walking interviews or co-produced research involving older people [48] Once these priorities and goals have been identified then cities are encouraged to devise their own action plans and monitor the subsequent implementation and progress of activities and initiatives [42]. Throughout these plans there is a focus on developing partnerships and collaborative working; involving older people in the decision-making process; and monitoring progress and evaluating the results.

4. Prisons and Age-Friendly Cities and Communities: Research, Policy, and Practice

4.1. Prisons as Urban Institutions

The published literature on age-friendly cities does not usually recognise prisons as significant urban institutions comparable, for example, with hospitals, shops, and leisure facilities, even though they may be large, visible buildings employing a significant local workforce. When prisons are physically and geographically located away from city conurbations, they are linked to cities and city communities via the backgrounds and relationships of prisoners, along with other individuals and organisations which engage with the prison and its residents. The city may be the home residence area of prisoners, or the locale in which their offending has taken place, or the area to which they are likely to be released. For some former prisoners, the city becomes their residence after release simply because they are unable to return to their previous home addresses, towns, or regions, sometimes because of the impact of their offending, associated stigma, or for the protection of the public, their victims or themselves.

The interactions between prisons, cities, and communities manifest themselves in a variety of ways. Prisoners themselves may be located in one geographical location (the prison); originate in a different location (e.g., their "home town" or city) and then engage with and be visited by people living in other places entirely. The nature of the isolation of prisoners from local communities, unless they are in open or semi-open conditions where, for example, they are allowed out to work or on other forms of release on temporary license (ROTL), means that they "belong" more to their home locale than where they may live, sometimes for many years.

4.2. Ageing, Prisons, Families, and Friends

When we discuss prisons, prisoners, and age-friendly cities and communities it is important to include non-imprisoned older people who, although they have not themselves been convicted, live within the "web of imprisonment" through their relationships with prisoners [51]. This can include most obviously the partners and spouses of prisoners, but can also include parents, children, other relatives and kin, and friends. As older offenders are themselves experiencing ageing, and demographic changes mean they are living longer, so may be their parents, meaning that older prisoners may themselves be visited by people who are even older. This is particularly significant in the light of the research into people who commit serious offences which attract high levels of media attention, such as some homicides and sexual offences, when after intimate and romantic relationships have ended, parents, especially mothers, continue to support their incarcerated adult (and elderly) child [51]. Thus, in the hypothetical situation of a man being convicted of multiple rapes and murders at the age of thirty, and being told at sentencing he will be subject to a whole-life tariff and die in prison, if his mother was 55 when he was thirty then by the time he is 60 his mother would be 85, and if he lives until he is 75 then his mother would be 100. Mothers are more likely than other friends or family members to continue to support their imprisoned adult children, and in most countries, women live longer than men, and thus this situation is not uncommon. If the prison is not conceptualised as part of the age-friendly city or community then these challenges experienced by non-imprisoned older visitors may go unnoticed.

4.3. The WHO Domains and Older Prisoners

The eight domains of age-friendliness set out by the WHO provide a useful starting point for exploring the age-friendliness of cities and communities for older prisoners and ex-prisoners.

4.3.1. Outdoor Spaces and Buildings

The first theme, that of age-friendliness of outdoor spaces and buildings, may not pose additional challenges beyond these experienced by non-imprisoned older people. However, criminal justice system agencies, including the police, probation, and other services for offenders, need to be as accessible to older people as younger people, even though the age profile of their client group may be younger.

4.3.2. Transportation

If the prison is located in a central urban setting then, as long as public transport is accessible for older people, or there are specific community transport resources which can be used, then visiting the prison may not pose a great transport challenge. However, if there is little availability of relevant transport, and the prison is, like many prisons, built on the edge of a city or, as in the US and some parts of the UK, in a rural area, then the problems of transportation to prisons for family members, as already identified in the literature on prisoners' families, may be magnified where older people are experiencing mobility difficulties, chronic illnesses and mental health issues, including dementia. Health challenges may make long journeys impractical or painful. The transport problems of visiting prisons in the UK are well-documented, and then if we add in the challenges of ageing then the problems may be magnified, and also have a disproportionate negative impact on members of the poorest communities, who may not have access to cars or be able to drive. We already know that in the UK female prisoners are held further away from their homes and families than male prisoners, and thus these transportation difficulties can be compounded.

4.3.3. Housing

For older people leaving prison, age-friendly appropriate housing may be difficult or impossible to access. Where individuals have aged in prison, their partners/spouses may have died or relationships broken down; children may have grown up, and the "family home" if it ever existed at all, may not be there as a place to which the released prisoner can return. There is also the core problem of the concept of "ageing in place" and what happens to people who have either never had a "place" in which to age, if they were previously homeless, for example, or where their place to age was the prison. As a carceral setting the prison is not intended to offer a long-term residential placement where prisoners' sentences have ended, or where their risk assessment indicates that parole/release on license is appropriate, but the question then is where they should go.

Residential care homes may not be willing or able to house ex-prisoners, and designated residential settings for ex-prisoners (such as approved premises in the UK) may be unsuitable as they are populated mainly by younger men and may not have appropriate care/nursing facilities or create opportunities for bullying and harassment. Older ex-prisoners may thus not be able to be housed within adult social care settings for older people, nor within criminal justice/probation settings. That said, in Canada, Haley House in Peterborough ON is a pioneering unique halfway house for formerly imprisoned older men run by a non-profit organisation and funded mainly by the Correctional Service Canada (CIC) [50]. Older people leaving prison who do not have specific care needs face difficulties accessing public and private housing due to background checks and the need for references, and those convicted of sexual offences face additional barriers to accessing housing. These barriers create a risk of homelessness, and on becoming homeless, may not be able to access homelessness services because of their criminal convictions and/or risk profile. For example, older people who are homeless after prison may find that even if they previously accessed homelessness services once they have become older these services may not be suitable for them and specific provision for older people who are homeless is very rare [52]. Where older age intersects not only with a prior record of crime and incarceration but also mental health issues and substance abuse, street homelessness may be experienced as inevitable due to a lack of appropriate accommodation and services, even though lack of a settled address creates additional challenges of offender and risk management [53]. Homelessness itself is a traumatic event and creates additional risks of victimisation, including violence [54]. Although nearly all of the published research focuses on formerly imprisoned men, older female former prisoners constitute a subgroup of a subgroup, or a minority within a minority, which is even more vulnerable [53].

4.3.4. Social Participation

Social participation is interlinked with social integration, which has been recognised as a very significant element of the process of release and successful community resettlement and reentry. Older people may well be at risk of social isolation and loneliness after release, not only because of stigma and hostility, but also because if they have aged in prison then they may no longer have any supportive family or friendship networks which can be beneficial in relation to the practical and emotional impacts of release and resettlement. Fear of hostility, and fear of stigmatisation, can be powerful behavioural influencers in themselves, even if there are no actual hostile incidents or interactions. Family ties may never have existed, or could have been lost as a consequence of the offending or the sentence, with older offenders sometimes severing ties themselves. Strong family ties have been linked to increased levels of desistance (for all age groups) and lower levels of reoffending: older offenders may not be able to benefit practically, mentally, or emotionally on release, and thus may experience high levels of perceived disconnectedness [55]. Loneliness is a common experience for many older people, and this is exacerbated by the stigma of a criminal conviction and prison sentence, along with offender management controls over managing risk by defining, for example, where people can go and when, and with whom they can (or cannot) associate.

The same challenges, marginalities and invisibilities can apply too in relation to non-residential settings and community programmes. There are related issues around long-term prisoners and institutionalisation: long periods in prison create challenges to community re-entry, and these are magnified for older people.

4.3.5. Respect and Social Inclusion

Respect and social inclusion are linked to social participation. To sentence someone to prison is inherently an act of social exclusion, a symbolic denunciation of someone's conduct and a statement that a person is not welcome within the community. The status of offender, especially that of a prisoner or ex-prisoner, is usually a stigmatised identity and means that prison itself denotes someone as undeserving of respect, beyond the basic requirements of respect for human rights. Whilst older offenders are not all sex offenders, a substantial proportion are, and risk management and safeguarding may make some forms of social participation impossible due to risk management considerations. For example, if a community wants to create opportunities for inter- and multi-generational engagement, bringing children into contact with an adult convicted of sexual offences against children can be very dangerous.

4.3.6. Civic Participation and Employment

In the UK, despite several challenges via the European Court of Human Rights, prisoners serving a custodial sentence after conviction are not eligible to vote in any elections, echoing archaic historical concepts of "civil death" as a consequence of conviction. Civic participation is particularly challenging in jurisdictions, including some US states, where some or all ex-prisoners are disenfranchised, sometimes for life, by reason of a felony conviction. These felony disenfranchisement laws mean that not only are some convicted offenders banned from voting and banned from seeking civic and political offices, but there is no political advantage to be gained by politicians and civic leaders if they engage with the views and needs of ex-offenders and ex-prisoners [56].

Ex-prisoners of all ages face barriers to employment as a consequence of conviction and sentence. This can be linked directly to the nature of the offending, which may mean that some forms of employment are no longer available due to safeguarding requirements and criminal records checks, and also to the reluctance of many employers to employ ex-prisoners. Age discrimination is also a concern [57]. For older people leaving prison, unless they have a previous job to which they can return, or have the capacity to set up their own business or become self-employed, finding employment is often impossible, especially in times of recession where there is a very high level of competition for any available jobs [58,59].

4.3.7. Communication and Information

Accessing information can be challenging for some older people leaving prison, especially as many governmental agencies and advice organisations have moved to online resources and delivery. This is even more visible due to the impacts of the COVID-19 pandemic, which has accelerated anticipated shifts towards online provision of information and advice. Governmental agencies (such as the DWP in the UK) require all new claims to be made via their online portal. However, older people leaving prison may struggle to access these portals, due to digital poverty and lack of access to smartphones and the internet, and also especially if they have been long-term prisoners, due to a lack of knowledge, skills, and experience of using IT technologies which have developed apace during their sentence. Prisons exercise strict controls on access to mobile telephones and the internet, and for some offenders post-release supervision requirements, such as specific offending and harm prevention orders for sex offenders, mean that accessing the internet is banned entirely.

4.3.8. Community Support & Health Services

Older people who leave prison may be marginalised within the provision of community support services because they constitute a minority within the client group of an organisation. For example, criminal justice agencies, including probation, manage a caseload which is predominantly young and male. For organisations supporting older people, the particular needs of older people after leaving prison can present unfamiliar challenges, especially if offending behaviour co-exists with mental health issues, substance misuse, and homelessness. Older ex-prisoners fall through the gaps in service provision by virtue of being a minority within every client group, especially at a time when health and social services budgets have been cut drastically.

5. Conclusions: Towards Inclusion

The invisibility of prisons and former prisoners within age friendly cities reflects the stigmatised identity of the prison as an establishment and as an institution, and ongoing stigmatisation of prisoners and ex-prisoners. At best, this reflects what Crawley [60] and Cadet [61] refer to as "institutional thoughtlessness" and at worst this reflects discrimination against older people who offend or have a history of offending. Research, practice and policies on Age-Friendly Cities and Communities promulgates a vision of a positive, friendly, accessible locale and community, including active, engaged, and participatory older citizens, and older ex-prisoners, especially those who become homeless or continue to offend, do not fit easily into this almost-utopian vision. The situation becomes even more complex for older ex-prisoners who carry multiple marginalised identities linked to poverty, mental health, race and ethnicity, sexuality, illness and disability, and offence type. In developing further research, policy and practice it is important to recognise and unpack diversity within and between older people, and not to assume homogeneity on the basis of age. Ageing intersects with other factors including ethnicity, gender, sexuality, and socio-economic status, although the nuances of how these factors influence experiences of imprisonment and release from prison are under-researched.

The WHO domains are of some relevance to older prisoners and ex-prisoners, but further research is needed so as to identify the specific aspects of age-friendliness which are most important to older prisoners and older ex-prisoners. This research could also explore whether elements of the work of Buckner et al. [62] would be of value too. Buckner et al. [62] aimed to identify an evidence-based approach cities could use that (i) can be applied in different contexts, (ii) reflects the complexity of the initiatives, (iii) draws on sound data to make assessments of potential or demonstrable effectiveness, and (iv) presents findings clearly to a mixed audience. Their work presents an evaluation tool which responds to these requirements, based on fieldwork in Liverpool, UK. In contrast with the WHO indicators, which are often very specific, this tool is designed to gather evidence on a wider scale. It can indeed accommodate the WHO indicators, but these can be subsumed within the broader input areas, especially those of "provision and involvement of older people". Buckner et al. [62] argue that applying the WHO indicators together with the tool can draw attention to very specific issues which would be less visible when assessed by the tool alone.

The evaluation tool developed by Buckner at.al. [62] evaluation tool includes ten "input areas" for which evidence is required to assess policy and practice initiatives which strive to be age-friendly. These input areas are shown in Figure 1.

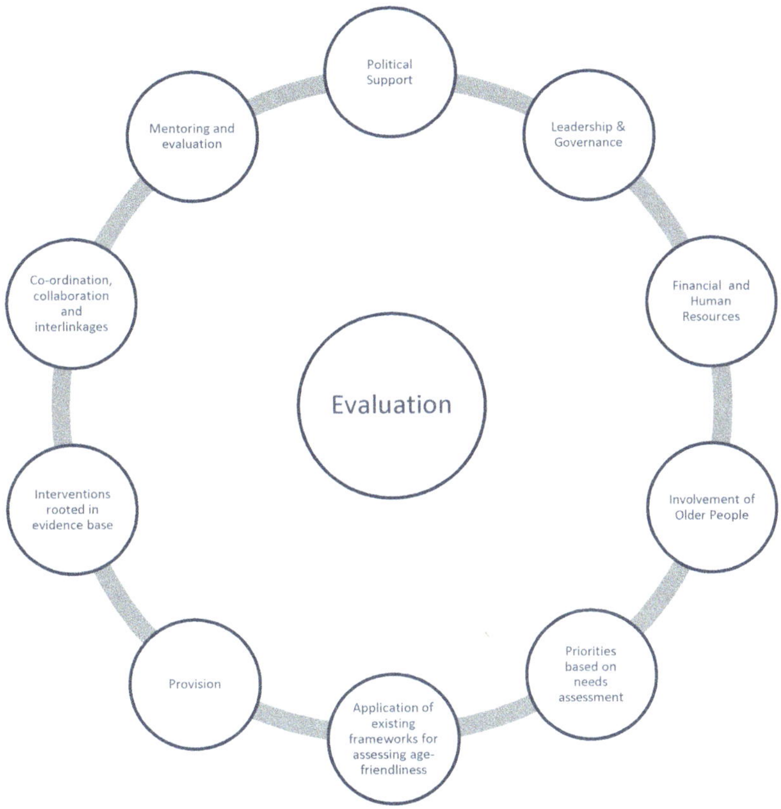
Political Support
Leadership & Governance
Financial and Human Resources
Involvement of Older People
Priorities based on needs assessment
Application of existing frameworks for assessing age-friendliness
Provision
Interventions rooted in evidence base
Co-ordination, collaboration and interlinkages
Mentoring and evaluation
Evaluation

Figure 1. Buckner et al.'s input areas.

In their conclusions they highlight the potential of the tool to act as, "an integrating framework for different city strategies that include an age-friendly agenda". They recognise that this might include adapting the ten input areas so that they can act as a generic guide and assessment framework "for and across diverse strategies", having discussed with stakeholders the potential relevance of the tool to other city-wide strategies including families, health promotion and housing.

With this in mind, future research which is co-produced with older prisoners and ex-prisoners could explore, adapt, and modify this framework, including reflection on the application of existing frameworks, so as to design and pilot a tool specifically for assessing the age-friendliness of cities and communities for prisoners, ex-prisoners and, indeed, for older people serving community penalties such as probation. This holistic, co-produced approach could gather data about older peoples' lived experiences during and after release from custody, and also prioritise the aspects of community re-entry and integration which are most important to older people, rather than focusing solely on the demands of offender management. This approach needs to adopt a realist approach, recognising that older people do not all reflect the characterisation of the positive, community-engaged older person as portrayed in the research literature, and recognising the nuances and dynamics of seeking age-friendliness. For example, whilst it is in many ways desirable to create opportunities for inter- and multi-generational contact, as exemplified in projects which build care homes and nurseries on the same site, safeguarding controls would mean that an exclusionary approach would have to be adopted for some older people if they have offended against children. A key question then is of how to create and enable beneficial inter- and multi-generational contacts within a framework of safeguarding. Conversely, some young people may themselves pose a risk to vulnerable older people, and thus again questions of how to manage inclusion come to the fore.

Buckner et al. [62] postulate that "it is the role of cities with an age-friendly agenda to create environments where higher-level influences interact with local-level policies and action in such a way as to foster active ageing and living as well as possible in older age". Some of the research literature refers to inclusion and marginalisation of some groups, including disabled older people, and a key challenge to the notion of an age-friendly city is the question of how the city includes people whom others may not want to be included, or who are socially, economically and politically marginalised. These issues go beyond questions of urban planning to become broader questions of social justice. For a city to be genuinely age-friendly it needs to be age-friendly for all older people, including those who experience imprisonment.

Funding: This research received no external funding.

Acknowledgments: Earlier versions of this paper were presented at the United Nations Celebration of the International Day of Older Persons at the UNHQ, NYC in October 2018; at the IFA Conference held in Toronto in August 2018, and at the TrentAging Conference at Trent University in May 2019. The author would like to thank the staff and residents of Haley House, Peterborough ON.

Conflicts of Interest: The author declares no conflict of interest.

References

1. Steels, S. Key characteristics of age-friendly cities and communities: A review. *Cities* **2015**, *47*, 45–52. [CrossRef]
2. Park, R.E.; Burgess, E.W. *The Cite*; University of Chicago Press: Chicago, IL, USA, 1925.
3. Shaw, C.R.; McKay, H.D. *Juvenile Delinquency and Urban Areas. A Study of Rates of Delinquents in Relation to Differential Characteristics of Local Communities in American Cities*; University of Chicago Press: Chicago, IL, USA, 1925.
4. Westwood, S. *Ageing, Diversity and Equality: Social Justice Perspectives*; Routledge: London, UK, 2018.
5. Davoren, M.; Fitzpatrick, M.; Caddow, F.; Caddow, M.; O'Neill, C.; O'Neill, H.; Kennedy, H.G. Older men and older women remand prisoners: Mental illness, physical illness, offending patterns and needs. *Int. Psychogeriatr.* **2014**, *27*, 747–755. [CrossRef] [PubMed]
6. Baidawi, S.; Turner, S.; Trotter, C.; Browning, C.; Collier, P.; O'Connor, D.; Sheehan, R. Older prisoners—A challenge for Australian corrections. *Trends Issues Crime Crim. Justice* **2011**, *461*, 421–440.
7. Human Rights Watch. *Old Behind Bars: The Aging Prison Population in the United States*; Human Rights Watch: New York, NY, USA, 2012.
8. Wahidin, A. Ageing Behind Bars with Particular Reference to Older Women prisoners in prison. *Ir. Probat. Serv.* **2011**, *8*, 109–123.
9. Aday, R.H.; Krabill, J.J. Older and Geriatric Offenders: Critical Issues for the 21st Century. In *Special Needs Offenders in Correctional Institutions*; SAGE Publications: Thousand Oaks, CA, USA, 2012; pp. 203–232.
10. Aday, R. *Aging Prisoners*; Praeger: Westport, CT, USA, 2003.
11. Hayes, A.J.; Turnbull, P.; Shaw, J.J.; Burns, A. Social and custodial needs of older adults in prison. *Age Ageing* **2013**, *42*, 589–593. [CrossRef]

12. Kim, K.; Peterson, B. *Aging Behind Bars: Trends and Implications of Graying Prisoners in the Federal Prison System*; Urban Institute: New York, NY, USA, 2014.
13. Fazel, S.; Baillargeon, J. The Health of Prisoners. *Lancet* **2011**, *377*, 956–965. [CrossRef]
14. Fazel, S.; Hope, T.; O'Donnell, I.; Piper, M.; Jacoby, R. Health of elderly male prisoners: Worse than the general population, worse than younger prisoners. *Age Ageing* **2001**, *30*, 403–407. [CrossRef]
15. Iftene, A. *Punished for Aging: Vulnerability, Rights, and Access to Justice in Canadian Penitentiaries*; University of Toronto Press: Toronto, ON, Canada, 2019.
16. Joyce, J.; Maschi, T. *In Here, Time Stands Still: The Rights, Needs and Experiences of Older People in Prison*; Irish Penal Reform Trust: Dublin, Ireland, 2016.
17. Cooney, F.; Braggins, J. *Doing Time: Good Practice with Older People in Prison—The Views of Prison Staff*; Prison Reform Trust: London, UK, 2010.
18. Ginn, S. Elderly Prisoners. *Br. Med. J.* **2012**, *345*, 24–27. [CrossRef]
19. Trotter, C.; Baidawi, S. Older prisoners: Challenges for inmates and prison management. *Aust. N. Zealand J. Criminol.* **2014**, *48*, 200–218. [CrossRef]
20. Hayes, A. Aging Inside: Older Adults in Prison. In *Emerging Issues in Prison Health*; Springer Science and Business Media LLC: Dordrecht, Germany, 2016; pp. 1–12.
21. Maschi, T.; Kaye, A. Responding to Crisis of Aging People in Prison: Global Promising Practices and Initiatives. In *Psychiatric Ethics in Late-Life Patients*; Springer Science and Business Media LLC: Cham, Switzerland, 2019; pp. 219–237.
22. Hayes, A.; Burns, A.; Turnbull, P.; Shaw, J. The health and social care needs of older male prisoners. *Int. J. Geriatr. Psychiatry* **2012**, *27*, 1155–1162. [CrossRef]
23. Forsyth, K.; Senior, J.; Stevenson, C.; O'Hara, K.; Hayes, A.J.; Challis, D.; Shaw, J. They just throw you out: Release planning for older prisoners. *Ageing Soc.* **2015**, *35*, 2011–2025. [CrossRef]
24. Brogden, M.; Nijhar, P. *Crime, Abuse and the Elderly*; Willan: Cullompton, UK, 2011.
25. Her Majesty's Inspectorate of Prisons. *No Problems—Old and Quiet: Older Prisoners in England and Wales: A Thematic Review by HM Chief Inspector of Prisons*; HMIP: London, UK, 2004.
26. HM Inspectorate of Prisons/Care Quality Commission. *Social Care in Prisons in England and Wales: A Thematic Report*; Her Majesty's Inspectorate of Prisons: London, UK, 2018.
27. Munday, D.; Leaman, J.; O'Moore, E. *Health and Social Care Needs Assessments of the Older Prison Population: A Guidance Document*; Public Health England: London, UK, 2017.
28. Eadie, T.; Grainge, P.; Jackson, J.; Safe, K.; Wilkes, J. *Good Practice Guide—Working with Older Prisoners*; RECOOP: Bournemouth, UK, 2016.
29. HM Prison & Probation Service. *Model. for Operational Delivery: Older Prisoners*; HMPPS: London, UK, 2016.
30. Prison and Probation Ombudsmen. *Learning from PPO Investigations: Older Prisoners*; HMSO: London, UK, 2017.
31. Howse, K. *Growing Old in Prison: A Scoping Study on Older Prisoners*; Prison Reform Trust: London, UK, 2003.
32. Cornish, N.; Edgar, K.; Hewson, A.; Ware, S. *Social Care or Systematic Neglect? Older People on Release from Prison*; Prison Reform Trust: London, UK, 2016.
33. Smoyer, A.B.; Madera, J.E.; Blankenship, K.M. Older adults' lived experience of incarceration. *J. Offender Rehabil.* **2019**, *58*, 220–239. [CrossRef] [PubMed]
34. Messinger, K. Death with Dignity for the Seeemingly Undignified. *J.Crim. Law Criminol.* **2019**, *109*, 633–674.
35. Bolger, M. *End of Life in Prison*; Winston Churchill Memorial Trust: London, UK, 2019.
36. Turner, M.; Peacock, M. Improving palliative care for prisoners: The 'both sides of the fence' study. *Prison Serv. J.* **2016**, *224*, 42–47.
37. Maschi, T.; Marmo, S.; Han, J. Palliative and end-of-life care in prisons: A content analysis of the literature. *Int. J. Prison. Heath* **2014**, *10*, 172–197. [CrossRef] [PubMed]
38. Merkt, H.; Haesen, S.; Meyer, L.; Kressig, R.W.; Elger, B.S.; Wangmo, T. Defining an age cut-off for older offenders: A systematic review of literature. *Int. J. Prison. Health* **2020**, *16*, 95–116. [CrossRef]
39. United Nations. *Handbook on Prisoners with Special Needs*; United Nations: New York, NY, USA, 2009.
40. Rémillard-Boilard, S. The Development of Age-Friendly Cities and Communities. In *Age-Friendly Cities and Communities: A Global Perspective*; Policy Press: Bristol, UK, 2018; pp. 13–32.
41. WHO. *Active Ageing: A Policy Framework*; WHO: Geneva, Switzerland, 2002.
42. WHO. *Global Age-Friendly Cities: A Guide*; WHO: Geneva, Switzerland, 2007.

43. Fitzgerald, K.; Caro, F.G. Introduction: International Perspectives on Age- Friendly Cities. In *International Perspectives on Age-Friendly Cities*; Routledge: Abingdon, UK, 2016; pp. 1–21.
44. Walsh, K.; O'shea, E.; Scharf, T.; Shucksmith, M. Exploring the Impact of Informal Practices on Social Exclusion and Age-Friendliness for Older People in Rural Communities. *J. Community Appl. Soc. Psychol.* **2014**, *24*, 37–49. [CrossRef]
45. Chonody, J.; Teatra, B. Livable and Age-Friendly Communities: A Scoping Review of Conceptual Concepts. *J. Aging Soc. Chang.* **2020**, *10*, 35–53. [CrossRef]
46. Plouffe, L.; Kalache, A.; Voelcker, I. A Critical Review of the WHO Age-Friendly Cities Methodology and Its Implementation. In *International Perspectives on Aging*; Springer Science and Business Media LLC: Cham, Switzerland, 2015; pp. 19–36.
47. Kashef, M. Urban livability across disciplinary and professional boundaries. *Front. Archit. Res.* **2016**, *5*, 239–253. [CrossRef]
48. Handler, S. *A Research & Evaluation Framework for Age-Friendly Cities*; UK Urban Ageing Consortium: Manchester, UK, 2014.
49. World Health Organization Centre for Health Development. *Measuring the Age-Friendliness of Cities: A Guide to Using Core Indicators*; World Health Organization Centre for Health Development: Kobe, Japan, 2015.
50. Balfour, G.; Boynton, T.; Byrne, D.; Cairns, C.; Colibaba, A.; Dieleman, C.; de Souza, H.; Skinner, M. *Community Reintegration of Aging Offenders Gaps in Knowledge Report*; Trent University: Peterborough, ON, USA, 2019.
51. Codd, H. *In the Shadow of Prison: Families, Imprisonment and Criminal Justice*; Willan: Cullompton, UK, 2008.
52. The Haven Toronto. Available online: https://www.haventoronto.ca/ (accessed on 1 May 2020).
53. Haesen, S.; Merkt, H.; Imber, A.; Elger, B.; Wangmo, T. Substance use and other mental health disorders among older prisoners. *Int. J. Law Psychiatry* **2019**, *62*, 20–31. [CrossRef]
54. Pope, N.D.; Buchino, S.; Ascienzo, S. Just like Jail: Trauma Experiences of Older Homeless Men. *J. Gerontol. Soc. Work* **2020**, *63*, 143–161. [CrossRef] [PubMed]
55. Wyse, J. Older Men's Social Integration After Prison. *Int. J. Offender Ther. Comp. Criminol.* **2018**, *62*, 2153–2173. [CrossRef] [PubMed]
56. Hodgson, J.; Roach, K. Disenfranchisement as Punishment: European Court of Human Rights, UK and Canadian Responses to Prisoner Voting. *Public Law* **2017**, *3*, 250–268.
57. Visher, C.A.; Debus-Sherrill, S.A.; Yahner, J. Employment After Prison: A Longitudinal Study of Former Prisoners. *Justice Q.* **2011**, *28*, 698–718. [CrossRef]
58. Ramakers, A.; Van Wilsem, J.A.; Nieuwbeerta, P.; Dirkzwager, A.J.E. Returning to a Former Employer: A Potentially Successful Pathway to Ex-prisoner Re-employment. *Br. J. Criminol.* **2015**, *56*, 668–688. [CrossRef]
59. Sheppard, A.; Ricciardelli, R. Employment after prison: Navigating conditions of precarity and stigma. *Eur. J. Probat.* **2020**, *1*, 34–52. [CrossRef]
60. Crawley, E. Institutional Thoughtlessness in Prisons and Its Impacts on the Day-to-Day Prison Lives of Elderly Men. *J. Contemp. Crim. Justice* **2005**, *21*, 350–363. [CrossRef]
61. Cadet, N. Institutional thoughtlessness and the needs of older probation clients. *Probat. J.* **2020**, *67*, 118–136. [CrossRef]
62. Buckner, S.; Pope, D.; Mattocks, C.; LaFortune, L.; Dherani, M.; Bruce, N. Developing Age-Friendly Cities: An Evidence-Based Evaluation Tool. *J. Popul. Ageing* **2019**, *12*, 203–223. [CrossRef]

International Journal of
Environmental Research and Public Health

MDPI

Case Report

Knowing, Being and Co-Constructing an Age-Friendly Tāmaki Makaurau Auckland

Judy Blakey [1,*] and Janet Clews [2]

[1] Comprehensive Care PHO, Auckland 0632, New Zealand
[2] The Trusts Community Foundation Ltd., Auckland 0650, New Zealand; jernie@xtra.co.nz
* Correspondence: judy.blakey@gmail.com

Received: 31 October 2020; Accepted: 30 November 2020; Published: 7 December 2020

check for updates

Abstract: A third of Aotearoa New Zealand's increasingly ageing population resides in Tāmaki Makaurau Auckland. This most populous cosmopolitan urban area in the country is also home to the largest Polynesian population of any global city. Sprawling across a North Island isthmus inclusive of Hauraki Gulf islands, 70% of the city region is rural, whilst almost 90% of the ethnically diverse residents live in urban areas. Members of Auckland Council's Seniors Advisory Panel (SAP) advocated for, and in 2018 secured unanimous support from the governing body to resource an Age-friendly City (AFC) Project. This case study inquiry applied bricolage methodology to provide diverse contextual perspectives of this unique Polynesian setting, prior to exploring interview narratives of three SAP members who served two consecutive terms (six years) as AFC advocates. Weaving insights gleaned from their interview transcripts responding to relational leadership prompts about their age-friendly advocacy with the findings from the council's AFC Community Engagement report highlighted the achievements and challenges of the evolving AFC Project. Service-learning recommendations include co-developing: (1) A sustainable co-governance framework for an independent steering group that embodies the values and principles of Te Tiriti o Waitangi to enable empowered active ageing for all residents; (2) A succession plan that enables the timely transfer of knowledge and skills to empower incoming SAP members.

Keywords: age-friendly; Tāmaki Makaurau Auckland; Polynesian population; relational leadership; Te Tiriti o Waitangi

---

1. Introduction

An increasing number of countries are responding to the challenges associated with demographic changes and population ageing; challenges that have been amplified by the disruptive impact of the coronavirus pandemic [1]. Planning for the diverse implications of these changes in longevity and age structure has highlighted the need for greater investment in improving how societies age [2].

Combining demographic, economic, health and social gerontology models that explore optimizing participation in various roles and domains of life [3], the multi-dimensional concept of Active Ageing [4] has provided the most useful contemporary policy response to demographic ageing [5]. Emphasizing the link between activity and health that challenges the deficit model [6], expectations related to the three original Active Ageing pillars of participation, health and security identified by the World Health Organization (WHO) [7] are typically framed by researchers and policy makers, rather than older people themselves [8]. An emergent "good active ageing" conceptual and policy framework has added learning, ethical and moral foundations prescient within the context of deep technological, economic and social change, to create an additional Active Ageing pillar [9].

To translate the Active Ageing policy agenda into urban environments [10] the WHO initially collaborated with partners in 35 cities from high, middle, and low-income countries [11]. Guided by the

Vancouver protocol's methodological requirements, the project identified eight core age-friendly features that supported the dynamic ecological interplay between individual adaptation and environmental alteration [12] to optimize residents functioning as they aged. The resulting WHO Global Age-friendly Cities Guide [13] and companion checklist [14] captured the imagination of planners and connected with the zeitgeist of ageing communities across the globe. Currently the WHO's Global Network comprises 1000 cities and communities in 41 countries that impacts the lives of 240 million people [15].

The growth in the WHO's Global Network of Age-friendly Cities and Communities (AFCC) [16] has in turn generated a vast number of research publications [17–20]. Torku et al.'s (2020) systematic review of 98 AFCC publications observed that although AFCC are driven by community-led processes, major initiatives demand strong and committed political leadership and "top-down" support for implementing the 'bottom-up' community development age-friendly action plans [20]. A review commissioned to support the implementation of AFCC in Aotearoa New Zealand concluded that AFCC processes and initiatives need to have in-built flexibility that recognize local geographic and demographic diversity, and include the needs of indigenous Māori, Pacific and other cultural groups [19]. The review also stated that older people should be involved in all stages of the development of processes and plans for AFCC, and that their voices should be heard with respect and dignity [19].

In the UK, a Manchester-based age-friendly movement manifesto articulated a new urban agenda that focused on issues concerned with inequality and empowerment [10]. This noted the need for creative participatory research methods [21] and the development of interdisciplinary networks to generate comparative insights [22] and critical awareness of those who may be socially marginalized in the face of urban change.

The global pandemic has highlighted the need to protect older people's health and wellbeing. However, in Aotearoa New Zealand the downstream impact of past and contemporary colonization has caused and sustained intergenerational social, economic and health equity disadvantages, that have resulted in higher hospitalization and death rates for Māori during previous pandemics [23]. Prioritizing mitigating COVID-19's impact without increasing existing health inequities, the current pandemic response has nudged health and wellbeing service providers to examine if continuation under a business-as-usual model will preferentially benefit Pākehā (European) New Zealanders, and fail to protect Māori from the worst outcomes [23]? That question informs this research, which embraces community-based participatory research methodology [24] to co-construct narratives of Tāmaki Makaurau Auckland's evolving Age-friendly City (AFC) Project from the perspectives of four older community leaders and AFC champions. The narratives offer contextual details of the city's sprawling location and demographic contours of her older residents; summarise achieving AFC Project milestones that challenged ageism and created visibility of the needs of older residents in Auckland Council's research, planning and policy work; and articulate the community leaders' perceptions of the challenges and risks (both personal and organizational) associated with the AFC Project.

2. Materials and Methods

Bricolage research methodology embraces the complexity of researching lived experiences by applying critical methods that address the plurality and power dynamics of knowledge production [25,26]. In this research context the authors-as-research-participants explore interpretive bricolage as an activist scholarship inquiry process [27] to develop and inform a fuller understanding of multiple perspectives and texts that reflect diverse voices and information sources pertinent to Tāmaki Makaurau Auckland's emergent Age-friendly Action Plan [19,28,29].

Six contiguous sections reveal the selected contextual and methodological layers within this bricolage inquiry [30]. The first section introduces Tāmaki Makaurau Auckland's unique Polynesian setting [31], including the city's governance framework [32], Aotearoa New Zealand's founding indigenous document, *Te Tiriti o Waitangi* [27,33] and salient demographic contours of the city's residents [19]. The second section provides historical insights about the evolving Age-friendly Auckland

Project [34,35] highlighting the two SAP's achievements. Section three situates and elaborates on methodological challenges associated with autoethnographic inquiries [36] as a segue to the fourth section describing the processes involved in using relational leadership interview prompts [37,38] to elicit the narratives of older co-researchers active in progressing Tāmaki Makaurau Auckland's evolving Age-friendly City (AFC) agenda [39]. Section five describes the research participants, and section six explains the methods used to analyse the interview transcripts.

2.1. The Place: Our Unique Polynesian Setting

Māori, who are the indigenous people (mana whenua) of Aotearoa New Zealand, have lived in Tāmaki Makaurau for over 1000 years [40]. Tāmaki is the Māori name for Auckland and means desired by many; a name that alludes to the desirable qualities of the land, volcanic cones, mountains, waters, harbours and 3700 km coastline that first attracted Māori to settle in the isthmus. Founded in 1840 as a colonial settlement by British naval officer William Hobson, the clusters of modest dwellings and trading ports have evolved over the intervening 180 years into one of the largest urban areas in Australasia [31].

Two harbours, an extensive volcanic field and two mountain ranges have shaped Auckland's urban morphology, which has been characterised by sprawling low-density development, with residents reliant on private motor vehicles for mobility [41]. The new millennium has ushered in more medium density housing developments and apartments, particularly in the city centre, but also in fringe areas. Transport infrastructure has also received considerable investment, bringing train into the city and a busway to Auckland's North Shore, with a significant increase in public transport patronage [31].

2.1.1. Auckland Council Governance Processes

In 2010 central government's Royal Commission on Auckland Governance recommended the amalgamation of eight existing territorial authorities into a single Auckland Council [42]. The resulting "Super City" shares governance functions across a governing body (comprising an elected mayor and 20 councillors) that focuses on regional strategic decisions and 21 local boards whose members focus on local issues, activities and facilities. In addition, a number of council controlled organisations deliver a range of services to residents and visitors (e.g., transport, water, property development and management, regional facilities, and tourism and events). An Independent Māori Statutory Board ensures the views of local Māori residents—inclusive of both mana whenua (residents who have ancestral relationships with at least one of the 19 designated tribal groupings within Tāmaki Makaurau) and matāwaka (residents whose tribal ancestors settled outside the region) —are taken into account [32].

Auckland is experiencing sustained population growth, and future projections indicate the 2018 Census measure of 1.6 million residents will exceed 2 million by 2030, maintaining the demand for equitable and accessible housing, transport and employment solutions [31]. Ethnically and culturally diverse, the city is currently home to people from over 120 ethnicities [43]. The Auckland Plan 2050 highlights the rapid growth in the numbers and proportion of older residents (included because of the strong advocacy of the Seniors Advisory Panel's March 2018 "Focus on the Future" forum, amongst other consultation feedback), which will impact on the demand for and provision of health, support, and transport services [44]. Auckland Council provides opportunities to engage diverse community perspectives on a range of regional policies, plans and strategies through meetings and workshops with demographic and sector advisory panels [45]. The panel members also advise the council about any matters of particular concern relevant to their respective communities [32].

The Auckland Plan 2050's shared values of Atawhai (Kindness, generosity), Kotahi (strength in diversity), Auaha (creativity, innovation), Pono (integrity) and Taonga tuku iho (future generations) [46] (p. 23) express the contemporary ethos of Auckland's unique cultural heritage. In addition, the explicit focus within the plan on developing and nurturing partnerships with local Māori to position Māori aspirations at the heart of ethical strategic actions breathes life into Auckland Council's statutory obligations to honour the principles articulated in Aotearoa New Zealand's founding document, *Te Tiriti o Waitangi (te Tiriti)/The Treaty of Waitangi (The Treaty)* [46] (p. 58).

2.1.2. Te Tiriti o Waitangi

Signed in 1840 by Māori leaders and representatives of the British Crown, the Auckland Plan 2050 acknowledges the specific obligations that Auckland Council has as a delegate of the Crown to Māori under *te Tiriti* [46] (2050 Print). Māori political action has ensured that *te Tiriti* has assumed a progressively significant place in legislation, jurisprudence, social and economic life in Aotearoa New Zealand [47] (Barnes). Treaty principles that have emerged have been expressed through a range of courts and the Waitangi Tribunal [46], however, integrating them into effective policies and strategies that identify and address the underlying social determinants of systemic inequalities resulting from colonization continues to challenge sector agencies [48,49].

The preamble to *te Tiriti* foreshadows the content of the articles that follow by focusing on authentic relationship building processes (whanaungatanga) which recognize each party's sphere of influence and ways of relating to facilitate power sharing, mutual respect and understanding [27]. Recognising the crucial links between *te Tiriti* and effective health promotion practice, Berghan et al. (2017) state: "*Te Tiriti o Waitangi (te Tiriti)* legitimises settler presence in Aotearoa New Zealand and governance by the British Crown. Therefore, *te Tiriti* must lie at the heart of ethical health promotion in this country." [27] (p. 8). They explain that health promotion practices enabling people to take control over their health align with strategic principles and values expressed in *te Tiriti,* particularly developing reciprocal partnerships, providing active protection, empowering informed decision making, enabling self-determination and evaluating equitable outcomes.

Building relationships through sharing experiences and working collaboratively provides a strong basis for an intercultural Auckland [46] (p. 32). In 2018, the neighbouring city of Hamilton, which is 130 km south of Auckland, became the first New Zealand and 600th global city to join the WHO's AFCC Global Network [16,50]. Similar social processes are implicit in the community development activities that preceded, informed and shaped the city of Hamilton's age-friendly action plan [51].

2.1.3. The People: Demographic Contours

The Auckland Plan 2050 reports that Tāmaki Makaurau Auckland has always been ethnically diverse, and that migration patterns in the past two decades have substantially increased the numbers of Asian People living in Tāmaki Makaurau Auckland [52]. Data presented in Table 1 reveal the comparative percentages of New Zealand and Tāmaki Makaurau Auckland residents who self-identified with one of the four main ethnic groups (European, Asian, Māori and Pacific Peoples) in the 2018 Census. The term "Asian people" is a very broad category that includes a range of national origins and ethnic identities with Chinese, Indian, Korean, Filipino and Sri Lankan communities comprising the five largest Asian groups in Tāmaki Makaurau Auckland [52]. The Middle Eastern/Latin American/African (2.3%) and "Other ethnicity" (1.1%) groups in Tāmaki Makaurau Auckland are not included in Table 1 due to the relatively small percentages of people included in these extremely diverse ethnic categories [53]. The adjacent Aucklanders' median ages column reveals that both the Māori (24.9 years) and Pacific Peoples' (24.0 years) are relatively youthful populations in comparison with the European (oldest at 39.4 years) and Asian (31.9 years) populations.

Table 2's presentation of median ages across Tāmaki Makaurau Auckland's 21 local boards alongside the percentage and numbers of residents aged 65 plus provides a more nuanced appreciation of the geographic dispersion of ethnic ageing across the region. The data reveal that larger numbers of older European and Asian residents reside on Auckland's Hauraki Gulf Islands and suburbs north and east of the central city [52]; while the more youthful Māori and Pasifika residents have gravitated to suburbs in the south and west. 2018 Census data show nearly a quarter (23.4%) of the total Māori population in Aotearoa New Zealand live in Tāmaki Makaurau, with one in nine (11.5%) city residents identifying as Māori. Only five percent of Māori were aged 65 years or older; however, the 45.9%

growth in that age group was considerably faster than the 26.9% growth rate for the overall usually resident Māori population [54].

Māori migration from rural to urban areas accelerated at the end of World War II, encouraged by government policies and incentives to stimulate post war industry and boost employment [55]. The downstream impact of these policies has meant that many urban Māori have had to face significant disadvantages such as inadequate housing, racial discrimination, unemployment and the erosion of their language, culture and identity when they were discouraged from speaking their language (Te Reo Māori) in schools or workplaces [56].

Barnes and McCreanor's (2019) essay addresses the stories of the historical trauma Māori experienced as evidenced in the trajectory of population health disparities over time, which reveal how migrant settler communities flourished at the expense of local Māori. They write: "The lived experience of injustice, brutality, deprivation, and marginalisation has been transmitted across multiple generations, aggravated by land loss, economic disempowerment, poverty, disease and racism that are reflected in diverse statistics of disparity and particularly as we have agreed, in health and wellbeing." [47] (p. 23). The accumulative impact of these traumatic multi-generational losses is evident in the lower life expectancy statistics for both Māori and Pacific Peoples compared with European and Asian groups in Aotearoa New Zealand (See Table 1).

Table 1. Comparative ethnic profiles in New Zealand and Tāmaki Makaurau Auckland showing ethnic groups' median ages for Auckland residents and population level life expectancy at birth.

Ethnic Groups	2018 Census % of New Zealanders Who Self-Identified [a]	2018 Census % of Aucklanders Who Self-Identified [b]	2018 Census Aucklanders' Median Ages (Years) [c]	2012–2014 NZ Female Life Exp. at Birth (Years) [d]	2012–2014 NZ Male Life Exp. at Birth (Years) [d]
European	70.2%	53.5%	39.4	83.9	80.3
Asian	15.1%	28.2%	31.9	87.2	84.4
Māori	16.5%	11.5%	24.9	77.1	73.0
Pacific Peoples	8.1%	15.5%	24.0	78.7	74.5

Data sources include: [a] Stats NZ 2018 Census population and dwelling counts [57]. [b] Stats NZ 2018 Census Place Summaries Auckland Region [53]. [c] Auckland Council Research and Evaluation Unit (RIMU): *Māori in Tāmaki Makaurau* [54]. [d] Ministry of Social Development: *Health Life expectancy at birth report* with 2012–2014 data [58].

Over the past 150 years Pacific Peoples have also settled in Tāmaki Makaurau Auckland. During that period of time two significant waves of migration in the 1960s and later the 1970s saw the initial small immigrant community in search of employment, educational opportunities and/or for family reasons, grow into one of considerable size and social significance [59]. Mainly from Polynesian islands with historical connections to Aotearoa New Zealand (such as Samoa, Tonga, the Cook Islands and Niue), the Pacific population is the youngest of all the main ethnic groups and continues to grow mainly through natural increase, but also migration. Depending on the future impact of climate change in the Pacific nations current migration projections could change. The 2018 Census data show that two thirds (63.9%) of Pacific Peoples live in Auckland, compared with a quarter (25.5%) of those who identified as European [60]. The nearly one quarter of a million Auckland residents who identified as Pasifika Peoples represented a 25.1% increase since 2013. As with Māori, a relatively small proportion of the Pasifika population (5.6%) is 65 years or older, but the 38.7% increase in older Pacific Peoples is much faster than the overall growth rate for the entire Auckland-based Pasifika population [60].

Salesa has observed that Auckland is often called the world's largest Polynesian city, but that in reality most residents lived next door to that city [61]. Table 2 data provide glimpses of why Salesa stated that Tāmaki Makaurau Auckland was heading towards a population of "old white people and young brown people: the fastest growing group of babies are Māori and Pasifika, and the caregivers for elderly Pākehā (Europeans) will be Pasifika, Māori and Asian" [61] (p. 2). Salesa concluded that policy implications for our shared Pacific future would require greater attention also be paid to young Māori and Pasifika People's education, training, health and wellbeing [62].

Table 2. Tāmaki Makaurau Auckland's 21 local boards ranked from oldest to youngest by median age, alongside the percentage and the actual numbers of residents aged 65+ years [1].

#	Local Board (Island/Location) (North/West/South/East/Central)		Median Ages (Years)	% of Residents Aged 65+	Residents Aged 65+
1	Aotea/Great Barrier	(Island)	52.9	24.5%	234
2	Waiheke	(Island)	46.5	20.9%	1893
3	Rodney	(North)	42.2	16.7%	11,088
4	Hibiscus and Bays	(North)	41.2	17.6%	18,357
5	Franklin	(South)	40.5	15.1%	11,304
6	Orakei	(East)	40.0	15.8%	13,329
7	Devonport-Takapuna	(North)	39.4	16.3%	9426
8	Howick	(East)	37.3	13.5%	19,086
9	Waitakere Ranges	(West)	36.8	10.4%	5403
10	Upper Harbour	(North)	35.7	12.1%	7605
11	Kaipatiki	(North)	34.8	11.6%	10,257
12	Whau	(West)	34.4	12.2%	9618
13	Albert-Eden	(Central)	34.2	10.1%	9945
14	Puketapapa	(West)	33.8	12.1%	7014
15	Henderson-Massey	(West)	33.1	10.4%	12,336
16	Maungakiekie-Tāmaki	(East)	33.0	10.6%	8115
17	Papakura	(South)	32.0	10.5%	6069
18	Waitematā	(Central)	31.4	7.9%	6546
19	Manurewa	(South)	29.5	8.3%	7980
20	Otara-Papatoetoe	(South)	29.1	8.2%	6963
21	Māngere-Otahuhu	(South)	29.0	8.5%	6642
	Tāmaki Makaurau Auckland		34.7	12.0%	189,210

[1] Auckland Council Research and Evaluation Unit (RIMU). 2018 Census Results, local board and special area information sheets [63].

2.2. *Ka Mua, Ka Muri (A Māori Proverb That Means "Walking Backwards into the Future"): Co-Constructing Our Age-Friendly Futures*

In 2014 Auckland Council convened the first Seniors Advisory Panel (SAP) (2014–2016). In their final report the SAP noted, "from the outset, the panel made it clear that Auckland should become part of the World Health Organisation (WHO) international network of Age-friendly Cities, if it was to be the world's most liveable city." [34] (p. 3). Despite encountering political and administrative roadblocks that thwarted them during their term the SAP advocated for the rapidly increasing number of seniors who were contributing to Auckland's expanding diversity. Their advocacy resulted in Auckland Council commissioning research to gauge seniors' wellbeing and the production of *Older Aucklanders: A Quality of Life Status Report 2017* [64]. The report reviewed domains and indicators in the New Zealand government's Positive Ageing Strategy [65,66] and the WHO's AFCC [16] and provided useful baseline evidence to cite in support of on-going age-friendly advocacy.

The eight seniors (three Māori and five European/Pākeha) selected to serve on the second SAP (2017–2019) were united in their quest to progress the age-friendly agenda, and on 10 July 2018 the governing body's Environment and Community Committee resolved unanimously to join the WHO's global AFCC network [35]. Subsequent resource allocation by the council enabled Auckland's AFC Project Community Engagement work to begin. Connected to the Belonging and Participation strategic outcomes in the Auckland Plan 2050 [46], the AFC Project's purpose was "to develop a region-wide cross sector action plan" [39] (p. 5). Engagement focused on eight policy domains comprising the WHO's Age-friendly framework, with an additional (ninth) Culture and Diversity domain. Written feedback from twenty community workshops and facilitated conversations attended by over 600 mainly older residents and staff from community organisations providing services for older adults was merged with responses to two different surveys.

Survey respondents aged 15–100 years included: 449 "Have Your Say" online and translated hardcopy survey (including Mandarin, Samoan and Tongan) respondents aged 55 years and older, but mostly in the 65–84 age group, with 19% Asian, 16% Pasifika and 3% Māori respondents; 2232 "People's Panel" online respondents, mostly European/Pākehā female, with 5% Māori, 4% Asian and 3% Pasifika respondents. The 21% People's Panel response rate was considerably higher than the usual 12% survey response rate and demonstrated the significance of the AFC Project for Aucklanders. Community feedback revealing the needs and aspirations of older residents is summarized in the Findings Report [39] and presented in Table 3 below.

Table 3. Age-friendly Auckland Project's Key Community Engagement Messages [1].

#	WHO Age-Friendly Framework Domains
1	Outdoor Spaces and Buildings: ■ Accessible and safe journeys from public transport or finding parking through to getting into buildings and accessing indoor and outdoor activities. ■ Public amenities in the places we go that are clean, accessible and well maintained. We feel more comfortable when both gender specific and unisex toilets are available.
2	Transportation: ■ Safe and accessible roads, footpaths, public transport, transport hubs and everything in between that accommodate different abilities and modes of transport. ■ Our transport journey to be seamless. We need accessible parking options, seating and weather protection at stops and drivers to wait until we are seated on public transport.
3	Housing: ■ Affordable housing for all, across Auckland. ■ We need housing options that are universally designed to allow us to age in place. Different housing types, models and sizes.
4	Social Participation: ■ We need barrier free access to transport, facilities, activities, outdoor spaces and events. ■ Affordable activities, programmes and venues for our groups.
5	Respect and Inclusion: ■ Visibility, positive images, diversity and stories of older Aucklanders. ■ Intergenerational respect and understanding—our lives, choices and diversity.
6	Civic Participation and Employment: ■ We need employment options and ways to transition from full-time employment to part-time work, flexible work, volunteering or retirement, which recognize our changing circumstances, abilities and the contribution we want to make. ■ Opportunities for lifelong learning.
7	Communication and Information: ■ Places to access information and get affordable support and training so we can keep up with technology. ■ Information and news about community matters, services, events and activities provided in a range of formats, across multiple channels and ideally in our own language.
8	Community Support and Health Services: ■ Accessible healthcare—services to be where we need them, when we need them. Mobile facilities that go to the places where we are. ■ We need affordable healthcare services and support, including dentistry.
9	Culture and Diversity: ■ An open, friendly and inclusive society of all cultures, where there is care, respect and all people are valued. ■ Opportunities for connection with our own culture, other cultures and intergenerationally.

[1] Compiled from pages 2–4 of the Age-friendly Auckland Project Community Engagement Findings Report [39].

The merged community feedback was condensed into four conceptual pathways that offer exploratory opportunities of working together for lasting change [67]. The four pathways included: (1) Enabling greater connection between older people and the world; (2) Recognising the individuality and diversity of older people; (3) Creating clear and accessible information pathways; and (4) Making everyday life easier for older people. Since the establishment of the inaugural SAP in 2014 Panel members have traversed each of these pathways in their advocacy and advice proffered to create and enhance awareness of the potential intergenerational and cross-cultural benefits throughout the life course associated with age-friendly communities [4,19].

2.3. Framing Autoethnographic Lived Experience

As the authors of this article traversed the boundaries between researchers and research participants, it is instructive to provide clarifying details about their social locations [68]. Firstly, this article's collaborative co-production processes involved discussing the ethical implications of participant involvement [24] and secured the informed consent of fellow two-term members of the Auckland Council SAP. Secondly, given the dearth of older co-researcher-participants in Age-friendly publications and the need to confront challenges associated with democratizing knowledge production [69], this bricolage inquiry weaves auto-ethnographic threads into the text [36]. Thirdly, the sudden and unexpected introduction of a maximum two-term limit at the start of 2020 for those serving on the council's six Demographic Advisory Panels raised concerns about the lack of continuity in community leadership on the SAP at a time when developing the AFC Action Plan would involve "Working with council teams, community partners and organisations, informed by the community engagement to develop a plan that will make a real difference to older Aucklanders" [39] (p. 9).

2.4. Interview Method

The dynamic flux of past, present and future collaborative interactions adds a temporal structure to this inquiry [30]. Temporal flux is apparent in the fifteen relational leadership interview prompts that were originally developed to glean how service-learning partnerships between community agencies and institutions of higher learning in New England (USA) evolved over time [37]. Enhancing understanding of community partnership processes and outcomes in organisations hosting tertiary students, the interview prompts focused specifically on revealing the voices of community partners to elucidate "their knowledge, attitudes and skills" so that "deeper insights can be mined about growing and sustaining partnerships" [38] (p. 2). Furthermore, three specific leadership proficiencies of: knowing (especially sharing a common purpose to facilitate empowering participatory citizenship through ethical decision making that promotes and supports community processes); being (especially expressing hopeful commitments to socially responsible power sharing that promotes equity, values integrity and develops systems thinking perspectives); and doing (especially involving others in co-creating visions to identify goals, build coalitions and nurture reflective learning capacities) proved to be foundational in collective cooperative relationships among people striving to achieve positive change [70].

The semi-structured interview guide development followed Kallio et al.'s (2016) recommended phases [71]. Doraldo and Giles' (2004) fifteen prompts were identified as suitable for the current research setting and adapted by the lead author who changed the generic reference in the prompts from "the project" to "Auckland Council's Age-friendly City (AFC) project" (refer Table A1 in Appendix A). The lead author then used these adapted prompts in semi-structured individual interviews of three fellow two-term SAP members, to elicit their in-depth responses about Auckland Council's AFC Project. The initial interview of the SAP (2017–2019) chairperson as a key informant affirmed the internal validity of the interview protocol. The subsequent two interviews demonstrated that the protocol was flexible enough to allow for clear differences and similarities to emerge and for the interviewer, who was very familiar with the topic, to probe further, where appropriate [71].

2.5. Participants

Participatory inquiry processes involved discussions amongst four older Pākehā (European) community leaders, who served two terms (2014–2016 and 2017–2019) on Auckland Council's Seniors Advisory Panel (SAP) over a period of six years. Aged between 71 and 93 years, two of the three female research participants (the oldest, J.L.R., and the youngest, lead author, J.B.) reside, respectively, in the Kaipatiki and Hibiscus and Bays Local Board areas on the North Shore; the third female (co-author J.C. who is 87 years) lives in the Waitakere Ranges Local Board area to the west of the central city and the male research participant (R.F.—aged 72 years) lives in the Māngere-Otahuhu Local Board area in the south (See Figure 1 below). J.C. and R.F. are New Zealand born, whilst J.L.R. and J.B. are South African born migrants who settled in Aotearoa New Zealand 30–40 years ago.

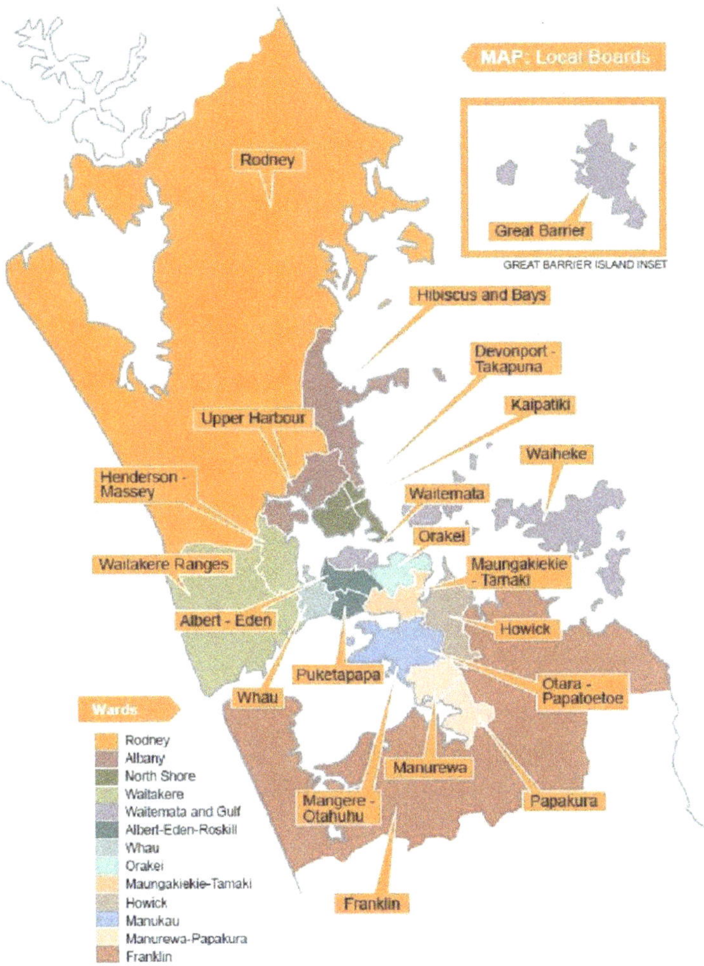

Figure 1. Map showing the locations of Tāmaki Makaurau's 21 local boards. Map source [72].

Face-to-face interviews were conducted in late February 2020 in J.L.R. and J.C.'s homes, and a telephone interview with the third community leader (R.F.) in early March 2020. The three audio-recorded interviews ranged in length from 33:58 to 48:22 minutes and were transcribed verbatim. Each participant received their verbatim transcript to verify and edit, prior to confirming their informed consent that the lead author apply a relational leadership model (RLM) lens [38] to extract evidence of leadership components and narrative themes from their transcripts.

2.6. Data Analysis

The visible expressions of older community leaders' ways of knowing, being and doing in the current inquiry context [38] are linked to the five core leadership components identified by Komives, Lucas and McMahon (2013) in their relational leadership model (RLM) [70].

A narrative analysis of the verbatim interview transcripts afforded the co-authors opportunities to explore how individual and collective community leadership experiences influenced and supported advancing the SAP's shared age-friendly vision for Tāmaki Makaurau Auckland [73].

The transcripts were initially read and explored individually to glean an understanding of their emergent structure and thematic content. That procedure offered valuable insights about collective collaborative processes and networks which established pragmatic strategic links [74] to set aside roadblocks and facilitate the activation of age-friendly initiatives within the council and across the region.

The three transcripts were then merged to create a combined (collective) transcript structured in question order, which was shared with the co-author. The lead author read through a printout of the combined transcripts and coded the text to identify the prevalence of five different RLM leadership components (purposeful, inclusive, empowering, ethical and process-oriented) in the transcribed responses. A framework analysis grid [75] comprising 15 columns (one for each interview prompt) and five rows (one for each RLM leadership component) was populated column by column with the initials of those participants whose responses revealed one or more of the five RLM leadership components. The resulting visual synopsis revealed the leadership component response profiles of each participant and the collective distribution of leadership components within and across the 15 interview prompts. A visual inspection of the patterns of collective leadership components across the 15 interview prompts offered evidence of the influence of dynamic temporal flux across the participant responses, which were grounded in the present but reflected on the past and anticipated a more age-friendly future [30].

3. Results

Despite sharing a common vision of an age-friendly Tāmaki Makaurau Auckland, noticeable differences emerged in the purposeful intent and focus of the three participants' interview responses; an observation that provides glimpses of the nuanced nature of diversity in later life [76,77]. Accordingly, the results initially focus on the differing community leadership experiences and divergent expressions of knowing, being and co-constructing age-friendly processes and initiatives [38]. The collective narrative offers shared insights about temporal flux and loss in momentum of the AFC Project, in addition to mitigating resistance to progressing an AFC agenda, and the generative value of lifelong learning [78]. Table 4 (below) summarises these findings.

Table 4. Heterogeneity and shared insights in the relational leadership interview narratives.

	Heterogeneity		Shared Insights
1.	Constructing purposeful and ethical leadership (J.C.)	1.	Dynamic temporal flux and loss in momentum of Tāmaki Makaurau Auckland's AFC Project
2.	Voicing hopeful optimism for more inclusive local age-friendly activities (J.L.R.)	2.	Mitigating resistance to progressing the AFC agenda
3.	Empowering more inclusive access to transport mobility (R.F.)	3.	Lifelong learning

3.1. Heterogeneity in the Age-Friendly Relational Leadership Interview Narratives

Participant narratives are presented in the chronological order the interviews were conducted. The narratives begin with the first two interview prompt responses (Q1 and Q2) that describe each participant's role/personal involvement and their motivation for participating in Auckland Council's AFC Project. The subsequent narrative structure reflects insights gleaned from participant descriptions of and reflections on their prior experiences in community projects similar to the AFC Project that mainly focus on their Q10 and Q11 responses. Details about relevant age-friendly contributions of community partners and networks (Q3 and Q12 responses) conclude and provide a backdrop for the subsequent focus on the dynamic temporal flux noted, especially when encountering and mitigating resistance to integrating AFC concepts within the council.

3.1.1. Constructing Purposeful and Ethical Relational Leadership

The Chair of the 2017–2019 SAP was the first participant interviewed. J.C.'s introductory responses revealed her purposeful, yet patient intent evident from the outset in her role as chair of the second SAP: *We both got involved at the very beginning, really, on the first panel* (which was advocating registration with the WHO's global network of Age-friendly Cities, but encountered political and administrative resistance) ... *and because of the way the (inaugural) panel was treated and the end point that first panel came to, we were so cross that we became absolutely determined to take that as our main plank forward; um, supposing they allowed us to remain on the panel.* This comment revealed J.C.'s appreciation of the fact that council processes and staff determined the SAP membership.

Referring to her prior experiences J.C. explained that she drew on a deep well of community involvement: In my 55 years or whatever it is of working in the community as an elected representative, it is a case again of conviction. I guess you have to say something about integrity, and by that, I mean having proved yourself to be able to walk the talk, as it were; come up with what you promised; never over promise. Well I had to fight for five years to make sure we got our new library ... We did get our new library in the end, but we also got a set of traffic lights ... there as a mark, as far as I see it, to the occasional bad things that happen in council because that was delayed; but, on the other side, by delaying it we actually got a better outcome all around. Ethical and process-oriented leadership components evident in the interview extract above typify J.C.'s open and transparent collaborative interactions to facilitate achieving empowering community outcomes.

Reflecting on any potential lessons learned from past experiences J.C.'s empathetic relational intelligence [79] and awareness of connecting with community members was readily apparent: *I think I just worked in my normal way of working, which is collaboratively. I've always tried to be empathetic where necessary. And I've had that comment made to me too, before, about the way I've worked with people. Because when you're chairing things like the annual plan or the long-term plan in committee and you see people coming in on a regular basis, you know what's going on sometimes in their lives. And that's where you can show that empathy without it looking like you're trying to be smart. Because you're not. You're only trying to help them cope with what's going on. ... And it's community. And community is so important. It doesn't matter what size it is. Start at the bottom; small and grow. That's where you go.*

J.C.'s deep knowledge of central and local government ecology and networks salient for progressing an age-friendly agenda was instrumental in developing and strengthening alliances and processes to mitigate the resistance the inaugural SAP experienced. She explained: *Well we were fortunate because the government had moved, with Hon. Tracey Martin (Minister for Seniors), and had already got themselves into the AFCC network on behalf of the country, which in theory should make it easier for others to follow. I'm not sure that's necessarily the case, but still it's a good point because we knew then that we had support from a ministerial level.*

J.C. went on to describe collaborative process-oriented doing actions the SAP took to ensure that the politicians and council staff were better informed about the WHO's AFCC network, and the staff appropriately resourced to deliver what was required: *The Mayor and council we felt had to be convinced, and so we set about putting in place a strategy to convince them. Staff were a different matter, because of course, their masters are the council. And we had no obvious way to change their role, because it's quite prescriptive—their work programme is set and funded. We were no longer in quite the right way included within their work programme. What we wanted to happen was not happening in the way we would like it to. As for the external partners, it depends I suppose who you're looking at? Service providers or "other stakeholders" in inverted commas, some of which are not actually service providers in the true sense, but I suppose they are providing a social service to their members. Grey Power is just a club, really, isn't it, with a special focus? But Age Concern is supposedly supplying services to the cohort that it should do.* Grey Power is a voluntary national organization founded in 1986 to support seniors' welfare and wellbeing [80]. Established in 1948, Age Concern New Zealand promotes wellbeing, rights, respect and dignity for older people [81]. J.C.'s comments about "other stakeholders" revealed her awareness of the need to be inclusive of a range of stakeholders within the sector.

Reflecting on the length of time J.C. had been in local government and the diversity of her extensive social network she observed: *Yes, my daughter-in-law used to say: "Somebody knows you wherever you go". But it's not really quite the same now, because I've moved sort of back a bit; but it does help. That sort of thing does help ... because you can join the dots.* When the interviewer (J.B.) cited the importance of crystal-clear communication to avoid projects failing J.C.'s response revealed a purposeful "can do" leadership component: *Exactly. Well, I've seen that happen too in other organisations, and wouldn't like that to happen to anything that I was involved with, because you don't put your energy into something for it to die.*

3.1.2. Voicing Hopeful Optimism for More Inclusive Local Age-Friendly Activities

The oldest participant's responses drew on over half a century of social work and community development roles setting up local projects; activities J.L.R. has previously described as similar to setting up Chinese spinning plates, as they require checking every so often to ensure they're still spinning [82]. Responding to the initial interview prompts J.L.R. remembered: *I was very much involved in thinking of what an Age-friendly City was.* She explained that well over a decade ago, when the AFC advocate Dr Alex Kalache visited Aotearoa NZ: *There was a group of men who were involved in the council and we put it (the AFC concept) to them. And they discussed it. It was just discussion at that time. But it was "What could we do to promote Age-friendly?". Meaning there would be activities which would be for older people and we felt not only for older people, but for everybody—that it would serve the community. And that I remember was the main thing.* In the interview J.B. responded, noting J.L.R.'s inclusive intergenerational approach was evident right from the start, and a characteristic feature of her feedback to council. J.L.R. explained that she had joined the SAP: *Because I have always been a member of the subsidiaries (that influence the council), and I knew my involvement was to represent the community.*

When asked to identify any factors that might contribute to the success and/or failure of the AFC Project (Q9) J.L.R. made the first of four references to the North Shore's Older Women's Network (OWN), which was established in 1990 by a group of older women and "seeks to enrich women's lives" [83]: *It's alright to say Auckland is an AFC but they've done nothing that says "Oooh look we've organised this group and we've organised that". We've got this Older Women's Network or OWN. OWN members went to the next city (Hamilton); we caught a boat and we did this, but we organised everything; whereas I think the council could have.* OWN featured again when J.L.R. described her prior experiences that were similar to the council's AFC Project (Q10): *Um, through OWN we have organised events, trips,* etc. *But nothing to do with Auckland Council.* Responding to the prompt about AFC Project partnerships (Q12), OWN again became the focal point: *I would take it as the Older Women's Network, OWN, that have kept meeting to do the things that we spoke about in those days. And in fact get it done.* J.L.R.'s comments revealed her expectations that an AFC should include council staff and processes supporting age-friendly community groups such as OWN to arrange relevant activities for older residents. In response to the Q11 prompt asking if any prior community project experiences influenced her current behaviour J.L.R stated: *I still don't think that Auckland is an AFC, but I haven't given up hope ... that's why I think, like having the Older Women's Network that are doing things and still having events, does give it (the AFC concept) a link.*

J.L.R.'s hopeful optimism about Tāmaki Makaurau Auckland becoming an AFC—*There's no reason not to*—was expressed in a number of her interview responses: *It's time to remember the very first time I heard (about) the AFC I felt invigorated. And um, I thought "Let's do THAT!" And the others weren't so enthusiastic.* (Response to Q5 prompt discussing initiating and/or securing commitment from partners to advance the AFC Project goals.)

3.1.3. Empowering More Inclusive Access to Transport Mobility

A retired director of the Māngere-East Community Learning Centre, R.F. explained his motivation to participate in Tāmaki Makaurau Auckland's AFC Project: *As one reaches the ripe old age into the 60s and 70s you start to realise that often senior citizens are nearly non-citizens; or nearly invisible, or not taken account of. And it's that stark reality that this isn't good enough; that our city and our society should be all inclusive and involve people from diverse backgrounds and ages.* R.F.'s introductory statement revealed his awareness of the need to challenge unconscious ageist assumptions [84,85].

When describing his involvement on the SAP, R.F.'s central focus on transport mobility and accessibility issues highlighted the significance of inclusive and process-oriented relational leadership components in his responses: *I was engaged with Auckland Transport's (AT's) Passenger Transport Accessibility Group (PTAG)—a disability group pushing for better and easier and safer access, mainly for public transport around the city.* Responding to the interview prompts about prior community leadership experiences (Q10 and Q11) R.F. reported: *Probably my experiences … with the community opposition to the proposed east-west motorway. To me that showed how well that people can get together and have a major impact on a major bad decision, if you like, from the government and AT. And I've been involved in many campaigns over the years.* R.F. described a recent campaign which re-established a Post Office and Kiwibank in Māngere's local shopping centre, only to discover the landlord (a supermarket chain) wanted to evict the two service organisations to establish a $2 shop. R.F.'s community activism focused mainly on being empowering and ensuring strategic "doing" actions achieved the identified goal. *We organised a big public protest. We had about 200 people rallying outside the shopping centre, and parked two of our community centre buses in the car park and announced that if the supermarket didn't rescind the eviction notice on our Post Office we'd be running a free bus service, an half hour bus service for their customers, to take them to a rival supermarket on the other side of Māngere to do their shopping and within 20 min I got a call from the supermarket to say they'd drop their eviction notice from our Post Office. So these examples of people power and campaigning gave me heart that when push comes to shove people can get together and have a major impact on, again, poor decision making, to put it mildly.* R.F.'s account included evidence of all five relational leadership components and revealed how an older community leader who exercised his citizen role in search of shared intergenerational objectives secured improved environmental and community outcomes [3].

Responding to the interview prompts about community partners, R.F. reported that he mostly communicated with those involved in PTAG and AT staff. Aware of R.F.'s passion for promoting the benefits of free public transport (PT), J.B. also inquired about that topic; R.F. responded: *Yes, well I wrote a paper around that, highlighting the Seniors' Super Gold Card* [86] *and how it had changed the lives of so many senior citizens being able to easily get around the city and do what they want to do; whereas previously that was a major hurdle for a lot of people, just getting out and about, socializing and engaging. So if free public transport was so successful, I argued, for senior citizens, why should it not be expanded throughout the rest of society? And perhaps starting with school students and tertiary students and slowly expanding it? I realise that free PT is not something that could be implemented over night; it will involve a lot of planning and probably be more successful if it was implemented stage by stage, and hence the suggestion of starting with students as the next stage after the successful gold card experiment with seniors. We discussed that on the SAP and that concept got warm endorsement and I took it further to AT, citing examples from overseas where free PT has been expanded to citizens successfully in other cities. And as we speak it's expanding now quite rapidly around the world, where more and more municipalities are introducing or considering introducing free PT across the board, to really get people mobile; not just senior citizens, but everybody—with a view of not just mobility and accessibility but also to seriously cut pollution, traffic congestion and as a way of combatting climate change.* The intergenerational focus in R.F.'s response demonstrated an inclusive leadership component, whilst the reference to combatting climate change provided process-oriented systems thinking perspectives. At the beginning of the 2017-2019 SAP the members identified "protecting our environment for future generations" as one of five priorities in their work programme [35].

R.F. concluded his responses about his prior experiences as a community leader with a statement discussing the benefits that accrue for seniors accessing free PT that revealed ethical and inclusive leadership components and expressed collectivist values: *It's not good enough to say "Oh well I'm all right Jack. This is great. I can get around". Instead of taking that attitude and saying "This is so good, and so beneficial; obviously beneficial, why should it not be spread across the board?".*

3.2. Dynamic Temporal Flux and Loss in Momentum

Research understanding older Aucklanders' attachment to their social spaces recommended that future inquiries explore their experiences of connections across time [87]. Temporal dimensions such as changes in rhythms and pace as people age [30] can be overlooked. For example, this response embedded in J.C.'s interview narrative reported above: *But it's not really quite the same now, because I've moved sort of back a bit* provides a glimpse of how an individual's reference to a change in pace can pass undetected if the text is scrutinized through a lens that ignores changes over time.

All three participants interviewed explicitly expressed their concerns about the loss in momentum of the AFC Project. For example, responding to the prompt that probed awareness of any personal or organizational risks associated with the AFC Project (Q7) J.C. commented: *The only risk now is that the momentum is kept up because we are not there yet by a long shot. We are only still at the beginning of working out the work programme that's got to go by the end of this year (2020) to the World Health Organization. And it worries me a little bit because it could have been done more quickly to have got the basic work programme there, and then expanded as you went along; each annual plan you could add to that, and so forth. But it didn't seem to be picked up that way. I think that it needs freeing up a little bit. It's a bit tightly held and I think the more important thing to make sure that happens is that they choose a governance set up which is not just service providers. You've got to have someone who is going to monitor what the service providers provide, and they can't monitor themselves. It cannot be just the SAP, because that has no full credence or life span. It will need to be a group of people, not randomly selected, but people with some knowledge of the life and times of people over sixty-five.* J.C.'s assessment of risks associated with the council's current top-down approach aligns with Torku et al.'s (2020) observation that previous top-down implementations have failed to support AFCC initiatives, whereas closer collaboration between partners at the flax roots and local levels have been effective, particularly in resource-scarce cities and communities [20]. J.C.'s insightful stock take included a strategically mindful consideration of the council being willing to share power with seniors and explore sustainable future governance options [88,89].

R.F. also raised his concerns when responding to the prompt asking about the AFC project's successes and possible failures: (Q13) *Yeah, I'm very disappointed with the decision to not allow members who have been involved for two terms because that has the effect of cutting the continuity ... To me this is like a movement: things grow, and to cut them short, you know, unnecessarily and artificially, has the risk of stopping that continuity; stopping the momentum if you like for age-friendly prospects in the city. And yeah, I see that as a major risk and I'd suggest that perhaps one way around that if council can't be persuaded to change that policy, which was again announced without any discussion (with panel members) that I'm aware of, that there should be consideration to setting up a vehicle to continue that momentum from the previous panels, and perhaps that could be in the form of setting up some sort of lobby group which would no doubt be independent from the council because it would no longer be a council body so to speak ... Yes that's a good start, but my worry is that it's just going to dissipate and fall away, again because of the likelihood that there's little or no momentum to carry it forward. These things don't happen just out of the blue. They happen because people want them to happen, and so there's got to be that ability to continue pushing for these ideals of an AFC and everything that goes with it, otherwise it's just going to end up as a lot of nice fuzzy words and no action.* Golant's (2014) critique of age-friendly communities warns of the dangers where the prime catalyst for initiatives is strong leadership and not community need [89]. R.F.'s involvement in his local community centre, and his activism within that community suggests he would be an ideal actor to participate in the development and implementation of age-friendly initiatives in South Auckland [90].

J.L.R. responded to the Q13 prompt asking how successful she felt the AFC Project was to date? So far as I know Auckland Council are not involved in age-friendly. Maybe they are and they contact younger people, but I don't know. The rationale that informed J.L.R.'s comment emerged when she responded to the next prompt asking that she indicate ways in which the AFC Project has or might yet fail to achieve its goals: I don't know who on Auckland Council of their staff is responsible (for the AFC Project), because if they were we would know and could try and contact them; but we don't know if there is anybody. We certainly haven't been told what they're considering. In fact I know very little of council, because they do not correspond with "outside". You know, there's just Auckland Council and that's all you know; but they don't contact groups. J.L.R. continued that response thread with a future focused suggestion about the opportunity for council staff to sustain reciprocal relationships with previous panel members: Especially if some of us have been involved, I would have thought that if you get people who have been involved, just for a meeting to say what could you suggest for the future? That would be something. And we'd feel that they'd take advantage of what we learnt and so on and so forth. J.L.R.'s reflective insights about paths of engagement in partnerships resonate with Doraldo and Giles' (2004) conclusions that partnerships evolve over time and that institutional factors mediate how committed partnerships are to their relationships and the degree to which actions and interactions reveal learning (e.g., finding out, discovering, understanding), aligning (e.g., reviewing, reconsidering, re-assessing) and nurturing (e.g., cultivating, cherishing, encouraging) behaviours [37].

3.3. Mitigating Resistance

The Q4 interview prompt asked the participants to describe any resistance they had encountered to the council's AFC Project, and what methods they used as AFC champions to overcome them? J.L.R.'s response focused on the reactions of the initial group of older men who had first been introduced to the AFC concept by Dr Alex Kalache over a decade ago: *I can't say they supported it. But they didn't, uh they didn't talk against it.* However, a few moments later she added: *I think there was (resistance), but I knew I was right. You know I'm very short, so people aren't scared of me, because I'm down here, and ...* Joan chuckled sharing this observation. J.B. asked "How do you overcome that? How do you grow in stature? Do you match them with a sharp mind?", J.L.R. responded: *No. I, I uh ask for their help.* J.L.R. 's community development experiences revealed her knowledge about ways of being and doing including forming alliances and building community partnerships to navigate operational pathways through entrenched power structures.

R.F.'s Q4 interview prompt was framed around accessible mobility in public transport (PT). His response explained how a few years ago Auckland Transport (AT) invited residents to send in contributions to what they called "The BIG Idea". *So I took that opportunity, after discussing it with the SAP and also with the disability panel, of taking my paper proposing free PT for all in Auckland ... and sent it to this quest for a BIG Idea at AT. And it got dismissed as being far-fetched.* R.F. did not mention any specific tactics to overcome the resistance he encountered at the time, but later noted how AT had subsequently changed their position and were now beginning to offer opportunities to access free PT (see for example AT's free child weekend fares action [91]). The Ministry of Transport's 2018 strategic outcomes framework [92] "to improve people's wellbeing and the liveability of places" (p. 3) currently facilitates implementing initiatives such as the "far-fetched" action that R.F. had proposed.

J.C. responded to the Q4 prompt by immediately introducing a pragmatic process-oriented way that the SAP had mitigated resistance in 2018: *Well the whole (AFC) Project—when we picked it up in that second term—was to bring the council around to seeing that they had made a wrong move in sticking just to do their internal work, and not become more linked to the world-wide problem of ageing citizens. So we set about proving that to them by showing there was great support; or we felt, greater support than they did, for AFCs to be embedded in council's work programmes on every single level and we've still got a really long way to go there. But that's what really drove us.* Asked to clarify whether her reference to council meant the elected representatives or the council staff, J.C. continued: *Both. I'm talking about both, because one leads the work of the other, so therefore we had to go to council to convince them to move in a certain direction, which was a little more structured than they had been. And then for the staff to pick that up; do the work, not only for the actual programme that we want to put in place which is to join the network, but also make sure that the whole staff of council and all its many off shoots, the CCOs (Council Controlled Organisations) and so on, have the same methods and that it is embedded in all their thinking that they must cater for the tsunami of aged people that are now going to sweep the world. And I don't think they realise what's coming at them. And young ones, not disparaging young people at all, they just don't understand because they're not there yet. And they probably have grandparents that have not yet reached there either.* J.C.'s response highighted the value of considerable lived experience in local government settings and reflective understanding of age-appropriate strategies required to assist older people navigate ways of being and doing in urban environments.

3.4. Lifelong Learning

Responding to the Q9 interview prompt about identifying any factors contributing to the success and/or failure of the AFC Project, J.C. observed: *I think that the failure last time (when we did, at the end of the first panel's term), when it was, well let's say it was side tracked, I think part of that was that there was not sufficient interaction with the political side of council to explain what the differences were (with an AFC); which brings us to why we (the SAP) had the forum (in March 2018)* [93]. J.B. noted that the 2018 "Focus on the Future" Forum seemed to be a great education tool for the elected representatives and multiple stakeholders who attended, to which J.C. responded: *Well it was good; it was good, and we did have some political buy in to that too. I think it was just unfortunate timing—right at the end of the council's term that it (the rejection) happened. Um and it goes to show that you really do need, although you're not there to be political in the sense of the council's workings, you do have to have engagement with political people so that they do understand what you're trying to achieve. ... We had a new mayor, one who had agreed that he thought becoming an AFC was a good idea, because he came to the forum and learnt. We were able to present that to him and to the chair of the committee with whom I'd worked for many years, and that certainly did no harm either. So it does help to have people who I guess know the ropes a little bit better, and can, without being over bearing, can work with people; because you get nowhere unless you have good team work. And I think that the SAP had pretty good team work, on the whole.*

The Q9 response extract above demonstrates the value of the lead author being embedded in the inquiry context and reflecting on J.C.'s knowledge of networking processes gleaned from "within" [30], which enabled beneficial partnership alignments to optimise her relational leadership influence and thereby gather political support for the AFC concept [73]. In his interview R.F. observed that under J.C.'s leadership the SAP had enjoyed *healthy democratic discussions ... that J.C. encouraged that open debate and discussion instead of stifling it (because) she could see the (AFC) vision and encouraged others to share that. J.C. also sees the bigger picture. Instead of having a narrow view, we've tended to adopt a broad and futuristic view.* R.F. also mentioned that he had attended two international conferences in Tallin, the capital city of Estonia and major flag bearer of free PT, to learn more about the topic.

The final three interview prompts elicited "Reflecting and learning" process-oriented leadership components. Responding to Q13 about the success of the AFC Project to date (i.e., the beginning of March 2020), J.C. observed: *Well, as I say, we've been successful up 'til now and now we've just got to make sure that people understand how to take it forward. I think that education is the key. Not just to—I mean old people themselves need educating, in some aspects, don't they? Lifelong learning—there's no question about that. None of us know it all, and we should be in a position where we can share and enhance the lives of our fellow travellers as much as we can.* Peter Kearns' (2018) focus on late life learning draws attention to the increasing importance of intergenerational learning together to nurture our "living and growing humanistic heritage" [94] (p. 44).

4. Discussion

Understanding the complex and dynamic relationships between the global phenomena of population ageing and urbanisation has captured the attention of public policy analysts [95] and spawned an impressive and expanding body of age-friendly research activities [22,96–98]. Influenced by activist scholarship and research within Aotearoa New Zealand that gathers and provides evidence to advance social justice and equity agendas [27,99], the inquiry's applied bricolage methodology has pieced together [100] contextual information [19] with lived experience perspectives of Tāmakai Makaurau Auckland's emergent and expansive age-friendly terrain [25].

Co-constructing Tāmaki Makaurau Auckland's evolving AFC Project narrative with fellow AFC champions has required careful attention be paid to meaning-making, as the participant-researchers were/are embedded in the inquiry setting. On the other hand, the co-authors have explored open collaboration as we/they coincidentally pursued later life learning activities. Adopting an interpretive bricolage approach within an activist scholarship paradigm [99] required that all four participant researchers understand the interactive nature of the inquiry processes [25], and that the co-authors in particular examine how their personal histories and commitment to advancing social justice agendas that support active ageing shaped their inquiry interactions [73]. Lived experience in their respective fields of local government, education and research informed reflexive scrutiny of their positioning within the current inquiry setting. Their reflections revealed a shared aim to co-produce knowledge that reported on the evolving AFC Project to date (until March 2020) so the text could be used to inform, support and, where appropriate, challenge on-going AFC Project processes [99].

Applying an equity lens to the layered bricolage pieces that describe Tāmaki Makaurau's whakapapa resulted in the lead author intentionally privileging the significant roles that indigenous Māori and Pacific Peoples play in the city [27,100]. Although 5.0% of Māori and 5.6% of Pacific Peoples were aged 65 plus in 2018, those numbers had increased considerably since the 2013 Census (by 45.9% and 38.7%, respectively). Cognizant of the future implications of these structural demographic features, Salesa recommended the audience at his 2018 Michael King Memorial lecture embrace Pasifika values including "speaking the language of others" [61]. The expression accentuates plurality by acknowledging the linguistically, culturally and geographically different island nations in the South Pacific [101]. However, an evaluation of three New Zealand AFCC case study sites highlighted the limited inclusion of engaging with Māori and migrant groups to develop age-friendly initiatives [102]. The Pasifika engagement process referred to as "Yavu" that acknowledges the importance of respect for Māori (Tangata Whenua) as indigenous to Aotearoa and Te Tiriti o Waitangi as the foundation for Pacific Peoples' relationship with Tangata Whenua, offers ways to engage with diverse ethnic communities in Tāmaki Makaurau [101]. Grounded in core Pacific values of family, collectivism, respect, spirituality and reciprocity in the engagement process, Yavu offers opportunities to co-create age-friendly arenas of convergence "where social identity, environmental cosmos, and the ancestral world meet and engage" [101] (p. 6). In the current inquiry 93-year-old J.L.R.'s interview comments revealed a lapse in communications with the council. She was unaware of what was happening with the AFC Project, because the council *do not correspond with "outside". You know there's Auckland Council, and that's all you know, but they don't contact groups.* J.L.R. had referred to the absence of any reciprocal engagement with the council earlier in her interview, when she wondered: ... *maybe they contact younger people*? The reference to "younger people" reflects J.L.R.'s awareness of her communication preferences (for hard copy text, phone calls or face-to-face meetings), and the invisibility of gauging the communication needs of residents in their 90s receiving information from and interacting with council. Given J.L.R.'s strong and active involvement with the Older Women's Network (OWN) activities, she was also aware that council had not contacted OWN to disseminate any updates about the AFC Project. Developing collaborative community partnerships and networks that enable manākitanga (welcoming reciprocity) to affirm and empower older residents and their families [103] should be a key priority when co-producing [104] a sustainable AFC Action Plan [88] for Tāmaki Makaurau Auckland.

To introduce the unique features of the inquiry's Polynesian setting the lead author observed Māori tikanga (processes) by exploring, selecting and "placing in layers" narrative text that revealed Tāmakai Makaurau's whakapapa (origins) [105]. Traversing space and time, the city's whakapapa revealed relationships with both the land and the people, and acknowledged the mana (prestige) held by the region's first people; mana that was ignored by colonial settlers [47,106]. Diverse information sources described the city's rapid urban development [31] and current local government governance processes [32]. They also revealed how contemporary statutary obligations to honour principles articulated in Te Tiriti o Waitangi [107] have been translated into values such as Atawhai (kindness, generosity), Kotahi (strength in diversity), Auaha (creativity, innovation), Pono (integrity) and Taonga tuku iho (future generations) in The Auckland Plan 2050 [46] (p. 23), to nourish residents' wellbeing [108]. Feedback to council planners from older residents, SAP members and organisations supporting seniors not only drew attention to the importance of including demographic ageing in the final draft of the Auckland Plan 2050, but highlighted the need for greater age-friendly awareness within and across council's organisations. Given the patronising face of ageism that has emerged during the COVID-19 pandemic [109], taking appropriate counter measures requires careful and considered attention. One possible way to respond is to involve older people in qualitative particpatory research which can be used to co-produce evidence that challenges and influences ways in which societies construct ageing [110]. Participatory research and engagement with older people requires that attention be paid to four key areas: Mahi tahi (collaborative and equitable involvement) to address and resolve issues of power imbalance; Kotahitanga (solidarity and capacity building) which may require co-learning through the exchange of knowledge and skills; Rangatiratanga (empowerment and action for social systems change) which is one of the purposes of participatory research and aims to inform and facilitate taking civic action because of increased community awareness [99] and Kaitiakitanga (sustainability) to optimise opportunities that develop supportive infrastructure for on-going participatory research [110]. Including process-related actions that improve council's engagement and communications with diverse community networks (including Māori and ethnic communities and those aged 85 years or older), should be included in Tāmaki Makaurau's evolving AFCC Action Plan.

Using RLM interview prompts to "hear" older voices [111] enabled the three AFC champions to share their lived experience as community leaders with the lead author [104]. Commenting on mitigating resistance within council to age-friendly concepts J.C. also drew attention to the need to develop on-going age-friendly awareness and training programmes that should be embedded in all council's thinking, services and processes *so they are ready to cater for the tsunami of aged people*. The *Age-Friendly Community Evaluation Report* prepared for New Zealand's Office for Seniors [102] concluded with a similar recommendation about the educative role the Office for Seniors could play "to ensure central and local government and communities understand what age-friendly means" (p. 2). Informed by community insights gleaned from the AFC Project's Key Community Engagement Messages (refer to Table 3) [39], the Office for Seniors and the council could partner with creative agencies to co-produce an innovative education programme that challenges invisible yet pervasive ageist assumptions within the community [109,112]. Developing an age-friendly accreditation for diverse organisations across the region (see for example the Arts Council England's Age-Friendly Standards [113]) could likewise ensure that venues hosting popular intergenerational events such as Auckland Conversations [114], the Auckland Writers Festival [115] and cultural or sports events are welcoming, accessible and age-friendly.

In his interview R.F. highlighted that a significant downstream impact of cutting the continuity of AFC leadership on the SAP has the risk of stopping the momentum for age-friendly prospects in the city. He added that there should be some consideration to setting up a vehicle to continue that momentum from the previous panels ... *which would no doubt be independent from the council, because it would no longer be a council body*. J.C. expressed similar concerns when she observed that she thought the evolving AFCC Action Plan needed to free up a little bit: *It's a bit tightly held and I think the more important thing to make sure that happens is that they choose a governance set up which is not just service providers.* J.L.R.'s comments that so far as she knew council are not involved in age-friendly because she had received no communication about what was happening highlights the need for council to develop a more outward focussed communications policy that is inclusive of our oldest residents. J.L.R.'s astute observation about council's loss of AFC relational leadership knowledge on the incoming SAP illustrated that council had failed to consider the need for succession planning that enabled knowledge transfer for the incoming SAP members: *Especially if some of us have been involved, I would have thought that if you get people who have been involved, just for a meeting to say what could you suggest for the future? And ... take advantage of what we learnt* (over the past six years). It is noticeable that the evaluation of the three NZ AFCC sites identified that "A committed steering group was central to the process of implementing an age-friendly programme" and that "managing community politics was a necessary skill required by the steering group leadership" [102] (p. 30). On-going collaborations with seniors to enable the co-production of flax roots age-friendly initiatives are important [20]. However, as the interview narratives have revealed, the top priority for the council is to create an appropriate AFCC governance structure that embraces the values articulated in the Auckland Plan 2050 [46], embeds the principles of Te Tiriti o Waitangi within the structures and processes [27,108], and empowers active ageing for all across their life span.

The theme of lifelong learning [116] emerged when "listening to hear" the voices of the SAP's AFC champions [111]. J.C. referred to the educational value of the SAP's 2018 "Focus on the Future" Forum, which was attended by over ninety older residents and encouraged expressions of active citizenship, through an agenda that included stimulating presentations on a variety of relevant age-friendly topics [3] and World Cafe group discussions [117] to elicit and shape feedback for the Auckland Plan 2050 [46]. "Opportunities for lifelong learning" was also a key Auckland Project community engagement message, under the AFC Project Framework's Civic Participation and Information Domain (refer Table 3). Commenting on the success of the AFC Project when she was interviewed at the end of February, J.C. expressed concerns about how to take the project forward? She recognised that not only council staff need to become better educated about AFCC, but older people themselves: *I mean old people themselves need educating, in some aspects, don't they? Lifelong learning—there's no question about that. None of us know it all, and we should be in a position where we can share and enhance the lives of our fellow travellers as much as we can.*

Kearns' vision of a learning city, where learning in later life is nurtured and community centred, recognises the possiblilties of seniors with lived experience, time and relationships developing into community leaders [94]. The vibrant growth in the network of "Third Age" U3A branches across the Auckland region since the establishment of the first branch in 1989 reveals how opportunities to extend personal learning through collaborative research, discussions and field trips provide personal and social benefits for members [118]. Kearns also predicted the increasing importance of enabling intergenerational learning to transfer shared cultural values [94], which is reflected in Auckland Libraries' strategic plans [119] and the ninth "Culture and Diversity" Domain of the AFC Project that was added to the WHO AFCC Framework [14]. In their roles as SAP members both J.L.R. and R.F. articulated strong support and advocacy for diverse intergenerational age-friendly initiatives. A successful intergenerational transmission of cultural values from grandmother to mother to child that was established in 1982 is currently regenerating Māori language through Kōhanga Reo "language nests", which provide total immersion in Māori language and values for preschool children and their families. This Māori-led initiative has not only increased the numbers of people speaking te reo, but also affirmed Māori identity and empowered Māori women to engage in on-going education [120]. Opportunities exist for the emergent AFCC Action Plan to support the continuing regeneration of te reo. Similarly, the highly acclaimed Pacific Heritage artists and cultural leaders who formed the Pacifica Mamas (and Papas) collective in the late 1980s, so first generation migrants could meet to exchange stories, extend their knowledge and strengthen their Pasifica arts practice, facilitate intergenerational transmission of Pasifika cultural values through diverse community activities and performances [121].

Recent research has described the specific challenges that Pasifika families in New Zealand faced when adjusting to coping with the pandemic's disruption, uncertainty and social distancing measures [122]. The explosion of virtual learning and demand for digital connections to access essential services such as healthcare and banking have in turn revealed that digital access and digital literacy are fundamental factors that determine older people's capacities to sustain their agency and wellbeing during pandemic lockdowns [123]. Clearly the evolving AFCC Action Plan will need to include strategic actions to improve digital inclusion [124].

5. Conclusions

The current inquiry has challenged normative expectations that traditionally seniors are the objects of Active Ageing research [8]. Knowing how to transform into being active participant-researchers required seeking and learning ways to apply innovative interpretive bricolage techniques [25,26], in order to convey the multiple complexities involved in co-constructing these age-friendly Tāmaki Makarau Auckland narratives [19,110]. Guided by activist scholarship principles [27,99,106] and the co-authors' concerns about equity and social justice, the research-participant narratives were curated to reveal past developments, capture present accomplishments and opportunities, and anticipate future priorities [19,30]. Developing co-constructed narratives of a dynamically evolving AFC Project during a global pandemic [2] has highlighted the challenges inherent in balancing the "top-down" versus "bottom-up" interactions that drive AFCC implementation processes [20].

The 2017 review commissioned to support the implementation of AFCC in Aotearoa New Zealand advised that processes and plans should have built-in flexibility, and older people should be involved in all stages of the development of AFCC processes and plans [19]. Developing a shared understanding of the implications of "being involved" in AFCC co-production processes requires greater attention be directed to clarifying where on the public participation spectrum the diverse AFC Project community engagement interactions lie [104,110]. The interview narratives of the three older community leaders and Tāmaki Makaurau Auckland AFC Project champions have provided insightful reflections on the milestones achieved as of March 2020. Their insights also offer thought-provoking case study material that could be included in service learning opportunities, to enhance ways of working together across all four conceptual pathways that were identified from the merged AFC Project community engagement feedback [67].

A number of service-learning recommendations were made when discussing the results. However, on reflection, two emerge as immediate priorities: (1) Co-develop a sustainable AFC Project Steering Group co-governance framework that embodies the values and principles of Te Tiriti o Waitangi to enable empowered active ageing for all residents across the region [27,108]; (2) Co-develop a succession plan that enables the timely transfer of knowledge and skills to empower incoming SAP members about the evolving AFC Project [125].

Author Contributions: Conceptualization, J.B. and J.C.; methodology, J.B.; validation, J.B. and J.C.; formal analysis, J.B.; investigation, J.B.; data curation, J.B.; writing—original draft preparation, J.B.; writing—review and editing, J.B.; visualization, J.B.; project administration, J.B. All authors have read and agreed to the published version of the manuscript.

Funding: This research received no external funding.

Acknowledgments: Fellow Auckland Council Seniors Advisory Panel members Joan Lardner-Rivlin and Roger Fowler provided lived experience accounts of their involvement as age-friendly champions in Tāmaki Makaurau Auckland's Age-friendly City Project. Vanessa Burholt read an earlier draft of the manuscript and provided helpful feedback.

Conflicts of Interest: The authors declare no conflict of interest.

Appendix A

Table A1. Auckland Council's Age-friendly City (AFC) Project interview prompts [1].

1	Describe your role/personal involvement in Auckland Council's AFC Project.
2	Discuss your motivation to participate in Auckland Council's AFC Project.
3	List the partners to Auckland Council's AFC Project and discuss the initial receptiveness and commitment of each partner.
4	Describe any resistance encountered and methods you used to overcome them as a champion of Auckland Council's AFC Project. (Please be as specific as possible providing anecdotes or stories.)
5	Discuss the use of any strategy that helped to initiate, implement, gain commitment from partners, and in general further the goals of Auckland Council's AFC Project.
6	Discuss any recognition you might have received for your role in Auckland Council's AFC Project.
7	Discuss the risks (both personal and organizational) associated with Auckland Council's AFC Project.
8	Discuss your perception of your effectiveness in facilitating the goals of achieving desirable outcomes for Auckland Council's AFC Project.
9	Identify any factors contributing to the success and/or failure of Auckland Council's AFC Project.
10	Describe any prior experiences you have had with any projects similar to the Auckland Council's AFC Project.
11	Did any of your prior experience(s) influence your behaviour in this project? How? Can you please provide some examples?
12	Discuss your relationship with partners in Auckland Council's AFC Project, and how those relationships influenced your behaviour in this project.
13	Say something about how successful you feel Auckland Council's AFC Project is to date.
14	Indicate any ways in which you think the Auckland Council's AFC Project has or might yet fail to achieve its goals.
15	Describe what factors have contributed to the success and/or failure of Auckland Council's AFC Project.

[1] Adapted from Dorado and Giles (2004) [37].

References

1. Mallapaty, S. The coronavirus is most deadly If you are old and male. *Nature* **2020**, *585*, 16–17. [CrossRef] [PubMed]
2. Scott, A.; Old, J. The Interaction Between Covid-19 and an Ageing Society. Available online: https://voxeu.org/article/interaction-between-covid-19-and-ageing-society (accessed on 10 October 2020).
3. Del Barrio, E.; Marsillas, S.; Buffel, T.; Smetcoren, A.-S.; Sancho, M. From active aging to active citizenship: The role of (age) friendliness. *Soc. Sci.* **2018**, *7*, 134. [CrossRef]
4. Kalache, A. Active ageing makes the difference. *Bull. World Health Organ.* **1999**, *77*, 299. [CrossRef] [PubMed]
5. Flores, R.; Caballer, A.; Alarcón, A. Evaluation of an age-friendly city and its effect on life satisfaction: A two-stage study. *Int. J. Environ. Res. Public Health* **2019**, *16*, 5073. [CrossRef]
6. Annear, M.; Keeling, S.; Wilkinson, T.; Cushman, G.; Gidlow, B.; Hopkins, H. Environmental influences on healthy and active ageing: A systematic review. *Ageing Soc.* **2014**, *34*, 590–622. [CrossRef]
7. World Health Organisation. *Active Ageing: A Policy Framework*; World Health Organisation: Geneva, Switzerland, 2002; Available online: https://extranet.who.int/agefriendlyworld/wp-content/uploads/2014/06/WHO-Active-Ageing-Framework.pdf (accessed on 13 October 2020).
8. Foster, L.; Walker, A. Active and Successful Aging: A European Policy Perspective. *Gerontologist* **2015**, *55*, 83–90. [CrossRef]
9. Kearns, P. Towards a conceptual and policy framework for good active ageing. In *Towards Good Active Ageing for All*; Kearns, P., Reghenzani-Kearns, D., Eds.; PIMA: Victoria, Australia, 2018; pp. 8–9.
10. Buffel, T.; Phillipson, C.A. Manifesto for the Age-Friendly Movement: Developing a New Urban Agenda. *J. Aging Soc. Policy* **2018**, *30*, 173–192. [CrossRef]

11. Plouffe, L.; Kalache, A. Towards global age-friendly cities: Determining urban features that promote active aging. *J. Urban Health Bull. N. Y. Acad. Med.* **2010**, *87*, 733–739. [CrossRef]
12. Lawton, M.P.; Nahemow, L. Ecology and the aging process. In *The psychology of adult development and aging*; Eisdorfer, C., Lawton, M.P., Eds.; American Psychological Association: Washington, DC, USA, 1973; pp. 154–196. [CrossRef]
13. World Health Organisation. *Global Age-Friendly Cities: A Guide*; World Health Organisation: Geneva, Switzerland, 2007; pp. 1–76.
14. World Health Organisation. *Checklist of Essential Features of Age-friendly Cities*; World Health Organisation: Geneva, Switzerland, 2007; pp. 1–4.
15. World Health Organisation. Age-friendly World. Available online: https://extranet.who.int/agefriendlyworld/network/ (accessed on 13 October 2020).
16. World Health Organisation. WHO Global Network for Age-friendly Cities and Communities. Available online: https://www.who.int/ageing/projects/age_friendly_cities_network/en/ (accessed on 15 September 2020).
17. Lui, C.-W.; Everingham, J.-A.; Warburton, J.; Cuthill, M.; Bartlett, H. What makes a community age-friendly: A review of international literature. *Aust. J. Ageing* **2009**, *28*, 116–121. [CrossRef]
18. Neville, S.; Napier, S.; Wham, C.; Jackson, D. An integrative review of the factors related to building age-friendly rural communities. *J. Clin. Nurs.* **2016**, *25*, 2402–2412. [CrossRef]
19. Davey, J. *Age-friendly Cities and Communities World experience and pointers for New Zealand*; Office for Seniors, Ministry of Social Development: Wellington, New Zealand, 2017; pp. 1–85.
20. Torku, A.; Chan, A.P.C.; Yung, E.H.K. Age-friendly cities and communities: A review and future directions. *Ageing Soc.* **2020**, 1–38. [CrossRef]
21. Dalbelko-Schoeny, H.; Fields, N.L.; White, K.; Sheldon, M.; Ravi, K.; Robinson, S.; Murphy, I.E.; Jennings, C. Using community-based participatory research strategies in age-friendly communities to solve mobility challenges. *J. Gerontol. Soc. Work* **2020**, *63*, 447–463. [CrossRef] [PubMed]
22. World Health Organisation. *Global Network for Age-friendly Cities and Communities Looking Back over the Last Decade, Looking Forward to the Next*; World Health Organisation: Geneva, Switzerland, 2018; pp. 1–35.
23. Jones, R. *Why Equity for Māori Must be Prioritized during the COVID-19 Response*; The University of Auckland: Auckland, New Zealand, 2020.
24. Durham Community Research Team. *Community-Based Participatory Research: Ethical Challenges*; Centre for Social Justice and Community Action, Durham University: Durham, UK, 2011; pp. 1–13.
25. Rogers, M. Contextualizing theories and practices of bricolage research. *Qual. Rep.* **2012**, *179*, 1–17.
26. Kincheloe, J.L. Critical pedagogy and knowledge wars of the twenty-first century. In *Key Works in Critical Pedagogy*; Hayes, K., Steinberg, S.R., Tobin, K., Eds.; SensePublishers: Rotterdam, The Netherlands, 2011; Volume 32, pp. 385–405.
27. Berghan, G.; Came, H.; Coupe, N.; Doole, C.; Fay, J.; McCreanor, T.; Simpson, T. *Te Tiriti o Waitangi-Based Practice in Health Promotion*; STIR: Stop Institutional Racism: Auckland, New Zealand, 2017.
28. Warne, T.; McAndrew, S. Constructing a bricolage of nursing research, education and practice. *Nurse Educ. Today* **2009**, *29*, 855–858. [CrossRef]
29. Wibberley, C. Getting to grips with bricolage: A personal account. *Qual. Rep.* **2012**, *17*, 1–8.
30. Vandenbussche, L.; Edelenbos, J.; Eshuis, J. Coming to grips with life-as-experienced: Piecing together research to study stakeholders' lived relational experiences in collaborative planning processes. *Forum Qual. Soc. Res.* **2019**, *20*, 1–17.
31. Hoffman, L. *A Brief History of Auckland's Urban Form*; Auckland Council: Auckland/Tāmaki Makaurau, New Zealand, 2019.
32. Auckland Council Governance Manual. Available online: https://governance.aucklandcouncil.govt.nz (accessed on 19 September 2020).
33. Health Promotion Forum of New Zealand. *Health Promotion Competencies for Aotearoa New Zealand*; Runanga Whakapiki Ake i te Hauora o Aotearoa Health Promotion Forum of New Zealand: Auckland/Tāmaki Makaurau, New Zealand, 2012.
34. Auckland Council Seniors Advisory Panel 2014–2016. *Collaborative Accomplishments: Brief. Reflections from the 2014–2016 Auckland Council Seniors Advisory Panel*; Auckland Council: Auckland/Tāmaki Makaurau, New Zealand, 2016.

35. Auckland Council Seniors Advisory Panel 2016–2019. *Auckland Council Seniors Advisory Panel Report 2016–2019 Term*; Auckland Council: Auckland Tāmaki Makaurau, New Zealand, 2019; Available online: https://knowledgeauckland.org.nz/media/1436/auckland-council-seniors-advisory-panel-report-2016-2019.pdf (accessed on 19 September 2020).
36. Olmos-López, P.; Tusting, K. Autoethnography and the study of academic literacies: Exploring space, team research and mentoring. *Trab. Linguística Apl.* **2020**, *59*, 264–295. [CrossRef]
37. Dorado, S.; Giles Jr., D.E. Service-Learning Partnerships: Paths of Engagement. *Mich. J. Community Serv. Learn.* **2004**, *11*, 25–37.
38. Goldberg, N.; Atkins, L.C. Community partners as service-learning co-leaders. *Collab. J. Community-Based Res. Pract.* **2020**, *3*, 1–11. [CrossRef]
39. Auckland Council Community and Social Policy. *Age-Friendly Auckland Project Community Engagement Findings Report*; Auckland Council: Auckland/Tāmaki Makaurau, New Zealand, 2020; pp. 1–62.
40. Auckland Plan, Strategy and Research Department. *Auckland Plan. 2050. Outcome: Māori Identity and Wellbeing. Māori Identity and Wellbeing Explained*; Auckland Council: Auckland, New Zealand, 2018.
41. Silva, C. Auckland's urban sprawl, policy ambiguities and the peri-urbanisation to Pukekohe. *Urban. Sci.* **2019**, *3*, 1. [CrossRef]
42. Royal Commission on Auckland Governance Website. Available online: https://www.dia.govt.nz/Decommissioned-websites---Royal-Commission-on-Auckland-Governance (accessed on 19 September 2020).
43. Office of Ethnic Communities Website. Available online: https://www.ethniccommunities.govt.nz/news/new-page-2/ (accessed on 23 September 2020).
44. Auckland Plan, Strategy and Research Department. *Auckland Plan. 2050. About the Auckland Plan. Auckland's Population*; Auckland Council: Auckland, New Zealand, 2018. Available online: https://www.aucklandcouncil.govt.nz/plans-projects-policies-reports-bylaws/our-plans-strategies/auckland-plan/about-the-auckland-plan/Pages/aucklands-population.aspx (accessed on 23 September 2020).
45. Terms of Reference Auckland Council Demographic Advisory Panels 2019–2022. Available online: https://www.aucklandcouncil.govt.nz/about-auckland-council/how-auckland-council-works/advisory-panels/Documents/terms-of-reference-for-demographic-advisory-panels-2019-2022.pdf (accessed on 23 September 2020).
46. Auckland Plan, Strategy and Research Department. *Auckland Plan. 2050 (full print version)*; Auckland Council: Auckland, New Zealand, 2018. Available online: https://www.aucklandcouncil.govt.nz/plans-projects-policies-reports-bylaws/our-plans-strategies/auckland-plan/about-the-auckland-plan/docsprintdocuments/auckland-plan-2050-print-document.pdf (accessed on 23 September 2020).
47. Barnes, H.M.; McCreanor, T. Colonisation, hauora and whenua in Aotearoa. *J. Royal Soc. New Zealand* **2019**, *49*, 19–33. [CrossRef]
48. Hobbs, M.; Ahuriri-Driscoll, A.; Marek, L.; Campbell, M.; Tomintz, M.; Kingham, S. Reducing health inequity for Māori people in New Zealand. *Lancet* **2019**, *394*, 1613–1614. [CrossRef]
49. Marmot, M. Social determinants of health inequalities. *Lancet* **2005**, *365*, 1099–1104. [CrossRef]
50. Hamilton City Council: Hamilton Age Friendly Plan—2018–2021. Available online: https://www.hamilton.govt.nz/our-city/community-development/Pages/Hamilton-Age-Friendly-Plan---2018-2021.aspx (accessed on 22 September 2020).
51. Hamilton, New Zealand an Age Friendly City: Plan and Process for Becoming a More Age-Friendly City, 2018–2021. Available online: https://www.hamilton.govt.nz/our-city/community-development/Documents/Community%20-%20Hamilton%20Age%20friendly%20city%20plan%20FINAL%20-%20March%202018.pdf (accessed on 22 September 2020).
52. Auckland Plan, Strategy and Research Department. *Auckland Plan. 2050. About the Auckland Plan. Auckland's Asian Population*; Auckland Council: Auckland, New Zealand, 2018. Available online: https://www.aucklandcouncil.govt.nz/plans-projects-policies-reports-bylaws/our-plans-strategies/auckland-plan/about-the-auckland-plan/Pages/aucklands-asian-population.aspx (accessed on 22 September 2020).
53. Statistics New Zealand 2018 Census Place Summaries Auckland Region. Available online: https://www.stats.govt.nz/tools/2018-census-place-summaries/auckland-region (accessed on 22 September 2020).

54. Auckland Council Research and Evaluation Unit (RIMU). *Māori in Tāmaki Makaurau*; Auckland Council: Auckland/Tāmaki Makaurau, New Zealand, 2020; Available online: https://knowledgeauckland.org.nz/media/1453/maori-2018-census-info-sheet.pdf (accessed on 22 September 2020).
55. Ryks, J.; Kilgour, J.; Whitehead, J.; Rarere, M. Te Pae Mahutonga and the Measurement of Community Capital in Regional Aotearoa New Zealand. In *New Zealand Population Review*; Kukutai, T., Hohmann-Marriott, B., Eds.; Population Association of New Zealand: Wellington, New Zealand, 2018; Volume 44, pp. 85–109.
56. Robson, B.; Harris, R. (Eds.) *Hauora: Māori Standards of Health IV. A Study of the Years 2000–2005*; Te Rōpū Rangahau Hauora a Eru Pōmare: Wellington, New Zealand, 2007.
57. Statistics New Zealand 2018 Census Population and Dwelling Counts. Available online: https://www.stats.govt.nz/information-releases/2018-census-population-and-dwelling-counts (accessed on 22 September 2020).
58. Ministry of Social Development. Health Life Expectancy at Birth Report. Available online: http://socialreport.msd.govt.nz/health/life-expectancy-at-birth.html (accessed on 22 September 2020).
59. Auckland Plan, Strategy and Research Department. *Auckland Plan. 2050. About the Auckland Plan. Pacific Auckland*; Auckland Council: Auckland, New Zealand, 2018; Available online: https://censusauckland.co.nz/files/Auckland%20area%202018%20Census%20info%20sheets%20(all%20local%20boards).pdf (accessed on 22 September 2020).
60. Auckland Council Research and Evaluation Unit (RIMU). *Pacific Peoples in Auckland*; Auckland Council: Auckland/Tāmaki Makaurau, New Zealand, 2020. Available online: https://www.aucklandcouncil.govt.nz/plans-projects-policies-reports-bylaws/our-plans-strategies/auckland-plan/about-the-auckland-plan/Pages/pacific-auckland.aspx (accessed on 22 September 2020).
61. Heritage, E. AWF18: Michael King Memorial Lecture—Ready or Not.—Damon Salesa. Available online: https://booksellersnz.wordpress.com/2018/05/21/awf18-michael-king-memorial-lecture-ready-or-not-damon-salesa/ (accessed on 23 September 2020).
62. Jackson, N. Introduction and overview. *Policy Q.* **2017**, *13*, 1–9. [CrossRef]
63. Auckland Council Research and Evaluation Unit (RIMU). *2018 Census Results Local Board and Special Area Information Sheets*; Auckland Council: Auckland/Tāmaki Makaurau, New Zealand, 2019.
64. Reid, A. *Older Aucklanders: A Quality of Life Status Report 2017. Summary Report*; Auckland Council: Auckland/Tāmaki Makaurau, New Zealand, 2017.
65. SuperSeniors The Positive Ageing Strategy—Background. Available online: http://www.superseniors.msd.govt.nz/about-superseniors/office-for-seniors/positive-ageing-strategy.html (accessed on 24 September 2020).
66. Davey, J.; Glasgow, K. Positive Ageing—A Critical Analysis. *Policy Q.* **2006**, *2*, 21–27. [CrossRef]
67. Innovation Unit an Age-friendly Tāmaki Makaurau. Available online: https://www.innovationunit.org/thoughts/an-age-friendly-tamaki-makaurau/ (accessed on 24 September 2020).
68. Tinkler, A.; Tinkler, B.; Hausman, E.; Strouse, G.T. Key elements of effective service-learning partnerships from the perspective of community partners. *Partnersh. J. Serv. Learn. Civ. Engagem.* **2014**, *5*, 137–152.
69. Buffel, T. (Ed.) *Researching Age-Friendly Communities. Stories from Older People as Co-Investigators*; The University of Manchester Library: Manchester, UK, 2015; pp. 1–143.
70. Komives, S.R.; Lucas, N.; McMahon, T.R. Strategies for change. In *Exploring Leadership: For College Students Who Want to Make a Difference*, 3rd ed.; Jossey-Boss: San Francisco, CA, USA, 2013; pp. 443–495.
71. Kallio, H.; Pietilä, A.; Johnson, M.; Kangasniemi, M. Systematic methodological review: Developing a framework for a qualitative semi-structured interview guide. *J. Adv. Nurs.* **2016**, *72*, 2954–2965. [CrossRef] [PubMed]
72. Thorne, H.; Bellringer, M.; Abbott, M.; Landon, J. *Brief. Literature Review to Summarise the Social Impacts of Gaming Machines and TAB Gambling in Auckland*; Technical Report; 2012; Available online: https://www.researchgate.net/publication/269875531_Brief_Literature_Review_to_Summarise_the_Social_Impacts_of_Gaming_Machines_and_TAB_Gambling_in_Auckland_Authors (accessed on 27 October 2020).
73. Endres, S.; Weibler, J. Towards a three-component model of relational constructionist leadership: A systematic review and critical interpretive synthesis. *Int. J. Manag. Rev.* **2017**, *19*, 214–236. [CrossRef]
74. Denzin, N.K.; Lincoln, Y.S. Introduction: The discipline and practice of qualitative research. In *The SAGE Handbook of Qualitative Research*, 5th ed.; Denzin, N.K., Lincoln, Y.S., Eds.; SAGE Publications: London, UK, 2018; pp. 1–26.

75. Ritchie, J.; Spencer, L. Qualitative data analysis for applied policy research. In *Analyzing Qualitative Data*; Burgess, R.G., Bryman, A., Eds.; Routledge: London, UK, 1994; pp. 173–194.
76. Zubair, M.; Norris, M. Perspectives on ageing, later life and ethnicity: Ageing research in ethnic minority contexts. *Ageing Soc.* **2015**, *35*, 897–916. [CrossRef]
77. Enßle, F.; Helbrecht, I. Understanding diversity in later life through images of old age. *Ageing Soc.* **2020**, 1–20. [CrossRef]
78. London, M. Trends and Directions for lifelong learning programs and research. In *The Oxford Handbook of Lifelong Learning*, 1st ed.; London, M., Ed.; Oxford University Press: London, UK, 2018; pp. 11–12.
79. Pless, N.M.; Maak, T. Relational intelligence for leading responsibly in a connected world. *Acad. Manag. Annu. Meet. Proc.* **2005**, *2005*, 11–16. [CrossRef]
80. Grey Power New Zealand Federation Inc. Aims and Objectives. Available online: https://greypower.co.nz/about-us/ (accessed on 17 October 2020).
81. Age Concern New Zealand Federation Vision, Mission and Values. Available online: https://www.ageconcern.org.nz/Public/About_Us/Who_We_Are/Vision__Mission_and_Values/Public/About/Who_are_we/Vision__Mission_and_Values.aspx?hkey=7053d22d-d5dd-45d9-b02d-97efcbb365f9 (accessed on 17 October 2020).
82. Powley, Y.; Greenaway, R.; Hutching, M.; Howard, R. *My Story Your Story Together Builds Communities*; Auckland North Community and Development Inc. (ANCAD): Takapuna, New Zealand, 2016; pp. 26–33.
83. Older Women's Network. Available online: http://own.org.nz/index.php (accessed on 7 October 2020).
84. Sweetland, J.; Volmert, A.; O'Neil, M. *Finding the Frame: An Empirical Approach to Reframing Aging and Ageism*; FrameWorks Institute: Washington, DC, USA, 2017.
85. Gendron, T.L.; Inker, J.; Welleford, E.A. A theory of relational ageism: A discourse analysis of the 2015 White House conference on aging. *Gerontologist* **2018**, *58*, 242–250. [CrossRef] [PubMed]
86. Super Gold Card. Available online: https://www.supergold.govt.nz (accessed on 17 October 2020).
87. Wiles, J.L.; Allen, R.E.S.; Palmer, J.; Hayman, K.J.; Keeling, S.; Kerse, N. Older people and their social spaces: A study of well-being and attachment to place in Aotearoa New Zealand. *Soc. Sci. Med.* **2009**, *68*, 664–671. [CrossRef] [PubMed]
88. Grantmakers In Aging. *Guiding Principles for the Sustainability of Age-Friendly Community Efforts*; GIA Grantmakers in Aging: Arlington, VA, USA, 2015; pp. 1–29.
89. Golant, S. Age-friendly communities are we expecting too much? In *IRPP Insight 5*; Institute for Research on Public Policy: Montreal, QC, Canada, 2014; pp. 1–20.
90. Auckland Council TSI. The Southern Initiative. *What Are We Learning?* Available online: https://www.tsi.nz/learnings (accessed on 21 September 2020).
91. AT GO on an adventure Free Child Weekend Fares. Available online: https://at.govt.nz/childweekendfares (accessed on 17 October 2020).
92. Ministry of Transport Te Manatū Waka. *A Framework for Shaping our Transport System: Transport Outcomes and Mode Neutrality*; Ministry of Transport Te Manatū Waka: Wellington, New Zealand, 2018; pp. 1–8.
93. Our Auckland Advisory Panels Provide Significant Input to Decision Making. Available online: https://ourauckland.aucklandcouncil.govt.nz/articles/news/2019/10/advisory-panels-provide-significant-input-to-decision-making/ (accessed on 17 October 2020).
94. Kearns, P. Harnessing learning cities and communities. In *Towards Good Active Ageing for All. Kearns, P., Reghenzani-Kearns, D., Eds.*; PIMA: Victoria, Australia, 2018; pp. 43–45.
95. Buffel, T.; Phillipson, C.; Rémillard-Boilard, S. Age-friendly cities and communities: New directions for research and policy. In *Encyclopedia of Gerontology and Population Aging*; Gu, D., Dupre, M.E., Eds.; Springer Nature: Cham, Switzerland, 2019; Volume 2, pp. 21–27. [CrossRef]
96. Buffel, T.; Handler, S.; Phillipson, C. Introduction. In *Age-Friendly Cities and Communities: A Global Perspective*; Buffel, T., Handler, S., Phillipson, C., Eds.; Policy Press: Bristol, UK, 2018; pp. 3–12.
97. Dikken, J.; van den Hoven, J.F.M.; van Staalduinen, W.H.; Hulsebosch-Janssen, L.M.T.; van Hoof, J. How older people experience the age-friendliness of their city: Development of the age-friendly cities and communities questionnaire. *Int. J. Envirn. Res. Public Health* **2020**, *17*, 6867. [CrossRef]
98. Xie, L. Age-friendly communities and life satisfaction among the elderly in urban China. *Res. Aging* **2018**, 1–23. [CrossRef]

99. Came, H.; MacDonald, J.; Humphries, M. Advocating for activist scholarship in New Zealand and beyond. *Contention* **2015**, *3*, 37–53. [CrossRef]
100. Yardley, A. Piecing together—A methodological bricolage. *Forum Qual. Soz./Forum: Qual. Soc. Res.* **2008**, *9*, 31.
101. Ministry for Pacific Peoples. *Yavu Foundations of Pacific Engagement*; Ministry for Pacific Peoples: Wellington, New Zealand, 2018; pp. 1–27.
102. Neville, S.; Adams, J.; Napier, S.; Shannon, K. *Age-Friendly Community Evaluation*; Ministry of Social Development Office for Seniors: Wellington, New Zealand, 2018; pp. 1–42.
103. Ocloo, J.; Matthews, R. From tokenism to empowerment: Progressing patient and public involvement in healthcare improvement. *BMJ Qual. Saf.* **2016**, *25*, 626–632. [CrossRef]
104. Rémillard-Boilard, S.; Buffel, T.; Phillipson, C. Involving older residents in age-friendly developments: From information to coproduction mechanisms. *In J. Hous. for the Elder.* **2017**, *31*, 146–159. [CrossRef]
105. Māori ki Te Whare Wānanga o Ōtākou Mihi—Introductions. Available online: https://www.otago.ac.nz/maori/world/te-reo-maori/mihi-introductions/index.html (accessed on 22 October 2020).
106. Tuhiwai Smith, L. *Decolonising Methodologies: Research and Indigenous Peoples*, 3rd ed.; Zed Books: London, UK, 2012.
107. Manatū Hauora. Te Tiriti o Waitangi and the Health and Disability System. Available online: https://www.health.govt.nz/our-work/populations/maori-health/te-tiriti-o-waitangi (accessed on 20 October 2020).
108. Parr-Brownlie, L.C.; Waters, D.L.; Neville, S.; Neha, T.; Muramatsu, N. Aging in New Zealand: Ka haere ki te ao pakeketanga. *Gerontologist* **2020**, *60*, 812–820. [CrossRef]
109. Fraser, S.; Lagacé, M.; Bongué, B.; Ndeye, N.; Guyot, J.; Bechard, L.; Garcia, L.; Taler, V. Ageism and COVID-19: What does our society's response say about us? *Age Ageing* **2020**, *49*, 692–695. [CrossRef] [PubMed]
110. Stephens, C.; Burholt, V.; Keating, N. Collecting qualitative data with older people. In *The SAGE Handbook of Qualitative Data Collection*; Flick, U., Ed.; SAGE Publishing: Thousand Oaks, CA, USA, 2018; pp. 639–642. [CrossRef]
111. McGloin, C. Listening to hear: Critical allies in indigenous studies. *Aust. J. Adult Learn.* **2015**, *55*, 267–292.
112. Stovell, J. *Challenging Assumptions on the International Day of Older Persons*; Help Age International: London, UK, 2020; pp. 1–3.
113. Age Friendly Standards Family Arts Campaign. Available online: https://www.familyarts.co.uk/age-friendly-standards/ (accessed on 20 October 2020).
114. Auckland Conversations Making Auckland an Age-friendly City. Available online: https://conversations.aucklandcouncil.govt.nz/events/making-auckland-age-friendly-city (accessed on 24 October 2020).
115. Auckland Writers Festival Continues Its Record-Breaking Run. Available online: http://www.writersfestival.co.nz/news/Page2/auckland-writers-festival-continues-its-record-breaking-run/ (accessed on 20 October 2020).
116. Findsen, B. Aotearoa New Zealand. In *Towards Good Active Ageing For All*; Kearns, P., Reghenzani-Kearns, D., Eds.; PIMA: Victoria, Australia, 2018; pp. 28–29.
117. World Café Method. Available online: http://www.theworldcafe.com/key-concepts-resources/world-cafe-method/ (accessed on 20 October 2020).
118. U3A New Zealand. Available online: https://www.u3a.nz/home.htm (accessed on 20 October 2020).
119. Dobbie, A. *Auckland Libraries Te Kauroa—Future Directions 2013–2023*; Auckland Council: Auckland Tāmaki Makaurau, New Zealand, 2013; pp. 1–58.
120. New Zealand History Te Kōhanga Reo 1982. Available online: https://nzhistory.govt.nz/women-together/te-kohanga-reo (accessed on 26 October 2020).
121. Pacifica Arts Who We Are. Available online: https://www.pacificaarts.org/who-we-are/our-story/ (accessed on 24 October 2020).
122. University of Canterbury Lockdown Study Sheds Light on Pasifika Achievement in Education. Available online: https://www.canterbury.ac.nz/news/2020/lockdown-study-sheds-light-on-pasifika-achievement-in-education-.html (accessed on 24 October 2020).
123. InternetNZ. *Solving Digital Divides Together An InternetNZ Position Paper*; InternetNZ: Wellington, New Zealand, 2018; pp. 1–21.
124. Digital Inclusion Map. Available online: https://digitalinclusion.nz/?regions=auckland#maptop (accessed on 25 October 2020).

125. Lipper, L.; Lazarus, W. Six Strategies for Nonprofit Leadership Transition. Stanford Social Innovation Review May 2017. pp. 1–5. Available online: https://ssir.org/articles/entry/six_strategies_for_nonprofit_leadership_transition?utm_source=Enews&utm_medium=Email&utm_campaign=SSIR_Now&utm_content=Title (accessed on 30 October 2020).

Publisher's Note: MDPI stays neutral with regard to jurisdictional claims in published maps and institutional affiliations.

International Journal of
Environmental Research and Public Health

MDPI

Article

Physical Environment vs. Social Environment: What Factors of Age-Friendliness Predict Subjective Well-Being in Men and Women?

Elena del Barrio [1,*], Sandra Pinzón [2], Sara Marsillas [1] and Francisco Garrido [3]

1 Matia Institute of Gerontology, C/ Orense 6, 28020 Madrid, Spain; sara.marsillas@matiafundazioa.eus
2 Andalusian School of Public Health, Cuesta del Observatorio, 4, 18011 Granada, Spain; sandra.pinzon.easp@juntadeandalucia.es
3 Department of Criminal Law, Philosophy of Law, Moral Philosophy and Philosophy, University of Jaen, Carretera Bailen, 12, 23009 Jaén, Spain; fpena@ujaen.es
* Correspondence: elena.barrio@matiafundazioa.eus

Abstract: "Age-Friendly Cities and Communities" is an initiative launched by the WHO in 2007 that has spread to more than 1000 cities and communities around the world. This initiative is based on an integrated physical and social environment for older people, and a model of participatory, collaborative governance. An enabling social environment setting is just as important as material conditions in determining well-being in later life. The objective of this study is to analyze the interaction between age-friendliness (physical and social) and subjective well-being in women and men aged 55 and over in the Basque Country. The methodology was based on a survey of a representative sample (n = 2469 individuals). In order to know the predictive power of age-friendliness over subjective well-being, linear regression models separated by gender were constructed. The predictive models of age-friendliness are composed by different variables for men and women. In both cases, the physical environment variables do not remain in the final model. Among the predictors of well-being in men, the coexistence stands out as a safety and support network. In women, the neighborhood has proved to be a very important resource. The conclusions of this study contribute to literature and interventions promoting more effective strategies that enhance older people well-being, considering the gender perspective.

Keywords: age-friendly cities; well-being; older people; participation; physical environment; social environment; gender

Citation: del Barrio, E.; Pinzón, S.; Marsillas, S.; Garrido, F. Physical Environment vs. Social Environment: What Factors of Age-Friendliness Predict Subjective Well-Being in Men and Women?. *Int. J. Environ. Res. Public Health* **2021**, *18*, 798. https://doi.org/10.3390/ijerph18020798

Received: 7 November 2020
Accepted: 15 January 2021
Published: 19 January 2021

1. Introduction

The development of age-friendly cities and communities, adapted to older people's needs, has become an important area of work in the fields of health, ageing, and public policy. This is the result of several trends, including the complexity of demographic change, the policy objective of supporting the maintenance of people in their homes for as long as possible [1] and the recognition of the role of the environment in active and healthy ageing [2].

In this sense, the "Age-Friendly Cities and Communities" initiative launched by the WHO in 2007 has been extended to more than a thousand cities and communities worldwide [3], highlighting the importance of the systematic and inclusive approach in generating enabling environments [4]. In the Basque Country, the age-friendliness movement began in 2009 with the adhesion of the capitals to the initiative launched by the WHO. In 2012 the Basque Government launched a project at territorial level (Euskadi Lagunkoia-Age-Friendly Basque Country), which currently includes more than 60 municipalities [5]. Since then, age-friendliness has become one of its political strategies on ageing [6].

An age-friendly community is defined as a place where older people are actively involved, valued, and supported with infrastructure and services that are effectively tailored to their needs [7].

Making cities and communities age-friendly ensures that they are inclusive and equitable places, leaving no one behind, especially the most vulnerable older people [4]. Age-friendliness is primarily characterized by the adaptation of mutually reinforcing social and physical environments, by a participatory model of collaborative governance and, above all, by inclusion [8]. This emphasizes an underlying assumption that is now widely shared by policymakers: An enabling social environment is as important as the material conditions in determining the well-being of older people's lives [9].

Research has shown that age-friendly environments are associated with higher levels of well-being and quality of life in older people [10–13]. It has even been concluded that older people who perceive their environments as age-friendly are almost four times more likely to report a better quality of life than those who report lower levels of age-friendliness [11]. Its positive association to well-being is not surprising, as the criteria for an age-friendly environment align almost perfectly with both concepts [13]. However, much existing environmental gerontological research has focused on the indoor settings, mainly homes and overlooked wider contexts such as neighborhoods and communities [14,15]. More recently, some studies have extensively examined the multidimensional aspects of the environment [15,16]. Van Dijk [15] explored the relationship of social characteristics of the neighborhood, such as social capital, social cohesion, and social support with well-being. Park and Lee [14] found that after controlling for demographic covariates, physical and social environment features are significantly related to the life satisfaction of older people in Korea. This finding is an empirical basis for identifying those aspects of the environment that can serve as modifiable resources and improve the psychological well-being of older people, in this case, particularly the most vulnerable ones.

Despite these conclusions, there is still insufficient understanding of the actual holistic effects of interventions on the physical and social environments [9,17]. More evidence needs to be generated about how improvements in both settings affect the health and well-being of older people [8]. One of the main challenges facing all community initiatives–either related to ageing or not-is how to assess their impact on individuals and groups [18]. The term "age-friendly" is used when considering how various aspects of a community promote or reduce the health and well-being of individuals as they age [19]. However, scientific research continues to investigate why some places are more age-friendly than others and how age-friendliness relates to the well-being of older people [8].

Focusing on well-being, there is a growing interest in the variables that influence the subjective well-being of older people. Some of the individual factors related to well-being in old age have been highlighted in previous research. Some of these studies conclude that well-being was strongly related to socio-demographic [20]; socio-economic [21,22]; health [23,24]; lifestyle [25,26]; psychological characteristics [27,28]; as well as social relations [22].

Gender is one of the most relevant socio-demographic characteristic in old age. Growing old is not the same for men and women [29]. Sex and gender are important determinants of health and wellbeing [30]. Gender is the characteristic with enough evidence to suggest that there is different wellbeing or survival relationships for older men and women [31]. To explain social phenomena, the Gender Perspective takes into account the differentiated or egalitarian situation, depending on belonging to one sex or the other [29]. Gender is an explanatory social category, also constructed, that helps to understand what lies behind biological sex. Gender, as a social construction, reveals differences in thinking, roles, health, economics, politics, and labor and in old age, these differences are even bigger. These inequalities do not appear in the last stages of life, but are nourished throughout the life cycle and are therefore continuous [32].

Although the Framework for Action on Active Ageing highlighted gender as a cross-cutting determinant, research on ageing from a gender perspective is still limited [29]. The gap in women's representation in human studies has been well documented [33].

Gender-based analysis is designed to identify the sources and consequences of inequalities between women and men and to develop strategies to address them [30].

In this context, the general objective of this study is to analyze the interaction between age-friendliness, subjective well-being, and gender, specifically regarding the perception of age-friendliness of the physical and social environment, among men and women aged 55 and over in the Basque Country. Variables of perception of the eight areas of age-friendliness, ranging from public spaces, housing, transport, social participation and employment, civic participation, respect and social inclusion, communication and information, and social and health services, are included.

2. Materials and Methods

Although the WHO has made several documents available to facilitate the measurement of age-friendliness [34,35], there is no official quantitative tool yet. One of the challenges in evaluating age-friendly city initiatives is to identify an evidence-based approach [36–38]. There is a great need for monitoring, evaluating, measuring and assessing the age-friendliness of cities and communities [38]. Despite these challenges, in recent years different researchers have developed a number of tools to measure and evaluate these initiatives in a quantitative way [38–44].

In this study, however, the tool for measuring friendliness is based on a survey of the living conditions of people aged 55 and over carried out periodically in the Basque Country. This means it does not count on a tool designed ad hoc, but it includes a series of relevant indicators related to the areas of age-friendliness indicated by the WHO [45].

The methodology of this study was based on a survey of a representative sample of community-dwelling residents aged 55 and over in Basque Country (739,231 people aged 55 and over, 33.8% of the total population). Structured interviews were conducted through face to face survey based on a questionnaire assisted by computer. Sampling selection was made through stratified random sampling considering geographic area and age group (55–64 years-old, 65–69, and 80 and over) as main criteria of stratification. Sample distribution followed a proportional method for territory strata and quotas according to age group (55–64, 65–79, and 80 and over) and gender were applied. Households in each stratum were chosen by random selection of those with one person aged 55 and over, only interviewing one person per household. Sample size was determined by required level of disaggregation. Statistics on ageing generally categorize older people as being above a certain age threshold. Indeed, the United Nations (UN) defined older people as those aged 60 years or more in World Population Ageing 2013, while the WHO states that older people in developed world economies are commonly defined as those aged 65 years or more. The WHO also uses an alternative definition, whereby an older person is defined as someone who has passed the median life expectancy at birth [46]. The age selected for analysis, 55 and over, is one of the most widely used cohorts for the study of the ageing population from research and public policy (for example: The Active Ageing Index). Although, there is still much debate about the redefinition of the threshold for the onset of old age because of its implications for the design of public policies and for the social perception of old age [47].

The sample was composed of 2469 individuals (1177 men and 1319 women). Their ages ranged from 55 to 102 years old, with 69.36 (SD = 9.9) being the average age. Regarding marital status, 61% of the participants were married, 9% were single, 6% were divorced, and 24% were widowed (Table 1).

Table 1. Demographics of participants (n = 2469).

	n	%
Gender		
Male	1115	45%
Female	1381	55%
Age		
Mean (SD)		69.4 (9.92)
55–64	974	39%
65–79	1044	42%
80+	478	19%
Educational level		
Less than primary education	847	34%
Complete primary studies	799	32%
Secondary and higher education	844	34%
Origins		
Basque Country	1477	59%
Others	1019	41%
Type of dwelling		
Owner-occupant	2314	93%
Private rent	145	6%
Others	34	1%
Marital status		
Single	231	9%
Married or living with a partner	1524	61%
Widowed	601	24%
Separated/Divorced	140	6%
Living together with a partner	1926	37%
Needs help DLAs	503	20%

Anonymity and confidentiality of the answers were guaranteed and participation in the study was voluntary. All subjects gave their informed consent for inclusion before they participated in the study and the protocol was approved by the Ethics Committee of University of Jaen (MAY.13/3.TES).

The questionnaire includes items and scales that explore perceptions in relation to areas of age-friendliness (age-friendliness components). The WHO's subjective well-being scale (WHO5 Well Being Index -1998) is also included for this analysis.

To find out the predictive power of the components of age-friendliness on the subjective well-being of men and women aged 55 and over in the Basque Country, two multiple linear regression models have been carried out, using the WHO5 Well Being Index as the dependent variable [48], and both the predictors of well-being according to the von Humboldt and Leal [49] categories (16 variables) and the selected components of age-friendliness (34 variables) as independent variables

Subjective well-being is a general term used to describe the level of well-being experience of people according to subjective assessments of their lives [49]. It was measured using the WHO-5 Well Being Index -1998 version, a five-item self-administered scale, Likert-type scale with response options of 0 to 5. This scale exclusively measures the positive aspects of the psychology of well-being in short non-invasive questions. It is one of the most widely used questionnaires to assess subjective psychological well-being [50].

The validity of construct of the WHO-5 was analyzed with the item response theory model formulated by Rasch (2012) in older people [51], which confirmed that the 5 items constitute a one-dimensional scale, where each item adds unique information on the level of well-being [50]. A total score can be obtained by adding up all items, with a range of scores from 0 to 100 covering from a total absence of well-being to the highest conceivable level of well-being [50].

In the field of later life, the WHO-5 scale has been validated in different studies for the detection of depression [52–54], apathy [55], or suicide [52]. An internal and external validation of the scale has also been carried out in the general older population [56], concluding that the WHO-5 is a useful instrument for the identification of people with reduced subjective quality of life.

This study analyzed the psychometric nature of the scale used to ensure the quality of the measurement. This was done through the analysis of internal consistency as well as through the performance of exploratory factor analyses of main components with Varimax rotation.

Regarding linear regression analyses, in order to control the predictive values of the age-friendliness components by the factors that has been identified by literature and evidence as predictors of wellbeing [49], some independent variables were included such as age, educational level, habitat, marital status, type of household, or health status, among others. These are drawn from several categories that are divided into: Social support; socio-demographic factors; health status; and psychological factors. Moreover, a total of 34 variables related to the 8 age-friendliness areas described by WHO have been included as age-friendliness components (Table 2). The number of indicators available in the survey related to each domain is different, which means that there are domains with 10 indicators and others where only one indicator has been found. The variables in this study encompassed within the physical environment are those included in the areas of outdoor spaces, housing, transport, communication, and health services (Areas 1, 2, 3, 7, and 8). The variables considered in the social environment are those in the areas of social participation, respect, and social inclusion, and citizen participation and employment (Areas 4, 5 and 6). The indicators corresponding to the age-friendliness components proposed by the WHO were included in the linear regression model to explore their association to wellbeing.

Table 2. Variables selected as components of age-friendliness.

Area 1. Outdoor Spaces and Buildings
1. Barriers in the immediate environment (yes/no) 2. Perception of crime, violence or vandalism (yes/no) 3. Difficulty of access to parks and green areas (yes/no) 4. Difficulty of access to supermarket or food shop (yes/no)
Area 2. Housing
5. Barriers inside the home (yes/no) 6. Access barriers to the building (yes/no) 7. Tenancy regime (property/other situation) 8. Adapted housing (yes/no)
Area 3. Transport
9. Difficulty in accessing public transport (bus, train, etc.) (yes/no) 10. Public transport barriers (bus, train, etc.) (yes/no)
Area 4. Social participation
Carrying out of activities: (performed/not performed) 11. Physical or sporting, 12. Domestic leisure, 13. Cultural, 14. Social, 15. Tourism, 16. Religious acts and 17. Educational activities
Area 5. Respect and social inclusion
18. Sense of belonging to a community or group of people (0–10)

Table 2. *Cont.*

Area 6. Civic participation and employment
Participation in voluntary activities: 19. Social and community services (participation/not participation) 20. Educational, cultural, sports or professional, gastronomic, choral and literary associations (participation/no participation) 21. Social or charitable movements (participation/no participation) 22. Neighborhood associations (participation/no participation) 23. Parish groups (participation/no participation) 24. Other organizations (participation/no participation) Political participation: 25. Union, political party or political action group meeting (participation/no participation) 26. Attendance at protest or demonstration (participation/no participation) 27. Contact with a politician or public official (participation/no participation) Employment 28. Relationship with work activity (working, not working).
Area 7. Communication and information
29. Availability of mobile phone (yes/no) 30. Availability of land line (yes/no) 31. Computer/Tablet availability (yes/no) 32. Internet access at home (yes/no) 33. Internet use (yes/no)
Area 8. Health services
34. Difficulty in accessing the health center (yes/no)

In a first phase, a descriptive analysis of the variables separated by men and women was carried out, following the recommendations of Calvente, Rodrigo, and Morante [57], to observe the gender gaps. For the analysis of the quantitative variables, the basic statistics (mean and standard deviation) were used. For categorical variables, the relative frequency distribution with 95% confidence intervals was used.

In order to know the relationship of subjective well-being with the rest of the variables, an analysis of variance was carried out to determine the predictors of subjective well-being, by gender. In order to know the predictive power of age-friendliness over subjective well-being, linear regression models separated by gender were constructed. Then, variables that did not contribute to explain this relationship were eliminated until the final models were obtained.

3. Results

3.1. Subjective Well-Being

Subjective wellbeing showed satisfactory psychometric properties, in terms of internal consistency (alfa: 0.87). Regarding construct validity (KMO: 0.85), a single factor has been obtained explaining 67.35% of the variance.

Considering descriptive results, the average well-being score was 64.12, with a standard deviation of 22.24 points (Scale of 0–100). Men have a higher well-being index ($\bar{x} = 67.9$) than women ($\bar{x} = 61.2$).

3.2. Factors Associated with Well-Being by Gender

The gender-segregated analysis showed that the factors associated with subjective well-being are different for men and women. However, most of these factors have statistically positive results in their relationship to subjective well-being in both genders ($p < 0.005$) (Table 3).

Table 3. Subjective well-being according to determinants by gender.

Variable	Male				Female			
	n	Mean	σ	*p*	*n*	Mean	σ	*p*
Total	**916**	**68.06**	**19.99**		**1170**	**61.45**	**22.98**	
Age								
55–64	406	69.26	19.7		452	65.09	22.2	
65–79	418	68.06	20.0	0.003	519	61.05	22.7	0.000
80+	109	61.92	22.7		215	53.23	24.8	
Educational Level								
Less than primary education	250	66.28	20.0	0.151	426	56.16	23.4	0.000
Primary education or higher	682	64.43	20.4		759	64.02	22.7	
Wealth level								
Low	34	61.32	25.99		47	45.00	27.90	
Medium	795	67.60	19.71	0.000	1040	61.70	22.33	0.000
High	59	77.98	15.33		62	73.67	20.74	
Habitat								
<20,000 inhabitants	312	70.00	19.2	0.022	366	66.46	21.9	0.000
20,000 inhabitants or more	621	66.79	20.8		820	58.81	23.5	
Origin								
Born outside the Basque Country	372	66.29	21.2	0.053	506	59.10	24.5	0.000
Born in the Basque Country	561	68.91	19.6		680	64.95	21.6	
Married or living together								
Yes	686	69.18	18.9	0.001	644	62.95	22.7	0.004
No	247	64.22	23.4		543	59.06	23.7	
Type of household								
Individual	158	61.94	24.6	0.000	309	58.28	24.5	0.011
Live with other people	775	69.07	19.1		878	62.19	22.7	
Non-presential contact								
No	58	64.71	22.3	0.227	71	49.23	24.9	0.000
Yes	870	68.03	20.2		1110	61.97	23.0	
Satisfaction of personal relationships								
Low	8	29.73	27.95		15	42.07	23.50	
Medium	398	63.69	20.60	0.000	500	53.67	22.67	0.000
Hight	510	72.10	17.90		655	67.83	21.09	
State of health								
Regular, bad or very bad	350	58.94	22.2	0.000	536	50.01	23.3	0.000
Good or very good	583	73.22	16.9		650	70.41	18.7	
Need for assistance DLAs								
No	846	69.07	19.6	0.000	953	65.00	21.5	0.000
Yes	87	56.23	23.1		233	45.58	23.5	
Satisfaction Achieved								
Low	12	32.56	26.13		27	31.26	19.56	
Medium	501	64.74	20.12	0.000	675	56.44	22.38	0.000
High	388	73.55	17.14		444	70.98	19.32	
Safe and secure satisfaction that you feel								
Low	16	40.82	29.74		13	49.68	26.39	
Medium	455	63.87	20.01	0.000	591	55.53	23.18	0.000
High	440	73.78	16.84		558	68.36	20.47	
Satisfaction and confidence in your future								
Low	38	53.75	26.74		64	46.11	27.20	
Medium	510	66.24	19.5	0.000	630	57.29	22.84	0.000
High	323	73.78	16.65		392	71.09	18.05	
Concern about old age								
No	549	69.19	18.9	0.013	524	65.35	21.8	0.000
Yes	367	65.81	21.9		638	57.80	23.9	

3.3. Subjective Well-Being and Age-Friendliness Components by Gender

The gender-segregated analysis showed that the components of age-friendliness are different for men and women (Table 4). For instance, more housing, social participation and communication, and information indicators related to subjective well-being in case of women compared to men. Concerning outdoors spaces, barriers in the immediate environment and difficulty of access to the supermarket or grocery shop are associated with subjective well-being in both women and men. In the latter, the difficulty of access to the park or green area is also associated, although with little significant relevance. In the area of housing, subjective well-being is related with barriers within the home for both men and women. For women, barriers to entry and tenure are also associated with well-being. In the area of social participation, there is a direct association between the performance of all activities and women's subjective well-being. Among men, no association was found with attendance at religious events or educational activities. In the area of citizen participation and employment, for men, subjective well-being is associated with the practice of activities in the field of social and community services, associations of all kinds and political parties. In the case of women, subjective wellbeing is associated with all kinds of these voluntary practices except participation in parish groups, and also participation in the labor market. In the area of communication, the outstanding gender difference is that compared to men, the case of women having a mobile phone is also associated with their well-being, in addition to having a computer/tablet and access to and use of the Internet, which are significant in both genders.

Table 4. Subjective well-being according to components of age-friendliness by gender.

	Males				**Females**			
	n	**Mean**	σ	p	n	**Mean**	σ	p
Outdoor Spaces								
Barriers in the immediate environment	94	63.10	22.5	0.015	180	51.59	27.8	0.000
Perception of unsafe environment	86	68.67	22.7	0.839	147	60.50	25.6	0.649
Difficulty of access to the park or green area	48	63.03	21.4	0.040	72	61.95	23.0	0.259
Difficulty in accessing a supermarket or grocery shop	46	55.7	24.2	0.000	95	48.73	25.8	0.000
Housing								
Home ownership	848	68.27	19.78	0.051	1120	61.51	23.10	0.024
Barriers inside the home	52	61.66	23.6	0.021	101	48.48	25.2	0.000
Barriers in the access to the building	93	64.34	21.5	0.072	186	53.12	27.6	0.000
Adapted housing	416	67.16	19.1	0.354	467	61.85	22.8	0.282
Transport								
Barriers in public transport	55	52.96	23.5	0.000	99	50.34	26.7	0.000
Difficulty in accessing public transport	67	59.91	23.1	0.001	134	45.65	27.6	0.000
Social participation								
Physical activity	875	68.92	25.1	0.000	1028	63.46	21.8	0.000
Domestic leisure activities	404	70.59	19.3	0.000	668	63.72	21.7	0.000
Cultural activities	443	71.68	17.4	0.000	613	67.24	19.8	0.000
Social activities	817	69.69	18.9	0.000	979	64.36	21.6	0.000
Tourism	640	71.14	18.1	0.000	714	67.03	21	0.000
Religious events	445	69.17	20.3	0.060	767	63.31	22.2	0.000
Educational activities	114	68.88	20.1	0.571	175	67.36	20.8	0.000
Respect and inclusion								
Sense of belonging to a community or group								

Table 4. *Cont.*

	Males				Females			
	n	Mean	σ	*p*	*n*	Mean	σ	*p*
Low	11	44.86	29.3		29	35.52	26.8	
Medium	461	64.83	21		571	55.81	22.6	
Hight	426	72.65	17.1	0.000	535	69.11	19.9	0.000
Citizen participation and employment								
Social and community services	50	73.84	19.66	0.032	68	69.82	22.99	0.002
ducational, cultural, and gastronomic associations	94	75.78	16.85	0.000	64	70.13	2084	0.001
Social or charitable movement	48	70.46	20.14	0.366	46	70.51	22.31	0.005
Neighborhood associations	47	74.87	16.53	0.015	58	72.00	20.68	0.000
Parish groups	32	66.95	21.52	0.795	65	63.11	24.89	0.492
Other Organizations	29	67.10	23.24	0.836	39	69.00	24.90	0.033
Participation in trade unions	65	73.90	19.20	0.012	38	63.10	25.80	0.591
Participation in events	116	72.10	20.70	0.015	90	65.41	20.50	0.074
Contact with a politician	47	73.41	21.20	0.052	41	60.79	27.90	0.927
Relationship with work activity: Working	167	70.32	18.99	0.084	167	69.22	19.80	0.000
Communication and information								
Mobile phone	834	68.30	20.0	0.059	1004	62.31	22.6	0.000
Land line	830	68.27	19.7	0.088	1095	61.11	23.0	0.738
Computer or tablet	500	70.75	19.0	0.000	562	63.47	22.6	0.002
Internet access	506	70.55	18.8	0.000	565	63.00	22.2	0.013
Internet use	514	64.93	21.3	0.000	776	57.96	23.7	0.000
Health Services								
Difficult access to the health center	46	54.60	24.0	0.000	87	45.80	28.2	0.000

3.4. Predictors of Subjective Well-Being by Gender

In order to identify the predictors of the subjective well-being in men and women, different regression models have been carried out. The same variables, selected by literature review, have been included in the initial models for each gender, but those that have obtained significant results for each have been maintained in the final models.

3.4.1. Predictors of Subjective Well-Being in Men

In order to identify the predictors of the subjective well-being in men, several regression analyses were carried out: Firstly, incorporating in the model the factors associated with well-being that had obtained significant results; secondly, the components of age-friendliness.

In the first of the regressions, 7 out of 12 variables were selected as potentials for the final model (corrected R square = 0.232). The variables selected were habitat (Beta −0.068; $p = 0.019$); type of household (Beta 0.065; $p = 0.026$); satisfaction with personal relationships (Beta 0.088; $p = 0.031$); health status (Beta 0.206; $p < 0.000$); need for help (Beta −0.071; $p = 0.017$); satisfaction with achievements (Beta 0.128; $p = 0.002$); and satisfaction with how safe and secure they feel (Beta 0.176; $p < 0.000$).

Regarding the components of age-friendliness, seven were selected to be introduced in the final model (corrected R square = 0.142). These were perform physical or sport activities (Beta 0.108; $p < 0.000$); perform leisure-housing activities (Beta 0.078; $p = 0.011$); perform social activities (Beta 0.114; $p < 0.000$); perform tourism, travel activities (Beta 0.114; $p < 0.000$); satisfaction with his/her feeling of belonging to the community or group of people (Beta 0.198; $p = 0.000$); participates in educational, cultural, gastronomic associations (Beta 0.071; $p = 0.021$); and having difficulty in accessing the health center (Beta −0.093; $p = 0.003$).

In the regression analysis for the final model, the variables resulting from the previous regressions were included. The final model in men was constructed with nine variables, four related to the components of age-friendliness (corrected R square = 0.247) (Table 5).

Table 5. Model weights of each predictor and their significance on the dependent variable for men.

	Beta	Sig.	95% CI	
Living with others	0.074	0.083	−0.508	8.249
Satisfaction with personal relationships	0.095	0.021	0.199	2.457
Good or very good health	0.211	0.000	6.048	11.087
Satisfaction with achievements in life	0.103	0.013	0.286	2.439
Satisfaction with how safe and secure his feel	0.162	0.000	1.034	3.274
Perform physical or sports activities	0.100	0.001	3.552	13.228
Perform leisure-housing activities	0.066	0.024	0.339	4.908
Perform social activities	0.062	0.039	0.191	7.713
Participate in gastronomic, educational, cultural or sports associations	0.063	0.032	0.337	7.643
Control variables				
Age (65+)	−0.007	0.809	−2.611	2.037
Wealth level	−0.042	0.166	−4.506	0.776
Educational level (Primary and higher)	0.027	0.409	−0.552	1.353
Marital status(married or living together)	−0.011	0.793	−4.222	3.228

Considering collinearity, two variables obtained high results in the indices but below the recommended threshold of 30, so they remained in the analysis [58].

By including age, marital status, educational level, and economic level as control variables in the final model, the variable "lives with others" leaves the model (Sig = 0.083; Beta 0.074); but none of these variables are significant in the final model

3.4.2. Predictors of Subjective Well-Being in Women

In order to identify the predictors of the subjective well-being in women, several regression analyses were carried out: Firstly incorporating in the model the factors associated to the well-being, which obtained significant results; secondly, the components of age-friendliness.

In the first of the regressions, 8 out of 15 variables were selected as potentials for the final model (corrected R square = 0.326). The variables selected were habitat (Beta −0.072; $p = 0.006$); origin (Beta 0.075; $p = 0.004$); social network contact (Beta 0.088; $p = 0.001$); satisfaction with personal relationships (Beta 0.098; $p = 0.003$); health status (Beta 0.242; $p < 0.000$); need for help for ADLs (Beta −0.130; $p < 0.000$); satisfaction with the achievements she is making in life (Beta 0.191; $p < 0.000$); and satisfaction with her security regarding her future (Beta 0.108; $p = 0.001$).

Considering the components of age-friendliness, seven were selected to be introduced in the final model (corrected R square: 0.234): Barriers in public transport (Beta −0.112; $p < 0.000$); performance of physical or sports activities (Beta 0.105; $p < 0.000$); social activities (Beta 0.076; $p = 0.011$); doing tourism and/or travel (Beta 0.142; $p < 0.000$); satisfaction with their feeling of belonging to a community or group of people (Beta 0.294; $p < 0.000$); participation in neighborhood associations (Beta 0.083; $p = 0.002$); and labor market participation (Beta 0.089; $p = 0.001$).

In the regression analysis for the final model, the variables resulting from the previous regressions were included. The final model in women was constructed with 11 variables, 4 of them related to the components of age-friendliness (corrected R2: 0.323) (Table 6).

Table 6. Model weights of each predictor and their significance on the dependent variable for women.

	Beta	Sig.	95% CI	
Municipality of more than 20,001 inhabitants (Habitat)	−0.075	0.002	−6.547	−1.549
Born in the Basque Country (Origin)	0.060	0.051	−0.006	4.691
Social network contact	0.067	0.005	2.068	11.828
Satisfaction with personal relationships	0.088	0.011	0.330	2.495
Good or very good health	0.237	0.000	7.835	13.095
Need for help for ADLs	−0.089	0.000	−9.768	−2.819
Satisfaction with the achievements in life	0.158	0.000	1.076	2.987
Perform physical or sport activities	0.091	0.001	2.696	9.945
Perform tourism, travel activities	0.101	0.000	2.091	7.194
Satisfaction with her sense of belonging to a community or group of people	0.089	0.020	0.173	1.998
Participation in neighborhood associations	0.065	0.017	1.128	11.684
Control variables				
Age (65+)	−0.022	0.417	−3.420	1.417
Wealth level	0.021	0.444	−1.540	3.514
Educational level (Primary and higher)	0.043	0.119	−0.199	1.741
Marital status(married or living together)	−0.025	0.346	−3.449	1.211

As in the male model, two variables obtained high results in collinearity indices but below the recommended threshold of 30, so they remain in the analysis [58].

By including age, marital status, educational level, and economic level as control variables in the final model, the variable "born in the Basque Country" leaves the model (Sig = 0.051; Beta 0.052); but none of these variables are significant in the final model.

4. Discussion

Gender is a characteristic with enough evidence, suggesting that there is different well-being or survival relationships for men and women [31]. For instance, Lennartsson and Silverstein [59] found that solitary activities reduced mortality risk for men but not for women, while Warr, Butcher, and Robertson [60] found that family and social relationships influenced more women's well-being compared to men. Agahi and Parker in Adams and colleagues [31] also found that women's mortality risk decreased with social activities, whereas men's risk was higher with solitary hobbies and gardening, for example. This previous evidence highlights the importance of analyzing subjective well-being in men and women separately in order to clarify what influences and predicts the well-being of both.

The final model obtained in men is composed of nine predictors, four of which are included in the components of age-friendliness, particularly social and citizen participation. The other variables included are relevant factors selected from scientific evidence where social support, health status, and psychological factors predominate. Thus, the variables predicting men's well-being are living with other people, being satisfied with personal relationships, being in good health, being satisfied with their achievements and with how safe and protected they feel, as well as carrying out physical exercise, domestic and social leisure activities, and participating in associations of a gastronomic, educational, cultural, or sporting nature.

Regarding women, the final model consists of 11 factors, 4 belonging to the components of age-friendliness within the areas of social participation, citizen participation, and social inclusion. The other includes socio-demographic, social support, health, and psychological variables. Living in a rural environment (less than 20,000 inhabitants); having been born in the Basque Country; maintaining contact with family, friends and/or neighbor; being satisfied with their personal relationships; being in good health; not needing help for the DLA; being satisfied with their achievements; doing physical exercise; tourism or travel; being satisfied with their feeling of belonging to the community; and participating in neighborhood associations, predicts higher levels of subjective well-being in women.

The results, therefore, have shown that only for women socio-demographic factors such as habitat or origin are relevant, leaving out other important variables such as age, marital status, wealth, or educational level. These findings contradict previous studies where some demographic variables, such as age, income, work status, marital status, and educational level [61] are associated with subjective well-being. However, these studies have also revealed that these variables only explain a partial amount of the variance in well-being [61]. This means that the weight of other variables is very important and could explain, to a greater extent, individual differences in levels of well-being and the subjective nature of the concept [61]. Additionally, subjective well-being as an overall measure does not seem to undergo significant changes associated with age, either in cross-sectional or in longitudinal studies [62]. On the other hand, educational level does not seem to be relevant either when controlling for other factors, and it is possible that education may exert indirect relations to subjective well-being through a mediating role [61]. With regard to the level of wealth or income, it has also been concluded that countries with the highest level of wealth have almost no correlation between this variable and well-being [61,63–66].

Sociodemographic variables have been maintained as predictors of subjective well-being only in women, being origin (place of birth) and rurality (less than 20,000 inhabitants). Regarding rurality, some researchers have analyzed the differences between urban and rural communities related to well-being, but scarce evidence is found in terms of ageing population [67]. According to Van Hoof and Kazak [67], some studies have corroborated that rural areas approach or exceed urban areas in terms of life satisfaction or well-being. However, the higher the density of urban settlement, the greater the proximity to public services, influencing the quality of life of people and being especially relevant for older people [67]. In the literature, findings about environment and health focus largely on urban areas, however, how the age-friendly community characteristics are related to rural environments is less known [39]. Research of well-being in rural women has also been relatively scarce [68]; for instance, some authors found a relationship between habitat and life satisfaction in women, in which rural women obtained higher life satisfaction than urban women, although not significantly [68]. In this study, women who live in areas with fewer than 20,000 inhabitants were more likely to report higher levels of well-being. A possible explanation may be related to the conclusions of previous research in which satisfaction with social relations is higher among older people living in rural environments [69], due to in less populated areas people know each other better. Neighbors are a very important type of relationships in villages, especially for women [62]. Studies such as Bosch and Gómez [70] show that women have a deeply rooted role and caring function, and in rural environments they find support to continue to carry out their role in "good neighbor" networks in an adequate and satisfactory way.

Origin, a socio-demographic predictor of women's well-being, refers to having been born in the Basque Country. This variable could be understood in relation to the importance of the community and belonging to the place, another predictor variable of well-being in women. As women age, their dependence on their neighborhood increases [71] and their residential stability is associated with attachment to the community [71,72].

Regarding men's well-being, socio-demographic variables have not remained as predictors. However, social support factors emerged as predictors, for instance, living with other people. For men, living in a household with other people, i.e., living together, has a positive effect on their well-being. This type of social support is very important because of their relative poorer performance and independence in leading an autonomous life on their own, at least compared to women [73]. The assignment of traditional gender roles leads to a men's higher level of dependence in domestic tasks, which implies the need to live with other people in order to perform them. Several studies show how living together as a couple entail higher life satisfaction, better emotions, physical and mental health, economic resources, and social integration, support, and relations [74]. Additionally, marriage is one of the strongest predictors of subjective well-being: Married people report a higher degree of life satisfaction than single, widowed, or divorced ones [61,65–67].

Another predictor of well-being, in this case for men and women, is satisfaction with personal relationships. Good relationships with family, friends, and other people in their social network provide higher indices of subjective well-being in both genders. Social support networks have been identified as important influences on the affective and cognitive components of well-being [75]. Furthermore, protective effects of social networks on morbidity and mortality have been strongly recognized [71,76]. This correlation between various types of social support and well-being in older people [19] is considered a consistent result.

Health predominates among other predictors of subjective well-being. The relationship between health and well-being has also been found in multiple studies [19,22,77,78]. Menec and Nowicki [39] found that perceived health had significant positive effects on the physical environment, social environment, opportunities for participation, and transport options. In our study, perceived health is the strongest predictor in the final models for men and women.

In addition, in women, the situation of dependence or autonomy remains together with health. For them, not needing help to carry out the daily life activities is also a clear predictor of higher subjective well-being. Functional limitations of older people have been found to be associated with it [61,78] and some studies have corroborated how this affects women more [61]. These results may be related to the importance of living together for men, but not for women. In this sense, older women, more "autonomous" in terms of not needing other people to run their home, can find greater obstacles in functional dependence situations, decreasing their subjective well-being.

On the other hand, in men, satisfaction with feelings of safety and protection is included as one of the psychological factors predicting well-being. These results can be analyzed in coherence with the previous ones on coexistence. For their greater well-being, men need to perceive a safety network that begins with live as a couple. In later life "the family becomes the great substitute for employment as a source of sociability, identity and self-esteem or time structuring" ([79], p. 115). When men retire, they move from a socially open relationship in a working environment, which provides them with references of identity, prestige, friendships, solidarity and so on, to a state that requires them to adjust to new developments in the world of marriage and the family [80]. In women, however, the continuity of the role can have positive consequences, with a better psycho-social adjustment at this life stage.

Moreover, satisfaction with the achievements made in life is one of the psychological factors emerged as predictor of well-being for both men and women. In this sense, self-esteem and self-efficacy have positive relationships with the highest level of well-being [61]. Regarding self-efficacy, Gómez et al. [81] indicate that the more confident a person feels in achieving their goals and objectives in life, the higher level of subjective well-being experiences. According to Diener et al. [65], the relationship between subjective well-being and goals is mediated not only by the fact that people have clear goals, but also by the progress made in achieving them [62]. At the individual level, the continuity or replacement of roles through participation in appropriate activities and with family support can contribute to the individual's sense of meaning or purpose and the maintenance of a sense of identity [31]. Participation in activities involves the pursuit or achievement of personal goals, thus adding a sense of personal mastery or achievement [31,82].

Therefore, the activities carried out by people take on special relevance for the perception of well-being. The other large group of variables included in the model presented in this study are those age-friendliness components described above. Of the eight areas of age-friendliness, only few remain in the model for predicting well-being in men and women, mainly social and citizen participation.

Among the social participation activities predicting well-being for men and women, physical or sporting activities such as doing sport or exercise, walking, going to the mountains, etc., predominate. Several studies have already confirmed this positive relationship between the practice of physical exercise and the feeling of well-being and personal satisfaction [61,83,84], and even effects have been found on physical and psychological health in older people [85].

In men, it has also been identified that participation in domestic leisure activities or hobbies, such as gardening, handicrafts, DIY, etc., is a predictor of well-being. These activities, commonly more solitary, have obtained contradictory results in previous research [86], although a recent study has found that "solitary-active" activity is associated with a reduction in mortality risk in men [59].

Other types of activities that favor the subjective well-being of men are those of a social nature such as going to the bar, meeting friends, going outdoors to have lunch or dinner, etc. These type of social participation and social contacts have positive correlations with personal well-being measures, as confirmed by previous research [86] and from which the ageing theory of activity emerges [87]. The review conducted by Adams et al. [31] confirms that informal social participation, such as visiting friends, has a positive outcome in relation to well-being in old age. According to these authors, strong evidence relating social activity with positive well-being, as inherent social intimacy seems, to be a very important, if not the most important, aspect of engagement that influences people's well-being [31].

However, for women, tourism, travel, and/or excursions are the social participation activities that predict subjective well-being. These results are corroborated by previous studies that have shown how travelling in old age affects physical, psychological, social, and spiritual dimensions such as integration, acceptance, contribution, updating, and coherence; and that this leisure activity offers opportunities for significant participation in adulthood [88,89]. The review done by Morgan et al. [90] finds that tourism can improve the well-being of older people and promote a renewed sense of purpose, facilitating their transition from work to retirement. Several authors have found that tourism has a positive psychological impact on older people, on their well-being, quality of life, perceived health, and life satisfaction, regardless of the type or length of travel [90]. However, few studies analyzed tourism in old age from a gender perspective [88,89]. Liechty et al. [88] found that group travel with other older women promoted a sense of belonging, empowerment, feelings of self-determination, personal growth, positive emotions and has well-being implications.

On the other hand, in the area of age-friendliness that encompasses social inclusion, the variable feeling of belonging was included. This predicts well-being in women, but not in men. Similar results were found in the study of Tiraphat et al. [11], including social trust as one of the predictors of age-friendly environments [11]. Recent studies have shown the positive effects of social capital, as measured by group participation, sense of belonging, and relationship with neighbors [91] on the perceived functional and psychological health of older people. Well-being is also closely related to a sense of community, and this acts as a predictor of social and psychological well-being [92]. With regard to gender, Phillipson et al. [93] found that women were more concerned about the deterioration of social capital, as they fulfil the role of "neighborhood keepers". So, as women get older, their dependence on their neighborhood increases [71]. The feeling of belonging seems to be related, in turn, to other predictors of well-being in women such as origin and rurality. In Young et al.'s study [76] another variable associated with a greater sense of belonging in women was living alone, that is, those women who lived alone had a greater sense of belonging to the community arguing that they may have developed social support networks to compensate for living alone.

Finally, for both men and women, the resulting regression models had variables from the civic participation component, although the specific indicator differs. For men, it is participation in educational, cultural, sporting, professional, gastronomic, choral, or literary associations, which predict well-being. Conversely, for women the predictor is participation in neighborhood associations. Several studies have found that participation of older people in socially productive activities is associated with well-being [94] as well as meet service needs in the community [15].

The differences between men and women in the type of civic participation are linked to the other predictor variables and the gender differences found throughout this study. Associations of a cultural, sporting, professional, choral, or gastronomic nature are traditionally made up of men in the Basque Country, something that is reflected today in their greater participation in this type of associations [95,96]. Neighborhood associations played a fundamental role in the recovery of areas of sociability in the Basque Country, not only in the field of self-management, the assembly movement, or the control of municipal management, but also in others such as the revitalization or recovery of popular festivals [95]. This type of associative participation being a predictor of women's participation is a result that is in line with the previous ones. The neighborhood is a space conquered beyond the home, which means many benefits for women, and which is related to other variables such as rurality, origin, or sense of belonging.

Therefore, none of the variables introduced as physical environment areas are kept as predictor variables in the resulting models, in contradiction to other studies that have found that the areas of "outdoor spaces and buildings", "transport", "housing", along with "community support and health services" [15], and "security" [97] seemed to be essential elements for older people and an important goal to prevent them from losing their social and physical well-being [97].

Despite the findings, our study also has some inherent limitations. First, it is based on the use of a survey not specifically designed for the purpose of measuring perceptions of friendliness. For this reason, some indicators may not fully reach to catch the multidimensionality of friendliness components. Even so, this survey has a wide variety of indicators related to this concept, so this limitation can become an opportunity by optimizing the use of this tool for different purposes and to test its potential in the research of this or other fields. Additionally, it is a cross-sectional study, which prevents capturing the dynamics of friendliness and well-being and extracting causal inferences. Therefore, it is not possible to determine their direction of the association based on the findings of this study. However, the results establish a significant association, which is an important step that encourages further studies to identify directionality. On the other hand, although the survey contains a variable to measure the habitat in which the respondent resides, which would allow a multilevel analysis to be made by looking at the differences between the more rural and more urban environments of men and women, the sampling conducted does not provide a sufficient number of people who meet these conditions for a detailed analysis of habitat of less than 20,000 inhabitants. Future research could indeed be developed in order to identify area level effects regarding friendliness.

5. Conclusions

Among the predictors of well-being in men, coexistence stands out as a safety and support network. In women, however, the neighborhood has been found to be a very important resource. Both for men and women, good health, satisfaction with personal relationships, achievements, and physical exercise are predictors of wellbeing.

Regarding age-friendliness components and areas, those related to the social environment (social participation, citizen participation, and social inclusion) are the fundamental elements in people's well-being. Conversely other aspects such as physical environment (outdoor spaces, housing, and transport) and municipal services (communication and information, and health services) seem to be less important. However, fewer variables on social and health services were included in this study compared to social environment ones, which may have influenced the results about their impact on people's well-being.

Finally, it is important to analyze separately the perceptions of men and women in order to advance in the knowledge of the different realities. This study has contributed to literature by providing regression models including predictors of well-being and age-friendly components separated by gender. In this way, action programs and policies can be designed more concretely, including the gender perspective, in order to promote more effective strategies that enhance their well-being.

Author Contributions: Conceptualization, E.d.B., S.P. and F.G.; Data curation, E.d.B.; Formal analysis, E.d.B. and S.M.; Investigation, E.d.B.; Methodology, E.d.B., S.P. and S.M.; Supervision, S.P. and F.G.; Visualization, E.d.B.; Writing—original draft, E.d.B.; Writing—review & editing, E.d.B., S.P., S.M. and F.G. All authors have read and agreed to the published version of the manuscript.

Funding: This research received no external funding.

Institutional Review Board Statement: The study was conducted according to the guidelines of the Declaration of Helsinki, and approved by the Ethics Committee of University of Jaen (MAY.13/3.TES).

Informed Consent Statement: Informed consent was obtained from all subjects involved in the study.

Data Availability Statement: Restrictions apply to the availability of these data. Data was obtained from Basque Country Government and are available from the authors with the permission of Basque Country Government.

Acknowledgments: The Basque Government is thanked for the availability of the survey data for use in this study.

Conflicts of Interest: The authors declare no conflict of interest.

References

1. Phillipson, C.; Buffel, T. Can global cities be age-friendly cities? Urban development and ageing populations. *Innov. Aging* **2017**, *1*, 745. [CrossRef]
2. Noordzij, J.M.; Beenackers, M.A.; Roux, A.V.D.; Van Lenthe, F.J. Age-friendly cities: Challenges for future research. *Bull. World Health Organ.* **2019**, *97*, 436–437. [CrossRef]
3. World Health Organization. Age-Friendly World. 2020. Available online: https://extranet.who.int/agefriendlyworld/ (accessed on 31 October 2020).
4. World Health Organization. *The Global Network for Age-Friendly Cities and Communities: Looking Back over the Last Decade, Looking Forward to the Next*; WHO: Geneva, Switzerland, 2018.
5. Del Barrio, E. *Guía de Implantación y Uso en Municipios: Euskadi Lagunkoia*; Departamento de Empleo Y Políticas Sociales-Gobierno Vasco: Vitoria-Gasteiz, Spain, 2014.
6. Gobierno Vasco, Matia Instituto. *Estrategia Vasca de Envejecimiento Activo 2015–2020*; Departamento de Empleo Y Políticas Sociales-Gobierno Vasco: Vitoria-Gasteiz, Spain, 2015.
7. Fitzgerald, K.G.; Caro, F.G. An Overview of Age-Friendly Cities and Communities Around the World. *J. Aging Soc. Policy* **2014**, *26*, 1–18. [CrossRef]
8. Lui, C.; Everingham, J.-A.; Warburton, J.; Cuthill, M.; Bartlett, H. What makes a community age-friendly: A review of international literature. *Australas. J. Ageing* **2009**, *28*, 116–121. [CrossRef]
9. Buffel, T.; Phillipson, C.; Scharf, T. Ageing in urban environments: Developing 'age-friendly'cities. *Crit. Soc. Policy* **2012**, *32*, 597–617. [CrossRef]
10. Toma, A.; Hamer, M.; Shankar, A. Associations between neighborhood perceptions and mental well-being among older adults. *Health Place* **2015**, *34*, 46–53. [CrossRef] [PubMed]
11. Tiraphat, S.; Peltzer, K.; Thamma-Aphiphol, K.; Suthisukon, K. The Role of Age-Friendly Environments on Quality of Life among Thai Older Adults. *Int. J. Environ. Res. Public Health* **2017**, *14*, 282. [CrossRef] [PubMed]
12. Nieboer, A.P.; Cramm, J.M. Age-Friendly Communities Matter for Older People's Well-Being. *J. Happiness Stud.* **2017**, *19*, 2405–2420. [CrossRef]
13. Gibney, S.; Zhang, M.; Brennan, C. Age-friendly environments and psychosocial wellbeing: A study of older urban residents in Ireland. *Aging Ment. Health* **2020**, *24*, 2022–2033. [CrossRef]
14. Park, S.; Lee, S. Age-friendly environments and life satisfaction among South Korean elders: Person–environment fit perspective. *Aging Ment. Health* **2016**, *21*, 693–702. [CrossRef]
15. van Dijk, H. Neighbourhoods for Ageing in Place. PhD Thesis, Erasmus University Rotterdam, Rotterdam, The Netherlands, 25 June 2015.
16. Wahl, H.-W.; Schilling, O.; Oswald, F.; Iwarsson, S. The home environment and quality of life-related outcomes in advanced old age: Findings of the ENABLE-AGE project. *Eur. J. Ageing* **2009**, *6*, 101–111. [CrossRef] [PubMed]
17. Scharlach, A.E.; Lehning, A.J. Ageing-friendly communities and social inclusion in the United States of America. *Ageing Soc.* **2012**, *33*, 110–136. [CrossRef]
18. Greenfield, E.A.; Oberlink, M.M.; Scharlach, A.E.; Neal, M.B.; Stafford, P.B. Age-Friendly Community Initiatives: Conceptual Issues and Key Questions. *Gerontologist* **2015**, *55*, 191–198. [CrossRef] [PubMed]
19. Greenfield, E.A. Age-Friendly Initiatives, Social Inequalities, and Spatial Justice. *Hast. Cent. Rep.* **2018**, *48*, S41–S45. [CrossRef] [PubMed]
20. George, L.K. Still Happy After All These Years: Research Frontiers on Subjective Well-being in Later Life. *J. Gerontol. Ser. B* **2009**, *65*, 331–339. [CrossRef]

21. Larson, R. Thirty years of research on the subjective well-being of older Americans. *J. Gerontol.* **1978**, *33*, 109–125. [CrossRef]
22. Pinquart, M.; Sörensen, S. Influences of socioeconomic status, social network, and competence on subjective well-being in later life: A meta-analysis. *Psychol. Aging* **2000**, *15*, 187. [CrossRef]
23. Jones, T.G.; Rapport, L.J.; Hanks, R.A.; Lichtenberg, P.A.; Telmet, K. Cognitive and psychological predictors of subjective well-being in urban older adults. *Clin. Neuropsychol.* **2003**, *17*, 3–18. [CrossRef]
24. Leung, B.W.-C.; Moneta, G.B.; McBride-Chang, C. Think Positively and Feel Positively: Optimism and Life Satisfaction in Late Life. *Int. J. Aging Hum. Dev.* **2005**, *61*, 335–365. [CrossRef]
25. Sasidharan, V.; Payne, L.; Orsega-Smith, E.; Godbey, G. Older adults' physical activity participation and perceptions of well-being: Examining the role of social support for leisure. *Manag. Leis.* **2006**, *11*, 164–185. [CrossRef]
26. Şener, A.; Terzioğlu, R.G.; Karabulut, E. Life satisfaction and leisure activities during men's retirement: A Turkish sample. *Aging Ment. Health* **2007**, *11*, 30–36. [CrossRef] [PubMed]
27. Ferguson, S.; Sue, J.; Goodwin, A.D. Optimism and Well-Being in Older Adults: The Mediating Role of Social Support and Perceived Control. *Int. J. Aging Hum. Dev.* **2010**, *71*, 43–68. [CrossRef] [PubMed]
28. Herero, V.G.; Extremera, N. Daily life activities as mediators of the relationship between personality variables and subjective well-being among older adults. *Pers. Individ. Differ.* **2010**, *49*, 124–129. [CrossRef]
29. Fernández-Mayoralas, G.; Schettini, R.; Sánchez-Román, M.; Rojo-Pérez, F.; Agulló, M.S.; João Forjaz, M. El Papel Del género En El Buen Envejecer. Una revisión sistemática Desde La Perspectiva científica. *Prisma Social* **2018**, *21*, 149–176.
30. Heidari, S.; Babor, T.F.; De Castro, P.; Tort, S.; Curno, M. Equidad según sexo y de género en la investigación: Justificación de las guías SAGER y recomendaciones para su uso. *Gac. Sanit.* **2019**, *33*, 203–210. [CrossRef]
31. Adams, K.B.; Leibbrandt, S.; Moon, H. A critical review of the literature on social and leisure activity and wellbeing in later life. *Ageing Soc.* **2010**, *31*, 683–712. [CrossRef]
32. García, R.I.C.; Fernández, C.C.; Cortés, C.C. Envejecer activamente desde una perspectiva de género. In *Identidades Culturales y Educación en la Sociedad Mundial [Recurso Electrónico]*; Universidad de Huelva: Pabellón, Huelva, 2012.
33. Coen, S.; Banister, E. *What a Difference Sex and Gender Make: A Gender, Sex and Health Research Casebook*; Canadian Institutes of Health Research: Ottowa, ON, Canada, 2012.
34. World Health Organization. *The Checklist of Essential Features of Age-Friendly Cities*; World Health Organization: Geneva, Switzerland, 2007.
35. World Health Organization. *Measuring the Age-Friendliness of Cities: A Guide to Using Core Indicators*; WHO: Geneva, Switzerland, 2015.
36. Buckner, S.; Mattocks, C.; Rimmer, M.; LaFortune, L. An evaluation tool for Age-Friendly and Dementia Friendly Communities. *Work. Older People* **2018**, *22*, 48–58. [CrossRef]
37. Buckner, S.; Pope, D.; Mattocks, C.; LaFortune, L.; Dherani, M.; Bruce, N. Developing Age-Friendly Cities: An Evidence-Based Evaluation Tool. *J. Popul. Ageing* **2019**, *12*, 203–223. [CrossRef]
38. Dikken, J.; Hoven, R.F.V.D.; Van Staalduinen, W.; Hulsebosch-Janssen, L.M.; Van Hoof, J. How Older People Experience the Age-Friendliness of Their City: Development of the Age-Friendly Cities and Communities Questionnaire. *Int. J. Environ. Res. Public Health* **2020**, *17*, 6867. [CrossRef]
39. Menec, V.; Nowicki, S. Examining the relationship between communities' 'age-friendliness' and life satisfaction and self-perceived health in rural Manitoba, Canada. *Rural. Remote Health* **2014**, *14*, 2594.
40. Handler, S. *A Research & Evaluation Framework for Age-Friendly Cities*; UK Urban Ageing Consortium: Manchester, UK, 2014.
41. Neal, M.B.; Wernher, I. Evaluating Your Age-Friendly Community Program: A Step-by-Step Guide. Available online: https://pdxscholar.library.pdx.edu/cgi/viewcontent.cgi?article=1012&context=aging_pub (accessed on 31 October 2020).
42. Orpana, H.; Chawla, M.; Gallagher, E.; Escaravage, E. Developing indicators for evaluation of age-friendly communities in Canada: Process and results. *Health Promot. Chronic Dis. Prev. Can.* **2016**, *36*, 214–223. [CrossRef] [PubMed]
43. Pinheiro, F.A.; Diogo, M.T.; Góis, J.E.S.; Paúl, C. Age-Friendly Cities Performance Assessment Indicators System Validation. *Psychology* **2015**, *6*, 622–632. [CrossRef]
44. Zaman, A.U.; Thornton, K. Prioritization of Local Indicators for the Development of an Age-Friendly City: A Community Perspective. *Urban Sci.* **2018**, *2*, 51. [CrossRef]
45. World Health Organization. *Global Age-Friendly Cities: A Guide*; World Health Organization: Geneva, Switzerland, 2007.
46. Europe, A. Looking at the Lives of Older People in the EU. 2019. Available online: https://ec.europa.eu/eurostat/statistics-explained/index.php/Ageing_Europe_-_looking_at_the_lives_of_older_people_in_the_EU (accessed on 28 December 2020).
47. Abellán García, A.; Ayala García, A.; Pujol Rodríguez, R. A Vueltas con el Umbral de Inicio de la Vejez. 2017. Available online: http://envejecimientoenred.es/vueltas-umbral-inicio-la-vejez/ (accessed on 28 December 2020).
48. WHO. *Promoting Mental Health: Concepts, Emerging Evidence, Practice: Summary Report*; World Health Organization: Geneva, Switzerland, 2004.
49. von Humboldt, S.; Leal, I. Qué influye en el bienestar subjetivo de los adultos mayores? Una revision sistematica de la literatura. *Rev. Argent. Clín. Psicol.* **2014**, *3*, 219–230.
50. Topp, C.W.; Østergaard, S.D.; Søndergaard, S.; Bech, P. The WHO-5 Well-Being Index: A Systematic Review of the Literature. *Psychother. Psychosom.* **2015**, *84*, 167–176. [CrossRef]

51. Lucas-Carrasco, R.; Allerup, P.; Bech, P. The Validity of the WHO-5 as an Early Screening for Apathy in an Elderly Population. *Curr. Gerontol. Geriatr. Res.* **2012**, *2012*, 1–5. [CrossRef]
52. Heun, R.; Bonsignore, M.; Barkow, K.; Jessen, F. Validity of the five-item WHO Well-Being Index (WHO-5) in an elderly population. *Eur. Arch. Psychiatry Clin. Neurosci.* **2001**, *251*, 27–31. [CrossRef]
53. Sibai, A.M.; Chaaya, M.; Tohme, R.A.; Mahfoud, Z.; Al-Amin, H. Validation of the Arabic version of the 5-item WHO well being index in elderly population. *Int. J. Geriatr. Psychiatry* **2008**, *24*, 106–107. [CrossRef]
54. Barua, A.; Kar, N. Screening for depression in elderly Indian population. *Indian J. Psychiatry* **2010**, *52*, 150–153. [CrossRef]
55. Awata, S.; Bech, P.; Koizumi, Y.; Seki, T.; Kuriyama, S.; Hozawa, A.; Ohmori, K.; Nakaya, N.; Matsuoka, H.; Tsuji, I. Validity and utility of the Japanese version of the WHO-Five Well-Being Index in the context of detecting suicidal ideation in elderly community residents. *Int. Psychogeriatr.* **2006**, *19*, 77–88. [CrossRef]
56. Heun, R.; Burkart, M.; Maier, W.; Bech, P. Internal and external validity of the WHO Well-Being Scale in the elderly general population. *Acta Psychiatr. Scand.* **1999**, *99*, 171–178. [CrossRef]
57. Calvente, M.D.M.G.; Rodrigo, M.L.J.; Morante, E.M. *Guía Para Incorporar la Perspectiva de Género a la Investigación en Salud*; Escuela Andaluza de Salud Pública: Granada, Spain, 2010.
58. Pardo, A.; Ruiz, M.A. *SPSS 11. Guía Para el Análisis de Datos*; Mc Graw Hill: New York, NY, USA, 2002.
59. Lennartsson, C.; Silverstein, M. Does Engagement With Life Enhance Survival of Elderly People in Sweden? The Role of Social and Leisure Activities. *J. Gerontol. Ser. B* **2001**, *56*, S335–S342. [CrossRef] [PubMed]
60. Warr, P.; Butcher, V.; Robertson, I. Activity and psychological well-being in older people. *Aging Ment. Health* **2004**, *8*, 172–183. [CrossRef] [PubMed]
61. Satorres, E. Bienestar Psicológico en la Vejez y su Relación con la Capacidad Funcional y la Satisfacción Vital. Ph.D. Thesis, Universitat de València, Valencia, Spain, 2013.
62. Triadó, M.C.; Villar, P.F. *Envejecer en Entornos Rurales*; Madrid: Imserso, Estudios, 2003.
63. Veenhoven, R. El estudio de la satisfacción con la vida. *Interv. Psicosoc.* **1994**, *3*, 87–116.
64. Diener, E. El bienestar subjetivo. *Psychosoc. Interv.* **1994**, *3*, 67–114.
65. Diener, E.; Suh, E.M.; Lucas, R.E.; Smith, H.L. Subjective well-being: Three decades of progress. *Psychol. Bull.* **1999**, *125*, 276. [CrossRef]
66. Barrientos, J. *Calidad de Vida: Bienestar Subjetivo*; Ediciones UDP: Santiago, Chile, 2005.
67. Van Hoof, J.; Kazak, J.K. Urban ageing. *Indoor Built Environ.* **2018**, *27*, 583–586. [CrossRef]
68. Mansfield, P.K.; Preston, D.B.; Crawford, C.O. Rural-urban differences in women's psychological well-being. *Health Care Women Int.* **1988**, *9*, 289–304. [CrossRef]
69. Bosch, P.M.; Gómez, A.D.V.; Ferrer, B.S. Los Grandes Olvidados: Las personas mayores en el entorno rural. *Psychosoc. Interv.* **2009**, *18*, 269–277. [CrossRef]
70. Bosch, P.M.; Gómez, A.D.V. Las personas mayores como actores en la comunidad rural: Innovación y empowerment. *Athenea Digit.* **2010**, *19*, 171–187.
71. Yasuda, N.; Zimmerman, S.I.; Hawkes, W.; Fredman, L.; Hebel, J.R.; Magaziner, J. Relation of Social Network Characteristics to 5-Year Mortality among Young-Old versus Old-Old White Women in an Urban Community. *Am. J. Epidemiol.* **1997**, *145*, 516–523. [CrossRef] [PubMed]
72. Bolan, M. The Mobility Experience and Neighborhood Attachment. *Demography* **1997**, *34*, 225–237. [CrossRef] [PubMed]
73. Ortiz, L.P. Jubilación, Género y Envejecimiento. In *Envejecimiento Activo, Envejecimiento en Positivo*; Universidad de La Rioja: Logrono, Spain, 2006.
74. Abellán, A.; Puyol, R. *Envejecimiento y Dependencia: Una Mirada al Panorama Futuro de la Población Española*; Mondial Assistance: Madrid, Spain, 2006.
75. Lu, L.; Shih, J.B.; Lin, Y.Y.; Ju, L.S. Personal and environmental correlates of happiness. *Pers. Individ. Differ.* **1997**, *23*, 453–462. [CrossRef]
76. Young, A.F.; Russell, A.; Powers, J.R. The sense of belonging to a neighbourhood: Can it be measured and is it related to health and well being in older women? *Soc. Sci. Med.* **2004**, *59*, 2627–2637. [CrossRef]
77. Ponce, M.S.H.; Rosas, R.P.E.; Lorca, M.B.F. *Social Capital, Social Participation and Life Satisfaction among Chilean Older Adults*; Revista de Saúde Pública: São Paulo, Brasil, 2014; pp. 739–749.
78. Román, X.A.S.; Toffoletto, M.C.; Sepúlveda, J.C.O.; Salfate, S.V.; Grandón, K.L.R. Factors associated to subjective wellbeing in older adults. *Texto Contexto Enferm.* **2017**, *26*. [CrossRef]
79. Pérez-Ortiz, L. Construcción social de la vejez: El sexo y la dependencia. *Rev. Española Geriatría Gerontol.* **2003**, *38*, 308–310. [CrossRef]
80. Fericgla, J.M. *Envejecer: Una Antropología de la Ancianidad*; Anthropos: Barcelona, Spain, 1992.
81. Gómez, V.; De Posada, C.V.; Barrera, F.; Cruz, J.E. Factores predictores de bienestar subjetivo en una muestra colombiana. *Rev. Latinoam. Psicol.* **2007**, *39*, 311–325.
82. Lawton, M.P.; Moss, M.S.; Winter, L.; Hoffman, C. Motivation in later life: Personal projects and well-being. *Psychol. Aging* **2002**, *17*, 539. [CrossRef]
83. Poon, C.Y.M.; Fung, H.H. Physical activity and psychological well-being among Hong Kong Chinese older adults: Exploring the moderating role of self-construal. *Int. J. Aging Hum. Dev.* **2008**, *66*, 1–19. [CrossRef]

84. García-Molina, V.A.; Carbonell-Baeza, A.; Fernández, M.D. Beneficios de la actividad física en personas mayores. *Rev. Int. Med. Cienc. Act. Fís. Deporte* **2010**, *10*, 556–576.
85. Campos, J.; Huertas, F.; Colado, J.C.; López, A.L.; Pablos, A.; Pablos, C. Efectos de un programa de ejercicio físico sobre el bienestar psicológico de mujeres mayores de 55 años. *Rev. Psicol. Deporte* **2003**, *12*, 7–26.
86. Menec, V.H. The Relation Between Everyday Activities and Successful Aging: A 6-Year Longitudinal Study. *J. Gerontol. Ser. B* **2003**, *58*, S74–S82. [CrossRef]
87. Havighurst, R.J.; Albrecht, R. Older People. *Population* **1954**, *9*, 357. [CrossRef]
88. Liechty, T.; Ribeiro, N.F.; Yarnal, C.M. Traveled Alone, but Never Felt Alone: An Exploration of the Benefits of an Older Women's Group Tour Experience. *Tour. Rev. Int.* **2009**, *13*, 17–29. [CrossRef]
89. Small, J. The Voices of Older Women Tourists. *Tour. Recreat. Res.* **2003**, *28*, 31–39. [CrossRef]
90. Morgan, N.; Pritchard, A.; Sedgley, D. Social tourism and well-being in later life. *Ann. Tour. Res.* **2015**, *52*, 1–15. [CrossRef]
91. Norstrand, J.A.; Glicksman, A.; Lubben, J.; Kleban, M. The Role of the Social Environment on Physical and Mental Health of Older Adults. *J. Hous. Elder.* **2012**, *26*, 290–307. [CrossRef]
92. Vega, M.T.; Pereira, M.A. Sentido de comunidad y bienestar en usuarios de asociaciones sociales de salud. *Glob. J. Community Psychol. Pract.* **2012**, *3*, 1–5.
93. Phillipson, C.; Bernard, M.; Phillips, J.; Ogg, J. Older people's experiences of community life: Patterns of neighbouring in three urban areas. *Sociol. Rev.* **1999**, *47*, 715–743. [CrossRef]
94. McMUNN, A.; Nazroo, J.; Wahrendorf, M.; Breeze, E.; Zaninotto, P. Participation in socially-productive activities, reciprocity and wellbeing in later life: Baseline results in England. *Ageing Soc.* **2009**, *29*, 765–782. [CrossRef]
95. Hess, A. Gastronomic Societies in the Basque Country. In *Learning Organizations*; Springer Science and Business Media LLC: Berlin, Germany, 2018; pp. 91–109.
96. Teixidor, F.L. Los marcos de la sociabilidad en el país Vasco contemporáneo. *Vasconia* **2018**, *33*, 139–157.
97. Nieboer, A.P.; Lindenberg, S.; Boomsma, A.; Bruggen, A.C.V. Dimensions Of Well-Being And Their Measurement: The Spf-Il Scale. *Soc. Indic. Res.* **2005**, *73*, 313–353. [CrossRef]

International Journal of
Environmental Research and Public Health

MDPI

Review

Quality of Life Framework for Personalised Ageing: A Systematic Review of ICT Solutions

Sabina Baraković [1,2,3,*], Jasmina Baraković Husić [3,4], Joost van Hoof [5,6], Ondrej Krejcar [7], Petra Maresova [7], Zahid Akhtar [8] and Francisco Jose Melero [9,10]

1 Faculty of Transport and Communications, University of Sarajevo, Zmaja od Bosne 8, 71000 Sarajevo, Bosnia and Herzegovina
2 American University in Bosnia and Herzegovina, Zmaja od Bosne 8, 71000 Sarajevo, Bosnia and Herzegovina
3 Little Mama Labs, Gradačačka 29, 71000 Sarajevo, Bosnia and Herzegovina; jasmina_barakovic@yahoo.com
4 Faculty of Electrical Engineering, University of Sarajevo, Zmaja od Bosne bb, 71000 Sarajevo, Bosnia and Herzegovina
5 Chair of Urban Ageing, Faculty of Social Work & Education, The Hague University of Applied Sciences, Johanna Westerdijkplein 75, 2521 EN Den Haag, The Netherlands; j.vanhoof@hhs.nl
6 Department of Spatial Economy, Faculty of Environmental Engineering and Geodesy, Wrocław University of Environmental and Life Sciences, ul. Grunwaldzka 55, 50-357 Wrocław, Poland
7 Faculty of Informatics and Management, University of Hradec Kralove, Rokitanskeho 62, 500 03 Hradec Kralove, Czech Republic; ondrej.krejcar@uhk.cz (O.K.); petra.maresova@uhk.cz (P.M.)
8 Department of Computer Science, University of Memphis, 234 Dunn Hall, Memphis, TN 38152, USA; zahid.eltc@gmail.com
9 Technical Research Centre of Furniture and Wood of the Region of Murcia, C/Perales S/N, 30510 Yecla, Spain; fj.melero@cetem.es
10 Telecommunication Networks Engineering Group, Technical University of Cartagena, 30202 Cartagena, Spain
* Correspondence: barakovic.sabina@gmail.com; Tel.: +387-61-265-615

Received: 7 April 2020; Accepted: 23 April 2020; Published: 24 April 2020

check for updates

Abstract: Given the growing number of older people, society as a whole should ideally provide a higher quality of life (QoL) for its ageing citizens through the concept of personalised ageing. Information and communication technologies (ICT) are subject to constant and rapid development, and can contribute to the goal of an improved QoL for older adults. In order to utilise future ICT solutions as a part of an age-friendly smart environment that helps achieve personalised ageing with an increased QoL, one must first determine whether the existing ICT solutions are satisfying the needs of older people. In order to accomplish that, this study contributes in three ways. First, it proposes a framework for the QoL of older adults, in order to provide a systematic review of the state-of-the-art literature and patents in this field. The second contribution is the finding that selected ICT solutions covered by articles and patents are intended for older adults and are validated by them. The third contribution of the study are the six recommendations that are derived from the review of the literature and the patents which would help move the agenda concerning the QoL of older people and personalised ageing with the use of ICT solutions forward.

Keywords: ICT; older adults; patent; personalised ageing; quality of life; review; smart ageing

1. Introduction

According to the latest statistics from the World Health Organization (WHO) and the United Nations (UN) [1,2], the number of people 60 years and over will increase from 900 million to 2 billion by 2050 [1]. Furthermore, it is shown that the population is ageing quicker than it used to, especially in developing societies compared to developed ones [2]. Older people are estimated to make up 22% of the entire world population. The ageing of society is not as straightforward as it seems. The usual approach to ageing is that of calendar years, which is an objective indicator of age, and which completely neglects biological, subjective, and sociological ageing, as well as many other aspects of it. What the world needs is a more nuanced approach that reflects the multidimensional aspects of ageing. Therefore, the societies that address ageing in a smart and multidimensional longevity-centred way will have vast economic and social opportunities before them.

Older adults require specific technological solutions that open a new market, which could stimulate the industry [3]. The creation of new products and services for older adults will, in turn, lead to new jobs and new companies in many innovative disciplines, such as electrical and software engineering, robotics, artificial intelligence, and so on. The economic potential of older adults should serve to change the ageing perception. Although ageing is usually connected with the loss of capabilities, older adults should stay active, since the professional experience and spending power of older adults could contribute to economic growth and development. Even more, in order to ensure sustainable society development in a future world where an average age is expected to be quite high, society as a whole must provide a high Quality of Life (QoL) for its ageing citizens [4]. In order to achieve a high QoL while ageing, one needs to have a personalised and individual approach regarding all its components. Personalised ageing refers to the fact that successful ageing is always connected to a person's unicity [5]. Achieving personalised ageing is a very challenging and time-consuming task, which requires reshaping our current social concepts and behaviours and producing effective models and frameworks.

Inevitably, intertwined personalised ageing and QoL as multidimensional concepts need to be treated differently in the ever-omnipresent digital environment, while at the same time, smart technology solutions need to be adapted to suit an ageing society and satisfy a high QoL [3,6]. Information and Communication Technologies (ICT) see a constant and rapid development, and provide a very powerful tool that can help in creating models and enable achievement of the ultimate goal, namely that of an age-friendly society with an improved QoL [7–9]. Yet, it is important that those ICT solutions are directed towards reaching the goal of personalised ageing and are initially designed and built to contribute to the QoL paradigm.

According to the abovementioned, at the centre of the vision on personalised ageing is the older adult who aspires to live independently and in safety. A good ICT solution that reaches this vision has to perceive an older adult's unique conditions and lifestyle. Therefore, the development of such an ICT solution should respect the older adult's way of living, so that one can perform daily routines undisturbed by the technology that contributes to one's QoL.

This also means that ICT should serve the need of the end-users, instead of being fancy gadgets with a finite lifespan and a limited applicability. Therefore, efforts and research activities should be directed towards making useful models and effective technologies that contribute to QoL and personalised ageing. This forms the foundation of the first of the three aims of this paper: the proposal of a framework for the QoL for older adults through a systematic review of relevant state-of-the-art articles and patents, i.e., personalised ageing which can further be utilised by various stakeholders on this path.

However, in order to utilise the future ICT solutions as parts of a smart environment that helps achieve personalised ageing with an increased QoL, one must first determine whether the existing ICT solutions are satisfying the needs of older people. In other words, are these solutions successful in their performance. The existing research shows that current ICT solutions are partly succeeding in the direct improvement of the QoL of older people [10]. Therefore, the second aim of this paper is to investigate to what extent ICT solutions directly improve QoL for older people by surveying the wider scope of research papers from the relevant databases and patents. The third aim is to draw conclusions and guidelines for future ICT solutions for older adults, so that we could optimise their implementation.

This paper is organised as follows: Section 2 describes the notions of smart ageing, QoL, and personalised ageing and their mutual interplay. Moreover, it presents a framework for the quality of life of older adults that shaped this review. Section 3 provides a detailed review methodology: data sources and search strategy, study selection processes (inclusion and exclusion criteria), and publications review and data abstraction. In other words, this part of the paper describes used methodology and provides meta-analysis. Section 4 gives the results of the conducted survey, while Section 5 discusses the obtained results, recognises the gaps and opens research questions for future studies, and describes study limitations. Finally, Section 6 provides the conclusions of the paper.

2. The Framework for Quality of Life and Personalised Ageing

This section introduces and elaborates the terms of quality of life and smart ageing, and discusses ICT solutions as building blocks that sync into the concept of personalised ageing, i.e., achieving quality of life for older adults. It provides the description of the proposed framework for achieving an increased QoL for older adults, i.e., personalised ageing, from the perspective of ICT solutions. This proposed framework is used for the structured review of the literature and patents, and serves as a basis for the presentation of the results of both reviews.

2.1. Quality of Life

Quality of life is a broad concept that has many definitions and meanings depending on the context under consideration. It is referred to as [11]: "a perception of one's position in life in the context of culture and value systems in which they live and in relation to their goals, expectations, standards, and concerns". The QoL is culturally built as a person's search to satisfy the three universal requirements, i.e., (1) safety and security, (2) a sense of integrity and meaning of life, and (3) a sense of belonging to a social network. As will be discussed below, this means that culture contributes to three QoL dimensions (i.e., economic and physical safety; overall experience of life; and leisure and social interactions). It is also specified in terms of well-being [12]: "a state of well-being which is a composite of two components: (1) the ability to perform everyday activities which reflect physical, psychological, and social well-being, and (2) patient satisfaction with levels of functioning and the control of disease and/or treatment related symptoms". Others use the term satisfaction with life [13]: "QoL is the degree of need and satisfaction within the physical, psychological, social, activity, material, and structural area". One can conclude that QoL is something like the overall enjoyment of life and a multidimensional concept which emphasises the self-perceptions of an individual's current state of mind, which is affected in a complex way by the person's physical health, psychological state, personal beliefs, social relationships, and their relationship to salient features of their environment [14].

According to the European Framework 8 + 1 [15], QoL constitutes the following eight dimensions: (i) material living conditions; (ii) health; (iii) education; (iv) productive and valued activities; (v) governance and basic rights; (vi) leisure and social interactions; (vii) natural and living environment; (viii) economic and physical safety; and lastly (ix) overall experience of life. Material living conditions cover the income, consumption, and material conditions of a person. Productive and valued activities relate to economic activity, i.e., quality and quantity of employment, as well as other activities, i.e., inactivity and unpaid work. Health is measured in outcomes, healthy and unhealthy behaviours, and access to healthcare. Education covers competences and skills, lifelong learning, and opportunities for education. Leisure and social interactions include quantity and quality of leisure, as well as access to leisure, and the social dimension, i.e., relations with people and activities for people together with social support and cohesion. Economic security and physical safety address wealth (assets), debt, and income insecurity from the economic side, and crime and a perception of physical safety from the physical side. Governance and basic rights cover institutions and public services, discrimination and equal opportunities, and active citizenship. Natural and living environments include pollution, access to green and recreation spaces, as well as landscape and built environments. The ninth dimension, i.e., overall experience of life, covers life satisfaction, effects (negative—being nervous or being depressed or down, and positive—being happy), and meaning and purpose of life.

2.2. Smart Ageing

Smart ageing is a term that is often used interchangeably with healthy ageing [16] or active ageing [17], but without an exact definition. One description explains it as a wide concept defined as technology and innovation usage in both the public and private sectors to produce products, services, solutions, and systems to improve the QoL of people who are 50 years old and over [18]. A similar definition is given by Varnai et al. in [19] and is as follows: smart ageing is using technology, innovation and design in both the public and private sectors to produce products, services, solutions, and systems to improve the quality of life for the older generation in three key areas: functional food, connected health, and assisted living. Moreover, Song et al. in [20] regards smart ageing as a concept for mitigating the effects of ageing and improving older peoples' life by managing various healthcare challenges with the utilisation of biomedical, computing, and communication technologies.

According to EuroHealthNet [16], the key determinants of smart ageing are: (i) access to services; (ii) employment and volunteering; (iii) physical activity; (iv) social inclusion and participation; (v) new technologies; (vi) diet and nutrition; (vii) long-term care; (viii) environment and accessibility; and (ix) education and life-long learning. Namely, appropriate health and social services should be accessible to all older people. It is important that older people are not excluded by a new means of delivering services (like a shift from personal care to online services). Being employed or involved in voluntary activities is a great way of maintaining health and avoiding social exclusion. In adults aged 65 years and over, physical activity includes leisure time; physical activity; transportation; occupations; household chores; play; games; sports; or planned exercise, in the context of daily, family, and community activities [21]. Social inclusion and participation in various activities enables older people to grasp opportunities to be active and breaks down barriers they face in their everyday lives, such as cognitive impairment and depression [22], a lack of stimulation and social interaction [23], lethargy, boredom, depression, and loneliness [24]. New technologies are developing at a rapid pace and affect every segment of our lives. ICT can and will play a key part in helping older people to be more independent and to lead healthier lives. In this regard, many ICT solutions are proposed to prolong and support the independent and active living of older adults. Therefore, those solutions contribute to long-term care by providing possibilities to monitor the activities and health of older adults. ICT solutions for activities monitoring are deployed at home to warn caregivers about any unusual behaviour in older adults or outside the home to control risky situations. On the other hand, ICT solutions for health monitoring combine ICT solutions for activity monitoring at home with the use of medical devices. However, those solutions have to address several challenges and barriers, i.e., (i) ease-of-use because many older adults are not comfortable with technologies; (ii) invisibility and disuse to isolate older adults; (iii) privacy and security to avoid older adults becoming vulnerable considering their health conditions; (iv) affordability of technology in terms of cost; and (v) supporting older people to stay in their homes or move in different environments independently. Ageing affects nutrition as well as lifestyle: adequate nutrition becomes increasingly difficult with increasing age, whereas physical activity usually decreases. Nutrition and lifestyle, however, are important determinants of health and outcome in older people, especially in those with multiple chronic conditions [25]. Nutritional status, dietary habits, and food patterns vary widely across Europe [26]. Moreover, the quality and accessibility of the environment in which an older person lives can have a significant bearing on how active they are in society. Finally, there is a strong connection between learning and better health for older people. The concept of life-long learning does not mean only obtaining employment-related qualifications, it also means promoting learning throughout the life course, for the well-being and enjoyment of all.

2.3. *The Framework—A Contribution of ICT Solutions*

The elaboration on quality of life and smart ageing provide the necessary building blocks to introduce the framework of personalised ageing. Figure 1 represents our framework for achieving personalised ageing, i.e., the QoL of older adults. The proposed framework has a horizontal and a vertical component.

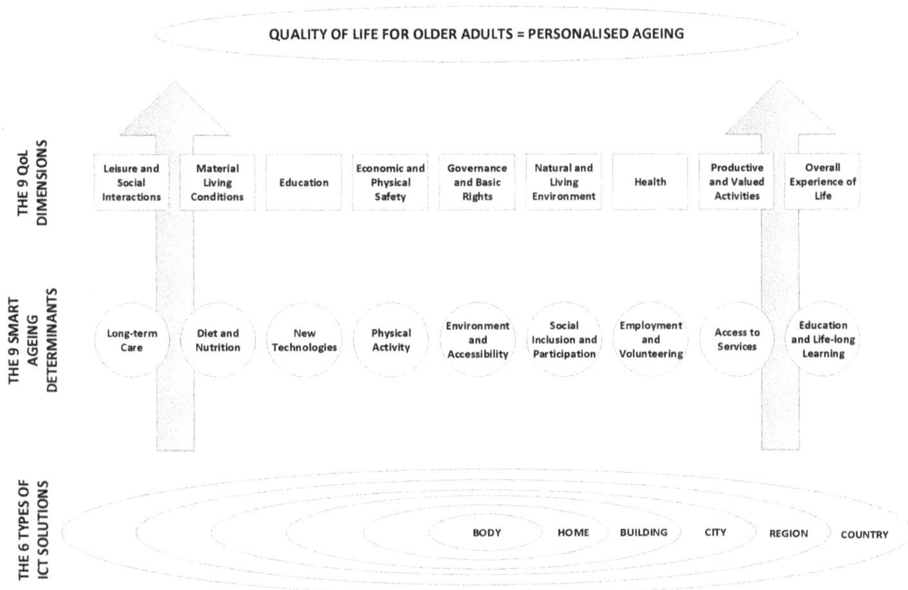

Figure 1. The framework for the Quality of Life (QoL) of older adults.

2.3.1. Horizontal Component

The horizontal component refers to and describes the environment in which the multiple ICT solutions will operate, further contributing to the smart ageing concept. As given in the framework, those can be the: (i) human body; (ii) home; (iii) building; (iv) city; (v) region; and (vi) country. Smart ICT body-worn solutions cover devices with installed tools, applications, or systems that will be placed on the human body, i.e., watches, glasses, bracelets, chips, and pacemakers. Smart ICT home solutions cover items that surround the older persons in their homes or narrow living environments such as smart furniture, phones, computers, spatial, and temporal sensors. Both types of solutions should aid older adults in their more confident and independent behaviour in the domestic environment. Furthermore, these solutions could be totally personalised to older individuals. Smart ICT building solutions include the rule of operation, and devices that older persons encounter and use as soon as they close their home doors, but before they are out in the streets and concern things such as stairs, elevators, keys, etc. Smart ICT urban solutions refer to solutions (logic, applications, systems, devices) that are placed anywhere in the city (or a village) and increase the ease the life of older adults when they come across environments that include public transport and public surfaces, various spatial and temporal sensors, and so on. ICT building solutions and city/urban solutions are ones that are used by other cohorts in the population too, but they need to be adjustable to older adults considering the fact that they will soon make up a quarter of the entire world population. Moreover, these solutions should encourage and support older adults to take their deserved place in society instead of withdrawing from it. Smart ICT regional solutions cover applications and systems that provide better governance of certain regions taking into account their specificities, while smart ICT country solutions refer to those that affect the country as a whole, and are mostly regulatory and policy related. The latter two also affect the other age groups in society, but they should be conceptualised in an adjustable fashion in order to satisfy the needs of older adults.

2.3.2. Vertical Component

Taking the bottom-top approach, the description of the vertical component of the framework aimed at the QoL of older adults is as follows: The first step on our way to a better QoL are ICT solutions (Figure 1). That is, the existing ICT solutions and ones that are to be developed in the (near) future should be designed to contribute to key smart ageing determinants.

The next level is having smart ageing determinants mapped out into QoL dimensions. A proposition for the mapping is given in Figure 2. The main aim of this mapping is to have a link between these two concepts. The knowledge of these connections, i.e., which smart ageing determinant influences which QoL dimension, gives better targeting opportunities and effective attainment of the ultimate goal—QoL for older adults, i.e., personalised ageing. The main aim of this mapping is to find a link between these two concepts (i.e., smart ageing determinants and QoL dimensions). For example, an ICT tool that is designed to satisfy the smart ageing determinant education and life-long learning can positively affect and improve the QoL for older adults by contributing to its following dimensions. First, leisure and social Interactions, because it allows older adults to entertain themselves and to get in touch with other learners. Second, material living conditions, because it allows older persons to increase their incomes by doing various paid jobs if they increase their knowledge in a specific domain. Third, education, because it allows them to have personal growth. Fourth, health, because it allows older adults to take better care of their physical and mental health if they constantly learn about the new medical improvements and health recommendations. Fifth, productive and valued activities, because it allows older adults to feel productive. Finally sixth, the overall experience of life, because it allows them to feel better if they enjoy learning.

On the other hand, QoL dimensions on material living conditions can be affected by the following smart ageing determinants: education and life-long learning; employment and volunteering; environment and accessibility; and access to services. For example, education and life-long learning allows older adults to gain knowledge they can monetise and improve their material status. Employment means that older adults can work and thereby improve their material living conditions. Environment and accessibility as well as access to services impact material living conditions as a QoL dimension in terms of providing opportunities to allow older adults to increase the level of their material living conditions.

It is also important to stress that in addition to the impact that these smart ageing determinants individually have on QoL dimensions, they can also have interdependent relations among each other. These interplays between them as well as constructs that they form which in the end can affect QoL dimensions should be additionally investigated in future research.

The final level is formed by the QoL constituents (in this framework called QoL dimensions (8 + 1) [15]) a contribution to the improvement of the overall QoL of older adults, which leads to personalised ageing. In case there are multiple ICT solutions designed to be personalised and satisfy multiple smart ageing determinants, which in combination contribute to multiple QoL dimensions, then those improved QoL dimensions jointly accomplish the goal of QoL while ageing or in personalised ageing.

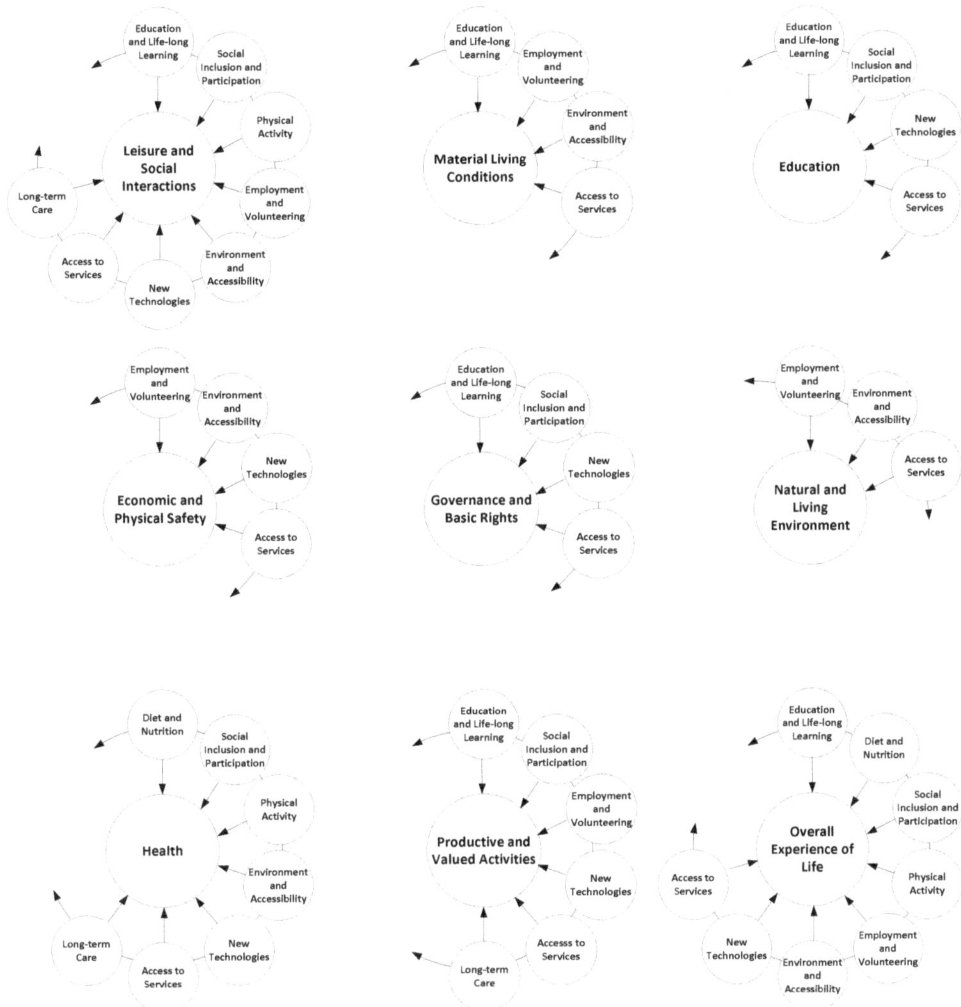

Figure 2. The proposed mapping of the smart determinants to QoL dimensions.

3. Methodology of the Review

The following paragraphs describe the methodology for the reviewing process, namely data sources and search strategy; the study selection process; the review of publications review and data extraction.

3.1. Data Sources and Search Strategy

As research on smart ageing and ICT solutions for QoL has been conducted in multiple scientific domains, and scientific findings have been published in different literature repositories, our search strategy focused on two data sources, i.e., scientific articles and intellectual property (IP) patents.

The article search was undertaken from January 2019 to March 2019 in order to identify published peer-reviewed articles in English. The databases searched included Web of Science (WoS), IEEE Xplore, and Scopus (the first source from 1999 until the last in 2019). The papers were extracted from databases using the following search phrases alone or in different combinations using logical operators of "AND" and "OR": smart elderly, smart aging, ambient assisted living, and ambient assistance living.

The patents search was performed in the ESPACENET database. The ESPACENET database was searched from November 2019 to March 2020 with the aim of finding relevant patents. The database search included the following keywords in "topic" search (title or abstract or claims): (smart AND elderly) OR (smart AND aging AND living AND elderly) OR (smart AND aging AND ambient AND assisted AND living AND elderly) OR (ambient assisted living) OR (ambient assistance living).

3.2. Study Selection Process

The titles and abstracts retrieved by the database search were analysed in order to select data sources (i.e., articles and patents) that satisfied the inclusion criteria. Two independent researchers (ZA and SB for articles, SB and JBH for patents) evaluated the titles and abstracts and compared them to the inclusion and exclusion criteria. They met in order to reach a consensus through discussion. In case of different opinions regarding the abstract's suitability, the given data source was included for further analysis. Further on, the two researchers surveyed the full texts of the selected data sources. In order to determine suitability for inclusion in further analysis, one researcher assessed all the articles and the other one evaluated all the patents. After data abstraction of the final selected data sources (i.e., articles and patents), two new researchers independently surveyed 20% of randomly selected articles and patents. If there was any disagreement on the suitability of data sources, advice was asked from a third researcher (JBH for articles, OK for patents) for an evaluation of the given data source. A third researcher was an interdisciplinary expert that provided a final decision whether or not to include the data source in the analysis. Figure 3 (inspired by [27]) shows the data source selection process in more detail.

3.2.1. Inclusion Criteria

The inclusion criteria were as follows:

- Articles and patents which included ICT solutions to achieve the QoL for older adults that:
    1. Addressed ICT solutions in home or supportive care environments for older adults with specific needs regardless of whether the ICT solution was embedded on the human body or in a home, building, city, region, and country;
    2. Addressed the physical and/or mental needs faced by older adults;
    3. Involved ICT solutions that have been implemented or deployed in pilot form contributing to the key smart ageing determinants (i.e., long-term care, diet and nutrition, new technologies, physical activity, social inclusion and participation, employment and volunteering, access to services, and education and life-long learning);
    4. Articles and patents which intend to understand various QoL dimensions (i.e., material living conditions, health, education, productive and valued activities, governance and basic rights, leisure and social interactions, natural and living environment, economic and physical safety, and overall experience of life) in terms of QoL for older adults;
    5. Articles and patents which are peer-reviewed and published in English within a 20-year period (i.e., 1999–2019).
    6. Articles that used any kind of research methodology with positive/negative results.

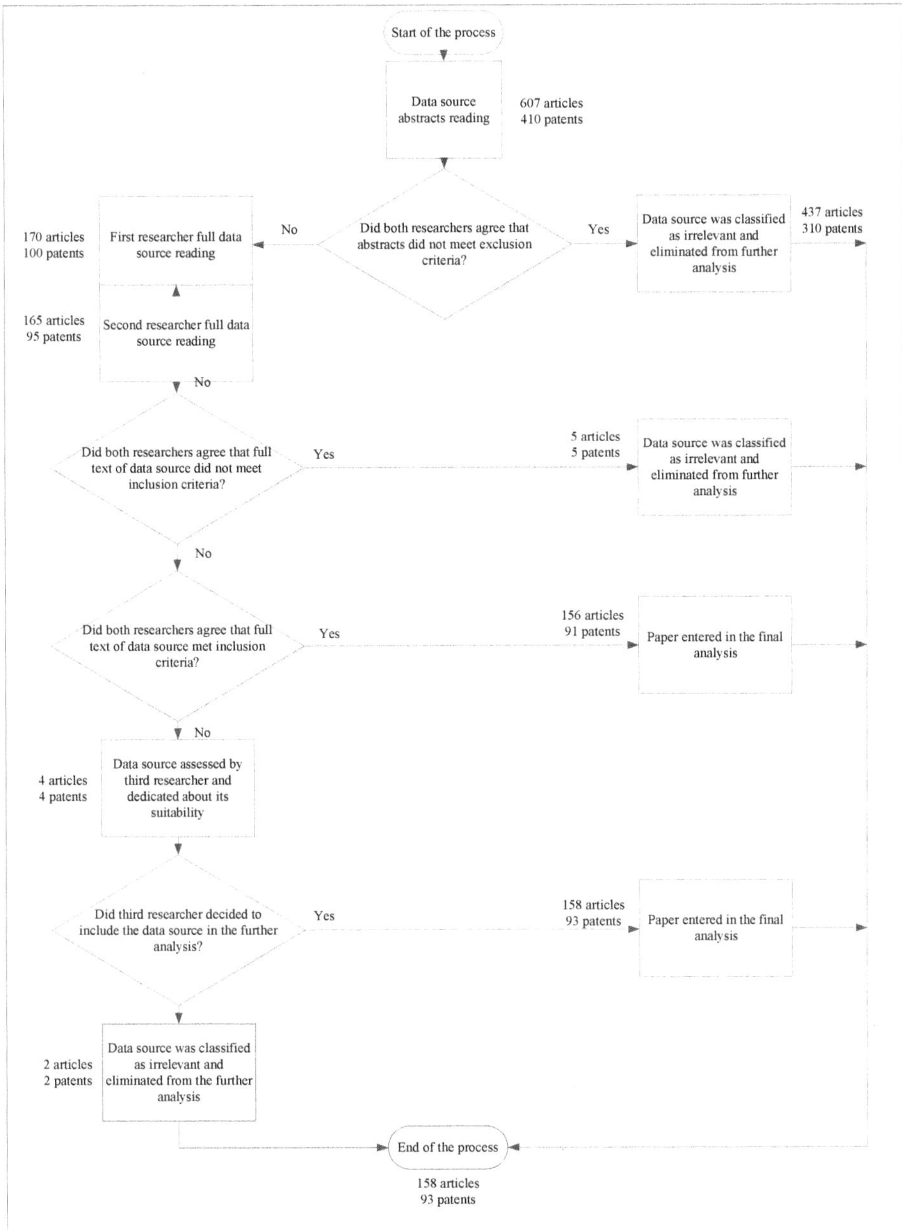

Figure 3. The data source selection process.

3.2.2. Exclusion Criteria

The exclusion criteria were as follows:

- Articles and patents written in a language other than English;
- Articles and patents that were unavailable or available with an abstract;
- Articles covering theoretical reviews, narrative reviews, meta-analyses, conference notes, and other types of literature reviews;
- Articles and patents that are about technology which differs from ICT for older people;
- Research published in conference proceedings, books, book chapters, and master's and doctoral theses;
- Articles and patents that consider ICT solutions contributing to smart concepts other than smart ageing and QoL for older adults;
- Articles and patents on assistive devices such as canes, wheeled walkers, hearing aids, etc.;
- Studies published before 1999;
- Research which focuses on ICT solutions contributing to the concept of smart ageing in developing countries, which are under different conditions to developed countries;
- Research with a focus on industry and production of ICT solutions;
- Research materials on telemonitoring, telemedicine or telehealth programs which include self-monitoring using low-complexity technologies;
- Research materials that reported combined interventions;
- Articles that did not provide enough information for categorising the data source.

3.3. *Publications Review and Data Extraction*

The analysis was conducted by an inductive approach. The results section was divided into two parts, i.e., an article analysis and a patent analysis. A detailed summary of each article and patent was provided. Throughout this process, the following items were systematically extracted: authors, titles, publication place, database (WoS, Scopus, Xplore), QoL dimensions (previously listed and described in Section 2.1), smart ageing determinants (previously listed and described in Section 2.2), service users (older adults, care members, family members, other), validation indication (has the solution been validated by the older adults?), and operating environment (body, home, building, city, region, and country). Then, the extracted fields were organised according to the framework in order to provide a structured overview of ICT studies contributing to QoL for older adults, i.e., personalised ageing. In addition, we used those fields to perform the meta-analysis of both selected articles and patents. The meta-analysis enabled the quantification of articles (in Section 4.1) and patents (in Section 4.2), which include ICT solutions to achieve the QoL for older adults in order to provide the input data for discussion and conclusions.

4. Results

In the following sections, the results of both the literature analysis and the patent analysis are described in more detail.

4.1. Literature Analysis

A total of 607 articles were identified during the initial search phase. After removing duplicates and applying the inclusion and exclusion criteria, only 158 studies were included in the final meta-analysis and data-abstraction phase (26%). Approximately 86% of them were found through the WoS database, while in Scopus and Xplore databases 11.5% and 2.5% of studies were found. It is important to note that the selected papers that are in WoS but also in other subject databases are categorised as WoS papers, while the ones that were only in Scopus or Xplore are marked accordingly. When it comes to the distribution by year, a total of 4.43% of articles were published between 1999 to 2009, and 31% between 2010 to 2014. Articles published in the period from 2015 to 2019 count for 12%, 14%, 18.4%, 16.5%, and 3.6% for each year respectively (Supplementary Materials).

Taking the bottom-up approach, the operational environment was addressed firstly (in accordance with Figure 1). The obtained results show that currently the most represented solutions are the ones for the home environment (66%, i.e., 104 articles out of 158 studies), followed by the ones that are related to the human body (24%, i.e., 38 articles out of 158 studies). Solutions categorised as building, city, region, and country count for a mere 1%, 4%, 0%, and 5%, respectively.

Further on, the addressed ICT solutions that are designed for smart ageing contribute to 7 out of 9 smart ageing determinants, which are represented in the following percentages: 36% for physical activity, 18% for new technologies, 16% for long-term care, 14% each for environment and accessibility and social inclusion and participation, and 1% each for diet and nutrition and access to services. Missing determinants are employment and volunteering and education and life-long learning. Moreover, the currently represented smart ageing determinants can be mapped to 7 out of 9 QoL dimensions, i.e., health (30%), overall experience of life (23%), economic and physical safety (17%), material living conditions (13%), natural and living environment (9%), leisure and social interactions (7%), and productive and values activities (1%). Missing QoL dimensions are education and governance and basic rights.

When it comes to the mapping of addressed smart ageing determinants to the addressed QoL dimensions, in accordance to the obtained results, the leisure and social interaction QoL dimension is impacted by ICT solutions designed to satisfy the following smart determinants: social inclusion and participation (7 studies), physical activity (2 studies), and environment and accessibility (1 study). Material and living conditions have been affected by ICT solutions for physical activity (7 studies), new technologies (6 studies), environment and accessibility (5 studies), and long-term care (3 studies). ICT solutions designed for physical activity (16 studies), long-term care (6 studies), environment and accessibility (2 studies), access to services, new technologies, social inclusion, and participation (1 study each) contribute to economic and physical safety. The natural and living environment is influenced by the ICT solutions for the next smart ageing determinants: physical activity (7 studies), environment and accessibility (5 studies), and long-term care and new technologies (1 study each). Physical activity related to ICT solutions (2 studies) are mapped to productive and valued activities as QoL dimensions. The QoL dimensions that the most diverse ICT solutions are mapped to are health and overall experience of life. Physical activity and long-term care (15 studies each), new technologies (10 studies), environment and accessibility (3 studies), social inclusion and participation (2 studies), and access to services; diet and nutrition; education and lifelong learning (1 study each) related to ICT solutions are mapped to health, while new technologies (12 studies), physical activity (9 studies), environment and accessibility (7 studies), social inclusion and participation (3 studies), and access to services; diet and nutrition; and long-term care (2 studies each) ICT solutions are mapped to the QoL dimension and overall experience of life.

Additional items that were investigated in this study were whether the addressed selected studies and the ICT solutions that they propose are made for older adults or for the care of a family member or other, and whether these solutions were validated by the aimed end users. Obtained results show that 60.8% of studies propose solutions for older adults, 24.7% for care members, 13.9% for others (such as scientists, data collectors, etc.), and only one study was exclusively for family members. We have found that 78.5% of the considered solutions are validated by the targeted group of end-users, while the remaining 21.5% are not.

4.2. Patent Analysis

A total of 410 patents were identified during the initial search phase. After removing duplicates and applying the inclusion and exclusion criteria, only 93 patents were included in the final meta-analysis and data-abstraction phase (22.7%). All of the patents were taken from ESPACNET. When it comes to the distribution by year, we found no relevant patents in the period 1999–2009. In the period 2010–2019, a total of 13% of the patents were published between 2010 and 2014, and patents published between 2015 and 2019 count for 3.2%, 6.4%, 14%, 32.2%, and 31.2% for each year respectively.

Applying the bottom-up approach again, the operational environment was firstly addressed. The obtained results show that currently, the most represented solutions covered by patents are the ones for the home environment (45.1%, i.e., 42 out of 93 patents). Second place is taken by the ICT solutions related to the human body (26.9%, i.e., 25 out of 93 patents). ICT solutions categorised as building, city, region, and country count for 3.2%, 0%, 1%, and 23.8%, respectively.

The addressed ICT solutions in patents designed for smart ageing contribute to 7 out of 9 smart ageing determinants. This is the same as for the literature review. Missing determinants are employment and volunteering and education and life-long learning as it was the case with the literature as well. The percentages are: long-term care with 50.5%; new technologies with 28%; physical activity with 7.5%; social inclusion and participation with 4.3%; and access to services, diet and nutrition, and environment and accessibility with 3.2% each. The currently represented smart ageing determinants in the patent analysis can be mapped to 6 out of 9 QoL dimensions, i.e., health (65.6%); leisure, social interactions, and economic and physical safety (8.6%); overall experience of life (7.5%); material living conditions (5.4%); and natural and living environment (4.3%). The missing QoL dimensions are education and governance and basic rights with added productive and valued activities. This corresponds to the outcomes of the literature review.

Regarding the mapping of the addressed smart ageing determinants to addressed QoL dimensions in patents analysis, in accordance to the obtained results, leisure and social interaction QoL dimensions are impacted by ICT solutions designed to satisfy the following smart determinants: social inclusion and participation (4 items); new technologies (2 items); and access to services (1 item). Material and living conditions have been affected by ICT solutions for new technologies (4 items) and physical activity (1 item). ICT solutions designed for new technologies (4 items), long-term care (2 items), and physical activity and access to services (1 item each) contribute to economic and physical safety. Natural and living environment is influenced by the ICT solutions for the following smart ageing determinants: environment and accessibility (3 items) and long-term care (1 item). Overall experience of life is covered by ICT solutions contributing to new technologies (6 items) and long-term care (1 item) smart determinants. The QoL dimension that the most diverse ICT solutions are mapped to is health. Long-term care (43 items), new technologies (9 items), physical activity (5 items), diet and nutrition (3 items), and access to services (1 item) related to ICT solutions are mapped to health.

An additional question that was addressed in this study is whether the addressed selected patents and the proposed ICT solutions are made for older adults or for carers or relatives or other persons. The obtained results show that 88% of patents propose solutions for the older adults (44%) and carers (44%), while 12% propose solutions for relatives. No evidence was found that the selected patents were validated by the targeted end-user groups.

Finally, the summary of joint literature and patent analysis results according to Figure 1 is given in Figure 4.

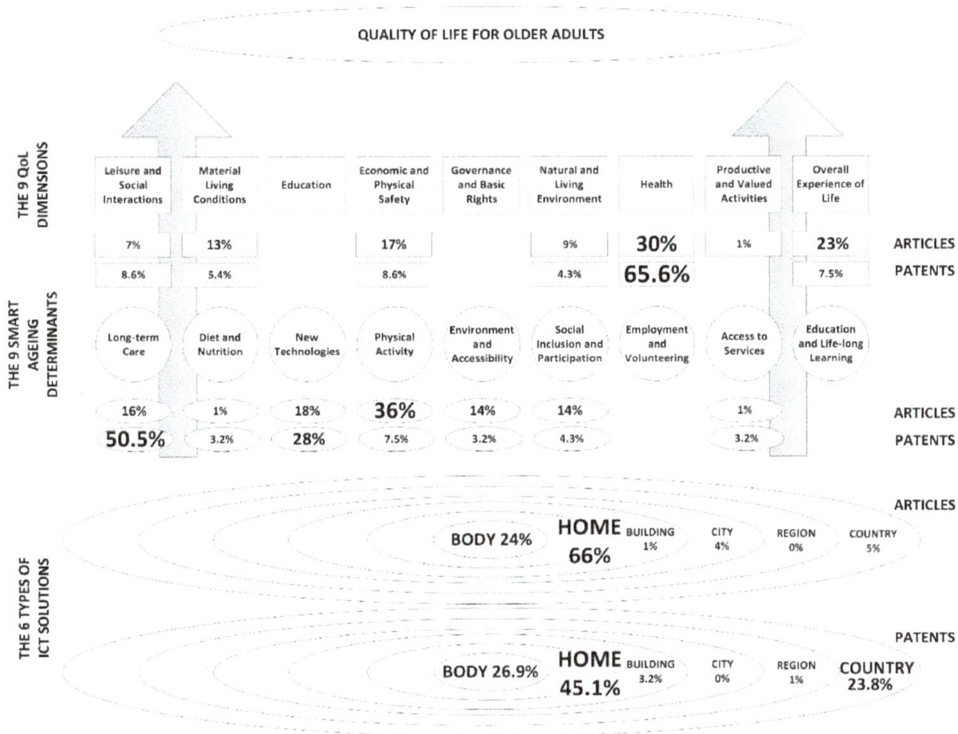

Figure 4. Summary of joint literature and patent analysis results in accordance with the framework on Figure 1.

5. Discussion

Results discussion is organised related to proposed framework consisting of horizontal and vertical components. From the horizontal component perspective, the proposed framework for achieving an improved QoL for older results and personalised ageing calls for a balanced distribution of ICT solutions across different application places such as body, home, city, building, region, and country (Figure 1). If the solutions are represented in a balanced manner, they create a basis for personalised ageing in combination. From the vertical component perspective, the framework advocates having ICT solutions which are designed to satisfy all nine different smart ageing determinants (Figure 1). This does not imply that one should have ICT solutions that simultaneously contribute to all nine determinants, but to one or several different ones if possible. Moreover, the framework proposes adequate mapping of smart ageing determinants to nine different QoL dimensions which ultimately would result in improved overall QoL for older adults (Figures 1 and 2). The following subsections elaborate these findings based on horizontal and vertical components of the proposed framework in more detail, as well as study flaws and limitations.

5.1. Horizontal Component

The obtained results of this structured review deviate from the horizontal component of the framework in several segments. Firstly, the article analysis shows that 90% of the ICT solutions are home- and body-focused, while the patent analysis shows that a lower percentage of patents of 72 is focused on such solutions. Very often, this is in connection with the monitoring of movement, certain body functions, and the spaces where a person moves around (bedroom, bathroom, and other selected parts of the apartment). Another finding of this study is that many ICT solutions can be identified in the field of motion tracking and monitoring of older people, in particular, in the domain of fall detection, tracking, and taking medication. When implementing these complex solutions, people run into the limits of the health care system's readiness to process the large amount of data that becomes available and can be shared.

The vast majority of existing body solutions are focused on solving a partial problem, as well as complex solutions where a home control unit is provided. Such home control units can be connected to, and interface with, a combination of health equipment, smart home appliances, smart medicine cabinets, a smart pantry, wearable sensors, motion detectors, video cameras, microphones, video monitors, speakers, smart thermostats, lighting, floor sensors, bed sensors, smoke detectors, glass breakage detectors, door sensors, and other perimeter sensors [28]. Similar findings are confirmed by other studies. For example, Haghi et al. [29] reviewed wearable health care devices, both in the literature as in commercial efforts. Their study showed that a vast array of wearables, with the help of improved technology, are considered to be reliable tools for long-term health monitoring systems. Furthermore, Yin et al. [30] showed that the rapidly advancing information technologies and the emerging Internet of Things (IoT) technology have provided great opportunities for developing smart healthcare information systems. Nevertheless, challenges still exist in achieving secure and effective telecare applications. In their view, identified areas for future improvement are listed as follows: self-learning and self-improvement; hardware; and standardisation or privacy and security. In terms of hardware, the question of how to achieve unobtrusiveness still poses a big challenge, as comfort is naturally a key concern. Actually, the need to integrate multiple sensors into one solution contradicts the goal of unobtrusiveness. Furthermore, a number of research teams and organisations have contributed to the deployment and standardisation of IoT technologies. Finally, the two main prerequisites of applying IoT-based systems are their utility and safety for users. The privacy of older adults must be ensured in order to prevent unauthorised identification and tracking. From this perspective, the higher the level of autonomy and intelligence of IoT items, the more challenges concerning the protection of identities and privacy would come to the fore [31,32]. Oude Weernink et al. [33] further distinguish between the settings in which such technologies are used, for instance, the nursing home or hospital environment versus the own home or on the street, and whether technologies are used to track or monitor older people, or even their belongings, as part of a maintenance protocol. In conclusion, a proper analysis of the goals, settings, and potential users (and their knowledge and awareness concerning technology, for instance, in the case of dementia) of technologies needs to be made before introducing technologies into the daily lives of older people.

Although the contribution of the selected ICT solutions to personalised ageing and improving QoL for older adults in body and home domains is not questionable, there seems to be a gap. What is currently missing from a more comprehensive approach to the topics of personalised ageing and QoL is a greater focus on urban-related ICT solutions, i.e., buildings, cities, regions, countries. The society as a whole should not consider older adults as individuals whose place is in their homes and controlled environments only. Ideally, older people should be given better conditions to cohabitate with younger representatives of society in all places worldwide and contribute accordingly. Therefore, the gap that should be covered by future research is the investigation and creation of ICT solutions for urban ageing, i.e., related to buildings, cities, regions, and countries. This recommendation further adds to the agenda of the WHO Age-friendly Cities and Communities programme [7].

5.2. Vertical Component

The existing ICT solutions deviate from the horizontal component of the framework in terms of a balanced contribution to different smart ageing determinants. The analysis of the literature shows the dominance of physical activity-related ICT solutions with a minor representation of solutions contributing to long-term care, new technologies, the environment and accessibility, and social inclusion and participation. The patent analysis is dominated by ICT solutions contributing to long-term care and new technologies. The lack of a balanced distribution of ICT solutions across all smart ageing determinants leads to a lack of a multidimensional contribution to different QoL dimensions, and ultimately, an improved overall QoL for older adults and personalised ageing. A second recommendation to be addressed in future investigation is the creation of a balanced representation of ICT solutions across different smart ageing determinants. For instance, there is a need for more work on ICT solutions focused on the underrepresented smart ageing determinants such as access to services, employment and volunteering, education, and life-long learning to name a few.

One can also conclude the same when it comes to the representation of the addressed QoL dimensions in the reviewed literature and patents. Current research and ICT solutions, as well as review studies, are mostly focused on health, overall experienced QoL, or economic or physical safety. Improved QoL, in general, is not improved by enhancing only these three dimensions, but all of them in interdependence of the personal preferences of an individual. Therefore, if one wants to have personalised ageing which assumes an improved QoL, it is suggested that the future research work provides ICT solutions covering a variety of QoL dimensions.

The mapping of smart ageing determinants to QoL dimensions that is in line with the proposed framework is another topic for discussion. The analysed literature has a better performance in terms of mapping in comparison to the reviewed patents. For example, our framework suggests enhancing the QoL dimension "overall experience of life" by eight different smart ageing determinants (Figure 2). In the literature, the overall experience of life is impacted by ICT solutions belonging to seven different smart ageing determinants (such as new technologies, physical activity, environment and accessibility, and so on), while in patents this dimension is influenced only by ICT solutions addressing new technologies and long-term care as smart ageing determinants (Figure 5). Although articles show a more innovative approach to improving QoL dimensions and overall QoL for older adults by influencing these domains by ICT solutions stemming from different smart ageing determinants, this approach needs major improvement. Future research activities should focus on ICT solutions that improve the QoL dimensions indirectly through a contribution to different smart ageing determinants.

It is important to note that it is hard to compare this part of the results, which are related to the proposed framework (the first aim of the study), to other studies given that the existing reviews and studies that have proposed frameworks [33–40] have not addressed personalised ageing and QoL improvement for older adults through the prism of ICT solutions. Many ICT solutions are proposed with the target to prolong and support the independent living of older adults and provide help for professional and informal carers [41]. In order to build an ecosystem that could satisfy the needs of carers, these ICT solutions should provide older adults with control over the timing and the place for monitoring their health [27], while at the same time reducing the stress on hospital capacity and care institutions [42,43]. However, there is a lack of standards, safety and interoperability of these ICT solutions, as well as methods for validation and verification methods in order to demonstrate the sustainability and reliability of ICT solutions for older adults [34]. Therefore, the awareness of the potential ICT solutions for personalised ageing among different stakeholders should be increased.

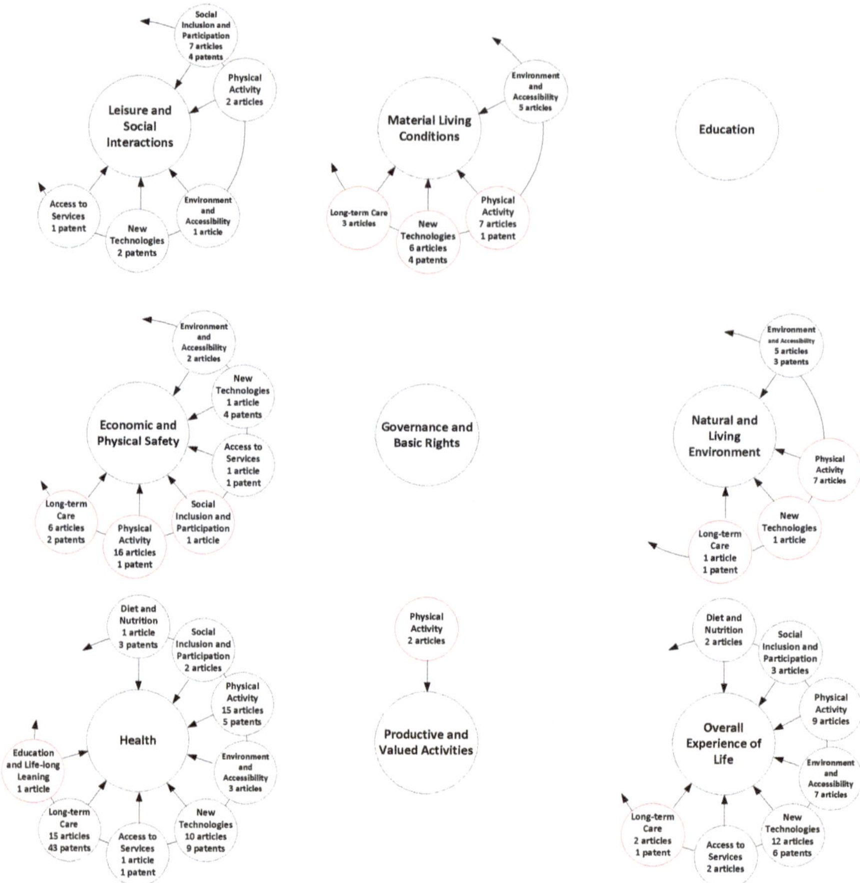

Figure 5. A superimposition of the results of the literature and patent review in terms of smart determinants to QoL dimensions show the gaps where scientific and R&D focus can be placed in the future, and where there is still room for scientific findings to be translated into potential patents. Newly added circles in red and omitted circles from the circle spoke diagram denote deviations from the proposed mapping.

The second aim of this paper was to investigate to what extent ICT solutions do directly improve QoL for older people by surveying a wider scope of the literature and patents. Both analyses show that the majority of ICT solutions are intended for older adults and that they are validated by them. As already indicated, this is opposite to the results obtained by Baraković Husić et al. [10]. The reason for opposite results is the variation in the selected articles and patents, i.e., ICT solutions. Therefore, depending on the reviewed items, the answer to the question of whether solutions are intended for older adults can be different. However, it is recommended for future research to continue to focus more on personalised ICT solutions that directly improve the QoL of older people and to provide older people with the means to enjoy the highest level of independent participation in everyday activities regardless of the place. In order to achieve this goal, the research community should focus on understanding the needs of older people in order to create scalable and flexible ICT solutions that could be adjusted in accordance with personal preferences. It is, therefore, very important to embed the commitment to create ICT solutions in line with the personal needs of older individuals into future research procedures.

5.3. Study Flaws and Limitations

Apart from the chosen application places represented in the framework for this study, there are additional application domains that could be considered, and which are derived from the taxonomy for gerontechnology by van Bronswijk et al. [44]. Gerontechnology aims at good health, full social participation, and independent living up to a high age, be it through research or the development or design of products and services to increase the QoL. According to the taxonomy, gerontechnology has five domains of application coupled with four types of technology impact. The application domains of the gerontechnology taxonomy include (i) health and self-esteem ("autonomy"); (ii) housing and daily living; (iii) mobility and transport; (iv) communication and governance; and (v) work and leisure. Technology impacts include (i) enhancement and satisfaction; (ii) prevention and engagement; (iii) compensation and assistance; and (iv) care support and organization [17]. These potential technology impacts especially could be investigated in more detail in future studies on ICT solutions and the improvement of QoL for older people. Contemporary examples of how technology can serve different communities and have various impacts can be found from the Technology In Later Life (TILL) study. This international, multi-centered, multi-methods study investigated how various technologies are used and impact on the leisure [45] and day-to-day activities of older adults living in both rural and urban geographic areas in the UK and Canada. Findings present two overarching themes: facilitators of technology use and detractors of technology; and numerous recommendations are proposed to move the existing debates forward in the area of gerontechnology and to reduce the notion of reinventing the wheel [46]. Age-friendly ecosystems relate to all citizens in society, and this includes dependent adults, careers, and children diagnosed with disabilities. Given the numerous technologies available at present and used by citizens, it is important to explore how such technologies can be used and deployed inside and outside of the home and across different communities in order to benefit the citizens in the respective age-friendly communities [47–49]. Whilst this framework was published by the World Health Organization in 2007 prior to significant technological developments, such technologies have been embraced by many citizens in their day-to-day lives and it illustrates the capabilities, forward thinking, and planning of existing and future ageing cohorts. There seems to be some implicit recognition of the role technology may play in realising the goals of the age-friendly cities and communities' movement [34].

Our study suffers from several limitations as well. There is the possibility that some relevant publications are not included in the systematic review due to the specificity of the search strings. Moreover, some publications may have not been identified in this literature and patent review due to exclusion criteria (previously listed in Section 3.2.2). This especially refers to publications considering ICT solutions contributing to smart concepts other than smart ageing and QoL for older adults. In addition, this systematic review has not covered research with a focus on the industry and production of related ICT solutions. Furthermore, the considered publications were categorised by publication year and database, QoL dimensions, smart ageing determinants, operating environment, service users, and validation indication. This categorisation served to provide the quantitative results, while the qualitative results are covered to a limited extent. Finally, there were a considerable number of parameters that could not be examined because the publications in the domain did not report them. In order to have more accurate results, various aspects of older people's QoL and personalised ageing need to be included in the equation of research activities.

6. Conclusions

As societies are ageing at a rapid speed, this research study aimed at contributing to the field of QoL for older adults and personalised ageing from an ICT perspective. The developments and the pace at which related solutions are brought to the marketplace, or are being implemented in the domain of healthcare and welfare, are ever-increasing. The main challenge is to put them into practice, thus taking a fundamental step towards improving the quality of life. This paper contributes to achieving this goal in three ways.

The first contribution is the proposition of a novel framework for QoL for older adults through a systematic review of the relevant state-of-the-art articles and patents, i.e., personalised ageing which can be further utilised by various stakeholders on this path. Namely, the framework advocates the approach in which if we have multiple ICT solutions designed to be personalised and satisfy multiple smart ageing determinants which in combination contribute to multiple QoL dimensions, then those improved QoL dimensions jointly accomplish the goal of QoL while ageing or relating to personalised ageing.

Furthermore, in order to utilise the future ICT solutions, the current ones need to be investigated for satisfying the needs of older people. The second contribution is the finding that they are intended for older adults and are validated by them. However, this can vastly depend on the selected samples.

The third contribution of the study are the guidelines for future ICT solutions, so we could optimise their implementation. There are six recommendations that are derived from the review of the literature and the patents covering them: a focus on urban ageing, i.e., relating to buildings, cities, regions, and countries; the creation of a balanced representation across different smart ageing determinants; the cover of a variety of QoL dimensions; an improvement in the QoL dimensions indirectly through a contribution to different smart ageing determinants; an increase in the awareness of personalised ageing among different stakeholders; and to continue to directly improve the QoL of older people and to provide older people with the means to enjoy the highest level of independent participation in everyday activities regardless of the place.

Supplementary Materials: The studies included in the literature analysis are available online at: https://drive.google.com/open?id=1qePpKiMK-4wkJzrm9b1FITRBtST17tuq. The patents included in the patent analysis are available online at https://drive.google.com/open?id=1qePpKiMK-4wkJzrm9b1FITRBtST17tuq.

Author Contributions: Conceptualisation, S.B. and J.B.H.; methodology, S.B. and J.B.H.; data collection, J.B.H. and O.K.; formal analysis, S.B., J.B.H., O.K. and Z.A.; investigation, Z.A., S.B. and J.B.H.; writing—original draft preparation, S.B., J.B.H, J.v.H., P.M. and F.J.M.; writing—review and editing, S.B., J.B.H. and J.v.H.; visualization, S.B., J.v.H., and F.J.M.; supervision, S.B., J.B.H., and J.v.H.; project administration, S.B. and J.B.H. All authors have read and agreed to the published version of the manuscript.

Acknowledgments: The networking activities leading to this publication are based upon work of COST Action CA16226 "Living Indoor Space Improvement: Smart Habitat for the Elderly" of the European Cooperation in Science and Technology—COST. COST is a funding agency for research and innovation networks. Our actions help connect research initiatives across Europe and enable scientists to grow their ideas by sharing them with their peers. This boosts their research, career and innovation. www.cost.eu. The authors would like to acknowledge Little Mama Labs research laboratory in Sarajevo, Bosnia and Herzegovina. Furthermore, authors acknowledge the internal research project Excellence 2020, Faculty of Informatics and Management, University of Hradec Kralove.

Conflicts of Interest: The authors declare no conflict of interest.

References

1. World Health Organization: 10 Facts on Ageing and Ealth. Available online: http://www.who.int/features/factfiles/ageing/en/ (accessed on 4 April 2020).
2. United Nations: World Population Ageing. 2017. Available online: https://www.un.org/en/development/desa/population/publications/pdf/ageing/WPA2017_Report.pdf (accessed on 23 April 2020).
3. Van Hoof, J.; Demiris, G.; Wouters, E.J. *Handbook of Smart Homes, Health Care and Well-Being*; Springer Science and Business Media LLC: Berlin, Germany, 2017.
4. Van Hoof, J.; Kolmer, D.M.B.G.; De Vlugt, E.; De Vries, S.I. Quality of Life: The Interplay between Human Behaviour, Technology and the Environment. *Int. J. Environ. Res. Public Health* **2019**, *16*, 5106. [CrossRef] [PubMed]
5. Irving, P.B. Personalized Aging: One Size Doesn't Fit All. In *The Upside of Ageing: How Long Life is Changing the World of Health, Work, Innovation, Policy and Purpose*; John Wiley & Sons, Inc.: Hoboken, NJ, USA, 2014; pp. 19–34.
6. Peek, S.T.M.; Luijkx, K.; Rijnaard, M.D.; Nieboer, M.E.; Van Der Voort, C.S.; Aarts, S.; Van Hoof, J.; Vrijhoef, H.J.M.; Wouters, E. Older Adults' Reasons for Using Technology while Aging in Place. *Gerontology* **2015**, *62*, 226–237. [CrossRef] [PubMed]

7. Marston, H.R.; van Hoof, J. "Who Doesn't Think about Technology When Designing Urban Environments for Older People?" A Case Study Approach to a Proposed Extension of the WHO's Age-friendly Cities Model. *Int. J. Environ. Res. Public Health* **2019**, *16*, 3525. [CrossRef]
8. Peek, S.T.M.; Kazak, J.K.; Perek-Białas, J.M.; Peek, S.T.M. The Challenges of Urban Ageing: Making Cities Age-Friendly in Europe. *Int. J. Environ. Res. Public Health* **2018**, *15*, 2473. [CrossRef]
9. van Hoof, J.; Kazak, J.K. Urban Ageing. *Indoor Built Environ.* **2018**, *27*, 538–586. [CrossRef]
10. Husic, J.B.; Baraković, S.; Dinarević, E.C. Smart Ageing: Are We Succeeding? In *Proceedings of the World Congress on Medical Physics and Biomedical Engineering 2006*; Springer Science and Business Media LLC: Banja Luka, Bosnia and Herzegovina, 2019; pp. 387–393.
11. The Whoqol Group Development of the World Health Organization WHOQOL-BREF Quality of Life Assessment. *Psychol. Med.* **1998**, *28*, 551–558. [CrossRef]
12. Gotay, C.C.; Moore, T.D. Assessing quality of life in head and neck cancer. *Qual. Life Res.* **1992**, *1*, 5–17. [CrossRef]
13. Hörnquist, J.O. The Concept of Quality of Life. *Scand. J. Soc. Med.* **1982**, *10*, 57–61. [CrossRef]
14. Theofilou, P. Quality of Life: Definition and Measurement. *Eur. J. Psychol.* **2013**, *9*, 150–162. [CrossRef]
15. Eurostat. Quality of Life (QoL). Available online: https://ec.europa.eu/eurostat/web/gdp-and-beyond/quality-of-life/data (accessed on 4 April 2020).
16. EuroHealthNet. Healthy Ageing. Available online: http://www.healthyageing.eu/sites/www.healthyageing.eu/files/featured/Healthy%20and%20Active%20Ageing.pdf (accessed on 4 April 2020).
17. Yang, Q.; Shen, Z. Active Aging in the Workplace and the Role of Intelligent Technologies. In Proceedings of the 2015 IEEE/WIC/ACM International Conference on Web Intelligence and Intelligent Agent Technology (WI-IAT), Singapore, 6–9 December 2015; Institute of Electrical and Electronics Engineers (IEEE): Piscataway, NJ, USA, 2015; Volume 2, pp. 391–394.
18. Department of the Taoiseach. Programme of Actions for Smart Ageing. Available online: https://www.taoiseach.gov.ie/eng/Publications/Publica-tions_2016/Programme_of_Actions_for_Smart_Ageing.pdf (accessed on 4 April 2020).
19. A Mapping of Smart Ageing Activity in Ireland and an Assessment of the Potential Smart Ageing Opportunity Areas. Available online: https://www.dcu.ie/sites/default/files/agefriendly/SmartAgingExecutiveSummary.pdf (accessed on 23 April 2020).
20. Song, I.-Y.; Song, M.; Timakum, T.; Ryu, S.-R.; Lee, H. The landscape of smart aging: Topics, applications, and agenda. *Data Knowl. Eng.* **2018**, *115*, 68–79. [CrossRef]
21. World Health Organization. Physical Activity and Adults. Available online: http://www9.who.int/dietphysicalactivity/factsheet_adults/en/ (accessed on 4 April 2020).
22. Ogita, M.; Okura, M.; Yamamoto, M.; Nakai, T.; Numata, T.; Arai, H. P101: Social participation is associated with physical frailty in Japanese older adults. *Eur. Geriatr. Med.* **2014**, *5*, S114. [CrossRef]
23. Cohen-Mansfield, J.; Marx, M.S.; Werner, P. Agitation in Elderly Persons: An Integrative Report of Findings in a Nursing Home. *Int. Psychogeriatrics* **1992**, *4*, 221–240. [CrossRef] [PubMed]
24. Buettner, L.L.; Fitzsimmons, S.; Atav, A.S.; Buettner, L.; Fitzsimmons, S.; Atav, S. Predicting Outcomes of Therapeutic Recreation Interventions for Older Adults with Dementia and Behavioral Symptoms. *Ther. Recreat. J.* **2006**, *40*, 12–14. Available online: http://libres.uncg.edu/ir/uncg/f/L_Buettner_Predicting_2006.pdf (accessed on 24 April 2020).
25. Granic, A.; Mendonça, N.; Hill, T.R.; Jagger, C.; Stevenson, E.J.; Mathers, J.C.; Sayer, A.A. Nutrition in the Very Old. *Nutrition* **2018**, *10*, 269. [CrossRef]
26. Volkert, D. Nutrition and lifestyle of the elderly in Europe. *J. Public Health* **2005**, *13*, 56–61. [CrossRef]
27. Liu, L.; Stroulia, E.; Nikolaidis, I.; Miguel-Cruz, A.; Ríos-Rincón, A.M. Smart homes and home health monitoring technologies for older adults: A systematic review. *Int. J. Med. Inform.* **2016**, *91*, 44–59. [CrossRef]
28. Haghi, M.; Thurow, K.; Stoll, R. Wearable Devices in Medical Internet of Things: Scientific Research and Commercially Available Devices. *Healthc. Inform. Res.* **2017**, *23*, 4–15. [CrossRef]
29. Yin, Y.; Zeng, Y.; Chen, X.; Fan, Y. The internet of things in healthcare: An overview. *J. Ind. Inf. Integr.* **2016**, *1*, 3–13. [CrossRef]
30. Van Hoof, J.; De Kort, H.; Markopoulos, P.; Soede, M. Ambient intelligence, ethics and privacy. *Gerontechnology* **2007**, *6*, 155–163. [CrossRef]

31. Van Hoof, J.; Verboor, J.; Weernink, C.O.; Sponselee, A.-M.A.-M.G.; Sturm, J.; Kazak, J.K.; Govers, G.; Van Zaalen, Y. Real-Time Location Systems for Asset Management in Nursing Homes: An Explorative Study of Ethical Aspects. *Information* **2018**, *9*, 80. [CrossRef]
32. Weernink, C.O.; Felix, E.; Verkuijlen, P.; Daele, A.D.-V.; Kazak, J.K.; Van Hoof, J. Real-time location systems in nursing homes: state of the art and future applications. *J. Enabling Technol.* **2018**, *12*, 45–56. [CrossRef]
33. Maresova, P.; Javanmardi, E.; Barakovic, S.; Husic, J.B.; Tomsone, S.; Krejcar, O.; Ramalho, T.C. Consequences of chronic diseases and other limitations associated with old age - a scoping review. *BMC Public Health* **2019**, *19*, 1431. [CrossRef] [PubMed]
34. Maresova, P.; Krejcar, O.; Baraković, S.; Baraković Husić, J.; Lemeski, P.; Zdravevski, E.; Chorbev, I.; Trajkovik, V. Health-Related ICT Solutions of Smart Environments for Elderly – Systematic Review. *IEEE Access.* **2020**, *8*, 54574–54600. [CrossRef]
35. Krejcar, O.; Maresova, P.; Selamat, A.; Melero, F.J.; Frischer, R.; Kuca, K.; Baraković, S.; Baraković Husić, J. Smart Furniture Definition and Specification. *IEEE Access* **2019**, *7*, 94822–94839. [CrossRef]
36. Frischer, R.; Krejcar, O.; Maresova, P.; Fadeyi, O.; Selamat, A.; Kuča, K.; Tomsone, S.; Teixeira, J.P.; Madureira, J.; Melero, F.J. Commercial ICT Smart Solutions for the Elderly: State of the Art and Future Challenges in the Smart Furniture Sector. *Electronics* **2020**, *9*, 149. [CrossRef]
37. Rocha, N.P.; Dias, A.; Santinha, G.; Rodrigues, M.; Queirós, A.; Rodrigues, C. A Systematic Review of Smart Cities' Applications to Support Active Ageing. *Procedia Comput. Sci.* **2019**, *160*, 306–313. [CrossRef]
38. Na Lee, L.; Kim, M.J. A Critical Review of Smart Residential Environments for Older Adults with a Focus on Pleasurable Experience. *Front. Psychol.* **2020**, *10*, 3080. [CrossRef]
39. Maskeliūnas, R.; Damasevicius, R.; Segal, S. A Review of Internet of Things Technologies for Ambient Assisted Living Environments. *Futur. Internet* **2019**, *11*, 259. [CrossRef]
40. Yang, P.; Lin, S.J. Digital Aging as an Essential Component of Active Aging: A Literature review. *Int. J. Lib. Arts Soc. Sci.* **2019**, *7*, 113–132.
41. Pal, D.; Funilkul, S.; Charoenkitkarn, N.; Kanthamanon, P. Internet-of-Things and Smart Homes for Elderly Healthcare: An End User Perspective. *IEEE Access* **2018**, *6*, 10483–10496. [CrossRef]
42. Vegesna, A.; Tran, M.; Angelaccio, M.; Arcona, S. Remote Patient Monitoring via Non-Invasive Digital Technologies: A Systematic Review. *Telemed. e-Health* **2016**, *23*, 3–17. [CrossRef] [PubMed]
43. Khan, S.; Ye, B.; Taati, B.; Mihailidis, A. Detecting agitation and aggression in people with dementia using sensors-A systematic review. *Alzheimer's Dement.* **2018**, *14*, 824–832. [CrossRef] [PubMed]
44. Van Bronswijk, J.; Bouma, H.; Fozard, J. Technology for quality of life: an enriched taxonomy. *Gerontechnology* **2002**, *2*, 169–172. [CrossRef]
45. Genoe, R.; Kulczycki, C.; Marston, H.R.; Freeman, S.; Musselwhite, C.; Rutherford, H. E-Leisure and Older Adults: Findings from an International Exploratory Study. *Ther. Recreat. J.* **2018**, *52*, 1–18. [CrossRef]
46. Marston, H.R.; Genoe, R.; Freeman, S.; Kulczycki, C.; Musselwhite, C. Older Adults' Perceptions of ICT: Main Findings from the Technology In Later Life (TILL) Study. *Healthcare* **2019**, *7*, 86. [CrossRef]
47. World Health Organization. Global Age-Friendly Cities: A Guide. Available online: https://www.who.int/ageing/publications/Global_age_friendly_cities_Guide_English.pdf (accessed on 23 April 2020).
48. Peek, S.T.M.; Wouters, E.J.; Van Hoof, J.; Luijkx, K.; Boeije, H.R.; Vrijhoef, H.J.M. Factors influencing acceptance of technology for aging in place: A systematic review. *Int. J. Med. Inform.* **2014**, *83*, 235–248. [CrossRef]
49. Van Hoof, J.; Dikken, J.; Buttiġieġ, S.C.; Hoven, R.F.M.V.D.; Kroon, E.; Marston, H.R. Age-friendly cities in the Netherlands: An explorative study of facilitators and hindrances in the built environment and ageism in design. *Indoor Built Environ.* **2019**, *29*, 417–437. [CrossRef]

International Journal of
Environmental Research and Public Health

MDPI

Communication

Smart Environments and Social Robots for Age-Friendly Integrated Care Services

Ionut Anghel, Tudor Cioara *, Dorin Moldovan, Marcel Antal, Claudia Daniela Pop, Ioan Salomie, Cristina Bianca Pop and Viorica Rozina Chifu

Computer Science Department, Technical University of Cluj-Napoca, Memorandumului 28, 400114 Cluj-Napoca, Romania; ionut.anghel@cs.utcluj.ro (I.A.); dorin.moldovan@cs.utcluj.ro (D.M.); marcel.antal@cs.utcluj.ro (M.A.); claudia.pop@cs.utcluj.ro (C.D.P.); ioan.salomie@cs.utcluj.ro (I.S.); cristina.pop@cs.utcluj.ro (C.B.P.); viorica.chifu@cs.utcluj.ro (V.R.C.)

* Correspondence: tudor.cioara@cs.utcluj.ro; Tel.: +40-264-202-352

Received: 14 April 2020; Accepted: 26 May 2020; Published: 27 May 2020

check for updates

Abstract: The world is facing major societal challenges because of an aging population that is putting increasing pressure on the sustainability of care. While demand for care and social services is steadily increasing, the supply is constrained by the decreasing workforce. The development of smart, physical, social and age-friendly environments is identified by World Health Organization (WHO) as a key intervention point for enabling older adults, enabling them to remain as much possible in their residences, delay institutionalization, and ultimately, improve quality of life. In this study, we survey smart environments, machine learning and robot assistive technologies that can offer support for the independent living of older adults and provide age-friendly care services. We describe two examples of integrated care services that are using assistive technologies in innovative ways to assess and deliver of timely interventions for polypharmacy management and for social and cognitive activity support in older adults. We describe the architectural views of these services, focusing on details about technology usage, end-user interaction flows and data models that are developed or enhanced to achieve the envisioned objective of healthier, safer, more independent and socially connected older people.

Keywords: social robots; ambient assisted living; machine learning; older adults care; daily life activities monitoring; technology limitation and acceptance; care services models

1. Introduction

According to the World Health Organization (WHO) the proportion of people over 60 years will double from 11% in 2006 to 22% by 2050 [1]. In this context, the world is facing major societal challenges because the aging population is putting increasing pressure on the sustainability of care. First, the demand for care and social services is steadily increasing while the supply is constrained by the decreasing workforce capacity. Second, as people grow older, the costs of care rapidly increase—mainly due to chronic diseases and comorbidities management.

To address this, WHO launched a worldwide initiative "age-friendly cities and communities" with a view of transforming and tailoring living spaces and cities to the needs of older adults [2]. The proposed age-friendly cities model guides the implementation of new services and policies in various domains from communication and information up to housing or community support and health services. The development of such a model was driven by several factors, such as improving the environments in which the older adults live and developing community-oriented policies promoting opportunities for enhancing the quality of life of older adults [3]. At the same time, recent technological advancements such as ambient intelligence and information and communication technology (ICT) mediated intervention, have supported the model implementation offering opportunities for older adults to be proactive in addressing age related challenges and co-producers of new services development. In fact, the model checklist of essential features of age-friendly cities provides lots of references to the adoption of new technological solutions [4].

Recent studies seek to extend the age-friendly cites model with the technology enablers needed to make it compatible with the smart and age-friendly ecosystems [5]. The direction of developing smart houses or indoor environments for older adult care [6] is identified as a relevant one as it optimally integrates the technology with the domain of housing defined by in the WHO age-friendly cities model [7]. In this context the implementation of smart, physical, social and age-friendly environments is a key intervention point for enabling older adults to stay as much possible in their residences and delay their institutionalization. Nevertheless, in this case, there is a high risk that older adults may become socially isolated and will not be able to care for themselves. If certain daily life activities (i.e., eat, drink, take medication as planned, move, etc.) are not properly carried out will significantly impact their condition, speeding up the deterioration of their health and wellbeing—especially in case of older adults suffering from comorbidities. However, the recent adoption of virtual personal assistants and/or socially assistive robots is advocated as a potential technological solution that may positively impact the older adults in society. Many of their features empower the older adults to remain socially engaged and at the same time they may successfully mediate the delivery of timely healthcare interventions [8]. Social robots may not only support older adults with daily activity, but at the same time they may contribute to emotional wellness by keeping older adults socially engaged and activating social interactions in communities [9]. Moreover, they may not only drive the implementation of new services in various domains defined by WHO's age-friendly model in which older adults perceive the social robots as helpful companions, but they also promote the human-to-human interactions.

Thus, although independent living reduces the demand and costs for care, it can also reduce the quality of care if not supported by innovative ambient assistive living (AAL) technologies and socially assistive robots. Efforts need to be committed to integrate and further develop such technologies to realize advanced care services for prolonging the autonomy and well-being of older adults. The implementation of technology-enabled supportive intelligent environments may offer opportunities to promote improved and more personalized care services into older age. Combined with care functionalities such as remote care support, medical reminders, behavioral monitoring and virtual coaching, they have the potential of delivering the right support to the end-users when help is needed. The combination of activity, safety, social and comfort functionality can lead to an extension of the time spent living in their own home by shifting or postponing parts of in-patient (i.e., care facility services) treatment, therapy and exercise training into the own home; thereby it will directly decrease or delay admissions into a care institution, diminishing the use of professionalized care services and/or lowering the burden of health care services and facilities.

In this context, the smart and 'age-friendly' environments will become fundamental pervasive technologies for supporting older adults care while the social robots may become important intervention tools due to their ability to provide support to older persons and open links with their community and professional caregivers and to cooperate and interact with older adults engaging them in the care process. Starting from the above identified challenges, the contribution of this study is twofold:

- A survey of smart environments and robot assistive technologies that have the potential of supporting the independent living of older adults at home by implementing age-friendly care services. In this process we identify the challenges in implementing the new care service models, existing technology limitations and its acceptance by the older adults;
- A discussion on how these technologies are used for the development of two care services for older adults centered and integrated care polypharmacy management and control of wellbeing decline by social and cognitive activity engagement.

The study is structured as follows: Section 2 reviews existing smart environments and social robots' technologies for older adult care, Section 3 analyses the application of the technology for new integrated care services and finally Section 4 presents the conclusions of the review.

2. Smart Environments and Assistive Robots' Technologies Review

In this section we provide an overview of state-of-the-art assistive technologies focusing on three main directions: objective monitoring using sensors devices, data analysis and machine learning for behavior assessment and finally delivering interventions using social robots. In the end, we discuss for each type of technology the limits, challenges and adoption from the perspective of older adults.

2.1. Monitoring Daily Life Activities

The development and deployment of sensors and smart devices for monitoring older adults' activities is a dynamic research and innovation area currently triggered by the advent of big data and machine learning technologies. On top of the monitoring devices, applications are developed for assisting the older adults' healthcare, improving the social communication and inclusion or for managing various activities targeting to prolong independent living. In [10] the most important dimensions of older adults' lifestyle that need to be properly monitored are identified as: the physiological parameters and the body functions, the changes in the daily life activities (DLAs) and daily routines, the social factors and the environmental factors. In [11] and [12] the data to be monitored and collected for older adults' support and intervention is classified in behavior, health, occupancy, lifestyle, home automation, environmental and personal safety. Similarly, in [13] the most common data types to be monitored and used in AAL systems are identified as: behavioral habit data, physiological information, healthcare information and environmental data.

On other dimension, there are several types of sensors which can be used to monitor and analyze different aspects of the older adults' healthcare and well-being, most frequently being classified in: (a) physical sensors, (b) virtual sensors and (c) logical sensors.

Physical sensors are the most frequently used type of sensors in collecting data about the older adults' healthcare and well-being. Table 1 presents an overview of various AAL physical sensors and the type of monitored data that was identified in the research literature [14]. These research approaches are classified and discussed below.

Wearable physical sensors are used to collect the data about (i) the physiological signs of a person (e.g., heart rate, blood pressure or temperature, blood cholesterol, blood oxygen saturation, respiratory rate, blood sugar level, etc.), (ii) the posture, gait and movement, (iii) the social interaction or (iv) the activities performed by a person during a day. All these data are analyzed to assess the health/wellbeing status of a person [15–19], the sleep quality [20–23] and the level of stress and cognitive decline [24–26] or to detect the falls [27]. Currently, the most important wearable sensors that can collect this type of data are embedded into wristbands, smart clothes, smartphones or smartwatches, arm bands or chest straps.

Monitoring the physiological signs and physical position provides valuable information regarding the health status of a person. Some of the main benefits provided by the wearable sensors in monitoring the health status of a person are the following [28]: (i) allow to continuously monitor the vulnerable patients, (ii) allow the medical specialist to have a better view on the patient's health issues and to make the most accurate diagnosis and (iii) offers the patients the opportunity to evaluate their health condition and consult a doctor when appropriate. In [15] the data collected to evaluate the health status of a patient is: physiological signs and physical position. The types of sensors used for collecting the data are airflow sensor, galvanic sensor, body temperature sensor, blood oxygen sensor, electroencephalogram (EEG)/ heart rate sensor and digital accelerometer. An Internet of Things (IoT)-based system for monitoring the health status of Cardiovascular disease(CVD) patients consisting of a sensing layer responsible for collecting the physiological signs of the patient (e.g., blood pressure, electrocardiogram (ECG), amount of oxygen in the blood (SpO2)) and the patient's location is proposed in [16]. Custom wristbands that integrate specific sensors (i.e., piezoelectret sensor) that can detect heartbeats are also proposed [29]. The piezoelectret sensor can help detecting the pulse waveform, which is similar to the one provided by an electrocardiogram. Similarly, arm-wearable ECG sensors are researched for monitoring the heart rate that integrates the main components of an ECG [17]. The sensor provides two functions, namely a monitoring function in which the signal is acquired and a Holter function in which the signal is stored in the internal memory. Authors of [18] develop a smart t-shirt for recording the ECG signals which integrates a set of active electrodes and an ECG Portable recorder. The accuracy of ECG signals recorded with the developed device was comparatively evaluated with a standard 12-lead Holter. A system for monitoring in real time the CVD patients' heart rate, blood pressure and body temperature which of multiple wearable sensors and collects medical information about patients with CVD, is connected to a web portal for displaying the acquired data from patients in [19].

Table 1. Ambient assistive living (AAL) physical sensors and data provided.

Available AAL Sensors	Type of Monitored Data	Approaches
	Wearable sensors	
Body temperature sensors, biosensors for monitoring vital signs	Body temperature, physiological attributes (e.g., heart rate, temperature, blood pressure, respiration rate, etc.)	[15–19,24,29]
Motion sensors such as accelerometers, gyroscope, magnetometers, passive infrared sensors, GPS, GSM, active badge systems	Movement, indoor/outdoor location, position, posture and gait	[15,16,21,22,25–27,30,32–37]
Photosensors, color sensors, acoustic sensors (i.e., microphones), etc.	Light levels, sound and audio	[22,24–26,30]
Body sleep sensors	Sleep levels, patterns, intensity, etc.	[20,22,23,30,31]
	Non-Wearable sensors	
Touch sensors	Touch (allow interaction with smartphones and tablets or home appliances)	[54–60]
Force/floor sensors	Falls and movement (walking, standing, sitting, etc.)	[14,45,47–50]
Pressure pad sensors	Surface pressure measurement (e.g., bed pressure mats)	[39–42,53]
Video sensors (e.g., various cameras)	Visual context (e.g., keep track of daily living activities performed by the older adult, locating the older adults in house)	[43–46]
Acoustic sensors	Fall-detection	[48–50]
Ambient sensors (temperature, appliances, toilet)	Ambient temperature, usage time duration of an equipment, Toilet-usage frequency	[14,38,51,52]
Contact sensors, magnetic switch	Open/close the office desk, open/close the TV, open doors, windows, etc.	[14,38,52]

Sleep quality is an important factor for a person's stage of health because it reduces the risk of developing chronic diseases and mental disorders. Most state-of-the-art approaches for monitoring sleep quality focus on comparative analyses and evaluation of the commercial devices available on the market [21,22,30], while only some of them present academic research solutions [20,23,31]. For example, in [21] commercial devices for monitoring the sleep quality are analyzed, the Up Move Jawbone (U) and the Withings Pulse accelerometers (monitor sleep duration, how many times s/he wakes up at night, etc.), the Bodymedia SenseWear Pro Armband actigraph (monitors the sleep quality by estimating the sleep duration and efficiency) and the home-polysomnography (collects data about thoracic and abdominal movements, airflow, etc.). Similarly, authors of [22] evaluate five wearable devices for recording the sleep quality, namely the Basis Health Tracker, the Misfit Shine, the Fitbit Flex, the Withings Pulse O2 and the Actiwatch Spectrum actigraph. The Basis Health Tracker is an actigraph embedded in a wristwatch, while the Misfit Shine is a sleep-tracking device provided with a strap to be worn on the hand. The Withings Pulse O2 is also a sleep-tracking device worn on the wrist, while the Actiwatch Spectrum is a wristwatch with an embedded accelerometer. In [30] the accuracy of a commercial device, namely, Fitbit Charge 2, compared to polysomnography, in measuring the sleep and the wake states is analyzed. This device can detect, besides the sleep and wake states, the time spent awake, in light or in deep sleep as well as to track the level of daily activities. In [23] it is proposed a wearable device for monitoring the abdominal and thoracic respiration that can be used to detect the obstructive sleep apnea by monitoring the breathing status. Chest-worn sensors collect data about the posture (during the day or the sleep), the position changes and body acceleration of a person in order to detect the sleeping and the waking periods to detect the quality of the sleep during the night and the time spend by the person in bed [20]. In [31] wearable sensors positioned on arms and chest are used to monitor the sleep quality. The sleep quality is evaluated based on the sleep posture and the sleep stages (awake, rapid eye movement (REM) sleep and non-REM sleep cycles).

Monitoring the level of stress is very important because, on long term, it has a negative impact on the cognitive functions of a person. Also, by monitoring the cognitive function, valuable information is obtained that can be used to improve the daily/detect early cognitive decline in the case of older adults. In [24] the physical attributes (e.g., galvanic skin response and skin temperature, EEG heart rate, respiration rate and voice data) are monitored and collected in order to assess in real time the emotional, physical and mental stress of a person. Data are acquired with a set of wearable biosensors integrated in smart clothing and with a microphone. In [25] a smartwatch which integrates a Global Positioning System (GPS) sensor, an ambient light sensor and an acceleration sensor, is proposed as a solution for monitoring wandering risk for older adults suffering from dementia. The developed smartwatch acquires the following types of data that are used to avoid the risk of the patient losing their way when they experience wandering episodes: the older adult position and the route in which s/he moves that is necessary to identify if the older adult moves outside the area considered to be safe, the sunlight exposure duration and the number of older adult's steps. In [26] the benefits of the physical activity on the cognitive functions of the older adults are inferred based on (i) the data (e.g., light/ moderate to vigorous physical activity) collected with an accelerometer and (ii) a set of questionnaires containing information about the cognitive ability of older adults. A platform for monitoring older adults at home in order to detect the early cognitive decline is researched in [32]. It integrates Infrared (IR) motion sensors with magnetic contact sensors and sensors for monitoring user computer interactions (e.g., mouse movements, computer usage time, etc.) and uses all the collected data to build the profile of changes in the activities performed by older adults, which are than analyzed in order to detect possible cognitive decline.

In the case of fall detection, most approaches from the research literature are based on accelerometers and gyroscopes. Accelerometers can provide information about the motion data during daily living activities (i.e., walking, running, stepping and falling), as well as the instability that can appear during these activities and can provide valuable information in predicting the risk of falling during walking [27,33]. Usually a wearable sensor feds data to a fall detection algorithm to identify the fall risk within the daily activities of a person [34]. In [35] the data about acceleration signals, postural instability and falls are recorded with a tri-axial seismic acceleration sensor placed on a belt while [36] presents an approach for detecting the fall, based on a smartphone which integrates a tri-axial accelerometer and a tri-axis gyroscope and is used to record the acceleration patterns, in the case of older adults, for the following types of daily activities: sitting, lying, jumping, running, walking and hitting the sensor. A fall monitoring system which integrates a portable sensor that can be placed on the person's shoulder, waist or foot and a mobile phone is proposed in [37]. The portable sensor records the data with a triaxis accelerometer, a triaxis gyroscope and a triaxis magnetometer and sends it to the mobile phone. The collected data are used to compute the acceleration and Euler angle which are provided as input to a fall detection algorithm.

In contrast with wearable sensors that need to be placed on the body of the person, ambient (non-wearable) sensors are positioned in different places of the older adult's home and are used to collect data regarding the behavior, the occupancy, the lifestyle, the environmental safety and the personal safety of a person. The non-wearable sensors can be used to detect the well-being/health status of a person as well as to monitor the sleep quality.

Ambient sensors can be used for monitoring the daily living activities performed by older adults as well as their daily routine and to detect behavior changes caused by the deterioration of the health state. In [14] the data that are monitored and collected in order to evaluate the wellness of the older adult in a controlled environment (i.e., his/her house) are: behavior, occupancy, lifestyle, environmental safety and personal safety. The monitored infrastructure integrates the following types of non-wearable heterogeneous sensing units installed in the older adult's houses: (i) movement sensors, (ii) electronics and electrical devices monitoring sensors placed on the electrical and electronic appliances, (iii) toilet sensors, (iv) contact sensors to monitor the opening/ closing of a door, office desk or and self-grooming table and (v) force sensors placed on sofa /bed/ armchair to monitor the sleeping or sitting activities. In [38] the solution proposed for detecting the deviation from the daily activity routine of older adults is based on a non-intrusive monitoring infrastructure consisting of low-cost sensors such as passive infrared (PIR) motion detectors and magnetic door contacts sensors located in each rooms of the house. The monitored data contains information about the older adults' lifestyle and is used to detect unusual activities performed by an older adult in a day or deviations from his previous routine.

Smart beds as well as cameras are an alternative to the wearable commercial devices for monitoring the sleep quality, beside the polysomnography and the videosomnography that can be used in clinical evaluations. Authors of [39] propose a non-intrusive monitoring infrastructure consisting of pressure sensors embedded in bed which is used for detecting sleep quality. The sleep quality is assessed based on the sleep position and the sleep stages. In [40] a microbend fiber optic mat embedded in the mattress of the bed is used to monitor the sleep quality. The sleep quality is evaluated based on the following types of data acquired from sensor: sleep duration, movements during the sleep, heart rate, awake stage duration, time spend in bed as well as the respiration rate. Similarly, in [41] a sensor integrating an Emfit foil electrode embedded in the mattress of the bed is used to measure the sleep quality. The sleep quality is evaluated based on the movement activity and the heart-rate fluctuations. Piezoelectric film sensors can be embedded in the bed mattress to monitor the sleep quality, based on the variation of the heart and respiration rate and the binary actigram [42]. Microsoft Kinect camera can be employed to detect the human shape and the body movements and a sensor tag that provides information about the sleep environment such as the temperature and humidity [43], while Near-Infrared camera can be used to analyze the sleep behavior, based on the collected videos/images [44].

Non-wearable sensors for fall detection approaches that are based on ambient sensors use cameras, infrared sensors, acoustic sensors or force sensors installed in the home environment to detect the fall. In [45], an approach for detecting the fall that is based on low-cost fall detector that integrates Raspberry Pi 2 and an universal serial bus (USB) camera and several algorithms (e.g., background subtraction, Kalman filtering optical flow) is proposed. The detector is developed as a portable device that can be moved from a room to another of the older adult's house and can detect the following positions: walking, standing, sitting and falling. Similarly, in [46] is presented a method of detecting the fall in the case of older adults. The method is based on a Microsoft Kinect sensor for collecting the images combined with an algorithm for background subtraction and an ensemble of decision trees. In [47] is proposed an approach for detecting the fall in the case of older adults that is based on a ground sensors network consisting of accelerometers and force sensors installed on the tiles from each room of the older adults' apartment while [48] proposes a classification method which is able to detect between human fall from non-fall, based on the acoustic waves transmitted on the ground collected with a floor acoustic sensor. A method to detect the fall in the case of older adults which combines acoustic sensors that collect the sound signals of the footsteps performed by older adults during the daily activities and a support vector machine algorithm is used to make distinction between fall and non-fall sounds is proposed in [49]. Authors of [50] develop a fall detection system that uses a circular array of 8—microphones to detect the older adult's fall in real time and sends alerts to the caregivers.

Wearable sensors can be combined with ambient sensors in complex monitoring infrastructures that can be used to obtain more accurate results in monitoring the heath/well-being status or sleep quality. In [51] the data that are monitored and collected in order to evaluate the wellness of the older adult in terms of functional and cognitive capacity can be classified in: vital sign, social interaction and physical activity. The monitoring infrastructure consists of a wireless sensor network integrating a collection of wearable and non-wearable heterogeneous sensors. eWall [52] is a holistic monitoring platform for home, which collects the following type of data in the case of older adults suffering of chronic obstructive Pulmonary disease, mild cognitive impairments or others age-related impairments: (i) health data (e.g., SpO2, pulse, heart rate), (ii) well-being state data (physical activity, sleep, mood), (iii) environmental data (e.g., temperature, luminosity). In [53] the sleep quality is monitored with a wearable three-axis accelerometer and a pressure sensor installed in bed. The accelerometer is used to determine the sleep pose and the sleep state (e.g., REM sleep and non-REM sleep cycles), while the pressure sensors are used to detect heart/respiration rate. Based on the collected data a novel algorithm is develop that is able to detect the sleep quality, based on the number of apneic episodes, the duration of sleep and the depth of sleep.

Virtual sensors are a source of data coming from software applications or services. For example, it is possible to determine an older adult's location not only by using tracking systems (physical sensors) but also by using a by browsing an electronic calendar, a travel-booking system, emails etc., for location information. Other attributes that can be sensed by virtual sensors include, e.g., the user's activity by checking for mouse-movement and keyboard input. Logical sensors are an extension of the virtual ones and make use of a couple of information sources and combine physical and virtual sensors with additional information from databases or various other sources in order to solve higher tasks. Pain Care is a healthcare app developed for iOS and Android device that allows older adults to keep a medical journal in which stores information about the medication that s/he take, specific symptoms/pains or side effects of medicine that could occur during the treatment [54]. Based on this medical journal, the causes of pain and treatment efficacy is estimated. All these data are transmitted to medical specialist that can adjusted the medical treatment according to the patient personal profile and his medical journal. Researchers have investigated the benefits of using computer or mobile applications (e.g., memory training application or brain training applications) in maintaining/ improving the cognitive functions of older adults [55–60]. In [55,56] specific smartphone applications for improving the cognitive function of older adults are comparatively analyzed. The attention and the working memory are improved by engaging the older adult in training tasks with different difficulty levels for concentration, speed, memory, visual and logic. HealtheBrain, is another smartphone application in which physical activities are combined with memorizing activities in order to improve the cognitive functions of older adults with and without mild cognitive impairment [57]. Similarly, in [58] the results of using the cognitive training game in improving the cognitive functions of older adults is analyzed. The game includes a set of tasks to be performed by the older adults which aim to train various cognitive functions of the older adult, such as attention, memory, visuospatial or language function. There are also studies that demonstrate the efficiency of using computer/smartphone applications in dementia treatment. For example, in [59] three smartphone applications are analyzed: EVO which is a cognitive training application that reduces the symptoms of depression, iPST which acts as a psychotherapy for depression and health tips which assists in the treatment control. In addition, in [60] the effect of playing action video games in increasing the cognitive ability in the case of the people suffering of with dementia is analyzed. Reference [61] presents SONOPA, a framework which combines ambient sensors with social networks to create social connection between older adults, based on their hobbies, localization or activity levels. The activity levels and the number of persons in a house (i.e., the level of occupancy) are determined based on the data collected with PIR and visual sensors, while the socialization interaction level of an older adult in a day is computed based on the level of the occupancy of the house and the information collected from the social network (the message communication, the visualized photograph, etc.). In addition, a matching algorithm is proposed that can identify new social connections for the older adults with low social level based on the data collected from sensors and from the social network (i.e., person profile, socialization level, etc.).

Considering the above, we have mapped the nowadays available sensing devices onto different type of assessments they enact aiming to determine their potential usage as reliable source of data for deciding on robot-based interventions (see Table 2).

Table 2. Potential usage of sensors.

Type of Assessment		Sensors	Potential Usage
Physiological	Stress/anxiety level	Wearable sensors for pulse rate, temperature, blood pressure	Stress or anxiety detection -> Play music as intervention
Daily life activities assessment	Sleeping	Bed Pressure Sensors	Sleeping problems detection
	General Activity level	Motion Sensors	Lack of physical activity -> individual training intervention
	Food intake	Devices embedded sensors	Intake problem -> intervention by reminding to eat, drink water, etc.
	Medication Intake	IoT Pillbox	Medication plan adherence problem -> intervention by reminding to take medication according to the prescription plan
Social Interaction	Physical interaction	Camera and image processing and Voice recognition	Video-based communication to support mediated connection
	Virtual interaction	Social network-based monitoring	
Cognitive	Automatic Reminders	Voice recognition	Memory stimulation using biography
		Personalized Information	News/weather feed
Safety	Safety Assistance	Fall detection sensors	Send of alerts/notifications

2.2. *ML for Behavior Assessment*

Machine learning (ML) techniques are an important component for building smart environments and associated technologies. Using the gathered monitored data, these techniques can be used for identifying and assessing certain situations in the older adults' behavior, situations that usually require personalized intervention from the caregivers or health professionals [62]. At the same time, the automatic recognition and classification of various daily life activities has the potential of reducing the costs associated with the healthcare of the older adults significantly, especially in the case of those cognitively challenged. By using sensors and advanced analytics over collected data, it is possible to extract information in real time about the monitored person and thus it is possible to detect anomalies and patterns that may indicate wellbeing, social and cognitive decline as well as healthcare problems that require intervention.

In this section we analyzed a selection of representative research articles which consider the application of ML techniques for various cases of behavior assessment for older adults. For each representative research article, the following characteristics are considered: the machine learning techniques used, their advantages and disadvantages and type of behavior assessment targeted. We have identified and classified the most important ML techniques that are used for building such smart AAL technologies:

- Classification techniques—The state-of-the-art literature features several methods based on different types of classifiers for monitored data streams out of which ensemble learning methods are considered the best techniques for the classification of the data streams. There are still a lot of challenges posed by the data streams in the case of the ensemble learning algorithms such as the temporal dependencies [63], the concept drifts [64] and the feature drifts [65] and those challenges may appear especially in the monitoring of the daily living activities that are situation-aware where similar monitored data can correspond to related activities such as ascending stairs or descending stairs;
- Regression techniques—The application of regression techniques for daily living activities recognition in context-aware AAL systems [66] is challenging because the identification of the activities should be performed after the beginning of the activities as soon as possible. A part of the limitations of the current approaches are the recognition of the activities after they are completed and the training of the models using offline historical data, a machine learning phase that leads to models which cannot predict the ongoing activities in a timely manner;
- Clustering techniques—The clustering of the data streams should be adaptable due to the fact that the underlying data streams may change and evolve significantly in time, like in the case of data that results from the monitoring of the older adults while they perform different types of daily living activities. In [67] are addressed in more details challenges regarding the clustering, the labeling and the interpretation of the IoT data streams dynamically, challenges that exist especially in those AAL systems that monitor the daily behavior of the older adults;
- Other ML techniques—This category considers techniques such as discovery of association rules, patterns detection, anomalies detection, etc. The abnormal human activities are very diverse [68] in nature due to a variety of aspects such as the way in which the anomalies are defined, the feature representations of the anomalies and the characteristics of the daily living activities data. The detection of the anomalies using various ML algorithms was approached in the research literature in a few studies such as the one presented in [69] where the analysis of the anomalies is not considered as the main subject of the study, but in relation with the recognition of the daily living activities, the discovery of the behavioral patterns and the decision support.

There are three types of older adult behaviors considered that is usually addressed in the research literature through ML techniques, namely daily activities behavior, agitated and aggressive behavior and medication adherence behavior.

Assessing the daily activity behavior of the older adults is relevant for the detection of the abnormal situations [70]. In [71] the authors propose a generic architecture for the monitoring of the activities in smart homes and approach a large variety of ML techniques such as the classification of the activities, the prediction and the reminding of various activities and the detection of the anomalous patterns. However, that review is focused on the basic daily living activities behavior of the older adults and it considers only partially or not at all other types of behavior such as the medication adherence behavior or dementia specific behavior. ML challenges related to the classification of frequent daily living activities (i.e., eating and drinking) are described in [72]. The authors consider data from three datasets collected using various types of monitoring sensors such as power meter sensors and motion, contact and audio sensors. The tested classifiers were support vector machines (SVM), random forest (RF), Fisher kernel learning (FKL) and hidden Markov model (HMM). A different classification approach in [73] considers classification techniques for the remote acoustic monitoring of the older adults in AAL scenarios of residential scale. The data were collected from wireless acoustic sensors and the decision to trigger or not an alarm is taken after the running of a two-stage ANN-based classification process for audio events. One ML usage in AAL systems is the prediction of the daily living activities of the older adults [74] ranging from regression techniques related to the prediction of the CO_2 consumed inside a room using an Artificial Neural Network (ANN) Levenberg–Marquardt (LMA) prediction model to other ML techniques related to the detection of the daily living activities from data collected by humidity, temperature or microphones [75]. The authors of [14] consider a smart aging system for distinguishing the variations from the baseline. The proposed ML method consists of preprocessing, segmentation, feature extraction, classification, pattern recognition and anomaly forecasting. Moreover, this approach also considers the medication activity with respect to the food intake activity. However, the performance results are affected by noise that can be generated by faulty sensors or by the presence of a visitor. Another approach, [76], proposes a method based on a deep convolutional neural network (DCNN) in order to classify ten types of activities. Even though that approach is based on one of the most preferred solutions for daily living activities monitoring, namely the unobtrusive activity recognition and returns a very high F1 score for eight out of ten activities that are monitored it may be more expensive in terms of computational resources than other approaches. The recognition of the activities was approached in [77] using data collected from public available datasets which are characteristic to smart home scenarios. In addition to classical daily living activities such as bathing, sleeping and eating, that approach also considers the medication intake activity. The proposed classifier is a long short-term memory (LSTM) model and compared to other existing machine learning models it returns better results while the performance of the approach is affected by various dimensions such as the number of residents, the number and the types of activities and the test days duration. The authors of [78] propose a fog-based deep learning fall detection system using data collected by a tri-axial accelerometer. The proposed architecture is based on three layers, namely a medical devices layer, a fog layer and a cloud layer. The results presented in that article show that the deep learning methods such as LSTM and gate recurrent unit (GRU) are better than the classical machine learning methods such as SVM and k-nearest neighbors (K-NN) for falls detection.

Agitated and aggressive behavior is one of the most challenging symptoms of dementia [79] and its automated detection using sensors is useful for the caregivers that can act quickly in these kinds of situations. In [80] the authors consider challenges related to the agitated behavior in the case of the people with dementia. The automatic detection of the agitation is approached considering data from various sensors placed around the bodies of the monitored subjects that collect information about the skin temperature, the skin response and the heart rate and that data are further analyzed using a SVM classifier. One drawback is that the approach requires the sensors to be placed on the bodies of the monitored older adults. The authors of [81] consider the application of novel technologies for the early Alzheimer disease (AD) detection. Some associated symptoms are the aggression, the anxiety, the aberrant motor behavior and the irritability. The data from the subjects was analyzed using an ANN with two classes (control subjects and AD), the approach is low cost and it does not have any side effects. Related to prediction of the agitative behavior for the patients with dementia an important challenge is overcoming weakly labeled and sparse data [82]. The goal is to infer proficiently the agitation episodes from data collected by wearable sensors using multiple-instance learning (MIL) models. However, that data comes only from 10 residential deployments, each with a duration of 30 days. In [83] the data collected from various sensors is used in order to detect the challenging behaviors in the advanced stages of dementia. K-means clustering was applied in order to cluster the residents in two groups, one group characterized by challenging behavior with more passive features, and the other group characterized by challenging behavior with more active features. However, the possibility to detect the disorientation using accelerometer data in different solutions based on assistive technologies is considered as a future research direction. The detection of the agitation behavior of the people with dementia using wearable devices is also approached in [84]. The combination of data from multiple sensors leads to better results than in the case when data from a single sensor is used. The applied classifiers are RF and SVM and the results show that the multi-model sensors are feasible for detecting agitation in the case of the people with dementia.

Medication adherence behavior of the older adults to specific medication plans is critical, especially when the older adults have special conditions such as dementia. The application of pervasive technologies [85] for the monitoring of the daily medication behavior may predict when the medication prompting is effective. The approach presented in [86] considers clustering challenges related to the medication adherence. Since the medication adherence behavior is correlated with other daily living activities such as drinking and eating, that approach also considers other activities. The proposed clustering approach is a k-means that is improved using fuzzy set. The authors of [87] consider the application of reminder-based interventions for the individuals with dementia as the memory limitations often lead to activities that are incomplete or not initiated. The article considers the application of the sensor technologies in combination with machine learning technologies in order to address those challenges. The classifiers considered in that approach are various such as decision trees (DT), K-NN, naïve Bayes (NB), SVM and logistic regression (LR). The approach presented in [88] assesses the medication adherence of 38 older adults with a mean age of approximately 87 years. The two measures of adherence proposed in that article are the percent of the days when the medications were missed and the spread in time when the medications were taken. The data were analyzed using three linear regressions and the medication intake habit was monitored continuously using a MedTracker 7-day pillbox. The medication adherence is approached in [89] in relation with other activities such as walking, drinking water, writing and texting. The applied classification algorithm is RF from Apache Spark. Even though the data were misclassified sometimes using that approach, the application of the near-field communication (NFC) sensors may improve the results. Medication intake behavior in relation with the eating and the drinking behavior is researched in [90]. The experiments were conducted using data collected from gyroscope and accelerometer sensors and the performance of various classifiers such as K-NN, NB, DT, multilayer perceptron (MPC), RF and HMM was evaluated. Moreover, two out of the five analyzed different users were seniors. The results presented in that article are very promising, and the system should provide an adequate basis for smart reminder triggering in the case of the autonomously living seniors. However, that approach was tested only on five seniors the method does not consider special characteristics of the older adults that may have dementia such as memory related problems or unpredictable behavior. The medication intake activities were considered in [91] using a solution based on data collected from a smartwatch in relation with other activities such as texting, writing, walking and bottled water intake. In terms of F1Score, the Gradient Boosted Trees (GBT)-based approach returned better results than the approaches based on LR, SVM and RF. One advantage compared to other approaches from literature that consider the medication intake activity is the fact that it considers at least two types of medication intake. In [92] the medication adherence is considered using a ML approach that is based on body worn sensors. The medication intake activity is analyzed considering correlated activities such as drinking, taking chocolate and eating and the applied machine learning classifier is the DT classifier.

2.3. Social Robots Driven Intervention

Social robots are nowadays seen as key technology for supporting older adults care at home or in care institutions. Even from the breakthrough of the assistive robot's technology two main advantages were identified: the functional capabilities and the affective aspects [93]. They can offer different care functions (physical activity, affective therapy, cognitive training, physiological therapy, etc.) while they can help to increase the quality of life of older adults through companionship and social interaction. There are basically two classes of social robots: physically assistive robots that are focused to perform physical tasks and socially assistive robots that can be used for the social and psychological needs of older adults [94].

Few literature studies offer a clear view over the current status and trends for social robots being focused most on old robot models and their potential application in the older adult care domain [93–95]. These studies highlight PARO as one of the first social robots with immediate applicability for older adult care. PARO is an interactive robot developed by Japanese AIST research institute that uses animal therapy as a care method. It has reached its 8th generation with a price around of €5000 and is successfully used in hospitals and care homes across the world, but it can be easily used in the older adult's home. PARO uses tactile, light, audition, temperature and posture sensors to learn the surrounding and interact with older adults and can dynamically adapt to the user's actions and preferences. As benefits, PARO can reduce patient stress and indirectly of their caregivers, stimulate patients and contribute to the socialization part of their life. A recent study has shown that PARO can be very useful for improving quality of life of older adults with dementia and Alzheimer, affection and social interaction, reducing depression and anxiety—even for reducing pain medication usage [96]. Another comprehensive evaluation study highlights the potential usage of PARO as a pet therapy for older people with dementia while identifying barriers for its wide usage such as the fact that users' needs and experiences are not properly taken into consideration and that it fails to meet the actual clinical needs [94]. Besides these, compared with nowadays social robots, PARO has no functionalities for requirements such as stimulating older adults' memory or cognitive functions, increasing physical activities or aiding the caregiver with care information.

The Pepper robot developed by SoftBank is a humanoid robot featuring multi-modal communication able to recognize faces and basic human emotions, is capable of human interaction directly through conversation [97]. It can also exhibit body language, perceiving and moving around and is currently used in schools for child education or different businesses mainly as information point for users. Pepper is priced around €15,000 (acquisition price and subscription fee for three years) and has spawned multiple projects for developing new instances of its basic features such as ASIMO, COMAN or Enon and EU research projects such as CARESSES, CROWD-BOT or ANIMATAS. As for its underlying technology, Pepper uses a six-axis inertial measurement unit (IMU) sensor, microphones, cameras and 3-D sensor, laser sensing modules, loudspeakers, sonar sensors, infrared sensors, tactile sensors, bumper sensors and features an attached tablet for direct interaction and configuration. For the specific use–case of older adult care, Pepper was successfully used in healthcare and older adult-care facilities mainly as narrative-memory-based human–robot companionship [98] and medicine taking reminding, encouraging older adults to keep active and helping them keep in touch with family and friends [99]. Recent research approaches have used Pepper as older adults' companion for suggesting personalized physical activities in the context of active aging [100]. The proposed solution uses deep learning methods on Pepper recorded information to classify the exercises and to schedule personalized physical activities. The robot is integrated in the context of a robot system named PHAROS which in addition to the robot component it contains a component for human exercises recognition which applies deep learning models on the data recorded by Pepper and a component which recommends physical exercises periodically considering the data from the agenda of the users. In [101] Pepper robot is used in the context of a system called Crowd of Oz (CoZ), an open-source system that allows conversational tasks. The objectives of CoZ are to enhance both the contextual and the social awareness of the workers, to manage the asynchronous nature of the workers during the conversational task and to support the task performance of the workers. The Pepper robot has also been used for the case of people that have special conditions such as schizophrenia or dementia during recreational or rehabilitation sessions [102]. Even though the humanoid robot can elicit simple instructions for simple activities such as physical exercises, numerous improvements are required in order to deploy the humanoid robots in the long-term care. Moreover, other aspects should be considered such as the motivation of the older adults or a sense of calmness from the clients' side. Some benefits of the application of Pepper in hospitals [103] are the lowering of the stress levels and the contacting of the family members when the older adults are unable to contact anyone especially in critical situations when something happens to them. However, there are still further research directions that should be considered such as the recognition of a wider range of emotions.

The Nao robot is reported in several approaches as useful coaching assistant [104–106]. In [104] a particular use case for Nao is presented as an illustrative scenario for social robot driven intervention, an autonomous exercise tutor. The robot is capable to learn from a human, to generate feedback situations such as speed and amplitude adjustment, mirroring detection and no motion. However, the older adult participants did not prefer the intervention of the robots due to the poor social skills and because they perceived the sessions with the robots as one-to-one instead as a social event. In [105] a Nao socially-assistive humanoid robot is tested in the context of a smart home environment. Even though the results presented there suggest that the interaction between the robot and the older adults is not characterized by anxiety, the maintenance of high levels of enjoyment for the older adults for prolonged time periods is still a challenge. Nao was also used to detect the behavioral disturbances of the people with dementia [106]. The authors aimed to evolve the role of the humanoid social robot to a technological support tool that functions autonomously, to drive to the resident and alert the staff or distract the resident temporarily when a behavioral disturbance is detected.

There are several other social robots that are reported in the literature as potential solution for older adult care intervention. Zora is one of these and can be used in interventions for the care personnel and for the older adult-care institutions [107]. The results show various types of impacts, ranging from negative to positive. A part of the participants suffered from memory disorders and others required round-the-clock care. The impact on the care personnel differs very much from the impact on the older adults. In the case of the care personnel the impact was on dimensions such as the working atmosphere, the professional development and the competences, while in the case of the older adults the impact was on the physical activities, the older adults' interaction and the sensory experiences. Authors of [108] consider a mini robot as support for a motivational decision-making system (DMS). The stimulating and the improvement of the interaction of the robot with the users is considered from various perspectives such as the performance of cognitive exercises and the performance of educational games. In the scenario described in that article the mini robot has two motivations, namely a social motivation and a relaxing motivation, and those two motivations must be in equilibrium while the robot interacts with a user. However, one drawback of that approach is that the robot is modeled using only two motivations and many other complex aspects should be considered when the users have specific health conditions. Another approach [109] proposes the learning of the social gestures through imitation through a humanoid robot called Tangy that is programmed to avoid the self-collisions and to generate arm trajectories that are collision-free. Even though the human demonstrators considered in that article do not have health conditions, the research considered in that article can be further adapted to stimulate the interactions of the older adults with the social robots. Another study that considers the application of social robots for older adults' intervention is presented in [110] where the authors propose Stevie robot that is tested and validated on different categories of users such as the residents of a retirement community and the healthcare personal of that community. However, the capabilities of the robot should be extended in order to apply that robot in the case of the people with dementia or with different types of physical disabilities. A combination of more than one robot for developing behavioral intervention systems but focused on the children with autism spectrum disorders is proposed in [111]. The approach uses iRobiQ and CARO robots for providing training and support.

Table 3 summarizes the main approaches analyzed in the context of older adults' robot driven coaching and intervention organized by the type of social robot intervention used.

Table 3. Social robots' intervention approaches in research literature.

Social Robot	Approach	Conditions	Older Adult Interventions
Nao	[104–106]	cognitively healthy older adults; persons with dementia/Alzheimer's	detection of behavioral disturbances; physical exercises tutoring, recreational activities; physical training
Pepper	[99–103]	cognitively healthy older adults; crowd workers; people with schizophrenia or dementia	detection and classification of physical exercises; stress management, companion for older adults; rehabilitation recreational activities; sentiment analysis; narrative-memory-based human–robot companion; medicine taking reminding, encouraging older adults to keep active and social stimulation
PARO	[94–96]	older adults with dementia	pet therapy; reduce patient stress; social interaction, reducing depression and anxiety
Stevie	[110]	care house residents and caregivers	care support, entertainment, cognitive engagement, social connectivity
iRobiQ & CARO	[111]	children that have autism disorders	social training, emotions analysis
Zora	[107]	older adults with memory disorders	stimulating older adults through exercises and interaction
mini & Tangy	[108,109]	cognitively healthy older adults	educational games; imitation learning

2.4. Technology Limitation and User Acceptance

Older adults are keen to continue living in their own homes rather than move into residential institutions and the assistive technologies reviewed in the above sections have the potential of providing the need support in managing various problems of their daily life. However, there are specific challenges that need to be addressed for both technological development perspective and integration with the care models as well as regarding its acceptance by the older adults.

From the technological perspective, the nowadays older adults assistive services are shifting towards the use of objective monitoring using IoT sensors and sensors networks, but in general, they lack in personalization when it comes to addressing the older adults wishes and needs and are relying on dedicated healthcare resources for assuring the intervention and continuity of care. The assistive service models in the area of managing and carrying of older adults are focused on providing general information and awareness of the specific disease. Being overwhelmed due to daily life activities and carrying duties the end-users are no longer interested in general-purpose information, but they want personalized target support. In addition, most of today's care process assessment is still relying on self-reporting of "perceived behaviors", but this kind of models are proven not to be viable in the case of elders who mostly deals with problems such as forgetfulness and confusion and chaining mood and behavior. Recent IoT advancements and the development of miniaturized sensors have the potential of changing this situation, by enabling the remote and daily monitoring of important care aspects such as adherence to recommended therapy and lifestyle changes delivering more coordinated innervation through the means of social robots. In addition, this has the potential of improving the older adults' engagement and adherence and timely communication among all parties involved in the care process. Moreover, there is a need of integrating within the nowadays care models novel technology solutions supporting the non-face-to-face interaction and follow-up of older adults, such as advanced robot-supported verbal communication tools with caregivers and patient and/or family/caretaker support for self-management, independent living and activities of daily living. All these limitations need to be systematically addressed to support the perspective shift for next-generation of coordinated care service models for older adults which are relying on ICT-based pervasive and objective monitoring of daily live functioning using advanced IoT sensors, quantifiable metrics of assessing the elders' deviations signaling conditions decline and timely interventions supported by robots/tablets/avatars.

Acceptance of these novel technologies well as their daily usage may be challenging for older adults. As shown in the literature, several technology acceptances factors can be correlated with aging ranging from technology costs, privacy implications and usability up to social aspects such as the implications for family or friends [112]. Several acceptance models can be used to support the process as technology acceptance model (TAM), unified theory of acceptance and use of technology (UTAUT) or senior technology acceptance model (STAM) [113] by assessing indicators such as technology perceived usefulness, ease of use, experience or social implications. However, even these models cannot capture aspects such as user acceptance in time and miss key aspects in the older adult life such as cognitive decline and social isolation [114,115].

Monitoring older adults' activities is the most common identified barrier for older adults' acceptance since it involves breaking their privacy by installing smart devices such as wearables or sensor networks in their homes and collecting sensitive data [116]. Even that at beginning the older adults may not trust in these technologies, after using them they start to perceive them as important. A key role for accepting in home remote monitoring is attributed to family, friend and caregivers that can assist, train and support the older adult in embracing the change. Passive monitoring-based on IoT devices is the most suitable approach for smart home data collection while wearables technology seems to have a good acceptance ratio especially to well-educated older adults that appreciate the possibility of self-monitoring their health status [117]. In contrast, active monitoring such as monitoring older adults with cameras in their environment is raising major privacy and ethical concerns and consequently it encounters their reluctance of using such systems even though they are useful for users that have health problems such as dementia [118,119]. In domestic environments, sensor-based monitoring infrastructures usually require combining heterogenous sensors and devices for capturing information regarding the older adult behavior leading to another major issue for developing smart AAL systems, namely data heterogeneity. However, this issue was thoroughly researched leading to different solutions ranging from involving web semantics and sharing a common context model for building smart objects in heterogenous IoT networks [120,121] to defining and using ML and big data technologies to process time-series-based heterogeneous and distributed streams of data in a unitary approach [62,122].

The benefits of assistive technologies come from their core Artificial Intelligence (AI) components that use advanced ML techniques for taking decisions, alerting or providing support for doctors and caregivers. The user acceptance for these technologies relates to their understanding of the brought benefits and potential improvement for their quality of life. In general, older adults, doctors and caregivers agree and seem to be comfortable to us AI/ML technologies for assisting and improving the care process [123,124]. They are usually adapted to particularities of older adult's health status such as mild dementia [83], medication and polypharmacy [88], cardiovascular problems [15] or physical activity [76]. However, the acceptance of such technology is usually influenced by factors such as age and education [125], while the adoption of intelligent technologies is corelated with the older adult loneliness and with the support provided by caregivers [114].

The use of social robots for older people care at home or in initialized care is a new technological trend for supporting the intervention in assistive care models. Existing studies for the social robots' acceptance are relatively new and conclude that further research is required for assessing acceptance rate, but in the same time clearly identify the care areas where the robots can be successfully used as physical assistance, safety/monitoring and social companionship for an older adult [124,126]. Other surveys show that older adults have positive thoughts regarding the usefulness, utility, safety and trust of a social robot, while doctors and caregivers consider that the robot is a useful tool for rehabilitation [127]. In general, more positive acceptance is found after the users interact with the robot after a period, while the acceptance level is directly influenced by the robot's social capabilities [128]. Other authors pinpoint that usefulness, adaptability, enjoyment, sociability, companionship and perceived behavioral control are important for the high acceptance rate of social robots [129]. One specific factor for accepting the social robot as a care companion is loneliness, the social robots may offer support and companionship especially at home [130].

3. Novel Integrated Robot-Based Care Services

In this section we discuss on the potential usage of the reviewed technologies for the development of advanced assistive and care services focusing on their features implemented and architectures.

3.1. Polypharmacy Management

Most older adults with comorbidities are taking several drugs per day being exposed to the negative effects of polypharmacy. Ensuring appropriate medication usage in this population is clinically important because of the significant risks for institutionalization and negative impact of drugs related problems on older adults' wellbeing. Polypharmacy management includes the review of medication intake, identification of medication side effects and lack of adherence of patents thus it tends to be challenging in case older adults. For medical professionals it is difficult to properly assess the behavioral and psychological symptoms of the older adult patient and distinguish them from medication side effects, since changing is gradually and is likely to be multifactorial (also because the patients have difficulty describing the changing situation) while for the patient it is difficult to take the appropriate medication at the right time. A medication review is utmost important because unfortunately, due to age-related drug metabolism and other problems related to frailty (low vision and reduced psychomotor functioning among others) or due to transitions towards home healthcare, the older adult is at risk of experiencing drug-related problems. These problems are usually caused by drug use, drug choice and adverse reactions, interactions or contraindications. Drug related problems may occur in various steps of the medication process (from prescription till evaluation) and they are dependent on various actors in the chain of pharmaceutical care such as the physician, nurse, pharmacists or their accountable assistants and off course the patient himself.

The polypharmacy management service (see Figure 1) aims improve the medication process for older adults by combining the objective monitoring by means of sensors with machine learning techniques to properly assess the medication use and potential side effects experienced and by leveraging on social robot/tablet to provide timely personalized support to older adult patients (i.e., medication reminders, direct link to caregivers or medical professionals, etc.). This service is related to the EU AAL MedGUIDE project [131], in which the authors are responsible to its technical implementation.

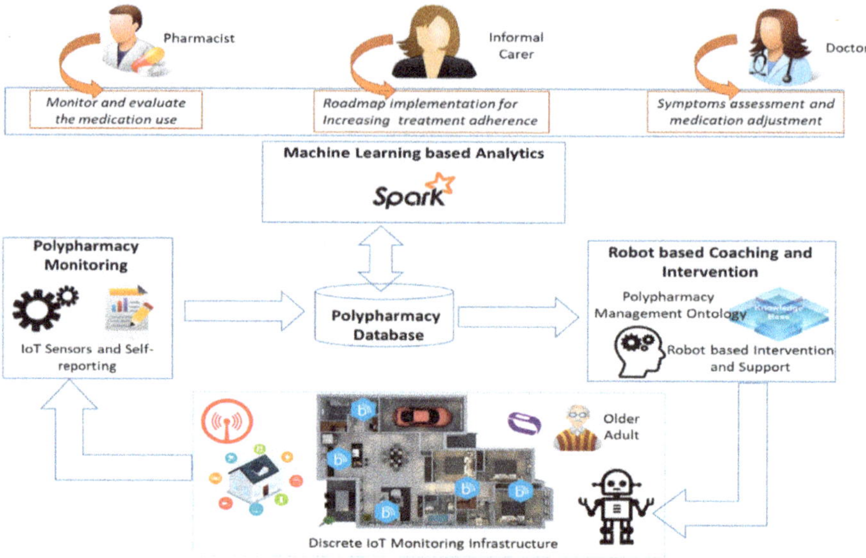

Figure 1. Assistive technologies use to implement the polypharmacy management service.

The polypharmacy monitoring deals with the acquisition of data from sensors that are deployed inside the older adult home targeting the monitoring of activity of daily life with a view of assessing the daily routine baseline and deviations and medication intake to asses adherence to the prescribed medication plan. The following types of activities of daily living were identified as relevant and on-the-shelf commercial sensors, including devices associated with the environment in which the older adult patient lives were used for their monitoring:

- Community mobility—refers to outdoor activities;
- Feeding—refers to the activities of preparing and eating food;
- Functional mobility—refers to indoor activities;
- Total hygiene—refers to the toilet visits and showering activities;
- Sleeping—refers to overnight sleeping and afternoon naps

Motion sensors and iBeacon tags are placed around the home such as on the refrigerator door or on the bed, to monitor and deduce older adults' activities (see Table 4).

Table 4. Types of sensors installed in the home and the monitored daily life activity.

Sensor Names	Installation Place	Monitoring of	Daily Life Activity
Bed sensor	Bedroom	Sleeping pattern of an older adult in terms of period and continuity	Sleeping
Fridge sensor	Kitchen	The number of times the fridge has been opened by the older adult	Feeding
Motion sensor	Kitchen	The older adult's activity in the kitchen	Feeding
Entrance sensor	Entrance	The number of times the entrance door has been opened or closed	Community mobility
Motion sensor	Entrance	Whether the older adult has left or entered the home	Community mobility
Motion sensor	Living room	How much physical activity is performed in the house	Functional mobility
Motion sensor	Bathroom	The number of times the older adult has been to the toilet	Hygiene

For medication intake monitoring on-the-shelf pillboxes is used. In this case, the pillbox will not be used as a simpler organizer or a locked box with a daily alarm but will enable the assessment of adherence level to the medication plan and the report that information back to a doctor, pharmacist or caregiver.

Machine learning-based analytics leverages on big data techniques to process the heterogeneous and distributed streams of monitored data to establish the baseline daily life activities of older adult and to detect in real time events that represent changes, either sudden or gradual, in patients' activity routines which may signal progression of his symptoms, wellbeing decline or side effects of medication [132]. The recent advancements in sensing technologies, IoT and the prevalence of miniaturized, affordable sensors and smart objects, will led to an "explosion" in contextual big data that may be used for improving the older adults with dementia care and treatment. To efficiently exploit the large amount of historical monitored data machine learning algorithms may be used to extract new knowledge and correlation between unrelated daily life activities events which may represent deviations from original older adult patient baseline.

The data sensor records collected throughout a day are further aggregated and the relevant features are extracted to identify the daily sequence of activities for each older adult (see Figure 2).

Activity	Start time	End time
Sleeping	00:00	05:30
Total hygiene	05:35	05:40
Sleeping	05:45	08:30
Total hygiene	08:37	08:50
Functional Mobility	08:51	09:45
Feeding	09:46	10:30
Functional Mobility	10:45	12:00
Total hygiene	12:05	12:10
Community mobility	12:15	14:00
Total hygiene	14:05	14:10
Feeding	14:10	15:00
Functional Mobility	15:05	15:30
Sleeping	15:50	18:30
Total hygiene	18:30	18:35
Functional Mobility	18:40	21:20
Total hygiene	21:25	21:40
Feeding	21:45	22:30
Total hygiene	22:30	22:35
Sleeping	22:40	24:00

(**a**)

Activity	Duration (hours:minutes)	Frequency
Community mobility	1:45	1
Feeding	2:19	3
Functional mobility	5:14	4
Total hygiene	53	7
Sleeping	12:15	4

(**b**)

Figure 2. (**a**) Example of monitored older adult activities in a day; (**b**) features extracted and used in machine learning.

The sensors data flow management is achieved using the following technologies (see Figure 3): (i) Zookeeper [133] as centralized service used for maintaining configuration information, distributed consistent states and synchronization, (ii) Kafka [134] for building real-time data streaming pipelines to be integrated in the master data set and (iii) Cassandra [135] database for storing time series data from sensors.

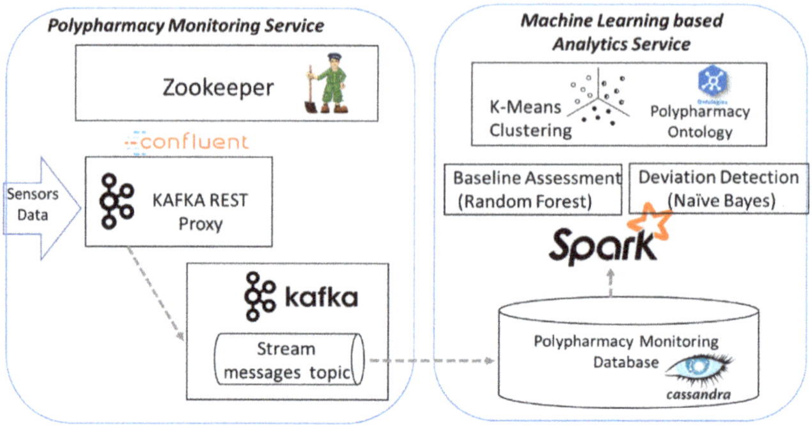

Figure 3. Sensor data management and machine learning (ML)-based analytics.

Baseline assessment techniques aim to identify the routine of an older adult for the entire day, i.e., the daily activities that s/he will normally carry out. Features are extracted from the daily monitored data, and for each type of activity considered, an input for the random forest classifier is provided, which works by building a set of decision trees. Each decision tree is trained on a subset of the training data set. During the testing phase, each decision tree part of the random forest votes for the class to which a test instance belongs (i.e., baseline or not); the class with the most votes is assigned to the associated test instance [136].

Deviation detection techniques seek to detect changes in older adult daily routines that may represent potential side effects of medications s/he had taken, as corelated with the information acquired using the Table 4 sensors infrastructure and pillbox monitoring. A significant deviation from the baseline may be classified, for example, if the total time and frequency corresponding to at least one activity type performed by the older adult on a specific day is higher or lower than a pre-defined threshold as compared to the same activity type registered in the baseline. For this technique, naïve Bayes classifiers can be applied to compute the probability of performing a specific type of activity at a given moment, considering the baseline behavior as a set of conditional probability models.

To correlate detected deviations from potential side-effects of drug–drug interactions, a drug–drug interactions domain ontology is used [137]. This ontology models the pharmacological effects of drugs; the pharmacodynamics actions of drugs; the mechanisms by which these actions are performed; the processes of absorption; transportation, distribution, metabolism and elimination of drugs; the recommended dose and the interactions between drugs. Concepts of the ontology are used to label and annotate the significant deviations detected with potential side effects of drug to drug interaction taken form ontology. Then, a clustering algorithm such K-means is trained and then used to cluster similar days containing significant deviations from the baseline and the results of the clustering algorithm are used to correlate future monitored days with potential drug–drug interactions. Each cluster will contain similar annotated days and the label of the cluster is given by the annotation (i.e., drug–drug interaction and its adverse effects) of the cluster's centroid.

Robot-based coaching and intervention provides personalized care and coordinated guidance, motivation and support for the older adult patient and associated informal caregivers aiming to increase their adherence to the medication plan. An interactive social robot may be used that can speak, respond and receive and send messages to any kind of electronic device (candidate robots: James robot [138], KOMP/AV1 robots [139], etc.). The output of the machine learning analytics will be used for personalizing the robot-based interventions. To achieve this, we pre-define and use robot activities configuration templates and scripts that are associated with each type of identified definition. They will be defined using drag and drop symbol-based programming language and will be integrated with the robot to automatically boot strap and setup the coaching processes fitting older adults' needs, wishes and post discharge recommendations. This will positively impact their adherence to medication plan and will overcome problems which may lead to re-hospitalization. At the same time, the robot can be used to deliver roadmaps and list of actions for better polypharmacy management by implementing the doctors and pharmacist recommendations. Predefined step-by-step video or audio instructions in conducting various lifestyle changes activities or reminders for taking medications delivered using the robot. This may include care feedback and anticipatory guidance for transitional care allowing the patient or the caregivers to repeat information back to confirm understanding ("teach-back"). In addition, personalized motivation slogans and sayings will be pre-registered and used to achieve a high degree of personalization of the care of older adults as the symptoms progress helping them to follow the doctors' recommendations. Social robot usage will increase the independence of the older adults allowing them to connect on-demand with the doctor or informal caregiver via scheduled virtual video meetings.

Figure 4 shows the main data flow among components as well as the interaction of end-users with the polypharmacy management service as well as the interactions between the service modules. The doctor/pharmacist may register the older adult with the service and introduce relevant information known routines, active drug prescriptions—including the drugs that the older adult takes, the dosage, the intake moments and the duration of the treatment. They may check the older adult's medication adherence for a selected date, the daily baseline and potential deviations as well as the machine learning-based suggestions for potential deviations. In addition, they play an important role in robot-based intervention configuration by annotating the deviations with potential side effects of the drug–drug interactions and providing personalized recommendations and content to be played by the robot. The older adult activities of the daily living are continuously monitored, may provide his/her wishes and needs concerning the service and receive the recommendations, instructions to follow via engaging with the social robot companion. The caregiver may supervise the interaction of an older adult with the robot and at the same time may view the recommendations to be implemented.

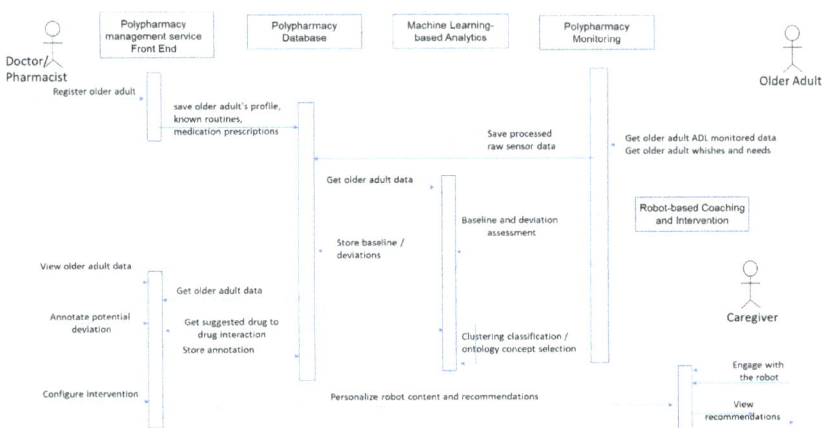

Figure 4. End-user interactions and data flows among modules of the polypharmacy management service.

3.2. Social and Cognitive Activity Engagement

Social assistive robot-based systems featuring sensor-based monitoring, activity and cognitive games and social networking capabilities can be used to stimulate the physical, cognitive and social conditions of people by consolidating their current condition and/or restraining deterioration of their cognitive state [140]. To improve their quality of life while independent living at home, a social robot can provoke the older adult in playing games and perform social activities considering their current state, wishes, needs and preferences.

The older adults' monitoring is based on a combination of seniors and virtual sensing devices (self-reporting condition or memories) used to determine the older adults' activity levels, sleeping patterns/quality and mood as well as their metal condition and relevant information to achieve a more personalized interaction with the robot. The robot device can be used as an intelligent hub for collecting and pushing data into the cloud for further analysis and assessment. The monitored data will be stored in a data storage enacting its future processing to allow contextualization of the robot-based activities.

The assessment will be centered on detecting older adults either sudden or long-term decline in physical, social or cognitive activities. Machine leaning techniques can be employed to mine the monitored data, for translate the older adult's past and present state into estimates of the future thus, obtaining a reference to the potential decline well-being (i.e., long-time trends, seasonal and irregular components, etc.). Motivation to conduct specific activity is challenging and will be implemented using gamification, providing goal and reward scores and social networking applications. Physical and mental stimulation and prevention of cognitive decline will be provided through interactive gamification.

A certain degree of personalization can make cognitive and physical activities more social and enjoyable for the older people by an innovative combination of visual games and applications and a robot companion. The robot modules will not be merely standalone applications, but will be contextualized, filtered and integrated to give personalized experience of a smart and seamless environment. The personalized filtering will facilitate social participation of the older person, reminding scheduled upcoming activities and visits, either through direct communication or through displaying them on tablet and/or flat screen TV. The robot will encourage them and follow-up on a wide range of activities, which can be performed individually or in groups and both indoors and outdoors. Publicly available exercise games and content will be used/adapted to interface with the robot and will not require log in from older adults being offered in a full-kiosk mode to avoid accidentally closing or exiting the application and improving the app has visible and clear appearance.

The conceptual architecture of this system, to be developed in the context of EU AAL ReMind project [141], is presented in Figure 5 and defines the two type of interaction paths between the older adult and the robot (Zora James robot): (i) individual personalized interaction—one-on-one interaction of an older adult with the robot and (ii) non-personalized interaction—more related to the group of older adults interaction with the robot (i.e., fitting the care facility scenarios).

The personalized interaction path is supported through the bibliography module, which is responsible to acquire and store various biography information (i.e., memories) to be used then for defining the older adult customized interaction. The biography data are stored in a personalization database, on top of which the user-engagement and support module will run analytics to detect the right social triggers for personalizing the older adult—robot interaction. The personalization will be carried out both with regards to the type of robot-based applications to be triggered at a specific moment of time and with the content the applications will leverage. As result personalized kiosk of robot-based applications will be created customized to the biography information of the older adult. The caregiver (CG) will be able to filter the inferred social triggers and using the caregiver application will set up appointments for robot driven activities using a calendar-based application. At the same time, it will be able to put in contact or connect the older adult with its social network (i.e., family members, friends, etc.) to carry out different social activities.

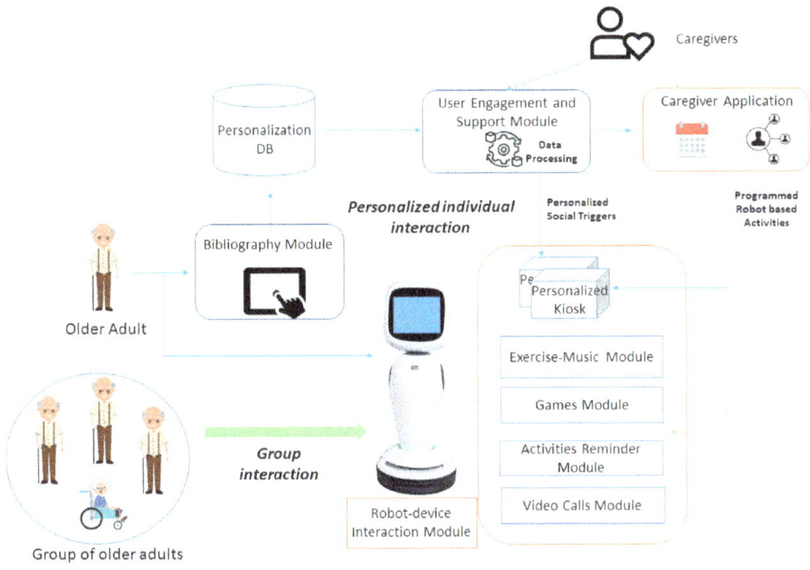

Figure 5. Personalization of the robot-based interaction.

On the robot various modules are implemented and used in correlation with the activities the older adult may conduct to increase its activities levels and timely address the potential cognitive decline. The exercise–music module will be able to play entertainment content such as music, video or TV or it will provoke the older adult to conduct physical activities such as follow the robot. In addition, it will be able to play videos of older adults performing physical activities tailored to the older adult's physical condition and will engage them in such in physical activities by providing instructions and encouragement. The games module will be featuring games that can be played with the help of the robot. Games such as bingo, proverb quiz, packing my suitcase, etc. will be considered with the robot being able to play the role of the game host or caller. The activities reminder module will be able to remind to drink water and take medication as planed and will provide reality orientation activities by providing information on weather, news, upcoming events and daily meals. The video calls module will be able to set up video calls for the older adult with members from its social network based on previously made appointments in calendar. The interaction between the older adult and the robot is facilitated by the robot–device interaction module, featuring vocal commands and tactile-based interaction.

The user-engagement and support module implements and runs analytics on top of the data collected by the biography module to understand the social triggers for older adult's engagement with the robot and to create personalized kiosks according to the older adult profile and biography, to be enforced on the robot. The personalization will be achieved both in regards with the type of robot-based applications to be triggered at a specific moment of time and with the content that the applications will use. Figure 6 presents the internal architecture and technologies used for implementing this module.

The following internal components will be implemented. Knowledge Base Management component is responsible for performing create/read/update/delete (CRUD) operations on the social triggers' knowledge base using the Model2OntologyLibrary [142]. It is also responsible for interacting with the Keosity application [143] through its dedicated representational state transfer (REST) application programming interface (API) to extract the biography of the older adult. The Model2Ontology Library it is a library defined by the authors is providing a very light interface for accessing the knowledge in the form of ontology and reduces the code complexity. It offers one-line methods for performing basic operations (create, update, delete, find). It uses reflection to parse the

Java entities, hiding in this way the code complexity needed by APIs like Jena [144] and Ontology Web Language (OWL) API [145] to perform operations on ontologies, at the same time, benefitting from the performance and scalability properties offered by these. Furthermore, it is the first library that offers the functionality of generating semantic ontological model from an object-oriented model.

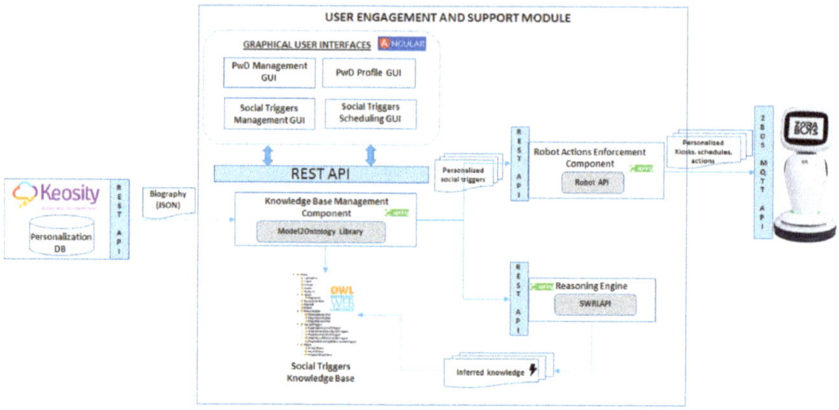

Figure 6. User-engagement and support module implementation.

The social triggers knowledge base is the data model of this module being implemented as an OWL ontology which contains the concepts and rules-based on which the older adult specific data are analyzed. The social triggers knowledge base will model four main facets of the older adults as core sub-ontologies (see Figure 7 for the ontology design model):

- Bibliography aspects—which may be familiar or unfamiliar and it is collected using the bibliography module;
- Personal profile aspects—which concern his/her preferences wishes and needs being also provided by the bibliography module;
- Robot-based Actions—potential actions in which the older adult may be engaged with the robot;
- Consequences—the actual and desired result of conducting a specific activity with the robot;

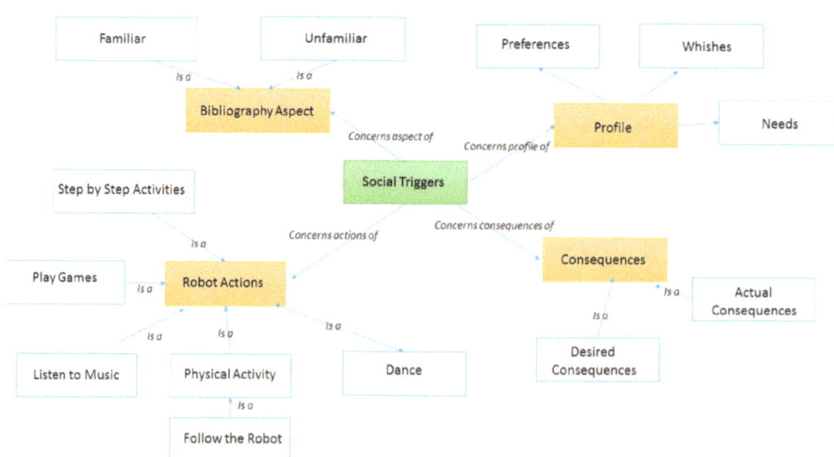

Figure 7. Proposed older adult–robot engagement and motivation ontology.

The reasoning engine is based on an inference engine allowing to run reasoning rules on the ontology considering the older adult specific data to infer personalized triggers that will be further enforced on the robot. It is based on tools like Pellet [146], Jena and D2RQ [147] and will run and evaluate the defined rules for assessing older adult specific triggers by using the data feed by the bibliography module. Two types of rules could be defined and used on the user-engagement and support ontology classes and associated individuals: reasoning rules and query rules. The reasoning rules are written in the semantic web rule language (SWRL) [148] language and used to infer new social triggers information or knowledge out of the ontology. The SWRL rules are injected into the ontology and used to reason about ontology individuals in terms of specific concepts, object and datatype properties. Rules are written in the form of an implication between an antecedent (body) and consequent (head). Both the antecedent and consequent consist of multiple atoms conjunctions. The SWRL rules are evaluated by a reasoning engine in our case the Pellet reasoner. The query rules are written in semantic query-enhanced web rule language (SQWRL) [149]. They are language is data-oriented in the sense that it only queries the individuals held in the ontological models and makes no inferences. In the case the reasoner is started, the queries can return not only data that exists physically in the ontology, but also data that is inferred.

For example, the SQWRL query from Table 5 selects the music content available on the robot to which the older adult is familiar with; in this case, a music file being loaded on the robot if the name of the singer associated to the music file is retrieved in the memories provided by the older adult using the biography module.

In the same table an example of SWRL rule is provided that infers whether an older adult has knowledge (i.e., is familiar) with some music content available on the robot by determining if the name of the singer associated to the music file is retrieved in the stored memories. By executing the rule, a correlation between the older adult and the specific singer is established using the has Knowledge of Music object property.

Table 5. Example of social triggers assessment rules.

Type	Social Trigger Assessment Rule
SWRL rule	Patient(?p) ^ hasId(?p, ?id) ^ swrlb:matches(?id, 1) ^ hasMemory(?p, ?m) ^ hasDescription(?m, ?d) ^ hasRobot(?p, ?robot) ^ hasPlayMusicAction(?robot, ?action) ^ hasMusic(?action, ?music) ^ hasSinger(?music, ?singer) ^ hasId(?music, ?musicid) ^ swrlb:contains(?d, ?singer) -> sqwrl:select(?musicid)
SQWRL query	Patient(?p) ^ hasId(?p, ?id) ^ swrlb:matches(?id, 1) ^ hasMemory(?p, ?m) ^ hasDescription(?m, ?d) ^ swrlb:contains(?d, \"Michael Jackson\") ^ hasRobot(?p, ?robot) ^ hasMusic(?robot, ?music) ^ hasSinger(?music, ?singer) ^ swrlb:contains(?singer, \"Michael Jackson\") -> hasKnowledgeOfMusic(?p,?music)

The robot actions enforcement component converts the older adult personalized triggers into specific robot actions and personalized kiosks that are further run on the robot. The communication with the robot is performed through a message queuing telemetry transport (MQTT) API [150]. To create a new kiosk, the inferred information about the personalized social triggers is used as a filter to search for specific content in the robot's files system by means of an executioner filter. The filtering result is sent to a kiosk builder that creates a new kiosk object which is sent using MQTT connection and uploaded to the robot.

4. Conclusions

This study provides a comprehensive survey of smart environments and robot assistive technologies by identifying the main research problems and technologies limitation and highlighting the current status of their development. The goal was to analyze the foundation for implementing age-friendly care services and for supporting the independent living of older adults at home. The study is organized in three directions: monitoring daily activities, machine learning for behavior assessment and social robots-based intervention. The survey shows that even though various technologies and techniques do exist in the AAL domain, future research is required for matching these onto the specific needs of older adults and their living context and increase their level of adoption. Finally, we discuss on potential usage of these technologies, in the context of two innovative care services, namely polypharmacy management and social and cognitive activity engagement. These care services are based on the findings and developments made in ongoing H2020 Ambient Assistive Living projects and showcase the potential of smart spaces, machine learning and social robot-based systems for improving the quality of life and care processes of older adults. As future steps, we plan to integrate the proposed big data polypharmacy management infrastructure into the H2HCare AAL project platform for developing an older adult post-discharge monitoring and follow-up service that will assess the adherence to the prescribed post discharge lifestyle changes recommendations and medication plan of an older adult and will offer support to him/her through the KOMP/AV1 social robots. In the same fashion, we plan to further develop and integrate the social and cognitive activity engagement service as part of the ReMember-Me and ReMIND AAL projects for developing solutions for stimulating the physical, cognitive and social conditions of older adults through the James robot.

Author Contributions: Conceptualization, I.A. and T.C.; methodology, I.S. and T.C.; investigation, D.M., C.D.P. and M.A.; writing—original draft preparation, I.A., T.C., V.R.C. and D.M.; writing—review and editing, C.B.P. and T.C.; visualization, I.A. and D.M.; supervision, I.S.; funding acquisition, I.A. and T.C. All authors have read and agreed to the published version of the manuscript.

Funding: This research was funded by the Romanian National Authority for Scientific Research and Innovation, CCCDI–UEFISCDI and of the AAL Program with co-funding from the European Union's Horizon 2020 research and innovation program Grant Number AAL59/2018 ReMIND, AAL159/2020 H2HCare and AAL162/2020 ReMember-Me within PNCDI III.

Conflicts of Interest: The authors declare no conflict of interest.

References

1. Age-Friendly Cities and Communities. Available online: https://www.who.int/ageing/projects/age-friendly-cities-communities/en/ (accessed on 1 April 2020).
2. Global Network for Age-friendly Cities and Communities. Available online: https://www.who.int/ageing/projects/age_friendly_cities_network/en/ (accessed on 1 April 2020).
3. Plouffe, L.; Kalache, A. Towards Global Age-Friendly Cities: Determining Urban Features that Promote Active Aging. *J. Hered.* **2010**, *87*, 733–739. [CrossRef] [PubMed]
4. World Health Organization. Global Age-Friendly Cities: A Guide. Available online: https://www.who.int/ageing/publications/Global_age_friendly_cities_Guide_English.pdf (accessed on 23 April 2020).
5. Marston, H.R.; van Hoof, J. "Who Doesn't Think about Technology When Designing Urban Environments for Older People?". A Case Study Approach to a Proposed Extension of the WHO's Age-Friendly Cities. *Model. Int. J. Environ. Res. Public Health* **2019**, *16*, 3525.
6. Stefanov, D.H.; Bien, Z.; Bang, W.C. The Smart House for Older Persons and Persons With Physical Disabilities: Structure, Technology Arrangements, and Perspectives. *IEEE Trans. Neural Syst. Rehabil. Eng.* **2004**, *12*, 228–250. [CrossRef] [PubMed]
7. Age Friendly Model, Housing. Available online: https://extranet.who.int/agefriendlyworld/age-friendly-practices/housing/ (accessed on 22 May 2020).
8. Marston, H.R.; Samuels, J. A Review of Age Friendly Virtual Assistive Technologies and their Effect on Daily Living for Carers and Dependent Adults. *Health* **2019**, *7*, 49. [CrossRef]
9. Breazeal, C.L.; Ostrowski, A.K.; Singh, N.; Park, H.W. Designing social robots for older adults. *Natl. Acad. Eng. Bridge* **2019**, *49*, 22–31.
10. Suzman, R.; Beard, J.; Boerma, T.; Chatterji, S. Health in an ageing world—What do we know? *Lancet* **2015**, *385*, 484–486. [CrossRef]

11. Almeida, A.; Mulero, R.; Rametta, P.; Urošević, V.; Andrić, M.; Patrono, L. A critical analysis of an IoT—aware AAL system for elderly monitoring. *Futur. Gener. Comput. Syst.* **2019**, *97*, 598–619. [CrossRef]
12. Alkhomsan, M.N.; Hossain, M.A.; Rahman, S.M.M.; Masud, M. Situation Awareness in Ambient Assisted Living for Smart Healthcare. *IEEE Access* **2017**, *5*, 20716–20725. [CrossRef]
13. Forkan, A.R.M.; Khalil, I.; Tari, Z. CoCaMAAL: A cloud-oriented context-aware middleware in ambient assisted living. *Futur. Gener. Comput. Syst.* **2014**, *35*, 114–127. [CrossRef]
14. Ghayvat, H.; Awais, M.; Pandya, S.; Ren, H.; Akbarzadeh, S.; Mukhopadhyay, S.; Chen, C.; Gope, P.; Chouhan, A.; Chen, W. Smart Aging System: Uncovering the Hidden Wellness Parameter for Well-Being Monitoring and Anomaly Detection. *Sensors* **2019**, *19*, 766. [CrossRef]
15. Miramontes, R.; Aquino-Santos, R.; Flores, A.; Rodríguez, G.; Anguiano, R.; Ríos, A.; Edwards, A. PlaIMoS: A Remote Mobile Healthcare Platform to Monitor Cardiovascular and Respiratory Variables. *Sensors* **2017**, *17*, 176. [CrossRef] [PubMed]
16. Li, C.; Hu, X.; Zhang, L. The IoT-based heart disease monitoring system for pervasive healthcare service. *Procedia Comput. Sci.* **2017**, *112*, 2328–2334. [CrossRef]
17. Villegas, A.; McEneaney, D.; Escalona, O. Arm-ECG Wireless Sensor System for Wearable Long-Term Surveillance of Heart Arrhythmias. *Electronics* **2019**, *8*, 1300. [CrossRef]
18. Boehm, A.; Yu, X.; Neu, W.; Leonhardt, S.; Teichmann, D. A Novel 12-Lead ECG T-Shirt with Active Electrodes. *Electronics* **2016**, *5*, 75. [CrossRef]
19. Kakria, P.; Tripathi, N.K.; Kitipawang, P. A Real-Time Health Monitoring System for Remote Cardiac Patients Using Smartphone and Wearable Sensors. *Int. J. Telemed. Appl.* **2015**, *2015*, 1–11. [CrossRef]
20. Razjouyan, J.; Lee, H.; Parthasarathy, S.; Mohler, J.; Sharafkhaneh, A.; Najafi, B. Improving Sleep Quality Assessment Using Wearable Sensors by Including Information From Postural/Sleep Position Changes and Body Acceleration: A Comparison of Chest-Worn Sensors, Wrist Actigraphy, and Polysomnography. *J. Clin. Sleep Med.* **2017**, *13*, 1301–1310. [CrossRef]
21. Gruwez, A.; Libert, W.; Ameye, L.; Bruyneel, M. Reliability of commercially available sleep and activity trackers with manual switch-to-sleep mode activation in free-living healthy individuals. *Int. J. Med. Inform.* **2017**, *102*, 87–92. [CrossRef]
22. Mantua, J.; Gravel, N.; Spencer, R. Reliability of Sleep Measures from Four Personal Health Monitoring Devices Compared to Research-Based Actigraphy and Polysomnography. *Sensors* **2016**, *16*, 646. [CrossRef]
23. Zhang, H.; Zhang, J.; Hu, Z.; Quan, L.; Shi, L.; Chen, J.; Xuan, W.; Zhang, Z.; Dong, S.; Luo, J.; et al. Waist-wearable wireless respiration sensor based on triboelectric effect. *Nano Energy* **2019**, *59*, 75–83. [CrossRef]
24. Seoane, F.; Mohino-Herranz, I.; Ferreira, J.; Alvarez, L.; Buendia, R.; Ayllon, D.; Llerena, C.; Gil-Pita, R. Wearable Biomedical Measurement Systems for Assessment of Mental Stress of Combatants in Real Time. *Sensors* **2014**, *14*, 7120–7141. [CrossRef]
25. Shin, D.; Shin, D.; Shin, D. Ubiquitous Health Management System with Watch-Type Monitoring Device for Dementia Patients. *J. Appl. Math.* **2014**, *2014*, 878741. [CrossRef]
26. Stubbs, B.; Chen, L.-J.; Chang, C.-Y.; Sun, W.-J.; Ku, P.-W. Accelerometer-assessed light physical activity is protective of future cognitive ability: A longitudinal study among community dwelling older adults. *Exp. Gerontol.* **2017**, *91*, 104–109. [CrossRef] [PubMed]
27. Hua, A.; Quicksall, Z.; Di, C.; Motl, R.; Lacroix, A.Z.; Schatz, B.; Buchner, D.M. Accelerometer-based predictive models of fall risk in older women: A pilot study. *NPJ Digit. Med.* **2018**, *1*, 25. [CrossRef] [PubMed]
28. Marston, H.R.; Hadley, R.; Banks, D.; Miranda-Duro, M.D.C. Mobile Self-Monitoring ECG Devices to Diagnose Arrhythmia that Coincide with Palpitations: A Scoping Review. *Health* **2019**, *7*, 96. [CrossRef] [PubMed]
29. Tajitsu, Y. Piezoelectret sensor made from an electro-spun fluoropolymer and its use in a wristband for detecting heart-beat signals. *IEEE Trans. Dielectr. Electr. Insul.* **2015**, *22*, 1355–1359. [CrossRef]
30. de Zambotti, M.; Goldstone, A.; Claudatos, S.; Colrain, I.M.; Baker, F.K. A validation study of Fitbit Charge 2™ compared with polysomnography in adults, Chronobiology International. *J. Biol. Med. Rhythm Res.* **2018**, *35*, 465–476.

31. Kwasnicki, R.; Cross, G.W.V.; Geoghegan, L.; Zhang, Z.; Reilly, P.; Darzi, A.; Yang, G.-Z.; Emery, R. A lightweight sensing platform for monitoring sleep quality and posture: A simulated validation study. *Eur. J. Med. Res.* **2018**, *23*, 28. [CrossRef]
32. Lyons, B.E.; Austin, D.; Seelye, A.; Petersen, J.; Yeargers, J.; Riley, T.; Sharma, N.; Mattek, N.; Dodge, H.; Wild, K.; et al. Corrigendum: Pervasive computing technologies to continuously assess Alzheimer's disease progression and intervention efficacy. *Front. Aging Neurosci.* **2015**, *7*, 232. [CrossRef]
33. Hsieh, C.-Y.; Liu, K.-C.; Huang, C.-N.; Chu, W.C.; Chan, C.-T. Novel Hierarchical Fall Detection Algorithm Using a Multiphase Fall Model. *Sensors* **2017**, *17*, 307. [CrossRef]
34. Huynh, Q.T.; Nguyen, U.D.; Irazabal, L.B.; Ghassemian, N.; Tran, B.Q. Optimization of an Accelerometer and Gyroscope-Based Fall Detection Algorithm. *J. Sensors* **2015**, *2015*, 1–8. [CrossRef]
35. Bagalà, F.; Becker, C.; Cappello, A.; Chiari, L.; Aminian, K.; Hausdorff, J.M.; Zijlstra, W.; Klenk, J. Evaluation of Accelerometer-Based Fall Detection Algorithms on Real-World Falls. *PLoS ONE* **2012**, *7*, e37062. [CrossRef] [PubMed]
36. Abbate, S.; Avvenuti, M.; Bonatesta, F.; Cola, G.; Corsini, P.; Vecchio, A. A smartphone-based fall detection system. *Pervasive Mob. Comput.* **2012**, *8*, 883–899. [CrossRef]
37. Mao, A.; Ma, X.; He, Y.; Luo, J. Highly Portable, Sensor-Based System for Human Fall Monitoring. *Sensors* **2017**, *17*, 2096. [CrossRef] [PubMed]
38. Susnea, I.; Dumitriu, L.; Talmaciu, M.; Pecheanu, E.; Munteanu, D. Unobtrusive Monitoring the Daily Activity Routine of Elderly People Living Alone, with Low-Cost Binary Sensors. *Sensors* **2019**, *19*, 2264. [CrossRef]
39. Barsocchi, P.; Bianchini, M.; Crivello, A.; La Rosa, D.; Palumbo, F.; Scarselli, F. An unobtrusive sleep monitoring system for the human sleep behaviour understanding. In Proceedings of the 2016 7th IEEE International Conference on Cognitive Infocommunications (CogInfoCom), Wroclaw, Poland, 16–18 October 2016; Institute of Electrical and Electronics Engineers (IEEE): Los Alamitos, CA, USA, 2016; pp. 000091–000096.
40. Sadek, I.; Bellmunt, J.; Kodyš, M.; Abdulrazak, B.; Mokhtari, M. Novel Unobtrusive Approach for Sleep Monitoring Using Fiber Optics in an Ambient Assisted Living Platform. In *Computer Vision*; Springer: Berlin/Heidelberg, Germany, 2017; Volume 10461, pp. 48–60.
41. Kortelainen, J.M.; Mendez, M.O.; Bianchi, A.M.; Matteucci, M.; Cerutti, S. Sleep Staging Based on Signals Acquired Through Bed Sensor. *IEEE Trans. Inf. Technol. Biomed.* **2010**, *14*, 776–785. [CrossRef]
42. Paalasmaa, J.; Waris, M.; Toivonen, H.; Leppäkorpi, L.; Partinen, M. Unobtrusive online monitoring of sleep at home. In Proceedings of the 2012 Annual International Conference of the IEEE Engineering in Medicine and Biology Society, San Diego, CA, USA, 28 August–1 September 2012; Volume 2012, pp. 3784–3788.
43. Lee, J.; Hong, M.; Ryu, S. Sleep Monitoring System Using Kinect Sensor. *Int. J. Distrib. Sens. Networks* **2015**, *2015*, 1–9. [CrossRef]
44. Wang, Y.-K.; Chen, H.-Y.; Chen, J.-R.; Chen, H.-Y. Unobtrusive Sleep Monitoring Using Movement Activity by Video Analysis. *Electronics* **2019**, *8*, 812. [CrossRef]
45. De Miguel, K.; Brunete, A.; Hernando, M.; Gambao, E. Home Camera-Based Fall Detection System for the Elderly. *Sensors* **2017**, *17*, 2864. [CrossRef]
46. Stone, E.E.; Skubic, M. Fall Detection in Homes of Older Adults Using the Microsoft Kinect. *IEEE J. Biomed. Health Inform.* **2015**, *19*, 290–301. [CrossRef]
47. Daher, M.; Najjar, M.E.B.E.; Khalil, M. Automatic Fall Detection System using Sensing Floors. *Int. J. Comput. Inf. Sci.* **2016**, *12*, 75–82. [CrossRef]
48. Droghini, D.; Principi, E.; Squartini, S.; Olivetti, P.; Piazza, F. Human Fall Detection by Using an Innovative Floor Acoustic Sensor. In *Advances in Theory and Practice of Computational Mechanics*; Springer: Berlin/Heidelberg, Germany, 2017; Volume 69, pp. 97–107.
49. Khan, M.S.; Yu, M.; Feng, P.; Wang, L.; Chambers, J. An unsupervised acoustic fall detection system using source separation for sound interference suppression. *Signal Process.* **2015**, *110*, 199–210. [CrossRef]
50. Li, Y.; Ho, K.C.; Popescu, M. A Microphone Array System for Automatic Fall Detection. *IEEE Trans. Biomed. Eng.* **2012**, *59*, 1291–1301. [CrossRef] [PubMed]
51. Palumbo, F.; La Rosa, D.; Ferro, E. Stigmergy-based Long-Term Monitoring of Indoor Users Mobility in Ambient Assisted Living Environments: The DOREMI Project Approach. In Proceedings of the Artificial Intelligence for Ambient Assisted Living 2016 co-located with 15th International Conference of the Italian Association for Artificial Intelligence (AIxIA 2016), Genova, Italy, 28 November 2016; pp. 18–32.

52. Kyriazakos, S.; Prasad, R.; Mihovska, A.; Pnevmatikakis, A.; Akker, H.O.D.; Hermens, H.; Barone, P.; Mamelli, A.; De Domenico, S.; Pocs, M.; et al. eWALL: An Open-Source Cloud-Based eHealth Platform for Creating Home Caring Environments for Older Adults Living with Chronic Diseases or Frailty. *Wirel. Pers. Commun.* **2017**, *97*, 1835–1875. [CrossRef]
53. Nam, Y.; Kim, Y.; Lee, J. Sleep Monitoring Based on a Tri-Axial Accelerometer and a Pressure Sensor. *Sensors* **2016**, *16*, 750. [CrossRef]
54. Pain-Care. Available online: http://myhealthapps.net/app/details/163/pain-care (accessed on 1 April 2020).
55. Oh, S.J.; Seo, S.; Lee, J.H.; Song, M.J.; Shin, M.-S. Effects of smartphone-based memory training for older adults with subjective memory complaints: A randomized controlled trial. *Aging Ment. Health* **2017**, *22*, 526–534. [CrossRef]
56. Hill, N.L.; Mogle, J.; Wion, R.; Kitt-Lewis, E.; Hannan, J.; Dick, R.; McDermott, C. App-based attention training: Incorporating older adults' feedback to facilitate home-based use. *Int. J. Older People Nurs.* **2017**, *13*, e12163. [CrossRef]
57. Shellington, E.M.; Felfeli, T.; Shigematsu, R.; Gill, D.P.; Petrella, R.J. HealtheBrain: An innovative smartphone application to improve cognitive function in older adults. *mHealth* **2017**, *3*, 17. [CrossRef]
58. Lu, M.-H.; Lin, W.; Yueh, H.-P. Development and Evaluation of a Cognitive Training Game for Older People: A Design-based Approach. *Front. Psychol.* **2017**, *8*, 1837. [CrossRef]
59. Areán, P.A.; Hallgren, K.A.; Jordan, J.T.; Gazzaley, A.; Atkins, D.C.; Heagerty, P.J.; Anguera, J.A.; Kauppi, K.; Schueller, S.; Ben-Zeev, O. The Use and Effectiveness of Mobile Apps for Depression: Results From a Fully Remote Clinical Trial. *J. Med. Internet Res.* **2016**, *18*, e330. [CrossRef]
60. Kühn, S.; Berna, F.; Lüdtke, T.; Gallinat, J.; Moritz, S. Fighting Depression: Action Video Game Play May Reduce Rumination and Increase Subjective and Objective Cognition in Depressed Patients. *Front. Psychol.* **2018**, *9*. [CrossRef]
61. Bilbao, A.; Almeida, A.; López-De-Ipiña, D. Promotion of active ageing combining sensor and social network data. *J. Biomed. Inform.* **2016**, *64*, 108–115. [CrossRef] [PubMed]
62. Moldovan, D.; Anghel, I.; Cioara, T.; Salomie, I. Adapted Binary Particle Swarm Optimization for Efficient Features Selection in the Case of Imbalanced Sensor Data. *Appl. Sci.* **2020**, *10*, 1496. [CrossRef]
63. Puschmann, D.; Barnaghi, P.; Tafazolli, R. Adaptive Clustering for Dynamic IoT Data Streams. *IEEE Internet Things J.* **2017**, *4*, 64–74. [CrossRef]
64. Zliobaite, I.; Bifet, A.; Read, J.; Pfahringer, B.; Holmes, G. Evaluation methods and decision theory for classification of streaming data with temporal dependence. *Mach. Learn.* **2014**, *98*, 455–482. [CrossRef]
65. Lin, C.-C.; Deng, D.-J.; Kuo, C.-H.; Chen, L. Concept Drift Detection and Adaption in Big Imbalance Industrial IoT Data Using an Ensemble Learning Method of Offline Classifiers. *IEEE Access* **2019**, *7*, 56198–56207. [CrossRef]
66. Barddal, J.P.; Gomes, H.M.; Enembreck, F.; Pfahringer, B. A survey on feature drift adaptation: Definition, benchmark, challenges and future directions. *J. Syst. Softw.* **2017**, *127*, 278–294. [CrossRef]
67. Wan, J.; Li, M.; O'Grady, M.; Gu, X.; AlAwlaqi, M.A.; O'Hare, G.M. Time-bounded Activity Recognition for Ambient Assisted Living. *IEEE Trans. Emerg. Top. Comput.* **2018**, *1*. [CrossRef]
68. Dhiman, C.; Vishwakarma, D.K. A review of state-of-the-art technologies for abnormal human activity recognition. *Eng. Appl. Artif. Intell.* **2019**, *77*, 21–45. [CrossRef]
69. Islam, S.M.R.; Kwak, D.; Kabir, H.; Hossain, M.; Kwak, K.-S. The Internet of Things for Health Care: A Comprehensive Survey. *IEEE Access* **2015**, *3*, 678–708. [CrossRef]
70. Botía, J.A.; Villa, A.; Palma, J. Ambient Assisted Living system for in-home monitoring of healthy independent elders. *Expert Syst. Appl.* **2012**, *39*, 8136–8148. [CrossRef]
71. Ni, Q.; Hernando, A.B.G.; De La Cruz, I.P. The Elderly's Independent Living in Smart Homes: A Characterization of Activities and Sensing Infrastructure Survey to Facilitate Services Development. *Sensors* **2015**, *15*, 11312–11362. [CrossRef]
72. Debes, C.; Merentitis, A.; Sukhanov, S.; Niessen, M.; Frangiadakis, N.; Bauer, A. Monitoring Activities of Daily Living in Smart Homes: Understanding human behavior. *IEEE Signal Process. Mag.* **2016**, *33*, 81–94. [CrossRef]
73. Navarro, J.; Vila, E.V.; Alsina-Pagès, R.M.; Hervás, M. Real-Time Distributed Architecture for Remote Acoustic Elderly Monitoring in Residential-Scale Ambient Assisted Living Scenarios. *Sensors* **2018**, *18*, 2492. [CrossRef] [PubMed]

74. Vanus, J.; Belesova, J.; Martinek, R.; Nedoma, J.; Fajkus, M.; Bilik, P.; Zidek, J. Monitoring of the daily living activities in smart home care. *Human-Centric Comput. Inf. Sci.* **2017**, *7*, 1–34. [CrossRef]
75. Pires, I.M.; Marques, G.; Garcia, N.M.; Pombo, N.; Flórez-Revuelta, F.; Spinsante, S.; Teixeira, M.C.; Zdravevski, E. Recognition of Activities of Daily Living and Environments Using Acoustic Sensors Embedded on Mobile Devices. *Electronics* **2019**, *8*, 1499. [CrossRef]
76. Gochoo, M.; Tan, T.-H.; Liu, S.-H.; Jean, F.-R.; Alnajjar, F.S.; Huang, S.-C. Unobtrusive Activity Recognition of Elderly People Living Alone Using Anonymous Binary Sensors and DCNN. *IEEE J. Biomed. Health Inform.* **2018**, *23*, 1. [CrossRef]
77. Liciotti, D.; Bernardini, M.; Romeo, L.; Frontoni, E. A sequential deep learning application for recognising human activities in smart homes. *Neurocomputing* **2020**, *396*, 501–513. [CrossRef]
78. Sarabia-Jácome, D.; Usach, R.; Palau, C.; Esteve, M. Highly-Efficient Fog-Based Deep Learning Aal Fall Detection System. *Internet Things* **2020**, 100185. [CrossRef]
79. Khan, S.; Ye, B.; Taati, B.; Mihailidis, A. Detecting agitation and aggression in people with dementia using sensors-A systematic review. *Alzheimer's Dement.* **2018**, *14*, 824–832. [CrossRef]
80. Sakr, G.; Elhajj, I.H.; Huijer, H.A.-S. Support Vector Machines to Define and Detect Agitation Transition. *IEEE Trans. Affect. Comput.* **2010**, *1*, 98–108. [CrossRef]
81. Lopez-De-Ipina, K.; Hernández, J.B.A.; Travieso-González, C.M.; Solé-Casals, J.; Eguiraun, H.; Faundez-Zanuy, M.; Ezeiza, A.; Barroso, N.; Ecay-Torres, M.; Martinez-Lage, P.; et al. On the Selection of Non-Invasive Methods Based on Speech Analysis Oriented to Automatic Alzheimer Disease Diagnosis. *Sensors* **2013**, *13*, 6730–6745. [CrossRef] [PubMed]
82. Alam, R.; Bankole, A.; Anderson, M.; Lach, J. Multiple-Instance Learning for Sparse Behavior Modeling from Wearables: Toward Dementia-Related Agitation Prediction. In Proceedings of the 2019 41st Annual International Conference of the IEEE Engineering in Medicine and Biology Society (EMBC), Berlin, Germany, 23–27 July 2019; Volume 2019, pp. 1330–1333.
83. Goerss, D.; Hein, A.; Bader, S.; Halek, M.; Kernebeck, S.; Kutschke, A.; Heine, C.; Krueger, F.; Kirste, T.; Teipel, S. Automated sensor-based detection of challenging behaviors in advanced stages of dementia in nursing homes. *Alzheimer's Dement.* **2019**, 1–9. [CrossRef]
84. Khan, S.S.; Spasojevic, S.; Nogas, J.; Ye, B.; Mihailidis, A.; Iaboni, A.; Wang, A.; Martin, L.S.; Newman, K. Agitation Detection in People Living with Dementia using Multimodal Sensors. In Proceedings of the 2019 41st Annual International Conference of the IEEE Engineering in Medicine and Biology Society (EMBC), Berlin, Germany, 23–27 July 2019; Volume 2019, pp. 3588–3591.
85. Wherton, J.P.; Monk, A.F. Technological opportunities for supporting people with dementia who are living at home. *Int. J. Hum. Comput. Stud.* **2008**, *66*, 571–586. [CrossRef]
86. Tang, L.; Zhou, X.; Yu, Z.; Liang, Y.; Zhang, D.; Ni, H. MHS: A Multimedia System for Improving Medication Adherence in Elderly Care. *IEEE Syst. J.* **2011**, *5*, 506–517. [CrossRef]
87. Das, B.; Cook, D.J.; Krishnan, N.C.; Schmitter-Edgecombe, M. One-Class Classification-Based Real-Time Activity Error Detection in Smart Homes. *IEEE J. Sel. Top. Signal Process.* **2016**, *10*, 914–923. [CrossRef] [PubMed]
88. Austin, J.; Klein, K.; Mattek, N.; Kaye, J. Variability in medication taking is associated with cognitive performance in nondemented older adults. *Alzheimer's Dement. Diagn. Assess. Dis. Monit.* **2017**, *6*, 210–213. [CrossRef] [PubMed]
89. Ma, J.; Ovalle, A.; Woodbridge, D.M.-K. Medhere: A Smartwatch-based Medication Adherence Monitoring System using Machine Learning and Distributed Computing. In Proceedings of the 2018 40th Annual International Conference of the IEEE Engineering in Medicine and Biology Society (EMBC), Honolulu, HI, USA, 17–21 July 2018; pp. 4945–4948.
90. Gomes, D.; Mendes-Moreira, J.; Sousa, I.; Silva, J.R. Eating and Drinking Recognition in Free-Living Conditions for Triggering Smart Reminders. *Sensors* **2019**, *19*, 2803. [CrossRef] [PubMed]
91. Fozoonmayeh, D.; Le, H.V.; Wittfoth, E.; Geng, C.; Ha, N.; Wang, J.; Vasilenko, M.; Ahn, Y.; Woodbridge, D.M.-K. A Scalable Smartwatch-Based Medication Intake Detection System Using Distributed Machine Learning. *J. Med. Syst.* **2020**, *44*, 1–14. [CrossRef]

92. Hezarjaribi, N.; Fallahzadeh, R.; Ghasemzadeh, H. A Machine Learning Approach for Medication Adherence Monitoring Using Body-Worn Sensors. In Proceedings of the 2016 Design, Automation & Test in Europe Conference & Exhibition (DATE); Research Publishing Services, Dresden, Germany, 14–18 March 2016; pp. 842–845.
93. Broekens, J.; Heerink, M.; Rosendal, H. Assistive social robots in elderly care: A review. *Gerontechnology* **2009**, *8*, 94–103. [CrossRef]
94. Hung, L.; Liu, C.; Woldum, E.; Au-Yeung, A.; Berndt, A.; Wallsworth, C.; Horne, N.; Gregorio, M.; Mann, J.; Chaudhury, H. The benefits of and barriers to using a social robot PARO in care settings: A scoping review. *BMC Geriatr.* **2019**, *19*, 232. [CrossRef]
95. Kachouie, R.; Sedighadeli, S.; Khosla, R.; Chu, M.-T. Socially Assistive Robots in Elderly Care: A Mixed-Method Systematic Literature Review. *Int. J. Hum. Comp. Interact.* **2014**, *30*, 369–393. [CrossRef]
96. Kang, H.S.; Makimoto, K.; Konno, R.; Koh, I.S. Review of outcome measures in PARO robot intervention studies for dementia care. *Geriatr. Nurs.* **2019**. [CrossRef] [PubMed]
97. Pandey, A.K.; Gelin, R. A Mass-Produced Sociable Humanoid Robot: Pepper: The First Machine of Its Kind. *IEEE Robot. Autom. Mag.* **2018**, *25*, 40–48. [CrossRef]
98. Dominey, P.F.; Paléologue, V.; Pandey, A.K.; Ventre-Dominey, J. Improving quality of life with a narrative companion. In Proceedings of the 2017 26th IEEE International Symposium on Robot and Human Interactive Communication (RO-MAN), Lisbon, Portugal, 28 August 2017; pp. 127–134.
99. Culture Aware Robots and Environmental Sensor Systems for Elderly Support. Available online: http://caressesrobot.org/en/ (accessed on 1 April 2020).
100. Costa, A.; Martinez-Martin, E.; Cazorla, M.; Julian, V. PHAROS—PHysical Assistant RObot System. *Sensors* **2018**, *18*, 2633. [CrossRef] [PubMed]
101. Abbas, T.; Khan, V.-J.; Gadiraju, U.; Barakova, E.; Markopoulos, P. Crowd of Oz: A Crowd-Powered Social Robotics System for Stress Management. *Sensors* **2020**, *20*, 569. [CrossRef] [PubMed]
102. Sato, M.; Yasuhara, Y.; Osaka, K.; Ito, H.; Dino, M.J.S.; Ong, I.L.; Zhao, Y.; Tanioka, T. Rehabilitation care with Pepper humanoid robot: A qualitative case study of older patients with schizophrenia and/or dementia in Japan. *Enfermería Clín.* **2020**, *30*, 32–36. [CrossRef]
103. Rozanska, A.; Podpora, M. Multimodal sentiment analysis applied to interaction between patients and a humanoid robot Pepper. *IFAC-PapersOnLine* **2019**, *52*, 411–414. [CrossRef]
104. Görer, B.; Salah, A.A.; Akın, H.L. An autonomous robotic exercise tutor for elderly people. *Auton. Robot.* **2016**, *41*, 657–678. [CrossRef]
105. Torta, E.; Werner, F.; Johnson, D.O.; Juola, J.F.; Cuijpers, R.H.; Bazzani, M.; Oberzaucher, J.; Lemberger, J.; Lewy, H.; Bregman, J. Evaluation of a Small Socially-Assistive Humanoid Robot in Intelligent Homes for the Care of the Elderly. *J. Intell. Robot. Syst.* **2014**, *76*, 57–71. [CrossRef]
106. Nauta, J.; Mahieu, C.; Michiels, C.; Ongenae, F.; De Backere, F.; De Turck, F.; Khaluf, Y.; Simoens, P. Pro-active positioning of a social robot intervening upon behavioral disturbances of persons with dementia in a smart nursing home. *Cogn. Syst. Res.* **2019**, *57*, 160–174. [CrossRef]
107. Melkas, H.; Hennala, L.; Pekkarinen, S.; Kyrki, V. Impacts of robot implementation on care personnel and clients in elderly-care institutions. *Int. J. Med. Inform.* **2020**, *134*, 104041. [CrossRef]
108. Gomez, M.M.; Castro-González, Á.; Castillo, J.C.; Malfaz, M.; Salichs, M.A. A Bio-inspired Motivational Decision Making System for Social Robots Based on the Perception of the User. *Sensors* **2018**, *18*, 2691. [CrossRef] [PubMed]
109. Zhang, T.; Louie, W.-Y.; Nejat, G.; Benhabib, B. Robot Imitation Learning of Social Gestures with Self-Collision Avoidance Using a 3D Sensor. *Sensors* **2018**, *18*, 2355. [CrossRef] [PubMed]
110. McGinn, C.; Bourke, E.; Murtagh, A.; Donovan, C.; Lynch, P.; Cullinan, M.F.; Kelly, K. Meet Stevie: A Socially Assistive Robot Developed Through Application of a 'Design-Thinking' Approach. *J. Intell. Robot. Syst.* **2019**, *98*, 39–58. [CrossRef]
111. Yun, S.-S.; Kim, H.; Choi, J.; Park, S.-K. A robot-assisted behavioral intervention system for children with autism spectrum disorders. *Robot. Auton. Syst.* **2016**, *76*, 58–67. [CrossRef]
112. Peek, S.T.M.; Wouters, E.J.; Van Hoof, J.; Luijkx, K.G.; Boeije, H.R.; Vrijhoef, H.J. Factors influencing acceptance of technology for aging in place: A systematic review. *Int. J. Med. Inform.* **2014**, *83*, 235–248. [CrossRef] [PubMed]

113. Klímová, B.; Poulová, P. Older People and Technology Acceptance. In *Lecture Notes in Computer Science*; Springer: Berlin/Heidelberg, Germany, 2018; Volume 10926, pp. 85–94.
114. Chen, K.; Chan, A. A review of technology acceptance by older adults. *Gerontechnology* **2011**, *10*, 1–12. [CrossRef]
115. Yusif, S.; Soar, J.; Hafeez-Baig, A. Older people, assistive technologies, and the barriers to adoption: A systematic review. *Int. J. Med. Inform.* **2016**, *94*, 112–116. [CrossRef]
116. Giger, J.T.; Pope, N.D.; Vogt, H.B.; Gutierrez, C.; Newland, L.A.; Lemke, J.; Lawler, M.J. Remote patient monitoring acceptance trends among older adults residing in a frontier state. *Comput. Hum. Behav.* **2015**, *44*, 174–182. [CrossRef]
117. Li, J.; Ma, Q.; Chan, A.H.S.; Man, S. Health monitoring through wearable technologies for older adults: Smart wearables acceptance model. *Appl. Ergon.* **2019**, *75*, 162–169. [CrossRef]
118. Matthews, J.T.; Lingler, J.H.; Campbell, G.B.; Hunsaker, A.; Hu, L.; Pires, B.R.; Hebert, M.; Schulz, R. Usability of a Wearable Camera System for Dementia Family Caregivers. *J. Health Eng.* **2015**, *6*, 213–238. [CrossRef] [PubMed]
119. Mann, W.C.; Marchant, T.; Tomita, M.; Fraas, L.; Stanton, K. Elder acceptance of health monitoring devices in the home. *Care Manag. J.* **2002**, *3*, 91–98. [CrossRef]
120. Modoni, G.E.; Veniero, M.; Trombetta, A.; Sacco, M.; Clemente, S. Semantic based events signaling for AAL systems. *J. Ambient. Intell. Humaniz. Comput.* **2017**, *9*, 1311–1325. [CrossRef]
121. Cioara, T.; Anghel, I.; Salomie, I.; Dinsoreanu, M. A Policy-Based Context Aware Self-Management Model. In Proceedings of the 2009 11th International Symposium on Symbolic and Numeric Algorithms for Scientific Computing, Timisoara, Romania, 26–29 September 2009; pp. 333–340.
122. Chifu, V.R.; Pop, C.; Cioara, T.; Anghel, I.; Moldovan, D.; Salomie, I. Identifying the Polypharmacy Side-Effects in Daily Life Activities of Elders with Dementia. In *Intelligent Distributed Computing XII. IDC 2018. Studies in Computational Intelligence*; Del Ser, J., Osaba, E., Bilbao, M., Sanchez-Medina, J., Vecchio, M., Yang, X.S., Eds.; Springer: Berlin/Heidelberg, Germany, 2018; Volume 798, pp. 380–389.
123. Singh, D.; Kropf, J.; Hanke, S.; Holzinger, A. Ambient Assisted Living Technologies from the Perspectives of Older People and Professionals. In *Applications of Evolutionary Computation*; Springer Science and Business Media LLC: Berlin, Germany, 2017; Volume 10410, pp. 255–266.
124. Sapci, A.H.; Sapci, H.A.; Yang, R.; Du, Y. Innovative Assisted Living Tools, Remote Monitoring Technologies, Artificial Intelligence-Driven Solutions, and Robotic Systems for Aging Societies: Systematic Review. *JMIR Aging* **2019**, *2*, e15429. [CrossRef]
125. Jarvis, M.-A.; Sartorius, B.; Chipps, J. Technology acceptance of older persons living in residential care. *Inf. Dev.* **2019**. [CrossRef]
126. Bharatharaj, J.; Krägeloh, C.; Kutty, S.K.S.; Nirmala, P.R.; Huang, L. Questionnaires to Measure Acceptability of Social Robots: A Critical Review. *Robotics* **2019**, *8*, 88. [CrossRef]
127. Casas, J.; Gómez, N.C.; Cifuentes, C.A.; Gutierrez, L.; Rincon, M.; Múnera, M. Expectation vs. Reality: Attitudes Towards a Socially Assistive Robot in Cardiac Rehabilitation. *Appl. Sci.* **2019**, *9*, 4651. [CrossRef]
128. Hameed, I.; Tan, Z.-H.; Thomsen, N.; Duan, X. User Acceptance of Social Robots. In Proceedings of the Ninth International Conference on Advances in Computer-Human Interactions (ACHI 2016), Venice, Italy, 24–28 April 2016; pp. 274–279.
129. De Graaf, M.M.; Ben Allouch, S. Exploring influencing variables for the acceptance of social robots. *Robot. Auton. Syst.* **2013**, *61*, 1476–1486. [CrossRef]
130. Heerink, M.; Krose, B.; Evers, V.; Wielinga, B. The influence of social presence on acceptance of a companion robot by older people. *J. Phys. Agents (JoPha)* **2008**, *2*, 33–40. [CrossRef]
131. MedGUIDE AAL Project. Available online: http://medguide-aal.eu/ (accessed on 1 April 2020).
132. Peek, S.T.M.; Kazak, J.K.; Perek-Białas, J.M.; Peek, S.T.M. The Challenges of Urban Ageing: Making Cities Age-Friendly in Europe. *Int. J. Environ. Res. Public Health* **2018**, *15*, 2473. [CrossRef]
133. Apache Zookeeper. Available online: https://zookeeper.apache.org/ (accessed on 10 April 2020).
134. Apache Kafka. Available online: https://kafka.apache.org/ (accessed on 10 April 2020).
135. Apache Cassandra. Available online: http://cassandra.apache.org/ (accessed on 10 April 2020).

136. Moldovan, D.; Visovan, A.; Bologa, M.; Pop, C.; Chifu, V.R.; Anghel, I.; Cioara, T.; Salomie, I. Random Forest and Sequential Model for Anomalies Detection in the Activities of the People with Dementia. In Proceedings of the World Congress on Medical Physics and Biomedical Engineering 2008, Cluj-Napoca, Romania, 17–20 October 2018; Volume 71, pp. 207–213.
137. DINTO Ontology. Available online: https://bioportal.bioontology.org/ontologies/DINTO (accessed on 1 April 2020).
138. James Social Robot Helps Children with Diabetes. Available online: https://robots.nu/en/newsitem/social-robot-helps-children-with-diabetes (accessed on 1 April 2020).
139. AV1 Robot. Available online: https://www.noisolation.com/uk/av1/ (accessed on 1 April 2020).
140. Martinez-Martin, E.; Escalona, F.; Cazorla, M. Socially Assistive Robots for Older Adults and People with Autism: An Overview. *Electronics* **2020**, *9*, 367. [CrossRef]
141. ReMind AAL Project. Available online: https://www.aalremind.eu/ (accessed on 1 April 2020).
142. Pop, C.; Moldovan, D.; Antal, M.; Valea, D.; Cioara, T.; Anghel, I.; Salomie, I. M2O: A library for using ontologies in software engineering. In Proceedings of the 2015 IEEE International Conference on Intelligent Computer Communication and Processing (ICCP), Cluj-Napoca, Romania, 3–5 September 2015; pp. 69–75.
143. Keosity Platform. Available online: https://www.keosity.com/ (accessed on 1 April 2020).
144. Jena. Available online: https://jena.apache.org/documentation/ontology/ (accessed on 1 April 2020).
145. OWL API. Available online: http://owlcs.github.io/owlapi/ (accessed on 1 April 2020).
146. Pellet Reasoner. Available online: https://github.com/stardog-union/pellet (accessed on 1 April 2020).
147. D2RQ. Available online: http://d2rq.org/ (accessed on 1 April 2020).
148. Horrocks, I.; Patel-Schneider, P.F.; Boley, H.; Tabet, S.; Grosof, B.; Dean, M. SWRL: A Semantic Web Rule Language Combing OWL and RuleML. World Wide Web. 2004. Available online: http://www.w3.org/Submission/SWRL/ (accessed on 19 October 2012).
149. SQWRL: A Query Language for OWL. Available online: https://github.com/protegeproject/swrlapi/wiki/SQWRL (accessed on 1 April 2020).
150. Zora Robot Interaction API. Available online: https://docs.zoracloud.com/mqtt-api/ (accessed on 1 April 2020).

International Journal of
Environmental Research and Public Health

MDPI

Article

Connecting at Local Level: Exploring Opportunities for Future Design of Technology to Support Social Connections in Age-Friendly Communities

Jennifer Liddle [1,2,*], Nicole Pitcher [3], Kyle Montague [2], Barbara Hanratty [1], Holly Standing [4] and Thomas Scharf [1]

1 Population Health Sciences Institute, Campus for Ageing and Vitality, Newcastle University, Newcastle upon Tyne NE4 5PL, UK; barbara.hanratty@newcastle.ac.uk (B.H.); thomas.scharf@newcastle.ac.uk (T.S.)

2 Open Lab, Newcastle Helix, Newcastle University, Newcastle upon Tyne NE4 5TG, UK; kyle.montague@newcastle.ac.uk

3 Assistance Publique – Hôpitaux de Paris, 75004 Paris, France; nicole.valtorta@gmail.com

4 Department of Nursing, Midwifery and Health, Coach Lane Campus East, Northumbria University, Newcastle upon Tyne NE7 7XA, UK; holly.standing@northumbria.ac.uk

* Correspondence: jennifer.liddle@newcastle.ac.uk

Received: 19 July 2020; Accepted: 28 July 2020; Published: 31 July 2020

check for updates

Abstract: Social connectedness in later life is an important dimension of an age-friendly community, with associated implications for individual health and wellbeing. In contrast with prior efforts focusing on connections at a distance or online communities where the digital technology is the interface, we explore the design opportunities and role of technology for connectedness within a geographically local community context. We present findings from interviews with 22 older adults and a linked ideation workshop. Our analysis identified shared concerns and negative perceptions around local relationships, connections and characteristics of the geographical area. However, local connectedness through technology was largely absent from day-to-day life and even perceived as contributing to disconnection. By uncovering how older adults use and perceive technology in their social lives and combining these findings with their ideas for improving local connections, we highlight the need for thoughtful consideration of the role of technology in optimising social connections within communities. Our research highlights a need for design work to understand the specifics of the local context and reduce emphasis on technology as the interface between people. We introduce an amended definition—'underpinned by a commitment to respect and social inclusion, an age-friendly community is engaged in a strategic and ongoing process to facilitate active ageing by optimising the community's physical, social and digital environments and its supporting infrastructure'—to conceptualise our approach. We conclude by suggesting areas for future work in developing digitally connected age-friendly communities.

Keywords: connectedness; social relationships; later life; ageing; older people; age-friendliness; community; digital technology; loneliness; isolation

1. Introduction

Social connectedness in later life is important for health and wellbeing. Consequently, making it easy for people to develop and maintain social relationships is a fundamental ambition of 'age-friendly' communities. This local, place-based, policy approach recognises that physical and social environments are key determinants of whether people remain independent, autonomous and healthy in later life.

Human–computer interaction (HCI) researchers are directing increasing attention towards the role of technology in shaping and supporting social relationships in later life. Much of this work focuses on online communities or connecting across geographical or generational distances, where digital technology is the interface or infrastructure for connection. In addition, approaches commonly place emphasis on addressing technological inexperience, or on physical or cognitive impairment and decline.

In this paper, we are interested in considering technology and connectedness in later life within a specific local context, and exploring how innovation in social connection can be age-friendly and embedded within such physical community settings. We consider older adults as a heterogeneous group, rather than a group marked by singular identities of health, cognitive status, or technological proficiency. Nevertheless, our place-based approach aims to identify common values and experiences shared by people living in the same geographical area. Life events such as retirement, along with experiences of building and maintaining social connections over the life course, will also have implications for how and why older adults wish to develop and sustain proximate relationships in particular ways.

We suggest that considering these topics enables a deeper understanding of how to design for a digitally connected age-friendly neighbourhood, where both the design process and its outputs are age-friendly. Our paper presents findings from a study comprising two phases: qualitative interviews with 22 older adults; and a linked workshop ideation process to engage interviewees in beginning to consider how connections within their local area might be enhanced over time. The contributions of our paper centre around a context-specific and bottom-up approach to designing for increased local connectedness in later life. The importance of this topic has since been emphasised by the COVID-19 pandemic, heightening awareness of the need to consider ways to maintain and create social connectedness, particularly at a local level.

Our aim is not to design a technological output. Instead, we see our approach as prioritising a crucial, and often neglected, stage in technology design, which provides important insights that would be required for any future stage of a design process that aimed to design or create an actual technology. Themes that emerged from our interviews suggest that participants viewed technology as acceptable when it filled a 'gap' and did not have too many negative impacts on everyday life. Our starting point for the linked workshop was to consider some of these 'gaps' in local connectedness that interview participants had described. The workshop activities were used to facilitate participants in thinking creatively about addressing specific local challenges, or 'gaps' in connectedness. In drawing together participants' ideas about spaces, processes and mechanisms that might address these local challenges, we conclude the paper with implications that offer scope for further exploration and consideration in terms of how technology might support the operationalisation of local people's ideas for improving face-to-face connections in age-friendly community settings.

Related Work

Growing interest in what makes places 'good' to grow old in has led to an increasing focus on the 'age-friendliness' of different types of environments [1]. Despite variation in emphasis between models of age-friendly environments, most approaches promote consideration of how policies, services and structures can integrate physical and social environments, supporting social engagement and connection [2]. Our work adopts the following conceptual definition, with its emphasis on age-friendliness as commitment to a process rather than a standard to be reached:

> *'Underpinned by a commitment to respect and social inclusion, an age-friendly community is engaged in a strategic and ongoing process to facilitate active ageing by optimising the community's physical and social environments and its supporting infrastructure'* [3].

The adopted definition of age-friendliness shapes our research design and methods, with its emphasis on community engagement and the participation of older people in processes to optimise the environment to support social connections. We also draw on concepts from environmental gerontology, such as 'ageing in place' to understand the importance of the local area in older people's lives. An overarching premise of an age-friendly community is that it is 'friendly for all ages and not just "elder-friendly"' [1]. Even so, the argument that older people are 'able to remain more independent by, and benefit from, ageing in environments to which they are accustomed' [4] makes it all the more important to consider how environments can support people 'ageing in place' to optimise their social connectedness within their local area. This has become even more apparent during the 2020 COVID-19 pandemic, which has exposed the need for digital connection as an alternative to face-to-face interactions. Similarly, finding new ways to connect, even with people in proximate locations, has become a greater priority.

There has also been a strong emphasis on tackling the counterparts of social connectedness—loneliness and isolation. Warnings of the 'loneliness epidemic' and its associated public health implications are prevalent in media discourse [5–7], and the UK government appointed the world's first minister for loneliness in 2018 [8]. Accordingly, responses to the drive for increased social connection have often focused on mitigating unpleasant experiences, risks and deficits at an individual level [9]. Efforts along these lines reflect and uphold persistent ageist stereotypes that fail to acknowledge the roles that older people (can) play in communities, or their potential to contribute innovative ideas or create a voice for themselves [10–12]. Indeed, technology is often presented as the ideal way of solving these 'problems' faced by older adults [13]. Ten Bruggencate et al. draw our attention to the predominant focus on loneliness and/or isolation in studies about social technology, ageing and relationships [14]. In contrast, a growing body of work on social connectedness in later life challenges the image of older people as lonely and isolated. Population ageing is leading to increasing numbers of older people, thereby increasing the number of older people in society who experience loneliness. However, loneliness affects only the minority of older people, including the oldest old [15–17]. The likelihood of reporting feeling lonely decreases with age, with younger adults (16–24 years) reporting loneliness more often than those in older age groups [18]. While older adults may have smaller social networks, they are often more involved in the community than younger adults—socialising with neighbours, participating in religious organisations and volunteering [19]. However, even if social reciprocity and meaningful interactions are desired and enacted by older people, infrastructural barriers can, and do, impede the quantity and quality of such connectedness [20].

Technology offers the potential for scalable and cost-effective interventions to address barriers to connectedness. The design, or adoption, of digital technology to support social relationships in later life often results in technology being the core interface for connection between people, rather than a route to facilitating face-to-face connections by overcoming barriers. For example, online communities are promoted as presenting opportunities for older people to meet and interact with peers [21–24]. In this interfacing role, technology is a bridge across distances. Lindley et al. comment that much HCI research related to relationships focuses on ways to maintain feelings of connectedness or express intimacy at a distance [25]. Distances being bridged may be geographical, for individuals living in remote areas or wanting to connect with people with whom they share interests, friendship or familial bonds. Distances may also be generational, where, despite intentions to the contrary, technology replicates asymmetrical family interactions [23,26,27].

Growing proportions of older people are now using digital technologies. In the UK, 83% of adults aged 65–74, and 47% of adults aged 75 and over use the internet [28]. Thus, the majority rather than a minority of older people are technologically connected, suggesting a need to understand more about how this diverse population uses, and feels about, technology for connecting with others. The few studies that have explored older people's attitudes towards, and perceptions about, communication and connection suggest that rich interactions are valued above lightweight connections offered by newer technologies [14,25,29]. Again, this work primarily considers the capacity of digital technology to bridge geographical or generational distances, where more traditional technologies such as telephone and email are often preferred. Thoughtful and meaningful interactions are the goal, and technology provides the interface. Research methods centre around questions about how older adults use, or would choose to use, technology in their social relationships. For instance, Sayago et al. report on research with 700 older people (across six studies) that examined situated technology use and the reasons why participants did, or did not, incorporate particular forms into their everyday lives [23]. In this way, technological interfaces are often in-built as fundamental foundations for designing for connection, diminishing considerations of technology in non-interfacing roles.

Research that has explored ways to improve geographically proximate connections has also tended to concentrate on a prominent role for technology, often studying online community networks. These include bespoke online communities for older adults, or those formed on more widely used social networking platforms. Righi et al. focussed on how older people's use of social networking sites could be used to promote their involvement in both online and offline local communities [30]. While participants used, for example, Facebook to find out information about the local area, most did not post or share information or send messages to others. Instead, these interactions took the form of face-to-face conversations. On this basis, the authors conclude that proximity and face-to-face contacts should be kept in mind when designing online community networks. We would extend this argument further, to suggest reversing the design process. Such a process would design for proximity and face-to-face contact in offline communities, with technology kept in mind in a background, less visible, role.

The research described above concentrates on technology as the interface for connection between people. While the potential of technology to foster involvement in local communities has been explored, less attention has been paid to understanding and drawing on context-specific factors to develop approaches to promote connection in local areas *with*, rather than *for*, older people. This would be a fundamental approach for any community engaged in the ongoing process becoming (more) age-friendly. An effective strategy in one community will not necessarily translate to a community with different geographical, social or structural features. Likewise, the attitudes of older people towards technology will vary individually and across communities and countries. In their 'manifesto for change' in age-friendly cities and communities, Buffel et al. emphasise the necessity of ensuring the empowerment and recognition of older residents in order to achieve age-friendliness [31]. For these reasons, we adopted a bottom-up, place-based approach that can be responsive to local needs, preferences and resources. We recognise community as an inclusive concept, with the participation and empowerment of members (particularly older people) being fundamental to its creation and functioning [3,32,33].

The following sections present the methods and findings of our study. Our research design (in-depth interviews followed by an ideation workshop) draws on key concepts, theories, gaps and definitions in the literature outlined above. It is a bottom-up place-based approach that focuses on local needs, preferences and resources. It prioritises the participation of older people in exploring context-specific routes to local connection that present opportunities for future design of technology. We see our participants as crucial to developing ideas to increase or improve connection. As residents within the local area, they have a wealth of knowledge and experience and are best placed to identify resources, ideas and options that can lead to context-specific routes to connection.

Our overall aim within this study is to begin exploring context-specific routes to local connection that do not start the design process with attempts to design technological interfaces. Discovering issues or opportunities for increased connection at a community level is the first step in this process. These opportunities and 'gaps' also need to be considered alongside insights into the current practices and perceptions of older people regarding technology in their social lives. Once opportunities for increasing connection have been identified, ways to address these can then be explored by older people with local expertise and knowledge. Therefore, in practice, the workshop methods were designed after analysis of our interview data so that we could draw on the interview findings as the starting point for workshop activities and discussions. However, for structural clarity, the methods for both the interviews and workshop are presented first in this paper, followed by the findings from our analyses.

2. Materials and Methods: Phase One Interviews

The first phase of our study aimed to explore opportunities for designing to improve proximate social connections for older people living within a geographically identified 'community'. We also wanted to know more about how and why research participants were using technology, or not, in their social lives. Qualitative interviews were an appropriate method for exploring these two topics, with their potential to elicit personal accounts that help people to 'make explicit things that have hitherto been implicit—to articulate their tacit perceptions, feelings and understandings' about their social lives and technology [34].

2.1. Participants and Context

The study setting was an electoral ward (district) within a city in the North of England, UK, chosen for its proximity to the research team's institutional location. Just over 10% of the around 13,600 people living in this geographical area are aged 60 or over (compared to 23% overall in England and Wales). It is also one of the most ethnically diverse and socially deprived wards in the region [35].

Following institutional ethical approval (Ref. 13284), we recruited 22 older adults (15 women, 7 men) to take part in audio-recorded interviews. Sixteen interviews were with individual participants and three interviews were with couples living in the same household who chose to be interviewed together. Our only inclusion criterion was that participants were aged 60 or over. However, we also sought to achieve a diverse sample in terms of age, gender, ethnicity, social connectedness and living arrangements. Table 1 summarises participant characteristics. Participants were aged between 60 and 84 and had been living in the area for between seven months and 84 years. One participant was Asian and the remaining 21 participants were White. Eight participants were living alone, and the others lived with at least one other person (a spouse/partner ± extended family). With the exception of one participant who was working part-time, all participants were retired. Recruitment was via face-to-face conversations at community events and locations (such as a weekly café held in a local church) and contact details shared by community groups and organisations based in the area. We made substantial efforts to achieve a sample with greater ethnic diversity, including seeking assistance from individuals running local organisations and groups for people from non-White backgrounds, and posters in local culturally diverse food and clothing shops. We also made provisions for language translation in interviews. However, in the time available, we were unable to identify additional people from different ethnic groups who were willing to take part in an interview. Longer-term development of relationships within the community would likely be needed to increase interest and trust, which was not possible in a study of this scale.

2.2. Procedure and Analysis

All potential participants were given an information sheet about the study and a copy of the consent form to read. Interviews were arranged at times to suit participants, and they were offered a choice of location. One participant chose to meet for their interview in a community building and all other interviews were conducted in people's own homes. After completing the consent form and giving an opportunity for the interviewee to ask any questions, we audio-recorded the interview with the participant's agreement. Interviews were conducted by JL, HS or NP. We initiated the interviews with a narrative approach, asking individuals to tell the story of their social lives since they had been living in the area. This facilitated the exploration of each individual's own concerns, meanings and priorities related to their social lives, rather than these being imposed by predetermined questions [36]. The same question was asked at the beginning of each interview: 'Can you please tell me the story of your social life while you've been living in [this area]; your relationships with family, friends, neighbours and other people?'. Participants were asked to talk about any events and experiences that were important for them, and invited to take as long as long as they needed to tell their story. This narrative section of the interview was followed by supplementary probing questions to explore areas of particular interest, including the role of technology in their social lives. These questions were not pre-defined in order that interviewers were free to explore anything that they felt was of interest and relevant to the overall aims of the study, maintaining a natural and spontaneous flow within the interview. Brief reflective field notes were made by interviewers after each interview.

Table 1. Sociodemographic characteristics of sample.

	Number of Participants $n = 22$
Age group (years)	
60–64	1
65–69	5
70–74	7
75–79	4
80–84	5
Sex	
Female	15
Male	7
Ethnicity/Nationality	
White British	21
Asian British	1
Living Arrangements	
Living alone	8
Living with one other person	13
Living with more than one other person	1
Marital Status	
Married/Long-term Partner	14
Single	2
Divorced/Separated	1
Widowed	5
Current Work Status	
Retired	21
Part-time Work	1
Recruitment Source	
Community café	14
Electoral ward annual public meeting	2
Local church	1
Local organisation run by, and for, older people	1
Local wellbeing charity	1
Sports club	1
Referred by another interviewee	1
Gardening association	1

Electronic data files were stored in password-protected folders in the University filestore. Interview recordings were transcribed and names were anonymised. We then completed initial inductive coding [37] of the data to explore (a) opportunities to improve connections at a local level, i.e., factors that had the potential to impact negatively on people's geographically proximate social relationships in terms of quality, quantity or satisfaction; and (b) participants' engagement with technology in relation to their social lives generally. Codes were organised under themes, following the process outlined by Braun and Clarke [37]. For example, codes such as 'places people used to socialise no longer exist', 'many buildings are not accessible', and 'there are few facilities' were grouped together under the theme 'few local places to socialise'. Coding and theme development were completed independently by two researchers (J.L., N.P.) and then discussed and refined with all members of the research team.

While all names used in this paper are pseudonyms, participants in photographs gave consent for their images to be included in research outputs.

3. Materials and Methods: Phase Two Ideation Workshop

The second phase of the study comprised an ideation workshop. We drew on the following conclusions from our interview analysis when designing the workshop:

- there were concerns and perceptions about local community connections and characteristics that offered opportunities for design;
- our participants predominantly used technology to connect with family, or friends at a distance; existing local technological connections in their social lives were less obvious;
- many participants were actively using a variety of technologies, but their willingness to do so depended on perceptions of unmet needs and balancing the negative aspects (additional work, potential contribution to face-to-face disconnection) in their everyday lives.

We designed the workshop to explore and generate ideas to improve and optimise social connections in the local area, focusing on four of the opportunities we identified in our interview analysis. Based on the in-depth understanding about participants' use and perceptions of technology that we gained from the interviews, we designed 'playful' workshop activities that deliberately did not ask participants explicitly to consider how technology could address issues in local social connections. Instead, we wanted to begin by eliciting participants' thoughts about the best ways to tackle these issues before considering any technological needs that arose from these suggestions. This approach avoids the tendency of previous research to foreground technology at the start of the design process. By deliberately *not* seeking to design a technology or technological interface in this study, we could instead reflect on the potential needs or roles for technology once we knew what type of interventions our participants had suggested. Our approach also fitted well with our desire to draw on participants' knowledge, experience and capacity for creative thinking, and was in keeping with our aim of developing approaches to promote connection with, not for, older people, prioritising their participation in a bottom-up design process.

3.1. Participants and Context

All interview participants were sent a postal invitation to the workshop. Eleven individuals initially confirmed their availability and nine attended on the day (6 women, 3 men). These individuals were aged between 68 and 84 and had been living in the area for between 30 and 69 years. The workshop was held in a church hall in the local area and refreshments were provided.

3.2. Procedure and Analysis

Participants were asked to read and complete the consent form on arrival. Consent to being photographed was optional.

The workshop was structured around four opportunities to improve local social connections that we identified as themes through our interview analysis. Each theme represented shared concerns and negative perceptions about local relationships, connections and characteristics of the area that participants had talked about. The four themes were 'few local places to socialise', 'not knowing neighbours well', 'absence of a shared community feeling', and 'activities on offer not always conducive to socialising or making new friends'. These themes were chosen to take forward in the workshop based on their content being both appealing and generic enough for all participants to engage with, regardless of their individual circumstances and experiences.

In line with age-friendly models, our aim was for a bottom-up approach in which workshop attendees' participation and contributions were fundamental to the resulting design ideas [38]. Confronting ageist stereotypes, we also wanted to capitalise on participants' creative abilities and ingenuity along with their knowledge and experience as residents within the local area. In line with these priorities and our aim to explore participants' thoughts about how to improve connections at a local level without a specific focus on technology, we designed a range of playful ideation (idea-generating) activities to scaffold workshop discussions. Choosing activities to maintain a 'playful mindset' was a central ambition in our design, as this has been identified as a key enabler when ideating [39].

Participants worked in small groups, with each group asked to choose one theme to focus on throughout the activities. We gave groups the option of completing one, some, or all of the activities, depending on which appealed to them and how much time they spent on each activity. All groups tried at least two of the three activities:

3.2.1. Reverse Brainstorming

Participants were asked to generate ideas about how to cause the issue/theme or how to make it worse. This generated a list of problems or criticisms that participants were then asked to reverse or convert into positive ideas or solutions (Figure 1). An example idea from participants was to remove the internet. They then converted this into an idea to provide free internet access alongside TV licences.

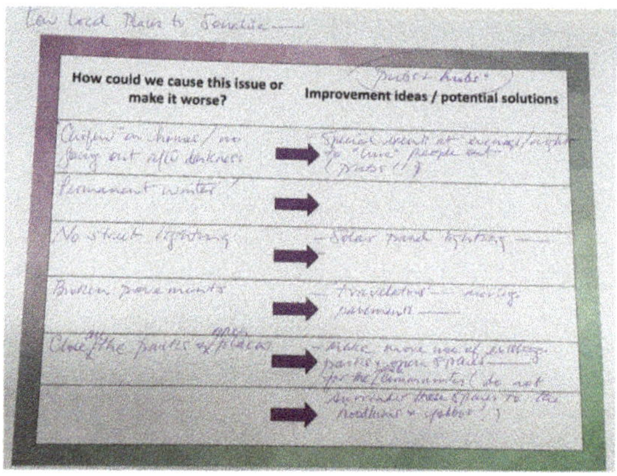

Figure 1. Example reverse brainstorming activity responses.

3.2.2. Character Activity

This activity involved imagining how a famous person or character (fictional or real) with a wealth of skills, resources or power might respond to the issue. One group chose Vladimir Putin, President of Russia, as their inspiration, with ideas that reflected their views on his leadership style, including mandatory socialising (e.g., meeting for a chat over a cup of tea or coffee) at particular times of day with street marshals to monitor and guarantee people's involvement.

3.2.3. Group Passing

The third activity began with each group member writing an initial idea on a piece of paper which was then passed around the group for others to contribute to, comment on, or develop the initial idea (Figure 2). An example of this process was an initial idea to have more benches and ice cream vans driving round parks to encourage families with children to stay and chat. This resulted in the suggestion that the vans could double-up to provide other services like newspapers or bread, which might attract a wider range of people.

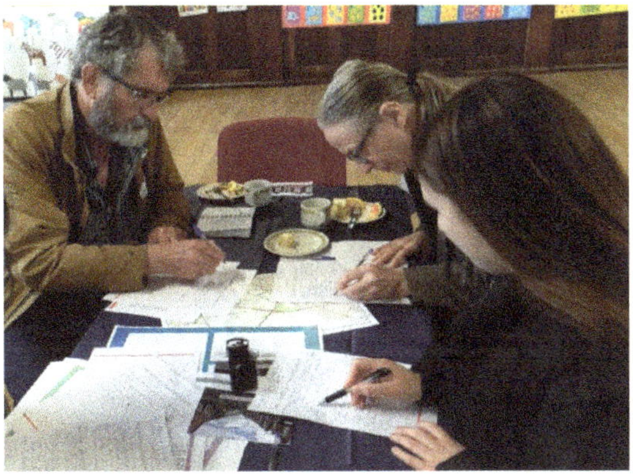

Figure 2. Participants developing ideas in the 'group passing' activity.

Data collection in the workshop comprised ideas written by participants on the templates provided (see Figure 1 for example data). All data were stored in a locked filing cabinet within an access controlled workspace. The workshop activities generated an extensive list of ideas and suggestions for facilitating social interaction within the immediate local area. Each group wrote down every idea that resulted from the activities they completed. After the workshop, we combined these ideas into one longer list and grouped and organised them under three overarching themes and 12 sub-themes that captured the overall range, content and types of ideas [37]. Themes and sub-themes were developed by two researchers (JL, TS) and then discussed with all members of the research team.

4. Findings: Phase One Interviews

As described earlier, the interview data were coded to explore (a) opportunities to improve connections at a local level, i.e., factors that had the potential to impact negatively on people's geographically proximate social relationships in terms of quality, quantity or satisfaction; and (b) participants' engagement with technology in relation to their social lives generally. The following sections outline the main findings in relation to each of these topics.

4.1. Opportunities to Improve Connections at a Local Level

In our interviews with participants, we adopted a place-based approach to focus in on social lives at a geographically local level. It soon became apparent that there were many aspects of the locality that participants were content with, or did not wish to change. For example, some described strong friendships and connections with local friends and neighbours that had endured over time. Others were actively involved in attending and/or organising local social events.

However, there were shared concerns and negative perceptions around local relationships, connections and characteristics of the area that offered opportunities for further exploration as topics to design around. Our analysis of the interview data specifically aimed to identify these opportunities to improve connections at a local level, by pinpointing factors that had the potential to impact negatively on people's geographically proximate social relationships in terms of quality, quantity or satisfaction.

We report here on the four of these themes that were taken forward to the ideation workshop. These were chosen from a larger number identified, based on the criteria that they would be both appealing and generic enough for all participants to engage with, whatever their individual circumstances and experiences. Table 2 outlines the four themes, along with linked examples from the interview data.

Table 2. Themes relating to concerns and negative perceptions about local relationships, connections and characteristics of the area.

Theme	Example Data
Few Local Places to Socialise	*"One of the things that's wrong with [this area], I would say, is that there aren't many 'getting out of your house and meeting people' places about."* (Claire) *"I think it's a shame that there isn't a hub, a community hub type thing, because I witness what seems to be the backend of beyond [. . .], where they have very, very active women's institutes and community centres. [Here, there's] a very small parade of shops and there's not the communal coffee shop type place like there is in [another local electoral ward in the city]."* (Liz) *"I often think it would be quite nice to live somewhere where if you wanted to in an evening, [. . .] just once a week, just a local pub you could pop into and meet people but of course that goes back to the covenant [. . .] that there can't be any public houses within a certain radius."* (Catherine) *"There are not an awful lot of facilities here. If we were religious, then yes, there are churches here, but we're not, either of us. [. . .] I wouldn't be interested if it was a church thing, no, no."* (Alan)
Not Knowing Neighbours Well	*"I've lived in this street for 48 years. So it's a street where there is a lot of movement. A lot of young couples come, they're working couples, with no family and they'll come for a couple of years. Then, there will be a baby come along and then they want a house with a garden. So they're always on the move."* (Sheila) *"I used to know people who lived in the next to end house. And I know the woman opposite, but I'm not particularly friendly with her. The busyness of the road doesn't make it that conducive to. . . You know like you can't really have a street party on this street. So I wouldn't say I know a lot of people well around here."* (Deborah)
Absence of a Shared Community Feeling	*"You can't talk about the [local area] community, you just can't, there isn't one. There are people living in [the local area]."* (Alan) *"I think in some ways this [area] between the east central motorway and even going up towards [one of the main roads], it kind of hasn't got a soul to it, it doesn't have a kind of focal point, so it's a bit of an amorphous area. I think an area that has a strong focal point seems to do better."* (Paul) *"The degree of integration is not great. [. . .] It is a source of concern that there is so little contact between the immigrant population and other folk."* (Christopher)
Activities on Offer not always Conducive to Socialising or Making New Friends	*"There's no friends, just had one lady who teaches me [. . .] I forget her name. (Laughter) I've never contacted anybody from my class."* (Rizwana) *"I've been attending a yoga class [. . .] for years and years and years. [. . .] But there is never an opportunity to have a chat to people. You might just be able to say, 'Are you alright?' as we're packing up, you know, 'I haven't seen you for ages', but there's not an opportunity to chat with people."* (Sally)

Beginning with the first of the four themes, most participants reported that there were few places in the immediate local area that they could use for socialising beyond their own homes. They described how there was no central community centre in the area, and no clearly distinguishable main high street. Perceptions about the lack of local options contrasted with participants' opinions about the venues, centres and cafés available in other areas where they felt that community spaces and cafés were prominent and actively used and adopted by people living there. Some participants were happy to socialise at home, but others saw this as too much of a burden or did not feel comfortable inviting people into their home. A noteworthy and unique characteristic of the local area highlighted by participants was the historic covenant on the land in the vicinity, preventing any licensed premises or pubs from operating. In the face of limited options in terms of usable spaces, local churches often hosted (or were booked to host) activities and events. However, this itself was a deterrent to some participants who felt uncomfortable attending events that had a religious connection—even if religion was not intended to be part of the event, such as a community café. Overall, the perspective was that the community's physical features and built environment did not facilitate face-to-face social activities and interactions.

The second theme (not knowing neighbours well) did not apply to all interview participants. In fact, some participants described their neighbours as good friends. These interviewees lived in quieter, more spacious streets, accommodating larger houses with gardens. Other interview participants felt very disconnected from their neighbours. Those living in particularly 'neighbourly' streets were aware that their situations were unusual in the wider local area where different road and housing types and tenures were more dominant, and fewer longstanding residents were living alongside the same neighbours for extended time periods. Population churn, the movement of people in and out of streets, was perceived as a factor influencing the extent to which participants knew their neighbours. Growing families and the number of properties available to rent in the area were cited as reasons behind this movement. Streets were often busy with traffic—a factor that participants identified as not being conducive to unplanned meetings or chats with neighbours. While the physical proximity of neighbours potentially offered the most geographically close opportunities for social interaction, this had not translated into actual interactions for many participants. In particular, participants indicated that local issues of population mobility and transport routes contributed to the under-development of these relationships.

The essence of the third theme (a lack of shared community feeling) was expressed by many participants. Some attributed the absence of community to the area's geographical characteristics and location within the wider city, including the proximity of a motorway and the absence of a central focal point, or main high street, in the area. Interview participants also commented on the lack of interaction between people of different ethnic and cultural backgrounds, despite the fact that the area was home to a diverse population. Some talked about how this had been a longstanding issue, first noticed when their children were at school. Together, both the physical environment and the population makeup of the area appeared to contribute to participants feeling that there were physical and cultural divisions within the geographical community.

The fourth theme illustrates the complexity of developing new connections and relationships that extend beyond acquaintanceship: activities on offer are not always conducive to socialising or making new friends. Even when participants were meeting people and seeking new friendships, these interactions did not often translate into deeper relationships. Some participants described attending regular or one-off activities where they felt that the type and format of sessions were not helpful for getting to know people. For example, the focus was on a particular activity so chatting was only possible during brief time periods while setting up or packing away. Another barrier was that some participants were more passive than others, and did not initiate conversations or connections themselves. In addition, participants mentioned that the same volunteers or people were often involved in several different groups and activities, resulting in a smaller pool of people to form friendships with. In other instances, it was simply that occasional casual conversations participants had with others did not result in deeper friendships or relationships that were sustained or developed beyond interactions at the events themselves, and individuals, therefore, remained acquaintances.

Taken together, these themes demonstrate clear barriers in, and characteristics of, local community connections. The themes capture issues that were impacting on the quality and quantity of participants' relationships in the local area, offering opportunities for participatory design processes to address these.

4.2. Technology and Social Lives

Alongside identifying opportunities to improve connections at a local level, the other focus of our analysis of the interview data was on understanding more about participants' existing engagements with technology in relation to their social lives. This engagement ranged from minimal (i.e., landline telephone only) to extensive (including social media, real-time audio/video interactions and applications).

We use eight central themes to capture participants' accounts of the existing roles that technology played, or did not, play in their social lives. These themes, and examples of the data that support them, are outlined in Table 3.

Table 3. Themes relating to the current roles of technology in participants' social lives.

Theme	Example Data
Connecting across Geographically Distant Locations	*"We do FaceTime our son a lot. And actually, a friend in Japan and these friends in Portugal. It's the easiest way. [. . .] Well, it is nice to see people. [. . .] Then we can show them that we've got the snow or whatever. I think it gives you more than talking on the phone, for sure. Yes. Especially looking at grandchildren and they [waving gesture], 'Hello, Nana'."* (Liz) *"But FaceTime, I love it. I really love that, because [Son] is in the States. And we must speak to him about four times a week actually. [. . .] I love the fact that you can see him. You really feel that the person is there. I think, basically, I'd would be kind of heart broken, because he's there, if it wasn't for that. I find that hugely, very enjoyable and very good. When we go to see him, I kind of feel – while it's lovely to see him in person – 'It's not been that long really' because of. . . "* (Claire) *"I heard about Airbnb and thought, 'I'll try that and, you know, I could use it as a stop gap until I find somebody suitable to live here.' Then I just liked it, [. . .] it's enjoyable, mainly nice people. I've made some friends. I've got invites to go. . . [. . .] people who came as Airbnb guests and who have invited me to go and stay with them."* (Deborah)
Connecting Family Members and Groups	*"Oh, WhatsApp all the time, with the family. We've got a family group. [. . .] It would be a strange day when I didn't get several WhatsApp messages from other members of the family, even if it's only pictures of what they're doing. 'Here's my dinner.' [. . .] I mean, I WhatsApp-ed them all last night when I'd been to the cinema, telling them what I'd seen and telling them to go and see it."* (Christopher) *"I know at Christmas time myself and [son 1] and [daughter] had a group to discuss what we were going to do about [son 2]'s Christmas present. My eldest son has got a little girl, 18 months old, and when she was coming up to a year he had a family group to discuss her birthday party. [. . .] So just anything where you want a group of you it's just handy."* (Catherine) *"We WhatsApp people all the time, we're on a WhatsApp group as a family, we've got two, one for just my wife and I and the kids, and one for the wife and I, the kids and my sister. I think that's great, because my sister's becoming more isolated, she's 82 with health problems, so she knows what's going on, because she gets the WhatsApps, she gets the pictures. She always thought she was being left out until that, and instead of having to ring people round asking what's happening or tell them about something, you just WhatsApp it."* (John) *"They basically log your life and your habits [. . .] for targeted advertising for people. [. . .] So it can be quite invasive [. . .] I reluctantly loaded the WhatsApp thing into my phone because of [son's name] going to Singapore, it was handy when he was wanting to check up on one or two things back and forth. [. . .] As soon as I downloaded it, it read all my contact list. [. . .] So when I opened up the WhatsApp app I see all my contacts so it was a bit scary."* (Paul) *"My sister, I talk to her, she lives down in the Midlands. I talk to her every now and then, every couple of weeks or so. Either she rings me, or I ring her."* (Martin)
Capturing and Sharing Images	Marie: *"It's got an excellent camera. I use it as a camera because I'm useless at taking photographs otherwise."* Simon: *"See, if Marie uses a camera to take somebody's photograph, and eventually either cuts them in half or chops their head off, you know, which is-But, with this phone, it's absolutely brilliant."* Marie: *"Yes, yes."* Simon: *"The pictures that she's taken when she's been on holiday and things, absolutely superb."*
	"I get loads of photographs of the children when they're opening birthday presents. Their mother takes a photograph and sends it with a comment on what they said when they were trying on things." (Lynne)
Sharing Information and Making Arrangements	*"Actually, it is more important than I'm making out because we're always making arrangements. [. . .] You have no idea how difficult it is making a weekend arrangement with people who are constantly out of the country. [. . .] That's another thing that's important, I don't know why I'm even saying it's not important. We do go away quite often, so I do use technology to organise where I'm going and what we're doing and what you can do while you're there, basically. So yes, I do use technology quite a lot at that. It's probably very important."* (Claire) *"Because, I'm not very good. If I have to make a phone call to somebody, I'm terrible. If I've got to make, like, a cold call to somebody, 'Can you phone so and so to ask them to do this?' I'm going, 'Do I have to? Do I have to?' [. . .] and I hate it. I've always hated the telephone for making phone calls out. Texting is a lifesaver. You can text whenever you want, when you feel like it, and you're not having to speak to somebody and say the wrong thing. So, that's what I like about that technology."* (Marie)

Table 3. *Cont.*

Offering an Alternative to Interactions with People	*"television is something [...] that is more personal than other electronic things."* (Jane) *"Well, probably a Sunday, unless on the odd occasion [son] is here, because there aren't any social things going on and most of the people here [in this housing development] probably have their children around them or their grandchildren, which I haven't got, plus the fact that sometimes just your general health, if you just feel down generally, that makes you feel lonely as well. [...] I put on music sometimes because I find it uplifting [...] or a Pam Ayres DVD, which is funny, something that just makes you laugh or the music uplifts you."* (Brenda)
Contributing to Disconnection	*"My friend had been [to a local activist/campaigning event] on the Friday, and because I don't use social media I just hadn't heard [...] It did make me think, 'What would I have to do not to miss the way information about things like that is circulated?' [...] To find out information about what's on, you can't really even Google, because if it's on social media it doesn't come up as a website. [...] So there is the issue of becoming more isolated because the information sharing is happening in a way that I'm not part of."* (Sally) *"[Our friend] has two phones and she's always on them. I find that quite difficult. When she's eating here, she's not allowed phones at the table. She obviously finds that really difficult because she lives her life on Twitter or whatever. And I just, I'm not criticising her. I just recognise it's a different way to be. But when I've read recently about if you've got a phone near you, you behave differently from if you hadn't. Even if it's not ringing. [...] If you carry it everywhere with you, you do actually behave differently. Your subconscious is aware that you might be interrupted. I can really recognise that, so it's very interesting."* (Liz)
Creating another 'Chore'	*"I'm not that keen on technology. [...] Whereas I've used it in the past for emailing friends, as a way of keeping in touch, I hardly have time... no that's not... [...] there are so many things that need attending to. You are just bombarded by people [...] and you've got to read it, or respond to it, or whatever. And [...] I don't have that long. I've got my tea cooking or I'm just doing a quick check. I am not sitting down to be chained to a desk for the next five hours [...] It does feel like a chore."* (Sally) *"In my social life? I suppose emails, texting... I'm going to be really honest with you. I find getting involved... These friends [...] they're on WhatsApp and constantly... I made a conscious decision, "I'm not joining it." I just can't be doing with constantly... [...] So yes, emails and texts, yes, heavily into despite myself because it seriously takes too much time. [...] It's the interactive ones that are... You just think, 'People text you for nothing, don't they?' You think, 'mmm...' So, yes I use it, but sometimes unwillingly."* (Claire) *"I keep saying to [husband], 'Emails are really like your post,' you don't get so many letters through the post now, they come* via *email, so you do have to look at them."* (Catherine)
Not Filling a 'Gap'	*"We have no need to use them. Interesting, locally, take, for example, the concerts arranged now by the church. [...] The church warden puts up a big poster on the railings, 'concert this week' [...] They have noticeboards, and she puts stuff up there, we put up notices inside the church when the café is on, on a Thursday [...] and we put flyers through each other's doors. Organising local things here is by word-of-mouth and that, sort of, contact."* (Christopher) *"I do not have a computer. I do not have a laptop. The family have always said, 'You should get one.' I said, 'No. If I need anything...' [...] When I need something, I get it from my son [...] and his wife, and my daughter and the grandchildren, you know, and they can all do it. So I said, 'What is the point of me having one?' [...] So, no, I have no regrets at not doing it."* (Judith)

The first theme about the role of technology in interviewees' social lives focuses on its use to connect participants with people in geographically distant locations. In fact, many of the digitally mediated interactions described by participants bridged geographical distances. Applications and platforms such as FaceTime, Facebook and WhatsApp (along with traditional landline phone calls) were commonly used to keep in touch with friends and family located in geographically separate locations. Grandchildren were frequently mentioned as being a priority in seeking to connect face-to-face at a distance. While the financial savings of free long-distance technological connection were noted and appreciated by some, interviewees also reflected on the emotional value of being able to stay visually connected with loved ones. For Claire, this connection even changed her perception of the duration of time passing between in-person interactions, making it feel like she had seen her son in person more recently than was the case in reality. In contrast to those using technology to bridge distances in order to maintain existing relationships, Deborah was unusual among interviewees in that she had formed long-lasting friendships with people she met initially through the use of an online marketplace. As someone living alone in later life, she was using technology designed for one purpose (financial/accommodation transactions) to initiate and facilitate face-to-face interactions with strangers from geographically distant locations, offering the potential for developing new social relationships.

Our next theme encapsulates the role of technology in connecting family members and groups. Family relationships were frequently discussed as examples of connections that were supported by technology, through informal chatting, sharing photographs or stories and news about day-to-day life events. Family connections using technology ranged from group chats to individual messages, and instant short communications as well as ongoing asynchronous conversations. WhatsApp was often highlighted in this context, particularly for its usefulness in communicating with a group, and across generations. Examples included WhatsApp groups with interviewees, their children and partners, and grandchildren. These were sometimes longstanding groups for general communication, but at other times were set-up for a specific purpose, such as organising a birthday party. Cross-generational interactions were also perceived as improving the connectedness of family members who had previously felt 'left out' of family communications. John described the example of his sister, who was previously less connected with other members of the family but could now see photographs and hear about what other members of the family were doing, without them needing to make a special effort to include her. Technology was seen, in cases like this, as a solution to the barriers to instantaneous communication with family members with diverse and busy lives and routines. However, telephone calls were also important to participants as a way of keeping in touch, particularly with others who were nearer in age such as siblings or friends. In addition, Paul expressed his unease at the invasive nature of commonly used apps and platforms which, for example, access lists of contacts from the device they are using or collect data to support targeted advertising. His use of WhatsApp was 'reluctant' on this basis, but he acknowledged its usefulness in keeping in touch when his son was abroad, highlighting the trade-off he had to negotiate between privacy and connection.

We did not ask participants explicitly about the ways in which they chose to record social interactions or events, but the use of in-built cameras in mobile phones featured in participants' accounts of the role of technology in their social lives. We have described this theme as 'capturing and sharing images'. The ease of taking photographs with a smartphone in comparison to using a camera was noted by some participants, facilitating them in documenting social occasions. Moreover, despite his privacy concerns about the invasiveness of technology more generally, Paul valued the fact that he was able to recover digital images from an automatic cloud backup after he accidentally deleted photos (documenting an international trip) from his mobile phone. Photographs as mementos of experiences in participants' social lives, like Paul's trip, were treasured. Additionally, the act of sharing and receiving images was a central feature of participants' digital interactions, connecting participants with events and experiences when they were not physically present.

After initially dismissing much technology (apart from FaceTime) as insignificant in her social life, Claire later reflected that it did play a large role in how she organised and arranged social events and interactions. The theme of 'sharing information and making arrangements' draws on these organisational uses of technology described by interviewees. Information was generally not necessarily shared on social networking sites or more visible platforms, but interactions commonly took place through instant messaging and other technological channels rather than solely in person. In fact, for Marie, there were additional benefits to using technology as a tool for organising or making arrangements with people. She preferred the control that it gave her in contrast with the unpredictability and social awkwardness she experienced when talking on the phone.

Technology was mainly described by interviewees in terms of its role as a tool for connecting, or supporting connections between, people. Conversely, several participants noted the ways in which technology itself was a dimension of their social life, offering an alternative to interactions with people. Perhaps because of its dominant focus on portraying human lives and activities, Jane felt that television was a more 'personal' type of technology. Patricia and Brenda watched television at times when other company or interaction was inaccessible. For Patricia, this was at 'silly hours' of the day or night, whereas Brenda described how she might watch television, DVDs or listen to CDs when she found herself alone or 'down'. There were particular times when others living in her housing development were more likely to be spending time with family, such as weekends, where she used music or television as a strategy to deal with loneliness. At the other end of the spectrum, Simon tended to avoid face-to-face social activities and events with other people, preferring to spend time playing games or reading on his computer.

There were two main ways that participants described technology as contributing to disconnection in terms of social interactions and events: its prevalence as a platform for information about events; and its disruptive potential during face-to-face interactions. Sally used the internet but chose not to engage with social media for privacy and security reasons, but felt that this was increasingly disadvantaging her when it came to finding out about local events. She reflected on her reliance on other people to keep her informed, and the difficulties of being separate from the dominant route of information sharing via social media. For Sally, information sharing was happening in a way that excluded her, meaning that she missed out on attending social activities and events that she would have chosen to go to otherwise. In contrast, Liz highlighted the capacity of technology to disrupt social interactions themselves. She described both a friend's extensive use of a smartphone, and purely the presence of a phone (in use or not), as disrupting face-to-face interactions and impacting on their quality. Sally's and Liz's accounts indicated a reluctance to allow technology to become pervasive in everyday life, balanced against a recognition that there were places and circumstances where it could be beneficial.

Along with concerns about the potential for technology to disrupt relationships, the positive impacts of technology in participants' social lives were also, in some cases, accompanied by additional unwanted work. Our penultimate theme, therefore, centres around experiences of technological interaction as an additional 'chore'. Sally described being 'bombarded' by messages, and she and others found their perceived continual need to respond and interact electronically to be a burden. The perpetual nature of communicating using interactive technologies such as email, texts and instant messages was also unpopular with some interviewees because of the amount of time it consumed. Responding was not perceived as an optional activity. Even if emails contained welcome content, the task of checking, opening and reading them was viewed as a compulsory individual task and responsibility. Catherine likened this to the responsibility to open letters that came through the post, rather than a choice or pleasurable activity.

Our final theme sums up participants' thoughts about not needing digital technologies. More traditional technologies such as the telephone or television were commonly accepted as integral to daily life. In fact, their deep-seated role in participants' social lives meant that they were often no longer considered or mentioned (by participants) when talking about technology. Instead, participants tended to focus on newer digital technologies such as social media, applications and email. Regarding these more modern technologies, there was a sense for some participants that they were unnecessary. For example, when talking about social media, Liz explained that she did not 'think there's a gap that I need them.' Christopher used the internet and email but did not consider it necessary to go online to find out about local social events as he was exposed to paper-based publicity, such as posters and flyers, as well as information via word-of-mouth. For Judith, the whole idea of using a computer or the internet was superfluous when she could instead rely on her family for support, asking them for anything she needed.

Overall, technological connections were predominantly bridging distances, with existing local technological connections less obvious. Technology was mainly seen as a tool to be used to make connecting easier where there were needs, barriers or 'gaps' (geographical or generational distances, difficulties sharing information, capturing images, avoiding uncomfortable face-to-face interactions), but not at the expense of disrupting desired face-to-face interactions or in situations where technology was seen as unnecessary (other strategies would suffice). In addition, the additional work required to use technology as an aid to connection was an unwanted consequence. Willingness to use technology depended on balancing the positive and negative aspects.

5. Findings: Phase Two Workshop

Exploring Ideas to Increase Opportunities for Local Social Interactions

As described earlier, the workshop was designed to build on the findings from our interviews. An extensive list of ideas was generated through our ideation activities, which we combined and organised under themes and sub-themes. Table 4 summarises the themes and sub-themes identified in our analysis of the written workshop data. Participants commented that the workshop had been enjoyable and thought-provoking—an outcome that supports us in challenging ageist stereotypes of older people as unable or unwilling to engage in creative, disruptive or wild thinking.

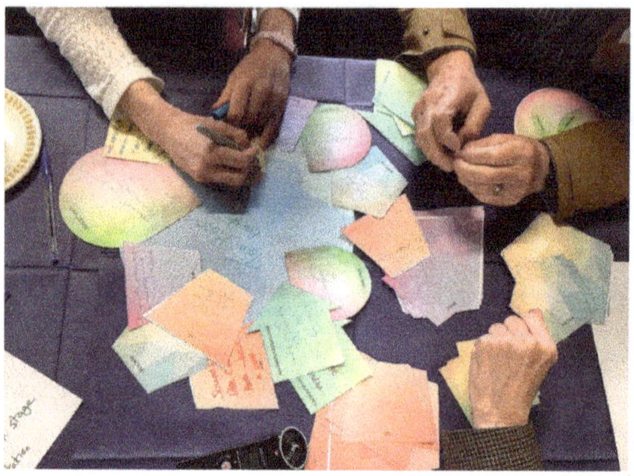

Figure 3. Participants generating an idea to develop a beach and water feature on an existing outdoor area of green space.

The three main themes we use to understand the workshop data are: social spaces and places; processes to promote social interactions; mechanisms to drive change. These themes capture different dimensions of participants' ideas for facilitating social interactions in the local area. Ideas varied in both scale and scope (see Table 4 for examples).

The first theme describes ideas that related to the physical environment and developing spaces and places to promote interactions. The proposed changes were either to directly provide locations for organised or informal activities to take place, or to change environmental factors to increase the likelihood of people meeting and connecting in their everyday lives. Ideas for developing locations for activities included making better use of existing spaces as well as creating new spaces or places. Residents suggested taking advantage of the large areas of green space that were nearby and using them in new ways. They also thought that new community premises, such as a community centre, would be helpful. Ideas to change other environmental factors included improving the environment for pedestrians and improving security of tenure to increase the length of time that people are resident in the same location before moving home. While some ideas residents suggested were more generic, others were particularly context-specific. Participants drew on their local knowledge to consider what resources in the local area could be used, and identified other resources that were lacking.

Table 4. Themes from workshop data analysis.

Theme	Sub-Themes	Example Data
Social Spaces and Places	*Making better use of existing geographical features and spaces* for social purposes, such as large areas of green space (e.g., Figure 3)	Longer opening hours e.g., library Marquees/undercover spaces in parks etc., for rainy days Make better use of open/green spaces for community activities e.g., exercise equipment, open a beach, more benches, ice cream vans to encourage use of parks
	Creating new spaces and places for social activities and events—organised and informal	New premises—big sports hall, comprehensive village/community centre
	Adapting the built environment to support pedestrians and encourage other non-car travel	Pedestrianise more areas/reduce speed limits to 20 mph, improve pavements, introduce more crossings and travellators/moving pavements
	Considering housing issues from a social and community perspective, including security of tenure and student accommodation	Social/community-focused strategy for housing e.g., reduce proportion of properties not for permanent residence, improve security of tenure/rent control, expand student halls of residence into area
Processes to Promote Social Interactions	*Improving communication strategies and publicity* within the local area	Improving communication strategy/publicity e.g., television appearances, community newspaper/flyers (with rotas for delivery), local council to focus on one ward in turn in Council magazine
	Making links across ethnic social groups	Link between ethnic groups to reduce divides along religious/ethnic lines in community
	Engaging with the wider community to share ideas and seek feedback	Wider community preference-seeking around how to solve issue of few places to socialise e.g., questionnaire and workshops Maximise work of existing social groups Monthly meetings for volunteers to pool ideas
	New transport options to support travel in the immediate local area and into the city centre	Frequent, small scale local transport e.g., minibus every 10 min Extend the metro into the area to improve access to city
	Focusing on proximate relationships i.e., at a street level or between those volunteering at the same events, as well as at the community level	Encourage greater walking in area e.g., parents taking children to school Encourage volunteers to build friendships/relationships outside volunteering activities/context Street level interventions e.g., street meetings/cups of tea, annual events
Mechanisms to Drive Change	*Community-driven/commissioned or cooperative initiatives* around social spaces, information provision, transport and learning/training	Community/cooperative/volunteer-run hospitality venues Buy a property on a co-operative basis and use as community resource/café/party venue Community uber-style, tandems/sidecars or other forms of 'fun' transport, bike sharing, motorcycle lessons—teaching/learning/using transport Cafes that also operate as training kitchen for cooking healthily, training in basic work skills by involvement in running community hub
	Incentives to: sustain and attract small catering and hospitality businesses to the local area; encourage local people to participate in social activities	Increase incentives for small catering/hospitality businesses e.g., no rates/taxes for first years after opening Happy hours in cafes etc., with free tea/coffee/cake, sponsored by local businesses Credits for free attendance at social activities for residents e.g., swimming pool on particular days/times/a month, extra credits could be earned through volunteering Dedicated time slots for social and/or physical activity/exercise time
	Finding ways of improving the commitment and contributions of individuals to the local area to create and sustain a sense of community	Commitment of individuals to community e.g., minimum number of community work hours/community service and strategy to deal with those who do not contribute, volunteers to supervise weekend sporting activities for children, create sense of community between residents/students

The second theme brings together ideas that participants had for processes and actions that could play a part in promoting social interactions. These included: prioritising engagement within the wider community to develop ideas; connecting different groups with each other; improving provision of information about events and activities in the local area; connecting people with locations and activities in the city centre; and focusing particularly on making use of proximity as a tool in the process of connection. Encouraging people to walk in the local area more often, and setting up hyper-local events such as street meetings, were examples of ideas to facilitate people in connecting with others living in close proximity. Participants' ideas emphasise the importance and desire for strong relationships at a local level, particularly building on the existing work and connections of volunteers and groups that they were aware of.

The third theme considers what types of mechanism could be used to drive change and engagement by local people, in order that involvement in supporting social connections is seen as an attractive opportunity. Participants' ideas included the use of cooperative initiatives to develop or run transport services or community spaces, and incentives for small businesses to make the local area an attractive place to set up or move to. They also suggested that incentive schemes for local residents (such as loyalty cards or credits) to participate in local activities would encourage people to maintain involvement. Participants proposed that making a public commitment to community work could not only increase the contributions made by individuals within the local area, but also contribute to an increased sense of community. Taken together, these ideas portray a community with actively engaged members working to make positive changes, that directly and indirectly lead to individual connections being strengthened.

We take forward one example sub-theme from each of these three main themes for further consideration in the second half of the discussion section of this paper, in order to begin thinking about how technology might contribute to supporting these types of initiative, as well as noting some of the challenges that would need to be addressed in designing such technologies.

6. Discussion

This paper makes a case for adjusting the design process to accommodate a bottom-up component that precedes design of technological outputs. We begin our discussion of the findings from this study by considering the interview data, and their position in relation to wider debates and literature around technology and social interaction in later life. We then move on to discuss what the ideas generated by workshop participants offer in terms of implications, scope and challenges for future technology design around social connectedness, particularly when considered in the context of the interview findings. We use three sub-themes from the workshop (making better use of existing geographical places and spaces; focusing on proximate relationships; community driven/commissioned or cooperative initiatives) as examples to avoid our discussion of implications and challenges for future technology design being too generic, and to ensure that our focus remains on designing in the particular context of our research community and participants.

Within an age-friendly context, our analysis of interview data identifies a number of opportunities to design for increased social connectedness within local communities. Participants felt that: there were few local places to socialise; they often did not know their neighbours well; there was an absence of shared community feeling; social activities on offer did not always lead to socialising or making new friends. In a policy and practice environment where technology-based initiatives are increasingly perceived as offering huge potential, our findings highlight the importance of age-friendly approaches that are grounded in the local context [1,2]. This has become even more apparent during the COVID-19 pandemic, which has exposed the need for digital connection as an alternative to face-to-face interactions. Similarly, finding new ways to connect, including with people in proximate locations, has become even more important in ways we did not anticipate when conducting this study. Every community is unique, so designing to optimise social connectedness at a local level requires understanding and recognition of context-specific characteristics. In addition, taking account of the social and structural particularities of places gives insight into meanings and functions that are the result of cumulative experiences over time [40]. In our study, the geographical layout of the community, restrictions on licensed premises and population churn were all factors that participants highlighted as playing a role in disconnection. However, these issues can also be seen as 'leverage points' where interventions could afford the greatest benefits within a specific local context [40].

Our interview data also contribute to understanding more about how older people use and perceive technology in their social lives. Unlike Dickinson and Hill's findings in 2009 that older people did not engage with instant messaging or other forms of computer technology aside from email [29], participants connected using a range of methods and formations of communication. Family connections using technology ranged from group chats to individual messages, and instant short communications as well as ongoing asynchronous conversations. Participants were not necessarily using social networking sites to share information, as Righi et al. [30] also found, but in our study these information-sharing interactions were commonly taking place through instant messaging and other technological channels rather than solely in person. These findings reflect changing levels of digital connection for older people in the UK [28] and emphasise the need for HCI to reconsider longstanding stereotypes of older people as digitally inexperienced or uninterested [13]. The COVID-19 pandemic has provided further evidence to counter these outdated stereotypes, with many older people embracing technology to facilitate connections with friends and family at a time when face-to-face meetings have been restricted.

Yet, while participants in our study made regular use of technology to support their connections with others, this use was carefully considered. Technology was not, in itself, an attractive prospect unless it was perceived to fill a 'gap' and the 'chore' of using it did not overly impact on everyday life. Similarly, Lindley et al. reported that older people were cautious of the time commitments required to use technologies, although they also used technology as a way to manage levels of contact and control their own availability to other people [25]. In addition, participants in our study were aware of the potential for technology to contribute to disconnection. Waycott et al. [41] reflect that the mismatching of values and assumptions guiding a technology-based social intervention with those of the older adults participating in the evaluation, noticeably contributed to individual decisions not to participate. In an increasingly digital society, our findings again indicate the importance of design processes that are in tune with the perceptions and values of older adults.

Marston and van Hoof draw our attention to the fact that the World Health Organization's age-friendly cities model does not explicitly consider the role of technology [1,42]. By adopting a lens of age-friendliness, studies like ours can ensure that methods and processes are rooted in opportunities, concerns and 'gaps' that are relevant and engaging to participants. Consequently, we put forward an amended definition that highlights the need for explicit and thoughtful consideration of the role of technology in an age-friendly setting:

> *Underpinned by a commitment to respect and social inclusion, an age-friendly community is engaged in a strategic and ongoing process to facilitate active ageing by optimising the community's physical, social and digital environments and its supporting infrastructure.*

Another contribution of our work comes from its findings about the potential for technology to contribute to building and strengthening connections in geographically-bounded communities. The combination of shared local concerns and opportunities for improving connections, combined with the knowledge that technology was infrequently used to sustain or support local connections, suggests this is a design space worth exploring. Participants in this study were comfortable using digital technology to stay in touch with friends and family in geographically distant locations, particularly to maintain close family connections. Kharicha et al. also found that engagement with the outside world by landline telephones and computers was an important strategy adopted by older people experiencing loneliness [43]. For this reason, it would seem plausible that technology to facilitate local, proximate, connections and social lives would also be acceptable, should it fill perceived gaps and not lead to unacceptable levels of additional effort.

The methods we used in the workshop were intended to encourage 'playful' creativity, and they were successful in their purpose of generating a wide range of ideas as well as being acceptable and enjoyable for participants. In future, we would consider adapting these methods to reduce their paper-based nature, further enhancing their potential for prompting creative thinking by participants. Exploring options beyond face-to-face participation may also be important in the context of COVID-19 and its aftermath.

Drawing the interview findings together with one sub-theme from each of the themes we used to organise the ideas generated by workshop participants, we suggest a number of ways in which technology might support greater face-to-face connection in local community contexts and operationalise local people's ideas. By deliberately not placing technology in the foreground in the workshop, we contend that participants' ideas (technological or otherwise) about how to tackle local issues are more likely to align with their own values and perceptions, meaning that any technological needs that arise from these suggestions will be filling 'gaps' rather than technology being introduced as the automatic interface in connection. We maintain that design processes and spaces should be context-specific and bottom-up, but summarise general implications that offer scope for further exploration and consideration in community settings.

6.1. Making Better Use of Existing Geographical Places and Spaces

Workshop participants expressed interest in re-purposing spaces in the local area that they felt were underused, or offered potential as social spaces. This ranged from using existing green spaces or buildings on a permanent or temporary basis, to creating new spaces and places for social activities and events. A real-life example of creative use of space by older people that challenges expectations and norms was the transformation (for one night only) of a nightclub in Manchester, UK, into a night-time venue reserved for older people [44]. In our study, there were suggestions that spaces could be acquired or managed by groups of local residents as cooperative initiatives. Such work is ongoing in virtual spaces by older people in the UK creating a radio network [45]. Other adaptations to the built environment were also suggested by participants to improve suitability for pedestrians. However, operationalising these ideas and coordinating the input of the local community presents challenges at many levels. While online platforms to facilitate community commissioning of digital services exist [46], it is not immediately clear that these tools and processes would translate to local community commissioning of resources and events. Moreover, it is unrealistic to expect the required intense interaction with such digital platforms, leading to the need for alternative situated means of participating and engaging in the processes. Given the interest by study participants in leveraging local infrastructures and spaces, it is plausible to consider situated artefacts that would mediate between local, physical, and online engagements. For example, PosterVote is an innovative electronic polling system aiming to provide easy electronic voting for communities [47]. A traditional poster is augmented with buttons that can be pressed by community members to register digital responses to questions on the poster. Providing infrastructure for residents to have greater input and control over the provision of their immediate local environments would facilitate their participation in the process of age-friendliness at a community level.

6.2. Focusing on Proximate Connections

While our workshop focussed on connections at a local i.e., electoral ward level, some discussions were about connecting with people who were located very close nearby or even physically 'connected' by living on the same street. In fact, two participants expressed surprise on discovering that they had both been living in the area for many years a few houses apart on adjacent streets, yet they had never interacted before. Concerns about safety, privacy and possible lack of interest by others were mentioned as barriers to interventions at a street level. In recent years, we have witnessed a surge in location-based and serendipitous dating/meet-up services and networks (i.e., Tinder [48]). The core functionalities of these technologies are the abilities to discover similar individuals in your local area; privately extend an invitation to initiate a conversation; whilst maintaining a degree of privacy and safety through the network's services (not revealing personal details such as address or phone number). Such solutions would have scope to support the hyper-local match-making of friendships within communities. However, our research showed that participants were not using existing online services designed to develop new relationships, indicating that these did not appeal. This is echoed by findings that older people who were lonely did not report using the internet to cultivate new friendships, despite using telephones and computers to engage with the outside world [43]. In fact, one participant, Deborah, had instead capitalised on the ability of an accommodation matching platform to facilitate face-to-face interactions in her home with strangers, who then had the potential to become friends. The opportunity for such encounters (through mutually beneficial financial, or other resource, transactions) to result in long-lasting friendships is an area for further exploration. In particular, it would be interesting to consider how these types of interaction could be translated into a purely local context, given that Deborah's formation of new friendships contrasts with experiences of those in our study who attended regular local activities but did not find them conducive to making friends.

6.3. *Community Driven/Commissioned or Cooperative Initiatives*

The findings from our study indicate an opportunity for design around community or cooperative ways of addressing local transport gaps. A number of ideas generated by workshop participants related to improving transport in the immediate local area in order to facilitate connection to physical spaces and locations to meet other people. Community or cooperative initiatives were suggested as one option, or mechanism, for driving new models of transport in the area. Volunteer-run minibus and car transport did exist in the local area, but these prioritised 'essential' travel such as hospital appointments and did not have the flexibility that participants thought important. While existing schemes (e.g., StreetBank [49]—a website that facilitates possession sharing and borrowing between neighbours) have been successful in meeting other needs at a very local level, hyper-local journeys in suburban communities outside busy city centres are unlikely to offer sufficient cost/profit ratios to be attractive to existing sharing economy or peer-to-peer services such as Uber. A small number of demand responsive transport (DRT) schemes are running in the UK, and in theory sound promising. However, it is notable that a DRT service actually operated in our study area in the past, but closed in 2011 [50,51]. Similarly, existing bicycle sharing schemes rely on scale of use within large communities or cities to remain profitable, but in contrast, restricted access to a smaller population might reduce the risk of damage and loss experienced by larger scale operations. Consideration of what a hyper-local transport system might look like would include questions about who might provide and use the service, and what their incentives would be. Participants in this study also suggested teaching, learning and training opportunities as potentially playing a role. This is another avenue for exploration in future technology design which could serve the dual purposes of creating new connections between those learning and teaching, as well as the transport itself facilitating connections between people living in the area.

7. Conclusions

Our study adopted an age-friendly, bottom-up approach to explore opportunities for facilitating social connectedness for older adults in a local community context. We focused on specific community issues that could be addressed and considered the physical, social and structural mechanisms (potentially mediated or supported by technology) that might offer routes to tackling these. By understanding more about our participants' current use and perspectives on the role of technology in their social lives, we highlight a need for design work to reduce emphasis on technology as the interface between people. In contrast to previous work, we focus on connection between people in geographically close locations. We also demonstrate the importance of understanding the specific local context within which any technological interventions will take place. Our findings reflect changing patterns of technology use among older adults in the UK, suggesting that adoption of new technology is acceptable when it fills gaps and does not create intrusive levels of additional work or contribute to disconnection. Our modified definition of age-friendliness highlights a need for the explicit and thoughtful consideration of the role of technology. We identify topics for consideration by those seeking to design with local communities, and make the case for an age-friendly approach to designing (digital) interventions to address social connectedness in later life.

Author Contributions: Conceptualisation, J.L., N.P., K.M., B.H., H.S. and T.S.; Interviewing, J.L., H.S. and N.P.; Workshop facilitation, J.L., B.H., T.S. and N.P.; Initial analysis, J.L. and N.P.; Writing—original draft preparation, J.L.; Writing—review and editing, J.L., N.P., K.M., B.H., H.S. and T.S.; Project administration, J.L., H.S. and N.P.; Funding acquisition, H.S., J.L., K.M., and N.P. All authors have read and agreed to the published version of the manuscript.

Funding: This research was supported by funding from the Newcastle University Institute for Ageing (NUIA) and the Newcastle University Institute for Social Renewal (NISR). The views expressed are those of the authors and not necessarily those of NUIA or NISR.

Acknowledgments: We thank all participants who took part in this research. Our appreciation also goes to Cathrine Degnen for her involvement in the design, planning and acquisition of funding for the study, and to Drake Long, Meena Nanduri and Marlo Owczarzak for their support in facilitating the workshop.

Conflicts of Interest: The authors declare no conflict of interest.

References

1. World Health Organization. *Global Age-friendly Cities: A Guide*; World Health Organization: Geneva, Switzerland, 2007.
2. Lui, C.-W.; Everingham, J.-A.; Warburton, J.; Cuthill, M.; Bartlett, H. What makes a community age-friendly: A review of international literature. *Australas. J. Ageing* **2009**, *28*, 116–121. [CrossRef]
3. Liddle, J.; Scharf, T.; Bartlam, B.; Bernard, M.; Sim, J. Exploring the age-friendliness of purpose-built retirement communities: Evidence from England. *Ageing Soc.* **2013**, *34*, 1601–1629. [CrossRef]
4. Rowles, G.D. Evolving images of place in aging and 'aging-in-place'. *Generations* **1993**, *17*, 65–70.
5. Easton, M. How Should We Tackle the Loneliness Epidemic? 2018. Available online: https://www.bbc.co.uk/news/uk-42887932 (accessed on 20 September 2018).
6. Klinenberg, E. Is Loneliness a Health Epidemic? 2018. Available online: https://www.nytimes.com/2018/02/09/opinion/sunday/loneliness-health.html (accessed on 20 September 2018).
7. Uotila, H.; Lumme-Sandt, K.; Saarenheimo, M. Lonely older people as a problem in society—Construction in Finnish media. *Int. J. Ageing Later Life* **2011**, *5*, 103–130. [CrossRef]
8. Prime Minister's Office; Office for Civil Society; The Rt Hon Theresa May MP. PM Commits to Government-Wide Drive to Tackle Loneliness. 2018. Available online: https://www.gov.uk/government/news/pm-commits-to-government-wide-drive-to-tackle-loneliness (accessed on 20 September 2018).
9. Carroll, J.M.; Convertino, G.; Farooq, U.; Rosson, M.B. The firekeepers: Aging considered as a resource. *Univers. Access Inf. Soc.* **2011**, *11*, 7–15. [CrossRef]
10. Rogers, Y.; Paay, J.; Brereton, M.; Vaisutis, K.L.; Marsden, G.; Vetere, F. Never too old. In *Proceedings of the SIGCHI Conference on Human Factors in Computing Systems (CHI'14)*; Association for Computing Machinery (ACM): New York, NY, USA, 2014; pp. 3913–3922. [CrossRef]
11. Reuter, A.; Bartindale, T.; Morrissey, K.; Scharf, T.; Liddle, J. Older voices: Supporting community radio production for civic participation in later life. In *Proceedings of the 2019 CHI Conference on Human Factors in Computing Systems—CHI '19*; Association for Computing Machinery (ACM): New York, NY, USA, 2019; pp. 1–13. [CrossRef]
12. Buffel, T. (Ed.) *Researching Age-Friendly Communities: Stories from Older People as Co-Investigators*; The University of Manchester Library: Manchester, UK, 2015.
13. Vines, J.; Pritchard, G.; Wright, P.; Olivier, P.; Brittain, K. An age-old problem: Examining the discourses of ageing in HCI and strategies for future research. *TOCHI* **2015**, *22*, 1–27. [CrossRef]
14. Bruggencate, T.T.; Luijkx, K.G.; Sturm, J. Friends or Frenemies? The Role of Social Technology in the Lives of Older People. *Int. J. Environ. Res. Public Health* **2019**, *16*, 4969. [CrossRef]

15. Brittain, K.; Kingston, A.; Davies, K.; Collerton, J.; Robinson, P.L.; Kirkwood, T.B.L.; Bond, J.; Jagger, C. An investigation into the patterns of loneliness and loss in the oldest old—Newcastle 85+ Study. *Ageing Soc.* **2017**, *37*, 39–62. [CrossRef]
16. Victor, C.; Scambler, S.; Bond, J.; Bowling, A. Being alone in later life: Loneliness, social isolation and living alone. *Rev. Clin. Gerontol.* **2000**, *10*, 407–417. [CrossRef]
17. Owen, T. The high cost of isolation. *Work. Older People* **2001**, *5*, 21–23.
18. Office for National Statistics. *Loneliness—What Characteristics and Circumstances are Associated with Feeling Lonely?* ONS: London, UK, 2018.
19. Cornwell, B.; Laumann, E.O.; Schumm, L.P. The Social Connectedness of Older Adults: A National Profile. *Am. Sociol. Rev.* **2008**, *73*, 185–203. [CrossRef]
20. Emlet, C.A.; Moceri, J.T. The Importance of Social Connectedness in Building Age-Friendly Communities. *J. Aging Res.* **2011**, *2012*, 1–9. [CrossRef]
21. Bradley, N.; Poppen, W. Assistive technology, computers and Internet may decrease sense of isolation for homebound elderly and disabled persons. *Technol. Disabil.* **2003**, *15*, 19–25. [CrossRef]
22. Kanayama, T. Ethnographic Research on the Experience of Japanese Elderly People Online. *New Media Soc.* **2003**, *5*, 267–288. [CrossRef]
23. Sayago, S.; Righi, V.; Ferreira, S.M.; Rosales, A.; Blat, J. Tales of the map of my mobile life: Intergenerational computer-mediated communication between older people and fieldworkers in their early adulthood. In *Intergenerational Mobilities: Relationality, Age and Lifecourse*; Murray, L., Robertson, S., Eds.; Routledge: London, UK; New York, NY, USA, 2017; pp. 54–64.
24. Xie, B. Multimodal Computer-Mediated Communication and Social Support among Older Chinese Internet Users. *J. Comput. Commun.* **2008**, *13*, 728–750. [CrossRef]
25. Lindley, S.E.; Harper, R.; Sellen, A. Desiring to be in touch in a changing communications landscape. In *Proceedings of the SIGCHI Conference on Human Factors in Computing Systems Empowering People—CHI '90*; Association for Computing Machinery (ACM): New York, NY, USA, 2009; pp. 1693–1702.
26. Miyajima, A.; Itoh, Y.; Itoh, M.; Watanabe, T. "Tsunagari-kan" Communication: Design of a New Telecommunication Environment and a Field Test with Family Members Living Apart. *Int. J. Hum. Comput. Interact.* **2005**, *19*, 253–276. [CrossRef]
27. Plaisant, C.; Clamage, A.; Hutchinson, H.B.; Bederson, B.B.; Druin, A. Shared family calendars. *ACM Trans. Comput. Interact.* **2006**, *13*, 313–346. [CrossRef]
28. Office for National Statistics. *Internet Users, UK: 2019*; ONS: London, UK, 2019.
29. Dickinson, A.; Hill, R.L. Keeping in Touch: Talking to Older People about Computers and Communication. *Educ. Gerontol.* **2007**, *33*, 613–630. [CrossRef]
30. Righi, V.; Sayago, S.; Blat, J. Older people's use of social network sites while participating in local online communities from an ethnographical perspective. In Proceedings of the CIRN Community Informatics Conference, Prato, Italy, 7–9 November 2012.
31. Buffel, T.; Handler, S.; Phillipson, C. Age-friendly cities and communities: A manifesto for change. In *Age-friendly Cities and Communities: A Global Perspective*; Buffel, T., Handler, S., Phillipson, C., Eds.; Policy Press: Bristol, UK, 2018; pp. 273–288.
32. Buffel, T.; Phillipson, C.; Scharf, T. Ageing in urban environments: Developing 'age-friendly' cities. *Crit. Soc. Policy* **2012**, *32*, 597–617. [CrossRef]
33. Warth, L. The WHO Global Network of Age-Friendly Cities and Communities: Origins, Developments and Challenges. In *Age-Friendly Cities and Communities in International Comparison*; Moulaert, T., Garon, S., Eds.; Springer: Cham, Switzerland, 2016; pp. 37–46.
34. Arksey, H.; Knight, P. *Interviewing for Social Scientists*; SAGE Publications: London, UK, 1999.
35. Office for National Statistics. 2011 Census Data. Available online: https://www.ons.gov.uk/census/2011census (accessed on 31 March 2017).
36. Mishler, G. *Research Interviewing: Context and Narrative*; Harvard University Press: Harvard, MA, USA, 1991.
37. Braun, V.; Clarke, V. Using thematic analysis in psychology. *Qual. Res. Psychol.* **2006**, *3*, 77–101. [CrossRef]
38. Garon, S.; Veil, A. Les villes amies des aînés au Québec: Un mouvement de changement à large échelle en faveur des aînés. *Vie Vieillissement* **2011**, *9*, 6–12.
39. IDEO. *From Ideas to Action Toolkit*; IDEO: San Francisco, CA, USA, 2016.

40. Buffel, T. *Experiences of Place and Neighbourhood in Later Life: Developing Age-Friendly Communities*; VUBPress: Brussels, Belgium, 2012.
41. Waycott, J.; Vetere, F.; Pedell, S.; Morgans, A.; Ozanne, E.; Kulik, L. Not for me: Older adults choosing not to participate in a social isolation intervention. In *Proceedings of the 2016 CHI Conference on Human Factors in Computing Systems*; Association for Computing Machinery (ACM): New York, NY, USA, 2016; pp. 745–757.
42. Marston, H.R.; Van Hoof, J. Hoof "Who Doesn't Think about Technology When Designing Urban Environments for Older People?" A Case Study Approach to a Proposed Extension of the WHO's Age-Friendly Cities Model. *Int. J. Environ. Res. Public Health* **2019**, *16*, 3525. [CrossRef] [PubMed]
43. Kharicha, K.; Manthorpe, J.; Iliffe, S.; Chew-Graham, C.A.; Cattan, M.; Goodman, C.; Kirby-Barr, M.; Whitehouse, J.H.; Walters, K. Managing loneliness: A qualitative study of older people's views. *Aging Ment. Health* **2020**. [CrossRef] [PubMed]
44. Handler, S. *An Alternative Age-Friendly Handbook*; The University of Manchester Library: Manchester, UK, 2014.
45. Later Life Audio and Radio Network. Available online: https://www.mixcloud.com/LLARN/ (accessed on 20 April 2020).
46. Garbett, A.; Comber, R.; Jenkins, E.; Olivier, P. App Movement. In *Proceedings of the 2016 CHI Conference on Human Factors in Computing Systems*; Association for Computing Machinery (ACM): New York, NY, USA, 2016; pp. 26–37. [CrossRef]
47. PosterVote. Available online: https://postervote.openlab.ncl.ac.uk (accessed on 20 April 2020).
48. Tinder. Available online: https://tinder.com (accessed on 20 April 2020).
49. StreetBank. Available online: https://www.streetbank.com (accessed on 20 April 2020).
50. Metro. *Good Practice Guide: Transport and Social Inclusion*; Pteg: Leeds, UK, 2005.
51. Demand Responsive Transport in the UK. Available online: https://en.wikipedia.org/wiki/Demand_responsive_transport#United_Kingdom (accessed on 20 April 2020).

International Journal of
Environmental Research and Public Health

MDPI

Article

Effects of Technology Use on Ageing in Place: The iZi Pilots

Helen A.M. Silvius [1,2,*], Erwin C.P.M. Tak [3], Dennis O. Mook-Kanamori [1,4], Hedwig M.M. Vos [1,2], Mattijs E. Numans [1,2] and Niels H. Chavannes [2,5]

1 Department of Public Health and Primary Care, Medical Center, Leiden University, Hippocratespad 21, 2333 ZD Leiden, The Netherlands; d.o.mook@lumc.nl (D.O.M.-K.); h.m.m.vos@lumc.nl (H.M.M.V.); M.E.Numans@lumc.nl (M.E.N.)

2 Medical Center-Campus The Hague, Leiden University, Turfmarkt 99, 2511 DC The Hague, The Netherlands; n.h.chavannes@lumc.nl

3 Department of Education, Culture and Wellbeing, Municipality of The Hague, 2542 ED The Hague, The Netherlands; erwintak2@gmail.com

4 Department of Clinical Epidemiology, Medical Center, Leiden University, Postbus 9600, 2300 RC Leiden, The Netherlands

5 National e-Health Living Lab, PO-Box 9600, 2300 RC Leiden, The Netherlands

* Correspondence: A.M.Silvius@lumc.nl; Tel.: +31-650-640-967

Received: 8 May 2020; Accepted: 26 June 2020; Published: 14 July 2020

check for updates

Abstract: In the iZi study in The Hague, use and acceptance of commercially available technology by home-dwelling older citizens was studied, by comparing self-efficacy and perceived physical and mental Quality of Life (QoL)-related parameters on an intervention location of 279 households and a control location of 301 households. Technology adoption was clinically significantly associated with increased perceived physical QoL, as compared with control group, depending on the number of technology interventions that were used. A higher number of adopted technologies was associated with a stronger effect on perceived QoL. We tried to establish a way to measure clinical significance by using mixed methods, combining quantitative and qualitative evaluation and feeding results and feedback of participants directly back into our intervention. In general, this research is promising, since it shows that successful and effective adoption of technology by older people is feasible with commercially available products amongst home-dwelling older citizens. We think this way of working provides a better integration of scientific methods and clinical usability but demands a lot of communication and patience of researchers, citizens, and policymakers. A change in policy on how to target people for this kind of intervention might be warranted.

Keywords: older citizens; ageing; technology; digital

1. Introduction

Increased life expectancy is posing a challenge on economies in general and the healthcare system because not all years gained are healthy years [1]. The increase of our ageing society is a positive yet challenging phenomenon, as population ageing, and urbanization are the culmination of successful human development [2]. The interaction of ageing and urbanism, which is termed urban ageing [3,4], raises issues for all types of communities in various domains of urban living [5]. The demographics of a society with an increasing number of older citizens asks for smart solutions to maintain quality of life and quality of care [6]. Policymakers and technology producers state that technology will help in providing these solutions. Evidence of effectivity of technology is present [7], however pilots are usually performed in closed communities or by means of single-platform tools. Solid proof of effects of technology in this field was currently lacking. In 2010, a review of reviews led to the conclusion that telemedicine is effective, but that evidence in a lot of studies is promising but incomplete and in a lot of other studies is limited and inconsistent. Major problems were found in economic analyses, benefit for patients, complexity of telemedicine, and ongoing collaborative achievement in unpredictable processes [8]. This inhibits investments of public and private parties in development and implementation of technology.

In the Netherlands, a transition has been made to shift the care for older citizens from centrally organized to municipally organized. The aim is to reduce formal and intramural care to promote healthy home-based aging. This necessitates another way of involvement of both formal and informal caretakers.

In the municipality of The Hague, the "iZi study", focusing on technology adoption by older citizens, aimed to experiment with introducing technology in a need-driven way. This provided opportunities to tailor those needs and connect them to possible technologic solutions. In this study, the municipality of The Hague has taken the initiative to experiment with technology introduction to establish how it can contribute to the transition soon.

In this study, we aim to evaluate whether need-driven introduction of technology in adult humans leads to improved self-reliance and a better perceived quality of life. We think that need-driven introduction and use of technology will lead to positive effects on aging in place.

2. Materials and Methods

2.1. Study Design

The iZi pilot is a prognostic controlled observational study and was performed in a community in the municipality of The Hague. The community consists of community-dwelling older citizens (55+). The total complex counted 279 households. Because the intervention was tailored to individual needs, and therefore differed for each participant, the intervention was evaluated based on intention-to-treat analysis. The participants on the iZi location were compared with citizens on a location in The Hague that was matched on relevant characteristics, to be comparable to the intervention location. This community consisted of four apartment buildings, with a total of 301 households.

The process of inclusion is depicted in a flow chart that is attached as Figure A1.

We have chosen to evaluate effects in this study by comparing the differences in effect between T0 and T12 of participants in the study with the control population.

On the intervention location, residents were matched to technology from a preselected list, based on previous needs assessment and selected together with participants in group sessions. All items were supplied for the pilot by technology producers and suppliers. This list is attached as Table A1.

On the intervention location, participants were included in a stepwise fashion. First, they were recruited by using several strategies such as group meetings, door-to-door-calls by the iZi team, and posters and messages on the (specifically installed) electronic bulletin board. Once residents participated in the technology trial, they were approached to participate in the effect evaluation by giving informed consent. Participants who had given informed consent for the evaluation were visited by a research nurse for evaluation at T = 0 and T = 12 months.

On the control location, participants were recruited by letters sent by the housing corporation. They could respond by sending an enclosed response form to a free mail address but were also provided with a telephone number and an e-mail address. After a resident responded, the research nurse called to provide information, and if people chose to participate, an appointment was made in which informed consent was obtained and evaluation at T = 0 and later T = 12 was performed.

The baseline characteristics of the intervention population and the control population are described in Table 1.

Table 1. Composition of intervention and control group at different timepoints.

Composition	Intervention T0	Intervention T12	Control T0	Control T12
n	83	56	77	48
Age	(%)	(%)	(%)	(%)
51–65	8.4	5.4	11.7	8.3
66–70	10.8	12.5	13.0	14.6
71–75	25.3	25.0	18.2	20.8
76–80	30.1	30.4	27.3	29.2
>81	25.3	26.8	29.9	27.1
Sex	(%)	(%)	(%)	(%)
Male	39.8	41.1	35.1	33.3
Female	60.2	58.9	64.9	66.7
Marital status	(%)	(%)	(%)	(%)
Living together	37.3	32.1	53.2	45.8
Single	62.7	67.9	46.8	54.2

During the study, the inclusion targets for the effect analysis were not met. Differences between two groups were seen in the composition of the households of the participants. On the intervention location, a higher number of singles participated than on the control location.

2.2. *Self-Reliance and Participation*

Self-reliance was measured using the "Impact on Participation and Autonomy Questionnaire" (IPAQ) [9,10]. The IPAQ consists of five domains: autonomy indoors, family role, autonomy outdoors, social relations, and work and educational opportunities. Each domain consists of a different number of items. Answers were scored on three- and five-point Likert scales. For each domain, the participation score and the problem experience score were calculated by summing the item scores. Higher scores denote more restrictions in participation and/or a higher problem experienced on the specific domain.

2.3. *Quality of Life*

Quality of life (QoL) was scored using the SF-12 health survey, a survey consisting of 12 items in which physical functioning, role limitations due to physical health, bodily pain, general health perceptions, vitality, social functioning, role limitations due to emotional problems, and mental health are scored [11]. The SF-12 scores were calculated using the general scoring system provided by the developers [12]. Since country-specific scoring did not differ much [13], the original scoring system was used to provide better external validity.

In the general population, the average score is set on 50, with 0 representing the worst possible health and 100 representing the best possible health. In the Dutch population, the physical component score on SF-12 tends to diminish with increasing age. The mental component score shows no such tendency. The mean score of Dutch women on both components is lower than that of men. This effect is consistent in all age groups [13].

2.4. *Establishing Statistical and Clinical Significance*

To get significant results, a certain number of participants are needed. Therefore, a power calculation was performed, using the IPA norm scores [14].

To detect statistically significant changes at a 5% significance level with 80% power, with two-sided testing, inclusion of at least 112 households on the intervention location and 120 households on the control location would be necessary to be able to detect a 10% change.

For clinical significance of measured effects, we could not do prior calculations of number of participants needed, however we call effects clinically significant if a change occurs that has consequences in the real-life world of participants. This practically means that the effect is seen after a relatively short amount of time and has a magnitude that is perceived either directly by the participants or can be picked up by the researchers by means of their measuring tools.

2.5. Statistical Analysis

For some participants, scores could not be calculated due to missing data. Linear regression analysis was used to establish whether possibly significant effects due to differences in age, gender, and marital status were missed. We compared the differences in the mean scores using paired *t*-test statistics in SPSS statistics 25 (IBM, New York, NY, USA).

First, we compared the differences in IPAQ score between T0 and T12 in both the iZi group and the control group separately, using paired *t*-tests. For this analysis, we examined the five main dimensions of the IPAQ score. Next, we compared the differences of the two scores (mental and physical) of the SF-12 between T0 and T12 in both the iZi group and the control group separately, using paired *t*-tests as well. The outcomes for both populations are described in Tables 3 and 4. Linear regression analysis, performed to establish whether possibly significant effects due to age, gender, and marital status were missed, yielded no significant effects.

After that, we subtracted the score of T0 from the score on T12 for each specific person on each specific location, thus creating the specific change on a dimension (delta) for each person on each location. We compared the median value of this delta for both locations, using the Mann–Whitney U for testing on significance.

Finally, we checked whether the significant changes that also had a clinical significance could be ascribed to the amount of technology offered. We also explored whether a specific kind of technology could be related to the statistical or clinical effect seen.

3. Results

The results of both groups at both timepoints on the different domains of the IPAQ are depicted in Table 2.

Table 2. Scores of intervention and control group on IPAQ at different timepoints.

IPAQ Domain	Intervention T0	Intervention T12		Control T0	Control T12	
	Mean (SD) *n*	Mean (SD) *n*	*p*	Mean (SD) *n*	Mean (SD) *n*	*p*
Autonomy indoors	0.97 (0.66) 76	0.98 (0.51) 48	0.02	0.97 (0.57) 82	1.10 (0.28) 56	0.24
Family role	1.32 (0.73) 73	1.19 (0.46) 47	0.60	1.34 (1.01) 78	1.30 (0.42) 56	0.68
Autonomy outdoors	1.37 (0.79) 74	1.17 (0.44) 47	0.90	1.30 (0.77) 79	0.32 (0.36) 56	0.84
Social relations	1.11 (0.58) 71	1.10 (0.32) 43	0.05	1.07 (0.59) 78	1.19 (0.18) 55	0.67

p-values calculated with paired *t*-test.

The results of both groups at both timepoints on the different domains of the SF-12 are depicted in Table 3.

Evaluation of IPAQ yielded statistical significant difference in the scores for autonomy indoors in the intervention group and social relations in the intervention group. However, the magnitude of the effect was so little that we did not see this as a workable starting point to perform further evaluation of these domains into subgroups.

Evaluation of SF-12 yielded statistical significant differences in the scores for physical health in the control group and statistical significant differences in the scores for mental health for both the control group and the intervention group.

Table 3. Scores of intervention and control group on SF-12 at different timepoints.

SF-12 Domain	Intervention T0	Intervention T12	*p*	Control T0	Control T12	*p*
	Mean (SD) n = 79	Mean (SD) n = 46		Mean (SD) n = 74	Mean (SD) n = 56	
Physical health	41.42 (12.15)	39.90 (4.81)	0.57	41.95 (11.61)	38.69 (6.21)	0.002
Mental health	43.42 (9.85)	39.78 (6.33)	<0.0001 *	43.72 (9,71)	42.29 (6,60)	<0.0001 *

p-values calculated with paired *t*-test. * Statistical and clinical significant.

We then compared the differences between T12 and T0 of both intervention and control group, to evaluate whether the differences observed could be related to the intervention. (Subtracting measurements of T0 does provide a "net" value that makes comparison possible if the groups are equal in composition).

The results of this comparison are depicted in Table 4.

Table 4. Comparison of differences in health scores of intervention group and control group.

IPAQ Domain	Intervention	Control	*p*−Value
	Delta Median (Interquartile Range)	Delta Median (Interquartile Range)	
Autonomy indoors	0.00 (−0.23, 0.75)	0.00 (−0.14, 0.57)	0.649
Family role	0.00 (−0.14, 0.29)	0.00 (−0.36, 0.50)	0.380
Autonomy outdoors	0.00 (−0.20, 0.40)	0.20 (−0.40, 0.55)	0.975
Social relations	0.00 (−0.29, 0.75)	0.07 (−0.14, 0.43)	0.315
Physical health	−7.85 (−12.70, 4.08)	−2.42 (−13.18, 7.91)	0.037
Mental health	−1.35 (−9.94, 9.03)	−4.79 (−9.65, 2.93)	0.124

p-calculated using Mann-Whitney U.

We assessed whether the effect on perceived physical health might be related to intensity of technology use. On the iZi location, participants were matched to between zero and seven different technologies. Distribution of technology is described in Table 5.

Table 5. Number of technologies matched to a household.

Number of Technologies	Number of Households	% of Households
0	203	69,0
1	30	10,2
2	28	9,5
3	19	6,4
4	8	2,7
5	4	1,4
6	1	0,3
7	1	0,3
Total	294	100,0

Because few participants had four or more technologies, for further analysis a division was made into four groups: participants with zero, one, two, and three or more technology matches. For practical reasons, we put all the people who did participate in the evaluation but did not get (control location) or did not get matched to technology (intervention location) in the "no technology" group.

This is depicted in Figure 1.

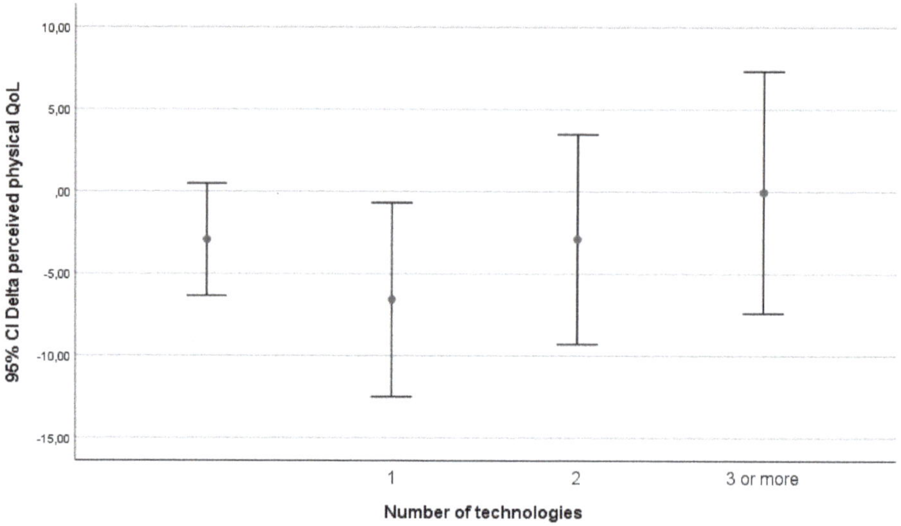

Figure 1. Relation between delta perceived physical health (SF-12$_{(\text{physical health T12})}$ − SF-12$_{(\text{physical health T0})}$) and number of technologies (1,2 or 3 or more) compared with those who did not get or did not get matched to technology.

What is seen is a decrease in perceived physical QoL when persons go from no technology to starting technology, but from there an almost linear trend of increasing QoL with increasing number of technologies can be seen.

Because a lot of different technologies were used, we performed a subgroup analysis based on two different classifying systems: a classification on technological level and a functional classification. We checked all classifications for subclasses that revealed useable patterns.

The classification of technological level was made in three groups: high-tech, low-tech, and in-house mechanical adaptations. The division high tech vs. low tech was made from the apparatus and user point of view, labelling high tech all those technological interventions that had complex operating systems or provided multiple functions or options.

The functional classification, with which the intervention originally started, divided technology into groups depending on the domain of life to which they were attributed and matched, and used the following classes: safety, mobility, communication. The classifications and the used technologies are depicted in Table A1.

We visually evaluated graphs for relevant results. Only the classification on technological level yielded possible relevant differences. These differences are depicted in Figures 2–4.

In our follow-up, being matched to technology was only associated with an increase in perceived physical health in the group that received in-house adaptations. In the high-tech and low-tech groups, there was a decrease in perceived physical health.

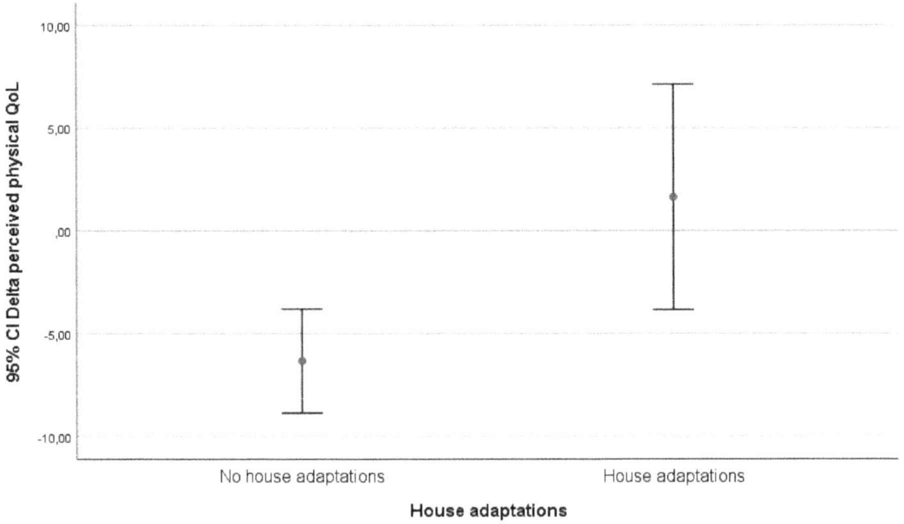

Figure 2. Relation between delta perceived physical health (SF-12$_{(physical\ health\ T12)}$ − SF-12$_{(physical\ health\ T0)}$) and match to in-house adaptations.

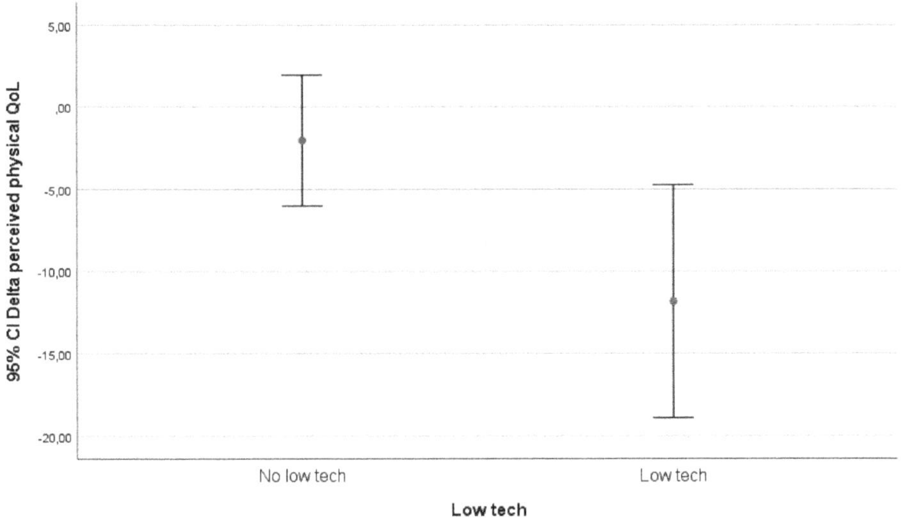

Figure 3. Relation between delta perceived physical health (SF-12$_{(physical\ health\ T12)}$ − SF-12$_{(physical\ health\ T0)}$) and match to low-tech technology.

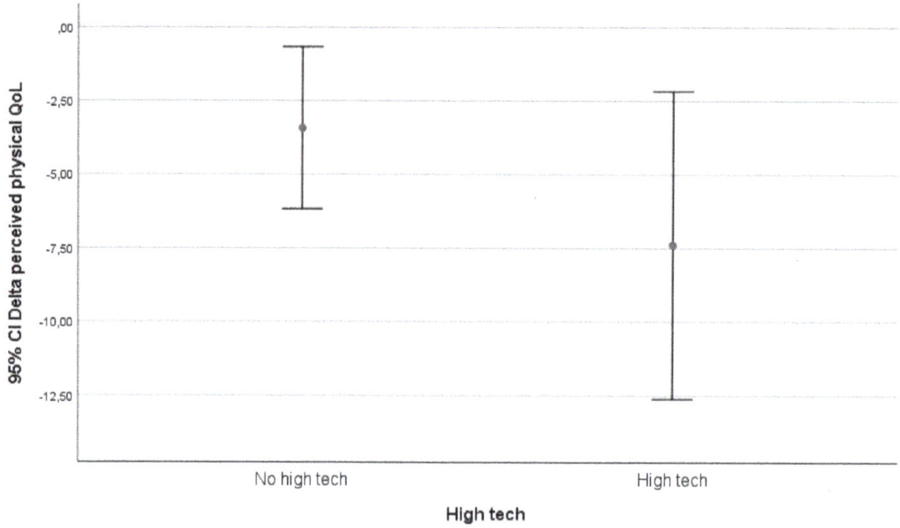

Figure 4. Relation between delta perceived physical health (SF-$12_{(\text{physical health T12})}$ − SF-$12_{(\text{physical health T0})}$) and match to high-tech technology.

4. Discussion

The goal of all long-term care arrangements is to reduce the disabling effects of physical impairments and functional limitations. However, the means with which individuals cope with disability may not be equivalent and these differences may influence self-reports of disability in surveys. Agree et al. [15] examined assistive devices and personal care as factors in the measurement of disability among persons aged 70 and concluded that the use of assistive technology differs from personal care on a fundamental level. They also concluded that it does not require the ongoing cooperation or coordination of other people and therefore increases the sense of independence with which a disabled individual can meet their long-term care needs. Their results indicate that older individuals can expect to spend most of their remaining years in good functional health, but up to two-thirds of disabled years will be spent with unmet needs. Among those who are disabled, those who use only equipment and no personal care report less residual difficulty with mobility than those who use personal assistance (either alone or in combination with equipment), but the use of equipment alone is most effective for those with the least severe limitations. This coincides with the finding in our study that in-house adaptations provide the largest shift in QoL.

A lot of technology is available for aging societies, but acceptance amongst older citizens is difficult [16], and there are also ethical dilemma's involved [17]. Technology introduction for older citizens is difficult, because the ability to learn new things usually wanes with age and might even be worse in those who might potentially benefit the most. However, effectiveness of technology in people with learning abilities has been shown [18]. Tailoring interventions to personal needs might help to improve acceptance, adoption, and use of technology [9]. Thus introduced, technology might enable older citizens to age at home [19]. Our study shows that in tailoring interventions, older citizens are accepting and adopting technology. The use of technology, be it high-tech or low-tech, is associated with a decrease in QoL. The effects on physical health seem in this study only to be associated with in-house adaptations and not with high-tech or low-tech solutions. However, the follow-up period was quite short, and a relative low number of high-tech and low-tech solutions were matched. What possibly might influence the results is the fact that in the prior consultation, most people rated accessibility as one of the most important domains. Therefore, most people have been matched to items in this range, and those were mostly low-technology items. The needs that require high-technology solutions are fewer and therefore do not contribute to a large component in the effect, but positive results are seen by researchers and reported by participants that have been exposed to high-technology solutions.

It turns out that technology might help in facilitating adaptive changes, but that implementing the right technology at the right moment for the right reason and the right person is quite difficult. Currently, tools are being developed to support this process [16]. What tool is suited for which problem is difficult to ascertain. Efforts have been made to devise a taxonomy describing essential features of interventions [13].

Most people prefer to age the way they have lived all their life, however, sometimes circumstances change. These changes in circumstances may be the result of a process that has been going on for years, but may also be provoked by an event (for example changes in living arrangements or illness). These changed circumstances may also affect the relationship with the informal caretaker (usually the partner, child, or other family member) and may disrupt the status quo, necessitating adaptive changes. It is important to identify people that may be prone to benefit from technology when these changes are to occur, to assess their needs, and to see if those needs can be met [9]. Since the needs within this population differ, communication about needs is vital.

The iZi study in The Hague shows that, contrary to earlier studies and beliefs amongst caretakers, older citizens are interested in the adoption of technology and once recruited and enabled to partake in the matching process, can successfully adopt technology. Technology adoption is associated with an increased perceived physical health as compared with the control group, depending on the number of technology interventions that are used.

Whether this is due to the technology or whether participants in this study were healthier at the start of the study is something that remains to be established. In general, this research clearly shows that successful and effective adoption of technology by older citizens is feasible with commercially available products amongst home-dwelling older citizens.

Unfortunately, from a point of view of cost-effectiveness the intervention cannot be implemented in the way it was researched on a larger scale, since on the intervention location a lot of people were involved in the matching process. From a funding point of view, cost-effectiveness can be evaluated by looking at it from both municipal and health insurance budgets, because at this point municipalities must pay for the intervention, while the gain is made on the health insurance budgets. Unfortunately, health insurers were not involved in this study.

During the intervention, the idea arose that the most vulnerable citizens were possibly not targeted by this specific recruitment. The intervention managed to reach only a part of the older citizens, and from analysis of subgroups that we did, we had the idea that especially older citizens from other cultures and people dealing with social issues or diseases tended not to participate. This leaves the question open whether, apart from the fact that this intervention shows a positive change in the intervention group as compared with the control group, this intervention (if there is a cause–effect relation) might have the potential to have an effect if it would access populations that could benefit from it in a better way. Therefore, it would be interesting to establish which older citizens stand to gain the most from which interventions, and how the matching and recruitment process can be improved in the future. Collaboration between GPs and municipality might be helpful in selecting and reaching out to older citizens who might benefit. More research on this subject is needed to establish if this indeed is a successful route.

The statistical significant increase in perceived autonomy indoors and social relations compared with the control population has a magnitude and therefore a clinical significance that is small. These results might be due to a lack of power, but it might also suggest that even if people want to use technology, getting used to using technology requires an effort and might also pose difficulties that are not so easily overcome [16]. It would be interesting to know what the effects are over a longer period, since a lot of time and effort was spent on getting used to the technology. The time lost on solving functionality issues and testing might have negatively influenced the perceived physical health, because getting to work with technology that helps solve physical issues requires that people do recognize and accept those issues. So paradoxically, for technology to be able to help people function in a better way, it might start by making them feel worse. If this is indeed the case, it is important to recognize and describe this process, to prevent premature abortion of potential successful interventions.

The statistically and clinically significant decrease in perceived mental health in both populations warrants further exploration.

Moreover, difficulty in reaching older citizens who might really benefit and difficulty in obtaining technology that was really tailored to the needs of these citizens might have given an underestimation of the real effect of technology. The initial results show that successful and effective adoption of technology by older citizens is feasible with commercially available products. The iZi project established a way to measure clinical significance by using mixed methods, combining quantitative and qualitative evaluation and feeding results and feedback of participants directly back into our intervention. We think this way of working provides a better integration of scientific methods and clinical usability but demands a lot of communication and patience of researchers, citizens, and policymakers. Given our results, this warrants further exploration. Especially, more research is needed to establish the existence of unmet care needs amongst this specific population to evaluate if the effect we see can be improved, thus making the intervention—if there is a causal relation between intervention and effect—possibly more cost-effective.

5. Conclusions

Though target inclusions were not met in this study, we were able to demonstrate a decrease in perceived physical health in the control population that was not seen in the intervention population. Both populations showed a decrease in perceived mental health, measured with the SF-12. Lastly, on the intervention location, an increase in perceived autonomy indoors and social relations compared with the control population was measured. The clinical effect of this change was however small.

An increase in the number of technology matches was associated with an increase in perceived physical health with three or more successful matches to technology. In our subgroup analysis, being matched to technology was only associated with an increase in perceived physical health in the group that received in-house adaptations. In the high-tech and low-tech groups, there was a decrease in perceived physical health.

Author Contributions: Conceptualization, H.A.M.S. and E.C.P.M.T.; methodology, H.A.M.S. and D.O.M.-K; software, M.E.N.; validation, H.A.M.S., M.E.N. and N.H.C.; formal analysis, H.A.M.S.; investigation, H.A.M.S.; resources, H.A.M.S.; data curation, H.A.M.S.; writing—original draft preparation, H.A.M.S.; writing—review and editing, H.A.M.S., D.O.M.-K, H.M.M.V., E.C.P.M.T., N.H.C., and M.E.N.; visualization, H.A.M.S.; supervision, N.H.C., M.E.N.; project administration, H.A.M.S.; funding acquisition, E.C.P.M.T. All authors have read and agreed to the published version of the manuscript.

Funding: This research was funded by a grant of the municipality of The Hague, grant number B01_L_17_670.001.01.380B01_L_17_UCB_tijdelijke_dekking_programma_zorg_innvoatie.

Acknowledgments: F. Büchner is acknowledged for writing the initial study protocol, E. Sucu for performing part of the interviews on location, the iZi team of the municipality The Hague for their unwavering enthusiasm, A.C.S. Felix is thanked for helping to sort out the massive amount of literature in the field of e-Health/health technology, R. Vos for helping to sort out the details of this study, and last but not least, the colleagues at LUMC-Campus The Hague are thanked for providing the right environment to finish this project.

Conflicts of Interest: The authors declare that since they are working in healthcare they might benefit from developments that improve delivery of care to older citizens in that it might improve their working conditions. The funders had no role in the design of the study; in the collection, analyses, or interpretation of data; in the writing of the manuscript, or in the decision to publish the results.

Appendix A

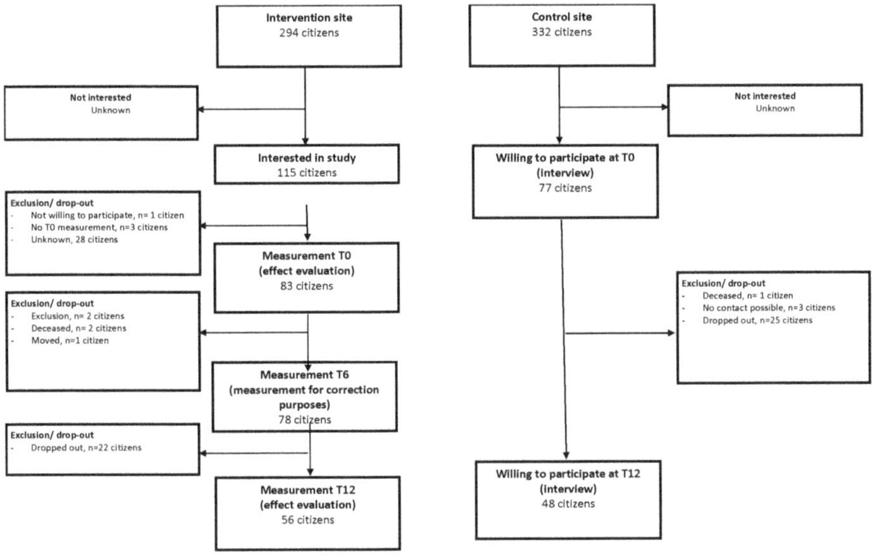

Figure A1. Flow chart inclusion.

Appendix B

Table A1. Available items in study and their classification.

Device	Functional	Technological
Alarms (carbon monoxide, carbon dioxide)	S	LT
Anti-slip tiling	M	IHA
Assistive chair	M	IHA
Automated lighting	S	LT
Balcony step	M	IHA
Dementia app	C	HT
Diverse ergonomic tools	S	IHA
Doorstep equalizer	M	IHA
Drawers kitchen/worktop	S	IHA
Electronically operated openers (door/window/curtain) **	S	LT
Electronic peephole	S	LT
Elevated washing machine	S	IHA
Emergency flashlight	S	LT
Faucets	S	IHA
Personal alarm	S	LT
LEA (electronic walking aid) */**	M	HT

Table A1. *Cont.*

Device	Functional	Technological
Lifestyle monitoring	S	HT
Robocat	C	LT
Robot vacuum cleaner	S	HT
Saddle stool	S	IHA
Shower chair	M	IHA
Smartphone	C	HT
Smoke alarm activated security stove	S	LT
Supportive handrails	M	IHA
Tablet computer	C	HT
Tessa (agenda with voice interface)	C	HT
Video intercom *	S	HT
Wash/dry toilet	S	LT

* limited availability; ** not available at start study. S = Safety; M = Mobility; C = Communication; LT = Low Tech; HT = High Tech; IHA = In House Adaptations.

References

1. WHO. *Global Health and Aging*; WHO: Geneva, Switzerland, 2011.
2. Plouffe, L.; Kalache, A. Towards global age-friendly cities. Determining urban features that promote active aging. *J. Urban Health* **2010**, *87*, 733–739. [PubMed]
3. Van Hoof, J.; Kazak, J.K.; Perek-Białas, J.M.; Peek, S. The challenges of urban aging: Making cities age-friendly in Europe. *Int. J. Environ. Res. Public Health* **2018**, *15*, 2473. [CrossRef] [PubMed]
4. Van Hoof, J.; Kazak, J.K. Urban Aging. *Indoor Built Environ.* **2018**, *27*, 283–286. [CrossRef]
5. Buffel, T. and Philipson, L. Can global cities be 'age-friendly' cities? Urban development and ageing populations. *Cities* **2016**, *55*, 94–100. [CrossRef]
6. Sonn, U.; Davegårdh, H.; Lindskog, A.C.; Steen, B. The use and effectiveness of assistive devices in an elderly urban population. *Aging* **1996**, *8*, 176–183. [CrossRef] [PubMed]
7. Raghunath, N.; Dahmen, J.; Brown, K.; Cook, D.; Schmitter-Edgecombe, M. Creating a digital memory notebook application for individuals with mild cognitive impairment to support everyday functioning. *Disabil. Rehabil. Assist. Technol.* **2019**, *15*, 421–431. [CrossRef] [PubMed]
8. Ekeland, A.G.; Bowes, A.; Flottorp, S. Effectiveness of telemedicine: A systematic review of reviews. *Int. J. Med. Inform.* **2010**, *79*, 736–771. [CrossRef] [PubMed]
9. Cardol, M.; De Haan, R.J.; De Jong, B.A.; Van den Bos, G.A.; De Groot, I.J. Psychometric properties of the Impact on Participation and Autonomy Questionnaire. *Arch. Phys. Med. Rehabil.* **2001**, *82*, 210–216. [CrossRef] [PubMed]
10. Andreoni, G.; Arslan, P.; Costa, F.; Muschiato, S.; Romero, M. Ergonomics and design for sustainability in healthcare: Ambient assisted living and the social environmental impact of patients' lifestyle. *Work-J. Prev. Assess. Rehab.* **2012**, *41*, 3883–3887. [CrossRef] [PubMed]
11. Haufe, M.; Peek, S.T.M.; Luijkx, K.G. Matching gerontechnologies to independent living seniors' individual needs: Development of the GTM tool. *BMC Health Serv. Res.* **2019**, *19*, 26. [CrossRef] [PubMed]
12. Ware, J.; Kosinski, M.A.; Keller, S.D. *How to Score the SF-12 Physical and Mental Health Summary Scales*; SF-12: Boston, MA, USA, 1998.
13. Schulz, R.; Czaja, S.J.; McKay, J.R.; Ory, M.G.; Belle, S.H. Intervention taxonomy (ITAX): Describing essential features of interventions. *Am. J. Health Behav.* **2010**, *34*, 811–821. [CrossRef] [PubMed]
14. Gandek, B.; Ware, J.E.; Aaronson, N.K.; Apolone, G.; Bjorner, J.B.; Brazier, J.E.; Bullinger, M.; Kaasa, S.; Leplege, A.; Prieto, L.; et al. Cross-validation of item selection and scoring for the SF-12 Health Survey in nine countries: Results from the IQOLA Project. International Quality of Life Assessment. *J. Clin. Epidemiol.* **1998**, *51*, 1171–1178. [PubMed]

15. Sapci, A.H.; Sapci, H.A. Innovative Assisted Living Tools, Remote Monitoring Technologies, Artificial Intelligence Driven Solutions, and Robotic Systems for Aging Societies: Systematic Review. *JMIR Aging 2019* *2*, e15429. [CrossRef]
16. Peek, S.T.; Luijkx, K.G.; Rijnaard, M.D.; Nieboer, M.E.; Van der Voort, C.S.; Van Hoof, J.; Vrijhoef, H.J.; Wouters, E.J. Older Adults' Reasons for Using Technology while Aging in Place. *Gerontechnology* **2016**, *62*, 226–237. [CrossRef] [PubMed]
17. Sanchez, V.G.; Taylor, I.; Bing-Jonsson, P.C. Ethics of smart house welfare technology for older adults: A systematic literature review. *Int. J. Technol. Assess. Health Care* **2017**, *33*, 691–699. [CrossRef] [PubMed]
18. Guillomia, M.A.; Falco, J.L.; Artigas, J.I.; Garcia-Camino, M. Time orientation Technologies in Special Education. *Sensors* **2019**, *19*, 2571. [CrossRef] [PubMed]
19. Agree, E.M. The influence of personal care and assistive devices on the measurement of disability. *Soc. Sci. Med.* **1999**, *48*, 427–443. [CrossRef]

International Journal of *Environmental Research and Public Health*

MDPI

Article

Smart and Age-Friendly Cities in Romania: An Overview of Public Policy and Practice

Loredana Ivan [1], Dorin Beu [2] and Joost van Hoof [3,4,*]

1 Department of Communication, National University of Political Studies and Public Administration, Bulevardul Expoziţiei 30A, 012102 Bucharest, Romania; loredana.ivan@comunicare.ro

2 Faculty of Building Services Engineering, Technical University of Cluj Napoca, Strada Memorandumului 28, 400114 Cluj-Napoca, Romania; dorin.beu@insta.utcluj.ro

3 Faculty of Social Work and Education, The Hague University of Applied Sciences, Johanna Westerdijkplein 75, 2521 EN Den Haag, The Netherlands

4 Institute of Spatial Management, Faculty of Environmental Engineering and Geodesy, Wrocław University of Environmental and Life Sciences, ul. Grunwaldzka 55, 50-357 Wrocław, Poland

* Correspondence: j.vanhoof@hhs.nl

Received: 12 June 2020; Accepted: 16 July 2020; Published: 18 July 2020

Abstract: The role of smart cities in order to improve older people's quality of life, sustainability and opportunities, accessibility, mobility, and connectivity is increasing and acknowledged in public policy and private sector strategies in countries all over the world. Smart cities are one of the technological-driven initiatives that may help create an age-friendly city. Few research studies have analysed emerging countries in terms of their national strategies on smart or age-friendly cities. In this study, Romania which is predicted to become one of the most ageing countries in the European Union is used as a case study. Through document analysis, current initiatives at the local, regional, and national level addressing the issue of smart and age-friendly cities in Romania are investigated. In addition, a case study is presented to indicate possible ways of the smart cities initiatives to target and involve older adults. The role of different stakeholders is analysed in terms of whether initiatives are fragmentary or sustainable over time, and the importance of some key factors, such as private–public partnerships and transnational bodies. The results are discussed revealing the particularities of the smart cities initiatives in Romania in the time frame 2012–2020, which to date, have limited connection to the age-friendly cities agenda. Based on the findings, a set of recommendations are formulated to move the agenda forward.

Keywords: age-friendly cities; smart cities initiatives; smart city; Romania; public policies on smart cities; evaluating smart cities initiatives; older people

---

1. Introduction

All over the world, societies are ageing and older people become increasingly visible in daily living. According to the Organisation for Economic Cooperation and Development (OECD) [1], the population share of those adults aged 65 years and over is expected to rise to 25.1% in 2050 across its member states. A similar pattern can be observed for Romania, a European Union member state which also has an intention to become an OECD member state and whose membership request is under consideration by the OECD Council. Cities in particular have large numbers of older inhabitants; over 40% of all older people live in urban areas. The relationships between ageing populations and urban change, in conjunction with the need to develop supportive urban communities, are a cause of issues and concerns for public policies and practise [2].

The understanding of these relationships led to the emergence of so-called age-friendly cities [3–6]. There are eight domains of an age-friendly city, namely Social participation; Communication and information; Civic participation and employment; Housing; Transportation; Community support and health services; Outdoor spaces and buildings; Respect and social inclusion. The WHO proposed that policies, services, and structures in an age-friendly city, which are related to the physical and social environment, are designed to support and enable older people to "age actively". In other words, to live in security, enjoy good health, and continue to participate fully in society [3,6–8].

Within the framework of age-friendly cities and communities, technology does not play an explicit role [9], but it needs to be noted that in the daily living of older people, technology is all around and cannot be ignored as a major source of support for activities, stimulation of social participation and the provision of care [10–13]. Given the numerous technologies available at present and used by citizens, it is important to explore how such technologies can be used and deployed in the home and across different communities in order to benefit the citizens in the respective age-friendly communities including those communities that are not categorised as age-friendly by the WHO [6,9,10,14]. The new smart age-friendly ecosystem framework proposed by Marston and van Hoof [9] considers the rapid pace in which technology develops but also to ensure all citizens in society are represented, and intersects with the current trends in the domain of smart cities.

Albino et al. [15] attempted to clarify the meaning of smart cities through a literature review, and found that it first emerged in the 1990s. They concluded that it is a multifaceted phenomenon, which includes, amongst others, qualities of people and communities as well as ICTs. There seems to be a lack of universality, both in its definition and in measures of performance [15,16]. Some of the definitions include references to healthcare, for instance, that a smart city is prepared to provide conditions for a healthy and happy community under the challenging conditions that global, environmental, economic, and social trends may bring. Or, the use of smart computing technologies to make the critical infrastructure components and services of a city, including healthcare, more intelligent, interconnected, and efficient [15]. In this paper, a smart city is an urban area that utilises and deploys various electronic Internet of Things devices and sensors [12], which have the ability to collect data and utilise the data in an attempt to provide efficient and smarter resources to residents and communities. A wide array of data can be collected from public and private sources, which can be processed for the better good of society [17]. In relation to advancing age-friendly interventions, the WHO touches upon the collaboration with transnational (city) networks, such as smart cities networks, for which addressing ageing will help advance their strategic priorities [9]. Podgórniak-Krzykacz et al. [18] also called for smart cities to seek to ensure meeting the needs of older citizens and promoting solutions tailored to their computer literacy, digital skills, and perception capabilities. A similar trend was also seen by Woolrych et al. [19] in relation to emerging technologies for the support of health and independence of senior citizens. In their study, many senior citizens were willing to use a wide range of technologies in the context of age-friendly smart cities. In a study on age-friendly city development in South Australia, Zaman and Thornton [20] identified a large set of priority indicators. One of the topics raised is the provision of training for older people on the latest technologies. Additionally, Gudowsky et al. [21] and Righi et al. [22] stated that smart cities need to adapt to ageing societies and that great hopes are projected on technology to support solutions for urban ageing.

A growing number of cities and communities worldwide are striving to better meet the needs of their older residents. The WHO Global Network for Age-friendly Cities and Communities was established to foster the exchange of experience and mutual learning between cities and communities worldwide (Figure 1). Cities and communities in the network are of different sizes and are located in different parts of the world. Their efforts to become more age-friendly take place within very diverse cultural and socioeconomic contexts. What all members of the Network do have in common is the desire and commitment to promoting healthy and active ageing and a good quality of life for their older residents. Romania does not have any cities or communities that are members of the WHO Global Network for Age-friendly Cities and Communities. At the same time, there are numerous smart city initiatives in the country, which may or may not intersect with the age-friendly cities movement and its strategic agenda.

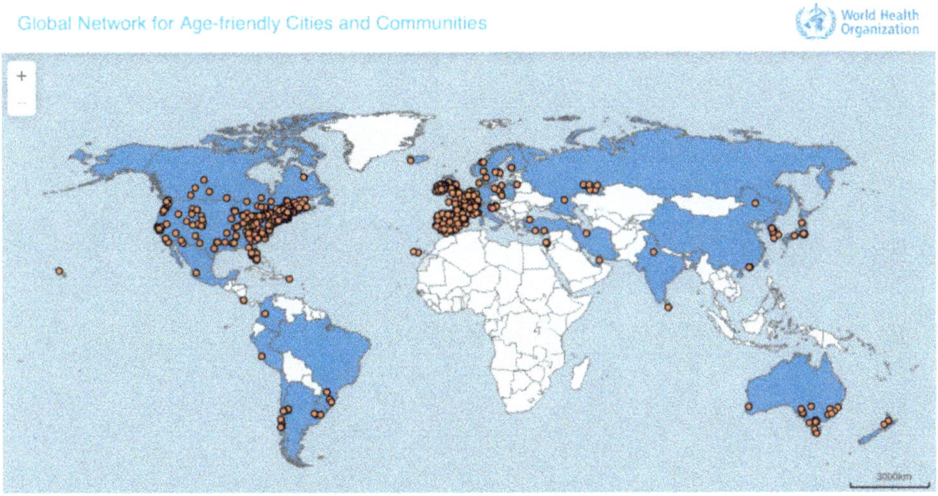

Figure 1. No city in Romania has yet joined the Global Network for Age-friendly Cities and Communities (status quo July 2020) [23].

The current study investigates smart city initiatives at the local, regional, and national level in Romania aiming to answer the following research questions:

Research Question 1: *What are the main characteristics of smart city initiatives in Romania during the past eight years*? The time period 2012–2020 is used as a time frame after exploring the moment such initiatives started to develop to a large scale, in several Development Regions around the country. The goal is to investigate whether the initiatives were mainly national or local, private or public, coherent or sporadic, short-term-oriented or long-term-oriented; what was the role of the industry and of the private operators, the type of projects (strategic, policy-oriented, concrete actions, etc.), and also what was the role of the transnational organisations in financing and promoting such initiatives?

Research Question 2: *To what extent do the smart cities initiatives in Romania, for the past eight years, have an age-friendly component*? This question investigates the extent to which the large-scale smart city projects developed in Romania had frail and vulnerable groups of people as an explicit objective, for instance, in terms of access to urban facilities and urban life in general. The main focus is on the older population and whether such initiatives took the older population into consideration in developing smart cities initiatives.

The paper starts with background information on the country of Romania and key cities. This is followed by an overview of the methodology and the results of the social document analysis on existing smart city initiatives and practices from Romania. Subsequently, the results are discussed revealing the particularities of the smart cities initiatives in Romania, in the time frame 2012–2020. This is followed by a conclusion and recommendations section for future steps that Romania could take to move the agenda forward, and how to connect the smart cities' and age-friendly cities' agendas for the future development of urban centres in Romania.

2. Outline of Romania

The Republic of Romania is divided into three major regions: Walachia (Southern part, with Bucharest the capital of Romania as the main city), Transylvania (Western part, with Cluj-Napoca and Brașov as main cities) and Moldavia (Eastern part—with Iași as the main city), and as well as some other minor regions (Figure 2). The Carpathian mountain range is the main natural barrier dividing these major regions. The territorial and administrative organisation of Romania is based on Law 2/1968, which is still valid today. There are seven so-called Development Regions (North-West, West,

Centre, North-East, South-East, South-West, and South) plus the Bucharest and Ilfov Region (Figure 3). Romania's demographics are split between Romanian nationals (22,204,507 in 2019) and actual residents (19,414,458 in 2019) due to the emigration of the population to other European Union member states (Table 1). The last census was held in 2011 when 21.4 million people were expected to live in the country. The final outcome of the census was a population of 20.1 million people, as many citizens are working abroad without a work permit, or by returning every three or six months from working abroad. Officially, between 1990 and 2018, 577,555 persons have emigrated permanently, but the actual number of people working abroad remains unclear. Some journalists mention a potential decline of the Romanian population by as much as 30% in 2050 based on international reports [24].

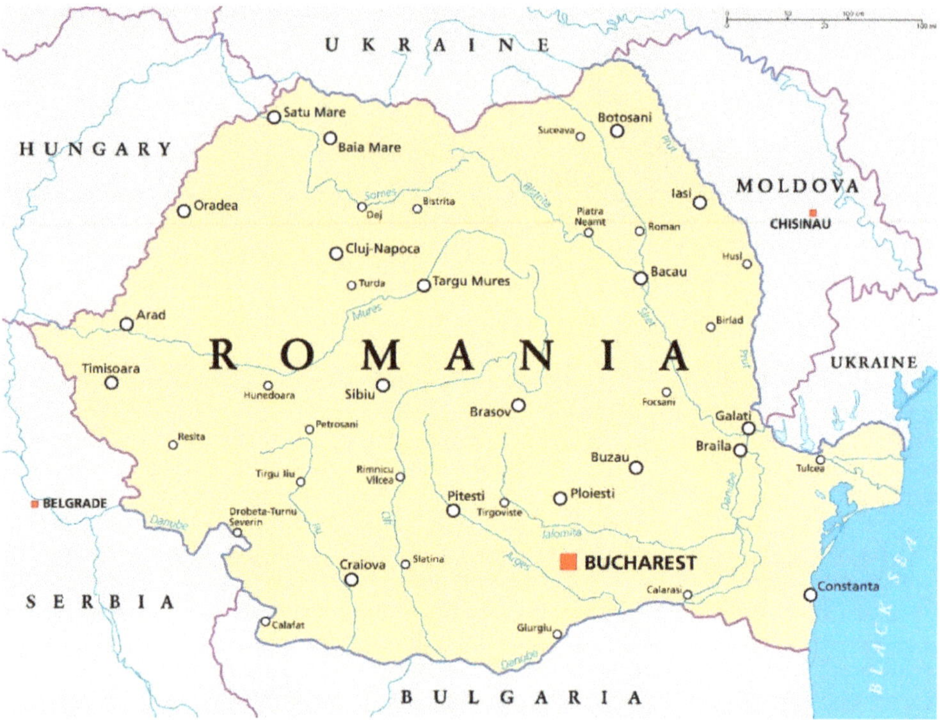

Figure 2. Map of Romania and its main population centres. Source: https://www.shutterstock.com/nl/image-vector/romania-political-map-capital-bucharest-national-321930074.

Table 1. Basic statistics of Romania [25,26].

Total Population (2017)	19,778,000
Gross national income per capita (EUR PPP international $, 2017)	18,800
Life expectancy at birth m/f (years, 2017)	72/79
Probability of dying under the age of five (per 1000 live births, 2018)	7
Probability of dying between the ages of 15 and 60 years m/f (per 1000 population, 2016)	191/77
Total expenditure on health per capita (Intl $, 2017)	1079
Total expenditure on health as % of GDP (2017)	5.0

According to official figures from the National Statistics Institute [26], where data is available for the years 1992 to 2019, there is a decline of around 4% of the population (Table 2). The percentage of the urban population has risen from 53.9 to 56.4%. When it comes to the ageing of the population, the percentage of older people has risen from 10.9% in 1992 to 16.5% in 2019 (for people over 85 years from

0.6 to 1.8%, Tables 3 and 4). This increase is mainly due to urbanisation, and the availability of better healthcare services.

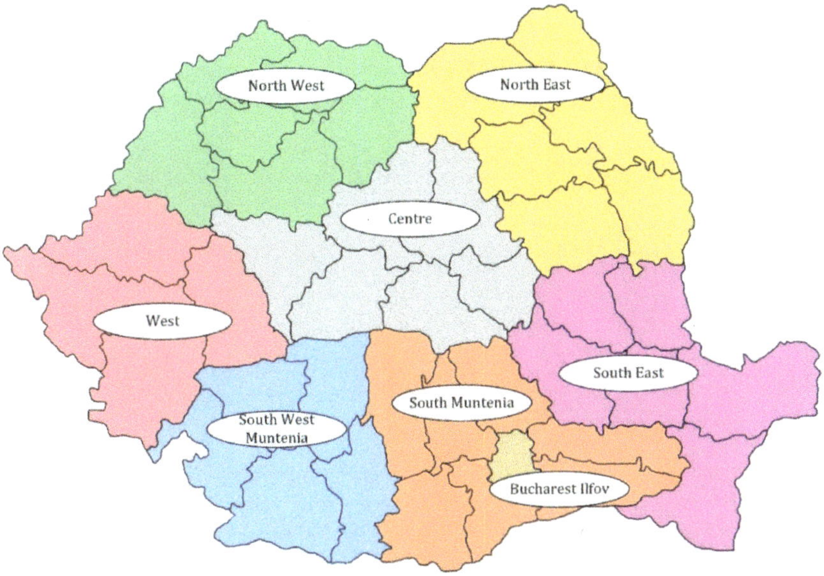

Figure 3. Map of Romania and its Development Regions. Taken and adapted from source: https://en.wikipedia.org/wiki/Development_regions_of_Romania#/media/File:Regiuni_de_dezvoltare.svg.

Table 2. The population of Romania and the main Development Regions [26].

	Total Population 1992	Total Population 2019
Romania	23,143,860	22,204,507
Urban Romania	12,478,618	12,520,160
Rural Romania	10,665,242	9,684,347
North-West Region	2,964,507	2,833,789
West Region	2,118,807	2,003,368
Centre Region	2,709,383	2,631,033
North-East Region	3,861,059	3,979,271
South-East Region	3,000,498	2,828,048
South-West Region	2,448,573	2,163,319
South Region	3,574,993	3,194,237
Bucharest and Ilfov Region	2,466,040	2,571,442

Table 3. The older population of Romania per age cohort [26].

Age Range	Romania		Urban Romania		Rural Romania	
	1992	2019	1992	2019	1992	2019
65–69	1,033,959	1,251,318	403,076	755,541	630,883	495,777
70–74	560,805	840,746	215,436	454,052	345,369	386,694
75–79	481,408	664,299	178,586	330,687	302,822	333,612
80–84	306,882	526,865	108,831	249,097	198,051	277,768
85+	141,672	389,476	49,506	185,201	92,166	204,275
Total	2,524,726	3,672,704	955,435	1,974,578	1,569,291	1,698,126

Take, for example, the city of Cluj-Napoca. In this city, there is a slight increase of the population with around 4%, but a major increase of the older population from 8.65% in 1992 to 17.14% in 2019 (Table 4). Like many Romanian cities, a large number of people moved from the rural area to towns during communist times, when there was a high demand for a labour force in the industry. This also explains the higher percentage of the older people in the countryside. Since 2000 a lot of new buildings have been developed in the area around Cluj-Napoca. Floreşti, a village in the suburban area of Cluj-Napoca, has seen its population increase from 5574 inhabitants in 1992 to 39,652 in 2019, which is more than seven times as much.

Table 4. The older population of main Romanian cities per age cohort [26].

Age Range	Cluj-Napoca		Constanţa		Braşov		Iaşi		Bucharest	
	1992	2019	1992	2019	1992	2019	1992	2019	1992	2019
65–69	11,033	19,728	10,938	22,422	10,400	20,494	8825	21,898	97,569	134,723
70–74	6902	13,349	5138	13,345	5739	11,781	4811	12,516	56,886	84,278
75–79	4409	10,110	4239	10,432	3911	8822	3711	8199	46,845	58,339
80–84	3295	7223	2593	7886	2524	7174	2450	6338	28,705	49,430
85+	1493	5504	1260	5591	1068	5240	1261	4558	12,891	49,211
Total	27,132	55,914	24,168	59,676	23,462	53,511	21,058	53,509	242,896	375,981

According to the OECD [25], the life expectancy of Romanians has increased from 71.2 in 2000 to 75.3 years in 2017, with a high gender gap of 7.4 years (71.7 years for men and 79.1 for women). The most important cause of death remains ischaemic heart disease (three times higher than in the European Union as a whole) and stroke. The proportion of people aged 65 years and over reported to be in good health is 23% (compared with a European Union average of 41.4%). A total of 46% of the population aged 65 years and over have one or more chronic diseases, and 31% of this population reports some limitations in their activities of daily living.

In 2017, Romania spent €1029 per capita for health and most of this amount was spent on hospital care (42%) and pharmaceuticals and medical devices (27%). There is a shortage of physicians and nurses in Romania, which is mainly due to the large-scale emigration of skilled workers to countries that offer higher salaries. There are also additional challenges concerning the availability of general practitioners (GPs) in Romania: 328 communities (villages) have no GP available. A total of 559,611 persons, or 2.52% of Romanians, have no GP in the village where they live. In a total of 1414 cities and villages, there is a shortage of 2187 GPs. Only 271 cities have sufficient or even excess GP capacity, such as Bucharest and other university cities [27].

In each of the Romanian cities, there is a Department of Social Assistance, which includes departments like child and family protection. This department also takes care of the provision of assistance for older people. The service was initiated after 1990, mainly for solving the problem of abandoned children in Romania. It is currently in a slow transition towards providing services for an ageing population. The Department offers services such as daycare and activities in activity centres for older people, but currently, no projects are running to support the use of technology by older people.

Smart and Sustainable Housing

According to the Buildings Performance Institute Europe (BPIE) [16], 47.5% of the dwellings are in the rural area (95% unfamiliar houses) and in the urban area, 72% of the dwellings are in large blocks of flats, with an average of 40 apartments per block. Additionally, according to BPIE [28], the average surface of a dwelling is 55 m^2, with a majority of them built between 1960 and 1990. As the comfort standard of homes built during this period was low, there is a clear need for investment to update the quality of living and the quality of the home itself. According to Eurostat [29], the housing market in Romania is largely in private hands. A total of 96.8% of people live in owner-occupied dwellings, of which a mere 47% are overcrowded. This limits the use of European, national or local funding schemes for the improvement of homes. In Romania, the use of European funds is limited to improvements of the outer shells of buildings, for instance, adding or improving thermal insulation, and installing new insulating windows. National programmes can be used to install photovoltaic panels. At present, there are no (structural) subsidies for upgrading existing homes with smart home technologies. When it comes to new residential developments, there is a local sustainable certification system called Green Homes, developed by Romanian Green Buildings Council—RoGBC [30], which encourages sustainable and smart housing. According to RoGBC, a total of 10,905 new apartments in 44 projects are Green Homes certified [30]. The domains of this certification that can be classified as age-friendly are as follows:

- Entrances (installation of ramps, lighting, and automated doors for wheelchair access);
- Lighting (better lighting for safer homes, avoidance of glare, dimming options and night orientation lighting from the bedroom to toilet, motion sensors in circulation areas);
- Circulation space (possibility for turning a wheelchair in all spaces of the home);
- Accommodation of mobility devices (wheelchairs);
- Toilet and bathroom walls (firm fixing and grab bars/rails);
- Location of control services (height band from 450 mm to 1200 mm above the floor level);
- Flooring materials in common spaces (soft and resilient materials to avoid falls and gentler underfoot);
- Installation of handrails (both sides of a wall at high and low levels);
- Way-finding in common areas (use of different colours and textures and Braille signage);
- Installation of an intercom which is easy-to-use with visual intercom for people with a hearing impairment.

All the features mentioned above are part of a set of hardware solutions for an age-friendly home, which can be supplemented by smart home solutions. At present, there is no national programme intended for the construction of smart homes and there are no regulations for the design of age-friendly homes.

3. Methodology

Document analysis [31], which is based on keyword clustering, was used as a method to evaluate the current state-of-the-art of smart city programmes and action plans in Romania (Figure 4). In addition, it was also investigated whether the smart city strategies and solutions were age-inclusive or had an age-friendly component. By clustering, documents based on the criteria of keyword similarity were grouped. Two keywords were used to cluster the documents: "smart city" and "age-friendly city" (in Romanian smart-city and age-friendly are neologisms, used as such in the current language). The frequencies of these two keywords were studied in the documents and potentially for the co-occurrence of the two terms.

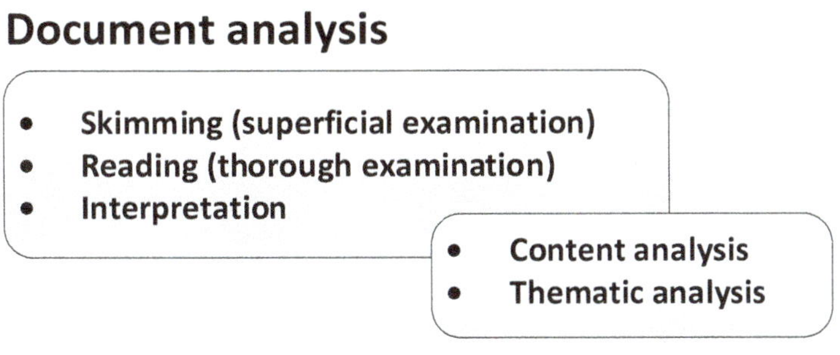

Figure 4. The process of document analysis [31].

3.1. Corpus of Analysis

A variety of policy papers, official documents, and websites presenting different initiatives both from the public institutions and from the industry, pieces of legislation and presentations in local conferences on the topic of smart city, were included. Programmatic documents and concrete projects were selected, which contained a set of measures impacting the community at the local, regional or national levels, affecting the lives of a sufficient number of people, and containing more than one single output, with a duration of at least one year.

In total, 53 documents were selected after searching on the main news portal in Romania [32], using the keywords: "smart city" and "age friendly city" and on the dedicated websites of the public institutions and professional organisations. These websites included those of The Romanian Association for Smart City and Mobility (RSCMA); The Ministry of Energy, The Ministry of Waters and Forests; The Chamber of Commerce and Industry of Romania; The Ministry of Regional Development and Public Administration of Romania; The Ministry of Telecommunication; and The Ministry of Health. Documents were selected for the time frame of 2012–2020, based on the fact that the year 2012 marks the year in which the first programmes labelled as "smart city" emerged in Romania. Once we identified the main cities in which such programmes were deployed (namely, Alba Iulia, Bucharest, Brașov, Baia Mare, Cluj-Napoca, Craiova, Iași, Suceava, Vaslui, Oradea, and Timișoara), the respective websites of these municipalities were also searched, as the particular municipality or local administration had a role in all local or regional initiatives that were encountered in this search.

3.2. Coding Procedure

In the first phase, initiatives belonging to the same programme and having the same stakeholders were grouped separately. In such cases, the main objective of the programme and the key action plan were used for clustering the documents. Programmatic documents were grouped as well (as, for example, national strategies), separately from the concrete projects containing a set of measures impacting the community at the local, regional, or national level.

In the final stage, documents were selected taking into account the following criteria: whether they affect the lives of a sufficient number of people, and contain more than one single output, with a duration of at least one year. In total, there were 30 initiatives, which were coded in line with the research questions. An axial coding system was used to code the documents on the following categories: (2) the organisation which initiated the programme and the key stakeholders (1) the type of action (local, regional, national); (3) the role of private/public sector; (4) type of document (programmatic documents, strategies, concrete actions, publicity, training, or other types of initiative); (5) the main objectives; (6) the age-friendly component—implicit or explicit; (7) the role of the industry (for example, in suggesting solutions/realising the actions); (8) the role of a transnational bodies/organisations—for example, in advising, promoting, financing, launching a particular initiative. The year (of the time frame) of the initiatives included in the analysis were recorded.

4. Results

This section presents the main characteristics of smart city initiatives in Romania in 2012–2020. The results from the coding process are presented in detail in Appendix A. The following subsections present the findings from this table in extenso. These subsections deal with (1) The regional disparities, and lock on inter-regional cooperation; (2) The governance; (3) The type of project, and the main objectives, (4) The role of transnational organisations; and (5) The age-friendly component of the projects. The final subsection deals with a short case study, which presents one the initiatives with an explicit age-friendly component (i.e., older people's access health services), namely the 4D Cities project from Baia Sprie.

The findings suggest the existence of a process of initiating and implementing smart city initiatives in Romania, in which some factors play an important role. For example, already existing economic disparities between the seven Development Regions in Romania create the context of different opportunities to contribute as local municipalities with local funds in cofinancing such projects. In addition, disparities in the economic development of the different regions create a chain in the process of implementing smart cities projects that would work in favour of the more advanced and developed regions: the ability to attract major private companies to invest in public–private partnerships for such initiatives is not equally distributed, and the human resources as well are concentrated in the most developed regions.

Regional disparities and the differences in the economic development between Development Regions favour the development of smart city initiatives in the three most developed regions of the country: Ilfov Region, North-West Region and West Region, whereas the other regions are left behind. The process perpetuates the cycle of inequalities (Figure 5).

Other important players with a decisive role in the chain of the implementation of smart city projects in Romania are the transnational organisations, mainly European Union programmes and grants, which are almost an exclusive source of financing of such projects for local and regional authorities. Consequently, the local authorities (most of the time municipalities) submit projects in line with those grants and not necessarily in line with the local priorities. This leads to a second vicious cycle (Figure 5), namely a gap between the local needs in terms of enhancing some of the "smart city" ideas, for example, the increased access for vulnerable persons to services and city opportunities) and the transnational priorities reflected in the European Union grants. On the one hand, local authorities initiate projects that are granted by the transnational bodies (for example, the Economic Competitiveness Sectorial Operational Program) and this would give them expertise in applying and implementing such projects and moving the "smart city" agenda forward. On the other hand, other opportunities to launch such projects (for example, through regional cooperation) are not sufficiently explored.

The chain of disparities (Figure 5) shows a tendency towards top-down approaches in terms of funding, with the transnational organisations having a central role in the "smart city" priorities set by the local authorities. In addition, there is also a tendency towards fragmentation and a poor articulation between smart city initiatives, due to their local implementation.

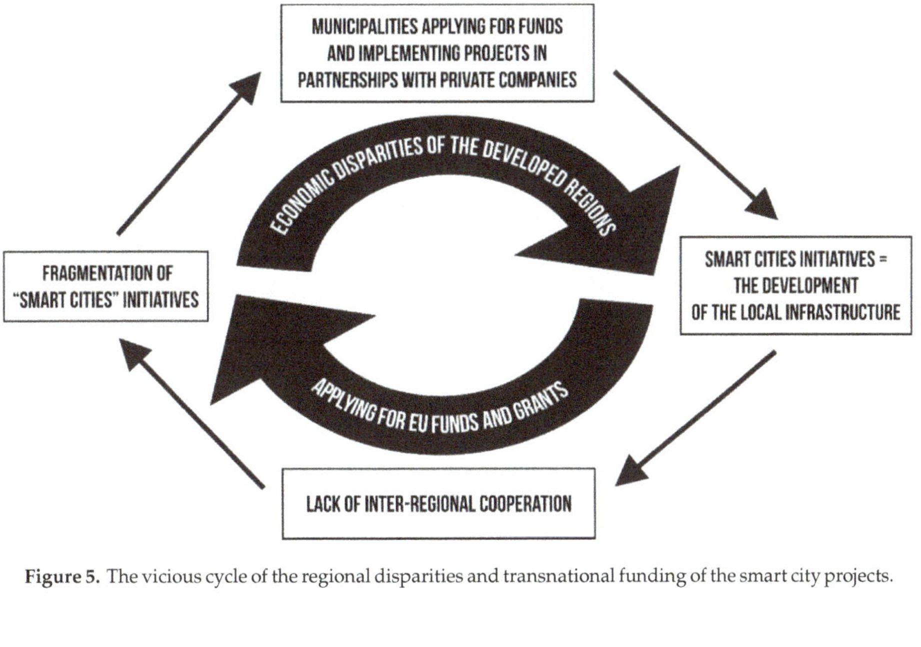

Figure 5. The vicious cycle of the regional disparities and transnational funding of the smart city projects.

4.1. The Regional Disparities and Lock on Inter-Regional Cooperation

Smart city solutions have been implemented in a few cities in Romania. The most important cities, in terms the number of citizens, the size of the industry and the economic power, are Bucharest (the capital city), Brașov, Sibiu, Timișoara, Craiova, and Cluj-Napoca. Most of the initiatives in these cities were local or regional initiatives, and the few national initiatives concerned mainly programmatic documents, policies, training activities or strategic action plans. Some of the national initiatives aimed to promote the smart city idea and smart city projects (such as the Annual Smart City Urban Projects Fair, since 2017).

Although the concrete smart-city actions were focused on the local and the regional levels, they accentuate the regional disparities at the country level, namely by be concentrated in the three most developed regions in Romania: the Bucharest-Ilfov Region, the North-West Region (around the cities Cluj-Napoca, Baia Mare and Oradea), the West Region (around the city of Timișoara), as well as in the Centre Development Region (around the cities of Brașov and Sibiu). The other four Development Regions (North-East, South-East, South-Muntenia, and South-West Oltenia) were less represented in regional initiatives and were represented more at the local level, as one-time and short-term projects. Only two large cities from the other four Development Regions were involved in smart-city initiatives in the 2012–2020 timeframes, namely Iași (located in the North-East region) and Craiova (located in the South-West Oltenia region).

This study also found that the regional economic disparities correspond with gaps in smart-city initiatives: more developed regions as the Bucharest-Ilfov Region and North-West Region have had more projects over the past eight years and have witnessed more articulated initiatives, whereas the other regions had fewer initiatives, saw more contextual projects (particularly related to calls for projects at the European Union level) and saw an actual lack of a long-term vision to the implementation of the "smart city" idea. Nevertheless, the already existing economic disparities between the Development Regions are reflected in the way smart cities projects were initiated and implemented. The lack of a strategic policy plan at the national level may eventually result in an increased regional gap.

In fact, the only regional cooperation that was found in the 30 analysed initiatives was the Western Alliance made up of the cities of Cluj-Napoca, Timișoara, Oradea, and Arad (Appendix A), launched in 2018, as a regional cooperation (North-West Region and West Development Region) aiming to improve the infrastructure in this part of the country. The agreement of the municipalities from the main cities in the two regions is focused on private–public partnerships through infrastructure projects, namely the support for the Transylvania Motorway project and Timișoara—Belgrade Motorway project, metropolitan underground transport systems, and tram projects, which are all positioned under the smart city umbrella (i.e., the ecological mobility).

Some of the medium-sized cities, such as Suceava and Vaslui (North-East Development Region), manage to have two large projects in the domain of smart cities: Suceava between 2012 and 2015, and Vaslui, between 2014 and 2020. In both cities, the idea of urban markets and sustainable food in urban communities (low carbon emissions) exploited the specificity of the region, such as the rural population, the presence of small farms, and an ageing/older population which is highly affected by emigration.

4.2. The Governance

Smart city solutions were only implemented in a few cities in Romania. With the exception of The National Strategy for Smart City, a programmatic document, the rest of the initiatives are private projects which with a mix of public–private governance: private companies in partnership with public authorities, most of the times municipalities, city halls, local authorities, but also national authorities such as The Ministry of Regional Development and Public Administration, and The Ministry of Energy. In the two operational programmes, Regional Operational Programme (version 1 for 2007–2013 and version 2 for 2014–2013), research institutes and universities were also involved. The role of private operators and the role of the industry, in general, seem to be very important in all the initiatives. Additionally, the number of economic operators is relatively large. For instance, over 600 economic operators contributed to the Regional Operational Programme. The industry participates in the activities and implementation stage of various programmes, as well as in training activities, in elaborating policies and action plans and in promoting different programmes related to the smart city concept. For example, The Romanian Association for Smart City and Mobility (RSCMA), a private body, forms a working group and takes part in the Smart City National Strategy. In addition, the RSCMA runs the Smart City Academy, a national training platform. The mission of this platform is to train smart city experts working for the participating companies, as well as from the central and local administrations. Moreover, as many activities from the smart city programmes in Romania consist of implementing digital solutions, Internet-based applications, free Wi-Fi in public transportation, and Internet-based technical solutions, the large multinational enterprises already existing on the Romanian market played a key role in the smart city initiatives. For example, in the Smart City Alba Iulia 2016–2018 pilot project, two large telecommunications' companies, which are key actors in the Internet and telephony industry on the Romanian market, played an important role. Additionally, some private companies offered developing grants, for example, in the case of Bucharest and the Smarter Cities Grants.

The role of the private enterprises in leading or implementing smart city projects in Romania comes along with accusations of corruption and potential distrust of the citizens in the partnership between the local administration (such as municipalities) and the industry. For example, Bucharest Smart City Development Strategy was based on a partnership between the Bucharest City Hall and an accountancy firm—in which the private enterprise provided consultancy in defining the strategy; this project was discussed in the local media because of alleged corruption [33]. Nevertheless, the partnership between private and public institutions is a relatively common aspect in all the smart city initiatives that were analysed for the time frame of 2012 to 2020.

4.3. Type of Projects and Main Objectives

Among the 30 analysed initiatives two were programmatic documents: Romanian Smart City Projects (a strategic plan started in 2016, aiming at the implementation of 320 Smart City projects in Romania, with a budget of €15 billion); and The National Strategy for Smart City (2018) developed under the supervision of The Ministry of Regional Development and Public Administration of Romania and experts from other ministries, including a working group from RSCMA. Both are strategic action plans, with a long-term approach. Three initiatives aimed to promote projects in the area of smart city concepts, and its activities were linked to the idea of promotion and awareness: Smart City Industry Awards (since 2016); Smart City Caravan (since 2017); Annual Smart City Urban Projects Fair (since 2017). Besides promotion, complementary projects have been developed, having publishing (Smart City Magazine, since 2016), training of experts (Smart City Academy, since 2017) and respectively lobbying (The Romanian Association for Smart City and Mobility working group, 2018) as objectives. Additionally, some of the initiatives remained in the stage of policies and strategic action plans, without any concrete actions or implementation (at least not in the mentioned initiative): Baia Mare USE ACT Urban Renewal (2015-policy plan); Bucharest IBM Smarter Cities Challenge grant (2010–2011, strategy and business analytics); Alba Iulia: City Logo (2010, a branding initiative focused on cultural tourism). The latter one was a contextual project aiming for a revival of the historical city of Alba Iulia, in anticipation of the 2018 centenary celebration of Romania becoming a unified state (The Great Union of 1918, at 1st December, Alba Iulia). Practically, one-third of the initiatives that were analysed were not followed by actual actions and implementation.

The rest of the initiatives required different actions and implementation of the various strategic plans. The main objectives of the actions (Appendix A) were coded, and it revealed that the smart city concept sphere is reduced to the following aspects: smart transport and ecological mobility (six initiatives); Free Wi-Fi and public safety using Internet solutions (six initiatives), recycling and garbage collection, and lower CO_2 emissions (six initiatives); saving energy including the control of lighting and public illumination (five initiatives); e-government (four initiatives), regeneration of small and medium-sized towns and disadvantaged neighbourhoods (four initiatives); sustainable development and land use (four initiatives); intelligent buildings and renewable and sustainable energy (four initiatives); and smart tourism such as a city app (four initiatives). The main objectives of the action plans in the different cities and small localities were focused on improving the infrastructure by applying ecological aspects and Internet-integrated applications. There was no particular regard to improving the daily lives of different categories of the Romanian population (such as older people or even peasants) that might be at risk of exclusion and marginalisation in the new "smart" living environment.

4.4. The Role of Transnational Organisations

The strategic programmes on smart cities have been initiated in Romania in close connection with programmes run by the European Union (Appendix A). Dedicated transnational bodies (for instance, European Union programmes and grants) played a key role in what type of projects was run through the country and which time frame they had. Particularly, The Smart City Association and Economic Competitiveness Sectorial Operational Program had a role in sustaining, financing, and promoting four of the analysed initiatives, and also the Economic Competitiveness Sectorial Operational Program (2007–2013; 2014–2020) supported some of the initiatives as a part of their grants. The same is valid for the Regional Operational Programme 2014–2020, which was also initiated by the European Union, who had a key role in the projects developed by the Bucharest Municipality and Bucharest-Ilfov Development Region. The European Union programmes created the opportunity of applying for grants in the smart city area, but also guidelines and standards of quality. The programmes also indicated specific smart city objectives, leaving some freedom to the regions, while prioritising some of the domains (as, for example, infrastructure and Internet-based technologies). In addition, the European Union programmes have contributed to fragmentation, as many of the projects run exclusively within the specific time frame of a specific European Union programme.

One important organisation, which plays a role in many of the actions concerning smart city initiatives, is URBACT (www.urbact.eu), a European Union organisation that promotes and monitors urban projects in the European Union member states. URBACT has a specific mission to help cities (including by financing programmes) in order to create sustainable development, by integrating environmentally friendly solutions. Seven out of the 30 analysed initiatives were supported, financed, and/or promoted through URBACT and this explains the focus of the programmes on the main objectives listed above. In addition, some private organisations have financed smart city initiatives. Still, the role of such private organisations in financing important, long-term strategies in the area of smart cities remains rather peripheral. Such enterprises are mostly involved in private–public partnerships with local municipalities or city halls.

4.5. The Age-Friendly Component

The age-friendly component is mostly absent in the most prominent smart city programmes and strategies in Romania for the past eight years. Still some initiatives (six out of 30) have an implicit age-friendly approach, as some of the initiatives address older people as a potential target group. For example, the RE-Block Disadvantaged Neighbourhoods initiative (Iași, 2018) was coded as an initiative that implicitly addresses the issue of age-friendliness. The initiative addressed disadvantaged communities in Romania (in Iași county and beyond), which are highly depopulated, with large segments of the population (particularly older population from rural areas and small localities) living in poor conditions, and with a lower quality of life. However, when going through the objectives and the action plans, such issues were addressed implicitly; not in explicit measures directed to the vulnerable cohorts of the population. The six initiatives were coded as implicit age-friendly programmes because they were implemented in the less economically developed Development Regions, which are highly affected by emigration and which have an increasingly older population. Still, neither of these initiatives explicitly addressed the age-friendly component, nor included age-friendly objects in the action plans.

By addressing the disadvantaged neighbourhoods, these initiatives had a more bottom-up approach and focused more on the disadvantaged local communities and their particular needs.

The lack of age-friendly components in the existing smart city initiatives in Romania is also linked with the type of programme objectives such initiatives had in recent years. As mentioned before, infrastructure, ecological aspects (such as recycling), smart transportation, and energy saving were among the most common priorities in the way "smart city" phenomena were operationalised during the past eight years. For instance, the project by the Western Alliance did not mention any age-friendly component as a goal of any trans-regional cooperation. The aforementioned projects in Suceava and Vaslui dealt with the idea of urban markets and sustainable food. These two cases are of interest because they had an implicit age-friendly component. In fact, only six out of 30 initiatives could be coded as having an explicit age-friendly component, all in relatively small-sized cities. Besides the two projects in Suceava and Vaslui, the project from Baia Sprie (4D Cities Baseline Study, Appendix A) is a project aiming to diversify the health services based on 4D tools, especially in emergency and safety situations. This project is used for the case study described below.

Case Study: Baia Sprie 4D Cities

The 4D Cities Baseline Study project (2012–2013; 2014–2020) was financed by URBACT, under the European Regional Development Fund of the European Union. The 4D Cities project aimed to promote innovative ways of delivering healthcare services and increase access to healthcare services of the vulnerable groups, including older people. Additionally, the projects aimed to stimulate social participation in providing innovative healthcare solutions (such as volunteering and crowdfunding), as well as for a public–private partnership involving the community in different action plans.

Baia Sprie is a small-sized town with 16,000 inhabitants, located 9 km from Baia Mare (a municipality and one of the largest cities of the North West Development Region of Romania). Traditionally, 50% of the local population worked in the mining industry and the percentage of people working has decreased over time, due to the closing of the local mines. The majority of the young population migrated to Baia Mare or moved abroad for work, whereas Baia Sprie became a typically small locality with an increasingly older population and poor living conditions. The high incidence of chronic diseases (as pulmonary diseases) is related to the miners' working conditions, thus, the importance of the health services for the local population was underlined in the project. The closure of the Chronic Disease Hospital pressed the City Council of Baia Sprie to create a partnership with private healthcare providers. In this context, the 4D Cities Baia Sprie project aims to diversify the health services through community involvement (social innovation tools). The initial focus was on professional medical care for emergency and safety situations. Furthermore, the project included the restoration of a local health centre for post-traumatic rehabilitation and regular treatment. Older people were involved as beneficiaries of the project but not in the project design and implementation.

An URBACT local support group was created to work in partnership with the city hall and the health centre. Still, not much information is publicly available about the results of this project, the success indicators and its sustainability. The municipality gives the same information as the URBACT website, meaning that there is only access to the main objectives, the source of financing, and the strategic plan. Information regarding the implementation, the success indicators, the evaluation of the project, possibilities of continuation, difficulties, and risks and also about the community involvement is not publicly available.

5. Discussion

Consistent with Bătăgan [34] and Rotună et al. [35], who previously analysed the dynamics of various indicators of the smart city concepts in Romania (such as e-governance [34]; smart cities ranking indicators [35]), this study also found that the regional economic disparities correspond with gaps in smart-city initiatives: more developed regions as the Bucharest-Ilfov Region and North-West Region have had more projects over the past eight years and have witnessed more articulated initiatives, whereas the other regions had fewer initiatives, saw more contextual projects (particularly related to calls for projects at the European Union level) and saw an actual lack of a long-term vision to the implementation of the "smart city" idea. In short, they were developed mainly in a few large cities: Bucharest (the capital city), Brașov, Baia Mare, Cluj-Napoca, Iași, and Timișoara. Some of the small to medium-sized cities where such programmes have been deployed (such as Alba Iulia, Suceava and Vaslui) benefitted from contextual European Union programmes and these cities got involved in a one-time initiative aiming at the revival of potential historical or cultural heritage. Manika [36] also found that in the case of smart cities, the European Union public procurement legislative framework encourages the deployment of innovation and sets the scene for a more strategic procurement for smart cities.

This study further found that smart city initiatives around the country accentuate the socioeconomic disparities between the eight Development Regions of Romania. For example, the South-Muntenia Development Region did not have a single smart city initiative within its borders. Four other Development Regions were hardly represented in the current sample of documents as well. Taking into account that The National Strategy for Smart City was launched in 2018, the regional disparities should have been considered when updating the strategy. Furthermore, only one initiative involving the cooperation between two Development Regions was identified. The transregional cooperation in such projects could be a goal to follow when planning the long-term strategy for smart cities in Romania.

Most of the smart city initiatives analysed had a mixed governance, consisting of public–private partnerships, usually between city halls or municipalities and different private enterprises. Costantino and Pellegrino [37] analysed how public–private partnerships have been adopted across the world and their characteristics, both in developed and developing countries, through a multiple case comparison methodology. The three most important aspects characterising a public–private partnership transaction are the risk transfer to the private partner, the use of private financing, and the use of private expertise and management skills. They found the same behaviour in their case studies in terms of risk transfer to the private party and use of private expertise and management skills in public–private partnership projects. Developed countries showed significantly greater use of private financing [37].

Although the key role of the industry in Romanian projects can be explained by taking into account the technical solutions required in the implementation of smart city projects, some of the initiatives, strategies, consultancy, policy documents, and training, could have benefitted more from the expertise of public research institutes. In only two out of 30 initiatives, research institutes and universities were involved. It was noted that some of the initiatives have created public debate concerning the potential risk of corruption and this might happen also due to the prominent role of various private operations in all the stages of smart city programmes, from the design stage all the way up to the stage of implementation.

Schipper and Silvius [38] looked at the characteristics of smart sustainable city development and the implications for project management. They stated that cities may require a centralised and comprehensive approach to strike an appropriate balance between diverse service exploration in different domains and intensive service exploitation. Publicly driven partnerships may help to accelerate smart city adoption at an early stage [38]. In the case of Croatian smart cities, Milenković et al. [39] showed how the government's role in public–private partnership projects is to evaluate and approve detailed execution plans of the concessionaire while the private partner's role is to design, build, finance, and operate the facilities.

The initiatives that were analysed for the Romanian context covered only some dimensions of the concept of a "smart city", particularly smart transport and ecologically-friendly mobility, free Wi-Fi and public safety, recycling and garbage and lower CO_2 emissions, energy savings, e-government, sustainable development and land use; regeneration of small and medium towns and disadvantaged neighbourhoods, intelligent buildings, renewable and sustainable energy, and smart tourism, which is in line with the societal aspects and key performance indicators of smart cities identified by other studies including Baltac [40] and Angelakoglou et al. [41]. Only one initiative was identified which addressed the access to services (health services) for vulnerable cohorts. Therefore, it is concluded that the "smart city" idea in Romania is strongly linked to the improvement of the country's infrastructure, saving energy and reducing CO_2 emissions, which is a relatively restrictive view of the concept of smart cities. The notion that some cohorts within the population, older people in particular, may benefit from the outcomes of some of the smart city programmes is not explicitly stated. The lack of age-friendly components in the Romanian smart city initiatives could be partially explained by the fact that local authorities have focused more on projects connected with the development of the infrastructure (for instance, infrastructure for recycling and saving energy), and to a lesser extent on the community needs. This is visible from the documents selected in the corpus and coded (Appendix A). The case of Romania could be typical for other middle-income countries in the European Union, as developing infrastructure, including Internet-based technologies, is seen as a sign of progress by the local authorities. Consequently, the smart city initiatives would not have a purpose in addressing people's needs but in enhancing economic development and local infrastructure. Such aspects need to be further analysed in other Eastern European countries and investigate whether similar patterns are to be found. Any smart city approach in Romania focusing on Internet-based technologies as a way of increasing people's quality of life may be a first step in connecting the agendas of the smart cities and the age-friendly cities movements. For instance, in the case of improving the energy efficiency of homes of older people, there could be an explicit connection between smart home technology to combat fuel and energy poverty among senior citizens [42]. In terms of environmental hazards such as floods or the protection of older people against climate extremes [43], both agendas may intersect. Here, the approach by Jiménez [44] could be of importance, who calls for new models of collaboration. Such models include collaboration with citizens, which leads the smart city communities beyond the approach of public–private partnerships. This should lead to a Quadruple Helix model defined by Public–Private–People Partnership or PPPP, in which citizens have a say about the design of solutions for their city. There are some positive exceptions, namely in projects conducted in small or medium-sized localities as Suceava, Vaslui, and Alba Iulia. In these cases, the initiatives are connected to the local potential (for example, the sustainable food and the renewal of the urban markets in Vaslui and Suceava). However, such initiatives are scarce and mostly contextual. The full potential of connecting the two agendas has not been achieved. The case of Romania could be typical for other middle-income countries in the European Union, as developing infrastructure, including Internet-based technologies, is seen as a sign of progress by the local authorities. Consequently, the smart city initiatives would not have a purpose in addressing people's needs but in enhancing economic development and local infrastructure. Such aspects need to be further analysed in other Eastern European countries and investigate whether similar patterns are to be found.

The strategic programmes in the domain of smart cities have been initiated in Romania in close connection with programmes run by the European Union. One important European Union organisation that promoted many of the actions of the smart city initiatives is URBACT, but also the sectorial operational programmes at the European Union level played an important role in dictating what type of initiatives were deployed, and which activities and main objectives to follow. Consequently, this study acknowledges the fact that European Union programmes and bodies played a key role in smart city strategies and projects developed in Romania during the past eight years. It also acknowledges that municipalities adjust their plans to apply for projects, and set their goals to fit the main programmes launched by the transnational organisations, without setting their own priorities for local development. The European Union rhetoric is in favour of developing infrastructure, recycling projects, renewable energy and sustainable transportation for a new member state as Romania. Therefore, municipalities are trying to fit into such rhetoric. European Union programmes are often seen as "the only alternative" for developing long-term initiatives at the regional level [45]. The risk, in this case, is to neglect other opportunities for financing and the role of the local resources, and to priorities some domains that are not in line with the local priorities and to pay little attention to inter-regional cooperation—an aspect that was already discussed.

Finally, the age-friendly component is missing in the analysed initiatives. In only six out of 30 analysed documents, the age-friendly component is implicit, such as the revival of small to medium-sized localities and the notion of improvements to disadvantaged neighbourhoods. In only one initiative, there was an explicit reference to the older people's access to the local health services and smart city solutions in order to increase access to, and the quality of, health services. In the future, the agendas for the further development of the age-friendly component in smart cities in Romania could start by connecting one or more of the eight domains of an age-friendly city, namely Social participation; Communication and information; Civic participation and employment; Housing; Transportation; Community support and health services; Outdoor spaces and buildings; Respect and social inclusion, to the strategic plans and programming of smart city initiatives. The new smart age-friendly ecosystem framework [9] could provide further guidance for a connection between both agendas. Given the nature of the smart city projects in Romania, a connection between the domains of Transportation and Housing could be a logical first step. For instance, the creation of healthcare smart homes [46,47], and the utilisation and deployment of ICT and networked technological solutions [11–13,48], with a specific focus on older people as a target group, would be concrete actions that the Romanians could engage in. As stated before, sufficient and adequate training for older users could be a key requisite. Co-creation, co-design and a structured approach to stakeholder involvement could be a stimulus for the active involvement of older people in the decision-making concerning age-friendly and smart cities [49,50]. Additional guidance could be found in the works by Peine and Neven [51,52], which could help overcome suboptimal investments by policy-makers and companies when failing to create scale and impact in the domain of older people and technologies.

One important issue that needs further analysis is the fact that the initiatives that were analysed in the present study are not transparent in the type of information they share with the general public. Even though these initiatives are run by public bodies (municipalities or the local authorities), they should have been more transparent in terms of the output achieved, as they are publicly accountable. Data regarding the success indicators of the action plans, risk evaluations, possibilities of continuation and the sustainability of those projects could not be found. Therefore, it is not possible to say how successful these initiatives were in achieving the initial goals and whether these initiatives have created a significant improvement in the lives of the communities and particularly in the lives of older people.

6. Conclusions

This study used the methodology of document analysis in order to investigate the characteristics of smart city initiatives developed in Romania over the past eight years (2012–2020). Such projects were often located in the Bucharest-Ilfov Region and the North-West Region. Smart city initiatives around the country accentuate the socioeconomic disparities between the eight Development Regions of Romania. Most of the smart city initiatives consisted of public–private partnerships. The initiatives covered only some dimensions of the concept of a "smart city". Only one initiative was identified which addressed the access to services (health services) for vulnerable cohorts. The "smart city" idea in Romania is strongly linked to the improvement of the country's infrastructure and sustainability, which is a rather restrictive view of the concept of smart cities. The notion that older people may benefit from the outcomes of some of the smart city programmes is not explicitly stated. In contextual projects conducted in small or medium-sized localities, there are age-friendly components to be identified. The full potential of connecting the agendas of smart cities and age-friendly cities, however, has not been achieved in Romania to date.

The case of the smart city initiatives presented here could be described as a typical case for the developing countries in the European Union. Though we can extend the conclusions of our research to other Eastern European countries, the mechanisms described in the findings have the potential for generalisation. Limitations of the current research lie in the absence of a comparative dimension, for example, in exploring what type of small cities projects have been developed in other European

Union member states, in the new member states as compared to the old members states and what factors are regulating the chains of implementation of such projects in countries other than Romania. Still, Romania can be considered as a typical case, at least for the new European Union member states, as the mechanisms suggested here are largely influenced by the opportunities to get funding through European Union programmes.

Additionally, the relative peripheral role of the age-friendly component in the smart city initiatives identified in the analysis might not be a feature typical of the Romanian context. In the absence of similar analyses on other Eastern European countries, the factors that lead to neglecting of the age-friendly component can only be speculated about. The condition that Eastern European countries have experienced a serious increase in the older population only during the last 20 years, the neglect of age-friendly cities by the national governments in long-term strategies and policies, and also the fact that those countries have been prioritising the development of infrastructure as an indicator of success for the local governance, may be part of the explanation.

Author Contributions: Conceptualisation, L.I. and J.v.H.; methodology, L.I.; formal analysis, L.I.; resources, L.I., D.B. and J.v.H.; writing—original draft preparation, L.I., D.B. and J.v.H.; writing—review and editing, L.I., D.B. and J.v.H. All authors have read and agreed to the published version of the manuscript.

Funding: This research received no external funding. The networking activities (December 2019 and February 2020) were funded through "THUAS meets East" (Grant Office of The Hague University of Applied Sciences).

Conflicts of Interest: The authors declare no conflict of interest.

Appendix A

Table A1. The corpus of analysis and the results of the coding process.

No Crt.	Name of the Initiative	Year	Initiated by	Type of Action	Governance	Documents/Activities/ Training/Promotion	Main Objectives	Age-Friendly Component?	Role of the Industry	Role of a Transnational Body/Organisation
1	Smart City Alba Iulia 2016–2018 pilot project	Since 2018	Regional Operational Program and local administration	Local	Private	Activities as part of a programmatic document	Energy consumption has been streamlined; local government controls the intensity of light; Buses with Wi-Fi, monitor air, projects to digitise education, and interact with public institutions	No	Telecom and Internet operator	Smart City Association and Economic Competitiveness Sectorial Operational Program, EU
2	Annual Smart City Industry Awards	Since 2016	RSCMA, High Patronage of the Ministry of Energy and local decision-makers; Ministry of Energy, Ministry of Waters and Forests, Chamber of Commerce and Industry of Romania	National	Private in partnership with public	Promotion	Awards and promotion	No	Key role	Idem above
3	Smart City Caravan	2017	RSCMA	National	Private in partnership with public	Promotion	Promotion of smart city solutions and education of decision-makers on new technologies, run in 12 regions of Romania.	No	Private association organising smart city courses	Idem above
4	Annual Smart City Urban Projects fair	Since 2017	RSCMA	National	Private in partnership with public	Promotion	Projects/fair-promotion	No	Key role	Idem above
5	Work group for Smart City National Strategy 2018	2018	RSCMA	National	Private in partnership with public	Documents	Lobby	National Strategy for Smart City does not have an explicit component	Key role	Not specified
6	Smart City Magazine	Since 2016	RSCMA	National	Private	Documents	Publication	No	Key role	Idem above
7	Smart City Academy, National training platform	Since 2017	RSCMA	National	Private in partnership with public	Training	Training; The mission of this platform is to train Smart City experts for both central and local institutions as well as companies that are active in the development of cities and communities in Romania.	No	Key role	Idem above

Table A1. *Cont.*

No Crt.	Name of the Initiative	Year	Initiated by	Type of Action	Governance	Documents/Activities/ Training/Promotion	Main Objectives	Age-Friendly Component?	Role of the Industry	Role of a Transnational Body/Organisation
8	Romanian Smart City Projects	Since 2016	RSCMA, High Patronage of the Ministry of Energy and local decision-makers; Ministry of Energy, Ministry of Waters and Forests, Chamber of Commerce and Industry of Romania	National	Private in partnership with public	Programmatic documents	320 Smart City projects in Romania (€15 billion available: 8 billion from national funds, 7 billion from EU funds)	No	Key role	Not specified
9	IASI Smart City	2016–2019	Municipality	Local	Private in partnership with public	Activities as part of a programmatic document	Smart transport and ecological mobility	Not specified	Key role	EU program
10	Cluj-Napoca Smart City	2013–2019	Municipality	Local	Private in partnership with public	Activities as part of a programmatic document	Smart transport and ecological mobility	Not specified	Key role	EU program
11	Cluj-Napoca – Timișoara – Oradea – Arad- the Western Alliance	Since 2018	Municipalities in the mentioned cities	Regional Region West and North-West	Public	Activities as part of a programmatic document	Development of motorway/road, trains, and air traffic infrastructures. The increase in ecological mobility through public transportation. Support of the public–private partnership through infrastructure projects	No	300 industry operators	No
12	www.e-guvernare.ro, Bucharest	2013	Bucharest City Hall	Regional-Region Bucharest-Ilfov	Private in partnership with public	Activities as part of a programmatic document	e-governance	No	Key role	No
13	Regional Operational Program EU	2007–2013	Region Bucharest-Ilfov and (Bucharest, Brasov, Sibiu, Timișoara, Craiova and Cluj-Napoca)	Regional, and large cities	Private in partnership with public	Activities	To create video T systems for areas with high criminality and to rehabilitate the public lighting system	Implicit component	Key role, 600 economic operators and research institutes and universities	Economic Competitiveness Sectorial Operational Program, EU
14	Regional Operational Programme, EU	2014–2020	Region Bucharest-Ilfov and Bucharest, Brasov, Sibiu, Timișoara, Craiova and Cluj-Napoca	Regional, and large cities	Private in partnership with public	Activities	Territorial cohesion in the urban regeneration of small and medium towns, especially those mono-industrial.	Implicit component	Key role, 600 economic operators and research institutes and universities	Idem above
15	Timișoara Smart City	2007–2013	Local municipality, Vest Region, Polytechnic University Timișoara	Local	Private in partnership with public	Activities	Smart transport, adaptive control system for traffic management, video surveillance	Implicit component	Key role	Idem above
16	Sibiu. ECRO, The Smart City Sibiu Project	2012–2015	Local municipality	Local	Private in partnership with public	Activities	Smart grid concept (energy efficiency and the reduction of CO_2 emissions)	No	Key role	Idem above
17	Craiova. Craiova Smart City. ARCA	2018–2021	Local municipality. Ministry of Energy	Local	Private in partnership with public	Activities	e-governance, digital public services, digital services (City app-for tourists)	No	Key role	EU POCA program

Table A1. *Cont.*

No Crt.	Name of the Initiative	Year	Initiated by	Type of Action	Governance	Documents/Activities/ Training/Promotion	Main Objectives	Age-Friendly Component?	Role of the Industry	Role of a Transnational Body/Organisation
18	Brașov, Smart City	Since 2008	Local municipality. Ministry of Energy	Local	Private in partnership with public	Activities	Telemetry system for public lighting (saving up to 35% during nighttime); intelligent containers for garbage and recycling	No	Key role	URBACT, EU. Other EU program
19	Alba Iulia: City Logo, Metropolitan Governance	2010	Alba Iulia municipality and URBACT, RO. The Ministry of Regional Development and Public Administration of Romania	Local	Private in partnership with public	Activities promotion, branding, action plan, local governance	A branding initiative focused on cultural tourism	No	Key role	URBACT, EU
20	Iași. RE-Block Disadvantaged Neighbourhoods	2018	Iași municipality and URBACT, RO. Ministry of Regional Development and Public Administration of Romania	Local	Private in partnership with public	Activities	Foster efficient regeneration of disadvantaged neighbourhoods' environmental quality, green neighbourhoods	Implicit component	Key role	URBACT, EU
21	Baia Mare USE ACT	2015	Baia Mare municipality and URBACT, RO. The Ministry of Regional Development and Public Administration of Romania	Local	Private in partnership with public	Documents and policies	Sustainable development and land use policy	No	Not specified	URBACT, EU
22	Baia Sprie. 4D Cities	2012–2013; 2014–2020	Baia Sprie local administration and URBACT, RO. The Ministry of Regional Development and Public Administration of Romania	Local	Private in partnership with public	Strategy, action plan	Diversifying the health services: professional medical act in emergency and safety situations, based on innovative tools	Explicit component	Not specified	URBACT, EU
23	Suceava. Urban Markets Renewal	2012–2015	Suceava municipality and URBACT, RO. The Ministry of Regional Development and Public Administration of Romania	Local	Private in partnership with public	Strategy, actions	Sustainable urban markets	Implicit component	Key role	URBACT, EU
24	Vaslui, Urban Markets. Sustainable Food in Urban Communities, Low Carbon Emissions	2014–2020	Vaslui municipality and URBACT, RO. The Ministry of Regional Development and Public Administration of Romania	Local	Private in partnership with public	Strategy, actions	Development of a competitive, safe, and healthy local food system, with low CO_2 emissions	Implicit component	Key role	URBACT, EU
25	Bucharest: Smarter Cities Challenge grants	2010–2011	Bucharest Municipality and IT international private Company	Local	Private in partnership with public	Strategy, analysis	Integrated Operations Centre and business analytics	No	The only role, private initiative	No

Table A1. *Cont.*

No Crt.	Name of the Initiative	Year	Initiated by	Type of Action	Governance	Documents/Activities/ Training/Promotion	Main Objectives	Age-Friendly Component?	Role of the Industry	Role of a Transnational Body/Organisation
26	Urban regeneration and Regional Operational Programme in Bucharest-Ilfov Region	2014–2020	Bucharest Municipality and Bucharest-Ilfov Region	Regional	Private in partnership with public	Actions	Measures dedicated energy-efficiency for buildings and urban mobility; Increase Energy Efficiency;	No	Key role	Regional Operational Program 2014–2020, EU
27	Bucharest Smart City Development Strategy	2018	City Hall Bucharest and accountancy private company	Local	Private in partnership with public	Document, strategy, consultation	Traffic management, lighting, infrastructure, e-government, public safety, telecommunications, environment – intelligent buildings, green energy, smart tourism	No	Key role	No
28	Bucharest Smart City projects	2017–2019	City Hall Bucharest and private sector (Telekom Romania and Cisco)	Local	Private	Actions	Smart city space in the Youth Park in Bucharest	No	Key role	No
29	Bucharest Smart City Map	2017	City Hall Bucharest and ANAGRAMA, software company	Local	Private in partnership with public	Actions	Intelligent City Map Application and City Drop. Software solution Incident Report; Free Wi-Fi; Accessibility; Local Recycle – Recycle locally; City Tourism – Tourism in town	No	Key role	No
30	National Strategy for Smart City	2018	The Ministry of Regional Development and Public Administration of Romania, other Ministries	National	Public	Programmatic document	Long-term strategy	No	Consultancy	No specify

Links:

- Smart City Alba Iulia 2016–2018 pilot project: https://hub.beesmart.city/city-portraits/alba-iulia-how-central-romania-quietly-created-a-smart-city-champion-in-europe.
- Smart City Industry Awards Annual Awards: https://scia2018.romaniansmartcity.ro/
- Smart City Caravan: https://caravana.romaniansmartcity.ro/
- Annual Smart City Urban Projects fair: https://scup2018.romaniansmartcity.ro/
- Work group for Smart City National Strategy 2018: https://businessforsmartcities.com/load/118/presentation/2_alexa_dimitrscu_1_28a81.pdf
- Smart City Magazine: https://smartcitymagazine.ro/
- SMART CITY ACADEMY, national training platform: https://academiasmartcity.ro/
- ROMANIAN SMART CITY PROJECTS: https://businessforsmartcities.com/load/118/presentation/2_alexa_dimitrscu_1_28a81.pdf
- IASI Smart City: https://iasismartcity.ro/
- Cluj Napoca Smart City: https://romaniansmartcity.ro/cluj-napoca-locul-3-smart-city/
- Cluj Napoca – Timișoara – Oradea – Arad- the WESTERN ALLIANCE: https://transylvanianow.com/four-romanian-cities-form-western-alliance/
- www.e-guvernare.ro, Bucharest
- Regional Operational Program, EU
- Timișoara Smart City: https://mysmartcity.ro/

Table A1. *Cont.*

No Crt.	Name of the Initiative	Year	Initiated by	Type of Action	Governance	Documents/Activities/ Training/Promotion	Main Objectives	Age-Friendly Component?	Role of the Industry	Role of a Transnational Body/Organisation

- Timișoara Smart City: http://www.primariatm.ro/epress.php?epress_id = 8288
- Sibiu ECRO, The Smart City Sibiu Project
- Craiova. Craiova Smart City. ARCA: https://caravana.romaniansmartcity.ro/craiova-implementeaza-proiecte-smart-city-caravana-smart-city
- Brașov, Smart City, https://romaniansmartcity.ro/brasov-smart-city-containere-inteligente/
- Alba Iulia: City Logo, Metropolitan Governance https://urbact.eu/sites/default/files/alba_iulia_an_ancient_capital_-local_action_plan.pdf
- Iași. RE-Block Disadvantaged Neighborhoods: https://urbact.eu/re-block-complete-overview
- Baia Mare. USE ACT. Urban Renewal: ttps://urbact.eu/sites/default/files/media/useact_lap_baia_mare_metropolitan_area.pdf
- Baia Sprie. 4D Cities: https://urbact.eu/sites/default/files/import/Projects/4D_CITIES/outputs_media/4D_Cities_Baseline_Study.pdf
- Suceava. Urban Markets Renewal: https://urbact.eu/sites/default/files/suceava_lap_long_version.pdf
- Vaslui, Urban Markets. Sustainable Food in Urban Communities, Low Carbon Emissions: https://urbact.eu/sites/default/files/sustainable_food_lap_summaries.pdf
- Bucharest. IBM Smarter Cities Challenge grants: http://www.smartercitieschallenge.org/city_bucharest_romania.html
- Urban regeneration and Regional Operational Program in Bucharest Ilfov Region. Regional Operational Program 2014-2020, EU
- Bucharest Smart City Development Strategy: http://2014-2020.adrbi.ro/media/3597/prezentare-smart-city_31-mai-2018.pdf
- Bucharest smart city projects: https://bucharestsmartcity.ro/
- Bucharest Smart City Map – Intelligent City Map Application and City Drop: http://2014-2020.adrbi.ro/media/3082/bucharest-steps-to-a-european-smart-city.pdf
- National Strategy for Smart City: https://magnanews.ro/2018/07/strategia-nationala-smart-city/
- URBACT, RO: https://urbact.eu/urbact-in-romania.

References

1. Organization for Economic Co-operation and Development. *Ageing in Cities*; OECD Publishing: Paris, France, 2015; ISBN 9789264231146.
2. Buffel, T.; Phillipson, C. Can global cities be 'age-friendly cities'? Urban development and ageing populations. *Cities* **2016**, *55*, 94–100. [CrossRef]
3. Plouffe, L.; Kalache, A. Towards Global Age-Friendly Cities: Determining Urban Features that Promote Active Aging. *J. Urb. Health.* **2010**, *87*, 733–739. [CrossRef] [PubMed]
4. Buffel, T.; Phillipson, C.; Rémillard-Boilard, S. Age-friendly cities and communities: New directions for research and policy. In *Encyclopedia of Gerontology and Population Aging*; Gu, D., Dupre, M.E., Eds.; Springer Nature: Cham, Switzerland, 2019. [CrossRef]
5. Rudnicka, E.; Napierała, P.; Podfigurna, A.; Męczekalski, B.; Smolarczyk, R.; Grymowicz, M. The World Health Organization (WHO) approach to healthy ageing. *Maturitas* **2020**, *139*, 6–11. [CrossRef]
6. World Health Organization. *Global Age-Friendly Cities: A Guide*; World Health Organization: Geneva Switzerland, 2007; ISBN 9789241547307.
7. Peek, S.T.M.; Kazak, J.K.; Perek-Białas, J.M.; Peek, S.T.M. The challenges of urban ageing: Making cities age-friendly in Europe. *Int. J. Environ. Res. Public Heal.* **2018**, *15*, 2473. [CrossRef]
8. Van Hoof, J.; Kazak, J.K. Urban ageing. *Indoor Built Environ.* **2018**, *27*, 583–586. [CrossRef]
9. Marston, H.R.; van Hoof, J. "Who doesn't think about technology when designing urban environments for older people?" A case study approach to a proposed extension of the WHO's age-friendly cities model. *Int. J. Environ. Res. Public Heal.* **2019**, *16*, 3525. [CrossRef]
10. Van Hoof, J.; Dikken, J.; Buttiġieġ, S.C.; van den Hoven, R.F.M.; Kroon, E.; Marston, H.R. Age-friendly cities in the Netherlands: An explorative study of facilitators and hindrances in the built environment and ageism in design. *Indoor Built Environ.* **2019**, *29*, 417–437. [CrossRef]
11. Peek, S.T.M.; Wouters, E.J.M.; van Hoof, J.; Luijkx, K.G.; Boeije, H.R.; Vrijhoef, H.J.M. Factors influencing acceptance of technology for aging in place: A systematic review. *Int. J. Med. Inform.* **2014**, *83*, 235–248. [CrossRef]
12. Baraković, S.; Baraković Husić, J.; van Hoof, J.; Krejcar, O.; Maresova, P.; Akhtar, Z.; Melero, F.J. Quality of life framework for personalised ageing: A systematic review of ICT solutions. *Int. J. Environ. Res. Public Heal.* **2020**, *17*, 2940. [CrossRef]
13. Baraković, S.; Baraković Husić, J.; Maraj, D.; Maraj, A.; Krejcar, O.; Maresova, P.; Melero, F.J. Quality of life, quality of experience, and security perception in web of things: An overview of research opportunities. *Electronics* **2020**, *9*, 700. [CrossRef]
14. Van Bronswijk, J.E.M.H.; Bouma, H.; Fozard, J.L. Technology for quality of life: An enriched taxonomy. *Gerontechnology* **2002**, *2*, 169–172. [CrossRef]
15. Albino, V.; Berardi, U.; Dangelico, R.M. Smart cities: Definitions, dimensions, performance, and initiatives. *J. Urban Technol.* **2015**, *22*, 3–21. [CrossRef]
16. Carli, R.; Dotoli, M.; Pellegrino, R.; Ranieri, L. Measuring and managing the smartness of cities: A framework for classifying performance indicators. In Proceedings of the 2013 IEEE International Conference on Systems, Man, and Cybernetics; Institute of Electrical and Electronics Engineers (IEEE), Manchester, UK, 13–16 October 2013. [CrossRef]
17. McLaren, D.; Agyeman, J. *Sharing Cities: A Case for Truly Smart and Sustainable Cities*; The Massachusetts Institute of Technology Press: Cambridge, MA, USA, 2015; ISBN 9780262029728.
18. Podgórniak-Krzykacz, A.; Przywojska, J.; Wiktorowicz, J. Smart and age-friendly communities in Poland. An analysis of institutional and individual conditions for a new concept of smart development of ageing communities. *Energies* **2020**, *13*, 2268. [CrossRef]
19. Woolrych, R.; Sixsmith, J.; Makita, M.; Fisher, J.; Lawthom, R. Exploring the potential of smart cities in the design of age-friendly urban environments. *Gerontechnology* **2018**, *17*, 67. [CrossRef]
20. Zaman, A.; Thornton, K. Prioritization of local indicators for the development of an age-friendly city: A community perspective. *Urban Sci.* **2018**, *2*, 51. [CrossRef]
21. Gudowsky, N.; Sotoudeh, M.; Capari, L.; Wilfing, H. Transdisciplinary forward-looking agenda setting for age-friendly, human centered cities. *Futures* **2017**, *90*, 16–30. [CrossRef]

22. Righi, V.; Sayago, S.; Blat, J. Urban Ageing: Technology, Agency and community in smarter cities for older people. In Proceedings of the ACM International Conference Proceedings Series, Limerick, Ireland, 27–30 June 2015; pp. 119–128. [CrossRef]
23. About the Global Network for Age-Friendly Cities and Communities. Available online: https://extranet.who.int/agefriendlyworld/who-network/ (accessed on 12 June 2020).
24. Bye-Bye, Balkans: A Region in Critical Demographic Decline. Available online: https://balkaninsight.com/2019/10/14/bye-bye-balkans-a-region-in-critical-demographic-decline/ (accessed on 12 June 2020).
25. Country Health Profile 2019. Available online: http://www.oecd.org/health/country-health-profiles-EU.htm (accessed on 12 June 2020).
26. Romanian National Institute for Statistics. Available online: http://statistici.insse.ro/ (accessed on 12 une 2020).
27. Harta Accesului Cetățenilor Români la Serviciile de Asistență Medical Primară Oferite de Cabinetele de Medicina Familiei. Available online: http://www.fnpmf.ro/images/harta-MF-2020.pdf (accessed on 12 June 2020).
28. Renovarea României. O Strategie Pentru Renovarea Durabilă A Fondului De Clădiri Din Romania. Available online: http://bpie.eu/wp-content/uploads/2015/10/Renovating-Romania_RO-Final.pdf (accessed on 12 June 2020).
29. Eurostat Statistics Explained. Available online: https://ec.europa.eu/eurostat/statistics-explained/index.php?title=Housing_statistics (accessed on 12 June 2020).
30. Green Homes Certified by RoGBC. Available online: http://www.rogbc.org/en/projects/green-homes (accessed on 12 June 2020).
31. Bowen, G.A. Document analysis as a qualitative research method. *Qual. Res. J.* **2009**, *9*, 27–40. [CrossRef]
32. Hotnews.ro. Available online: http://www.hotnews.ro (accessed on 12 June 2020).
33. Bucharest Mayor Signs Contract with Deloitte for Drafting Smart City Strategy. Available online: https://www.romania-insider.com/bucharest-deloitte-smart-city-strategy (accessed on 12 June 2020).
34. Bătăgan, L. The use of intelligent solutions in Romanian cities. *Informa. Econ.* **2012**, *16*, 37–43.
35. Rotună, C.I.; Cîrnu, C.E.; Gheorghiță, A. Implementing smart city solutions: Smart city map and city drop. *Qual. Life* **2017**, *28*, 313–327.
36. Manika, S. Mechanisms for innovative-driven solutions in European smart cities. *Smart Cities* **2020**, *3*, 527–540. [CrossRef]
37. Costantino, N.; Pellegrino, R. Public–private partnership implementation: Cross-case analysis. *Proc. Inst. Civil. Eng. Managm. Procure. Law* **2015**, *168*, 164–176. [CrossRef]
38. Schipper, R.P.J.R.; Silvius, A.J.G. Characteristics of smart sustainable city development: Implications for project management. *Smart Cities* **2018**, *1*, 75–97. [CrossRef]
39. Milenković, M.; Rašić, M.; Vojković, G. Using public private partnership models in smart cities—proposal for Croatia. In Proceedings of the 2017 40th International Convention on Information and Communication Technology, Electronics and Microelectronics (MIPRO), Opatija, Croatia, 25–26 May 2017; pp. 1412–1417.
40. Baltac, V. Smart cities—A view of societal aspects. *Smart Cities* **2019**, *2*, 538–548. [CrossRef]
41. Angelakoglou, K.; Nikolopoulos, N.; Giourka, P.; Svensson, I.-L.; Tsarchopoulos, P.; Tryferidis, A.; Tzovaras, D. A methodological framework for the selection of key performance indicators to assess smart city solutions. *Smart Cities* **2019**, *2*, 269–306. [CrossRef]
42. Boerenfijn, P.; Kazak, J.K.; Schellen, L.; van Hoof, J. A multi-case study of innovations in energy performance of social housing for older adults in the Netherlands. *Energy Build.* **2018**, *158*, 1762–1769. [CrossRef]
43. Szewrański, S.; Świąder, M.; Kazak, J.K.; Tokarczyk-Dorociak, K.; van Hoof, J. Socio-environmental vulnerability mapping for environmental and flood resilience assessment: The case of ageing and poverty in the city of Wrocław, Poland. *Integr. Environ. Assess. Manag.* **2018**, *14*, 592–597. [CrossRef]
44. Jimenez, C.E. Smart Cities, open innovation and open government: Towards "Public-Private-People Partnership" (PPPP) Models? In Proceedings of the 2015 Second International Conference on eDemocracy & eGovernment (ICEDEG), Quito, Ecuador, 8–10 April 2015. [CrossRef]
45. Hollands, R.G. Will the real smart city please stand up? *City* **2008**, *12*, 303–320. [CrossRef]
46. Stefanov, D.H.; Bien, Z.; Bang, W.-C. The smart house for older persons and persons with physical disabilities: Structure, technology arrangements, and perspectives. *IEEE Trans. Neural Syst. Rehabil. Eng.* **2004**, *12*, 228–250. [CrossRef]

47. Van Hoof, J.; Demiris, G.; Wouters, E.J.M. *Handbook of Smart Homes, Health Care and Well-Being*; Springer Science and Business Media LLC: Rotterdam, The Netherlands, 2017.
48. Marston, H.R.; Genoe, R.; Freeman, S.; Kulczycki, C.; Musselwhite, C. Older adults' perceptions of ICT: Main findings from the technology in later life (TILL) study. *Healthcare* **2019**, *7*, 86. [CrossRef]
49. Van Hoof, J.; Verkerk, M.J. Developing an integrated design model incorporating technology philosophy for the design of healthcare environments: A case analysis of facilities for psychogeriatric and psychiatric care in The Netherlands. *Technol. Soc.* **2013**, *35*, 1–13. [CrossRef]
50. Van Hoof, J.; Rutten, P.G.S.; Struck, C.; Huisman, E.R.C.M.; Kort, H.S.M. The integrated and evidence-based design of healthcare environments. *Arch. Eng. Des. Manag.* **2014**, *11*, 243–263. [CrossRef]
51. Peine, A.; Neven, L. From intervention to co-constitution: New directions in theorizing about aging and technology. *Gerontologist* **2018**, *59*, 15–21. [CrossRef]
52. Peine, A.; Neven, L. The co-constitution of ageing and technology—A model and agenda. *Ageing Soc.* **2020**. [CrossRef]

International Journal of
Environmental Research and Public Health

MDPI

Article

Intergenerational Effects on the Impacts of Technology Use in Later Life: Insights from an International, Multi-Site Study

Shannon Freeman [1,*], Hannah R. Marston [2], Janna Olynick [3], Charles Musselwhite [4], Cory Kulczycki [5], Rebecca Genoe [5] and Beibei Xiong [6]

1. School of Nursing, University of Northern British Columbia, Prince George, BC V2N 4Z9, Canada
2. Health and Wellbeing Strategic Research Area, School of Health, Wellbeing and Social Care, The Open University, Milton Keynes MK7 6AA, UK; Hannah.Marston@open.ac.uk
3. School of Nursing and Department of Psychology, University of Northern British Columbia, Prince George, BC V2N 4Z9, Canada; Janna.Olynick@unbc.ca
4. Centre for Innovative Ageing, Swansea University, Swansea SA2 8PP, UK; c.b.a.musselwhite@swansea.ac.uk
5. Faculty of Kinesiology and Health Studies, University of Regina, Regina, SK S4S 0A2, Canada; cory.kulczycki@uregina.ca (C.K.); rebecca.genoe@uregina.ca (R.G.)
6. School of Health Sciences, University of Northern British Columbia, Prince George, BC V2N 4Z9, Canada; bxiong@unbc.ca

* Correspondence: shannon.freeman@unbc.ca

Received: 7 July 2020; Accepted: 5 August 2020; Published: 7 August 2020

check for updates

Abstract: As the use of technology becomes further integrated into the daily lives of all persons, including older adults, it is important to investigate how the perceptions and use of technology intersect with intergenerational relationships. Based on the international multi-centered study Technology In Later Life (TILL), this paper emphasizes the perceptions of older adults and the interconnection between technology and intergenerational relationships are integral to social connectedness with others. Participants from rural and urban sites in Canada and the UK (n = 37) completed an online survey and attended a focus group. Descriptive and thematic analyses suggest that older adults are not technologically adverse and leverage intergenerational relationships with family and friends to adjust to new technologies and to remain connected to adult children and grandchildren, especially when there is high geographic separation between them. Participants referenced younger family members as having introduced them to, and having taught them how to use, technologies such as digital devices, computers, and social networking sites. The intergenerational support in the adoption of new technologies has important implications for helping older persons to remain independent and to age in place, in both age-friendly cities and in rural communities. The findings contribute to the growing literature in the fields of gerontology and gerontechnology on intergenerational influences and the impacts of technology use in later life and suggest the flexibility and willingness of older persons to adopt to new technologies as well as the value of intergenerational relationships for overcoming barriers to technology adoption.

Keywords: digital; intergenerational communication; gerontology; aging; family; cross-cultural research; qualitative research

1. Background

From monitoring personal health and wearable devices to playing online games and using social media to connect with friends and family, technology has become a valued component of daily life for many individuals. Interest in technology has steadily increased over the past decade, associated with unprecedented growth and innovation in information and communication technologies (ICTs) [1,2]. There has been an increase in the proportion of older adults (persons aged over 65 years) in countries across the world utilizing technology [3]. As the use of technology and associated ICTs increases, there is a greater need to expand the understanding of the intersection of technology, ageing, and intergenerational relationships. A particular gap in knowledge exists regarding the role of intergenerational elements in motivating older adults to learn how to use technology and associated ICTs.

Across the globe, societies are aging rapidly due to increased life expectancy as a result of better health and social care, and lower birth rates [4]. Recent United Kingdom (UK) population estimations suggest the proportion of those aged 65+ years in rural and urban environments will increase by 50% between 2016 and 2039, whilst those aged <65 years are projected to increase by eight percent in urban areas and to stagnate in rural locations [5]. In 2014, 15.6% of the Canadian population, equating to over 6 million persons, were aged 65, and it is predicted that by 2030, older adults will exceed 9.5 million persons, accounting for 23% of the Canadian population [6]. In Canada, the majority of older adults (56.4%) lived with a spouse or a common-law partner in 2011 while about one-quarter (24.6%) lived alone [6,7].

The increase in the migration of younger cohorts from rural to urban areas and of older adults from urban to rural areas leaves an increased proportion of older adults in rural areas who prefer to "age in place" [8,9]. Research focused on aging in urban areas has emphasized the challenges older adults face in accessibility, especially in access to public transportation, shopping, and green space [10]. As geographic separation between family members increases, the role of ICTs in helping to strengthen and maintain family bonds becomes more important [11]. However, the extent to which older adults use technologies for this purpose remains unclear. Although, in the future, aged cohorts may be more "tech savvy" [12], having used technologies regularly across their life course, new technologies may still arrive that could be disproportionately challenging for older people to adopt.

Technology (e.g., digital devices, the Internet, digital gaming, and mobile apps) use in later life is a growing field of research, with much new exploration and study [13–16]. Technology and associated ICTs are often aimed towards improving the health, wellbeing and quality of life of older adults, whether through applications for home healthcare and connected health services [17], medication reminders [18,19], mirrors that display health data [20], or wearable technology [21]. Technology use to enhance communication is routine practice for many older adults, with home computers being used to create a common interest among older and younger family members and improve family ties [22].

Technology use among older adults is growing [3]. For example, in Canada, between 2007 and 2016, Internet use increased from 32% to 68% among those aged 65 and older [23]. In 2016, 85% of people aged 65–69 used the Internet compared to 62% of those aged 70–79 and 40% of those aged 80 years and older [23]. Challenges with technology have been linked to age, evidenced by differences in use [24,25] and variation in the learning of technology (computers and Internet) between older and younger adults [12,26–31]. Older adults in Canada were less likely than younger adults to perceive technology as useful for communicating with others, making informed decisions, and saving time [23]. Several studies reported that Internet use is lower among older-aged cohorts than younger cohorts [32–34]; however, there is evidence of a cohort effect as there has been an increase in technology use within older-aged cohorts over time [2]. Older adults who do use the Internet report lower confidence in their ability to do so than younger adults [35], which may be tied to challenges older adults experience with technology use (e.g., visual difficulties and cognitive declines) [36,37]. Older adults are likely to make more errors and require assistance when learning computer systems and software [36,37].

Previous research suggests that older adults may be "technophobic" [38,39] and struggle to use technology [2], as they embrace technology differently and at a slower pace than younger adults [2], [32,40]. As the Canadian and UK populations age, differences in technology adoption and use across age cohorts may increase, amplifying the "generational gap" [41]. While learning to use technology serves as a rite of passage for today's youth, playing an important role in the self-definition of young adults [42], this may not be the case for older generations. Individuals not born into the current rapidly evolving digital age, sometimes referred to as "digital immigrants", must find ways to adapt to a changing society [43]. Rama noted that each "technology generation" may have been affected by common experiences during their formative years that influence behaviours towards and the use of technology [44]. However, these notions are challenged by Bennett and Maton, who note the diverse range of experience and engagement with technology among youth, as well as by Loos, who describes technology use as a spectrum affected not only by life stage but also by socialization and degree of age-related functionality [16,45]. Technology use is complex and can no longer simply be split into user vs. non-user groups. Instead, the heterogeneity in the use of technology includes not only use of the technology for an intended purpose but also the meaning and value that the use of technologies has in mediating social relationships and connection to the external world [46]. Existing research highlights differences in technology use between the generations; however, research on the connection between intergenerational factors, social variables, and technology use among older adults is less prevalent, with notable exceptions including [26–28]. However, other research suggests that age is not a consistent driving factor associated with aversion to technology such as computer anxiety [24]. As such, it remains less clear how factors such as intergenerational intelligence, solidarity, and adaptiveness apply to the learning and use of technology, especially by older adults [47–51].

Younger generations are the dominant early users and adopters of social networking sites [12,52], with few older adults (between 10% and 27%) using this form of technology [2,3]. Social networking and other technologies present opportunities for older generations to connect with younger generations and individuals in diverse geographic locations [22,53–55]. Technology has been shown to enhance an older adult's quality of aging [56], independence [57], social status [56], interpersonal relationships, control, self-esteem, and integration into society [57,58]. To understand how to meet the needs of an aging population in a technology-suffused society, it is useful to understand why older adults choose (or not) to use technology and whether (or not) they perceive the reasons driving their choice as constraints requiring negotiation or benefits to everyday life. The challenges to acquiring new technology skills and strategies for connecting with younger generations to overcome them suggest the importance of intergenerational influences on older adults' understanding and use of technology, which must be further explored.

The above findings are concerning in light of research reports that older adults are more likely to experience loneliness and isolation [34]. There is, to date, a growing body of scholarly work exploring the relationships between intergenerational relationships and technology [27,28], offering insight into how technology and associated ICTs lay within and across intergenerational networks. Taipale and colleagues [27] discuss ICT use through various lenses including both older and younger adults—a generational perspective, the family, and the home. To further extend research in this area, we describe further the relationship between technology use and interpersonal relationships—more specifically, the how older adults' understanding and use of technology is affected by their intergenerational relationships.

2. Methods

2.1. Aims and Objectives

The Technology In Later Life (TILL) study examined the experiences of older adults aged 70+ years with technology, exploring how they adopted, accepted, and used various types of technology. Subsequently, the team sought to identify the implications of using ICTs for current and future aging populations in rural and urban locations.

2.2. Study Location

The Technology In Later Life (TILL) study was an exploratory study conducted in Canada and the UK across four study sites. Canada and the UK were selected for this study as they both have aging populations and exposure to technology and contain different rural and urban populations. In each country, two sites were selected: one rural and one urban. The rural site in Canada was the town of McBride (BC), and the urban site selected was the city of Regina (SK). The rural sites in the UK included the village of Cwmtwrch and the village of Ystalyfera in Wales, and the urban site was the town of Milton Keynes (Buckinghamshire) in England.

2.3. Procedure

Participants were recruited through the use of posters and mailing list scripts tailored to each site distributed to local organizations including the Older People's Forum, seniors' centers, public libraries, seniors' community newsletters, and local public radio. Participants were also recruited through word of mouth in the community. Participants each voluntarily contacted the lead investigator for the research site closest to them to request to participate in the study. Upon contact, the participants were sent an email containing a link to the online survey, information on the study and a request for written consent to participate, and an invitation to set a date to join a focus group interview.

All participants completed the online survey prior to participation in a focus group. The survey was an iteration of an earlier survey [14,59], which covered eight domains: (1) technology use, (2) internet ownership and use, (3) social networking, (4) digital device ownership, (5) purchasing patterns, (6) quantified self- and life-logging, (7) information sharing and privacy issues, and (8) demographics. Bivariate analyses of the survey data were conducted using SPSS version 24. An inductive approach was taken to generate new knowledge from the qualitative data. A descriptive approach is beneficial for an initial study, as such an approach allows the researchers to richly describe the phenomenon being studied.

Focus group discussions, led by the lead researcher from each site, lasting between 40 and 60 minutes, were digitally audio-recorded and then transcribed verbatim in Microsoft Word by a UK-based transcription company. All the lead researchers were experienced in conducting qualitative research analyses and in leading focus groups. A semi-structured interview guide containing questions and probes was used to facilitate discussion (Supplementary Materials). The questions examined several areas including the ownership of technology, the purpose for using technology, internet social media use, life-logging, privacy issues and the sharing of information (e.g., what type of information and rationale for sharing), and willingness to embrace new technology (Supplementary Materials).

Content and inductive analyses [60] were conducted across all the transcripts. Given the exploratory nature of this analysis, the transcriptions were read closely for familiarization with the data, coded, and analyzed thematically. The data were classified into categories as a way of describing key themes [61]. In addition, areas of concordance and discordance were examined through the analysis. Specifically, open coding, with the creation of categories and abstraction, was undertaken. Coding was first conducted independently by a research assistant, trained in qualitative research methodologies and experienced in conducting analysis, and by a co-investigator, both of whom then came together to come to a consensus on the coding. Discrepancies were addressed by recoding areas of discordance, and then, the transcripts were reanalyzed by the research assistant and reviewed by a co-investigator of the study to promote accuracy and trustworthiness [62]. Ethics approval was granted by all four institutions.

3. Findings

Thirty-seven participants both completed an online questionnaire and attended a focus group discussion. This included 20 rural participants (McBride, Canada, $n = 10$, Cwmtwrch and Ystalyfera, UK, $n = 10$) and 17 urban participants (Regina, Canada, $n = 6$ and Milton Keynes, UK, $n = 11$) from 2015 to 2016. Most participants were female (67.6%), retired/not employed (86.5%), and in their late 70s (mean age, 77.4 years). Five themes were identified relating to intergenerational relationships. Three themes focused on the benefits of intergenerational relationships to support use of technology including 1) Motivation for older adults to use technology, 2) Use of technology as a facilitator of intergenerational connection and 3) Technology use for safety reasons. Additionally, two themes focused on the impediments of intergenerational relationships to use of technology including 1) Using technology to appease younger family members; and 2) Learning how to use technology in later life.

All participants used technology, the majority of whom did so on a regular basis (Table 1). Nearly all participants used a computer (97.3%) and owned a computer (89.2%). Most participants had used a computer for at least 10 years (75.7%) and used a computer more than once per day (62.2%). All participants used a digital device, typically a mobile/cell phone (70.3%), and to share information (82.7%). Nearly all participants identified having internet at home (94.3%) and most had used the internet for more than 10 years (75.8%). Participants used technology for a variety of tasks including e-mail, word processing, playing games, making telephone calls, online shopping, online banking, sharing information, social networking, searching/checking information, instant messaging, reading, uploading content, and lifelogging. Over half reported using social media (54.1%, $n = 20$) with more Canadian participants' self-reporting use of social media when compared to participants from the UK (62.5% vs. 47.6%) (Table 2).

Table 1. Characteristics and overview of technology use for all participants ($n = 37$).

Characteristics	Total Population 100% ($n = 37$)	Canada 47.2% ($n = 16$)	United Kingdom 56.8% ($n = 21$)
Mean age, years ±SD	77.4 ±6.4	79.3 ±5.9	75.9 ±6.6
Age range in years	67–89	70–89	67–89
Gender			
Female	67.6 (25)	87.5 (14)	52.4 (11)
Male	32.4 (12)	12.5 (2)	47.6 (10)
Have used a computer	97.3 (36)	93.8 (15)	100.0 (21)
Own a computer	89.2 (33)	93.8 (15)	85.7 (18)
Own a cell phone	70.3 (26)	50.0 (8)	85.7 (18)
Technology use/ownership			
Play video games	56.3 (18)	50.0 (8)	47.6 (10)
Own a digital/video game console	8.1 (3)	6.3 (1)	9.5 (2)
Have the internet at home	89.2 (33)	81.3 (13)	95.2 (20)
Use social media sites	35.1 (13)	50.0 (8)	23.8 (5)
Email	78.4 (29)	81.3 (13)	72.6 (16)

Note: SD denotes standard deviation; unless noted otherwise, responses are presented as percentages of total responses with the numbers of participants in brackets.

Table 2. Characteristics of social media use among participants who reported using social media (n = 20/37).

Characteristics	Participants Who Use Social Media 54.1% (n = 20/37)	Canada 62.5% (n = 10/16)	United Kingdom 47.6% (n = 10/21)
Person who introduced participant to social media			
Spouse/partner	5.0 (1)	10.0 (1)	-
Adult child	20.0 (4)	20.0 (2)	20.0 (2)
Friend	40.0 (7)	20.0 (2)	80.0 (5)
Relative	20.0 (4)	40.0 (4)	-
Other	5.0 (1)	10.0 (1)	-
Reasons to use social media			
Connect with friends	70.0 (14)	70.0 (7)	70.0 (7)
Connect with children/grandchildren	70.0 (14)	80.0 (8)	60.0 (6)
Share information with friends/family	50.0 (10)	60.0 (6)	40.0 (4)
Share photos with friends/family	60.0 (12)	60.0 (6)	60.0 (6)
Organize events	20.0 (4)	20.0 (2)	20.0 (2)
Participate in events/groups	15.0 (3)	20.0 (2)	10.0 (1)
Keep up to date with news	40.0 (8)	20.0 (2)	60.0 (6)
Express opinions/views	15.0 (3)	10.0 (1)	20.0 (2)

Note: Responses are presented as percentage of total responses with the number of participants in brackets.

3.1. Benefits of Technology Use—Motivation for Older Adults' Use of Technology

A primary motivation for participants to use technology was as a "digital gathering place" to communicate with family, especially adult children and grandchildren, and friends. Participants communicated through technology in a variety of ways including Skype, Facetime, e-mail, social networking sites (e.g., Facebook), and texting through cellular networks or WhatsApp. Interestingly, it was common that participants who used technology were taught how to do so by younger family members. The value of digital communication was enhanced when participants' children and/or grandchildren lived far away.

"Skype is brilliant. I've got a daughter in Spain, I've got a granddaughter in Spain, I've got a son in the West Indies and a daughter in London, and Skype is one of the most brilliant things that's happened because you can see, you can talk." [MK6, male].

"I've used Skype because my daughter lives in South Africa, but it's an atrocious service because South African broadband is atrocious. We now use Apple FaceTime and that is far superior." [MK3, male].

Given the time difference across geographic distances, technology afforded both parties the flexibility to schedule face-to-face communication at a convenient time. Social networking platforms including "Facetime with other members of the family" [Wales1, female] as well as e-mail, Facebook, and WhatsApp were used to engage with family to " … keep track of the grandkids and great grandkids" [McB4, male]. Participants connected across the generations as noted by one participant who shared, "I go on Facebook and I go on Skype with my daughter in Australia and I do research things. Last night I was talking to my grandson, who's seven" [MK2, female]. It is also useful to note that participants adjusted the platforms they used not only due to personal preferences but also in response to the variance in the infrastructure and broadband support across the locations.

3.2. Benefits of Technology Use—Technology as a Facilitator of Intergenerational Connection

Older adults reported using technology to connect with friends and family members, and to share information, also likely with family members. Participants often used computers for email (85.3%) and social networking (38.2%), most often in their own home (97.1%) and occasionally at an adult child's home (17.1%). Social networking sites were used to stay connected with children and/or grandchildren and friends, to share photos and information with friends and/or family, and to keep up to date with news. The Internet was used for sending/receiving e-mails, social media, making phone calls through Skype/Viber, and instant messaging. Older adults both created and sent content (e.g., photos and emails), as well as receiving content. It was both older adults and their family members/friends who took turns initiating contact.

Most participants identified that they used technology to write or speak with other family members; there were a few instances where participants reported using technology to partake in and share the hobbies of younger family members. Older adults were keen to try new things with their grandchildren such as interactive videogames and immersed themselves in the flow of the games. One participant noted, "[...] Jumping up and down to the things that they've got on the screen when you play tennis or jump up and down and dance, or whatever you're chasing, something. Yes. Video games, I suppose. Childish ones." [McB2, female]. Another participant used her daughter and granddaughter's iPad to take pictures of the community garden. Participants suggested that technology is not only used to connect and communicate with younger family members but also to learn about and actively participate in activities with younger generations.

3.3. Benefits of Technology Use—Technology Use for Safety Reasons

Of the participants using technology to stay in contact with family, some also acknowledged having started using a digital device for safety reasons at the suggestion of another family member, commonly an adult child. Most participants reported owning a mobile device or cell phone, many of whom owned these devices for "safety" [Regina2, Female] and "emergencies only" [MK5, female]. One participant living in rural British Columbia described how they started using a digital device specifically for driving purposes as well as feeling the need to maintain a sense of peace with their adult children.

"I got the cell phone because my kids kept thinking something was going to happen to me. I said, "Well you know if I have a breakdown on the highway, we managed for 70 years for God's sake by just stopping someone and they'd help you. But now, "Oh my God they could murder you." So, this was supposed to be a safety element to keep peace in the family." [McB1, female].

This participant further described displeasure with the cell phone because it cost them money each month and they never used the device. Several participants identified that they got digital devices at the suggestion of an adult child after having suffered a health scare. For example, when asked why they got a cell phone, one participant replied, "Oh, well it was the bright idea of my son. I had a mini stroke ... ever since, but they're [kids] always frightened ... of a recurrence. So, my son gave me a cell phone, his old one, which I used right away, or more or less. I think, they decided that I should have one, because I did get a few dizzy spells. So, now I just use it" [McB2, female].

Even though it was often a younger family member, such as an adult child, who suggested the participant carry a digital device for safety-related reasons, most participants had positive perceptions of using technology for such reasons. For example, one participant spoke positively of how they wore a certain piece of technology that they can press in an emergency situation to notify a family member or emergency service that help is needed. While it seems that most participants use technology to keep in touch with younger family members, the reasons for this contact vary, from safety and emergency situations to routine check-ins with children and grandchildren.

3.4. Impediments to Technology Use—Using Technology to Appease Younger Family Members

In some instances, participants seemed to use technology to make a younger relative happy even if they did not seem to need the technology. For example, "I don't even have an iPhone or iPad so I'm really out of date ... I will get more modernized so that my children will be happy" [Regina2, Female]. Another participant stated, "I've got a tablet that I was to take away with me because my grandchildren said it would be useful to have and I wouldn't be using theirs whenever I'm away on holiday with them. I don't get on terribly well with a tablet ... " [MK2, female].

Common responses for why participants owned technology included similar motivations, stemming from the children: " ... the kids decided we should have one [computer]" [McB4, male] and that their grandchildren were putting pressure on them to keep up with the latest technology. Furthermore, one participant explained that they were learning technology because the " ... grandchildren push me and they go, 'Oh Nana, you're so far behind, you should be up to date and you should be doing this and doing that.' So, they want me to be up to date with all the latest technology and I'm not." [Regina3, female].

In certain cases, younger family members purchased technology for older family members as gifts. One participant reflected on a life logging device they owned, explaining, "My daughter bought it for my birthday ... " [Wales1, female] after her husband began experiencing a health decline. These examples illustrate, across the different study sites, how the respective participants felt about technology and how digital devices had been implemented into their lives without consideration of their respective feelings, needs, and choice.

3.5. Impediments to Technology Use—Learning How to Use Technology in Later-Life

Many participants used computers as integral components of their jobs decades ago and were among the early adopters of computing technologies. One participant who was familiar with computers explained that they used to do IT at Milton Keynes College. Similarly, a participant from McBride learned the fundamentals of using a computer for their accounting position, explaining that they learned about spreadsheets. However, with the rapid pace of technology development, the technological skills participants had employed prior to retirement became quickly outdated.

Participants described that the challenges in keeping up with the rapid pace of changes in the technology itself were compounded by their frustrations in keeping up to date on the expanded language used to describe the technologies. Participants described the complexity in language and terminology used in technology tutorial classes and instruction manuals as too complicated and inhibiting their ability to adopt new technologies. One participant identified that instructors at computer classes "go way too fast for me. I can't keep up; there is too much new information ... the language like computer and technological language is totally different from what we were raised with" [McB2, male]. Another participant identified similar grievances about learning to use technology, such as the fact that they "can't understand technology words" [McB1, female] in instruction manuals and that when speaking with information technology (IT) specialists, the IT specialist would explain too quickly.

Although participants noted how they were confused about how to use technology, they still managed to do so, most commonly with assistance from younger family members. Participants were frequently introduced to digital devices and to social networking sites by a relative or adult child. Participants alluded to younger family members playing a key role in the learning process, saying things such as "My son set it [Skype] up ... " [MK2, female] and "Oh, my daughter is the one that does all the computerizing. She helps ... " [McB2, female]. They emphasized that they were not technophobic or averse to use of the technology itself but felt outpaced by the speed of change of technology. For many, they were unable to overcome the language barriers created to adapt and adjust to changes in technology on their own or with those of a similar age. Instead, they would connect with younger generations for help. Where confusion over technology existed, younger family members took on a teaching role, especially for newer technologies such as digital devices and social networking programs. "I ask my grandchildren. 'Okay, how do I do this?' They say, 'Don't you know?' But they will help me eventually" [Regina3, female]. Younger generations were able to bridge the technology gap and communicate complex language in lay language that was non-threatening. "Anything I want to know, I have to phone up my sons or my grandchildren because they're a lot more knowledgeable than I am ... " [MK1, female].

Even after being introduced to technology and learning how to use it, participants continued to contact their adult children and other relatives for assistance when faced with difficulties. For instance, one participant stated that "My son is an IT expert. If I have any problems, 'Can I speak to the IT man please.' He knows it's me. He sorts my problems" [MK3, female]. Some participants seemed to solely rely on younger family members for information when necessary. For instance, one participant concluded, "If I need to know something, I will get my daughter to look it up on her, whatever thing she packs in her pocket" [McB4, male].

4. Discussion

For many older adults, intergenerational relationships are leveraged to support the understanding and use of technology. The challenges in the adoption of and adaptation to the rapid developments in digital technologies facilitate opportunities and meaningful purposes for participants to connect and communicate with younger generations. The leveraging of technologies, including social media and virtual communication platforms, supported older adults in maintaining and enhancing social connections, especially with adult children and grandchildren who lived in different cities and countries. These findings support the idea that the use of digital technologies can enhance social connectedness across generations; as Taipale noted, "[...] distributed families can today nevertheless remain connected and feel a sense of togetherness, even when their members are not physically close to one another" [28].

The benefits of intergenerational relationships for technology, including motivation for older adults' use of technology and the use of technology as a facilitator of intergenerational connections, underlie each domain of the WHO Checklist of Essential Features of Age-Friendly Cities [63]. Furthermore, this reinforces the need for a revised smart age-friendly ecosystem framework as coined and posited by Marston et al. [10], who proposed an extension, noting that these features also apply to the rural, and non-urban, context. The desire to mitigate the digital divide fuels older adults' motivation to invest time in building and fostering intergenerational digital connections. Previous research similarly suggests that computers are commonly used by older adults as a method of communication with younger generations, serving as a gateway to the world of younger family members and a means to strengthen relationships [64]. Studies show that individuals will often play games, not because of enjoyment of the game itself, but because of the social interaction with others with whom they are playing [65]. Therefore, when creating an age-friendly environment or helping older persons to age in place, it is worthwhile to challenge those designing built environments to consciously address how they may seize opportunities to effectively and efficiently leverage ICTs to facilitate intergenerational engagement.

Older adults leveraged technology to connect, communicate, and actively participate in the interests and hobbies of their adult children and grandchildren in online formats, including digital gaming and photography. Participants encouraged and enjoyed interacting with younger family members to learn about different technologies (e.g., digital games) as a way of immersing themselves in the culture of younger generations. As previous research illustrates, participants in this study were using digital games as a "computational meeting place" that supported meaningful social interactions and shared motivation for group gaming [66]. Further evidence shows that gaming technologies foster intergenerational group interactions of up to four generations, including adult children and extended families [67]. Our study revealed findings similar to those noted above but for multiple digital technologies, which suggests a more universal and generalizable use of technologies among older adults to increase intergenerational family social interactions as a "digital gathering place". Health limitations, the costs of transportation, and social isolation can create barriers for travel, all of which might explain why communication technologies such as Skype were often used to connect with family members. These technologies can come close to replicating the face-to-face experience of conversing with another person and are an effective communication method to use when travel is not an option. The extended value of the support of intergenerational connection may be further amplified given the context of COVID-19 and in the post-COVID-19 context.

Language and terminology often impede the ability of older adults to learn how to use technology. This disconnect and incomplete understanding of technological language could explain why few respondents identified using social media/networking sites but went on to further indicate they do in fact use this form of technology. This discrepancy in responses may stem from a lack of clarity in the question about what social networking entails for the respective participants, or this may reflect a lack of recognition by older adults that they did in fact use social media/networking platforms. Despite these complications, participants were able to use technology and associated ICTs by learning to do so with their adult children and grandchildren, who were able to translate the jargon and technical terms used in information technology courses into a language that older adults could understand within the context of intergenerational relations. This is consistent with the findings from previous studies showing that adult children often initiate the technology use process for older adults and that extended family members (such as grandchildren) are important educators for older adults as they learn to use technology [64–69].

Intergenerational informal education between those with existing relationships may be more effective for knowledge/information exchange. When considering why adult children and grandchildren were common educators, there are a few ways to explain this finding. First, older adults might feel more comfortable learning from family members due to feelings of trust. Second, as it was often adult children and other relatives who introduced participants to technology, it makes sense that they would be the ones providing the lessons and education. Third, participants may have been learning from younger generations because they may have a greater knowledge of technology, having grown up in the information age. Fourth, older adults might choose to learn from younger family members as they use less confusing terminology (compared to user manuals or classes) and they are comfortable enough to ask questions. Many older adults in the present study used technology comfortably and were among the early adopters of computers and technology. The role younger generations play in guiding and motivating older adults to use technology may contribute to family cohesion and strengthen relationships. This supports the notion of the "change in family roles" put forward by Taipale [28], who highlighted the variance of perception between Italian and Slovenian contexts.

Nearly all participants reported using a computer at their own home, but other locations such as an adult child's home were also identified. Studies have shown that, among older adults who use computers, a majority do so in the comfort of their own home, although computers are also used in public locations such as at work, in a library, or at a friend's/family member's home [14,37,53,70]. Computers might be used at an adult child's home because this is where the learning and introduction to technology take place. However, this pattern of usage could also be indicative of locational convenience, access to computers, privacy issues, what the computer is being used for, or another combination of variables. These preliminary findings point to the importance of investigating further how these intergenerational factors influence the location of technology use.

Even though participants highlighted the many benefits and uses of technology, some participants remarked on the drawbacks and risks of living in the digital age. The finding that older adults often chose to use computers for leisure to share information and communicate, whereas cell phones were often used to appease worried children, suggests both positive and negative associations of technology. For instance, surveillance and privacy issues, along with digital crime, are risks of using certain technologies [71]. Despite the existence of privacy legislation, there exist privacy threats with the use of technology, such as the tracking of personal information, profiling, and privacy-violating interactions [72]. Despite voiced concern over privacy issues, participants continued to use technologies because of the benefits, such as bridging geographical distances to communicate with younger family members. As such, it seems the rewards outweigh the risk for older adults to use technology. Nonetheless, the acknowledgment of such risks by participants draws attention to the importance of providing clear education communicated in lay language on how to safely use technology.

This research specifically addressed intergenerational elements of technology use among individuals in both rural and urban areas in two countries. Research often overlooks social elements of technology use, viewing technology engagement as a solo activity. A strength of this study is the combination of an in-depth online survey and focus groups, which allowed for a deeper understanding of the topics being studied. Upon further validation, the survey could be used in future studies as a standard measure of technology use, social media habits and behaviour, information sharing, and privacy issues. Given the exploratory nature of the study, a small sample was acceptable as the aim was for each site to recruit 10 participants. Although our sample sizes enabled us to reach saturation of information, a larger sample is needed to confirm our findings. Differences in the recruitment methods across sites may have contributed to the difficulties of achieving the targeted number of participants. Future studies should recruit participants who use and who do not use technology to compare and contrast their behaviours and identify further barriers to and enablers of technology use in later life. Further investigations may extend this work to examine the intersection of technology and intergenerational relationships among older adults who are aging without family to expand the understanding of the roles that peers, friends, or even siblings play in comparison to that of adult children [73,74].

5. Conclusions

At a time when technology development and population aging research are prevalent, it is vital to capitalize on opportunities to learn about how technology can be used and deployed to increase social connectedness, improve the quality of life of older adults, and support aging in place. With rapid technological developments occurring, there are great opportunities to expand the understanding of gerontechnology and human–computer interaction from a multi-disciplinary standpoint. Technology has the potential to play an integral role in ensuring all attributes complement each other and keep knowledge up to date. Many participants used technology to maintain social connectedness with younger family members who were geographically dispersed. The findings from this study provide insight into the strengths and opportunities that technologies provide to older adults. Understanding how intergenerational relationships impact technology use in later life can inform further research and technological and social practices.

Supplementary Materials: The following are available online at http://www.mdpi.com/1660-4601/17/16/5711/s1.

Author Contributions: Conceptualization, S.F., H.R.M., C.M., and R.G.; data curation, C.K.; formal analysis, S.F., H.R.M., J.O., and C.M.; methodology, S.F. and H.R.M.; writing—original draft, S.F., H.R.M., J.O., C.M., C.K., R.G., and B.X.; writing—review and editing, S.F., H.R.M., C.M., C.K., R.G., and B.X. All authors have read and agreed to the published version of the manuscript.

Funding: We gratefully acknowledge the financial assistance for transcription from the Engineering and Physical Sciences Research Council (EPSRC) grant [Monetize Me] [Grant Agreement: EP/L02185/1].

Acknowledgments: We would like to thank all participants who agreed to take part in this study across the different study sites.

Conflicts of Interest: The authors declare no conflict of interest.

References

1. Anderson, M.; Perrin, A. Tech Adoption Climbs among Older Adults. Pew Research Center. 2017. Available online: https://www.pewresearch.org/internet/2017/05/17/tech-adoption-climbs-among-older-adults/ (accessed on 1 July 2020).
2. Standard Eurobarometer 78. Media Use in the European Union. Available online: https://ec.europa.eu/commfrontoffice/publicopinion/archives/eb/eb78/eb78_media_en.pdf (accessed on 6 August 2020).
3. Smith, A. *Older Adults and Technology Use*; PEW Research Center: Washington, DC, USA, 2014.
4. Nations United. *World Population Prospects: The 2017 Revision, Key Findings and Advance Tables*; Department of Economics and Social Affairs PD: New York, NY, USA, 2017.
5. Office ONS. Living Longer: How Our Population Is Changing and Why It Matters. 2018. Available online: https://www.ons.gov.uk/peoplepopulationandcommunity/birthsdeathsandmarriages/ageing/articles/livinglongerhowourpopulationischangingandwhyitmatters/2018-08-13 (accessed on 1 July 2020).

6. Government of Canada. Action for Seniors Report. 2014. Available online: https://www.canada.ca/en/employment-social-development/programs/seniors-action-report.html (accessed on 1 July 2020).
7. Statistics Canada. Living Arrangements of Seniors. 2012. Available online: https://www12.statcan.gc.ca/census-recensement/2011/as-sa/98-312-x/98-312-x2011003_4-eng.cfm (accessed on 1 July 2020).
8. McCracken, M.; Tsesto, K.; Jean, B.; Young, K.; Huxter, D.; Halseth, G.; Green, M. Seniors in Rural and Remote Canada: Position Paper. Available online: http://publications.gc.ca/collection_2008/statcan/21-006-X/21-006-x2007008-eng.pdf (accessed on 1 July 2020).
9. Dandy, K.; Bollman, R. Seniors in Rural Canada; Rural and Small Town Canada Analysis Bulletin. Statistics Canada: Ottawa, Canada, 2008. Available online: http://www.statcan.gc.ca/pub/21-006-x/21-006-x2007008-eng.pdf (accessed on 1 July 2020).
10. Marston, H.R.; van Hoof, J. Who doesn't think about technology when designing urban environments for older people? A case study approach to a proposed extension of the WHO's age-friendly cities model. *Int. J. Environ. Res. Public Health* **2019**, *16*, 3525. [CrossRef] [PubMed]
11. Mickus, M.A.; Luz, C.C. Televisits: Sustaining long distance family relationships among institutionalized elders through technology. *Aging Ment. Health* **2002**, *6*, 387–396. [CrossRef] [PubMed]
12. Marston, H.R. Millennials and ICT—Findings from the technology 4 young adults (T4YA) project: An exploratory study. *Societies* **2019**, *9*, 80. [CrossRef]
13. Marston, H.R.; Freeman, S.; Bishop, A.K.; Beech, C.L. Utilization of digital games for older adults aged 85+ years: A scoping review. *Games Health J.* **2016**, *5*, 157–174. [CrossRef] [PubMed]
14. Marston, H.R.; Kroll, M.; Fink, D.; de Rosario, H.; Gschwind, Y.J. Technology use, adoption and behavior in older adults: Results from the iStoppFalls project. *Educ. Gerontol.* **2016**, *42*, 371–387. [CrossRef]
15. Haddon, L.; Mante-Meijer, E. *Generational Use of New Media*; Routledge: Abingdon, UK, 2016.
16. Loos, E. Senior citizens: Digital immigrants in their own country? *Observatorio* **2012**, *6*. [CrossRef]
17. Gschwind, Y.J.; Eichberg, S.; Ejupi, A.; de Rosario, H.; Kroll, M.; Marston, H.R.; Drobics, M.; Annegarn, J.; Wieching, R.; Lord, S.R.; et al. ICT-based system to predict and prevent falls (iStoppFalls): Results from an international multicenter randomized controlled trial. *Eur. Rev. Aging Phys. Act.* **2015**, *12*, 10. [CrossRef]
18. Marston, H.R.; Samuels, J. A review of age friendly virtual assistive technologies and their effect on daily living for carers and dependent adults. *Healthcare* **2019**, *7*, 49. [CrossRef]
19. Purington, A.; Taft, J.G.; Sannon, S.; Bazarova, N.N.; Taylor, S.H. Alexa is my new BFF. Social roles, user satisfaction, and personification of the amazon echo. In Proceedings of the 2017 CHI Conference Extended Abstracts on Human Factors in Computing Systems, Denver, CO, USA, 6–11 May 2017.
20. Marston, H.R.; Hadley, R.; Banks, D.; del Duro, M.M. Mobile self-monitoring ECG devices to diagnose arrhythmia that coincide with palpitations: A scoping review. *Healthcare* **2019**, *7*, 96. [CrossRef]
21. European Commission. *Information Society and Media. 2010: Independent Living for the Ageing Society*; Office for Official Publications of the European Communities: Luxembourg, 2007.
22. Cotton, S.R.; Anderson, W.A.; McCullough, B.M. Impact of internet use on loneliness and contact with others among older adults: Cross-sectional analysis. *J. Med. Internet Res.* **2013**, *15*, e39. [CrossRef]
23. Schimmele, C.; Davidson, J. Evolving Internet Use among Canadian Seniors. No. 2019015e. Available online: https://www150.statcan.gc.ca/n1/pub/11f0019m/11f0019m2019015-eng.htm (accessed on 1 July 2020).
24. Fernández-Ardèvol, M.; Ivan, L. Why age is not that important? In *An Ageing Perspective on Computer Anxiety. Design for Aging. Lecture Notes in Computer Science, Proceedings of the Human Aspects of IT for the Aged Population, Los Angeles, CA, USA, 2–7 August 2015*; Zhou, J., Salvendy, G., Eds.; Springer: Cham, Switzerland, 2015.
25. Hargittai, E.; Dobransky, K. Old dogs, new clicks: Digital inequality in skills and uses among older adults. *Can. J. Commun.* **2017**, *42*. [CrossRef]
26. Ivan, L. Elders and the use of mobile phones in romania: First results of semi-structured interviews. In Proceedings of the 2nd Open Workshop A-C-M BCN at the Interdisciplinary Internet Institute (IN3), Bacelona, Spain, 17–18 October 2012.
27. Taipale, S.; Wilska, T.-A.; Gilleard, C. *Digital Technologies and Generational Identity: ICT Usage across the Life Course*; Routledge: Abingdon, UK, 2017.
28. Taipale, S. *Intergenerational Connections in Digital Families*; Springer: Berlin/Heidelberg, Germany, 2019.
29. LoBuono, D.L.; Leedahl, S.N.; Maiocco, E. Older adults learning technology in an intergenerational program: Qualitative analysis of areas of technology requested for assistance. *Gerontechnology* **2019**. [CrossRef]

30. Broady, T.; Chan, A.; Caputi, P. Comparison of older and younger adults' attitudes towards and abilities with computers: Implications for training and learning. *Br. J. Educ. Technol.* **2010**, *41*, 473–485. [CrossRef]
31. Olson, K.E.; O'Brien, M.A.; Rogers, W.A.; Charness, N. Diffusion of technology: Frequency of use for younger and older adults. *Ageing Int.* **2011**, *36*, 123–145. [CrossRef] [PubMed]
32. Berry, R. *Older People and the Internet: Towards a 'System Map' of Digital Exclusion*; The International Longevity Centre: London, UK, 2011; pp. 1–18.
33. MacFarlane, H.; Kinirons, M.T.; Bultitude, M.F. WWW. Do not forget older people. *Age Ageing* **2012**, *41*, 807–810. [CrossRef]
34. Sinclair, D.; Creighton, H. *Opportunity Knocks: Designing Solutions for an Ageing Society*; The International Longevity Centre: London, UK, 2015.
35. OfCom. Adults' Media Use and Attitudes Report. 2014. Available online: https://www.ofcom.org.uk/__data/assets/pdf_file/0020/102755/adults-media-use-attitudes-2017.pdf (accessed on 1 July 2020).
36. Friemel, T.N. The digital divide has grown old: Determinants of a digital divide among seniors. *New Media Soc.* **2016**, *18*, 313–331. [CrossRef]
37. Xie, B. Older adults, computers, and the internet: Future directions. *Gerontechnology* **2003**, *2*, 289–305. [CrossRef]
38. Heinz, M.; Martin, P.; Margrett, J.A.; Yearns, M.; Franke, W.; Yang, H.I.; Wong, J.; Chang, C.K. Perceptions of technology among older adults. *J. Gerontol. Nurs.* **2013**, *39*, 42–51. [CrossRef]
39. Nimrod, G. Technophobia among older internet users. *Educ. Gerontol.* **2018**, *44*, 148–162. [CrossRef]
40. Duggan, M. *Mobile Messaging and Social Media 2015*; Pew Research Center: Washington, DC, USA, 2015.
41. Bailey, A.; Ngwenyama, O. Bridging the generation gap in ICT use: Interrogating identity, technology and interactions in community telecenters. *Inf. Technol. Dev.* **2010**, *16*, 62–82. [CrossRef]
42. McMillan, S.J.; Morrison, M. Coming of age with the internet: A qualitative exploration of how the internet has become an integral part of young people's lives. *New Media Soc.* **2006**, *8*, 73–95. [CrossRef]
43. Prensky, M. Digital Natives, Digital Immigrants. Available online: https://www.marcprensky.com/writing/Prensky%20-%20Digital%20Natives,%20Digital%20Immigrants%20-%20Part1.pdf (accessed on 1 July 2020).
44. Rama, M.D.; de Ridder, H.; Bouma, H. Technology generation and age in using layered user interfaces. *Gerontechnology* **2001**. [CrossRef]
45. Bennett, S.; Maton, K. Beyond the 'digital natives' debate: Towards a more nuanced understanding of students' technology experiences. *J. Comput. Assist. Learn.* **2010**, *26*, 321–331. [CrossRef]
46. Fernández-Ardèvol, M.; Sawchuk, K.; Grenier, L. Maintaining connections: Octo-and nonagenarians on digital 'use and non-use'. *Nord. Rev.* **2017**, *38*, 39–51. [CrossRef]
47. Biggs, S.; Haapala, I.; Lowenstein, A. Exploring generational intelligence as a model for examining the process of intergenerational relationships. *Ageing Soc.* **2011**, *31*, 1107–1124. [CrossRef]
48. Knodel, J. Is intergenerational solidarity really on the decline? Cautionary evidence from Thailand. *Asian Popul. Stud.* **2014**, *10*, 176–194. [CrossRef]
49. Lendon, J.P. A decade of love and hate: Trajectories of intergenerational ambivalence experienced by two cohorts of older parents and adult children. *J. Fam. Issues* **2017**, *38*, 336–357. [CrossRef]
50. Lowenstein, A. Approaching generational intelligence: Complexity and agency in an intergenerational world. In Proceedings of the XVIII ISA World Congress of Sociology, Yokohama, Japan, 13–19 July 2014.
51. Fernández-Ardèvol, M.; Ivan, L. Older people and mobile communication in two European contexts. *Rom. J. Commun. Public Relat.* **2016**, *15*, 83–98. [CrossRef]
52. Lloyd, J. *Retirement Capital and Online Social Networking*; International Longevity Centre: London, UK, 2007.
53. Marston, H.R.; Genoe, R.; Freeman, S.; Kulczycki, C.; Musselwhite, C. Older adults' perceptions of ICT: Main findings from the technology in later life (TILL) study. *Healthcare* **2019**. [CrossRef]
54. Tacken, M.; Marcellini, F.; Mollenkopf, H.; Ruoppila, I.; Szeman, Z. Use and acceptance of new technology by older people. Findings of the international MOBILATE survey: 'Enhancing mobility in later life'. *Gerontechnology* **2005**, *3*, 126–137.
55. Barbosa Neves, B.; Franz, R.; Judges, R.; Beermann, C.; Baecker, R. Can digital technology enhance social connectedness among older adults? A feasibility study. *J. Appl. Gerontol.* **2019**, *358*, 49–72. [CrossRef]
56. McConatha, D. Aging online: Toward a theory of e-quality. In *Older Adults, Health Information and the World Wide Web*; Morrell, R.W., Ed.; Lawrence Erlbaum Associates Publishers: Avenue Mahwah, NJ, USA, 2002; pp. 21–41.

57. Robinson, P.K.; Livingston, J.; Birren, J.E. *Aging and Technological Advances*; Springer Science & Business Media: Berlin/Heidelberg, Germany, 2012; Volume 24.
58. Severs, M. Will the information technology revolution improve services to elderly people in the new millennium. *Age Ageing* **1999**, *28*, 5–9.
59. Marston, H.R. Older adults as 21st century game designers. *Comput. Games J.* **2012**, *1*, 90–102. [CrossRef]
60. Patton, M.Q. *Qualitative Evaluation and Research Methods*; SAGE Publications, Inc.: Newbury Park, CA, USA, 1990.
61. Elo, S.; Kyngäs, H. The qualitative content analysis process. *J. Adv. Nurs.* **2008**, *62*, 107–115. [CrossRef]
62. Guba, E.G.; Lincoln, Y.S. *Fourth Generation Evaluation*; Sage: Newbury Park, CA, USA, 1989.
63. World Health Organization. *Global Age-Friendly Cities: A Guide*; World Health Organization: Geneva, Switzerland, 2007.
64. Khvorostianov, N. Thanks to the internet, we remain a family: ICT domestication by elderly immigrants and their families in Israel. *J. Fam. Commun.* **2016**, *16*, 355–368. [CrossRef]
65. Lazzaro, N. Why We Play Games: Four Keys to More Emotion without Story. 2004. Available online: http://www.xeodesign.com/xeodesign_whyweplaygames.pdf (accessed on 1 July 2020).
66. Voida, A.; Greenberg, S. Wii all play: The console game as a computational meeting place. In Proceedings of the SIGCHI Conference on Human Factors in Computing Systems, Boston, MA, USA, 4–9 April 2009.
67. Voida, A.; Greenberg, S. Console gaming across generations: Exploring intergenerational interactions in collocated console gaming. *Univers. Access Inf. Soc.* **2012**, *11*, 45–56.
68. Derboven, J.; van Gils, M.; de Grooff, D. Designing for collaboration: A study in intergenerational social game design. *Univers. Access Inf. Soc.* **2012**, *11*, 57–65. [CrossRef]
69. Selwyn, N. The social processes of learning to use computers. *Soc. Sci. Comput. Rev.* **2005**, *23*, 122–135. [CrossRef]
70. Keenan, T. *Internet Use among Midlife and Older Adults: An AARP Bulletin Poll*; AARP: Washington, DC, USA, 2009.
71. Taylor, R.W.; Fritsch, E.J.; Liederbach, J. *Digital Crime and Digital Terrorism*; Prentice Hall Press: Upper Saddle River, NJ, USA, 2014.
72. Ziegeldorf, J.H.; Morchon, O.G.; Wehrle, K. Privacy in the internet of things: Threats and challenges. *Secur. Commun. Netw.* **2014**, *7*, 2728–2742. [CrossRef]
73. Hadley, R. The lived experience of older involuntary childless men. In *Annul Journal of the British Sociological Association Study Group on Auto/Biograpghy*; BSA Auto/Biography Group: Durham, UK, 2017; pp. 93–108.
74. Hadley, R.A.; Westwood, S. Ageing without children, gender and social justice. In *Ageing, Diversity and Equality: Social Justice Perspectives*; Routledge: Abingdon, UK, 2018; pp. 66–81.

International Journal of
Environmental Research and Public Health

MDPI

Article

Combining the Digital, Social and Physical Layer to Create Age-Friendly Cities and Communities

Sonja Pedell [1,*], Ann Borda [2], Alen Keirnan [3] and Nicole Aimers [4]

1 School of Design, Faculty of Health, Arts and Design, Swinburne University of Technology, Hawthorn, VIC 3122, Australia
2 Centre for Digital Transformation of Health, Faculty of Medicine, Dentistry and Health Sciences, University of Melbourne, Parkville, VIC 3010, Australia; aborda@unimelb.edu.au
3 Life Without Barriers, Richmond, VIC 3121, Australia; alen.keirnan@lwb.org.au
4 Summer Foundation, Box Hill, VIC 3128, Australia; nicole.aimers@summerfoundation.org.au
* Correspondence: spedell@swinburne.edu.au; Tel.: +61-3-9214-6079

Abstract: This qualitative investigation makes suggestions about creating age-friendly cities for older adults focusing on three domains of the World Health Organization (WHO) age-friendly city framework namely "Communication and Information", "Outdoor Spaces and Buildings" and "Social Participation". The authors present two case studies, the first one focusing on older adults using activity wearables for health self-management in the neighborhood, and the second one focusing on older adults engaged in social prescribing activities in the community. The authors then reflect on the relationships of the domains and future opportunities for age-friendly cities. These case studies apply a co-design and citizen-based approach focusing within these larger frameworks on emotions, values and motivational goals of older adults. Results suggest how the convergence of the often siloed age-friendly city components based on older adults' goals and input can lead to better social participation and longer-term health outcomes. The authors propose that the digital, physical and social aspects need to be considered in all domains of age-friendly cities to achieve benefits for older adults. Further work involving older adults in the future shaping of age-friendly neighborhoods and cities, and identifying barriers and opportunities is required.

Keywords: age-friendly cities; active ageing; social prescribing; wearable technology; digital data layer; age-friendly communities; older adults; citizen science

Citation: Pedell, S.; Borda, A.; Keirnan, A.; Aimers, N. Combining the Digital, Social and Physical Layer to Create Age-Friendly Cities and Communities. *Int. J. Environ. Res. Public Health* **2021**, *18*, 325. http://doi.org/10.3390/ijerph18010325

Received: 3 November 2020
Accepted: 28 December 2020
Published: 5 January 2021

1. Introduction

Physical activity is key for active and healthy ageing, but the main barriers, such as lack of information about appropriate activities or about the environment, prevent older adults from pursuing these activities in a comfortable and safe manner. We propose that access to physical activities through the support of environmental and community infrastructure and digital information is important for older adults to remain independently active as long as possible with opportunities for social participation.

Our work looks at active ageing determinants—social and health determinants and their relationship to the physical environment connected through digital technology. The World Health Organization (WHO) launched a world-wide programme for initiating Age-Friendly Cities and Communities in 2007 which includes eight domains or 'petals' [1]. We bring together the two domains of "Communication and Information" and "Outdoor Spaces and Buildings" to create a convergent infrastructure that enables "Social Participation" a third domain named in the WHO framework (see Figure 1). We see social participation within a broad context in that actively engaging in the city environment and community spaces can facilitate social encounters and support the choice to socialize. We suggest initiatives are more usefully aligned to older adults when they are enabled to pursue physical activities in their neighbourhood and can take up more easily council services and community offerings tailored to them for active ageing. Such an approach is not easy to achieve as government, health care and research operate in a siloed manner [2] and even the age-friendly domains themselves are looked at separately by councils. However, we suggest collaboration needs to be sustained across different domains and stakeholder groups with a focus on older adults' needs through a bottom up citizen-based approach. We investigate age-friendly cities for active ageing through the lens of two case studies using qualitative research methods—the first one using activity wearables in the neighbourhood and the second one focusing on social prescribing in the community.

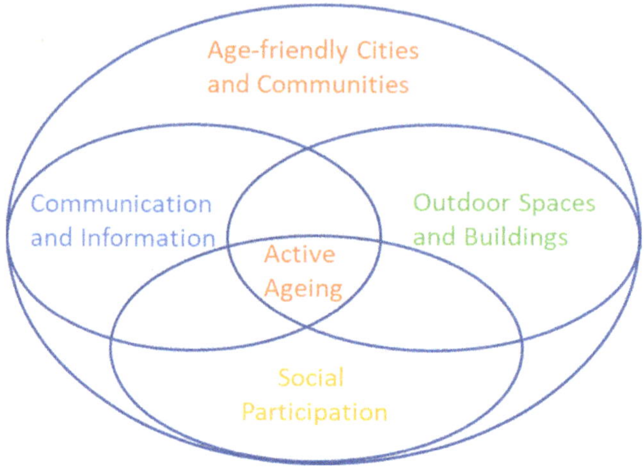

Figure 1. Convergence of age-friendly domains.

2. Case Study 1: Wearing the Smart City: Supporting Older Adults to Exercise by Combining Age-Friendly Environments and Tailored Digital Public Data

In response to the call for more age-friendly cities, this research focused on wearable health technology overcoming some challenges posed by the environment for older adults to be active. Due to the global trend of population ageing, there has been great emphasis placed on 'healthy ageing' which is defined as a "lifelong process of optimising opportunities for improving and preserving health and physical, social and mental wellness, independence, quality of life and enhancing successful life-course transitions" [3] (p. 1). In particular, an urgent need has been highlighted to develop strategies to ensure that older people enjoy life in their years and not just extra years in their life [4]. This gives rise to the question of how we can better support the parameters of healthy ageing.

Firstly, there needs to be an understanding of the parameters of digital literacy, without which older adults will experience limitations of the immense potential of the Internet, such as access to public services [5], and other information and communication technology (ICT) such as wearable devices for health self-management [6]. Several studies have revealed the positive effects of internet use and technologies not only on the wellbeing and quality of life of seniors [7], but also in the ability for them to engage in 'smart' forms of healthcare [6,8].

Secondly in response to this question, the WHO developed the concept of 'age-friendly cities' in order to optimise opportunities for preserving and improving wellness and quality of life [1,9]. As identified by Alley and colleagues [4], age-friendly cities should ideally provide a supportive environment, enabling residents to grow older actively within their families, neighbourhoods, and civic society and present opportunities for their participation in the community.

The convergence of ageing, residing within cities, and age-friendliness, is rapidly producing new modalities to better identify the challenges, such as the notion of 'urban ageing', defined as the population of older people living in cities [10]. Such challenges include the creation of inclusive neighbourhoods and the implementation of technology for ageing-in-place and independent living.

According to Kestens and colleagues [11], few studies have considered older adults' daily mobility to better understand how local urban and social environments may contribute to healthy aging. However, one way in which a better understanding can be gained is through the use of wearable sensors and software applications as they can offer novel means for gathering information on mobility and levels of physical activity [11]. In line with Kestens and colleagues [11], the use of wearable devices in the support and management of independent older adults is becoming more widely advocated [12] and a growing number of seniors are using wearable devices to self-monitor and manage their health [13].

2.1. Materials and Method

This case study was part of a larger project building an evidence base focusing on independently living older adults who are using or have used consumer wearable device(s) to self-manage or self-monitor their health [14]. From among the initial cohort of survey respondents, those opting to be interviewed were followed up and comprise this subsequent study. The present study involved a total of eight older adults aged 65 years or older actively using a wearable device(s). The group comprised two male and six female participants, seven of whom fell within the age range 65–69 at the time of the interview, and one in the age range over 80. Among the chronic conditions being 'managed' by wearable use included high blood-pressure, arthritis, and obesity. No specific or personal identifying medical information were sought and personal interview data on wearers' experiences were anonymised. Semi-structured interviews of approximately 60 min were conducted with participants via Skype, phone and/or email. Interview questions were centred around participant experiences and aspirations towards self-management of health using wearable devices.

We applied motivational modelling [15] as the analysis framework. In order to maximise uptake of wearable devices, we propose that more research needs to take place to better understand the functional, quality and emotional goals of older adults when using this technology to maximum benefit within their urban environment. Collectively, these goals form the basis of motivational modelling which not only focuses upon the functionality of solution concepts such as technology (i.e., what it should do) but also considers the social context in which the solution concept is being used. As such, by also modelling the quality goals (i.e., what it should be) and the emotional goals (i.e., how should it feel) of the solution concept, the holistic needs of the end users can be identified which will enable products, systems and services to better support people in their everyday lives [15–17]. A thematic analysis of interview transcripts was conducted through the lens of these three thematic frames: The individual user emotions (i.e., how the wearable technology should feel), the qualities of the wearable technology (i.e., what the wearable technology should be) and the functional aspects of the wearable technology (i.e., what the wearable technology should do).

The research reported on in this case study has received ethics approval by the University of Melbourne Human Research Ethics Committee (Ethics ID: 1646991.2).

2.2. Findings

2.2.1. Motivational Goals for Active Ageing

A common emotion experienced across all users was a feeling of motivation afforded by the wearable health technologies. This finding aligns with comparable studies [18]. Here, motivation was described by participants as the core driver to use their technology.

While a feeling of motivation was expressed as a core emotion when using wearable health technology, participants described the technology as being a reference point or providing feedback on their participation in exercise which attributed to their motivation.

This was seen as the key quality of the wearable device use tied in with motivational behaviour as the following quote shows:

> *"And then I found that I'd be sitting there till 10:00 or 11:00 in the morning doing some work. And then I realized I'd only done a thousand steps tonight and that would horrify me. So, I'd be out there and make sure [. . .] I did some activity after work and I was much more motivated knowing that I was needing to do more activity."*

The primary functional aspects for which participants described their wearable health technology is to manage their health. Managing one's health ranged from gaining insights into sleeping behaviours, blood pressure, weight and pain [19].

2.2.2. Wearable Health Technology and the Urban Environment

Several participants directly discussed their interactions with the urban environment. This took various forms. For example, the use of wearable health technology was a motivator for more city walking.

> *"If we don't have much on and we need to go into the city my husband and I will walk into the city so that is 3.5 km. You know I just like to record that."*

In two cases wearable health technology was a motivator in urban mobility in combination with other interventions, for example.

> *"The minimum exercise I have every day is walking to the bus stop and I get off the bus a few stops early and walk up the back streets to the hospital. And that's even more now because of the changes with the roadworks. Sometimes I'll get the bus in the morning and walk home at night. I just have to monitor how my hip [is doing] and bail out if it it's not up to it."*

In a unique case, one participant who took part in the study from outside Australia (Sweden) became increasingly involved in the use of multiple wearable health devices for health self-management, including the use of a chip implanted in his hand. The latter enabled the participant to engage in a smart city scenario.

> *"We use it in our office to open doors and get the printers running and I can use it when I check in to the gym. I can use it when I travel by Swedish railroad. The railroad company can read the chip with their Android phones. The motivational goals in this case are also tempered by emotional ones and perhaps due to the uncommon nature of the adoption of the technology."* and *"I have it [the chip] in my hand. So that's sort of a real—you know—discussion starter. Half of the people—no, one third, say "oh that's terrible". I would never do that. And it's really very emotional. It's not like you know they thought about the pros and cons."*

This quote demonstrates not only the potential for interacting in more substantial ways with the environment, but also the importance of emotional aspects for uptake.

2.3. Discussion

Through three thematic frames of analysis, it was identified that participants wanted to feel motivated when using the technology and, in addition to being a reference point, they wanted the wearable to aid in the management of their health and wellbeing in subtle and controllable ways.

The results show that while the potential design for future wearable health technologies can consider the emotional, quality and functional needs, the environment in which older people experience these attributes is paramount [20]. For example, consider an older person who requires access to public toilets. Their motivation to walk may be present but following through with the action (of walking) may be limited in environments where there are few public conveniences. Likewise, consider an older person who would like to rest under shaded areas on a sunny day. Using their wearable device as a reference point to compare how many steps they did for the day before becomes impractical because again, they are unlikely to go for a walk within environments where there are few shaded areas. Within the present study context, the emotional, quality and functional goals become obsolete when there are environmental barriers within the community, resulting in activity goals unable to be fully achieved. Supporting studies have shown that safe, walkable, and aesthetically designed neighbourhoods, with access to specific destinations and services positively influenced older adults' physical activity participation [12,21].

It is argued that more research needs to take place to better understand the holistic goals of older adults when using wearable devices within their urban environment and how to overcome barriers posed through the environment. By doing so, insights into framework development for the design of age friendlier cities can be gained.

The present study highlights the opportunities in considering the potential relationship of urban environmental factors within a digital health and urban ageing context. This 'lens' has inevitably considered that there are also differing definitional boundaries across individual preferences, health and wellbeing technologies and determinants of health, which require a larger cohort to determine the extent and measures of correlates providing more guidance for age-friendly city strategies. In this study we focused on independently living adults who already were using wearable devices—greater attention also needs to be paid to lower the threshold and increase digital literacy for a wider group of older adults to experience the benefits of wearable devices to be more active in their neighborhoods.

3. Case Study 2: Social Prescribing Supporting Social Connectedness in Age-Friendly Communities

Originating in Europe, social prescribing aims for a more holistic health approach to increase social integration while supporting a person's interests. Through a feasibility study on introducing social prescription in Australia we demonstrate that a bottom-up, neighbourhood-oriented approach is necessary to understand how to overcome barriers to designing a social prescribing service. Social prescribing shows the potential of supporting people to access social activities in the community they are interested in and create new opportunities for combining social and physical activity. We suggest that within the social prescribing concept digital technology can play a key role for people who are vulnerable and easily excluded. People who are digitally and socially connected are safer. Enabling social connections building resilient healthy communities is the responsibility of a holistic health system. Social prescribing is not only relevant for older adults but they have been identified as a main stakeholder group [22].

'Social prescribing' is a non-medical referral that links community services with people who are at risk, or experiencing isolation or depression [23]. The person or role prescribing the service can differ from country to country as well as within one country depending on the organisation. Prescribed activities can fall within 'social', 'physical' or 'economic' categories [24] and aim to improve self-care within the community [25]. The literature describes the characteristics of social prescription, stakeholders and models of delivery [23–26]. Accordingly, the health client journey involves general practitioners working with health clients to determine their level of wellbeing and social interests. In a holistic model of social prescribing, allied health clinicians also play a role in referring health clients to community services. Next, a community connector in collaboration with the health client develops an action plan detailing goals and schedules. Community connectors [25] are people who locate community services for health clients also develop care and well-being plans. A community connector will have strong relationships with umbrella organisations and use their interpersonal skills to help build their health clients' confidence and independence.

The literature shows promising evidence to the benefits of social prescribing, primarily in the United Kingdom [23–26] and in Canada [27]. Social prescribing can involve a variety of activities designed to support people with a wide range of social, emotional or practical needs. Services often focus on improving mental health and physical well-being; for example, volunteering, arts activities, group learning, gardening, healthy eating advice and sports [28–30]. 'Nature-based' social prescribing programs are expanding their reach rather than contracting, despite COVID-19 limitations [31]. In countries such as the UK, U.S., and Canada, there is a grass roots movement among healthcare providers and community and parks services to prescribe physical activity in greenspaces [32], such as Parkrx (https://www.parkrx.org/) managed by the Golden Gate National Parks Conservancy in the San Francisco area and the U.S. National Parks Service. In addition to the physical park spaces and park-based activities around San Francisco which encourage age-friendly activities, there is an openly accessible digital presence as an information hub for "Park Prescriptions" and community resources.

Building spaces also have the potential to draw on social capital and social participation opportunities in a more integrated way, such as museums and cultural venues. Cultural programming is integral to social prescribing referral schemes and they show documented benefits in the involvement of older adults with outcomes of improved psychological wellbeing and social connection [33].

Consequently, social prescribing is located at the crossroads of holistic health, community care and social engagement. Models are still in their infancy and yet to be adopted in Australia but there are strides towards adoption in some form. The COVID-19 predicament in particular has been seen as a timely catalyst for Australia to consider the emerging practice of social prescribing in responding to some of the harmful mental health outcomes of isolation that may not be suitably addressed with conventional medical care [34]. Here, we summarise some key findings on our research for a social prescribing service to be tailored for and piloted in Australia. We focus on the aspects relevant for age-friendly cities and communities.

3.1. Materials and Method

The community health provider we collaborated with already offers different portfolios (medical, clinical and community portfolio) of services and hence is uniquely positioned to use existing portfolios as springboard to deliver a social prescribing to their clients. However, the partner was unsure how such a service should be set up and introduced to the community to receive acceptance and longer-term adoption as well as how its success can be determined.

The study recognized the importance of health clients as citizens and co-researchers in the design of holistic healthcare solutions in the community. Co-design, as a participatory design process used in citizen science, collectively involves participants and stakeholders working together through active participation from the design stage of research to the interpretation of research results and to their transformation into concrete actions. This process makes full use of participants' knowledge, resources and contributions, to achieve better outcomes or improved efficiency in health research or service design (for example [35,36]).

We wanted to ensure representation from different departments, and using the literature about social prescribing highlighted departments and/or job functions that were previously described in the different UK equivalents. These included intake officers, community connectors, physicians and specialist therapist groups. With our selection criteria, we sent targeted emails to these groups for the purpose of recruitment for the first staff workshop. Staff in relevant service areas identified in this workshop were invited to the second workshop.

During the staff workshops, there was a thread describing who in the community were likely to be service users. These included people who were new parents, people who are migrating from one country to another, social technology-dependent people, night shift workers and older adults. These themes formed the basis of our selection criteria. Leveraging the Future Self and Design Living Lab community pool, six key community members who fit within these themes were contacted and asked to participate (age range in their twenties to nineties). As a result, a new parent (1), recently migrated (2), and older adults (3) participated in the workshop. More details on the recruitment process can be found in [22].

Michael Schrage [37] notes: "Innovation is not innovators innovating but customers adopting" (p. 91). Innovation should only be measured by the value it creates to people's lives. Hence, what often is missing is an approach that spans from designing to impact measurements of holistic health and community services that include the voice of the users. This is a key motivator of the present study and in the selection of methodologies. Also, interventions, as well as decision-making, are more effective when the target group is engaged in an equitable partnership [35]. The co-design process took place over the course of several iterative engagements through interviews and workshops.

Aims (with stakeholders and methods in brackets) were to:

1. Explore resources, enablers and barriers for a social prescribing service in the community (interviews and focus group with staff);
2. Explore emotions, values, qualities and goals of a social prescribing service with potential clients (focus group with community members);
3. Co-design a conceptual scenario-based service model with key stakeholders (focus group with staff);
4. Use citizen science as a model to maintain participatory approaches to shape social prescribing services as part of a bigger learning system (outlook on evaluation and sustainability)

We conducted seven interviews with the organisation's staff from different service areas to better understand the whole existing ecosystem. Building on the interviews and knowledge of the ecosystem gained two co-design workshops with health practitioners and one client workshop were facilitated to understand the goals of the respective stakeholder groups and the user journey throughout the social prescribing service. All three workshops were designed for the results to cascade into the next, ensuring the co-design process was open and flexible. The research for this case study has received ethics approval by the Swinburne Human Research Ethics Committee (ID 2016/144).

3.2. Findings

3.2.1. Barriers within the Community Health Provider's Ecosystem

The data collected with staff confirmed three portfolios which should 'ideally' refer services to each other and barriers preventing communication and client transfers where revealed. The rapid growth of the organisation was pointed out as a potential barrier to communication among the three portfolios creating silos. Established and one-directional pathways within the organisation prevented the clients from moving from one portfolio to another. In particular, the lack of mental health awareness was discussed as a whole of organisation barrier which also would affect the referral onward to a social prescription service in the community. Other barriers included time poor staff, broken pathways and channels, but also an assumed limited motivation and interest of clients.

The staff interviews reinforced the literature findings that social prescribing is not based on a traditional medical model, but needs to be tied in with the community structures:

> *"Social prescribing is looking at someone as a whole. It's a holistic approach to talking about someone's care"* and *"Ways they can prescribe things for them to do socially that will assist them for their health rather than just drugs they can take."*

Importantly its success is determined on how people want to feel and engage:

> *" ... ways that people can help themselves to improve their wellbeing or engage in an activity to help them benefit their mood."*

Consequently, the involvement of future service recipients is key to the social prescription concept. A client workshop with community members was organised to address this. A two-hour workshop with six potential clients revealed important insights about emotions, goals, tangible aspects of social prescription and, importantly, underlying values.

3.2.2. Values and Goals Expected from a Social Prescribing Service (Community Member Workshop)

The workshop with clients produced two main outcomes. The first outcome is describing the different values of a social prescription. It shows the different characteristics and values of a social prescription that clients would like to have embedded into their experience. The second outcome, a goal model, accompanies the values demonstrating the preferred emotions, qualities and functions that a health client would like to interact with during their social prescription service (see Figure 2).

Four values were deemed necessary if clients were to engage with a social prescription offering by the community health provider. A sense of connection (i) to the greater community was described as integral to the social prescribing journey. This might be a simple referral to a wider network of activities outside the organisation after a period of time. Clients also wanted to feel safe and comfortable (ii) with their clinicians and not stigmatised. This also included to be able to determine their own course of action.

The clinician should feel trustworthy (iii) that the clients could feel confident in their abilities e.g., a sense of knowing that the health provider is aware of mental health illness and how to diagnose and treat such illnesses were important. Finally, clients wanted a real sense of having a tailored approach (iv) to their social prescription. This included that their interests should be known. Upholding these values were associated emotions, qualities and functions as shown in Figure 2. Across all goals it is apparent how digital technology can play a key role in a successful community service achieving qualities such as being accessible in also providing information online and non-dismissive in taking on board needs and feedback over time. Functional goals such as the community service provider staying in touch that service recipients are feeling connected and supported could also be facilitated by technology.

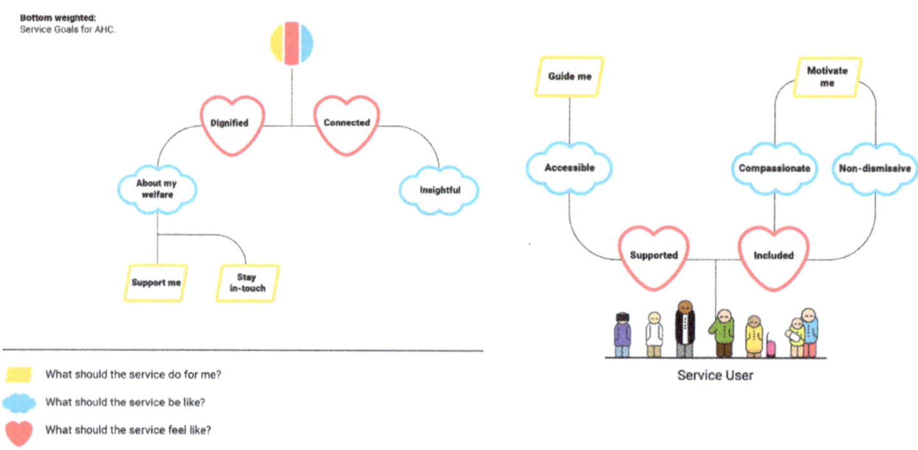

Figure 2. Goals (do/be/feel) that a social prescribing service should do according to the community.

A final co-design workshop with staff confirmed the values and goals collected with the service recipients. This led to a service concept based on the goals and values of the community.

3.3. Discussion

We framed the involvement of the multiple stakeholder groups as one informed by citizen science to understand how to overcome organisational and environmental barriers. The result is a concept proposal that suggests service pathways for a social prescription based on the healthcare providers' and their stakeholders' values and needs.

Older adults were identified as key stakeholder group. Our approach can inform other health-related services in the community giving older adults a stronger voice in the design, implementation and maintenance of wellbeing services that extend the traditional medical model of health and lead to more age-friendly cities.

The aim of the program logic (part of the service blueprint) was to capture whether the inputs, activities and outputs will lead to the desired outcomes according to the results from the client and staff consultation. To evaluate the outcomes of a social prescription trial service, and refine the service to a sustainable model, meaningful data, capturing the successes, failures, and positive or negative journey experiences for all stakeholders are necessary. Values and client goals become key to the evaluation over time.

A learning healthcare system (LHS) is broadly defined as: " ... one that is designed to generate and apply the best evidence for the collaborative healthcare choices of each patient and provider; to drive the process of discovery as a natural outgrowth of patient care; and to ensure innovation, quality, safety, and value in health care" [38].

Since this original definition, there has been increasing recognition of the need to engage with various stakeholders including patients, participants, health care providers, and policy-makers among others to understand how to drive a sustainable LHS [39]. The bottom-up approach of citizen science involving diverse stakeholders and localised problem-solving is an effective way to translate knowledge to a broader audience and to support iterative evaluation processes within an LHS [40]. A post-implementation stage of evaluation, for example, offers opportunities to engage citizens to monitor problems, and to facilitate an open exchange of various perspectives, and thereby improve mutual understanding without some of the limitations of formal research methods.

In this way, citizen science participation can be more open among other methodological approaches in that the citizens do not always need to be pre-selected by researchers or healthcare providers [41,42]. This allows for an agile model that focuses on evolving community needs rather than producing generalisable knowledge and which closely aligns with the notion of an LHS [39,43].

4. Discussion on Converging Perspectives

Taken together the two case studies illustrate a convergence of the three domains or petals of age-friendly cities, "Communication and Information" and "Outdoor spaces and buildings", leading to better "Social Participation" which are collectively undergoing a dramatic digital transformation as a result of the challenges created by COVID-19 [44,45]. These challenges present a unique opportunity to understand the future ways wearable technologies and communication technologies that can be integrated into digitally enabled age-friendly cities and community context and support the immediate social needs of older adults.

4.1. Communication and Information

Going forward, there is an urgent need to enable equitable access to the Internet, and digital enabling technologies, such as wearable technologies, especially if these are socially or medically prescribed [46]. The recently published Topol Review [47] notes that technology has the potential to worsen health inequality if not used correctly. In a move towards smarter cities and communities, in particular, there is a universal recognition that vulnerable people often are those who are not digitally literate [48], and thereby become excluded from accessing health interventions and community services increasing the digital divide in particular for older adults. Digital literacy requires the embedding of digital skills and accessible training, for instance, in a dedicated social prescribing program which can be available to intergenerational communities [49].

With this potential, citizens, such as older adults, can leverage smart cities with its digital technologies and Internet of Things (IoT)-enabled infrastructure to provide actionable insights that help improve their health and well-being [8]. Older adults, for instance, can use ICT to gather and share information about themselves and the environment that surrounds them. Projects like the European funded PULSE (Participatory Urban Living for Sustainable Environments) is developing a public health observatory, with the participation of intergenerational citizen scientists using wearable devices [50] across seven cities: Paris, Singapore, Birmingham, Barcelona, New York, Pavia, and Keelung.

4.2. Outdoor Spaces and Buildings

Our ability to connect spaces with people and healthy communication is key in this direction. Social prescribing, for instance, offers a capability to join up aspects of this—especially if a programme can integrate both physical and digital access—e.g., digital apps and wearables supporting older adults in their interactions in the built environment or local neighbourhood, whether for increased exercise, lower level mental health issues such as mild anxiety, and social isolation through chat applications and smart walking guides, for example, den Haan et al. [51].

In line with the 'age friendly' cities framework in which outdoor spaces and buildings are identified as a domain of city life which can assist with active and healthy ageing, it is argued that there is a further need for public infrastructure data sets. Specifically, if a digital city layer showing, for example where facilities such as public toilets, water fountains and shaded rest stops were located on exercise routes in communities, it is possible that this would support older people in achieving their exercise goals and ultimately, optimise opportunities for preserving and improving wellness and quality of life. This could be available as an app which would allow older people to download directly to their smart wearable device and customise the information, depending on where they are located and their preferences to show the information needed [11,52]. Given the continual advancements in wearable technology, the ability to tailor this information for each older person and integrate this information in an easy to understand way on their smart device is becoming achievable [53]. However, this means that the digital information layer about the environment needs to exist along with connectivity to the wearable device. Critically, a framework is required to be in place in which the individual and community can responsibly share the data, as well as govern it [6].

4.3. Social Participation

Studies show that sustained community engagement requires creative approaches to promote the wellbeing and social involvement of older adults and vulnerable individuals [54]. The co-design of community apps and the use of digital storytelling are among the effective ways of supporting age-friendly cities and communities [55]. An acknowledged gap is how technologies can be used and deployed across different communities and how these can be improved, adopted and innovated by communities of older adults [21]. There are untapped areas of technology adoption, for instance, such as gamification which may lend itself to support different social interactions in outdoors and building spaces, beyond what might be assumed as stereotypically a younger generational platform [56].

Partnerships of researchers and community agencies are integral in collaborating directly with communities so that social solutions can move beyond the generic and placeless, and become embedded into specific locally relevant programming to better connect the individual and community to a place in age-friendly ways.

Here we argue that in the context of age-friendly cities, there is a need to connect to the smart city discussion by breaking up silos of technology, the environment and human-centred design. In putting forward the goals of older adults, we acknowledge the existence of different needs and how they can be accomplished through knowledge about the environment and through forms of social participation. Given that wearable devices are increasingly being used by older adults, it is important to take the next step to connect the environment, socio-technological considerations, and the user in order to create a holistic system that supports the quality of life of an ageing person.

4.4. Limitations

This present study was limited to three domains of the Age-Friendly Cities and Communities Framework and the relationships across these. It was not intended to provide a comprehensive approach to the topic—but rather an exploratory one that highlights the opportunities in considering the potential relationships across the environment and ICT factors within a digital health and age-friendly context. This lens has inevitably taken into account the outcomes of the two case studies that highlight differing definitional boundaries across individual and community preferences, technologies and determinants of health. For instance, there were potential differences in the adoption of wearable technologies and literacies in health self-management. Subsequent studies will require a larger sample cohort to determine the extent and measurements of correlates. Visual analyses would further provide a means to examine social determinants of health, urban and geolocative features in more detail in order for these to translate into concrete recommendations for age-friendliness city and community strategies.

5. Conclusions

This paper has focused on three age-friendly city components and the benefits of their convergence to potentially help activate changes that can improve older peoples' health and support their social participation in neighbourhoods and communities. Through case study examples, the significance of place in the lives of older people and how they can participate underpin the importance of their surrounding environments as sources of meaning and self-identity.

In particular, support for active participation through digitally-enabled platforms can lead to sustained independence and reduced risk of isolation, for example, through the availability of appropriate communication and information to help maintain relationships and networks, as well as providing safer access to services and amenities. Thus, the reasons for such convergence are not only about creating an age-friendly environment, but they are also necessarily linked to increasing the years of quality of life.

Notwithstanding this, there needs to be much further work in building up real-world examples of interventions involving older adults in the future that shape age-friendly neighbourhoods and cities, as well as in identifying barriers to and opportunities from their participation. This can be in the form of the application of assistive technology in the community to navigate local environments as time spent outdoors or to reach amenities, or other supporting forms of social interaction and the development of social networks with consequential benefits for physical and mental health. The need for places where citizens regardless of their age will feel secure and capable is a significant challenge not least in terms of the range of experiences by different groups and their social determinants of health—but this is the start of the basis for re-designing age-friendly and smart communities directly and collaboratively with those affected communities in order to achieve such a goal.

Author Contributions: Conceptualization, A.B. and S.P.; methodology, A.B. and S.P.; formal analysis, N.A., A.B., A.K., S.P.; investigation, A.B., A.K., S.P.; resources, A.B. and S.P.; data curation, A.B. and S.P.; writing—original draft preparation, N.A., A.B., A.K., S.P.; writing—review and editing, A.B. and S.P.; project administration A.B. and S.P.; funding acquisition, A.B., A.K. and S.P. All authors have read and agreed to the published version of the manuscript.

Funding: For case study 1 Ann Borda received an Expert Visit grant in 2019 as part of the EPIC project funded under the EU Horizon 2020 programme (ICT) to explore advancing approaches to citizen science in health and medical research. The research of case study 2 was funded by Access, Health and Community, Melbourne Victoria and conducted in collaboration with Sonja Pedell and Alen Keirnan.

Institutional Review Board Statement: The Study was conducted according to the guidelines of the Declaration of Helsinki. Case Study 1 approved by the University of Melbourne Human Research Ethics Committee (Ethics ID: 1646991.1, 18 July 2016). Case Study 2 approved by the Swinburne Human Research Ethics Committee (ID 2016/144 and 23 August 2016).

Informed Consent Statement: Informed consent was obtained from all subjects involved in the study.

Data Availability Statement: The data presented in this study are available on request from the corresponding author. The data are not publicly available due to ethical approvals at the time.

Acknowledgments: We would like to thank all participants in case study 1 and staff and clients of Access Health and Community involved in the research of case study 2 and for the open discussion and their valuable insights during the co-design workshops.

Conflicts of Interest: The authors declare no conflict of interest.

References

1. World Health Organization. Global Age-Friendly Cities: A Guide; Report. 2007. Available online: https://www.who.int/ageing/publications/Global_age_friendly_cities_Guide_English.pdf (accessed on 23 December 2020).
2. Greenfield, E.A.; Oberlink, M.; Scharlach, A.E.; Neal, M.B.; Stafford, P.B. Age-friendly community initiatives: Conceptual issues and key questions. *Gerontologist* **2015**, *55*, 191–198. [CrossRef] [PubMed]
3. Health Canada. Workshop on Healthy Aging. 2001. Available online: http://publications.gc.ca/collections/Collection/H39-612-2002-1E.pdf (accessed on 23 December 2020).
4. Alley, D.; Liebig, P.; Pynoos, J.; Banerjee, T.; Choi, I.H. Creating elder-friendly communities: Preparations for an aging society. *J. Gerontol. Soc. Work* **2007**, *49*, 1–18. [CrossRef] [PubMed]
5. Caruso, L. Digital innovation and the fourth industrial revolution: Epochal social changes? *AI Soc.* **2018**, *33*, 379–392. [CrossRef]
6. Cosco, T.D.; Firth, J.; Vahia, I.; Sixsmith, A.; Torous, J. Mobilizing mHealth data collection in older adults: Challenges and opportunities. *JMIR Aging* **2019**, *2*. [CrossRef]
7. Gustafson, D.H.; McTavish, F.; Gustafson, D.H.; Mahoney, J.E.; Johnson, R.A.; Lee, J.D.; Quanbeck, A.; Atwood, A.K.; Isham, A.; Veeramani, R.; et al. The effect of an information and communication technology (ICT) on older adults' quality of life: Study protocol for a randomized control trial. *Trials* **2015**, *16*, 1–12. [CrossRef]
8. Cook, D.J.; Duncan, G.; Sprint, G.; Fritz, R.L. Using Smart City Technology to Make Healthcare Smarter. *Proc. IEEE* **2018**, *106*, 708–722. [CrossRef]
9. WHO. The Global Network for Age-friendly Cities and Communities: Looking Back over the Last Decade, Looking forward to the Next. 2018. Available online: https://www.who.int/ageing/publications/gnafcc-report-2018/en/ (accessed on 23 December 2020).
10. van Hoof, J.; Kazak, J.K.; Perek-Białas, J.M.; Peek, S.T.M. The challenges of urban ageing: Making cities age-friendly in Europe. *Int. J. Environ. Res. Public Health* **2018**, *15*, 2473. [CrossRef]
11. Kestens, Y.; Chaix, B.; Gerber, P.; Desprès, M.; Gauvin, L.; Klein, O.; Klein, S.; Köppen, B.; Lord, S.; Naud, A.; et al. Understanding the role of contrasting urban contexts in healthy aging: An international cohort study using wearable sensor devices (the CURHA study protocol). *BMC Geriatr.* **2016**, *16*, 96. [CrossRef]
12. Barnett, D.W.; Barnett, A.; Nathan, A.; Van Cauwenberg, J.; Cerin, E. Built environmental correlates of older adults' total physical activity and walking: A systematic review and meta-analysis. *Int. J. Behav. Nutr. Phys. Act.* **2017**, *14*. [CrossRef]
13. McMahon, S.K.; Lewis, B.; Oakes, M.; Guan, W.; Wyman, J.F.; Rothman, A.J. Older adults' experiences using a commercially available monitor to self-track their physical activity. *JMIR mHealth uHealth* **2016**, *4*, 35–45. [CrossRef]
14. Borda, A.; Gilbert, C.; Gray, K.; Prabhu, D. Consumer wearable information and health self management by older adults. In *Studies in Health Technology and Informatics*; Van den Berg, M., Maeder, A., Eds.; IOS Press: Amsterdam, The Netherlands, 2018; pp. 42–61. ISBN 9781614998440. [CrossRef]
15. Sterling, L.S.; Taveter, K. *The Art of Agent-Oriented Modeling*; MIT Press: Cambridge, MA, USA, 2018. [CrossRef]
16. Miller, T.; Pedell, S.; Sterling, L.; Vetere, F.; Howard, S. Understanding socially oriented roles and goals through motivational modelling. *J. Syst. Softw.* **2012**, *85*, 2160–2170. [CrossRef]
17. Marshall, J. Agent-Based Modelling of Emotional Goals in Digital Media Design Projects. *Int. J. People-Oriented Program.* **2014**, *1*, 44–59. [CrossRef]
18. Kononova, A.; Li, L.; Kamp, K.; Bowen, M.; Rikard, R.V.; Cotten, S.; Peng, W. The use of wearable activity trackers among older adults: Focus group study of tracker perceptions, motivators, and barriers in the maintenance stage of behavior change. *J. Med. Internet Res.* **2019**, *7*, e9832. [CrossRef] [PubMed]
19. Kim, B.Y.B.; Lee, J. Smart devices for older adults managing chronic disease: A scoping review. *JMIR mHealth uHealth* **2017**, *5*, e69. [CrossRef]
20. Ehn, M.; Johansson, A.C.; Revenäs, Å. Technology-based motivation support for seniors' physical activity—A qualitative study on seniors' and health care professionals' views. *Int. J. Environ. Res. Public Health* **2019**, *16*, 2418. [CrossRef]
21. Tuckett, A.G.; Freeman, A.; Hetherington, S.; Gardiner, P.A.; King, A.C. Older adults using our voice citizen science to create change in their neighborhood environment. *Int. J. Environ. Res. Public Health* **2018**, *15*, 2685. [CrossRef]
22. Pedell, S.; Borda, A.; Keirnan, A. Social Prescribing in Australia: How the Bottom-up Model of Citizen Science Can Facilitate Stakeholder Engagement in Health Service Design. In *Proceedings of DLLD 2020*; eBook; European Network of Living Labs (ENoLL): Brussels, Belgium, 2020; pp. 76–94. ISBN 9789464078923.
23. Carnes, D.; Sohanpal, R.; Frostick, C.; Hull, S.; Mathur, R.; Netuveli, G.; Tong, J.; Hutt, P.; Bertotti, M. The impact of a social prescribing service on patients in primary care: A mixed methods evaluation. *BMC Health Serv. Res.* **2017**, *17*. [CrossRef]

24. Woodall, J.; Trigwell, J.; Bunyan, A.M.; Raine, G.; Eaton, V.; Davis, J.; Hancock, L.; Cunningham, M.; Wilkinson, S. Understanding the effectiveness and mechanisms of a social prescribing service: A mixed method analysis. *BMC Health Serv. Res.* **2018**, *18*. [CrossRef]
25. Moffatt, S.; Steer, M.; Lawson, S.; Penn, L.; O'Brien, N. Link Worker social prescribing to improve health and well-being for people with long-term conditions: Qualitative study of service user perceptions. *BMJ Open* **2017**, *7*, e015203. [CrossRef]
26. Kimberlee, R. What Is Social Prescribing? *Adv. Soc. Sci. Res. J.* **2015**, *2*. [CrossRef]
27. Mulligan, K.; Hsiung, S.; Bhatti, S.; Rehel, J.; Rayner, J. *Rx: Community Social Prescribing in Ontario. Final Report*; Alliance for Healthier Communities: Toronto, ON, Canada, 2020.
28. Polley, M.; Fleming, J.; Anfilogoff, T.; Carpenter, A. *Making Sense of Social Prescribing*; University of Westminster: London, UK, 2017; Available online: https://uwe-repository.worktribe.com/preview/882260/Making-sense-of-social-prescribing-2017-PRINT.pdf (accessed on 23 December 2020).
29. Husk, K.; Blockley, K.; Lovell, R.; Bethel, A.; Lang, I.; Byng, R.; Garside, R. What approaches to social prescribing work, for whom, and in what circumstances? A realist review. *Health Soc. Care Community* **2020**, *28*, 309–324. [CrossRef] [PubMed]
30. Buck, D.; Ewbank, L. What Is Social Prescribing? Available online: https://www.kingsfund.org.uk/publications/social-prescribing (accessed on 23 December 2020).
31. Kondo, M.C.; Oyekanmi, K.O.; Gibson, A.; South, E.C.; Bocarro, J.; Hipp, J.A. Nature prescriptions for health: A review of evidence and research opportunities. *Int. J. Environ. Res. Public Health* **2020**, *17*, 4213. [CrossRef] [PubMed]
32. Leavell, M.A.; Leiferman, J.A.; Gascon, M.; Braddick, F.; Gonzalez, J.C.; Litt, J.S. Nature-Based Social Prescribing in Urban Settings to Improve Social Connectedness and Mental Well-being: A Review. *Curr. Environ. Health Rep.* **2019**, *6*, 297–308. [CrossRef] [PubMed]
33. Thomson, L.J.; Lockyer, B.; Camic, P.M.; Chatterjee, H.J. Effects of a museum-based social prescription intervention on quantitative measures of psychological wellbeing in older adults. *Perspect. Public Health* **2018**, *138*, 28–38. [CrossRef]
34. Wells, L. 'Iso'—A Spur to Think about Social Prescribing. *Croakey*. 13 May 2020. Available online: https://croakey.org/iso-a-spur-to-think-about-social-prescribing/ (accessed on 23 December 2020).
35. Den Broeder, L. Citizen Science for Health in All Policies. Ph.D. Thesis, Engaging Communities in Knowledge Development, VU University, Amsterdam, The Netherlands, 2017. Available online: http://library.wur.nl/WebQuery/wurpubs/529909 (accessed on 23 December 2020).
36. Wiggins, A.; Wilbanks, J. The Rise of Citizen Science in Health and Biomedical Research. *Am. J. Bioeth.* **2019**, *19*, 3–14. [CrossRef]
37. Ubiquity staff An Interview With Michael Schrage On Ubiquity. *Ubiquity* **2008**. [CrossRef]
38. Olsen, L.; Aisner, D.; McGinnis, J.M. The learning healthcare system: Workshop summary. *IOM Roundtable Evid. Based Med.* **2007**. [CrossRef]
39. Platt, J.E.; Raj, M.; Wienroth, M. An analysis of the learning health system in its first decade in practice: Scoping review. *J. Med. Internet Res.* **2020**, *22*, e17026. [CrossRef]
40. Van Brussel, S.; Huyse, H. Citizen science on speed? Realising the triple objective of scientific rigour, policy influence and deep citizen engagement in a large-scale citizen science project on ambient air quality in Antwerp. *J. Environ. Plan. Manag.* **2019**, *62*, 534–551. [CrossRef]
41. Borda, A.; Gray, K.; Downie, L. Citizen Science Models in Health Research: An Australian Commentary. *Online J. Public Health Inform.* **2019**, *11*, e22. [CrossRef]
42. Sauermann, H.; Vohland, K.; Antoniou, V.; Balázs, B.; Göbel, C.; Karatzas, K.; Mooney, P.; Perelló, J.; Ponti, M.; Samson, R.; et al. Citizen Science and Sustainability Transitions. Available online: https://ssrn.com/abstract=3511088 (accessed on 23 December 2020).
43. Petersen, C.; Austin, R.R.; Backonja, U.; Campos, H.; Chung, A.E.; Hekler, E.B.; Hsueh, P.-Y.S.; Kim, K.K.; Pho, A.; Salmi, L.; et al. Citizen science to further precision medicine: From vision to implementation. *JAMIA Open* **2020**, *3*, 2–8. [CrossRef] [PubMed]
44. Capolongo, S.; Rebecchi, A.; Buffoli, M.; Appolloni, L.; Signorelli, C.; Fara, G.M.; D'Alessandro, D. COVID-19 and Cities: From Urban Health strategies to the pandemic challenge. A Decalogue of Public Health opportunities. *Acta Biomed.* **2020**, *91*, 13–22. [CrossRef] [PubMed]
45. Ogden, J. Social Prescribing In A Time Of Covid-19 And Social Isolation. *Prog. Neurol. Psychiatry* **2020**, *24*, 4–5. [CrossRef]
46. Jungmann, S.; Mistry, P.; Conibear, T.; Gray, M.; Jani, A. Using technology-enabled social prescriptions to disrupt healthcare. *J. R. Soc. Med.* **2020**, *113*, 59–63. [CrossRef] [PubMed]
47. Topol, E. Preparing the Healthcare Workforce to Deliver the Digital Future The Topol Review. An Independent Report on Behalf of the Secretary of State for Health and Social Care. Available online: https://topol.hee.nhs.uk (accessed on 23 December 2020).
48. OECD. Smart Cities and Inclusive Growth. Available online: https://www.oecd.org/cfe/cities/OECD_Policy_Paper_Smart_Cities_and_Inclusive_Growth.pdf (accessed on 23 December 2020).
49. Good Things Foundation (GTF) Socially Prescribing Digital Skills: A How to Guide for Digital Inclusion in Health. Available online: https://www.onlinecentresnetwork.org/sites/default/files/how_to_socially_prescribing_digital_skills_in_health_v2.pdf (accessed on 23 December 2020).
50. Ottaviano, M.; Beltrán-Jaunsarás, M.E.; Teriús-Padrón, J.G.; García-Betances, R.I.; González-Martínez, S.; Cea, G.; Vera, C.; Cabrera-Umpiérrez, M.F.; Waldmeyer, M.T.A. Empowering citizens through perceptual sensing of urban environmental and health data following a participative citizen science approach. *Sensors* **2019**, *19*, 2940. [CrossRef]

51. den Haan, M.C.; Brankaert, R.G.A.; Lu, Y. What moves you? Designing a walking app for and with older adults. In Proceedings of the Design4Health, Sheffield Hallam University, Sheffield, UK, 4–6 September 2018; Christer, K., Craig, C., Wolstenholme, D., Eds.; Systemic Change: Sheffield, UK, 2018.
52. Cuignet, T.; Perchoux, C.; Caruso, G.; Klein, O.; Klein, S.; Chaix, B.; Kestens, Y.; Gerber, P. Mobility among older adults: Deconstructing the effects of motility and movement on wellbeing. *Urban Stud.* **2020**, *57*, 383–401. [CrossRef]
53. Baraković, S.; Husić, J.B.; Van Hoof, J.; Krejcar, O.; Maresova, P.; Akhtar, Z.; Melero, F.J. Quality of life framework for personalised ageing: A systematic review of ICT solutions. *Int. J. Environ. Res. Public Health* **2020**, *17*, 2940. [CrossRef]
54. Cinderby, S.; Cambridge, H.; Attuyer, K.; Bevan, M.; Croucher, K.; Gilroy, R.; Swallow, D. Co-designing Urban Living Solutions to Improve Older People's Mobility and Well-Being. *J. Urban Health* **2018**, *95*, 409–422. [CrossRef]
55. Marston, H.; Van Hoof, J. Who Doesn't Think about Technology When Designing Urban Environments for Older People? *Int. J. Environ. Res. Public Health* **2019**, *16*, 3525. [CrossRef]
56. Marston, H.R.; Kroll, M.; Fink, D.; Poveda, R.; Gschwind, Y.J. Digital Game Technology And Older Adults. In *Mobile e-Health. Human*; Computer Interaction Series; Marston, H., Freeman, S., Musselwhite, C., Eds.; Springer: Cham, Switzerland, 2017; pp. 149–171. [CrossRef]

International Journal of
Environmental Research and Public Health

MDPI

Article

How does a (Smart) Age-Friendly Ecosystem Look in a Post-Pandemic Society?

Hannah Ramsden Marston [1,*], Linda Shore [2] and P.J. White [3]

1 Health & Wellbeing Strategic Research Area, School of Health, Wellbeing & Social Care, The Open University, Milton Keynes, Buckinghamshire MK7 6HH, UK
2 Mi:Lab, Department of Design Innovation, Maynooth University, W23 F2H6 Co. Kildare, Ireland; Linda.Shore@mu.ie
3 DesignCORE, Humanities, Institute of Technology Carlow, R93 V960 Carlow, Ireland; PJ.WHITE@ITCARLOW.IE
* Correspondence: Hannah.Marston@open.ac.uk

Received: 28 September 2020; Accepted: 3 November 2020; Published: 9 November 2020

check for updates

Abstract: COVID-19 has impacted not only the health of citizens, but also the various factors that make up our society, living environments, and ecosystems. This pandemic has shown that future living will need to be agile and flexible to adapt to the various changes in needs of societal populations. Digital technology has played an integral role during COVID-19, assisting various sectors of the community, and demonstrating that smart cities can provide opportunities to respond to many future societal challenges. In the decades ahead, the rise in aging populations will be one of these challenges, and one in which the needs and requirements between demographic cohorts will vary greatly. Although we need to create future smart age-friendly ecosystems to meet these needs, technology still does not feature in the WHO eight domains of an age-friendly city. This paper extends upon Marston and van Hoof's 'Smart Age-friendly Ecosystem' (SAfE) framework, and explores how digital technology, design hacking, and research approaches can be used to understand a smart age-friendly ecosystem in a post-pandemic society. By exploring a series of case studies and using real-life scenarios from the standpoint of COVID-19, we propose the 'Concept of Age-friendly Smart Ecologies (CASE)' framework. We provide an insight into a myriad of contemporary multi-disciplinary research, which are capable to initiate discussions and bring various actors together with a positive impact on future planning and development of age-friendly ecosystems. The strengths and limitations of this framework are outlined, with advantages evident in the opportunity for towns, regions/counties, provinces, and states to take an agile approach and work together in adopting and implement improvements for the greater benefits of residents and citizens.

Keywords: older adults; community; aging; technology; digital; e-health; urban planning; smart ecosystem; gerontechnology; age in place; coronavirus; COVID-19; design hacking; internet of things; human-centered design; smart cities

1. Introduction

A Tale of Two Snows

The name Jon Snow (house of Stark) for many people will resonate with the fictional character from the television series Game of Thrones (GOT). The eighth season of GOT and the preceding seasons weave narratives featuring (dis) loyalty, treachery, war, passion, and history across various geographic locations or across the seven Kingdoms (e.g., the Kingdom of the North, the Kingdom of the Isles and the Rivers, the Kingdom of Mountain and Vale, the Kingdom of the Rock, the Kingdom of the Storm, the Kingdom of the Reach, and the Kingdom of the Dorne). Each Kingdom is represented by a 'House' (i.e., the Kingdom of the North) and in this example, House Stark of Winterfell—the ancestral home of Eddard (Ned) Stark; the landed gentry, including their families and the surrounding communities who are loyal to Winterfell, are depicted through the lens of fantasy and medieval history, illustrating the different cultures, expectations, loyalty, and behavior(s) of communities in different rural, urban, and city environments [1–9].

However, there is another John Snow, a real person who played a non-fictional part in the lives of city dwellers located in London, UK. John Snow (b.1813–d.1858) was a physician, a leader in the development of anesthesia and medical hygiene, and was most importantly known for identifying cholera as the 'hot spot' or outbreak in 1849 [10] in Broad Street (now known as Broadwick Street) located in an area of Soho, London.

Between 1846 and 1860, this was the third cholera epidemic, and Robert Koch, a German physician, is known to have said how cholera was "our best ally" [10] (p. 169) to improve the hygiene and sanitation of the citizens. The cholera epidemic broke out in England and Wales and lasted for two years; this resulted in 52,000 deaths, while John Snow is known as the physician to have identified a specific water pump—accessible to the public and located in Soho, as the primary source for this third cholera pandemic [10] (p. 170).

Although previously it was thought that the cause of this outbreak was miasma—also known as airborne particles [11,12], and as depicted in Figures 1 and 2 [13,14] created by Snow, he was able to identify the source of cholera as a waterborne disease instead. Given this location and accessibility of the water pump (Figure 2), citizens in this locality who were living or visiting the area for work would drink from the pump, which in turn facilitated the disease to travel, resulting in an increase in deaths. However, some of the workmen in the area chose not to drink from the water pump but instead chose to drink alcohol from the local brewery (including men who worked at the breweries); this choice led to the bacteria found in the waterborne disease to be killed [15]. The workhouses in the area also had their own water supply, and this too resulted in fewer deaths from cholera [15,16].

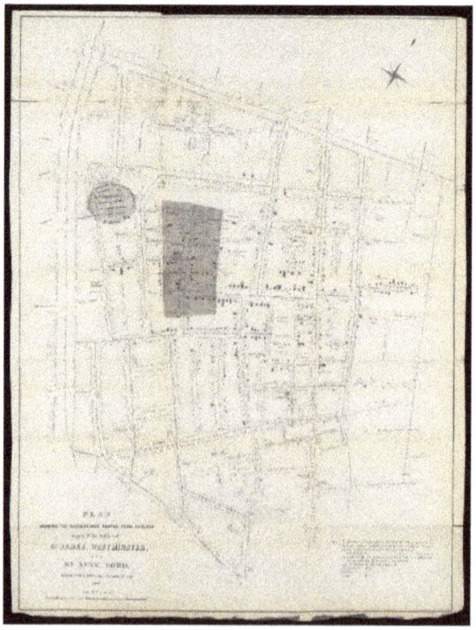

Figure 1. A map of Soho, London, created by John Snow to record the number of cholera deaths. Source: Wellcome Library, via Wellcome Images [13,14]. Permission granted via Creative Commons.

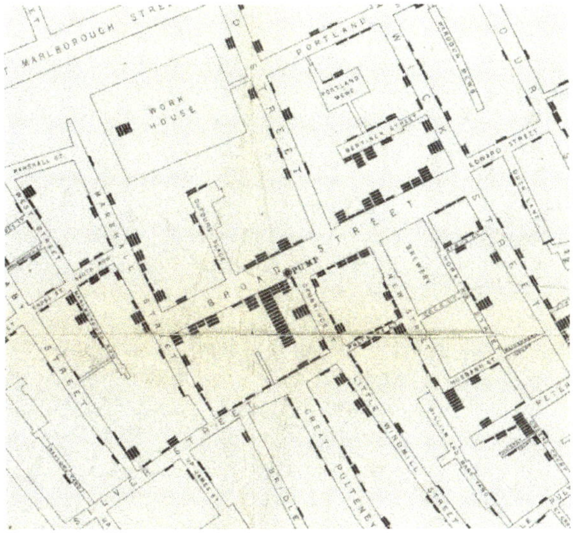

Figure 2. A map of Soho, London, created by John Snow to record the number of cholera deaths. Source: Wellcome Library, via Wellcome Images [13,14]. Permission granted via Creative Commons.

However, Snow conducted an experiment using two water sources located across London in two specific areas: (1) The Southwark Vauxhall Company and (2) The Lambeth Waterworks Company, whereby water was drawn directly from the river Thames, but from different locations. The location of Site 1 was closer to the city's sewage and Snow considered this area to be contaminated more than Site 2, which was located further up the river Thames.

Data taken from the two sites was compiled and coupled with the number of deaths in these two areas; it was noted in the location of Site 1 (Southwark Vauxhall water company) that there were 315 deaths associated to cholera per 10,000 homes, while in Site 2 (Lambeth Waterworks Company), there were only 37 deaths [17]. Having this information and data, the findings were shared and lobbied with the public health authority, which both resulted in and impacted a change to both social and sanitation across areas of London, also known as the slums. These changes were not solely conducted in London but across the country, leading to a greater improvement in health, and in turn resulting in a reduction in poor health and death of citizens [18]. This work conducted by Snow during this third cholera epidemic in the UK impacted science as well, and with the recording of deaths paved the way towards the field of epidemiology, understanding and identifying patterns [17,18].

Similarly, in the ongoing COVID-19 (SARS-CoV-2) pandemic, the first since the last global pandemic (1918–1920) that was caused by the H1N1 influenza A virus [19,20] which infected 500 million people across four successive waves. The field of epidemiology has played a key role in modelling and predicting the behavior(s) of this coronavirus [21,22], which attacks respiratory organs. Pandemics do not solely impact upon the health of citizens, but affect various "social, cultural, economic, and political," factors [23], (p. 1), which in turn, make-up our respective society and communities. The notion of pathogen mutation was, as Ironstone notes, sounded by scientists and experts in the field of biomedicine in the latter part of the 20th century [23].

Across UK Media outlets, citizens have been informed by their respective governments that they are following the science [24,25] presented by the SAGE (Scientific Advisory Group for Emergencies) committee. SAGE includes scientists from various Russell Group Universities, public agencies (e.g., Public Health England (PHE), Food Standards Agency (FSA)), funding agencies (e.g., Wellcome Trust, and UKRI), representation from devolved governments (e.g., Welsh Government, the Northern Ireland Executive, and the Scottish Government), the National Health Service/Digital, and UK Government offices (e.g., Foreign and Commonwealth Office, Department of Education) [26]. Additionally, the Scientific Pandemic Influenza Group on Behaviours (SPI-B) also advises the Government in "anticipating and helping people adhere to interventions that are recommended by medical or epidemiological experts" [26]. The SPI-B committee have also offered advice to the Government in an attempt to deal with the various stages of the pandemic unravelling across society, at both local, national, and global perspectives [26].

Considering what Ironstone [23] notes of the impact a pandemic can have on society at various levels of the ecosystem, Jayakumar and colleagues [27] provide a series of 'lessons learned' from the COVID-19 pandemic. These include: (1) transformation of the healthcare section, (2) working from home is highly possible, (3) online education, (4). growth of online business, (5) need for good network communication, (6) cybersecurity is a priority, and finally (7) reconnecting with oneself and loved ones. Furthermore, this relates to the myriad of factors outlined by Ironstone [23], while also acknowledging how societal behavior has changed at present, and possibly forever.

Digital technology and social media have played an integral role in the pandemic to date across various sectors of the community. Digital technology has and is enabling (vulnerable) citizens to shop online via protected delivery slots to children receiving online education via various communication platforms (e.g., Zoom), continuing and enhancing social interaction with family members, friends, and work colleagues [27–29]. We have seen via (social) media posts, advertisements, and interviews, that there are many community groups (e.g., churches and choirs) and organizations have been meeting online to conduct their (leisure) activities. Many communities up and down the country organically and in a rapid response to the pandemic, have created specific community groups to provide assistance to the vulnerable people in their respective communities and areas, including those people who became ill to the virus [27–29].

Previously, Marston and van Hoof [30] coined the term "smart age-friendly ecosystem" (SAfE) when presenting an alternative age-friendly framework, which incorporates and acknowledges the impact that technology and physical space plays within 21st century society. As has been witnessed and experienced since March 2020, technology and its associated devices and software have and are continuing to play a critical role in the lives of citizens and society—to maintain some sense and level of normality.

The purpose, aims, and objectives of this paper are to explore how digital technology, design hacking, and research approaches can be used to understand a (smart) age-friendly ecosystem in a post-pandemic society. We provide an insight into a myriad of contemporary multi-disciplinary research, which can initiate discussions and bringing various actors (e.g., planners, scholars, health practitioners, educators, residents, developers, local, national, and international governments) together. This will, in turn, narrate future planning and development of age-friendly environments and housing in the coming decades.

The outline of this paper follows an overview of global aging in Section 2, Section 3 explores the notion of smart cities, and Section 4 discusses social isolation and loneliness followed by a series of case studies in Section 5, whereby we discuss design hacking. Section 6 explores a series of case studies from the standpoint of the COVID-19 pandemic and Section 7 proposes the 'Concept of Age-friendly Smart Ecologies (CASE)' framework, using real-life scenarios, and Section 8 proposes recommendations and conclusions. We aim to offer an alternative blueprint, one which incorporates technology that has been largely ignored since the conception of the first framework.

2. Global Aging Societies

In 2019, the United Nations (UN) reported that 16% of the global population will reach the age of 65 years and older by 2050. From a global standpoint, the UN reported in 2018 that citizens who are aged 65 years and over will outnumber children who are aged five years and under [31]. Similarly, The Organization for Economic Co-operation and Development (OECD) [32] estimate that there will be an increase of 25.1% in adults aged 65 years by 2050 across the OECD member states [32].

Furthermore, with these estimated growing projections, incurred with incredible societal shifts associated to a rise in aging populations, coupled with low birth rates, access to amenities and ensuring a community ethos that caters for all citizens across the lifespan is critical for positive age-in-place.

The relationship and engagement between aging and urbanism has been termed urban aging [33,34], in conjunction with additional attributes such as the stresses, concerns, and matters contributing to local, regional and national communities across a variety of domains of urban living [35]. Therefore, given the rise in population aging, urban change, technology innovation, societal behavior, and the need for services in conjunction with the adaptation of existing physical spaces, these factors present several challenges for many actors at local, regional, and national levels in society.

In the following sections, we provide an overview of contemporary literature surrounding the notion of smart cities and age-friendly initiatives. The work presented here is significant because it contributes to the fields of gerontology, geography, social sciences, architecture, design, social policy, design, and health by building on existing scholarly activity, policies, and is pushing the narrative of the age-friendly movement forward in an attempt to open and enhance discussions more.

Additionally, the work presented in this paper has the potential to impact societies on both a national and international landscape, because we build on the existing and contemporary literature of the World Health Organisation (WHO) age-friendly framework [36] and the proposed extended SAfE framework posited by Marston and van Hoof [30]. The former framework was published 13 years ago, and at the time did not include technology [36], and with the recent extended SAfE framework [30], various technologies and exemplars are provided. Furthermore, given the rise in aging populations, and the differences between different cohorts (e.g., Baby Boomers, Gen X, Millennial's, Gen Z), the barriers, challenges, needs, requirements, and expectations will vary greatly across different cohorts. The living, physical, and urban environments must be agile and flexible to adapt for the various changes that will likely be experienced now and in the future by different societal populations.

In the following section, we provide an overview and insight on contemporary literature surrounding smart cities located across different regions and countries.

3. Creating a Smart City for the 21st Century

3.1. Smart Cities

In this next section, we explore the domain of smart cities, whereby we explore and discuss contemporary literature and research.

The concept/term of smart cities has been around for over two decades [37] whereby, members of the Academy have been conducting various scholarly activity intersecting at the fields of computer science, planning, and development. Firstly, Praharaj and Han [38] provide an extensive overview of the various global debates surrounding the smart city concept, including the various terms that have previously been used and are still interchangeable in current narratives and discourses. Such terms include digital city [39], tech city [40], wired city [41], ubiquitous city [42], intelligent city or information city [43], knowledge city [44], smart community [45], creative city [46], and sustainable city [47]. For this paper, we will use the term 'smart city'.

Smart cities [48–54] can offer great opportunities to reduce carbon emissions, while increasing sustainability targets, enhancing resilience, improving livability, and economic growth, coupled with the notion of increased populations [48–54].

Smart cities have the ability to collect and generate a vast amount of data, especially now more so than ever, given the phenomenal technological developments that have been conducted over the last 20 years. Technology innovation coupled with the notion of generating data is vast, enabling the coupling of technopoles, digital cities, and intelligent cities, affords various actors, organizations, and governments greater opportunities to exploit the generated data [50]. This, in turn, offer urban planners and other key actors the opportunity to respond to the myriad of societal challenges posed in the modern 21st century society.

Allam [48] provides an overview of the various concepts and differences surrounding digital, smart, and intelligent cities. The concept of a digital city is compounded by the integration of digital technology into the mainframe of the cities' infrastructure and systems, in conjunction with transport and buildings, which are seen as areas of the societal 'fabric' woven and embroidered to facilitate the process by which the data can be collected and processed.

However, the concept of a 'knowledge city' by Edvardsson, Yigitcanlar, and Pancholi [50] is associated with a greater breadth of dissemination and knowledge translation within the segments of the 'urban fabric', including both the public and private sectors of the societal ecosystem. This notion at the time of conception (1990s) relied on what is now referred to as 'big data'; yet, in the 1990s, this type of data was not available [53]. Since the 1990s, the term and concept of 'technopoles', coined by Allen J. Scott [53,54], relates to regions that are primarily focused on technological innovation [53,54], comprising of different components such as local business, educational institutes (e.g., universities), financial institutions, and public research organizations. Such developments are usually created either by the: (1) private sector, or (2) in partnership with both public and private sectors [55]. Moreover, the 'smart city' concept varies differently from the other concepts because it relies on the intelligence of digital devices and deployment across the physical space to improve the 'urban fabric', the economy, and the lives of the citizens [56–59].

The smart city [60,61] concept, in conjunction with the deployment of sensors, devices, and cameras that are interwoven across the infrastructure and mainframe of a city, has the potential and capability to generate various forms of data [60,61]. There are several examples of how the Internet of Things (IoT) can and are being integrated into real-world environments, such as the home, which include security systems—doorbells, smart heating, and lighting devices. Previously, Marston and van Hoof [30] described several IoT devices in their respective paper, describing various scenarios illustrated by existing real-life examples. Additionally smart/virtual devices assistants such as the Amazon Alexa or the Google Mini [62] can provide further information to citizens in the home environment, including medication reminders, calendar reminders, and leisure activities (e.g., selecting and listening to music) [62,63].

More recent application of smart devices and IoTs are starting to be integrated into kitchen appliances, such as washing machines, dishwashers, and coffee machines [64], enabling automatic reordering of washing machine powder/tablets, dishwasher tablets, and coffee beans when stocks are running low. Furthermore, smart cities provide regional, national municipalities/governments, citizens, and residents the opportunity to meet challenges surrounding carbon emissions, energy consumption, and traffic infrastructure [61]. While these examples are primarily focusing on the smart home environment, and in the context of smart cities, real-life examples of IoTs include reservation of car parking spaces or tracking usage of bicycles across a city (e.g., Copenhagen, Denmark) [62]. Coupled with the growing body of literature and research, which is exploring how cycling can be utilized in the context of big data, IoT, monitoring fleets, connected programs proposes programs such as the 'Smart Velomobility', which explores and considers both political and practical approaches to smart cycling [57–59,61,65–68].

Moreover, IoTs and associated technologies can be implemented into the context of 'Innovative Smart Grid Technologies' [57–59,61,65–68], which facilitates sensors and components to be integrated into the infrastructure of a city to track the energy consumption of residents [69]. While automation can play a role in detecting and changing power consumption, blackouts, and fuel loads, which, in turn, facilitate safety and economic savings to residents [69]. In towns such as Milton Keynes (along with other towns and cities), there are charging stations for drivers of electronic vehicles (EV), which enable EV owners/drivers the opportunity to 'recharge' their EV as well as continue to use their respective smart technologies should power outages or accidents occur [69].

Shin [70] provides a detailed understanding of the IoT ecosystem in the context of Korea, comprising of a multi-level analysis, which incorporates users, the wider society, and ecology. Findings from this in-depth study, which implemented the social construction of technology (SCOT) approach as a means of understanding how useful IoTs could be within a multi-level society, was studied. However, employing a socio-technical theory facilitated the intervention of appropriation as a social construction within society, which is interwoven and intersects at the differing levels within a respective ecosystem [70]. To date, Shin notes how there has been "too much emphasis on technology in IoT project" (p. 92) and by taking the respective study as a means of unpacking this statement, Shin highlights how there are many obstacles within projects, which lean more towards the social rather than the technical, and this includes privacy, universal service, and the digital divide. Shin purports that the technological lag of Korean development may not be related to the availability of technology but instead could be due to the lack of user/resident demand, which in turn transfers to a greater price increases for products [70].

Conversely, Shin [70] describes several negative concerns identified from the study, which includes the perceived understanding of IoTs from a top-down approach by the Government and the impact this may have on citizens. However, citizen concerns were noted and include the security and privacy concerns of the information exchanged from within the confines of a safe and secure socio-technical ecosystem, resulting from a potentially less secure external ecosystem and network(s). Additional concerns were highlighted by citizens in the respective study relating to existing wearable and IoT devices executing covert behavior or harvesting and sharing data unbeknown to the citizens/user(s) [70]. This concern leads to the ethical considerations of using, and implementing such devices not only on an individual level, but across wider spectrums of the ecosystem; Shin states that "without adequate and timely policies regarding these matters [...] smart cities cannot be successfully developed in future" (p. 92) [70–72].

Seven recommendation points are proposed by Shin [70] to move the narrative forward and gain a congruence associated to both ethical and socio-technical frameworks. The recommendations include: 1. Consider people before local context; consider local context before technology, 2. Demonstrate sustainability, scalability, and resilience over a long-term timeframe, 3. IoT of any new development should conform to the best available current standards for interoperability between IT systems in general, 4. New developments should demonstrate that they have considered the commercial viability of providing digital civic infrastructure services, 5. The government should support a meaningful IoT literacy program and raise awareness to empower self-regulation and enhance individuals' interactions with IoT, 6. Social demands should not be identified and addressed solely by the market. The boundary between the social and the economic must blur, and society must be reshaped into a more participatory arena, and 7. Users must be empowered to utilize IoT technologies to turn the physical environment into a socio-technical environment, where appropriate policies are shaped around them.

Concluding from his study, Shin [70] states that "Deployment of IoT is not far from reality. Unlike previous smart city initiatives, IoT will, and should, exist for a long time. For the time being, however, IoT remains more of an untested promise than a reality." (p. 97). Furthermore, and based on the findings from the respective study, and existing literature [71,72], Shin notes that there is still a lack of understanding of the positive and prospective benefits that IoTs can bring to society and ecosystems alike; and suggests Korea "may need a series of socio-technical experiments that emphasize both the sociological and technological aspects of development" [70] (p. 98). Emphasizing further, Shin describes how the infrastructure of an ecosystem should be perceived as an 'artifact' and taking an ethnographic approach is appropriate when designing and developing IoT sensors and devices. This though in turn will afford interested parties from industry, government, stakeholders, researchers, and designers the opportunity to identify and understand the impact of IoT via different user narratives [70].

Taking into account the proposed recommendations by Shin [70] local, regional and national governments, stakeholders, and actors have the opportunity to purvey big data which can in turn offer insight into and provide guidance to urban planners; for example, when expanding the smart city infrastructure into different locations [71–74]. Furthermore, Allam [75], Allam and Dhunny [76] notes such a concept of a smart city offers various actors the opportunity to collaborate, and utilize the various data from across the infrastructure to reach optimal usage, including the maximization of resources and technologies available within the infrastructure, buildings, and the urban fabric. Potentially, this in turn offers sustainability, feeding into outlets of the ecosystem.

In today's society, we have seen the potential possibilities of integrating technology and IoTs IoT into various urban developments, towns, and cities, as described by Marston and van Hoof [30], who posited the notion and integration of technology into the urban environment and physical space of Milton Keynes (MK). The MK: Smart project [77] (2014–2016) aiming to focus on the new town Milton Keynes, located in the county of Buckinghamshire, UK, was a consortium comprising of various partners, including Milton Keynes Council, Anglia Water, British Telecom (BT), consultancy partners, civil engineering, charities (e.g., Community action: MK), academic partners (i.e., University of Bedfordshire, University of Cambridge), and Catapult hubs. The concept of the MK: Smart project was to bring together various actors intersecting across the areas of education, business and community engagement, and service providers.

Given the growing technological developments, this notion is conceivable based on the existing IoTs/digital devices/sensors, and potential AI capabilities, which in turn offers compliance with sustainability targets and data generation [70–77]. Platforms facilitating IoTs and machine learning offer the interwoven sensors the ability to be connected [70–77], resulting in data transfer across the mainframe of a city. Allam and Dhunny [78] note how cloud computing affords data storage from the data generated across a smart city; while blockchain technology offers data security during transfer between nodes installed on the mainframe [79–83]. Data privacy is key in all aspects of society, and a smart city is no different; therefore, it is key to ensure the data that is generated within the infrastructure and mainframe of a smart city, during the different processes or generation, transfer and usage, is secure. This is imperative in ensuring for actors, residents, and citizens alike that the privacy of data is maintained, and no data breaches occur [80–83].

Obedait and colleagues [84] posits the concept of a smart city in the UAE and provide an overview of contemporary literature surrounding technology implementation within the smart city concept, development, and citizen centric governance. The former concept explores the various technologies that can be integrated into such developments, including:

- Internet of Things (IoT): which facilitates the interconnections of physical devices (e.g., sensors) with buildings and other digital devices, which in turn affords data to be exchanged.
- Augmented Reality (AR) and Virtual Reality (VR): offers specific businesses such as retail and real estate according to Obediat et al. [84]. While Alkhamisi and Monowar [85] posit how AR and VR have the potential to impact and redefine the governance of business.
- Big data: refers to the large data collected through various technologies and devices. The processing of big data has the potential to provide predictive insight into user behavior analytics, which in turn can provide information relating to service provisions—health, crime/policing, and business. This in turn has the potential to impact local, regional, and national policies, agendas, and governance [86].
- Blockchain: utilizes cryptography (e.g., Bitcoin) to ensure that the verification and storage of data is safe and ensures security is maintained at all levels. Transactions between governments, regional councils, service providers, and citizens could be streamlined via the implementation and use of Blockchain.
- Artificial Intelligence (AI): utilizes machine learning techniques [87] and has the potential to refine the customer experience via local, regional, national governments, and council agencies.

The scholarly work by Obedait and colleagues [84] relates to the concept of a smart city in the UAE, as a "pioneer and leader in providing best in class citizen services utilizing technology" (p. 78). Such a location as the UAE, which includes many citizens from residents to tourists, non-residents, expatriates, and workers, needs to ensure all needs are met. Many residents and workers are younger and mobile, having arrived in the UAE for employment purposes and reasons [84] coupled with the diversity of citizens. Obedai and colleagues [84] note how this variance within their society adds additional complexities to service provision of governance for all citizens, not solely one category of citizen. Therefore, the government of the UAE has rolled out an e-government portal in Abu Dhabi, enabling citizens, tourists, and businesses the opportunity to access government services in a cost-effective approach, which also enables answers to be provided to questions and complaints can be shared [84].

Within this portal [88], there are several elements that have been implemented and include: (1) UAE national identity card, (2) happiness meter, (3) Electronic Land Management System, (4) smart district guidelines (e.g., for developers expanding the across the city), (5) smart Dubai index (gauges impact relating to the implemented initiatives), (6) Dubai data (all key information collected will be shared with citizens and government(s) moving towards a participatory government), (7) Smart Dubai Platform—which relates to the integration of IoTs across the city infrastructure, and captures data in real time, and citizens are notified via dashboards, and (8) the Dubai Blockchain, which will offer secure and improved data transactions across the city, between the various service providers, government, citizens, and tourists.

The UAE 2021 vision [89] and the UAE Government strategy [90] have provided their vision and roadmap to transform the UAE into a smart ecosystem, which encompasses a livable and resilient city that aims to be achieved by improving the connectedness of the city. This vision aims to connect citizens in Dubai via the various services, as well as enhancing the quality of life via technology, which may enable greater streamlining of different societal aspects (e.g., social, cultural, education, and healthcare) [88,89].

In summary of this section, we have provided a contemporary overview of research and insight into scholarly activity surrounding smart cities and associated technologies that have been implemented and trialed across both Western and Eastern societies. In the next section, we discuss the contemporary literature surrounding the age-friendly initiatives.

3.2. Age-Friendly Initiatives

Contemporary literature surrounding the age-friendly initiative has previously been discussed at length by Marston and van Hoof [30]. However, one review by Lim, Edelenbos, and Gianoli [90] aimed to explore the development of a smart city, and this piece of research reviewed 55 papers, comprising of 12 positive and four negative results.

The positive results highlighted six papers primarily relating to theoretical concepts, which did not include evidence, while the other six papers included six themes: (1) enhancing citizen involvement, (2) protecting environment, (3) facilitating social development, (4) facilitating sustainable development, (5) fostering innovation, and (6) increasing social capital. Regarding the negative results, two of the four papers were categorized as theoretical in relation to privacy and security issues, and secondly, the notion of moderating freedom of speech and democracy.

Additional reviews and research within this domain include the work conducted by Cocchia [91], who explored the concepts of a smart city and of a digital city between 1993 and 2012. The Anthopoulos and colleagues [92] review highlighted seven applied domains in relation to smart cities: (1) resource, (2) transportation, (3) urban infrastructures, (4) living, (5) government, (6) economy, and (7) coherency, describing in some instances the notion and relationship between smart cities and sustainability. Furthermore, Traindade and colleagues [93] conducted work within the area of sustainability and smart cities, and more recently Komninos and Mora [94,95] reviewed the literature between 1992 and 2012, which purported and described the development of a smart city.

Ruza and colleagues [96] conducted research in the area relating to the age-friendly factor, specifically focusing on the Palo Alto area of California; this in turn resulted in the development of a framework, encompassing several criterion and assessments deployed by a web-based geographical information system (GIS).

The rationale by Ruza and colleagues [96] for choosing the Palo Alto area was based on the regional population characteristics (i.e., high income, greater proportion of older adults in comparison to the USA overall), and providing the opportunity for this particular population to continue living in this community. One further reason for this choice of research area was the ease of access for the research team.

Findings from this research highlighted three key elements that should be taken into consideration when aiming to improve the respective community and physical space: (1) open spaces, (2) public transportation, and (3) services for an aging population/community [96]. Furthermore, Ruza and colleagues [96] note how their results align with findings from the 'Community Services Department of the City of Palo Alto' [97]. Coupled with the additional changes to this region of California, they have the potential to reduce the existing marginalization of community members from lower socioeconomic status [96]. From the standpoint of enhancing public transport in this region, members of the Palo Alto region own at least one car per household. However, the findings from this respective study note the need for greater improvement and accessibility of public transportation services based on prospective health and wellbeing issues in later life [96]. Ruza et al. [96] acknowledge that this region of California is an urbanized area, and previous planning developments were conducted without the considerations and issues surrounding an aging population, and with this mind, purport the following:

> "[...] urge planners and decision makers to act on the items high-lighted in this study, as a lack of action will translate to escalating unmet needs and make Palo Alto unsustainable with respect to its healthcare resources and provision for its residents to age in place" (p. 395) [96].

The scholarly activity by Meijer and Bolivar [98] focused on the concept of smart urban governance and concluded this notion was between the collaboration of citizens and technology. The Centre for Ageing Better [99] based in the UK highlights the number of towns and cities that have received age-friendly status (n = 40) via support and engagement from stakeholder organizations, residents, and the leadership of respective towns and cities. Taking the lead from the eight domains (Figure 3) published by the WHO age-friendly framework [36], 1. Outdoor spaces and buildings, 2. Transportation, 3. Housing, 4. Social participation, 5. Respect and social inclusion, 6. Civic participation and employment, 7. Communication and information, and 8. Community and health services (Figure 3), the Centre for Ageing Better state, "Together, the eight domains and programme cycle create the framework for how places become increasingly age-friendly" [36].

Therefore, given how the notion, narrative, and discourse surrounding the age-friendly movement has continued for over a decade, utilizing the existing eight domains as a blue print, there is still little discourse to providing alternative, extended frameworks to the existing WHO age-friendly [36] with the exception of the work proposed by Marston and van Hoof [30].

Figure 4 illustrates the extended proposed framework by Marston and van Hoof [30], which at the time did not drill down into the different types of technology and peripheral solutions that could or should be considered in future smart age-friendly ecosystems. However, technologies and their associated software solutions (e.g., big data, Blockchain) do have a place in the design and revamping of existing and future proposed age-friendly ecosystems. It is also suggested by the authors that the adoption of new and smart technologies should consider age, gender, and personality traits [100], taking into consideration standpoints from both contemporary and post-pandemic societies. Therefore, such frameworks would differ and interact greatly or not when citizens globally have had their lives and society turned upside down during this pandemic.

In 2007, the age-friendly framework [36] was published by the WHO, and at this time, the Internet was accessible, videogame technology (hardware and software) was being used and tested for rehabilitation purposes, as well as exploring its use and medium with non-traditional audiences (e.g., older adults) in regard to cognition [101,102] and fun, [103–108]. Mobile technologies were developing at a phenomenal rate, whereby now we see the use of smartphones alongside mobile apps (mApps) and mobile health apps (mHealth Apps) [109], which are accessed and used by many citizens in their own respective ecosystems for a myriad of reasons [110].

This in turn has resulted in the field of gamification [111] and while Deterding and colleagues [111] discuss gamification from the standpoint of videogames and design, it has been part of our society through the activity of reward points (e.g., groceries, air miles, or petrol consumption) for many years. Much of the scholarly activity was published after the WHO age-friendly framework [36] was published, although at the time of designing this framework, there should have been some acknowledgement and/or theoretical discussion posited to the future and potential impact and role(s) played by technology within society.

Moreover, one of the areas that was not discussed by Marston and van Hoof [30] or by the WHO [36] was privacy and the surrounding issues associated to citizen's data and confidentiality [112–115]. In the first decade of the 21st Century, technology developments were witnessed and experienced in society (e.g., social media platforms, videogames, mobile, and smartphones) [116,117], including research and development of mobile apps (mApps), mHealth Apps [104], virtual assistants (VA) [62,117–120], and robots [121,122]. These technologies hold a user's data and thus privacy should also be taken into consideration when a technology is implemented.

The concept of a living lab (LL) is not new, and LLs allow multiple actors to collaborate with regard to design, development, testing, and evaluation phases to reach the goal(s) of innovation situated within a real-life environment [123,124]. The LL approach ensures full inclusivity of users who are driving the innovation, across the different phases, taking a co-creation approach aimed at services, products, and/or societal infrastructures such as smart cities [123].

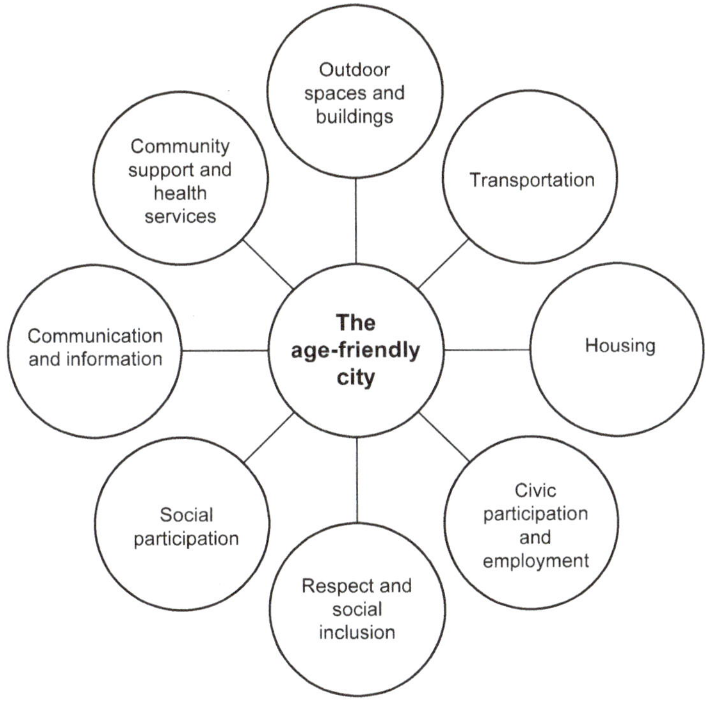
Outdoor spaces and buildings
Community support and health services
Transportation
Communication and information
The age-friendly city
Housing
Social participation
Civic participation and employment
Respect and social inclusion

Figure 3. The eight domains of an age-friendly city [36].

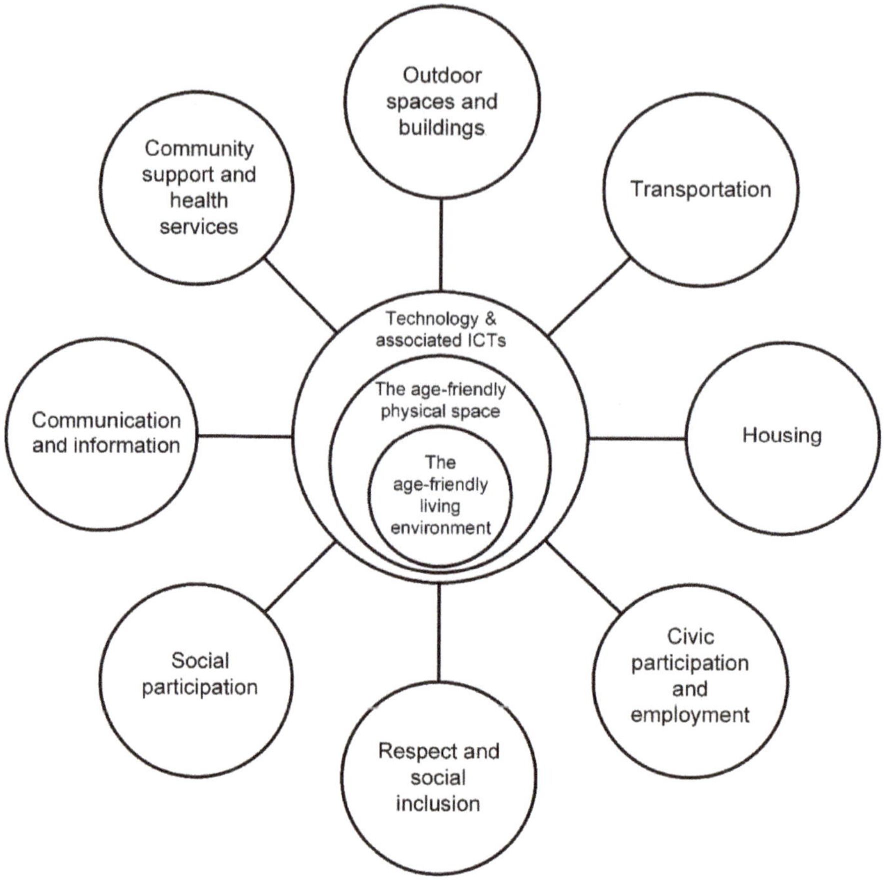

Figure 4. Smart age-friendly ecosystem framework (SAfE) [30].

Indeed, the work by Shin and Park [124] presents the concept of LL as an approach to understand the implementation of IoTs across three levels: 1. *Macro LL:* Constellation (ecosystem surrounding IoT), 2. *Meso LL:* innovation project and 3. *Micro LL:* user experience and acceptance. Ng and Wakenshaw [125] note how design and development is based on the needs of the user(s), established around a human-centered approach and system [70,126]. Moreover, the findings of the work by Shin and Park [124] who describe Bukchon Village in Korea as a real-life LL (the municipality implemented a top-down approach and did not initially consider user participation at its core) may be problematic for technology appropriation. Furthermore, Shin [70] notes how IoT implementation into a LL ecosystem can have several challenges, while taking a socio-technical approach does afford user participation from the conception stage. This allows users, stakeholders, industry, business, policy makers, and government officials to contribute across the three levels of a LL, while learning and understanding the different and meaningful experiences within this ecosystem. Lidtke and colleagues [127] note how the use and implementation of LLs have not been evaluated by academics, to ascertain whether this is a suitable approach to understanding the use and acceptance of technology and IoTs while implementing a co-design approach [128–131].

At the beginning of the pandemic outbreak and as the months continue, technology and communication tools have become integral features, playing a significant role in what the authors of this paper are coining the 'Concept of Age-friendly Smart Ecologies (CASE)' framework.

For many digital technologies and citizens, digital technologies have become an integral component within various ecosystems, as a means of continuing social engagement, reducing loneliness and isolation, in addition to maintaining and delivering a level of stability in education, support, and employment.

Finally, a recent review by Torku and colleagues [132] identified 81 publications and selected 39 papers for inclusion based on criterion relating to the "barriers that hinder the implementation of age-friendly initiatives in smart cities" (p. 1). Findings from the review identified several facets associated with 1. physical, 2. environmental, 3. technological, 4. social, 5. Financial, and 6. political barriers that smart cities currently experience or may experience by employing initiatives from the age-friendly cities narratives. The respective authors provide implications of this work for policymakers by suggesting that this review "would support policy makers in formulating policy recommendations to improve age-friendliness in cities" [132] (p. 1). Finally, Torku and colleagues [132] detail that the work presented in this systematic review compounds a myriad of features that may provide existing age-friendly initiatives into smart cities.

In summary, this section has explored and discussed contemporary research surrounding different age-friendly initiatives, frameworks, and research, highlighting that there is no one-size-fits-all model. We have also described various technologies that have become integral within contemporary society and offered an insight into how taking a user-centered approach to understanding technology through LLs can be a positive way of agile research, understanding how a piece of technology may or may not work within different settings.

In the following section, we explore the notion of social isolation and loneliness, which can affect both young and older adults, at various times of one's life.

4. Social Isolation and Loneliness

Loneliness and social isolation [133–139] have been known to be key contributors to one's poor quality of life and life expectancy and can be serious for older citizens with pre-existing chronic health conditions [140]. Scholars [139,140] note how the impact of chronic social isolation and loneliness are related to one's poor physical and mental health, while the experience of temporary or transient social isolation and loneliness posits fewer risks relating to the long-term negative impact on one's health and wellbeing.

Social isolation and loneliness can affect anyone across different age cohorts and throughout the life course. Be it a young person who has moved to a new region or country for employment or education purposes or older citizens who have continued to live in their home/ area, yet members of their family such as children or grandchildren have moved away, or the older person experiences a sense of loss through bereavement.

Dinkins [141] notes how socially engaging and interacting with friends, family members, and the wider community ecosystem forms part of being a human and is underpinned through positive health and wellbeing. Therefore, it should be ensured that interaction and social engagement can be accessed, in an attempt to reduce loneliness and social isolation, which in turn improves and/or enhances the overall health and wellbeing of citizens in society (including friends and family).

Contemporary research [142,143] demonstrates the importance and role that technology can play in reducing loneliness and social isolation. Schlomann and colleagues [142] ascertained positive findings from their quantitative study aimed at understanding ICT use by adults aged 80+ years. Adults in this study used ICTs in conjunction with their daily activities and reported a decrease in loneliness. However, Schlomann et al. [142] concluded how there is still an age-related digital divide and proposed the recommendation of further ICT training to reduce this difference.

Cotton and colleagues [144] conducted a study to understand the impact of Internet use on loneliness and perceived social isolation. This study was conducted in two living environments: 1. assisted living and 2. independent housing environments. Findings by Cotton and colleagues [144] ascertained participants who were recruited from one of the two living environments located in

Alabama, USA, showing how technology can facilitate older adults to stay connected and meet new people. The amount of communication with other people increased and offered comfort to the older adults who experienced greater connection with friends and family. This in turn, resulted in an increase in quality of communication, and feeling less isolated.

Another study using the 'Personal Reminder Information and Social Management (PRISM)' system was conducted by Czaja, Boot, Charness, Rogers, and Sharit [145]. This multi-site randomized field trial was conducted across three locations and recruited 300 people who were living independently and were identified at been at risk from social isolation. Findings showed, over the course of six months, that the sense of loneliness was reduced significantly, and an increase in perception of social support and wellbeing was noted. Czaja and colleagues reported that for participants who were using the PRISM system, the findings showed improvements from baseline and at 12 months, with further increases and improvements in computer self-efficacy, proficiency, and comfort of using computers at both six- and 12-months phases. Similarly, these findings support the growing body of evidence as presented by Cotton and colleagues [144], Schlomann, and colleagues [142]; whereby the notion and access to technology and its associated applications have the potential to support social connectedness and reduce loneliness and social isolation.

Conversely, there is the need to start exploring and understanding the challenges and issues surrounding future aging cohorts (for instance, Generation X, Millennials, and Generation Z) [108, 146–151]. This is important because, for various cohorts who have grown up in a digital society, with differing mental models [62] to those of existing older populations, it is important to understand the various mental models employed by different users during technology adoption as well as in earlier stages, such as the design process [62].

Citizens build and expand their mental models through various lens and experiences, which in turn impact their perception of adopting new technology into their lives and individual ecosystems. For example, citizens categorized as Generation X will still be able to remember what society was like prior to the use and integration of the Internet, and mobile/smartphone devices. However, Millennials and Generation Z do not have this previous experience and therefore, for these younger cohorts, it could be very difficult to comprehend not accessing or using such technologies. Therefore, while starting to understand the behavior, needs, and challenges that currently face younger citizens in society, there is the opportunity to plan and react efficiently to these future aging populations who may or may not have different expectations to our existing aging populations (e.g., Baby Boomers, Oldest Old) [147–151].

In summary, this section has presented research surrounding the use of technology by older adults in a bid to alleviate loneliness and social isolation. Although respective studies reported positive findings, technology is not a quick fix solution or replacement for face-to-face interaction. Technology should be perceived as an accompaniment to the user and/or older person, as a means of adding another layer of connectivity. Furthermore, we discuss how Generation X should be considered in future research to understand the appropriation of technology and user experiences from the standpoint of a different cohort, who has different experiences to Baby Boomers, Millennials, and Generation Z. Presently, Generation X has little attention from scholars across the fields of gerontology, gerontechnology, and human computer interaction (HCI). However, given the intersection of these fields within this multi-and-inter-disciplinary domain, we believe it is important to commence exploration of what the exact needs, challenges, and barriers are faced from Generation X [148–151].

In the following section we discuss a myriad of design hacks, which can afford citizens, businesses, academe, policy makers, and stakeholders the opportunity to retrieve rich information that in turn can be implemented into practice.

5. Design Hacks 2020

Societal and environmental sustainability relies on design approaches [152] and a universal design [152–155] approach is recommended when designing for older adults. This approach has been applied previously as a means of gaining user insights early on in the process [153] and highlights the importance of taking three facets into consideration: 1. design requirements, 2. user comfort, and 3. ease into account. Likewise, the challenges and experiences of aging can be understood by the implementation of this design approach, whereby this approach aims to solve and address unmet needs [156,157]. Furthermore, design fiction enables us to speculate and critique current and future scenarios about how things could be [158]. Employing universal design approaches and participatory design tasks enables designers, researchers, and users the opportunity to be innovative, while understanding unmet needs, barriers, and challenges, which may or may not be experienced. Furthermore, these approaches also afford the research team understanding, which highlights the positives and benefits of innovative technology design, while becoming less reliant on 'self-reporting' of environment experience (e.g., walkable neighborhoods or social drift) [158,159]. This collaborative approach draws on existing universal design principles between design teams and various age-friendly stakeholders, including older adults who have the potential to collaborate in a co-creation process successful and satisfying products, systems, and environments [145,156–159].

5.1. Case Studies

Design hacking is all around us; it is how we can personalize or adapt technologies or products to offer greater experiences or enhance our existing understanding and perceptions. This, in turn has the potential to increase and enhance our health, wellbeing, and quality of life. In contemporary fieldwork and research activities, design hacking has become an integral component of enquiry, and can give multi-and-inter-disciplinary teams the opportunity to facilitate this approach as a way of understanding appropriate pathways and routes to revaluating and reframing age-friendly environments and experiences [158,159].

The following case studies, which share the experiences and narratives of four older adults, describe and illustrate how they have overcome product challenges by 'hacking, adapting or preparing'. Names have been changed to maintain agreed anonymity between the participant and the researcher.

5.1.1. Case Study A—Mary (2016)

Mary lives alone and has been separated from her spouse for several years; she has two adult children. Mary still works as an art teacher/therapist on a part-time basis. Her front room is a studio, which is full of materials, paints, and books. Mary has macular degeneration and arthritis and takes daily medication for various health conditions. During one of the fieldwork sessions, the following information was revealed: *Marys' arthritis medication has consistently managed her condition well and she has not experienced any challenges or difficulty, until she received her last prescription from the pharmacy. Although the medication was not changed by the pharmaceutical manufacturer, the manufacturer did decide to 'update' the packaging which includes a blister pack which holds each of the pills. The material of the blister pack is made of a harder, tougher type of material than previous packaging. The font on the packaging has also been changed and is presented diagonally rather than horizontally (left to right) as previously printed. Additional changes have also been made to the style of the font, which is now presented in a less bold and readable font style. This in turn has led Mary to experience difficulty reading the information as she expresses, "If I didn't know this was my medication, I wouldn't be able to read it".*

These small changes by the manufacturer have led to greater difficulties for patients such as Mary, which in turn has led to greater difficulties and confusion because of her health condition—macular degeneration. Furthermore, Mary is experiencing greater issues in relearning or recalibrating her mental models to recognize the new pill packaging alongside her other existing medications. Additionally, due to the changes in the physical packaging of the medication, Mary expresses how she experiences increased pain from the pressure of trying to open/access the tablet through the blister pack.

The solution to ease both discomfort when accessing the tablets is that Mary's daughter will remove each of the tablets (1-month supply) from the packaging and store them in a jam-jar, which in turn enables Mary to easily access her medication. Mary has tried another option to access her medication, which includes using a spoon to burst or 'pop' open the blister packaging.

5.1.2. Case Study B—Joan (2014)

Joan's home has a colorful entrance with flowers blooming on each side of the pathway leading to her entrance door. Joan is an avid gardener and loves any opportunity to work outdoors making her garden look beautiful. Joan is widowed and lives alone. Her adult children and grandchildren visit regularly, and the family ties are close.

The maintenance and access of various systems in the home were discussed. Joan highlighted how her central heating timer and immersion switch to heat her water are in her 'hot-press' (Figure 5), which is the key source within her home for hot water supply. This hot press has no light, and the dials can be difficult to read and see. As a solution, Joan keeps a torch in the 'hot-press' (Figure 6), which affords her to see and read the visual setting of the central heating timer and immersion more easily. As an additional back-up as well as forming part of the consideration of this important aspect of comfort and hygiene, Joan keeps a supply of batteries to ensure the torch consistently works. This planning and consideration to tasks and home management is an example of challenge and opportunity to retro fit and update older homes with newer technologies that can offer improved ease of access.

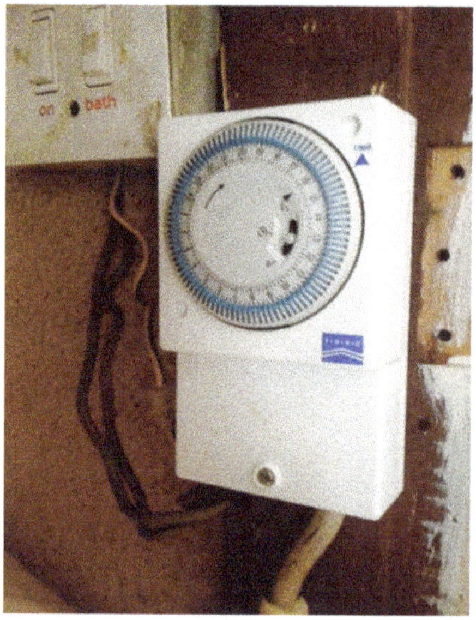

Figure 5. The interior of Joan's 'hot-press', displaying the central heating timer and immersion heater on the left, and torch on the right. Permission granted by Dr. L Shore.

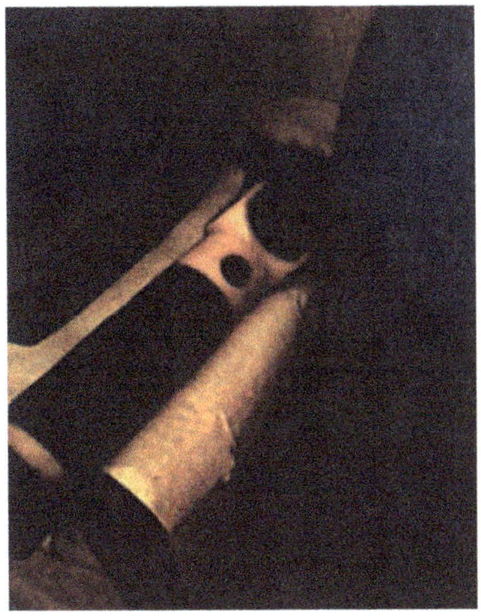

Figure 6. The interior of Joan's 'hot-press', displaying the central heating timer and immersion heater on the left, and torch on the right. Permission granted by Dr. L Shore.

5.1.3. Case Study C—William (2014)

William lives in a cottage with his wife in a rural area of Ireland. Several years ago, the cottage was extended with extra rooms and a new entrance doorway. This construction was started pre-retirement and because the planning commenced alongside active discussions regarding the type of home improvements, workflow and accessibility was required in their home.

At the beginning of this construction project, William and his wife considered their future selves and how the new rooms and access would impact their mobility, while also considering how they could implement an appropriate physical space to benefit and support them in later life, through their aging experience.

During this process, they factored in the idea that at some stage, either William or his wife could lose or encounter mobility challenges. This thought led them to consider the 'what if' question(s), relating to 'what if they were spending time in a wheelchair' or 'what if I was using a walking stick', or how easy would it be to live at 'home'.

With these types of questions in mind, they considered one significant feature, which they introduced into the physical space outside of their home, and this was to ensure that they had access to footpaths surrounding their home. This was important also in case they needed a level or ramp built to assist either of them, should they be in a wheelchair. This type of thought and consideration helps in maneuvering the device independently or ease the strain of pushing a wheelchair should a family member or friend be helping either of them onto the pathway.

Additionally, they were also intending to offset the potential 'disruption' of 'reactive home updates/renovations after an event has occurred, by actioning this foresight—the familiar pathway features would age with the building and not appear as a reminder to the experience of reduction in mobility.

These thoughts, considerations, and expressions were important conversations between William and his wife, which he relayed to the researcher. Furthermore, this thought process, and planning for the future, endorsed how as we age in place [159], acknowledging the physical and mobile aspects of aging, and can be prevented by exploring alternative considerations to enhance comfort within the individual home ecosystem. Furthermore, conducting physical changes to the home prior to retirement will ensure less disruption and construction works in the future when life and respective situations are more sensitive.

5.1.4. Case Study D—Jane and Remote Sunday Service

Jane who is 67 years old is now having to come to terms with empty nest syndrome, after her youngest daughter left the family home 12 months ago. Jane lives in a housing estate in a village located four kilometers from a busy Irish city center. She does not own a car, and given the proximity to the city center, she is able to travel quite easily via public transport. Her activities in the city center are weekly grocery shopping and seeing her grandchildren. Additionally, Jane likes to ride her bike or walk at least twice a week and attends her local place of worship, which she enjoys and has increased her involvement over recent years in because she has the time as well as is growing older. Jane believes it is important to foster and nurture a connection in the community and enjoys a range of activities, including being a member of the local organizing committee to grow organic produce with her friends on their allotments.

Jane admits to not being a regular user of technology; she tends to avoid the use of computers unless it is necessary and is usually assisted by a family member. Jane is a not a smartphone user; therefore, she chooses to stay in contact with friends and family via her home telephone or her basic mobile phone. However, over the last three years, Jane has learnt to send text messages, which has resulted in her growing in confidence. She now finds this engagement as a great way to keep in touch with friends and family. Although technology is a barrier for Jane, but when it comes to providing important communication touchpoints (i.e., contacting family members), she will try to overcome her fears and adapt accordingly. This is true of the recent COVID-19 pandemic situation, whereby Jane and many other citizens, old and young, have experienced limited face-to-face contact with friends, family, and community organizations. Technology has, for Jane, offered an alternative solution to maintaining existing relationships.

One example of the use of technology as a solution for Jane to maintain her community involvement and friendships is attending the weekly church service Figures 7 and 8). During the first lockdown, there were severe restrictions put in place, which resulted in members of the church not been able to attend their weekly Sunday service. For Jane to attend her weekly service online, her daughter helps set up a tablet device, which in turn presents the church service online church service, while she sits at her kitchen table. Jane accepts that technology in this instance is not a replacement for the church service but admits that it has brought a level of comfort and routine.

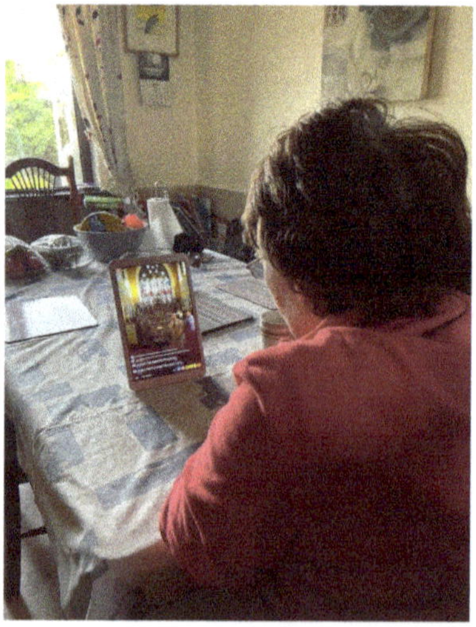

Figure 7. An older lady remotely attending church service in her community.

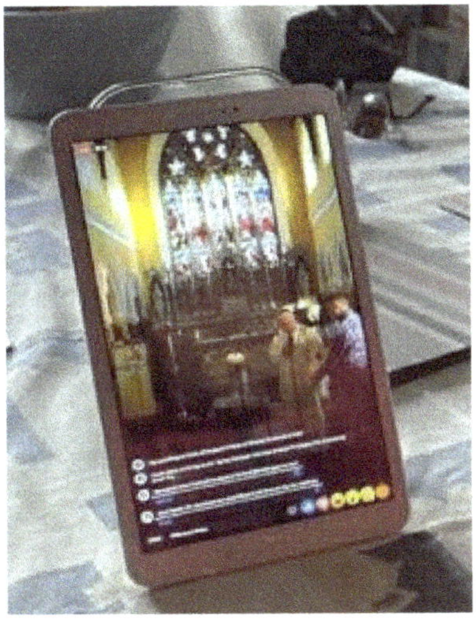

Figure 8. Interface of the church service via Facebook, coupled with comments and emoticons from fellow members of the congregation. Permission granted by Dr P. J. White, taken 2020.

There are two important messages, which can be taken and concluded from this adaptation: 1. the perceived barriers of use are overcome with her daughter's assistance; and 2. the comfort and routine gained from the online church service outweigh her technology fears.

In summary we have described and presented four various case studies that reflect real-world situations, and solutions for older adults who continue to live independently in their own homes. In the next section, we explore several case studies surrounding the COVID-19 pandemic.

6. Pandemic Case Studies

From a UK standpoint and context, lockdowns have varied and were introduced into British society on the March 25, 2020 [160]. This approach was taken by the UK Government and is continuing to impact the society from the standpoint of education, economy, mental health, social engagement, and business. Coupled with various societal changes occurring in the 21st century, the UK has been recovering from the 2008 recession, which involved 10 years of austerity, and now with the outbreak of the coronavirus pandemic, which has to date killed 41,988 thousand people in the UK [161], with a further 434,969 cases reported [161].

The week commencing August 10, 2020, the Chancellor of the UK Government (Rishi Sunak) announced [14.08.2020] that the UK was in the biggest recession in 100 years [162], with unemployment reaching approximately 730,000 people [163,164], since the lockdown commenced in March 2020. Furthermore, it is anticipated within a UK context and in conjunction with the furlough scheme ceasing in the autumn of 2020 that the level of unemployment is likely to increase [163,164]. Moreover, citizens and the society does not know what the future holds, as Marston and colleagues note in their blog [29]:

> "As the bells struck the stroke of midnight, ringing in 2020, citizens were smiling, pouring another glass of rosé, red wine or supping from their pint of Guinness from the confines of their local pub, house parties, restaurants, or clubs; while singing auld lang syne, shaking each other's hands, giving a kiss on the cheek to the person next to them or a hearty smooch with a loved one. The biggest challenge of a generation ahead, at this moment in time in the UK was Brexit, little did we know this was about to be surpassed by something even bigger." [29]

This is true. At the start of 2020, the Western world could not have imagined a change to their existing ecosystems, daily routines, lives, employment, health, and wellbeing. For many citizens, the use, integration, and acceptance of digital technologies into their individual smart age-friendly ecosystems is the norm, while for many citizens, this is not the case. For many citizens, what was the norm, the regular routines, and expectations of socializing and day-to-day activities, has now been turned upside down.

With regards to these unexpected changes faced and experienced by many citizens, we have provided a variety of scenarios below, building on previous exemplars posited by Marston and van Hoof [30], and in turn represent various ecosystems and sub-groups of populations currently in society.

Scenario #1: Middle-aged family

In contemporary society, it is not uncommon for young and middle-aged adults to have children but also be geographically displaced due to employment commitments which in turn result in having fewer support networks due to their extended families (e.g. grandparents) living elsewhere in the same country or even abroad.

Frederik is a 38-year old man who lives with his partner Zoe, and their two children, Johan (7) and Eva (3). Usually, the children go to school and nursey, respectively, while Zoe and Frederik work. During the week, their home life can be very busy—they have active careers with a limited support network (their families live in the Netherlands). However, their leisure activities are varied, and include playing football for a local team, while Zoe and the children go and watch sometimes. As a family, they like the outdoors—walking, canoeing, and nature. Zoe has recently started exploring the arts and crafts scene, while Johan likes reading, Lego, and watching cartoons with his sister. As a family, they eat freshly cooked meals, and will bake where possible.

The family do not have underlying health conditions, and they usually order their groceries online from a national retailer, while they purchase their fruit and vegetables from the local market stall on a weekly basis.

Since the lockdown, their home environment has changed considerably. They are still expected to work, while the children are not able to attend school/nursery, and Johan's school is conducting online classes throughout the day. Zoe is wondering how she is going to manage her job, while homeschooling Johan and ensuring Eva is occupied and learning too. Frederik is logging into the computer system so he can continue with his tasks and responsibilities.

Scenario #2: Intergenerational family

In society, there are many families who choose to live together under one roof. Intergenerational living has many benefits, such as sharing household responsibilities, (e.g., caring responsibilities of both young children and older adults), cleaning, cooking, learning, and social interaction. This scenario is rather complex, due to the various generations and situations.

The Smith family currently comprises of three generations living under one roof. They live in the South East of England and due to several changes in circumstances with different members of the family, are now practicing intergenerational living and have been for the last 18 months. The members of the family include Mabel (85 years) and Arthur (90), their daughter Alison (55) and son-in-law Stuart (57), who have three children: their daughter Jennifer (28) and her husband Michael (31), their second child Gareth (24), a local entrepreneur and businessman in town, and his girlfriend Sabine (24), who is from Germany, and their youngest daughter Heidi (19), who is supposed to be returning to university in the autumn, in the North of England.

As a family, they enjoy socializing with each other, playing boardgames, BBQing, watching movies, and sport.

Jennifer and Michael are expecting their first child in the summer. Arthur has been diagnosed with dementia and although Mabel is able to care for him, she relies on her family for support. The pandemic has highlighted the vulnerability of both Mabel and Arthur, who are now shielded because of their ages and health conditions, following the guidance and directive by the government.

Both Alison and her husband Stuart are keyworkers, while Stuart is now working shifts.

Gareth and Sabine had been living abroad, and while he had the opportunity to run his multiple businesses from afar, they chose to move back to his parent's home prior to purchasing their own house. Now that the pandemic has been declared, Sabine assists the family with tasks such as grocery shopping and caring for Mable and Arthur. Gareth has been looking for ways to retain his staff and is considering the furlough scheme.

Heidi is studying at a university in the North of England. She is excited to be returning for her second year of studies but accepts that her second year will be very different to her first. She has been working part-time and will usually transfer her employment to another site when she returns to University. Currently, she is continuing to study her subjects and continue with her assessments; she acknowledges that she is playing a pivotal role in the family ecosystem, alongside Sabine, in caring for her grandparents, and volunteering in the community.

Scenario #3—COVID-19 community support groups

Within weeks of lockdown having been announced in the UK, there were many communities taking an organic approach, by organizing online/social media support groups. Such groups facilitated the community and its residents to assist those most vulnerable or ill with certain requests, such as groceries and collecting prescriptions, among others.

Additionally, specific contacts/residents were also highlighted for streets/areas in that respective community, which in turn would enable a vulnerable resident to directly contact that point of contact and request assistance. This approach was invaluable for those who were shielding/isolating because of illness/health conditions, or who had been diagnosed with the coronavirus.

These support groups facilitated information to be shared relating to opening times, local grocery deliveries (e.g., fruit and vegetables), and regular updates. In some instances, such groups facilitated suggestions to parents who were/are homeschooling children, with the provision of ideas for activities.

Scenario #4—Older adults

Many older adults are continuing to live independently or with their spouses. The notion of death and facing widowhood can be daunting for many older adults, who have spent a significant amount of time together; in some instances, sharing both happy and tough memories and experiences.

The pandemic highlights the vulnerability of older adults in various situations, and this scenario will focus on older adults who are (a) still married, (b) widowed, and (c) live on their own and are aging without children.

Older adults—still married: Margaret (67 years) and Stan (70) have been married for 50 years; they have two children, six grandchildren, and 1 great-grandchild. They survive on their state pensions, and Stan has a small private pension. Their children (Kathryn—49 years, and Martin 47 years visit regularly throughout the week, popping in for a cup of tea and a catchup. The grandchildren range between 17 and 25 years; their great-grandchild is one year old.

Older adults—widowed: Derrick is 65 years old and recently widowed. His wife Stella died 8 months ago from a neurological condition at the age of 62 years. Derrick is adjusting to life on his own; he has a daughter who lives approximately 2 hours away, and who tries to visit her father on the weekend. Derrick still has friends and tried to maintain the odd social event at his local club, where he could still interact.

Older adults—live on their own: Suzanne is a 57-year old woman who recently took a severance package from her employer. She has never married, is aging without children, and her extended family are scattered across the UK and abroad. She enjoys cooking, growing vegetables, volunteering at the local charity shop and church, and arts and crafts.

Scenario #5—Resident/assisted living/care home(s)

The pandemic has cruelly highlighted the vulnerability of citizens residing in environments such as residential, assisted living, and/or nursing/care homes [165]. Early in the pandemic across the UK, it was reported that many staff (e.g., carers, chefs, management) chose to live in, in the respective home to 1. shield the residents, 2. reduce the risk of catching COVID-19 and passing it on to colleagues and residents, 3. similar to point two, but passing the coronavirus on to their families [166]. How will such environments operate in a post-pandemic society from the standpoint of carers/support staff, residents, and family members?

Scenario #6—Young person living on their own

There are many young people who move away from their friends and family for employment and/or studies. The pandemic is highlighting social isolation and loneliness, and mental health issues are impacting not only older adults, but young people as well.

Carl is a thirty-something professional who lives in a different County, approximately 6 hours from where he grew up. He has been living alone, renting an apartment in this area for some time but has found it difficult to form a solid friendship/social network. One of the reasons for this is because Carl has been on fixed-term contracts with his employer, which has hindered his ability to make friendships in the town. Carl's personality is outgoing—he enjoys watching sports, enjoys his job, and runs regularly with a running club. However, he has tried to form a social network through the running club, work colleagues, and his neighbors, but to no avail. Carl usually spends his down time reading, watching Netflix, and cooking.

Scenario #7—Family who has a member with serious health condition(s)

For many citizens who themselves suffer from or have family members with serious health conditions—cancer or a life-limiting or life-threatening health condition—the pandemic has added additional pressures to their home environment.

Darren (35) and his wife Roberta (33) have two children, James (7) and Amelie (11). Darren has been in the military for 15 years, while Roberta usually works part-time in the community. They live off base, which affords the family a greater level of freedom and gives them the opportunity to socialize with friends and colleagues on the base, enjoy BBQs, annual parties, and other events. Amelie has just finished junior school and is starting high school in September; she is looking forward to this transition and enjoys learning and making new friends.

James has a life-limiting health condition, which was diagnosed when he was toddler. Due to his health condition, Roberta attends various meetings with health and social care practitioners to ensure all his needs are being met, and his progress is recorded. Darren attends when he can; due to his work responsibilities, he finds it difficult to attend all the appointments and this at times means Roberta is caring for their children as a single parent. Although she has a social network in the community and amongst friends on the military base, their familial support networks are geographically displaced because her and Darren's parents live several hours away.

Since the pandemic and during lockdown, Darren has been away on exercise, which has led Roberta to be on her own, homeschooling the children, attending to the physio exercises for James, and furloughed from her job in the community. Her social interaction has thus been reduced considerably, and due to James's health condition, she and Amelie have had to shield themselves. Their friends from the military base have come by, dropping groceries off, and chatting through the window. Usually, Roberta is not troubled by the absence of Darren, because they have been together for over 10 years, and when they married, she knew this would be part of their life. Roberta communicates with hers and Darren's parents, but she is experiencing the additional stresses of homeschooling, social isolation, and loneliness while Darren is away, which is exacerbated by James' health condition and the pandemic. Appointments that had been scheduled for several months/weeks are not taking place or have been reduced.

These scenarios aim to illustrate the different circumstances of citizens across various age cohorts and home environments, in an attempt to reflect the everyday life for many citizens. Playing out such scenarios offers greater opportunities in identifying what type of technology, IoTs, support, and research can be roleplayed.

Taking into account the scenarios presented above, we propose and discuss the 'Concept of Age-friendly Smart Ecologies (CASE)' framework in the following section. The CASE framework is built on the WHO [36] framework and the extended framework by Marston and van Hoof [30].

7. Proposal of New Post-Pandemic Age-Friendly Ecosystems

Based on contemporary literature surrounding existing age-friendly frameworks [30,36], in conjunction with earlier discussions posited in this paper (i.e., design hacks, and the various case studies and scenarios), we believe a new 'Concept of Age-friendly Smart Ecologies (CASE)' framework (Figure 9) can be proposed to offer a myriad of actors the opportunity to adapt the 'Concept of Age-friendly Smart Ecologies (CASE)' framework to suit their needs and requirements, or to various situations.

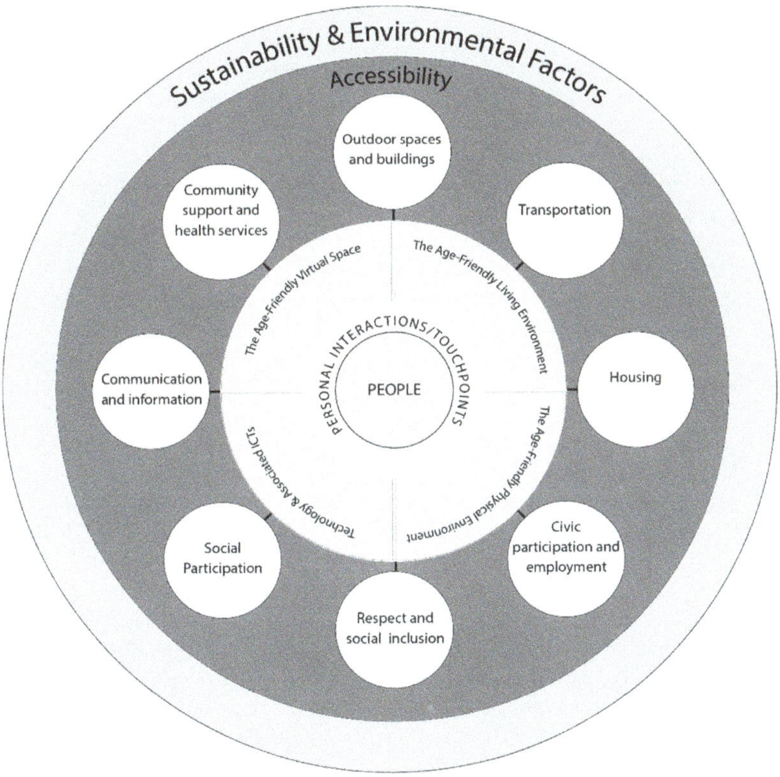

Figure 9. The newly proposed 'Concept of Age-friendly Smart Ecologies (CASE)' framework.

Furthermore, taking into consideration the rapid pace at which technology develops while ensuring all citizens in society are represented, the coining and positing of this term 'Concept of Age-friendly Smart Ecologies (CASE)' offers a myriad of actors the flexibility to adapt and future proof respective environments, where necessary.

The 'Concept of Age-friendly Smart Ecologies (CASE)' framework is an extension of the Marston and van Hoof [30] and WHO [36] frameworks.

In the CASE framework, we added several new sections to reflect on and consider existing as well as new areas of interest. The CASE framework is as follows: 1. The outer sphere is *'Sustainability, and Environmental Factors'* which relates to ensuring that all citizens, companies, organizations, educational institutions, etc. can and are contributing to a greener, more efficient, and sustainable environment. This could relate to local, regional, and national environments. This sphere can aid policy makers in assisting with this transition by including not only environmental benefits to adoption of sustainable approaches, but also economic advantage [166], which can initially appear high, but over time reduces. This, in turn, can benefit economies and budgets. Furthermore, by taking a co-creation approach in conjunction with a universal design approach, this outer sphere facilitates a wide variety of opportunities for many actors to co-design, co-create, and co-produce existing physical environments.

2. *Accessibility* is reflected by the inner sphere and relates to the accessibility of the intersection occurring between the relationships of the physical and digital ecosystems conducted and experienced by citizens, business, educational institutes, community hubs, etc. Because accessibility relates to and is interwoven through differing features of the infrastructure within our cities or towns, it is important that there is a strong relationship and understanding of how accessibility intersects our daily lives. Accessibility is incorporated through (a) buildings and transport, (b) business, educational institutes and community hubs and services, (c) packaging (including pills/medications), and (d) technology. This in turn is a necessary consideration to facilitate and adapt to the age-friendly concept for all citizens. It is apparent in the previous age-friendly framework [30] that accessibility is an important factor for all eight hubs, highlighted in case studies discussed in this article and illustrating how citizens can be hurt by poor accessibility design considerations.

3. The eight hubs represent various aspects in society and are taken from the 2007 WHO age-friendly framework [36].

4. As we become more technologically immersed in the current and future experiences of our respective ecosystems, both in contemporary and future societies, technology will continue to play a key role. The CASE framework ensures a notion of future-proofing the approach to design considerations of smart age-friendly cities by introducing four separate sections in the inner sphere, which are explained in Section 7.1 and highlight the beneficial outputs and scenarios to: (a) The *Age-Friendly Virtual Space*, (b) The *Age-Friendly Living Environment*, (c) The *Age-Friendly Physical Environment*, and (d) *Technology and Associated ICTs*.

5. The inner hub—*Personal Interactions/Touchpoints*—represents interactions and experiences that can be personal or shared with an individual. In contemporary society both pre-and-during COVID-19, many citizens are experiencing loneliness and social isolation because of both geographically displaced families as well as governmental lockdowns or cocooning [62]. The purpose of this inner hub aims is to afford citizens the emotional and social needs that are central to positive health, wellbeing, and age-in-place.

6. The central hub represents the citizens in both our current and future societies. Acknowledging the needs of citizens needs to remain central in ensuring that all that is offered, through various interactions within respective environments and operating systems, and with the use of products, has the potential to offer positive experiences for all—both young and old citizens. Furthermore, it is intended within the inner hub that there will be support afforded via human interventions and supportive networks and systems to those in need.

Indeed, while we are discussing the CASE framework from the standpoint of contemporary society, we should also take into consideration the future and what or how society will look in a post-pandemic society. While the *CASE* framework can reflect existing societal mechanisms, would differences occur for several actors relating to interaction and engagement at various micro and macro levels in respective ecosystems, which in turn may afford greater agility, adaptability, and scalability [70,124]?

For example, in a city, this diagram represents a district or a suburb depending on the size of each of the eight hubs: 1. Transport, 2. Housing, 3. Civic participation and employment, 4. Respect and social inclusion, 5. Social Participation, 6. Communication and information, 7. Community support and health services, and 8. Outdoor spaces and buildings.

The size of each of these hubs or domains may vary based on the positive and negative impacts indicative within each district or suburb. Similarly, this notion could be adapted and scaled up to reflect municipalities or provincial regions within countries. Therefore, the greater is the hub associated to one of these eight domains, the greater is the positivity or service(s) offered (e.g., public transport, ICT infrastructure, health service provision etc.). Alternatively, the smaller the hub, the lesser or negativity of services are afforded.

In summary, the *CASE* framework displays an innovative approach to amalgamating both the WHO [36] and SAfE [30] frameworks, while also recognizing that there are additional factors at play within the ecosystem that were not implemented or acknowledged in previous iterations. Furthermore, the *CASE* framework affords various actors the opportunity to evaluate their respective ecosystems given the increase in technologies and the potential changes and behaviors in the future, in a post-pandemic society.

In the following section, we describe a series of scenarios and provide solutions based on point 4 of the *CASE* framework.

7.1. Design Hacks, Technology, and IoT Solutions

In this section, we will revisit the different scenarios described in the previous section and suggest suitable solutions.

Scenario #1—Middle-aged family

Regarding scenario 1, the *CASE* framework accommodates the personal interactions that everyone has, in this instance, in conjunction with other family members (e.g., partner to partner, parent to children and them to their parents). In both a pre-and-post-pandemic society, the relationship between the user, technology, and the environments involves lived experiences within the eight domains. However, the new *CASE* framework central quadrants provide an insight into potential and specific interactions and touchpoints to these domains.

The Age-friendly Living Environment: As this family has not experienced aging, it may seem strange to explore age-friendly environments. However, the living spaces we reside in, both currently and in the future, may be modular or adaptable spaces that can consider areas for collective calm—they include features based on soundproofing and adequate sensory ambience, which in turn can encourage relaxation and to recharge oneself while facing the challenges of living through both a contemporary and post-pandemic society. Additionally, all family members can benefit from these spaces and there can be a shared space too, in addition to family members retreating to their bedrooms. Growing up in this type of space, children may have the opportunity to perceive this space as a form of relaxation as a part of a daily ritual, while learning valuable means to relax in stressful or worrying times.

The Age-friendly Physical Space offers this family the option of outdoor sharing or single activities, such as walking, canoeing, and enjoying the experience of time surrounded by nature. However, beyond these experiences, life in both a contemporary and post-pandemic society continues to have the additional requirements, such as shopping, waste, and health management.

This brings to the fore the possibility of sustainability and environmental features. It is apparent that people's view on fast fashion has changed to exploring 'slow fashion' or repurposing clothing, furniture, and sharing economies [167,168]. Zoe's interest in the arts and crafts scene endorses this and creates an opportunity to create items for the home, as gifts, or garments to wear. 'Crafting' is a hobby that is shared and interweaves generations, and an age-friendly community network of crafters was visited pre-pandemic [158]. Networks such as this can reopen in a post-pandemic society. However, visitors will be presented with hygiene and virus management challenges, ensuring each member is protected. To overcome this, there is the possibility of ensuring that materials are maintained and not shared, unless appropriately sanitized. These community craft times could perhaps provide greater comfort and opportunity for parents such as Zoe to attend alone or encourage a smaller group of children to explore various art-and-craft activities. There is also the possibility of intergenerational activities, whereby similar to the old 'punch and Judy' model, the players are behind the scenes and the audience can safely socially distance in new open spaces in towns, cities, or parks.

The Age-friendly Virtual Space is an exciting space to speculate a post-pandemic society. The possible solutions both encourage and include interactions with people and families with mobility or physical limitation. Relating to scenario one, the solution could offer interactive augmented reality spaces for education and play time for Johan and Eva. These spaces could be pods similar to how children played in a pre-pandemic society, whereby locations such as ball pit, play zones or trampolines and playgrounds facilitated free play.

Technology and Associated ICTs: this scenario considers the competencies of both Frederick and Zoe, who have busy lives, careers, and personal ambitions. In this case, it is imperative that various service systems, for example, health, energy, and home/banking management, can operate in a usable, friendly efficient way. Service providers have adapted greatly by increasing offerings, such as online shopping for groceries or financial transactions becoming increasingly contactless payment. Considering the post-pandemic world, some of these new behaviors will be maintained (e.g., contactless payment, increased from £30 to £45 in the UK). However, new forms of behavior, such as hybrid working—encompassing greater affordances and approaches to work from home—will rely on existing and innovative technologies to be accessible, and not being restricted due to network or server issues and difficulties.

Scenario #2—Intergenerational family

The Age-friendly Living Environment: The intergenerational family outlined in this paper has multiple needs for the current living environment they share. In a post-pandemic society, it is apparent that there is going to more changes and it is likely that Gareth and Sabine will seek to move home, while Heidi is anticipating her return to college in the autumn or experience a mix of online and face-to-face teaching.

The future experiences for Gareth and Sabine are normal events for most families as they grow. In a post-pandemic society, should a request for 'shielding' or 'cocooning' be advised, they may also include home adaptability or receive new responsibilities of care and support. Perhaps, not so much that Arthur and Mabel isolate, but for keyworkers such as Alison and Stuart to be reassured that they are able to continue their work, yet taking into account that they will not present any greater risk to the members of their own home environment.

It is suggested that perhaps an entry point is agreed in the home with a specific space for sanitizing, undressing, and showering to reduce the risk of spreading the virus to vulnerable members of their own household. Sabine appears to be at home to provide care and support, but this may change as the baby is born and how this will affect the family dynamic and use of comfort and spaces is unknown.

As per scenario 1, one solution could be to live in a modular housing development/unit, which in turn could support this family to allow for temporary move-ins (Gareth and Sabine) or connected living spaces that present a gathering opportunity or shielding for Arthur and Mabel.

The Age-friendly Physical Space: Accessibility has been noted as a feature within the domains of the age-friendly network (outdoor spaces and buildings). Health conditions and lifespan events (e.g., giving birth) can impact how we move from one location to another.

Currently, and during the lockdown in the UK and Ireland, public transport was restricted because of limitations on the numbers of passengers or services operating. As the months continued, users of public transport had to comply with governmental legislation relating to facemasks. Should a person wish to use public transport, they are required to wear a facemask. In a post-pandemic society, envisioning how society will behave could afford municipalities, governments, academics the opportunity to purvey alternative forms of transport/hubs. For example, the use of autonomous vehicles, bicycles programs (as found in Copenhagen) or shared transport networks could prove to be beneficial, because this would facilitate health and wellbeing, physical activity, and reduce the risk of any further contagion.

The Age-friendly Virtual Space can have a positive impact on connected health developments, such as interactive spaces between healthcare professionals or care workers and patients such as Mabel and Arthur. Likewise, additional connectedness could be experienced from within the home ecosystem by differing technologies, such as virtual assistants, alert systems, or apps accessible and even controlled remotely via a smartphone. This, in turn, would offer reassurance to family members if a vulnerable family member is alone, or should assistance be required, they can respond quickly.

Technology and Associated ICTs can be associated and connected to both healthcare and transport hubs and links, which, in turn, could provide supportive networks that facilitate and enable the autonomy and responsibility of lifestyle and independence. The monitoring of symptoms and testing facilitated by track-and-trace capabilities during the pandemic can be potentially done in a post-pandemic society. Furthermore, the integration of Blockchain and AI capabilities has the potential to afford healthcare providers, municipalities, business, and citizens the opportunity to engage both directly and indirectly within respective ecosystems. Additionally, promotions or campaigns across various modes of digital devices, social media platforms, and physical spaces (e.g., advertisement boards) can assist in reminding citizens to maintain regular hygiene practices, which, in turn, may reduce the opportunity of further susceptibility in a post-pandemic society. The recent progress made in Africa whereby the elimination of polio has progressed [169] is a good example of this.

Scenario #3—COVID-19 community support groups

Scenario #3 explores the activism conducted by people within communities to be supportive and helpful to those with needs such as those 'shielding' or in fact frontline workers who may have very little personal time to refresh.

The Age-friendly Living Environment: For an individual living alone or deemed vulnerable, they may still have requirements and needs that must be supported by neighbors or people within the community. Apps or simply creating a WhatsApp/phone group that supports images, videos/video conferencing, and voice share could continue to assist vulnerable people in a post-pandemic society. Likewise, the mobilization of smaller factories responded rapidly to the call for clothing to be worn by frontline workers should be maintained as a network that could be mobilized, should there be another outbreak of COVID-19 or another coronavirus/ emergency.

The Age-friendly Physical Space: Community 'hubs' could be encouraged and implemented by either utilizing existing structures such as community halls or creating new purpose built hubs, which, in turn, could provide leisure activities and work spaces, but also double up as an emergency area, should similar pandemics occur in the future.

The Age-friendly Virtual Space: Virtual and interactive opportunities could be made possible by applying AR in conjunction with social media and communication platforms, to enable and ensure group activities, as well as the delivery of education, health, and business meetings, are continued. This would be fruitful because if all members of the respective outlets are not available to attend in person, they can still attend virtually.

Technology and Associated ICTs can be implemented in community and connected activities to enable reliance on existing hardware and devices such as mobile phones and computer applications, which, in turn, will support contacts and updates to mobilize or stand down, should there be emergencies in the future. One prospective solution is to create a volunteer registry, which would facilitate and reassure each user/member of the security of their information and personal details; one that is transparent but yet, easily accessible via instant messaging, to ensure accessibility for all.

Scenario #4—Older adults living independently

The Age-friendly Living Environment relates to age-in-place [170,171] and is perceived as a beneficial approach to aging in later life, with a view to building on and sharing positive aging experiences [159].

Living independently highlights the opportunity to explore the home environment with a view on accessibility, which, in turn, could be easily adaptable, if necessary. Furthermore, new homes could be built with the view for positive and successful age-in-place, whereby doorways are wheelchair-friendly, light switches are placed at an accessible height, rather than at a height for a person standing up. Staircases and landings on the first floor are to be of suitable width, which enables wheelchair access and/or mechanical stairlifts to successfully transfer an individual from the ground floor without ruining the decoration. These approaches could be considered by William and his wife – as discussed in Case Study C. Luckily, there are building recommendations that support accessible a universal design in new builds, and retro fitting grants to adapt homes, typically after a need (e.g., home access ramps) is identified, can be made available. Additionally, we would suggest further features that support autonomy and security in the home. Whether from the standpoint of the pandemic or a post-pandemic society, the consideration of built environments to support a form of socializing but still maintain shielding could be explored in future developments [149]. Finally, what has been highlighted here is the essence of greater opportunities for the construction industry, developers, planners, architects, and academics in the fields of gerontology, gerontechnology, social sciences, and HCI. This could take a co-creation, co-design, and universal design approach to understanding the needs, challenges, issues, experiences, as well as positives of this type of living and development [62].

The Age-friendly Physical Space: Maintaining social connections appears to be a significant factor for older adults living independently and who are ageing without children (AWOC) [29]. This can be emphasized in a post-pandemic society by more activities that can be conducted in public spaces, such as green spaces, streets, community hubs, or gyms. Additionally, there could be the option for intergenerational spaces, which, in turn, could cater to all ages; they could have giant chess, boule, and table tennis tables. Implementing sensory spaces could afford residents and citizens the opportunity to relax outdoors, whereby seating is surrounded by different sounds, images, and touch and scent of the flora and fauna within the space. These spaces would include energizing areas that capture sunshine and places that are more serene and shaded.

The Age-friendly Virtual Space relates to various activities and energy we have, and which can change during the aging process. We may develop new health conditions (e.g., arthritis) or experience more severe and impactful diseases, such as a stroke or a heart problem. Recuperation and recovery programs in a post-pandemic society may be a feature of a new connected health service, and interactive screenings and appointments could be considered by municipalities or local health care providers.

Technology and Associated ICTs relates to maintaining one's independence as we age and move forward in a post-pandemic society, while creating new opportunities to explore robotic assistive devices that can enhance the independence and autonomy of an individual. IoTs and wearable technologies can provide reassurance (e.g., monitoring or alerts to falls, or sudden increase in body temperature) to neighbors, family members, and friends of the individual. These types of sensors and devices can also relate to alternative, new connected health programs that includes relevant professional and trusted members of an older adults' network (e.g., support network, health professionals, family, friends etc.). Blockchain and AI technologies have the potential to offer this type of service delivery, with focus on data privacy and security.

Scenario #5—Resident/Assisted living/Care Home(s)

The Age-friendly Living Environment: This scenario is similar to intergenerational living [62] and their respective needs. However, unlike an intergenerational family, bonds may not be emotionally strong. An example of this could relate to the care assistant or nurse, who choose to be a live-in, and who may also still be juggling her own family responsibilities, albeit remotely. Therefore, the resident/care home may require the assurance of staff calm spaces, where they can adequately support social interactions with other staff members or likewise have zones of relaxation and calm, where energies can be renewed.

The Age-friendly Physical Space, from a post-pandemic standpoint associated to residents of care homes, may renew shopping trips or outings that involve groups or sometimes outings with family that were enjoyed in a pre-pandemic society.

It is apparent that while there is no vaccine for COVID-19, it is not yet stated how long society will be continuing with differing variations of lockdowns and legislation. Therefore, wearing facemasks and using hand sanitization will become integral in day-to-day rituals (e.g., going into a grocery store, touching public artifacts, etc.).When we consider some aging factors, such as reduced hearing, vision, and ambulation, facemasks may present a challenge, not just in how they are worn, but also potentially interfering with hearing aids and/or glasses. Additionally, a facemask may also have an impact on the proprioception and/or spatial awareness of a person within the physical space, and this in turn may lead to them losing their balance and falling/tripping over. In turn, this requires assurances that features such as lighting or access is optimized to cater for all abilities and citizens.

The Age-friendly Virtual Space is important for the residents and staff of residential facilities and care homes. Technology for some of these facilities may be limited, coupled with the digital skills/literacy of the staff. However, technology and appropriate broadband networks are needed to ensure that features such as video calls or classes can still be conducted and experienced via communication platforms, which also facilitate a virtual space to socialize and engage with community activities, such as attending church services, as demonstrated in Case Study D, Section 5.1.4.

Technology and Associated ICTs can assist residents and staff in care homes with maintaining social and familial connections by taking a deep dive into technology and using the various features accessible in different social media and communication platforms, such as video calling, looking at photographs, listening and watching music and television programs, as well as communicating via email. Voice assistants may be helpful to provide social engagements for residents who are alone and may need to alert a member of staff for assistance. Additionally, with virtual assistants, there is the potential to be connected to wearable devices, which may also offer a feeling of safety to the resident and their family members.

Scenario #6—Young person living on their own

The Age-friendly Living Environment: For Carl, who is a healthy and fit person, this environment in both a contemporary and post-pandemic society may afford greater opportunities to enhance interactions that have been 'held back' due to geographic distances, detached meetings, and social outings.

The living environment has at times offered little comfort to people like Carl, who experience loneliness and social isolation. A suggested enhancement to the living environment would be greater accessibility on a long-term lease, which, in turn, would facilitate someone like Carl to feel 'at home' or 'in place'. The possibility to 'embed' or feel at home could build and enhance confidence to pursue more robust friendships or social networking opportunities through the living and/or communal spaces within these new environments. There might be a choice to have a 'pet' that does not require full responsibility of one person but offering a 'pet share' plan could enhance further social interactions with the partners of the pet.

The Age-friendly Physical Space lends itself to home working pods that are not coffee houses or linked with commercial brokers, but instead could be developed in a way that could retrofit unused or redundant spaces in localities. This type of example could work for neighbors who may be working from home, but could then congregate in a mimicked work environment, a 'Work-Gym'. Furthermore, this concept may also encourage new friendships, relationships, and broaden social networks.

The Age-friendly Virtual Space could support working from any geographical location; for Carl, this could mean he remains living in his hometown, surrounded by all things familiar, whilst working remotely, connecting through digital applications to engage in meetings or updates regarding projects or team collaborations. Alternatively, should Carl choose to work or relocate to a new geographical location, he could mirror certain behaviors, experiences, and views from home through ambient and responsive AR scenarios.

Technology and Associated ICTs can include virtual assistants and social robotic pets to enhance one's quality of living experience although it would not be a replacement for face-to-face contact. This proposal encourages a 'kit' whereby you build and include your preferences to personalize the type of home you wish, and the robotic pet could, for example, be a replica of a childhood pet. The benefits to people like Carl are the freedom to still take trips or visits to his hometown without planning or having the responsibility to find a suitable pet sitter or the cost of kennels.

Scenario #7—Family who has a member with serious health condition(s)

The Age-friendly Living Environment: More so than ever, people have experienced various impacts and difficulties during COVID-19. Family life can be challenging during normal times and it is apparent how Darren and Roberta rely on social scaffolding to enable a positive quality of life, socializing and interacting with friends and members of the community.

The work responsibilities Darren has impacts on Roberta's ability to make sense of day-to-day family living and time management. Additional support to the family could be further respite care for James, which allows for moments of refresh for Roberta, particularly when Darren is away. However, during the pandemic, this opportunity may not be possible. However, as James grows up and his needs become more complex, a respite facility may afford all family members the opportunity to relax. Furthermore, identifying appropriate networks within their existing social and familial networks and organizations could afford Roberta the opportunity to take time out for a walk in the green space close to their home and enjoy some time with their daughter Amalie before she starts high school. One of the support networks could assist by taking over homeschooling duty with James. This system could perhaps be encouraged and reversed during term time (e.g., one-to-one time with James, while a member of the support network homeschools Amalie).

The Age-friendly Physical Space: During the initial lockdown in the UK, there was a regular/weekly clap for frontline workers every Thursday evening at 7 pm. This was an important action to acknowledge all those citizens who were and continue to work on the frontline (e.g., medical professionals, health and social care providers, etc.) who are compromising their own health, their time with family, and personal lives to support those who fell ill.

Perhaps in a post-pandemic society, there could a way we should look at ways of remembering to take time to value those close to us and state it in a subtle way. Instead of purchasing items of 'stuff', it could simply be a gesture that is on a physical living space in a neighborhood. A thank you wall/park/space might work, whereby an assigned space affords the provision to allow for blocks or ornaments to be attached to this space to be purchased on behalf of someone by another person. This space would be accessible to all and could be shared and offer a space for reflection, while focusing on the gratitude for those individuals and keyworkers who served their communities during this time. This essentially could be a funded arts project that could be updated over time but is always changing and reflective of where life might be at that given time.

The Age-friendly Virtual Space could offer families and couples such as Darren and Roberta a specific space to spend some quality time together, while also being connected to specific health technologies. This, in turn, would allow healthcare professionals, patients, and family members to interact and share progress or prognosis updates securely, while not necessarily being together in any specific location. Sharing of information would be facilitated via the implementation of Blockchain and AI solutions, and securely accessed via an App and/or via a communications platform, or virtual assistant. Additionally, wearable devices and analytics could offer efficient updates and insights in real-time for James' parents, and his healthcare team. The design outcomes that are desirable in this prospective solution relate to data security, comfort, and ease of use for all key people involved in the health, wellbeing, and service delivery for James.

Technology and Associated ICTs: Accessibility and ease of use of service systems are necessary aspects to gain fully functioning optimization. Technology requirements would need to be supported on secure networks (e.g., via Blockchain) and future-proofed to ensure that the lifespan of the design for patients such as James is maintained and updated, where necessary. Additionally, the family could engage and manually update the system with personal additions/observations to the health system 'App', thereby allowing for random or surprise changes to James' prognosis to be captured. If Darren is away with work, he can still access, view, or add thoughts relating to the information presented on the App.

In summary, this section has provided possible solutions to the differing scenarios presented in Section 6 and relates to the four quadrants of the *CASE* framework. These theoretical solutions afford readers the opportunity envisage how different technological solutions could be implemented into different ecosystems.

In the following section, we discuss the work presented in this paper and provide our recommendations, strengths, and limitations.

8. Recommendations and Conclusions

This paper proposes an innovative smart age-friendly framework for existing sites that house previously purpose-built buildings and institutions, which, historically as well as currently, serve citizens from across the region and further afield.

Building on an existing model by the WHO [36], and the extended model proposed by Marston and van Hoof [30], we proposed an alternative framework called the 'Concept of Age-friendly Smart Ecologies (CASE)', which considers an age-friendly society, taking both a contemporary and post-pandemic approach for citizens in the Western world. The various scenarios and case studies illustrate real scenarios that citizens are currently experiencing. Marston and van Hoof [30] stated in their extended 'Smart Age-friendly Ecosystem' (SAfE):

> "Within and across society, and the lives of citizens, the relationships and engagement between the central, inner, and outer hubs/spheres will vary, based on users' needs, expectations, access to services, facilities and amenities. Sharing information via a closed, select group of friends/acquaintances is not unfamiliar and offers members of that group the opportunity to share information in real time and very quickly." (p.26)

With this in mind, the 'Concept of Age-friendly Smart Ecologies (CASE)' greatly expands this notion, whereby we have integrated and added additional spheres, hubs, and segments to represent engagement within various ecosystems by citizens and different actors at various intervals within the ecosystem, depending upon the activity and rationale.

Limitations of this proposed work and framework is the lack of qualitative and quantitative data to support the 'Concept of Age-friendly Smart Ecologies (CASE)' framework across society and its lifespan. The proposed *CASE* framework is theoretical and aims to reach out to multiple actors who are interested in transforming existing towns and cities into Smart Age-friendly Ecosystems (SafE) [30]. Evaluation of the *CASE* framework is needed, and this could be conducted through a living lab approach, as described by Shin [70], Shin and Park [124], while implementing universal design principles to evaluate the framework. These principles would facilitate the evaluation of future case-studies with a defined metric. The newly published 'Design for All' standard I.S. EN 17161:2019 [172] has appropriate measures to help commence this research.

The strengths of the 'Concept of Age-friendly Smart Ecologies (CASE)' framework includes the opportunity for towns, regions/counties, provinces, and municipalities to take an agile approach and work together in a locality approach to adopt and implement improvements aimed at making their existing environments into a SAfE, which, in turn, could afford residents and citizens greater benefits across the various hubs and infrastructures, by employing innovative technologies, such as Blockchain, AI, EVs, and digital portals and Apps.

Furthermore, these changes could be in the form of parish councils, regional councils, or from the perspective of the UK, regional mayors such as the position in Manchester—where at present, the Mayor of Manchester is a former member of parliament (MP)—Andy Burnham [173]. Additionally, we believe that this proposed 'Concept of Age-friendly Smart Ecologies (CASE)' framework is timely, given the global pandemic and how citizens in society, businesses, educational institutes, and health services are currently having to adapt and work in a more agile approach. At present, we do not know how long this pandemic will continue, and with this in mind, we have structured solutions in Section 7.1 from both the perspectives of contemporary society as well as looking into the future—in a post-pandemic society.

This position paper opened up with the narrative of the last epidemic and pandemics experienced in the 20th century, and it is possible that this pandemic of the 21st century will be around for some time, maybe forever, or until a vaccine is found. Either way, citizens globally are now having to adapt to the day-to-day changes and expectations set out by respective governments, based on the science of respective government advisors such as the SAGE (Scientific evidence supporting the government response to coronavirus (COVID-19)) committee for the UK/England [26].

At the time of writing this paper, the UK has various directives set out by respective devolved governments (Wales, Scotland, Northern Ireland, and England). As of 17–18 September 2020, the region of the North East (i.e., Northumberland, North and South Tyneside, Newcastle-upon-Tyne, Gateshead, Sunderland and County Durham) [174–176] and the North West (i.e., Lancashire, Merseyside, and Warrington) [177] of England have been informed of greater sanctions, which include a curfew between 10 p.m. and 5 a.m.—pubs are to be closed by this time and households are not allowed to mix and socialize outside of their social bubble/household [176,177], because of the rise of recorded COVID-19 cases.

Furthermore, from Tuesday 22 September 2020, additional regional lockdowns have been imposed across the Midlands, West Yorkshire, and further areas of the North West [177]. In Wales, the areas of the Rhondda Cynon Taf (RCT) and Caerphilly counties have had additional restrictions imposed on the citizens. Residents in the RCT area not permitted to enter or leave the area without a valid reason, facemasks must be worn indoors in public spaces, households are not allowed to continue socializing in their extended bubbles, and meet-ups must be outside and all pubs should be closed by 11 p.m. (1 h difference for England) [178].

For residents who have family members living in care homes, visits are now suspended in these respective areas, acting as a precautionary measure to keep all care home residents safe [179]. Yet, from the standpoint of Northern Ireland, the areas of Ballymeana, postcode areas of Belfast (BT43, BT28 and BT29—Glenavy, Lisburn and Crumlin) face restrictions on visiting friends and family indoors, and no more than six people from two different households can meet in a private garden. While essential visits to care homes and hospitals are permitted, there are restrictions on the number of visitors, and it is likely these tighter restrictions will be in place for two weeks [180].

Additionally, another area of Northern Ireland—BT60—which covers areas of the County of Armagh will have sanctions imposed from 5 p.m. on Friday 18 September 2020 [181]. Northern Ireland will commence 'drink-only' pubs from 23 September and this includes no dancing, table service only, only six people are allowed to sit at the same table as long as they are from the same household, track and trace (all customers to provide contact details), and face masks should be worn on entering/leaving the premises [181]. There is no restriction to closing time, unlike England (10 p.m.) and Wales (11 p.m.). From the standpoint of Scotland [182], indoor spaces that facilitate soft play, theatres, live music, and contact sports for young people aged 12+ years are prohibited from reopening until 5 October.

Residents in Scotland can meet both indoors and outdoors to a maximum of six people from two different households, while there are exceptions for specific events (e.g., funerals, weddings, organized sports, and civil partnerships), and physical spaces such as places of worship, which include a maximum of 20 people, been allowed to attend receptions and wakes at venues (e.g., hotels); in England, it is a maximum of 30 people. Additionally, specific areas, including Glasgow, North and

South Lanarkshire, East and West Dunbartonshire, Renfrewshire, and East Renfrewshire have been informed of tighter restrictions and include not meeting other households indoors. Police Scotland have the power to break up both house parties and parties held within university student accommodation. The British media are reporting how the Prime Minister Boris Johnson is not ruling out another national lockdown, based on the request of the Chief Medical Officer who wants the UK government to impose a two-week national lockdown [183]. The Mayor of London Sadiq Khan has already announced celebrations for New Year's Eve cancelled [184].

With these ever-changing directives during this pandemic, frameworks such as the 'Smart Age-friendly Ecosystem' [30] and the newly proposed 'Concept of Age-friendly Smart Ecologies (CASE)' framework illustrates how a myriad of actors across various levels of society can adapt respective ecosystems accordingly. This can be from the physical space of the individual home to the community space, or a specific organization/community hub (e.g., place of worship, educational institute, or business). Taking a locality approach may afford all respective and key actors the opportunity to share knowledge, evidence, and use and implement the voice of the residents/users with those who are playing key roles (e.g., councils, teachers, construction companies, and health practitioners).

Earlier on in this paper, we provided an array of frameworks that should be considered for future work, which could consider a combination of frameworks and universal design measures [173] as a means of assessing the framework presented here and by the respective work by Marston and van Hoof [30], Shin [70], Shin and Park [124] to afford this work to be taken to the next phase(s), while advancing the discussion of respective ecosystems and age-friendly narratives forward.

This may include a mixed-method approach comprising of qualitative and quantitative data collections—the former whereby various actors are interviewed to understand the needs, expectations, requirements, and impacts of the different hubs and spheres that make up the 'Concept of Age-friendly Smart Ecologies (CASE)' framework and/or 'Smart Age-friendly Ecosystem' (SAfE) [30] frameworks, while ensuring there is a co-production approach with stakeholders, business(es), users/residents, policy makers, technologists, gerontechnologists, social scientists, urban planners, geographers, economists, health practitioners, and gerontologists. Incorporating such a broad breadth of actors who represent different areas within the various levels of this framework has the potential to provide a rich amount of qualitative data.

The latter—quantitative data can provide similar affordances to these actors, as demonstrated by Dikken and colleagues [185], who recently published their validated age-friendly survey, the 'Age Friendly Cities and Communities Questionnaire (AFCCQ)'. This survey comprises of 23 items in the domains of: 1. Housing, 2. Social participation, 3. Respect and Social inclusion, 4. Communication and information, 5. Community support and health services, 6. Outdoor spaces and buildings, 7. Transportation and 8. Financial situation. The development and validation of this age-friendly survey has been tested on older adults and their experiences relating to the eight domains of the WHO age friendly cities model, with one extra domain—financial situation. It is anticipated and expected that the AFCCQ survey will help practitioners and researchers to understand and capture the level of age-friendly elements within a community in a quantified manner. Furthermore, there is the likelihood that this newly developed and validated tool will assist many interested researchers who are keen to understand the impact and potential benefits of age-friendly directives, policies, and social programs in the Western world.

The proposed 'Concept of Age-friendly Smart Ecologies (CASE)' framework is a working framework and one that can be adapted as technologies, developments, and society evolves and changes in the future. Future work should consult residents and users from various regions and communities, including areas that are both wealthy and deprived.

Torku and colleagues [132] note how both the WHO and the European Union (EU) have spearheaded the narratives of age-friendly cities and smart cities concepts and purport how these two "concepts are perceived as separate concepts" (p. 4). Yet, implementing and executing a co-design and co-producing approach to future research in this domain with actors, residents, and users from diverse populations not only produces a rich set of data, but also provides greater insight into the challenges, barriers, and enablers that various populations are faced with on a day-to-day level. Moreover, by taking a co-production approach in conjunction with the principles of universal design from both a philosophical and practical standpoint, there is the opportunity to centralize and knot together these two concepts (age-friendly cities and smart cities) [132]. We believe that the *CASE* framework can facilitate this nexus and afford future evaluations to be conducted using the framework presented here.

Understanding the challenges, barriers, and enablers which citizens are currently facing and may face in the future can offer research teams, policy makers, technologists, planners, and developers the opportunity to tailor areas specifically needed by residents in a town, city, or region [186].

To ensure that the voice of residents and users is heard, research and development (R&D) teams should aim to build strong and trustworthy relationships with communities that may or may not be hard to reach, and who may be skeptical of the intentions of policy makers, and R&D teams in delivering their needs, requirements, and expectations appropriately.

We would like to open this discussion further with various actors, policy-makers, researchers, and developers in a bid to move the debate of age-friendly forward to ensure a lasting legacy can be achieved and also adapted in an agile way.

Author Contributions: Conceptualization, H.R.M., L.S. and P.J.W.; writing—original draft preparation, H.R.M. and L.S.; writing—review and editing, H.R.M., L.S. and P.J.W. All authors have read and agreed to the published version of the manuscript.

Funding: This research received no external funding.

Conflicts of Interest: The authors declare no conflict of interest.

References

1. A Game of Thrones: Analysis of "Jon Snow". SparkNotes. Available online: https://www.sparknotes.com/lit/a-game-of-thrones/character/jon-snow/ (accessed on 24 August 2020).
2. Martin, G.R.R. *A Game of Thrones*; Bantam Books: New York, NY, USA, 1996; ISBN 0-553-10354-7.
3. Grossman, L.; George, R.R. Martin's Dance with Dragons: A Masterpiece Worthy of Tolkien. *Time*, 7 July 2011. Available online: https://web.archive.org/web/20130823230000/http://www.time.com/time/arts/article/0%2C8599%2C2081774%2C00.html(accessed on 24 August 2020).
4. Guillaume, J. This Game of Thrones. Fan Theory Will Blow Your Mind. *BuzzFeed*, 16 July 2014. Available online: https://www.buzzfeed.com/jennaguillaume/this-game-of-thrones-fan-theory-will-blow-your-mind? (accessed on 22 August 2020).
5. Pallotta, F. Fans Have A Crazy Game of Thrones Theory About Jon Snow' s True Parentage. *Business Insider*, 17 July 2014. Available online: https://www.businessinsider.com/game-of-thrones-jon-snows-parents-theory-2014-7?r=US&IR=T(accessed on 22 August 2020).
6. Wigler, J. This Game of Thrones Theory Will Blow Jon Snow Fans' Minds. *MTV New*, 15 July 2014. Available online: http://www.mtv.com/news/1868295/game-of-thrones-jon-snow-mother/(accessed on 22 August 2020).
7. Graham, D. Did Game of Thrones Just Confirm One of the Biggest Jon Snow fan Theories. *Metro*, 5 May 2015. Available online: https://metro.co.uk/2015/05/05/did-game-of-thrones-season-5-just-confirm-one-of-the-biggest-fan-theories-5180404/(accessed on 22 August 2020).
8. Robinson, J. All the Times Game of Thrones. Tried to Tell You Who Jon Snow's Parents Are. *Vanity Fair*, 26 June 2016. Available online: https://www.vanityfair.com/hollywood/2016/06/game-of-thrones-jon-snow-parents-lyanna-stark-rhaegar-targaryen(accessed on 22 August 2020).
9. Yglesias, M. Game of Thrones just Revealed Jon Snow's Real Parents. *Vox*, 26 June 2016. Available online: https://www.vox.com/2016/6/26/12029644/winds-of-winter-recap-jon-snow-parents(accessed on 22 August 2020).
10. Ackerknecht, E.H. *A Short History of Medicine*; Johns Hopkins University Press: Baltimore, MD, USA, 2016; ISBN 10:1421419548.
11. Eyeler, W. The changing assessments of John Snow's and William Farr's Cholera Studies. *Soz. Präventivmedizin* **2001**, *46*, 225–232. [CrossRef] [PubMed]

12. Paneth, N.; Vinten-Johansen, P.; Brody, H.; Rip, M. A rivalry of foulness: Official and unofficial investigations of the London cholera epidemic of 1854. *Am. J. Public Health* **1998**, *88*, 1545–1553. [CrossRef] [PubMed]
13. Snow, J. Plan showing the Ascertained Deaths from Cholera. Welcome Library Welcome Images. Available online: https://wellcomecollection.org/works/dx4prdbj (accessed on 18 August 2020).
14. Snow, J. A Map Taken from a Report by Dr John Snow. Welcome Library, Welcome Images. Available online: https://wellcomecollection.org/works/uxgfjt62/images?id=d4gnqhwy (accessed on 18 August 2020).
15. Roger, S. John Snow's Data Journalism: The Cholera Map that Changed the Word. 2013. Available online: https://www.theguardian.com/news/datablog/2013/mar/15/john-snow-cholera-map (accessed on 5 August 2020).
16. Your Genome. Science in the Time of Cholera. 2017. Available online: https://www.yourgenome.org/stories/science-in-the-time-of-cholera (accessed on 5 August 2020).
17. Zielinski, S. Cholera, John Snow and the Grand Experiment. *Smithsonian Magazine*, 18 August 2010. Available online: https://www.smithsonianmag.com/science-nature/cholera-john-snow-and-the-grand-experiment-33494689/(accessed on 5 August 2020).
18. Scally, G. Public health profession. In *Encyclopedia of Health Economics*; Elsevier: Amsterdam, The Netherlands, 2014; pp. 204–209. ISBN -9780123756787.
19. Spreeuwenberg, P.; Kroneman, M.; Paget, J. Reassessing the global mortality burden of the 1918 influenza pandemic. *Am. J. Epidemiol.* **2018**, *187*, 2561–2567. [CrossRef]
20. Gagnon, A.; Miller, M.S.; Hallman, S.A.; Bourbeau, R.; Herring, D.A.; Earn, D.J.; Madrenas, J. Age-specific mortality during the 1918 influenza pandemic: Unravelling the mystery of high young adult mortality. *PLoS ONE* **2013**, *8*, e69586. [CrossRef]
21. Ribeiro, S.P.; Dáttilo, W.; Barbosa, D.S.; Coura-Vital, W.; Chagas, I.A.D.; Dias, C.P.; Silva, A.V.C.C.dE.; Morais, M.H.F.; Góes-Neto, A.; Azevedo, V.A.C.; et al. Worldwide COVID-19 spreading explained: Traveling numbers as a primary driver for the pandemic. An. Acad. Bras. Ciênc. *An. Acad. Bras. Ciênc.* **2020**, *92*. [CrossRef] [PubMed]
22. Ribeiro, S.P.; Castro e Silva, A.; Dáttilo, W.; Reis, A.B.; Góes-Neto, A.; Alcantara, L.C.J.; Giovanetti, M.; Coura-Vital, W.; Fernandes, G.W.; Azevedo, V.A.C. Severe airport sanitarian control could slow down the spreading of COVID-19 pandemics in Brazil. *PeerJ* **2020**, *8*, e9446. [CrossRef]
23. Ironstone, P. The pandemic is (extra) ordinary. *TOPIA Can. J. Cult. Stud. COVID 19 Essays* **2020**. [CrossRef]
24. King-Hill, S.; Powell, M. What Does it Mean When the Government Say it is 'Following the Science'? *The Conversation*, 29 April 2020. Available online: https://theconversation.com/coronavirus-what-does-it-mean-when-the-government-says-it-is-following-the-science-137109(accessed on 6 August 2020).
25. Peck, T. The Government Claims It's Been 'Led by the Science'. So Why Has It Led to a Place Far Worse than Elsewhere? *Independent*, 13 April 2020. Available online: https://www.independent.co.uk/voices/coronavirus-uk-deaths-lockdown-boris-johnson-nhs-testing-a9462951.html(accessed on 6 August 2020).
26. UK Government. Scientific Advisory Group for Emergencies (SAGE): Coronaviurs (COVID-19) Response—Participant. 4 May 2020; Updated 17 July 2020. Available online: https://www.gov.uk/government/publications/scientific-advisory-group-for-emergencies-sage-coronavirus-covid-19-response-membership/list-of-participants-of-sage-and-related-sub-groups (accessed on 18 September 2020).
27. Jayakumar, P.; Brohi, S.N.; Zaman, N. Top 7 lessons learned from COVID-19 pandemic. *TechRxiv Prepr.* **2020**. [CrossRef]
28. Freeman, S.; Marston, H.; Olynick, J.; Musselwhite, C.; Kulczycki, C.; Genoe, R.; Xiong, B. Intergenerational effects on the impacts of technology use in later life: Insights from an international, multi-site study. *Int. J. Enviorn. Res. Public Health* **2020**, *7*, 5711. [CrossRef] [PubMed]
29. Marston, H.R.; Musselwhite, C.; Hadley, R.A. COVID-19 vs. Social Isolation: The Impact Technology Can Have on Communities, Social Connections and Citizens. *Ageing Issues*, 18 March 2020; The British Society of Gerontology. Available online: https://ageingissues.wordpress.com/2020/03/18/covid-19-vs-social-isolation-the-impact-technology-can-have-on-communities-social-connections-and-citizens/?fbclid=IwAR1sUsffKNd_G5u6d_oc0Z56u4Es7HyoCJYKr0qSnqFxX68pD3PY5JaSl7g(accessed on 6 August 2020).
30. Marston, H.R.; van Hoof, J. Who Doesn't Think about Technology When Designing Urban Environments for Older People? A Case Study Approach to a Proposed Extension of the WHO'S Age-Friendly Cities Model. *Int. J. Enviorn. Res. Public Health* **2019**, *16*, 3525. [CrossRef]

31. United Nations. World Population Ageing 2019. Available online: https://www.un.org/en/development/desa/population/publications/pdf/ageing/WorldPopulationAgeing2019-Report.pdf (accessed on 9 August 2020).
32. Organisation for Economic Co-operation and Development (OECD). *Ageing in Cities*; OECD Publishing: Paris, France, 2015; ISBN 9789264231146.
33. Van Hoof, J.; Kazak, J.K.; Perek-Białas, J.M.; Peek, S.T.M. The challenges of urban ageing: Making cities age-friendly in Europe. *Int. J. Environ. Res. Public Health* **2018**, *15*, 2473. [CrossRef] [PubMed]
34. Van Hoof, J.; Kazak, J.K. Urban ageing. *Indoor Built Environ.* **2018**, *27*, 583–586. [CrossRef]
35. Buffel, T.; Phillipson, C. Can global cities be 'age-friendly cities'? Urban development and ageing populations. *Cities* **2016**, *55*, 94–100. [CrossRef]
36. World Health Organization. *Global Age-Friendly Cities: A Guide*; World Health Organization: Geneva, Switzerland, 2007; ISBN 9789241547307.
37. Harrison, C.; Donnelly, I.A. A theory of smart cities. In Proceedings of the 55th Annual Meeting of the ISSS-2011, Hull, UK, 17–22 July 2011.
38. Praharaj, S.; Han, H. Cutting through the clutter of smart city definitions: A reading into the smart city perceptions in India. *City Cult. Soc.* **2019**, *18*, 100289. [CrossRef]
39. Yovanof, G.S.; Hazapis, G.N. An architectural framework and enabling wireless technologies for digital cities & intelligent urban environments. *Wirel. Pers. Commun.* **2009**, *49*, 445–463. [CrossRef]
40. Foord, J. The new boomtown? Creative city to tech city in east London. *Cities* **2013**, *33*, 51–60. [CrossRef]
41. Batty, M. Smart cities, big data. *Environ. Plan. B Plan. Des.* **2012**, *39*, 191–193. [CrossRef]
42. Anthopoulos, L.; Fitsilis, P. From digital to ubiquitous cities: Defining a common architecture for urban development. In Proceedings of the 6th International Conference on Intelligent Environments, Kuala Lumpur, Malaysia, 19–21 July 2010; pp. 301–306. [CrossRef]
43. Sairamesh, J.; Lee, A.; Anania, L. Information cities. *Commun. ACM* **2004**, *47*, 29–31. [CrossRef]
44. Yigitcanlar, T.; O'Connor, K.; Westerman, C. The making of knowledge cities: Melbourne's knowledge-based urban development experience. *Cities* **2008**, *25*, 63–72. [CrossRef]
45. California Institute for Smart Communities. Smart communities guide book. 2001. Available online: http://www.smartcommunities.org/guidebook.html (accessed on 8 November 2020).
46. Florida, R. *Cities and the Creative Class*; Routledge: New York, NY, USA, 2005. [CrossRef]
47. UN. Sustainable Development Goals, Goal 11: Make Cities Inclusive, Safe Resilient and Sustainable. Available online: https://www.un.org/sustainabledevelopment/cities/ (accessed on 9 August 2020).
48. Allam, Z. *Cities and the Digital Revolution: Aligning Technology and Humanity*; Palgrave Macmillan: London, UK, 2020; ISBN 978-3-030-29799-2.
49. Lee, M.; Yun, J.J.; Pyka, A.; Won, D.; Kodama, F.; Schiuma, G.; Park, H.; Jeon, J.; Park, K.; Jung, K.; et al. How to respond to the Fourth Industrial Revolution, or the Second Information Technology Revolution? Dynamic new combinations between technology, marker, and society through open innovation. *J. Open Innov. Technol. Mark. Complex.* **2018**, *4*, 1–24.
50. Edvardsson, I.R.; Yigitcanlar, T.; Pancholi, S. Knowledge city research and practice under the microscope: A review of empirical findings. *Knowl. Manag. Res. Pract.* **2016**, *14*, 537–564. [CrossRef]
51. Carrillo, J.; Yigitcanlar, T.; Garcia, B.; Lonnqvist, A. *Knowledge and the City: Concepts, Applications and Trends of Knowledge-Based Urban Development*; Routledge: New York, NY, USA, 2014.
52. Quan-Haase, A. *Technology and Society: Social Networks, Power, and Inequality*; Oxford University Press: Don Mills, ON, USA, 2012; p. 61.
53. Miller, J.C. The Geography of Technopoles: Computer and Electronic, Manufacturing by MSA 2005. Master's Thesis, The University of North Carolina at Greensboro, Greensboro, NC, USA, 2007. Available online: https://libres.uncg.edu/ir/uncg/listing.aspx?id=1180 (accessed on 23 September 2020).
54. Caves, R.W. *Encyclopedia of the City*; Routledge: New York, NY, USA, 2004; p. 662. ISBN 978-0415862875.
55. Allam, Z. Building a conceptual framework for smarting an existing city in Mauritius: The case of Port louis. *J. Biourbanism* **2017**, *2*, 47–61.
56. Meloa, A. How Smart City Technology & the Internet of Things Will Change Our Apartments, Grids and Communities. *Business Insider*, 16 January 2020. Available online: https://www.businessinsider.com/iot-smart-city-technology?r=US&IR=T#:~{|:text=Smart%20cities%20use%20Internet%20of,utilities%20and%20services%2C%20and%20more(accessed on 14 October 2020).

57. Piramuthu, O.B. Connected bicycles—State-of-the-art and adoption decision. *IEEE Internet Things J.* **2017**, *4*, 987–995. [CrossRef]
58. Romanillos, G.; Austwick, M.Z.; Ettema, D.; de Kruijf, J. Big data and cycling. *Transp. Rev.* **2015**, *1647*, 1–20. [CrossRef]
59. Behrendt, F. Cycling the smart and sustainable city: Analyzing EC policy documents on internet of things, mobility and transport, and smart cities. *Sustainability* **2019**, *11*, 763. [CrossRef]
60. Juarez, A.V.; Cook, M.; Potter, S. Roadmaps to Utopia: Tales of the Smart City. *Urban Studies* **2018**, *55*, 3385–3403.
61. Cook, M. Product service system innovation in the Smart City. *Int. J. Entrep. Innov.* **2018**, *19*, 46–55. [CrossRef]
62. Marston, H.R.; Samuels, J. A review of age friendly virtual assistive technologies and their effect on daily living for carers and dependent adults. *Healthcare* **2019**, *7*, 49. [CrossRef]
63. White, P.J.; Marston, H.R.; Shore, L.; Turner, R. Learning from COVID-19: Design, age-friendly technology, hacking and mental models [version 1; peer review: Awaiting peer review]. *Emerald Open Res.* **2020**, *2*, 21. [CrossRef]
64. Pantri. Available online: https://pantri.net/ (accessed on 5 October 2020).
65. Rjab, A.B.; Mellouli, S. Smart cities in the era of artificial intelligence and internet of things. In Proceedings of the 19th Annual International Conference on Digital Government Research: Governance in the Data Age, Delft, The Netherlands, 30 May–1 June 2018; pp. 1–10.
66. Kiefer, C.; Behrendt, F. Smart e-bike monitoring system: Real-time open source and open hardware GPS assistance and sensor data for electrically-assisted bicycles. IET Intell. *Transp. Syst.* **2016**, *10*, 79–88. [CrossRef]
67. Jenkins, M.; Duggan, D.; Negri, A. Towards a connected bicycle to communicate with vehicles and infrastructure: Multimodel alerting interface with Networked Short-Range Transmissions (MAIN-ST). In Proceedings of the 2017 IEEE Conference on Cognitive and Computational Aspects of Situation Management (CogSIMA), Savannah, GA, USA, 27–31 March 2017; pp. 2–4.
68. Behrendt, F. Why cycling matters for Smart Cities. Internet of Bicycles for Intelligent Transport. *J. Transp. Geogr.* **2016**, *56*, 157–164. [CrossRef]
69. Digiteum. The Role of IoT in Smart Grid Technology. 10 September 2019. Available online: https://www.digiteum.com/iot-smart-grid-technology#:~{}:text=Smart%20grid%20based%20on%20IoT,consumption%20on%20the%20consumer\T1\textquoterights%20side (accessed on 14 October 2020).
70. Shin, D. A living lab as socio-technical ecosystem: Evaluating the Korean living lab of internet of things. *Gov. Inf. Q.* **2019**, *36*, 264–275. [CrossRef]
71. Lee, C.; Lee, B.; Kong, Y. Privacy protection for a secure u-city life. *Lect. Notes Comput. Sci.* **2007**, *4490*, 685–692.
72. Shin, D. A critique of Korean national information strategy: A case of national information infrastructures. *Gov. Inf. Q.* **2007**, *24*, 624–645. [CrossRef]
73. Chang, Y.; Dong, X.; Sun, W. Influence of characteristics of the internet of things on consumer purchase intention. *Soc. Behav. Personal.* **2014**, *42*, 321–330. [CrossRef]
74. Shin, D. A socio-technical framework for internet-of-things design: A human centered design for the internet of things. *Telemat. Inform.* **2014**, *31*, 519–531. [CrossRef]
75. Allam, Z. Achieving neuroplasticity in artificial neural networks through smart cities. *Smart Cities* **2019**, *2*, 118–134. [CrossRef]
76. Allam, Z.; Dhunny, Z.A.; Siew, G.; Jones, D. Towards smart urban regeneration: Findings of an urban footprint survey in Port Louis Mauritius. *Smart Cities* **2018**, *1*, 121–133. [CrossRef]
77. The Open University. 2014–2016. MK Smart Project. Available online: http://www.mksmart.org/ (accessed on 21 September 2020).
78. Allam, Z.; Dhunny, Z.A. On big data, artificial intelligence and smart cities. *Cities* **2019**, *89*, 80–91. [CrossRef]
79. Blanco, J.L.; Fuchs, S.; Parsons, M.; Ribeirinho, M.J. Artificial Intelligences: Construction Technology Next Frontier. McKinsey Website. 2018. Available online: https://www.mckinsey.com/industries/capital-projects-and-infrastructure/our-insights/artificial-intelligence-construction-technologys-next-frontier# (accessed on 9 September 2020).
80. Guo, K.; Lu, Y.; Gao, H.; Cao, R. Artificial intelligence-based semantic Internet of Things in a user-centric smart city. *Sensors* **2018**, *18*, 1341. [CrossRef]

81. Bibri, S.E. The IoT for smart sustainable cities of the future: An analytical framework for sensor-based big data applications for environmental sustainability. *Sustain. Cities and Soc.* **2018**, *38*, 230–253. [CrossRef]
82. Reyna, A.; Martin, C.; Chen, J.; Soler, E.; Diaz, M. On blockchain and its integration with IoT: Challenges and opportunities. *Future Gener. Comput. Syst.* **2018**, *88*, 173–190. [CrossRef]
83. Perera, C.; McCormick, C.; Bandara, A.K.; Price, B.A.; Nuseibeh, B. Privacy-by-design framework for assessing internet of things applications and platforms. In Proceedings of the 6th International Conference on the Internet of Things, Stuttgart, Germany, 7–9 November 2016.
84. Obedait, A.A.; Youssef, M.; Ljepava, N. Citizen-centric approach in delivery of smart government Services. In *Smart Technologies and Innovation for a Sustainable Future*; Advances in Science, Technology & Innovation (IEREK Interdisciplinary Series for Sustainable Development); Al-Masri, A., Curran, K., Eds.; Springer: Cham, Switzerland, 2019. [CrossRef]
85. Alkhamisi, A.; Monowar, M. Rise of the augmented reality: Current and future application areas. *Int. J. Internet Distrib. Syst.* **2013**, *1*, 25–34. [CrossRef]
86. Mircea, R.T.; Ivan, M.L. Big data: Present and future. *Database Syst. J.* **2014**, *5*, 32–41.
87. De Montjoye, Y.A.; Farzanehfar, A.; Hendrickx, J.; Rocher, L. Solving Artificial Intelligence's Privacy Problem. Field Actions Science Reports, Special Issue [Artificial Intelligence and Robotics in the City] 17. 2017. Available online: https://journals.openedition.org/factsreports/4494 (accessed on 4 May 2020).
88. Smart Dubai 2021. Available online: https://2021.smartdubai.ae/ (accessed on 5 May 2020).
89. United Arab Emerites. UAE Government Strategy. Last Updated 17 September 2019. Available online: https://u.ae/en/more/uae-future/2021 (accessed on 5 May 2020).
90. Lim, Y.; Edelenbos, J.; Gianoli, A. Identifying the results of smart city development: Findings from systematic literature review. *Cities* **2019**, *95*. [CrossRef]
91. Cocchia, A. Smart and Digital City: A Systematic Literature Review. In *Smart City*; Springer: Berlin, Germany, 2014; pp. 13–43.
92. Anthopoulos, L.G. Understanding the smart city domain: A literature review. In *Transforming City Governments for Successful Smart Cities*; Springer: Berlin, Germany, 2015; pp. 9–21.
93. Trindade, E.P.; Hinnig, M.P.F.; da Costa, E.M.; Marques, J.S.; Bastos, R.C.; Yigitcanlar, T. Sustainable development of smart cities: A systematic review of the literature. *J. Open Innov. Technol. Mark. Complex.* **2017**, *3*, 11. [CrossRef]
94. Komninos, N.; Mora, L. Exploring the big picture of smart city research. *Sci. Reg. Ital. J. Reg. Sci.* **2018**, *1*, 15–38.
95. Komninos, N.; Pallot, M.; Schaffers, H. Special issue on smart cities and the future internet in Europe. *J. Knowl. Econ.* **2013**, *4*, 119–134. [CrossRef]
96. Ruza, J.; Kim, J.I.; Leung, I.; Kam, C.; Ng, S. Sustainable age-friendly cities: An evaluation framework and case study application on Palo Alto, California. *Sustain. Cities Soc.* **2014**. [CrossRef]
97. Community Services Department of the City of Palo Alto. Available online: https://www.cityofpaloalto.org/gov/depts/csd/default.asp (accessed on 12 August 2020).
98. Meijer, A.; Bolívar, M.P.R. Governing the smart city: A review of the literature on smart urban governance. *Int. Rev. Adm. Sci.* **2016**, *82*, 392–408. [CrossRef]
99. Centre for Ageing Better. UK Network Age Friendly Communities. Available online: https://www.ageing-better.org.uk/uk-network-age-friendly-communities (accessed on 5 May 2020).
100. Adapa, A.; Nah, F.F.H.; Hall, R.H.; Siau, K.; Smith, S.N. Factors influencing the adoption of smart wearable devices. *Int. J. Human Comput. Interact.* **2018**, *34*, 399–409. [CrossRef]
101. Pallavicini, F.; Ferrari, A.; Mantovani, F. Video Games for Well-Being: A Systematic Review on the Application of Computer Games for Cognitive and Emotional Training in the Adult Population. *Front. Psychol.* **2018**, *9*, 2127. [CrossRef]
102. Simons, D.J.; Boot, W.R.; Charness, N.; Gathercole, S.E.; Chabris, C.F.; Hambrick, D.Z.; Stine-Morrow, E.A.L. Do "Brain-Training" Programs Work? *Psychol. Sci. Public Interest* **2016**, *17*, 103–186. [CrossRef] [PubMed]
103. De Schutter, B. Never too old to play: The appeal of digital games to an older audience. *Games Cult.* **2011**, *6*, 155–170. [CrossRef]
104. De Schutter, B.; Brown, J.A. Digital games as a source of enjoyment in later life. *Games Cult.* **2015**, *11*, 28–52. [CrossRef]

105. De Schutter, B.; Roberts, A.R.; Franks, K. Miami six-O: Lessons learned from an intergenerational game design workshop. In *Game-Based Learning Across the Lifespan*; Advances in Game-Based Learning; Romero, M., Sawchuk, K., Blat, J., Sayago, S., Ouellet, H., Eds.; Springer: Cham, Switzerland, 2017; pp. 13–27. [CrossRef]
106. De la Hera, T.; Loos, E.; Simons, M.; Blom, J. Benefits and factors influencing the design of intergenerational digital games: A systematic literature review. *Societies* **2017**, *7*, 18. [CrossRef]
107. Brown, J.A.; De Schutter, B. Game design for older adults: Lessons from a life course perspective. *Int. J. Gaming Comput. Mediat. Simul. (IJGCMS)* **2016**, *8*, 1–12. [CrossRef]
108. Marston, H.R.; Duro, M.d.C.M. Revisiting the twentieth century through the lens of generation X and digital games: A scoping review. *Comput. Game J.* **2020**, *9*, 127–161. [CrossRef]
109. Cao, Y.; Li, J.; Qin, X.; Hu, B. Examining the effect of overload on the Mhealth application resistance behavior of elderly users: An SOR perspective. *Int. J. Environ. Res. Public Health* **2020**, *17*, 6658. [CrossRef]
110. Marston, H.R.; Hall, A.K. Gamification: Application for health and health information technology engagement. In *Handbook of Research on Holistic Perspectives in Gamification for Clinical Practice Hershey*; Novak, D., Tulu, B., Brendryen, H., Eds.; IGI Global: Hershey, PA, USA, 2015; pp. 78–104. [CrossRef]
111. Deterding, S.; Dixon, D.; Khaled, R.; Nacke, L. From game design elements to gamefulness: Defining gamification. In Proceedings of the MindTrek Conference 2011, Tampere, Finland, 28–30 September 2011.
112. Kang, R.; Dabbish, L.; Fruchter, N.; Kiesler, S. My data just goes everywhere: User mental models of the internet and implications for privacy and security. In Proceedings of the Symposium on Usable Privacy and Security (SOUPS), Ottawa, ON, Canada, 22–24 July 2015; USENIX Association: Berkeley, CA, USA, 2015; pp. 39–52.
113. Renaud, K.; Volkamer, M.; Renkema-Padmos, A. Why doesn't Jane protect her privacy ? In *Privacy Enhancing Technologies PETs 2014*; Lecture Notes in Computer, Science; De Cristofaro, E., Murdoch, S.J., Eds.; Springer: Cham, Switzerland, 2014; Volume 8555.
114. Ray, H.; Wolf, F.; Kuber, R.; Aviv, A.J. Woe is me: Examining older adults' perceptions of privacy. In Proceedings of the CHI Conference on Human Factors in Computing Systems Extended Abstracts (CHI'19 Extended Abstracts), Glasgow, UK, 4–9 May 2019; ACM: New York, NY, USA, 2019; p. 6.
115. Lorenzen-Huber, L.; Boutain, M.; Camp, L.J.; Shankar, K.; Connelly, K.H. Privacy, technology, and aging: A proposed framework. *Ageing Int.* **2011**, *36*, 232–252. [CrossRef]
116. Smith, A.; Page, D.U.S. *Smartphone Use in 2015*; Pew Research Center: Washington, DC, USA, 2015; Available online: https://www.pewinternet.org/2015/04/01/us-smartphone-use-in-2015/ (accessed on 5 May 2018).
117. Fox, S.; Duggan, M. *Mobile Health 2012*; Pew Internet: Washington, DC, USA, 2012; Available online: https://www.pewinternet.org/wp-content/uploads/sites/9/media/Files/Reports/2012/PIP_MobileHealth2012_FINAL.pdf (accessed on 21 November 2019).
118. Krämer, N.C. Social effects of virtual assistants. A review of empirical results with regard to communication. In *Intelligent Virtual Agents*; Lecture Notes in Computer, Science; Prendinger, H., Lester, J., Ishizuka, M., Eds.; Springer: Berlin/Heidelberg, Germany, 2008; Volume 5208. [CrossRef]
119. Rawassizadeh, R.; Sen, T.; Kim, S.J.; Meurisch, C.; Keshavarz, H.; Mühlhäuser, M.; Pazzani, M. Manifestation of virtual assistants and robots into daily life: Vision and challenges. *CCF Trans. Pervasive Comp. Interact.* **2019**, *1*, 163–174. [CrossRef]
120. Cohen, P.; Cheyer, A.; Horvitz, E.; El Kaliouby, R.; Whittaker, S. On the future of personal assistants. In Proceedings of the 2016 CHI Conference Extended Abstracts on Human Factors in Computing Systems, San Jose, CA, USA, 7–12 May 2016; pp. 1032–1037.
121. Breazeal, C. Toward sociable robots. *Robot. Auton. Syst.* **2003**, *42*, 167–175. [CrossRef]
122. Šabanović, S. Robots in society, society in robots. *Int. J. Soc. Robot.* **2010**, *2*, 439–450. [CrossRef]
123. European Commission Information Society and Media, Unit F4 New Infrastructure Paradigms and Experimental Facilities. Living Labs for User-Driven Open Innovation. An Overview of the Living Labs Methodology, Activities and Achievements. January 2009. Available online: https://www.eurosportello.eu/sites/default/files/Living%20Lab%20brochure_jan09_en_0.pdf (accessed on 14 October 2020).
124. Shin, D.-H.; Park, Y.J. Understanding the internet of things ecosystem: Multi-level analysis of users, society, and ecology. Digit. Policy Regul. Gov. *Digit. Policy Regul. Gov.* **2017**, *19*, 77–100. [CrossRef]
125. Ng, C.L.; Wakenshaw, Y.L. The internet-of-things: Review and research directions. *Int. J. Res. Mark.* **2017**, *34*, 3–21. [CrossRef]

126. Shin, D. User centric cloud service model in public sectors. *Gov. Inf. Q.* **2013**, *30*, 194–203. [CrossRef]
127. Liedtke, C.; Welfens, M.J.; Rohn, H.; Nordmann, J. Living lab user-driven innovation for sustainability. *Int. J. Sustain. High. Educ.* **2012**, *13*, 106–118. [CrossRef]
128. Vaziri, D.D.; Aal, K.; Ogonowski, C.; von Rekowski, T.; Kroll, M.; Marston, H.R.; De Rosario, H.; Poveda, R.; Gschwind, Y.; Delbaere, K.; et al. Exploring user experience and technology acceptance for a fall prevention system: Results from a randomized clinical trial and a living lab. *Eur. Rev. Aging Phys. Act. (EURAPA)* **2016**, *13*. [CrossRef]
129. Lindsay, S.; Jackson, D.; Schofield, G.; Olivier, P. Engaging Older People Using Participatory Design. ACM Press, 2012 [cited 7 November 2014]. p. 1199. Available online: http://dl.acm.org/citation.cfm?doid=2207676.2208570 (accessed on 15 September 2020).
130. Hartswood, M.; Rouncefield, M.; Procter, R.; Slack, R.; Vob, A.; Buscher, M.; Rouncefield, M.; Rouchy, P. Corealisation: Towards a principled synthesis of ethnimethodology and participatory design. *Scand. J. Inf. Syst.* **2002**, *14*, 2003.
131. Schumacher, J.; Feurstein, K. Living labs—A new multi-stakeholder approach to user integration. In Proceedings of the 3rd International Conference on Interoperability of Enterprise Systems and Applications (I-ESA'07), Funchal, Madeira, Portugal, 27–30 March 2007.
132. Torku, A.; Chan, A.P.C.; Yung, E.H.K. Implementation of age-friendly initiatives in smart cities: Probing the barriers through a systematic review. *Built Environ. Proj. Asset Manag.* **2020**. [CrossRef]
133. Marston, H.R.; Morgan, D.J. Technology & social media during COVID-19 pandemic. Special issue: COVID-19 & geriatric mental health worldwide. *IPA Bulletin* **2020**, *37*, 3. Available online: https://www.ipa-online.org/publications/ipa-bulletin/featured-articles/covid-19-bulletin-articles/technology-social-media-during-covid19 (accessed on 7 August 2020).
134. Victor, C.; Scambler, S.; Bond, J. *The Social World of Older People: Understanding Loneliness and Social Isolation in Later Life. Growing Older*; Open University Press: Maidenhead, UK, 2009.
135. Victor, C.R.; Scambler, S.J.; Bowling, A.N.N.; Bond, J. A survey of older people in Great Britain. *Ageing Soc.* **2005**, *25*, 357–375. [CrossRef]
136. Aartsen, M.; Jylhä, M. Onset of loneliness in older adults: Results of a 28 year prospective study. *Eur. J. Ageing* **2011**, *8*, 31–38. [CrossRef]
137. Utz, R.L.; Swenson, K.L.; Caserta, M.; Lund, D.; de Vries, B. Feeling lonely versus being alone: Loneliness and social support among recently bereaved persons. *J. Gerontol. Ser. B Psychol. Sci. Soc. Sci.* **2014**, *69*, 85–94. [CrossRef]
138. Burholt, V.; Windle, G.; Morgan, D.J. CFAS Wales team. A social model of loneliness: The roles of disability, social resources, and cognitive impairment. *Gerontologist* **2017**, *57*, 1020–1030. [CrossRef]
139. Holt-Lunstad, J.; Smith, T.B.; Baker, M.; Harris, T.; Stephenson, D. Loneliness and social isolation as risk factors for mortality: A meta-analytic review. *Perspect. Psychol. Sci.* **2015**, *10*, 227–237. [CrossRef]
140. Valtorta, N.K.; Kanaan, M.; Gilbody, S.; Ronzi, S.; Hanratty, B. Loneliness and social isolation as risk factors for coronary heart disease and stroke: Systematic review and meta-analysis of longitudinal observational studies. *Heart* **2016**, *102*, 1009–1016. [CrossRef]
141. Dinkins, C.S. Seeing oneself in the fact of the other: The value and challenge of human connectedness for older adults. *J. Psychosoc. Nurs. Ment. Health Serv.* **2017**, *55*, 13–17. [CrossRef]
142. Schlomann, A.; Seifert, A.; Zank, S.; Woopen, C.; Rietz, C. Use of Information and Communication Technology (ICT) devices among the oldest-old: Loneliness, anomie, and autonomy. *Innov. Aging* **2020**, 4. [CrossRef]
143. Francis, J.; Ball, C.; Kadylak, T.; Cotten, S.R. Aging in the digital age: Conceptualizing technology adoption and digital inequalities. In *Ageing and Digital Technology*; Neves, B.B., Vetere, F., Eds.; Springer: Singapore, 2019; pp. 35–49. [CrossRef]
144. Cotten, S.R.; Anderson, W.A.; McCullough, B.M. Impact of internet use on loneliness and contact with others among older adults: Cross-sectional analysis. *J. Med. Internet Res.* **2013**, *15*, e39. [CrossRef]
145. Czaja, S.J.; Boot, W.R.; Charness, N.; Rogers, W.A.; Sharit, J. Improving social support for older adults through technology: Findings from the PRISM randomized controlled trial. *Gerontologist* **2018**, *58*, 467–477. [CrossRef] [PubMed]

146. Brown, J.A.; Marston, H.R. Gen X and digital games: Looking back to look forward. In *Human Aspects of IT for the Aged Population. Applications in Health, Assistance, and Entertainment*; Lecture Notes in Computer, Science; Zhou, J., Salvendy, G., Eds.; Springer: Cham, Switzerland, 2018; Volume 10927. [CrossRef]
147. Marston, H.R. Millennials and ICT—Findings from the Technology 4 Young Adults (T4YA) Project: An Exploratory Study. *Societies* **2019**, *9*, 80. [CrossRef]
148. Tondeur, J.; Sinnaeve, I.; van Braak, J. ICT as cultural capital: The relationship between socioeconomic status and the computer-use profile of young people. *New Media Soc.* **2010**, *13*, 151–168. [CrossRef]
149. Carroll, J.; Howard, S.; Vetere, F.; Peck, J.; Murphy, J. Just what do the youth of today want? Technology appopriation by young people. In Proceedings of the 35th Annual Hawaii International Conference on System Sciences, Big Island, HI, USA, 10 January 2002; pp. 1777–1785.
150. Tully, C.J. Growing up in technologicalworlds: How modern technologies shape the everyday lives of young people. *Bull. Sci. Technol. Soc.* **2003**, *23*, 444–456. [CrossRef]
151. Hynan, A.; Murray, J.; Goldbart, J. Happy and excited: Perceptions of using digital technology and social media by young people who use augmentative and alternative communication. *Child Lang. Teach. Ther.* **2014**, *30*, 175–186. [CrossRef]
152. Chick, A.; Micklethwaite, P. *Design for Sustainable Change—How Design and Designers can Drive the Sustainability Agenda*; AVA Publishing SA: Lausanne, Switzerland, 2011.
153. Czaja, S.; Boot, W.R.; Charness, N.; Rogers, W.A. *Designing for Older Adults-Principles and Creative Human Factor Approaches*, 3rd ed.; CRC Press: Boca Raton, FL, USA, 2019.
154. Kaya, B.Y.; Dağdeviren, M. Selecting occupational safety equipment by MCDM approach considering universal design principles. *Hum. Factors Ergon. Manuf. Serv. Ind.* **2016**, *26*, 224–242. [CrossRef]
155. Jones, M.; Marsden, G. *Mobile Interaction Design*; John Wiley & Sons: Chichester, UK, 2006.
156. Dunne, A.; Raby, F. *Speculative Everything—Design Fiction and Social Daydreaming*; MIT Press: Cambridge, MA, USA, 2013.
157. Cooper, R.; Burton, E.; Cooper, G.L. *Wellbeing: A Complete Reference Guide, Wellbeing and the Environment*; John Wiley & Sons: Chichester, UK, 2014; Volume 2.
158. Shore, L.; Kiernan, L.; de Eyto, A.; Bhaird, D.N.A.; White, P.J.; Fahey, T.; Moane, S. Older Adult Insights for age-friendly environments, products and service systems. *Des. Technol. Educ.* **2018**, *23*, 40–58.
159. Shore, L. Developing the Concept of Shared Usability in Product Design for Older Adults. Master's Thesis, Institute of Technology Carlow, Carlow, Ireland, 2015.
160. UK Government. Prime Minister's Statement on Coronavirus (COVID-19). In *Speech*; 23 March 2020. Available online: https://www.gov.uk/government/speeches/pm-address-to-the-nation-on-coronavirus-23-march-2020 (accessed on 15 August 2020).
161. Worldometer. Coronavirus Cases in the United Kingdom (2020)—Worldometer. Available online: https://www.worldometers.info/coronavirus/country/uk/ (accessed on 28 September 2020).
162. Chan, S.P.; Plummer, R. Recession is unprecedented, says Chancellor Rishi Sunak. *BBC News, Business*, 12 August 2020. Available online: https://www.bbc.co.uk/news/business-53753189(accessed on 14 August 2020).
163. Available online: https://www.cityam.com/uk-unemployment-730000-lose-jobs-since-march/ (accessed on 20 September 2020).
164. ONS. Labour Market Overview, UK. August 2020; Published 11 August 2020. Available online: https://www.ons.gov.uk/employmentandlabourmarket/peopleinwork/employmentandemployeetypes/bulletins/uklabourmarket/august2020 (accessed on 20 September 2020).
165. Murray, J. We Did What We Set Out to Achieve: The Staff Who Moved Into Care Homes. *The Guardian News Paper*, 28 April 2020. Available online: https://www.theguardian.com/society/2020/apr/28/we-did-what-we-set-out-to-achieve-the-staff-who-moved-into-care-homes(accessed on 15 August 2020).
166. Akande, A.; Cabral, P.; Casteleyn, S. Understanding the sharing economy and its implication on sustainability in smart cities. *J. Clean. Prod.* **2020**, *277*, 124077. [CrossRef]
167. Liang, J.; Xu, Y. Second-hand clothing consumption: A generational cohort analysis of the Chinese market. *Int. J. Consum. Stud.* **2018**, *42*, 120–130. [CrossRef]

168. UNREICH, R. Slowing Down Fast Fashion. *Sunday Age*, 13 October 2019. Available online: https://www.smh.com.au/lifestyle/fashion/slow-approach-in-the-era-of-fast-fashion-20191009-p52z5t.html(accessed on 6 November 2020).
169. Leke, R.G.F.; Kaboré, B.J.; King, A.; Pallansch, M.A.; Tomori, O.; Jack, A.D.; Kironde, N.E.; Lopes-Feio, R.J.; Chunsuttiwat, S.; Maiga, Z.; et al. Certifying the Interruption of Wild Poliovirus Transmission in the WHO African Region on the Turbulent Journey to a Polio-Free World. *Lancet* **2020**, *8*, 1345–1351.
170. Oswald, F.; Jopp, D.; Rott, C.; Wahl, H.-W. Is aging in place a resource for or risk to life satisfaction? *Gerontologist* **2010**, *51*, 238–250. [CrossRef]
171. Sixsmith, A.; Sixsmith, J. Ageing in place in the United Kingdom. *Ageing Int.* **2008**, *32*, 219–235. [CrossRef]
172. NSAI. EN 17161:2019 Design for All. Accessibility Following a Design for all Approach in Products, Goods and Services. Extending the Range of Users. In Dublin, Ireland: National Standards Authority of Ireland. 2019. Available online: https://www.nsai.ie/about/news/a-design-standard-that-works-for-all/ (accessed on 28 October 2020).
173. What the Mayor Does. Greater Manchester Combined Authority. 2020. Available online: https://www.greatermanchester-ca.gov.uk/the-mayor (accessed on 28 September 2020).
174. Heffer, G. Coronavirus: North East Lockdown Begins as Curfew For Bars and Pubs and Ban on Household Mixing Brought. *Skye News*, 18 September 2020. Available online: https://news.sky.com/story/coronavirus-curfews-for-bars-and-pubs-among-new-lockdown-restrictions-in-northeast-england-12073858(accessed on 18 September 2020).
175. Ridler, F. Last Orders! Newcastle Sinks its Final Pints Before Curfew Comes in Across North-East from 10pm Tonight as Revellers in Leeds Make the Most of Their Final Days of Freedom with City Also on the Brink of a Local Lockdown. *Daily Mail*, 18 September 2020. Available online: https://www.dailymail.co.uk/news/article-8746837/Newcastle-sinks-final-pint-curfew-comes-North-East-10pm-tonight.html(accessed on 18 September 2020).
176. Parveen, N. Stricter Covid Restrictions Imposed in Lancashire, Merseyside and Warrington. *The Guardian*, 18 September 2020. Available online: https://www.theguardian.com/world/2020/sep/18/stricter-covid-restrictions-imposed-in-lancashire(accessed on 18 September 2020).
177. Tapsfield, J. North West, Midlands and West Yorkshire will go into Lockdown from Tuesday Amid Fears Ministers 'Could Extend Autumn Half-Term by a Week' as Part of NATIONWIDE 14-day 'Circuit-Breaker' to Stem Spread of Covid. *Daily Mail*, 18 September 2020. Available online: https://www.dailymail.co.uk/news/article-8747257/Is-England-heading-HALF-TERM-lockdown.html(accessed on 18 September 2020).
178. BBC News. Coronavirus: Newport and Merthyr Tydfil. *Under Close Watch*, 18 September 2020. Available online: https://www.bbc.co.uk/news/uk-wales-54202858(accessed on 18 September 2020.).
179. BBC News. Coronavirus: New rules and lockdowns 'could be too late'. 18 September 2020. Available online: https://www.bbc.co.uk/news/uk-wales-54144564 (accessed on 18 September 2020).
180. Sproule, L.; McCormack, J. Coronavirus Q&A: What has Changed in NI? *BBC News, Northern Ireland*, 15 September 2020. Available online: https://www.bbc.co.uk/news/uk-northern-ireland-53007269(accessed on 18 September 2020).
181. BBC News. Coronavirus: Local Restrictions on BT60 Begin this Evening. *BBC News*, 18 September 2020. Available online: https://www.bbc.co.uk/news/uk-northern-ireland-54202059(accessed on 18 September 2020).
182. Esson, G. Coronavirus in Scotland: What are the Latest Lockdown Rules? *BBC News*, 14 September 2020. Available online: https://www.bbc.co.uk/news/uk-scotland-53166816(accessed on 18 September 2020).
183. Pyman, T. Chris Whitty 'Wants a New Two-Week NATIONAL Lockdown and True UK Cases are as High as 38,000-a-day', ex-WHO Expert Who Sits on Independent Safe Panel Claims. *Daily Mail*, 17 September 2020. Available online: https://www.dailymail.co.uk/news/article-8741417/Professor-Chris-Whitty-wants-new-two-week-national-lockdown-ex-expert-claims.html(accessed on 18 September 2020).
184. Marsh, S. London New Year's Eve Fireworks Cancelled, Says Sadiq Khan. *The Guardian*, 18 September 2020. Available online: https://www.theguardian.com/uk-news/2020/sep/18/london-new-years-eve-fireworks-display-cancelled-sadiq-khan-coronavirus(accessed on 18 September 2020).

185. Dikken, J.; van den Hoven, R.F.; van Staalduinen, W.H.; Hulsebosch-Janssen, L.M.; van Hoof, J. How older people experience the age-friendliness of their city: Development of the age-friendly cities and communities questionnaire. *Int. J. Environ. Res. Public Health* **2020**, *17*, 6867. [CrossRef]
186. Van Hoof, J.; Dikken, J.; Buttiġieġ, S.C.; van den Hoven, R.F.M.; Kroon, E.; Marston, H.R. Age-friendly cities in The Netherlands: An explorative study of facilitators and hindrances in the built environment and ageism in design. *Indoor Built Environ.* **2020**, *29*, 417–437. [CrossRef]

Publisher's Note: MDPI stays neutral with regard to jurisdictional claims in published maps and institutional affiliations.

International Journal of
Environmental Research and Public Health

MDPI

Article

Digitalising the Age-Friendly City: Insights from Participatory Action Research

Arlind Reuter [1,*], Jennifer Liddle [1,2] and Thomas Scharf [2]

1 Open Lab, Newcastle University, Newcastle upon Tyne NE4 5TG, UK; jennifer.liddle@newcastle.ac.uk
2 Population Health Sciences Institute, Newcastle University, Newcastle upon Tyne NE2 4AX, UK; thomas.scharf@newcastle.ac.uk
* Correspondence: a.reuter2@newcastle.ac.uk

Received: 19 October 2020; Accepted: 2 November 2020; Published: 9 November 2020

check for updates

Abstract: The World Health Organization's age-friendly city initiative emerged as a response to the intersecting global trends of population ageing and urbanisation. However, a third global trend—digitalisation—has largely been overlooked in research and policy making relating to age-friendly cities and communities. Within the context of a general shift towards online civic participatory activities, this article explores older adults' digital citizenship in an age-friendly city in the North of England. Drawing on interviews, observations and field notes from design workshops as part of an ongoing participatory action research project, we consider two key questions. First, how does an age-friendly city stakeholder organisation of older adults make use of digital technologies in order to provide digital information and communications? Second, what is the potential of digital audio to increase civic participation in later life and local engagement with age-friendly issues? Our analysis focuses on two domains of the World Health Organization's age-friendly city framework: Communication and information and civic participation. First, we report on the stakeholder organisation's efforts to re-design their digital newsletter in order to provide information and communications to older residents about local work on ageing projects. We then outline the organisation's efforts, in a public setting, to engage with digital audio as a way to increase the participation of older residents with age-friendly topics. We conclude by suggesting the need to re-frame the role of digital technologies within the age-friendly city, broadening the scope from accessibility towards enhancing digital citizenship opportunities.

Keywords: ageing; digital citizenship; age-friendliness; urbanisation; participatory action research

---

1. Introduction

The World Health Organization (WHO) age-friendly city (AFC) initiative emerged in 2005 as a response to the intersecting global trends of population ageing and urbanisation [1]. Supporting cities to become more age-friendly by promoting active ageing and creating accessible and inclusive city structures, the AFC initiative has since become a global program that has also been extended to include rural communities [2]. While some countries, such as Ireland [3], have established national age-friendly initiatives, others have created national networks that seek to harness learning and share best practice between age-friendly cities and communities. In the United Kingdom (UK), 41 cities, towns and counties currently belong to a network of age-friendly communities [4]. Rooted in the discourse on healthy and active ageing, age-friendly cities aim to provide a space to promote and maintain physical and mental health across the life course [2]. The AFC initiative is based on a framework that emerged from an empirical project involving focus groups of older people in cities around the world. Participants identified the following eight domains as important: Social participation; communication and information; civic participation and employment; housing; transportation; community support and health services; outdoor spaces and buildings; and respect and social inclusion [5]. These domains comprise core features that can be used to assess the relative age-friendliness of different cities and communities [1]. Despite the checklist format developed by the WHO to capture these core features, some researchers regard it as more helpful to frame age-friendliness as an ongoing process and commitment to improve the physical and social environment of a city in response to the challenges and opportunities arising from demographic ageing [2,6]. The process to become an age-friendly city or community is based on a cyclical model for continuous improvement that is driven by older people themselves. It involves four stages: Engage and understand; plan; act; and measure [2]. While the age-friendly concept can be implemented in different ways across the domains, underlying the framework is a life-course perspective that acknowledges diversity at all life stages and promotes citizen contributions to all areas of community life [1].

Accompanying the global age-friendly agenda has been the rapidly increasing digitalisation of cities and communities. While there is a growing evidence base that highlights the need to explore digital aspects of later life, including, for example, re-framing stereotypes on ageing and information and communication technologies (ICT) use [7,8] or using the internet for civic or social participatory purposes in later life [9,10], the intersections between the WHO age-friendly domains and widespread digitalisation remain under-explored within the age-friendly city framework [11]. Within the domain of communication and information, for example, the WHO AFC checklist includes a brief mention of ICTs, but the information is limited to the accessibility of certain technological devices, such as mobile phones or public computers. Digital technologies are entirely absent from the civic participation domain of the checklist, thus ignoring the increasing role played by digital approaches in different forms of citizen engagement.

In this paper, we respond to the challenge of integrating digitalisation trends into existing debates about demographic ageing and urbanisation that underpin the global age-friendly initiative. Our approach entails exploring and positioning the concept of digital citizenship within the context of a medium-sized city in the North of England that belongs to the UK network of age-friendly communities. Working within the AFC domains of communication and information and civic participation and drawing on interview data, observations and field notes from a participatory action research project involving an AFC stakeholder organisation of older adults, we add to the current understanding of age-friendly cities and communities by providing practical examples of digital citizenship in later life. We seek to highlight the value of extending the WHO's age-friendly initiative beyond a narrow focus on digital accessibility and inclusion issues to incorporate the growing importance of digital citizenship in later life and the potential of digital approaches to facilitate active ageing by reducing the risks of digital exclusion faced by ageing adults.

2. Background

Digital Citizenship

Within the discourse on age-friendly cities and civic engagement lies the concept of 'urban citizenship', which recognises older adults as active agents who have a right to make full use of the city [12]. In their 'Manifesto for the Age-Friendly Movement', Buffel et al. argue that the concept of the 'right to the city' includes appropriating urban spaces, participating in decision making and influencing strategies of urban planning and regeneration. Urban spaces are characterised by growing inequalities within and between cities, including a trend towards increasing age-segregation. Preventing the exclusion of older people from participation in age-friendly initiatives, especially people belonging to disadvantaged groups, involves ensuring that all older people have opportunities to exercise their right to have their voice heard [13]. In terms of older adults' civic involvement at a local level, Buffel et al. highlight the paradox of neighbourhood participation: Even though older adults spend more time than younger people within the immediate neighbourhood of their homes, they are often the least, or last to be, engaged in civic decision making [13]. Moreover, in increasingly digitalised cities and communities, there is a fundamental need to reconsider what 'urban citizenship' entails and to reframe the potential role to be played by older adults as 'digital citizens' in shaping age-friendly cities and communities.

Whilst ICTs have been acknowledged as resources that might support older adults' involvement in local decision making [13], approaches are often solutionist [8]. A consideration of the role of digital technologies is also lacking within the WHO AFC framework [11], prompting responses to address this gap. For example, Marston and van Hoof have proposed a revision to the WHO framework to include technology as part of a smart age-friendly ecosystem that supports older adults' daily lives through ubiquitous and assistive technologies [11]. More recently, a revised definition of age-friendliness has emphasised the role of digital technologies within age-friendly settings:

> *Underpinned by a commitment to respect and social inclusion, an age-friendly community is engaged in a strategic and ongoing process to facilitate active ageing by optimising the community's physical, social and digital environments and its supporting infrastructure [14] (p. 19).*

Adopting the above definition of age-friendliness to reflect the crucial role of the digital environment as a facilitator of active ageing in age-friendly cities and communities, our research explores the use of digital technologies for a civic purpose, which is a concept that has been under-theorised and largely overlooked in relation to the AFC. We want to expand this discourse on technology within the age-friendly city by highlighting the concept of urban citizenship and its digital aspects, proposing a shift from technology as a solution in the age-friendly city towards a focus on the digital civic contributions of older adults. Digital citizenship is broadly defined as the ability to participate digitally within society on a regular basis [15]. In research, the subject of Digital Civics has been considered in the discipline of Human–Computer Interaction (HCI) [16,17]. It seeks to understand how technologies can be designed in the context of civic interactions and experiences. This can be done by turning to participatory systems that enable citizen engagement and the creation of counter narratives in a relational rather than transactional way [18], thus opening up a space for activism [19]. By recognising and acknowledging the effects of the digital divide, a digital civics research approach supports (marginalised) communities in co-producing political thinking, action and dialogue through relational technologies [16].

The focus on digital civics is especially important within the context of demographic ageing. Older adults have been shown to be at a heightened risk of exclusion from civic participatory activities [20]—a problem which is exacerbated by the digital divide [21]. However, as opportunities for civic participation increasingly shift from offline to online (e.g., creating and signing petitions online or engaging with local government services), more older adults are using technological tools in order to participate in digital civic activities [22]. Indeed, the number of older adults who are using the internet has been increasing in recent years and 83% of adults aged 65–74 and 47% of adults aged 75 and over use the internet in the UK [23]. In addition, 98% of UK premises have access to broadband and internet [24]. Buffel et al. propose that "information and communication technologies may support the involvement of older residents in navigating and designing their environment" [11] (p. 281). This aligns with the recent movement within the HCI community towards recognising forms of older adults' engagement with civic technologies in community settings [25,26]. Regarding the design of participatory systems or technologies, the field of social computing has progressed from designing for older adults [27] towards involving older users in the design of services [28] and reflecting on co-design methodologies, specifically within the context of ageing research [29–31]. An example of a co-design process was provided by Clarke et al., who used participatory media to explore older adults' engagement with the city in the context of urban planning [25,32]. In particular, the interdisciplinary design team considered "how technology can support documentation and re-envisioning of the age-friendly city of the future" [30] (p. 2). The study outlines how technology could be a mediating factor in urban planning contexts, facilitating discussions between local councils and older citizens. The contribution of Clarke et al. is important in demonstrating that digital media in particular can support older adults in making active contributions within their neighbourhood, highlighting key concerns for ageing beyond accessibility.

The COVID-19 pandemic has reinforced the imperative for the active participation of older adults in public debates. Given ongoing digitalisation processes, a stronger focus on "technology" as a key feature of the age-friendly city concept has become inevitable. However, the pandemic has focused attention on the need for individuals to be online in order to participate fully in social and civic life. The pandemic has also emphasised the importance of digital activity among older adults, with the digital inclusion of older adults gaining greater attention in government initiatives and within third sector organisations [33,34]. To date, local council digital inclusion strategies, in the UK at least, predominantly adopt a needs-based framework that addresses factors of access and accessibility (e.g., the ability to connect to the internet or "knowing where to start online") [34]. We distinguish between this form of digital inclusion and the concept of digital participation, which encompasses the active use and contributions of older adults in the digital space [35]. Indeed, older adults are increasingly participating in and actively contributing to digital spaces by creating their own content in the form of blogs, videos and radio/audio broadcasts [10,36,37]. Recent studies have examined older adults' content creation [9,10,38,39], suggesting that one of the key motivations for producing content lies in "being advocates for older people" [9]. While such developments emphasise the civic purpose of older adults' digital participation, this idea has yet to be directly picked up by government or age-friendly initiatives.

The body of work described above highlights the current, somewhat limited, discourse on technology and its role in supporting citizenship in age-friendly cities and communities. Given the pace with which the digitalisation of society is progressing, there is a need for a more differentiated perspective on age-friendly initiatives that can benefit from insights drawn from different scientific fields. Our work sits at the intersection of research on age-friendly environments within the field of social and environmental gerontology and related work undertaken in HCI. While the WHO age-friendly program has operated in an increasingly digitalised environment, linked policies and initiatives have, to date, not sufficiently addressed the concept of digital citizenship. Digital inclusion strategies have focused on access and accessibility, neglecting a consideration of older adults as active digital contributors. In this paper, we explore and position the concept of digital citizenship within the context of a medium-sized age-friendly city in the North of England by examining the civic use of digital technologies. We provide detailed qualitative insights into how a community organisation of older adults engages with digital communications and digital audio in order to facilitate and promote their engagement in the process of making their city more age-friendly. More specifically, we consider how the organisation operates within two of the eight domains identified in the WHO AFC framework: Communication and information and civic participation. As a result, our research seeks to contribute to discourse around digital participation and digital citizenship, making the case for the central role of these activities in age-friendly city and community programs. We present the methods and findings of our study in the following sections.

3. Methods

Our paper draws on an empirical study, which set out to explore digital citizenship of older adults within the context of a medium-sized city in the North of England that belongs to the UK network of age-friendly communities. As with other medium-sized cities in the UK and internationally participating in the WHO AFC program, the city is actively engaged in responding to the combined opportunities and challenges associated with demographic ageing and urbanisation [40,41]. Working with an AFC stakeholder organisation of older adults in the city, and reflecting where we saw evidence gaps in existing literature on age-friendly cities and communities, we sought to respond to two key research questions:

1. How can stakeholder organisations of older adults best exploit digital technologies to provide digital information and communications to support age-friendly city initiatives?

2. What is the potential of digital audio to promote civic participation in later life and to facilitate public engagement with age-friendly issues?

We draw on interviews, observations and field notes from design meetings collected as part of an ongoing participatory action research project, working collaboratively with an AFC stakeholder organisation. The project received institutional ethical approval (Ref. 8659/2018) and our work is being conducted in line with the ethical guidelines of the British Society of Gerontology [42], valuing a collaborative research process guided by the collaborators' experience. Pseudonyms are used to refer to all collaborators named in this paper.

3.1. Research Context

In early 2018, we (an interdisciplinary research team of HCI and social gerontology researchers) approached an organisation of older adults in the North of England, whose members are heavily involved in shaping the discourse around age and ageing in their city at a social and political level. The organisation has been a key stakeholder in the city's AFC group since the group was established. We engaged with the organisation using participatory action research (PAR), which is a highly contextual and localised approach to community-based research that typically aims to generate sustainable social change [43]. Reflecting its democratic and collaborative ethos, PAR requires constant communication between researchers and collaborators working with a cycle of "planning, acting and reflecting" [43]. Having engaged with the wider organisation in line with PAR principles, this paper reports on a specific collaboration with the organisation's communications team leaders, who self-selected and approached the authors for this project. We implemented the PAR process by using co-design methods and interviews at several stages throughout the project, as outlined below. In this paper, we report on one specific component of the broader PAR project, which is investigating how the organisation and its members engage with digital technologies in order to increase older adults' civic participation in age-friendly work across the city. Reflecting a commitment to promoting age-friendliness in multiple spheres of city life, the collaborating organisation engages in regular campaigning. In order to increase the impact of their activities, they use both digital and non-digital strategies to engage with older people across the city. In this paper, in line with the research questions specified above, we report on how the organisation works digitally within two of the WHO's AFC domains: (1) Information and communication, by communicating age-friendly work digitally, and (2) civic participation, by using digital audio to engage citizens in public spaces on the age-friendly agenda.

3.2. Working within the Information and Communication Domain

One element of the organisation's digital engagement takes place through its digital communications. Throughout the PAR project, it became clear that members of the organisation wished to restructure some of their digital output, in particular, their online newsletter. The newsletter had previously been prepared using Microsoft Word and circulated as a pdf file attached to an e-mail. In order to allow a more collaborative workflow and, more importantly, gather, for the first time, statistical information about user engagement, the organisation's communications team wished to shift their newsletter to the Mailchimp platform instead. Mailchimp allows content creators to manage mailing lists, newsletters and other digital content, whilst also providing users with insights into how content is accessed by its audience. In response to our first research question, we now report on the design process of shifting the organisation's newsletter to Mailchimp with the aim of exploring digital communications within the AFC context.

Research Methods and Analysis

Our analysis of this design process draws on two types of data (see Table 1). First, four interviews were conducted with the organisation's three communication leads (Sarah, Iris and Dora, who are older people themselves). Interviews took place at different stages throughout the project.

Second, observations and field notes from nine design meetings (average duration of 90 min) were made throughout the year 2019. The semi-structured interviews openly explored the organisation's information and communications work, as well as asked specific questions about the organisation's digital engagement within the AFC context (e.g., "What is the commitment of the AFC stakeholders regarding digital technology?"). All interviews were audio recorded and transcribed verbatim. The design meetings with the purpose of re-designing the organisation's e-mail newsletter were attended by A.R., a professional content creator and two of the organisation's communications leads (Iris and Dora). Field notes were taken contemporaneously and the researchers added further observations after each meeting as part of their research diaries. The design meetings provided an opportunity to collaboratively explore the organisation's existing media output and actively support the design of their e-mail newsletter in terms of content, functionality and layout. This design process was both guided by specific milestones that were important to the organisation (e.g., initiating a name change for the newsletter), and unstructured, as an open space for feedback, suggestions and ideas (e.g., personal challenges with the technology). We tried to create an informal atmosphere, as the meetings took place at the research facility. The aim was to signal that sufficient space and time were available to discuss any technical topics that emerged, despite being located in a school of computing. We provided tangible design materials, such as paper and pens, as well as tablets and laptops, to demonstrate ideas on a big TV screen.

Table 1. Interviews and design meetings timeline.

Members	Time	Topic
Iris and Dora	February 2019, Design Meeting 1	General ideas for the newsletter layout
Iris and Dora	February 2019, Design Meeting 2	Developing a Mailchimp concept to be presented to the wider organisation
Iris and Dora	March 2019, Design Meeting 3	Setup of Mailchimp account
Iris and Dora	March 2019, Design Meeting 4	Template setup and content layout
Iris and Dora	April 2019, Interview 1	Creating efficient workflows
Iris and Dora	April 2019, Design Meeting 5	Ideas for cover stories and name of newsletter
Iris, Dora and Sarah	May 2019, Interview 2 as part of Design Meeting 6	Re-design of newsletter to Mailchimp
Iris and Dora	September 2019, Design Meeting 7	Technical Advice
Sarah	September 2019, Design Meeting 8	Creation of mailing list and campaign
	October 2019: first digital Newsletter	
Iris	December 2019, Design Meeting 9	Increase audience engagement
Iris and Dora	February 2020, Interview 3	Evaluation of use of Mailchimp
Sarah	February 2020, Interview 4	Digital AFC and communications

We used reflexive thematic analysis [44] to analyse the interviews and field notes. Thematic analysis is a way to make patterns of shared meaning visible within a dataset, acknowledging the active role of the researcher as part of this process [44]. It is a flexible approach to qualitative data analysis and can be used within different theoretical frameworks [45]. We approach this analysis from a critical realist perspective, acknowledging the experience of our interviewees whilst at the same time contextualising these experiences in how they are shaped within a broader social context [46]; in our case, the age-friendly city's dynamics. We carried out the analysis in two stages. First, A.R. applied codes to the transcribed interviews in NVivo 12 software (QSR international, Burlington, MA, USA). The first stage of coding was carried out inductively to explore the transcript in its entity. In stage two, we repeated the coding process with a deductive focus to hone in on digital aspects whilst also integrating the field notes. All codes were discussed and the theme we derived in relation to the information and communication AFC domain is "communicating age-friendly work digitally". The theme is based on codes that consider audience engagement, collaborative work and the intersection of digital and non-digital aspects, all of which are presented in the findings section.

3.3. Working within the Civic Participation Domain

Our second research question aims to consider the role of digital technologies within the AFC civic participation domain. We explored this domain in collaboration with the same AFC stakeholder organisation, given the organisation's aim to advocate for older persons and their rights. Throughout 2019, for one day each month, the organisation was able to secure a unit in the city's centrally-located, historic covered market, in order to promote themselves and their work. The market is a popular destination for shopping and a space for intergenerational encounters. As the venue was offered to the organisation free of charge, no alternative was considered. The organisation's first day at the market generated only a low level of public interest. Reflecting the principles underlying the ongoing PAR project, one member of the organisation's communications team, Sarah, felt able to subsequently initiate two exploratory meetings with A.R. to discuss the potential of using digital media as a method to increase public engagement.

Research Methods and Analysis

The exploratory meetings were conducted as a combination of informal discussions and structured ideation. The sessions were spent exploring the goals of using digital technology as part of the organisation's engagement sessions at the market in an informal discussion, namely (1) engaging citizens in age-friendly work and (2) demonstrating impact (as outlined in the results section). We subsequently developed a digital engagement strategy for the organisation's market unit.

The organisation had previously completed a listening exercise in which they sought older people's opinions on various issues across the city, presenting the results as a written report. The members now voiced interest in replicating this listening exercise in a digital form. A.R. adopted a 'user scenarios' [47] approach as an ideation technique to co-design a digital engagement strategy to generate interactions in the market. Talking through different imaginary user scenarios, such as "What do people think when they pass the market unit?", "Why would people want to give their opinion?" or "How can we attract the interest of older people who are shopping in the market?", Sarah decided that using audio was an interesting and privacy-aware way of engaging people through technology, as well as capturing voices on a range of age-friendly topics. Despite wanting to create a more tangible evidence base on how older people respond to certain topics, the organisation wanted the audio to predominantly "spark discussions, rather than being too rigorous or methodological" (Sarah), emphasising the importance of using technology-based designs as a scoping tool to elicit topics of interest. As a topic for their listening exercise, the organisation was especially keen to explore opinions on intergenerational cohesion within the city. Through iterations of the ideation approach described above, we developed the idea to collaboratively create recordings of intergenerational provocative discussion starters. Six younger people and six older people were asked to respond to statements such as "I am proud of my generation", "I am grateful to the older generation" or "I am annoyed with my generation because ... ". The responses were audio recorded. We used the organisation's iPad to play these provocative statements. Even though we planned to use the audio recordings at the market as a playful way to engage people in discussions, we also wanted to provide a non-digital option to gather feedback. As an alternative for people who would prefer not to be audio recorded, we created small postcards that would encourage people to express their opinions (see Figure 1).

We analysed the findings from the ideation activities, as well as from the actual process of using digital audio in the market setting. A.R. analysed the field notes using reflexive thematic analysis, as previously described in the research methods of Section 3.2.

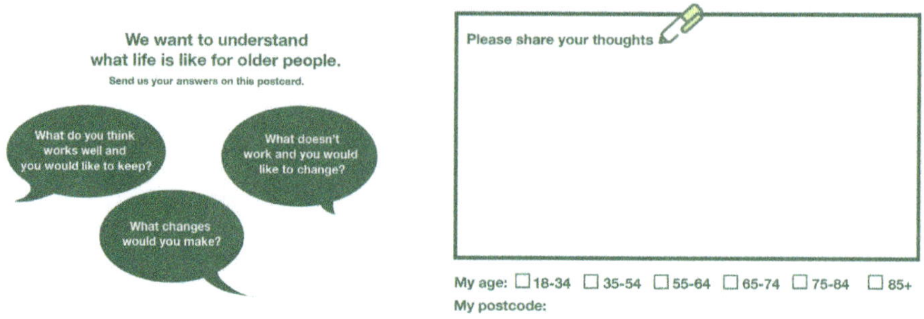

Figure 1. Front and back of feedback postcard.

4. Findings

We now report our findings on how a specific AFC stakeholder organisation operating in a medium-sized city in the North of England works digitally within the two AFC domains addressed as part of our research questions. We start with the communication and information domain, before moving on to the civic participation domain. These two aspects of the organisation's digital interactions provide an example of how the concept of digital citizenship is already addressed within an AFC. First, based on interview data and the re-design of their online newsletter, we report on how the organisation communicates their age-friendly work in a digital form. Second, drawing on results from the organisation's market engagement, we present the results on their use of digital audio as a way to engage older people with age-friendly topics in public spaces.

4.1. Communicating Age-Friendly Work Digitally

In this section, we present findings on how the organisation works towards communicating age-friendly work digitally regarding the AFC information and communication domain. Thematic analysis (TA) of the fieldnotes and interviews in relation to the organisation's communications and, especially, the re-design of their online newsletter suggested that the organisation perceived the potential to reach and engage a wider audience as the main benefit to be derived from engaging with digital communications. We present an overview of the themes and how they were derived in Table 2.

Table 2. Themes, example codes and data from the thematic analysis (TA) exploring the digital newsletter.

Themes	Example Code	Data
Reaching wider audiences	Retrieving audience statistics	*It went out to 569 people, had a 45% open rate and an 8.3% click rate. (Dora)*
	Getting personal feedback	*There was a lovely comment yesterday. A lady had sent a message in. (Dora)*
Showcasing AFC collaborations	Networking organisations	*So, we find a lot of organisations are using what we're putting out. (Iris)*
	Strategically distributing information between AFC members	*I've been at a meeting this morning and both the ladies that were there said 'We read the articles and we share with our members' (Dora)*
Creating efficient workflows	Committing time	*It's capacity timing, isn't it. That's the problem with that. (Iris)*
	Learning from each other	*I would like us to sit down together with the newsletter and email page and have a look at how you use it and how I use it. (Iris)*
Balancing digital and non-digital interactions	Connecting socially and reaching out	*We like face-to-face, we like paper, we like all of that, we've got to have, but, actually, we also need this other dimension, which is both about trying to get broader engagement, but, also, about how we present ourselves to the world. (Sarah)*
	Delivering online and offline information	*You can go on the website and you can find one there, but actually, have one delivered to you too. (Iris)*

Building on the organisation's previous discussions about the need to offer digital communications to older people across the city, the team emphasised the importance of using online communications in order to reach older adults, in particular, people in their 50s. Approximately 15 years ago, as part of the city's age-friendly efforts, the organisation was involved in developing an online platform to provide information for older adults. Sarah and other members of the AFC initiative advocated for the platform to be developed digitally at the time:

> *"When we did that back in 2006, 2007, we got a huge amount of flak because people said that older people don't go online. Thanks very much to a colleague of mine, who really said, 'No, we've got to do this as a digital platform, this has got to be online' we really stuck to our guns. So,* [the website] *is a key information resource for people in the city, but alongside that, we then tried in a small way, I guess, to create opportunities for older people to improve their digital skills." (Sarah)*

The struggle that Sarah and other older people's advocates faced when suggesting a digital platform highlights a lack of awareness relating to the topics of technology and ageing at that time. Sarah emphasises that using a digital platform can be an inclusive way to communicate age-friendly work to a wider audience, not just older adults themselves. The organisation aims to use their online communications and, in particular, their digital newsletter, which is mainly produced by the volunteers Iris and Dora, to engage older people across the city. The organisation wished to change the format of their newsletter from a pdf document to electronic content managed within a platform (Mailchimp) that merges design tools with audience management, in order to increase the marketing effectiveness. During the process of changing the format, we developed a structure within the newsletter that first emphasises the organisation's achievements within the AFC and other ongoing activities, before providing general information on activities across the city. This structural design choice was made by the organisation in order to heighten awareness of their work as older people's advocates across the city.

The development of the Mailchimp newsletter was driven by the desire for obtaining insight into audience statistics. Indeed, within a few months following the format shift, the organisation gained feedback as to how their newsletter was received by the public:

> *Iris: "We also know, from looking at the analysis, what's happening with it, which we didn't know from Word. We knew nothing from Word at all, we just knew how many people were getting it. So, it's about a 50% opening rate."*

> *Dora: "I can give you the facts and figures. The first one we did was on 4th October and it went out to 569 people, had a 45% open rate and an 8.3% click rate."*

This shows that both Iris and Dora are keen to stay updated with their audience statistics, tracking their opening rates and trying to understand user experience and engagement with the content that they distribute. The organisation uses the free version of Mailchimp rather than the paid options, which would allow for more detailed statistical insights. However, for the time being, they emphasise that having at least some limited insights is more useful than having none, as was the case when producing the newsletter in its earlier format. Despite this, the team continues to be interested in establishing correlations between specific topics addressed in the newsletters and user engagement:

> *"Because it would be helpful if we knew what was in the highest rating clicks, rather than look at the ones where ... you know, so we don't have to do every one, but if we get a really positive reaction to a particular* [newsletter]*, what was it in that* [newsletter] *that really attracted people's attention. That would be valuable." (Dora)*

This highlights the group's intention to tailor the content of the digital newsletter based on their audience's interests and to further analyse the impact of their activism. In addition to this digital feedback on audience engagement, the team had also received personal feedback from people across the city. However, despite originally aiming their newsletter at older individuals, the team noticed that other local organisations were also making use of the information presented in the newsletter:

> *"We always knew how many people it was going to. We have picked up more people, but they're organisations, rather than individuals. So, we find a lot of organisations are using what we're putting out, which is an interesting thing." (Iris)*

This engagement with the newsletter outside of their own membership shows the power of digital communications within a network of AFC stakeholders. Our findings suggest that by creating a cycle of information, in which different organisations promote each other, age-friendly topics and events can gain much wider attention. This heightened engagement through cross-promotion also reflects the importance of being strategic about promoting the work carried out as part of the AFC initiative. When the city initially joined the WHO's global age-friendly initiative, Sarah, as a stakeholder within the AFC, *"tried quite hard to get a communications strategy going* [...] *but ended up not pursuing it, which probably was a very bad mistake."* Our findings highlight that something as complex as a communications strategy cannot easily be organised and executed by an individual person and requires specific digital communications skills, insight into the AFC group and collaboration between the stakeholder organisations, as well as a time commitment. Time constraints and the need to increase the production efficiency served as additional reasons to re-design the organisation's newsletter:

> *"I would like us to sit down together with the newsletter and email page and have a look at how you use it and how I use it. Because I think that I don't use it in the most efficient way." (Iris, Interview 1)*

Throughout the design meetings, Dora and Iris agreed that, by working collaboratively as a team, the organisation's media output could be maximised. However, despite developing the concept and design of the newsletter together with the aim of increasing collaborative work, the interview in February 2020 revealed that the team members ended up taking the production in turns. We asked them to outline their reasons for continuing to work individually and Dora said:

> *"From my point of view, the commitment with that is quite different because, if you were both doing it at the same time, you're not actually having a break from it. I mean, I might put something in, or Iris might put something in and I might go, "That's not suitable. Take it out." So, there's the different interest, different ... and Sarah could come along and do something completely different. I'm happy with doing it two, four, however many issues and then having a break and it gives you time to think of other things as well and to read it when somebody else has done it and see, pick up different things." (Dora, Interview 4)*

This reflects the considerable time commitment that is associated with digital communications and the importance of being independent in the editorial process. Viewing the production of the newsletter as a process towards collaborative work, rather than an immediate new state of working, reflects the busy nature of the organisation's team of volunteers, who are learning new digital skills in order to advocate for their organisation online. In addition to working towards collaboration within their digital outputs, the communications team was mindful of creating face-to-face and non-digital interactions:

> *"So, some of it needs to be face-to-face, we still like that, we like face-to-face, we like paper, we like all of that, we've got to have, but, actually, we also need this other dimension, which is both about trying to get broader engagement, but, also, about how we present ourselves to the world." (Sarah)*

Valuing both face-to-face interaction and digital engagement is a relevant factor for Sarah, as the group's organiser. Being connected physically is crucial for running a network, such as the AFC group and its stakeholders, whilst using digital means can connect the group to the wider public and showcase the wider collaborations within the AFC group.

To summarise this component of our findings, we have outlined the importance of communicating age-friendly work digitally in terms of reaching wider audiences, showcasing collaborations across the city and creating efficient workflows. We have also reported on the importance of balancing digital and non-digital interactions within the age-friendly city. The next section discusses an example of digital work organised by the collaborating organisation, using digital audio to increase public engagement on age-related topics.

4.2. Using Digital Audio to Increase Civic Participation

In this section, we present findings from the organisation's digital work within the AFC domain of civic participation. We describe two themes (see Table 3), which outline why the organisation chose to experiment with digital audio as a way of heightening their civic impact: (1) The opportunity to engage citizens more widely, and (2) as a way to demonstrate the impact. We then report on findings from the activity of using digital audio in the local market hall.

Table 3. Themes, example codes, and data from the thematic analysis exploring digital audio.

Themes	Example Code	Data
Engaging citizens	Reaching different age groups	*Why is it* [that people] *are not interested? I'm sure they are but we're certainly not reaching them. The younger cohort. People in their 60s. (Sarah)*
	Inviting public feedback	*For the moment, everything is very hidden. I put this out and wait for people to tell us what they think... (Iris)*
Demonstrating impact	Creating digital evidence	Digital technologies are a creative way of evidencing work that had been done. (Author 1, field notes)
	Tracking audience engagement	Engaging digitally offers the opportunity to diagnose trends and be more responsive to the audience. (Author 1, field notes)

In April 2019, the organisation and A.R. used the digital audio statements as a way to engage older citizens on age-friendly and civic issues in the local market hall. As the first few exhibition days in the market unit were characterised by a notable lack of interest from passers-by, Sarah reflected that the issue lay in the way they were trying to reach their audience:

> *"Why is it [that people] are not interested? I'm sure they are, but we're certainly not reaching them. The younger cohort. People in their 60s." (Sarah)*

She perceived, in particular, younger cohorts of older adults as being more tech-savvy, concluding that it is important to use digital channels in order to promote the organisation's political and civic work. Using digital audio as a way to capture people's attention in the market unit and to invite feedback was seen as an opportunity to engage passers-by in deeper discussions (as opposed to paper-based leaflets that are handed out) and to learn more about residents' opinions, in order to reflect them in their activist work. Technology was also seen as a novel and interesting way to attract people to visit the unit, in particular, people who might not previously have heard about the organisation or the AFC work.

The second reason that underlay the organisation's motivation to engage with digital audio was the possibility to demonstrate the impact. As a third sector organisation, the group is partly dependent on external funding for their projects. As an advocacy organisation, "evidence" is often deemed necessary to have an influence on policy development. Presenting more tangible and creative insights into older residents' experiences in a digital format compared to a written report can provide a starting point for discussions on age-friendliness in more formal political settings. Sarah assumed that involvement with digital audio could transform the reputation of the AFC stakeholder organisation from *"inward looking to knowing what a range of older people in the city are actually interested in [by listening to them]"*, thus being more responsive to older citizens. This reflects the potential of digital audio to be a communications tool within the AFC that supports bottom-up citizen engagement. Using digital audio within the local market was seen as an opportunity to capture diverse opinions from older local citizens.

Over a duration of four hours, members of the organisation used the iPad to play the pre-recorded statements by older and younger people to passers-by (see Figure 2). A.R.'s field notes recorded that "many members of the organisation joined the team on the day, eager to promote their organisation's work". The setup of the iPad with the headphones caught many people's interest as they were passing by. The organisation's members actively approached and prompted people in the market to join them and listen to the recordings. Indeed, over the course of the morning, around 15 people listened and engaged with the group as a response. However, despite this heightened level of interest, only four people were willing to record their own responses. These responses were on average 1.26 min long and, despite our prompts to share opinions on intergenerational cohesion or raise local issues, the responses included a variety of topics: Food banks and social inequalities within the city; personal health issues; an interest in the history of the city; and a general political critique. Indeed, many of the people who chose not to be recorded were triggered by the intergenerational provocations to voice their concerns about or agreement with national issues. The experience showed that despite prompting for a certain topic, using audio sparked highly emotive discussions on a variety of topics and, in particular, on the wider political landscape. As an evaluation, the organisation and researchers jointly agreed that the approach of using audio as a way to collect evidence on a specific topic in a public space had its limitations. These were mainly due to people's concerns or shyness about being recorded and the wide variety of unanticipated topics raised by members of the public. We concluded that the pre-recorded statements needed to be refined and less provocative, in order to generate responses on topics that are relevant to the organisation and that can be used specifically for advocating for age-friendly work within the city. However, the intervention was not followed up directly, as the organisation decided to pursue a different strategy for their market unit in the following months.

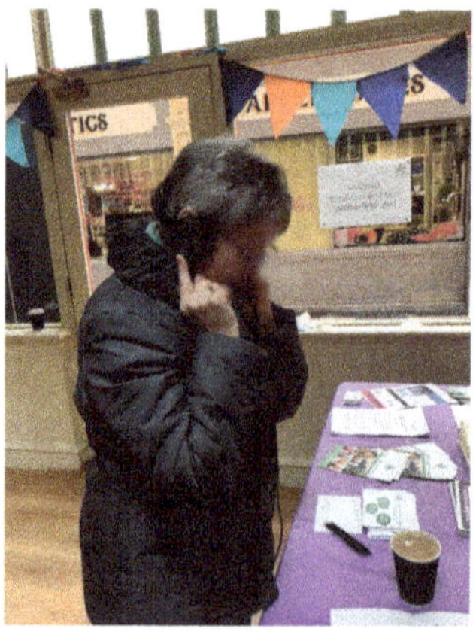

Figure 2. Listening to the audio statements.

Additionally, the organisation and authors prepared non-digital materials (see Figure 1), which most people who engaged with the organisation's members at the market unit also filled out. Approximately 15 postcards were collected, outlining different issues of relevance to AFC domains, such as parks and green spaces, historic tours and personal health issues. Overall, the researchers questioned whether the activity aimed to engage people in too many different things at once (listening to audio, handing out leaflets, and filling in postcards), which led to a loss of focus on the information that the organisation wanted to capture. Nonetheless, the range of formats provided numerous opportunities for engagement and resulted in an overall heightened engagement and interest compared to the organisation's initial experience at the market.

To summarise, the AFC stakeholder organisation used digital audio provocations as a way to spark discussions on intergenerational cohesion and capture older residents' voices on other age-friendly topics. The use of a very basic digital technology (iPad with audio) proved to be an effective way to engage people and attract people's attention to the organisation's market unit. However, the project provoked discussions on a wide range of topics, not necessarily reflecting age-friendliness, but nonetheless giving an opportunity to older adults to share with an AFC stakeholder what was going on in their lives. In addition, privacy concerns and the shyness of participants were underestimated in our design, resulting in an unwillingness of members of the public to be audio recorded. We concluded that, due to those reasons, audio might be a way to spark discussions, but despite its benefits to promote civic participation, it might not be the optimal route to capturing age-friendly interests in contexts such as the market setting.

5. Discussion

In this paper, we have explored different aspects of digital citizenship within the age-friendly city. Our research questions investigated (1) how organisations of older adults can best exploit digital technologies to provide digital information and communications to support age-friendly city initiatives, and (2) the potential of digital audio to promote civic participation in later life and to facilitate public engagement with age-friendly issues. We responded to these questions by illustrating how one AFC stakeholder organisation of older adults works within the age-friendly domains of communication and information and civic participation. Reporting on those two domains, we have outlined how the organisation makes use of digital communications in order to promote age-friendly work across the city. Additionally, we have reported on how the organisation used digital audio as a way to capture older people's voices at the local market as an effort to engage older citizens and provide evidence for older adults' civic participatory work.

Before discussing key insights of our research, such as the need to create digital visibility around age-friendly projects and to consider the importance of digital citizenship for older adults by looking at civic opportunities in online and offline spaces, it is useful to address some of the limitations of our approach.

5.1. Limitations

Our qualitative and participatory methods give insight into the practices of one particular age-friendly city in the North of England. Facing high inequalities in the wider region, age-friendly initiatives are highly dependent on the goodwill of local activists and politicians as other political issues have been prioritised over the years. Whilst our findings are limited to this particular local context and constrained by the obvious limitations of a small-scale empirical study, this is also a feature of other work on age-friendly cities and communities [48]. Moreover, the points raised in regard to digital citizenship as one aspect of promoting age-friendliness and, in particular, the importance of using digital media as a way to achieve this, are likely to be of wider interest to researchers and policy stakeholders engaged in AFC work in other geographic locations. Whilst some age-friendly cities have created an "AFC brand" for themselves and work with professional communications strategies, we, in contrast, report on how older adults themselves are acting in ways that can advocate for a stronger focus on age-friendliness in their cities and communities. As a result, we believe that our approach and findings are of importance to other age-friendly cities and communities who might not have the financial resources to advocate for AFC work professionally, but rely on older activists to communicate and engage citizens in age-friendly actions [49,50].

5.2. Creating Digital Visibility of Age-Friendliness

Throughout the research reported in this paper, we noticed that digital engagement was predominantly perceived and used as a tool to discuss social issues or collect "evidence" for opinions on political issues, therefore offering a way to uncover issues that are of importance to local older residents. Returning to the idea expressed by Buffel et al. in their manifesto for age-friendly cities of having a 'right to the city' [12], we associate this right with the opportunity to be able to use digital technologies as a means to achieve civic expression and a mechanism to actively contribute to civic debates in later life. We found that communicating AFC work through digital means is an important factor in how age-friendly a city is perceived to be by a public audience. Our research, conducted in a single location, highlights that cities which have not invested in a professional communications strategy might therefore be perceived as being less age-friendly than those whose work is more digitally visible, despite ongoing efforts and a great amount of activity around the topic. Echoing the findings of Clarke et al. on using digital media as a way to advocate for older people's issues at a neighbourhood planning event [25], we also established that using digital audio recordings to create evidence for political purposes was not always successful. However, while creative approaches may not necessarily produce measurable AFC outcomes, our study suggests that using digital audio may be useful as a conversational prompt. This points to the potential of using digital technologies as a creative way to engage people in discussions around the AFC and to initiate the dialogue with older adults that is necessary to underpin the development of age-friendly policies and practices in the future.

5.3. Considering Digital Citizenship in Later Life

As a main contribution of this study, we highlight the importance of considering the intersection between digital technologies and citizenship in later life as a pathway to supporting age-friendly cities and communities. Technology is often incorporated into cities with a focus on accessibility, supporting older adults' daily lives through smart assistive technology [11]. Our study extends this focus by contributing to the discourse on digital and civic forms of participation within the context of a burgeoning, global age-friendly movement. In the literature review, we identified a push within the field of Human–Computer Interaction towards recognising older adults' diversity [8] and towards evaluating how older adults make use of digital technologies within their community settings [26]. We add to this line of argument by blending gerontological and HCI research approaches and by highlighting the civic opportunities that the use of digital technologies offers as part of an AFC initiative. Indeed, as far as we are aware, based on our review of existing literature and policy documents, there are currently no guidelines in the public domain that would support older adults' digital citizenship. Our particular focus has been on the importance of having a voice in later life and the need for citizens to be adequately informed about age-friendly topics. The research reported here emphasises the crucial need to re-frame the (rather limited) concept of digital inclusion and to focus instead on supporting the active digital participation of older adults, strengthening their digital citizenship. Supporting older adults' digital participation, not only their inclusion, could be an asset for age-friendly city initiatives. Acknowledging a more active civic contribution of older adults in online spaces has the potential to challenge ageism in relation to digitalisation and expand the diversity of online discourse by supporting different voices to be heard. While the COVID-19 pandemic has been associated with an increase in older adults' visibility in online spaces, we suggest that AFC initiatives should prioritise activities that support older adults in becoming more active in digital civic activities. Using a combination of digital and non-digital tools, such as supporting offline efforts to encourage civic participation with digital media, can be a way of creating spaces for meaningful civic participation.

6. Conclusions

The research presented in this paper explored digital citizenship within the age-friendly city context. It adds to key debates on technology and ageing by highlighting a need to include digital citizenship as a factor within discourse on the role of technology in the age-friendly city. We have shown that while digital communications are crucial for informing the public about age-friendly work, older adults often face specific challenges in creating those communications. We have also demonstrated that digital audio can be a creative way to engage the public in discussions on a range of age-friendly topics. These findings have implications for the delivery of age-friendly projects, highlighting a need to incorporate digital and non-digital elements.

Our work also points to an important research agenda that exists at the intersection of the global trends of ageing, urbanisation and digitalisation. There is ample scope for future research to consider how different digital technologies can support an increasingly diverse population of older adults in urban settings in engaging with the age-friendly cities and communities agenda. Adding a civic participatory element to the predominantly needs-based narrative on ageing and assistive technologies is key to achieving the objectives of the global age-friendly movement. In this context, it will be of particular interest to discover new and creative ways through which digital technologies can facilitate a dialogue with older residents and age-friendly city groups. Equally relevant are studies that explore how age-friendly initiatives can be supported further to heighten awareness for their work in digital spaces. This is an exciting research agenda that necessarily cuts across scientific disciplines, engages with multiple methods of enquiry, and benefits from close collaboration between researchers and citizens.

Author Contributions: Conceptualisation, A.R., J.L. and T.S.; Interviewing and design workshops, A.R.; Formal analysis, A.R. and J.L.; Writing—original draft preparation, A.R.; Writing—review and editing, A.R., J.L. and T.S.; Supervision, J.L. and T.S. All authors have read and agreed to the published version of the manuscript.

Funding: This research was funded by the EPSRC CDT in Digital Civics (EP/L016176/1). Data supporting this publication is openly available under an 'Open Data Commons Open Database License'. Additional metadata are available at: https://doi.org/10.25405/data.ncl.13181981. We thank our collaborators from the AFC stakeholder organisation.

Conflicts of Interest: The authors declare no conflict of interest. The funders had no role in the design of the study; in the collection, analyses, or interpretation of data; in the writing of the manuscript, or in the decision to publish the results.

References

1. WHO. *World Health Organization Global Age-Friendly Cities: A Guide*; World Health Organization: Geneva, Switzerland, 2007; p. 87.
2. World Health Organisation. *The Global Network for Age-Friendly Cities and Communities*; WHO: World Health Organization: Geneva, Switzerland, 2018; p. 48.
3. Age Friendly Ireland. 10 Years Delivering For Ireland | A Decade Of Progress Listening to the Voice of Older People—The Driving Force of Change at Local Level. Available online: https://www.meath.ie/system/files/media/file-uploads/2019-12/Age%20Friendly%20Meath%2010%20Year%20Report%20210x210mm%20FINAL.pdf (accessed on 4 October 2020).
4. Centre for Ageing Better UK Network of Age-Friendly Communities. Available online: https://www.ageing-better.org.uk/uk-network-age-friendly-communities (accessed on 4 October 2020).
5. Buffel, T.; Phillipson, C.; Rémillard-Boilard, S. Age-Friendly Cities and Communities: New Directions for Research and Policy. In *Encyclopedia of Gerontology and Population Aging*; Springer: Cham, Switzerland, 2019.
6. Liddle, J.; Scharf, T.; Bartlam, B.; Bernard, M.; Sim, J. Exploring the age-friendliness of purpose-built retirement communities: Evidence from England. *Ageing Soc.* **2014**, *34*, 1601–1629. [CrossRef]
7. Neves, B.B.; Waycott, J.; Malta, S. Old and afraid of new communication technologies? Reconceptualising and contesting the 'age-based digital divide'. *J. Sociol.* **2018**, *54*, 236–248. [CrossRef]

8. Vines, J.; Pritchard, G.; Wright, P.; Olivier, P. An Age-Old Problem: Examining the Discourses of Ageing in HCI and Strategies for Future Research. *Tochi* **2015**, *22*, 1–27. [CrossRef]
9. Brewer, R.; Piper, A.M. "Tell It Like It Really Is": A Case of Online Content Creation and Sharing Among Older Adult Bloggers. In Proceedings of the 2016 CHI Conference on Human Factors in Computing Systems, San Jose, CA, USA, 7–12 May 2016; ACM: New York, NY, USA, 2016; pp. 5529–5542.
10. Celdran, M.; Serrat, R.; Villar, F. Older Adults as Internet Content Producers: Motivations for Blogging in Later Life. In *Perspectives on Human-Computer Interaction Research with Older People*; Springer: Cham, Switzerland, 2019; pp. 169–182, ISBN 9783030060763.
11. Marston, H.R.; Van Hoof, J. "Who doesn't think about technology when designing urban environments for older people?" A case study approach to a proposed extension of the who's age-friendly cities model. *Int. J. Environ. Res. Public Health* **2019**, *16*, 3525. [CrossRef]
12. Buffel, T.; Phillipson, C.; Scharf, T. Ageing in urban environments: Developing "age-friendly" cities. *Crit. Soc. Policy* **2012**, *32*, 597–617. [CrossRef]
13. Buffel, T.; Handler, S. *Age-Friendly Cities and Communities: A Global Perspective*; Policy Press: Bristol, UK, 2018; ISBN 144733132X.
14. Liddle, J.; Pitcher, N.; Montague, K.; Hanratty, B.; Standing, H.; Scharf, T. Connecting at Local Level: Exploring Opportunities for Future Design of Technology to Support Social Connections in Age-Friendly Communities. *Int. J. Environ. Res. Public Health* **2020**, *17*, 5544. [CrossRef]
15. Mossberger, K.; Tolbert, C.J.; McNeal, R.S. Defining Digital Citizenship. *Digit. Citizsh.* **2019**. [CrossRef]
16. Vlachokyriakos, V.; Crivellaro, C.; Le Dantec, C.A.; Gordon, E.; Wright, P.; Olivier, P. Digital Civics: Citizen Empowerement With and Through Technology. In Proceedings of the 2016 CHI Conference Extended Abstracts on Human Factors in Computing Systems, San Jose, CA, USA, 7–12 May 2016; pp. 1096–1099.
17. Olivier, P.; Wright, P. Digital Civics: Taking a Local Turn. *Interactions* **2015**, *22*, 61–63. [CrossRef]
18. McCarthy, J.; Wright, P. *Taking [a] Part: The Politics and Aesthetics of Participation in Experience-Centered Design*; MIT Press: Cambridge, MA, USA, 2015.
19. Asad, M.; Le Dantec, C.A.; Nielsen, B.; Diedrick, K. Creating a Sociotechnical API: Designing City-Scale Community Engagement. In Proceedings of the 2017 CHI Conference on Human Factors in Computing Systems, Denver, CO, USA, 6–11 May 2017; pp. 2295–2306.
20. Walsh, K.; Scharf, T.; Keating, N. Social exclusion of older persons: A scoping review and conceptual framework. *Eur. J. Ageing* **2017**, *14*, 81–98. [CrossRef]
21. GSMA Digital Inclusion 2014. 2014. Available online: http://www.gsma.com/mobilefordevelopment/wp-content/uploads/2014/11/GSMA_Digital-Inclusion-Report_Web_Singles_2.pdf (accessed on 4 October 2020).
22. Bloch, N.; Bruce, B.C. Older adults and the new public sphere. In Proceedings of the 2011 iConference, Seattle, WA, USA, 8–11 February 2011; pp. 1–7.
23. Office for National Statistics UK. Internet Users UK; 2019; pp. 1–11. Available online: https://www.ons.gov.uk/businessindustryandtrade/itandinternetindustry/bulletins/internetusers/2019 (accessed on 4 October 2020).
24. Office of Communications UK. Connected Nations 2018: UK Report; 2018; pp. 1–49. Available online: https://www.ofcom.org.uk/__data/assets/pdf_file/0020/130736/Connected-Nations-2018-main-report.pdf (accessed on 4 October 2020).
25. Clarke, R. Tinkering in Cities: Aging and Careful Technology Design for Participation in Urban Infrastructures. *Des. Cult. Care* **2018**, 85–100. [CrossRef]
26. Righi, V.; Sayago, S.; Blat, J. When we talk about older people in HCI, who are we talking about? Towards a 'turn to community' in the design of technologies for a growing ageing population. *Int. J. Hum. Comput. Stud.* **2017**, *108*, 15–31. [CrossRef]
27. Lindley, S.E.; Harper, R.; Sellen, A. Designing for elders: Exploring the complexity of relationships in later life. In *People and Computers XXII Culture, Creativity, Interaction*; British Computer Society: London, UK, 2008; pp. 77–86.
28. Essén, A.; Östlund, B. Laggards as innovators? Old users as designers of new services & service systems. *Int. J. Des.* **2011**, *5*, 89–98.

29. Frohlich, D.M.; Lim, C.; Ahmed, A. Co-designing a Diversity of Social Media Products with and for Older People. In Proceedings of the 7th International Conference on Software Development and Technologies for Enhancing Accessibility and Fighting Info-Exclusion, Vila Real, Portugal, 1–3 December 2016; pp. 323–330.
30. Vines, J.; Blythe, M.; Lindsay, S.; Dunphy, P.; Monk, A.; Olivier, P. Questionable concepts: Critique as a resource for designing with eighty somethings. In Proceedings of the SIGCHI Conference on Human Factors in Computing Systems, Austin, TX, USA, 5–10 May 2012; pp. 1169–1178.
31. Leong, T.; Robertson, T. Voicing values: Laying foundations for ageing people to participate in design. In *Proceedings of the 14th Participatory Design Conference: Full Papers-Volume 1*; ACM: New York, NY, USA, 2016; pp. 31–40.
32. Clarke, R.; Crivellaro, C.; Di Mascio, D.; Wright, P. Re-configuring participatory media for citizen elders in urban planning. In Proceedings of the 3rd Conference on Media Architecture Biennale, Sydney, Australia, 1–4 June 2016; pp. 1–10.
33. Davidson, S. Digital Inclusion Evidence Review. *Age UK* **2018**, 1–30. Available online: https://www.ageuk.org.uk/globalassets/age-uk/documents/reports-and-publications/age_uk_digital_inclusion_evidence_review_2018.pdf (accessed on 4 October 2020).
34. UK Government Digital Skills and Inclusion Policy Paper. Available online: https://www.gov.uk/government/publications/uk-digital-strategy/2-digital-skills-and-inclusion-giving-everyone-access-to-the-digital-skills-they-need (accessed on 8 July 2019).
35. Seifert, A.; Rössel, J. *Digital Participation—Encyclopedia of Gerontology and Population Aging*; Gu, D., Dupre, M.E., Eds.; Springer International Publishing: Cham, Switzerland, 2019; pp. 1–5, ISBN 978-3-319-69892-2.
36. Ferreira, S.M.; Sayago, S.; Blat, J. Older people's production and appropriation of digital videos: An ethnographic study. *Behav. Inf. Technol.* **2017**, *36*, 557–574. [CrossRef]
37. Reuter, A.; Bartindale, T.; Morrissey, K.; Scharf, T.; Liddle, J. Older voices: Supporting community radio production for civic participation in later life. In Proceedings of the 2019 CHI Conference on Human Factors in Computing Systems, Glasgow, UK, 4–9 May 2019.
38. Waycott, J.; Vetere, F.; Pedell, S.; Kulik, L.; Ozanne, E.; Gruner, A.; Downs, J. Older adults as digital content producers. In Proceedings of the SIGCHI Conference on Human Factors in Computing Systems, Paris, France, 27 April–2 May 2013; pp. 39–48.
39. Ferreira, S.; Sayago, S.; Blat, J. Older People Positive, Active and Creative ICT Use: A Study in Three Countries. In *Perspectives on Human-Computer Interaction Research with Older People*; Springer: Cham, Switzerland, 2019; pp. 183–197, ISBN 978-3-030-06076-3.
40. Buffel, T.; De Donder, L.; Phillipson, C.; Dury, S.; De Witte, N.; Verté, D. Social participation among older adults living in medium-sized cities in Belgium: The role of neighbourhood perceptions. *Health Promot. Int.* **2014**, *29*, 655–668. [CrossRef]
41. Buffel, T.; Phillipson, C. Can global cities be "age-friendly cities"? Urban development and ageing populations. *Cities* **2016**, *55*, 94–100. [CrossRef]
42. British Society of Gerontology Ethical Guidelines. Available online: https://www.britishgerontology.org/about-bsg/bsg-ethical-guidelines (accessed on 13 August 2018).
43. Hayes, G.R. Taking action in your research. *Interactions* **2012**, *19*, 50. [CrossRef]
44. Braun, V.; Clarke, V. Reflecting on reflexive thematic analysis. *Qual. Res. Sport. Exerc. Health* **2019**, *11*, 589–597. [CrossRef]
45. Braun, V.; Clarke, V. Using thematic analysis in psychology. *Qual. Res. Psychol.* **2006**, *3*, 77–101. [CrossRef]
46. Houston, S. Prising open the black box: Critical realism, action research and social work. *Qual. Soc. Work* **2010**, *9*, 73–91. [CrossRef]
47. Tomitsch, M. User Scenarios. Available online: http://designthinkmakebreakrepeat.com/methods/scenarios/ (accessed on 4 October 2020).
48. Buckner, S.; Pope, D.; Mattocks, C.; Lafortune, L.; Dherani, M.; Bruce, N. Developing Age-Friendly Cities: An Evidence-Based Evaluation Tool. *J. Popul. Ageing* **2019**, *12*, 203–223. [CrossRef]

49. Lehning, A.J.; Greenfield, E.A. Research on Age-Friendly Community Initiatives: Taking Stock and Moving Forward. *J. Hous. Elder.* **2017**, *31*, 178–192. [CrossRef]
50. Russell, E.; Skinner, M.W.; Fowler, K. Emergent Challenges and Opportunities to Sustaining Age-friendly Initiatives: Qualitative Findings from a Canadian Age-friendly Funding Program. *J. Aging Soc. Policy* **2019**, 1–20. [CrossRef]

Publisher's Note: MDPI stays neutral with regard to jurisdictional claims in published maps and institutional affiliations.

MDPI
St. Alban-Anlage 66
4052 Basel
Switzerland
Tel. +41 61 683 77 34
Fax +41 61 302 89 18
www.mdpi.com

International Journal of Environmental Research and Public Health Editorial Office
E-mail: ijerph@mdpi.com
www.mdpi.com/journal/ijerph